Equine Wound Management

To our families and friends.

To Aotearoa, for a warm welcome during the preparation of this book – Mauruuru koutou.

Equine Wound Management

Third Edition

Edited by

Christine Theoret, DMV, PhD, Diplomate ACVS

Director, Comparative Veterinary Tissue Healing Laboratory (http://theoretlab.com/index.php/en)
Professor, Département de biomédecine vétérinaire
Faculté de médecine vétérinaire
Université de Montréal
Québec, Canada

Jim Schumacher, DVM, MS, Diplomate ACVS, MRCVS

Professor, Equine Surgery
Department of Large Animal Clinical Sciences
College of Veterinary Medicine
University of Tennessee
Knoxville, Tennessee, USA

WILEY Blackwell

V.W.M.S.
VETERINARY WOUND MANAGEMENT SOCIETY

Editorial Offices
1606 Golden Aspen Drive, Suites 103 and 104, Ames, Iowa 50010, USA
The Atrium, Southern Gate, Chichester, West Sussex, PO19 8SQ, UK
9600 Garsington Road, Oxford, OX4 2DQ, UK

For details of our global editorial offices, for customer services and for information about how to apply for permission to reuse the copyright material in this book please see our website at www.wiley.com/wiley-blackwell.

Library of Congress Cataloging-in-Publication Data

Names: Theoret, Christine, editor. | Schumacher, Jim, 1948– editor.
Title: Equine wound management / edited by Christine Theoret, Jim Schumacher.
Description: Third edition. | Ames, Iowa : John Wiley & Sons, Inc., 2017. | Preceded by Equine wound management / [edited by] Ted S. Stashak, Christine Theoret. 2nd ed. 2008. | Includes bibliographical references and index.
Identifiers: LCCN 2016026519 (print) | LCCN 2016030764 (ebook) | ISBN 9781118999257 (cloth) | ISBN 9781118999233 (pdf) | ISBN 9781118999226 (epub)
Subjects: LCSH: Horses–Wounds and injuries–Treatment. | Horses–Surgery. | MESH: Horses–injuries | Horses–surgery | Wounds and Injuries–veterinary | Wounds and Injuries–therapy
Classification: LCC SF951 .S77 2017 (print) | LCC SF951 (ebook) | NLM SF 951 | DDC 636.1/08971–dc23
LC record available at https://lccn.loc.gov/2016026519

A catalogue record for this book is available from the British Library.

Wiley also publishes its books in a variety of electronic formats. Some content that appears in print may not be available in electronic books.

Cover image: zaricm/Gettyimages

Set in 9.5/12pt Minion by SPi Global, Pondicherry, India

1 2017

Contents

About the Editors

Christine Theoret

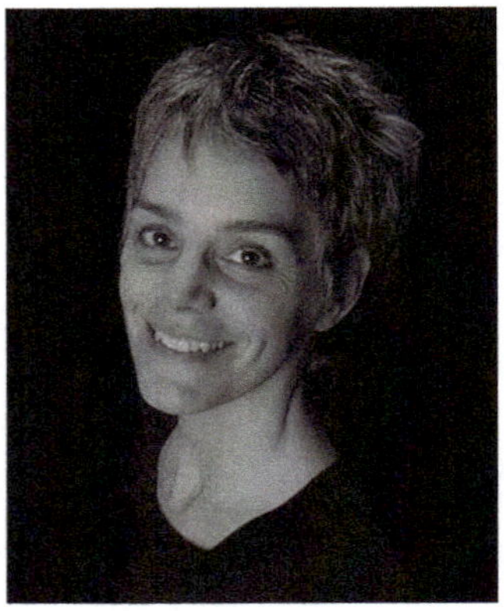

Dr. Christine Theoret is a full professor at the University of Montreal where she teaches veterinary anatomy and surgery in the DVM program. She received a DVM degree from the University of Montreal (1991) and completed an internship in equine medicine/surgery at the same institution in 1992. She then undertook a joint residency/MSc program in surgery at the Western College of Veterinary Medicine (1992–1995). She became a diplomate of the American College of Veterinary Surgeons in 1997. In 2000, Dr. Theoret received her PhD degree, studying the molecular mechanisms that govern healing and scarring, from the University of Saskatchewan.

Dr. Theoret founded the Comparative Veterinary Tissue Healing Laboratory in 2002, where she has since trained more than 30 highly qualified personnel, mostly MSc and PhD students. Her research has led to the publication of numerous articles in peer-reviewed, scientific journals. In 2008 she co-edited the second edition of the textbook *Equine Wound Management*. Dr. Theoret has served on the advisory boards of various national and international associations, including a term as President of the Veterinary Wound Management Society.

Jim Schumacher

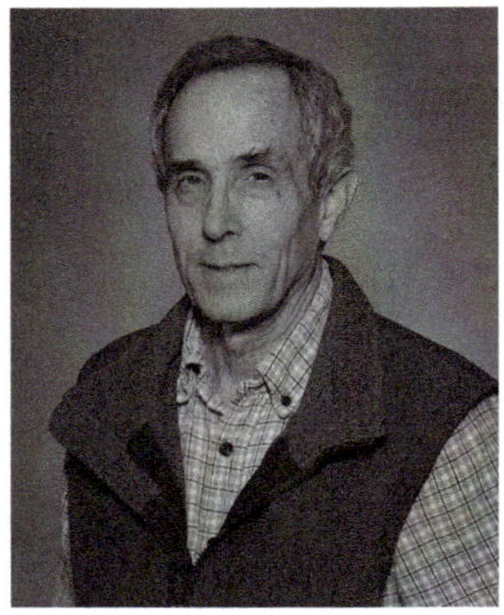

Jim Schumacher graduated from Kansas State University in 1973. He worked in equine and food animal practices in Texas, California, and Kansas for 5 years after graduation. Most of this time in private practice was spent working in feedyards in Kansas. He completed an MSc degree and a residency in large animal surgery at Texas A&M University in 1980.

He was a member of the faculty at Texas A&M University until 1997. Since then he has worked at the University of London, Auburn University, the University College Dublin, and the University of Tennessee, where he has been a member of the faculty of the Department of Veterinary Clinical Sciences since 2003. He is a diplomate of the American College of Veterinary Surgeons and a member of the Royal College of Veterinary Surgeons. He has lectured students about surgery for the past 35 years.

List of Contributors

Spencer Barber, DVM, Diplomate ACVS
Professor, Equine Surgery
Western College of Veterinary Medicine
University of Saskatchewan
Saskatoon, Saskatchewan
Canada

Gary M. Baxter, VMD, MS, Diplomate ACVS
Associate Dean for Clinical Services
College of Veterinary Medicine
University of Georgia
Athens, Georgia
USA

Christophe Celeste, DrVet, PhD, Diplomate ACVS, Diplomate ECVS
Clinique Vétérinaire Sagamie
Alma, Quebec
Canada

Linda A. Dahlgren, DVM, PhD, Diplomate ACVS
Associate Professor, Large Animal Clinical Sciences
Virginia–Maryland College of Veterinary Medicine
Blacksburg, Virginia
USA

Andrew J. Dart, BVSc, PhD, Diplomate ACVS, ECVS
Professor, Equine Veterinary Science
Director of the Research and Clinical Trials Unit
Veterinary Medical Teaching Hospital, Camden
The University of Sydney
Australia

Yvonne A. Elce, DVM, Diplomate ACVS
Associate Professor, Equine Surgery
Faculté de médecine vétérinaire
Université de Montréal
Montréal, Québec
Canada

R. Reid Hanson, DVM, Diplomate ACVS, ACVECC
Professor, Equine Surgery
College of Veterinary Medicine
Auburn University
Auburn, Alabama
USA

Stine Jacobsen, DVM, PhD, Diplomate ECVS
Professor, Large Animal Surgery
Department of Large Animal Sciences
Faculty of Health and Medical Sciences
University of Copenhagen
Denmark

Derek C. Knottenbelt, OBE, BVM&S, DVMS, Diplomate ECEIM, MRCVS
Emeritus Professor, Equine Internal Medicine
University of Liverpool
Neston, Wirral
United Kingdom

Beth Kraus, DVM, Diplomate ACVS
Chadds Ford, Pennsylvania
USA

Amelia S. Munsterman, DVM, MS, Diplomate ACVS, ACVECC
Clinical Lecturer, Equine Critical Care Medicine and Surgery
College of Veterinary Medicine
Auburn University
Auburn, Alabama
USA

James A. Orsini, DVM, Diplomate ACVS
Associate Professor, Equine Surgery
School of Veterinary Medicine
University of Pennsylvania
Kennett Square, Pennsylvania
USA

Jim Schumacher, DVM, MS, Diplomate ACVS, MRCVS
Professor, Equine Surgery
Department of Large Animal Clinical Sciences
College of Veterinary Medicine
University of Tennessee
Knoxville, Tennessee
USA

John Schumacher, DVM, MS, Diplomate ACVIM
Professor
Department of Clinical Sciences
College of Veterinary Medicine
Auburn University,
Auburn, Alabama
USA

Kathryn A. Seabaugh, DVM, MS, Diplomate ACVS, ACVSMR
Assistant Professor
College of Veterinary Medicine
University of Georgia
Athens, Georgia
USA

Albert Sole-Guitart, DVM, Diplomate ACVS
Clinician, Equine Surgery
Camden Equine Center
The University of Sydney
Australia

Ted S. Stashak, DVM, MS, Diplomate ACVS
Professor Emeritus, Equine Surgery
Colorado State University
Santa Rosa, California
USA

Christine Theoret, DMV, PhD, Diplomate ACVS
Director, Comparative Veterinary Tissue Healing Laboratory (http://theoretlab.com/index.php/en)
Professor, Département de biomédecine vétérinaire
Faculté de médecine vétérinaire
Université de Montréal
Montréal, Québec
Canada

Ferenc Toth, DVM, PhD, Diplomate ACVS
Assistant Professor
Department of Veterinary Population Medicine
College of Veterinary Medicine
University of Minnesota
St. Paul, Minnesota
USA

Jacintha M. Wilmink, DVM, PhD
Woumarec
Hamsterlaan 4
6705 CT Wageningen
The Netherlands

Preface

Wounds are among the most common medical conditions seen by veterinarians in their equine patients and one of the topics least addressed during the veterinary curriculum or at continuing education meetings. Because the horse's response to wounding differs from that of man, laboratory animals or even other veterinary patients, wound-management textbooks used in the human healthcare field or in small animal practice cannot be relied on to provide appropriate/specific therapeutic guidelines. Moreover, the general-purpose textbook covering equine medicine and surgery cannot possibly address the topic with the required depth because of the abundance of information on wound physiology and management now available. Consequently, the Equine Wound Management textbook is an essential reference for equine veterinarians because it provides readers with state-of-the-art theoretical and practical information, enhanced by an abundance of helpful tables, line drawings, and color figures.

With Dr. Ted Stashak firmly embracing a well-earned retirement, I (Dr. Theoret) was faced with the choice of a new co-editor willing to fill big shoes. Dr. Jim Schumacher courageously accepted the challenge and, due to his vast clinical experience and his familiarity with editorship, he has been an inestimable asset to the smooth execution of the task at hand. Together, we have striven to create a well-balanced book that addresses the needs of students, practitioners, postgraduate veterinarians in training programs (research- or clinically-oriented), and specialists (surgeons). Moreover, with the aim to make the book more reader-friendly, practical information has been highlighted in the text in easy-to-spot, quick-to-read "tips", and a companion interactive website posts text, questions/answers, figures, case series, "how to" videos, etc.

Since the second edition of this textbook was published in 2008, hundreds of new, relevant studies have been performed, and summaries of these findings and practical applications thereof have been included in the third edition. The wound-care market for human patients has grown in leaps and bounds over the past few years; consequently, countless new topical medications and interactive dressings have appeared on the market. In many cases, the use of these products in horses has not yet been thoroughly investigated. Despite the aforementioned differences in healing of wounds of horses, veterinarians may be tempted to extrapolate data from human or lab animal trials to the horse. Consequently, Chapters 5 and 6 have been thoroughly updated, and the author presents evidence for the effects of selected products specifically on healing tissues of the horse. Another important change since the previous edition is the increased awareness of antibiotic resistance. Accordingly, a concerted effort has been made by all contributing authors to promote responsible antimicrobial stewardship by better describing the infection continuum and reviewing the premise of antibiotic resistance and biofilms. These topics are particularly well addressed in chapters 3, 4, and 19. Finally, it seemed appropriate to add a section on dog-bite wounds and gunshot wounds to Chapter 20 and to add an entire chapter on innovative adjunctive therapies, discussing the most recent developments.

In closing we wish to express our gratitude to the authors for their willingness in bringing to this textbook all their valuable experience. We are pleased that we were able to include many world-renowned specialists to produce the highest-quality material. We are indebted to these people who generously contributed their clinical insight and current research data.

Acknowledgment

The third edition of *Equine Wound Management* is here today thanks to Ted Stashak's vision and commitment to serve the equine veterinary community.

About the Companion Website

This book is accompanied by a companion website:

www.wiley.com/go/theoret/wound

The website includes:

- a webliography from chapter 17 in the book;
- case studies;
- figures from the book as PowerPoint slides, to download;
- interactive multiple choice questions and answers;
- videos.

CHAPTER 1

Physiology of Wound Healing

Christine Theoret, DMV, PhD, Diplomate ACVS

Chapter Contents

Summary

Prior to undertaking the management of a wound, the underlying biology of wound healing must be understood so that the best approach at the correct time can be selected, and so that problems with healing, if they arise, are recognized.

This chapter aims to provide an update on the physiologic, cellular, biochemical, and molecular aspects of wound repair.

Introduction

A vital trait of living organisms, continually subjected to insults from the environment, is their capacity for self repair. Whether the injury is from surgery or accidental, it generates an attempt by the host to restore continuity to tissue. Two processes are involved in healing: regeneration and repair. Regeneration entails the replacement of damaged tissue with normal cells of the type lost and is only possible in tissues with a sustained population of cells capable of mitosis, such as epithelium, bone, and liver. Conversely, repair is a "stop-gap" reaction designed to re-establish the continuity of interrupted tissues with undifferentiated scar tissue. Repair is, therefore, an inferior method of healing, producing scar tissue that is less biologically useful than the tissue it replaced, and that may adversely affect adjacent normal tissues. When complications of wound healing arise, the final result is even worse.

Accidental wounds occur commonly in horses and exert a significant welfare concern and financial burden on the equine industry. A large study by the United States Department of Agriculture's National Animal Health Monitoring System found, in 2006, that injury/wound/trauma was the most common medical condition affecting horses, with a prevalence of 4.7% in equids 6 months of age and older.[2] Injury/wound/trauma was the leading cause of death of foals less than 6 months old, accounting for 24% of deaths, while for horses at least 6 months old, it accounted for 16% of deaths and was the leading cause of mortality, after old age.[2] A study in Mexico conducted specifically on a population of working equids found a prevalence of 20.6% for cutaneous pathologic conditions; among these, skin wounds (abrasions, lacerations, abscesses) were the most prevalent (6.8%).[3]

Figures are also concerning in Europe. A study conducted in the UK found that wounds were the most common type of injury reported by horse owners, accounting for roughly half of all injuries occurring over a 12-month period.[4] Another study found that wounds accounted for 21.6% of veterinary

This chapter is reprinted, in a modified form, from *Equine Surgery, 3rd edition*, Theoret CL, Wound repair, pp. 44–62, Copyright (2005),[1] with permission from Elsevier.

Equine Wound Management, Third Edition. Edited by Christine Theoret and Jim Schumacher.

Companion website: www.wiley.com/go/theoret/wound

treatments of injured polo ponies in the UK.[5] Horses in the southern hemisphere do not seem to fare any better: wounds ranked as the third most common medical condition encountered by equine practitioners in Australia and New Zealand and ranked second, after colic, as the most common cause of death or euthanasia.[6,7]

Finally, skin trauma/wounds are a frequent cause of morbidity in athletic horses. A study in Thoroughbred racehorses has shown that 70% of injuries leading to early retirement are the result of a musculoskeletal injury, of which 7% are associated with wounds or lacerations.[8]

The objective of repair is to re-establish an epithelial cover and to recover the integrity, strength, and function of the skin. Partial-thickness cutaneous wounds (e.g., abrasions and erosions) heal primarily by migration and proliferation of epidermal cells from the remaining underlying epithelium, as well as from the adnexal structures (i.e., hair follicles and sweat and sebaceous glands), with little participation of inflammatory or stromal cells. In contrast, second-intention repair of full-thickness cutaneous wounds hinges on four coordinated and interrelated phases (Figure 1.1). Partitioning the process into discrete phases suggests simplicity while, in reality, healing is exquisitely complex. The phases rely on interactions between multiple cellular types, their surrounding matrix, and the soluble mediators that govern the numerous activities required to rebuild the tissue. Moreover, the interactions are not static but rather in a state of constant flux, resulting in a microenvironment that is continually evolving as the wound heals.[10]

Before veterinarians can positively influence wound healing, they must understand its mechanisms so that they select the appropriate techniques of wound management. In fact, Hippocrates once said, "Healing is a matter of time, but it is sometimes also a matter of opportunity."[11]

Skin anatomy

The skin is the largest organ and serves key functions including physical protection, sensation, temperature regulation, and insulation. It is composed of two compartments – the epidermis and the dermis (Figure 1.2a). In the horse, the epidermis consists of five layers of keratinocytes: the *stratum basale*, *stratum spinosum*, *stratum granulosum*, *stratum lucidum*, and *stratum corneum* (Figure 1.2b). Additional epidermal components, referred to as skin appendages, include hair follicles, sweat glands, sebaceous glands, and hooves/nails. Although 90–95% of the cells populating the epidermis are keratinocytes, this compartment also includes melanocytes, Langerhans cells, and Merkel cells. Epidermis is attached to the dermis at the level of the basement membrane, a thin, glycoprotein-rich layer composed primarily of laminin and type IV collagen. This attachment is through hemidesmosomes, which physically attach the basal cells of the epidermis to the underlying dermis, as well as by vertically oriented type VII collagen anchoring fibrils, which bind the cytoskeleton.[12]

The dermal compartment consists of two regions, the papillary dermis and the reticular dermis. This compartment is composed of dense, fibroelastic connective tissue and constitutes the bulk of the skin. The epidermis projects into this underlying connective tissue via extensions known as rete pegs or ridges. A network of collagen fibers provides tensile strength to the dermis, and elastin and glycosaminoglycans (GAGs) ensure resilience. Collagen type I is the major collagen of the dermis (~62%) whereas collagen type III comprises ~15% of the dermis.[13] The fibroblast is the principal type of cell found in the dermis; perivascular mast cells and tissue macrophages are also found within the dermis. The connective tissue supports these cells and also a network of nerves, epithelial glands, keratinizing

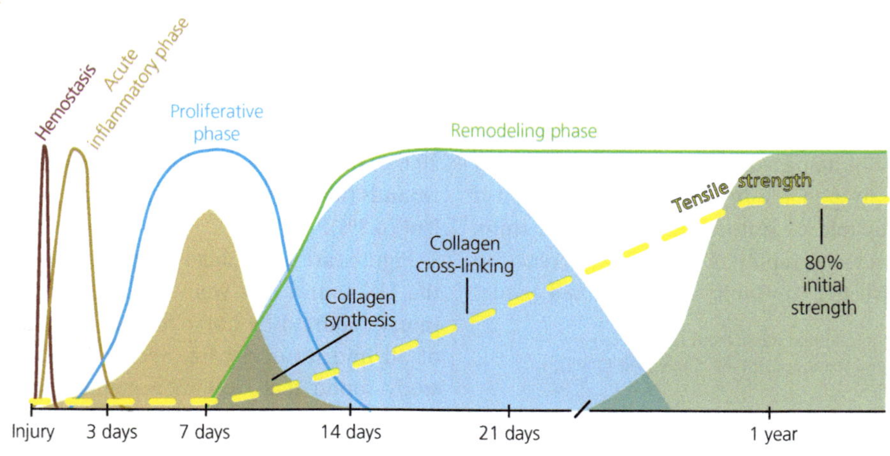

Figure 1.1 Temporal profile of synchronized phases and gain in tensile strength of healing cutaneous wounds. Solid lines show the healing profile of laboratory animals while superimposed shaded areas show the profile of healing full-thickness wounds on the limb of horses. It should be noted that the timescale is suggestive and depends on the size and extent of the wound. Source: Modified by Marco Langlois (Faculté de médecine vétérinaire, Université de Montréal) from Stashak & Theoret 2014.[9] Reproduced with permission of Elsevier.

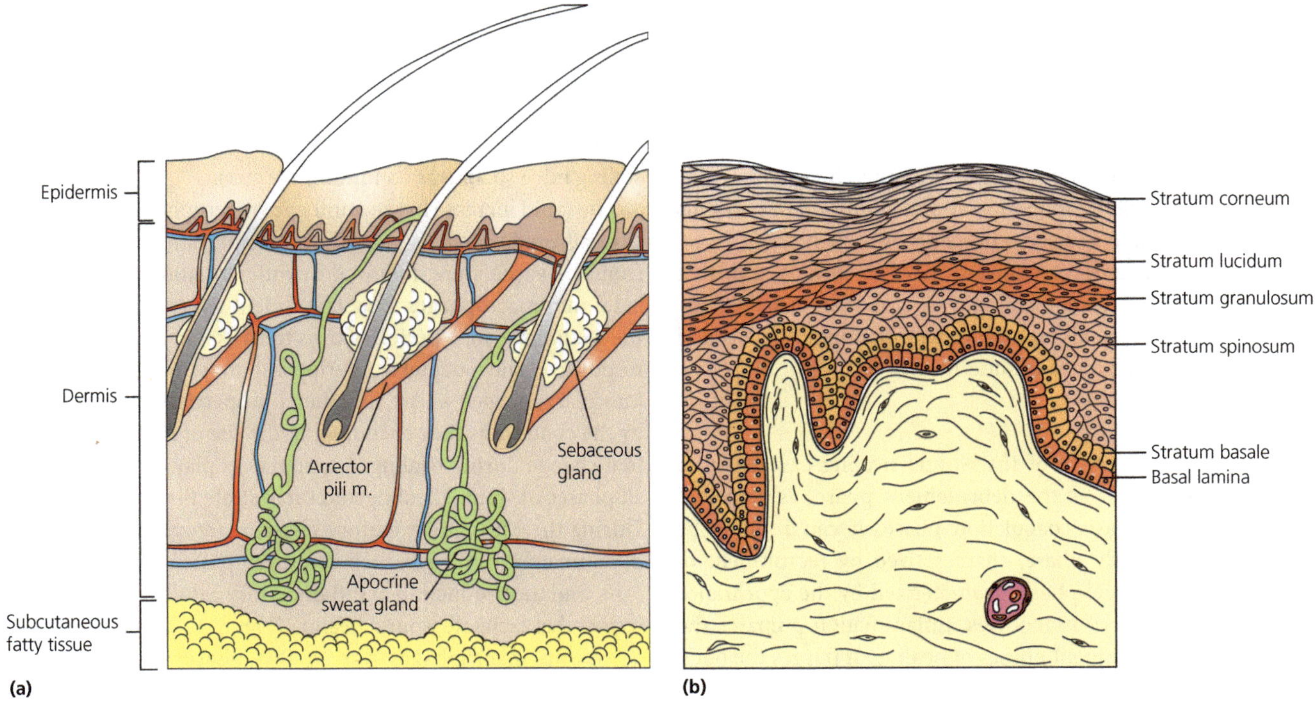

Figure 1.2 **(a)** Diagram of a cross-section of skin, showing the epidermal and dermal compartments. **(b)** Diagram of the layers of the epidermis of horse skin. Source: Stashak & Theoret 2014.[9] Reproduced with permission of Elsevier.

appendages, and a microvascular and lymphatic system. Indeed, only the dermal compartment is vascularized; nutrients reach the epidermis by diffusion.

In the horse, the thickness of the skin varies according to body site. For example, in the Dutch warmblood, the skin on the head, neck, and ventral abdomen is relatively thin, measuring between 1.73 mm (±0.16) and 2.03 mm (±0.2) whereas the skin on the limbs is slightly thicker, measuring an average of 2.83 mm (±0.27) for the forelimb and 2.89 mm (±0.24) for the hindlimb, depending on the specific anatomic location (e.g., the skin over the dorsal coffin joint is particularly thick, measuring 4.54 mm [±0.39]).[14]

The subcutaneous tissue (i.e., tissue just deep to the skin) is also known as the hypodermis or superficial fascia and is not considered part of the skin. It is comprised of loose connective tissue; approximately half of the body's fat stores are located in this region. The hypodermis anchors the skin to the underlying organs and allows the skin to move relatively freely. It also acts as a shock absorber and insulates the deeper body tissues from heat loss.

Phases of wound repair

Hemostasis/coagulation

The first phase of wound healing begins immediately upon injury, is completed within hours, and is dedicated to hemostasis and the formation of a provisional wound matrix. Hemostasis was long considered to be a component of the inflammatory phase, and only recently has its individual significance to wound healing been recognized. Many of the processes that occur during the ensuing phases rely on the normal execution of this short, but critical, initial phase.

Wounding traumatizes blood vessels, which results in hemorrhage. The injured endothelial cellular membrane releases phospholipids that are transformed into arachidonic acid and its metabolites that mediate vascular tone and permeability. Peripheral vasoconstriction, lasting 5–10 minutes, limits bleeding but simultaneously starves the surrounding tissues of oxygen and nutrients normally carried by the blood. The resulting transitory hypoxia and increased glycolysis, as well as pH changes, are beneficial because, along with the effects of the original vascular trauma, they enhance the activation, adhesion and aggregation of platelets, thereby initiating the intrinsic coagulation cascade, ultimately leading to the formation of a blood clot that seals the vessel.[15]

This clot, besides providing a small amount of strength to the wound, has multiple roles. It forms a provisional matrix, rich in fibrin, fibronectin, vitronectin, and thrombospondin, that fills the space created by the wound and serves as a scaffold for migrating cells. Special surface receptors (integrins) on inflammatory and stromal cells recognize binding sites on the proteins within the scaffold, ensuring ingrowth of cells involved in healing. This cellular influx is mediated by chemoattractants released by degranulating platelets, among other cells, present in the scaffold. Indeed, activated platelets are amongst the earliest promoters of inflammation, via the release of potent chemoattractants and mitogens from their storage granules.[16] Mediators released not only by platelets but also by mast cells modify vascular tone and permeability, which increase within 5–10 minutes of wounding (apparent clinically as a localized redness, heat and swelling of the wound), and thereby facilitate the aforementioned cellular migration and the diffusion of nutrients and oxygen required to sustain these newly arriving cells.

Over time, the surface clot desiccates to form a scab that protects the wound from infection. This scab is, in turn, lysed by plasmin and sloughs, along with dead inflammatory cells and bacteria, as healing proceeds underneath.

Inflammation

The inflammatory phase of the wound healing cascade (also referred to clinically as the debridement phase) is activated during the hemostasis/coagulation phase. It can roughly be divided into an early phase, characterized by recruitment of neutrophils, and a late phase, characterized by the appearance and transformation of monocytes. Inflammation prepares the wound for the subsequent phases of healing. It purges the body of alien substances and disposes of dead tissue, while the participating cellular populations liberate mediators to amplify and sustain the events to follow. The intensity of the inflammatory response is strongly correlated to the severity of trauma and determines the extent of scarring.

Leukocytes are recruited from blood circulating to the site of injury by the numerous vasoactive mediators and chemoattractants supplied by the coagulation and activated complement pathways, by platelets, by mast cells,[10] and by injured or activated stromal cells.[17] These signals initiate the processes of rolling, activation, tight adhesion, and, finally, transmigration of inflammatory cells through the microvascular endothelium. Chemoattractants also stimulate the release of enzymes by the activated neutrophils, expediting their penetration through vascular basement membranes. Diapedesis of neutrophils is further facilitated by increased capillary permeability brought about by the release of a spectrum of vasodilatory agents. Cellular influx begins within minutes and the concentration of neutrophils at the wound progressively increases to reach a peak 1–2 days after injury. Neutrophils act as a first line of defense in contaminated wounds by destroying debris and bacteria through phagocytosis and subsequent enzymatic and oxygen-radical mechanisms. Neutrophil migration and phagocytosis cease when contaminating particles are cleared from the site of injury. Most cells then become entrapped within the clot, which is sloughed during the later phases of repair. The neutrophils remaining within viable tissue die in a few days and are phagocytized by the tissue macrophages or modified wound fibroblasts, marking the termination of the early inflammatory phase of repair.[17] Although neutrophils help create a favorable environment within the wound and serve as a source of pro-inflammatory cytokines, they are not essential to repair of non-infected wounds. Indeed, a classic series of experiments in the 1970s showed that, as long as conditions were kept sterile, depletion of neutrophils in a guinea pig wound model seemed not to perturb tissue repair.[18] More recent knockdown experiments in mice support the depletion studies of the 1970s and go further, showing that repair is even more rapid than in wild-type sibling mice so long as conditions are sterile.[19]

The rapid increase in the number of macrophages in inflamed tissue is predominantly caused by the emigration of monocytes from the vasculature, followed by differentiation of the monocytes into macrophages to assist resident tissue macrophages at the wound site for a period of days to weeks. In this manner, the responsive and adaptable pluripotent monocytes can morph into macrophages whose functional properties are determined by the conditions they encounter at the site of mobilization and that change during healing. Macrophages play a central role in all phases of wound healing and orchestrate the overall process. During the early inflammatory phase, macrophages exert pro-inflammatory functions, such as antigen presentation, phagocytosis, and the production of inflammatory cytokines and growth factors that facilitate wound healing (Figure 1.3). The phenotype of wound macrophages during this phase is probably the classically activated or so-called "M1 phenotype." Later, during the proliferative phase of healing, macrophages stimulate proliferation of dermal, endothelial, and epithelial tissue to complete formation of the extracellular matrix (ECM), angiogenesis, and epithelialization. Macrophages can then change the composition of the ECM during the remodeling phase by releasing degradative enzymes (Figure 1.4). This suggests an important role for alternatively activated macrophages (also known as "M2 phenotype") in this phase of wound healing.[20,21]

More recent studies using genetically modified neonatal mice have shown that, like neutrophils, macrophages might not be essential for tissue repair.[22] Nevertheless, they probably play an important role in the regulation of fibrosis and scarring by degrading matrix.[23]

In spite of this new, somewhat conflicting evidence, acute inflammation is still considered crucial to the normal repair of wounds in adult mammals exposed to infective agents. When inflammation fails to resolve, however, and a chronic inflammatory response is established, the process can become dysregulated, resulting in pathologic wound repair and the accumulation of permanent fibrotic scar tissue at the site of injury. This fibrosis is characterized by the excessive accumulation of ECM components, including collagens, fibronectin, and hyaluronic acid at the site of injury, leading to a decrease in organ function and, in some cases, organ failure and death. In humans, an estimated 45% of deaths in the western world are now attributed to diseases in which fibrosis plays a major etiologic role.[24] One such "fibroproliferative disorder" encountered in full-thickness cutaneous wounds of the horse and that leads to increased scarring is the development of exuberant granulation tissue (the reader is referred to Chapter 15).

After injury, once infection has been countered and repair completed, all the inflammatory cells disperse from the wound.

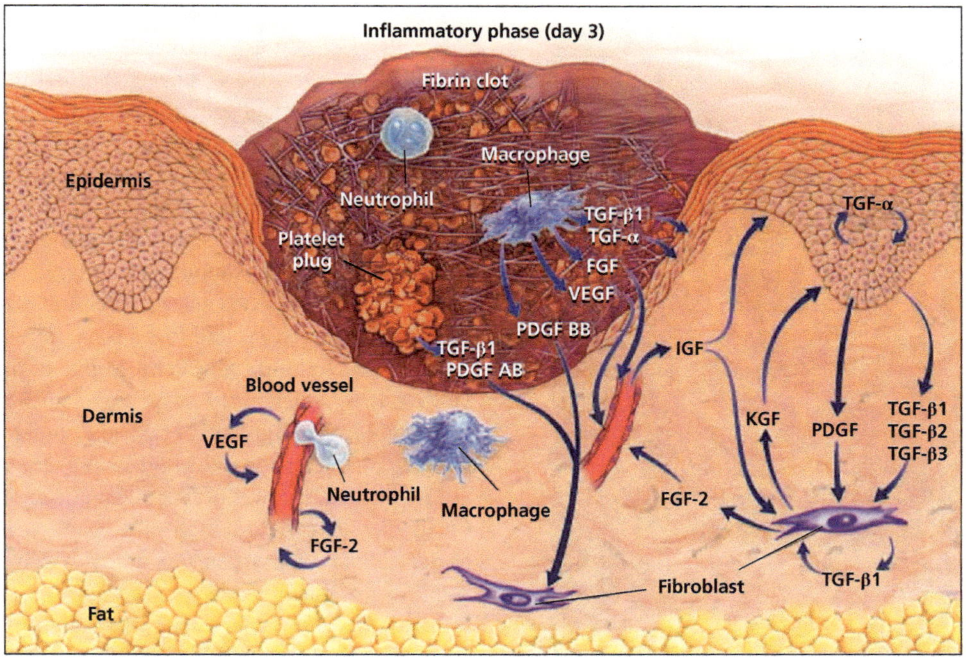

Figure 1.3 Illustration of a full-thickness cutaneous wound showing the cellular and molecular components present 3 days after injury. FGF, basic fibroblast growth factor; IGF, insulin-like growth factor; KGF, keratinocyte growth factor; PDGF, platelet-derived growth factor; TGF, transforming growth factor; VEGF, vascular endothelial growth factor. Source: Singer 1999.[17] Reproduced with permission of NEJM.

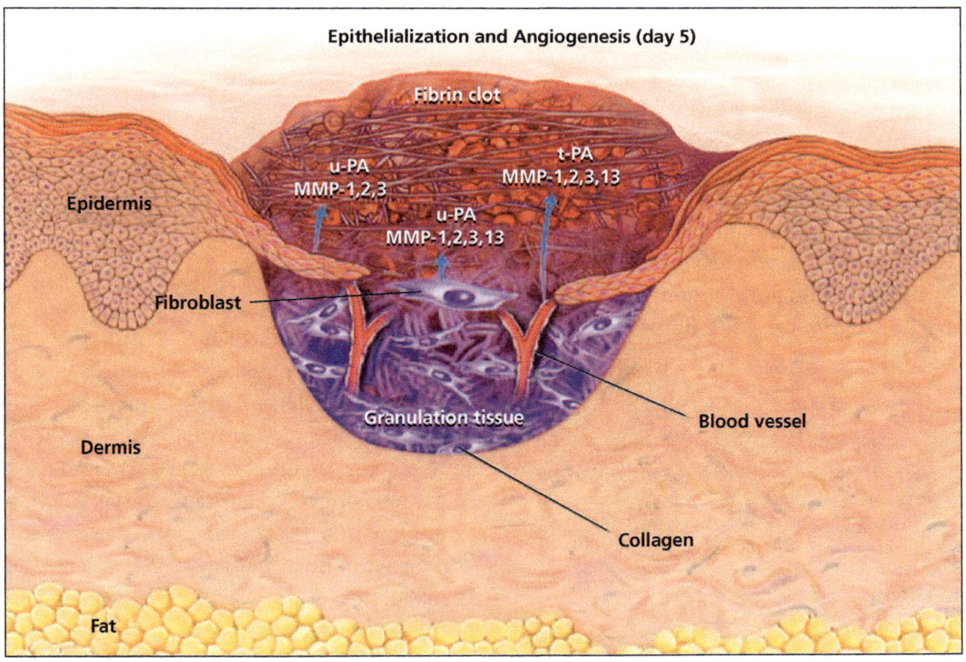

Figure 1.4 Illustration of a full-thickness cutaneous wound 5 days after injury showing angiogenesis, fibroplasia, and epithelialization. uPA, urokinase-type plasminogen activator; tPA, tissue-type plasminogen activator; MMP, matrix metalloproteinase. Source: Singer 1999.[17] Reproduced with permission of NEJM.

For inflammation to resolve, each of the events that initiated it must be halted or even reversed. Apoptosis, or programmed cellular death, is the universal pathway for eliminating unneeded cells in a phagocytic process that does not elicit additional inflammation.[25] This mechanism prevails during all phases of wound repair because each phase relies on rapid increases in specific cellular populations that prepare the wound for repair (inflammatory cells) or deposit new matrices and mature the

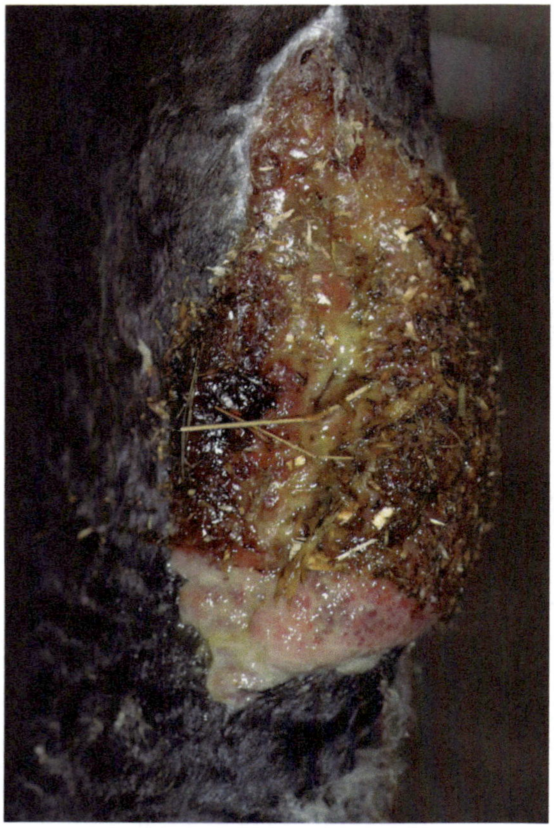

Figure 1.5 This metatarsal wound failed to heal for 7 months as a result of chronic low-grade inflammation due to exposure as well as superficial and deep infection. The wound in fact became larger rather than smaller, illustrating suspension of the healing process. Courtesy of Dr. Derek Knottenbelt.

wound (stromal cells), but then must be eliminated prior to progression to the next phase of repair. Indeed, a mature scar is typically acellular. There are several steps at which the process of resolution could go astray, leading to suppuration, chronic inflammation (Figure 1.5), and/or excessive fibrosis.

Tip

- Clinicians have the greatest influence on the acute inflammatory phase of healing: proper surgical debridement and irrigation, good hemostasis, and adequate drainage can greatly hasten wound healing.

Cellular proliferation

The main objective of the proliferative phase (also referred to clinically as the repair phase) is to achieve protection of the wound's surface via the formation of granulation tissue and a new epithelial cover and to restore the vascular network to nourish the new tissues.

Fibroplasia

The proliferative phase of repair comes about as inflammation subsides and is characterized by the appearance of red, fleshy granulation tissue, which ultimately fills the defect. Although the earliest part of this phase is very active on a cellular level, this activity does not immediately translate into a gain in the wound's strength. Indeed, during the first 3–5 days following injury, fibroblasts and endothelial and epithelial cells rapidly invade the wound in preparation for synthesis and maturation of the matrix or for wound coverage; however, these latter reinforcing mechanisms lag somewhat. Granulation tissue is formed by three elements that simultaneously move into the defect created by the wound: *macrophages*, which debride and produce mediators, such as cytokines and growth factors, that stimulate angiogenesis and fibroplasia; *fibroblasts*, which proliferate and synthesize new components of the ECM; and *new blood vessels*, which carry oxygen and nutrients necessary for the metabolism and growth of cells, and confer to the granulation tissue its characteristic red, granular appearance.

This stroma, rich in fibronectin and hyaluronan, replaces the fibrin clot to provide a physical barrier to infection and, importantly, provides a surface across which cells can migrate. A number of matrix molecules as well as cytokines and growth factors released by inflammatory cells are believed to stimulate fibroblasts from adjacent uninjured dermis and subcutaneous tissue to proliferate and express integrin receptors to assist their migration into the defect. Integrins are transmembrane proteins that act as the major cell-surface receptors for ECM molecules and thus mediate interactions between cells and their environment. They are particularly critical to the migratory movements exhibited by cells involved in wound healing, such as epithelial and endothelial cells and fibroblasts.[26] Migration of fibroblasts immediately precedes advancing capillary endothelial buds but follows macrophages that have cleared a path by phagocytizing debris. Fibroblasts themselves also possess an active proteolytic system, comprising proteinases, such as plasminogen activator (PA), various collagenases, gelatinase, and stromelysin,[27] to aid their migration into the fibrin blood clot.

After fibroblasts have arrived within the defect created by the wound, they proliferate then switch their function to protein synthesis and commence to gradually replace the provisional matrix with a collagen-rich one, probably under the influence of various cytokines and growth factors. As the wound matures, the ratio of type I (mature) to type III (immature) collagen markedly increases; proteoglycans also become abundant within the mature matrix. The greatest rate of accumulation of connective tissue within the wound occurs 7–14 days after injury, at least in the laboratory rodent, which translates into the period of most rapid gain in tensile strength (see Figure 1.1). Thereafter, the collagen content within the wound levels off as fibroblasts down-regulate their synthetic activities; this corresponds to a much slower gain in tensile strength as the wound remodels. The fibroblast-rich granulation tissue is subsequently replaced by relatively avascular and acellular scar tissue, as the capillaries within the wound regress and fibroblasts either undergo apoptosis[28] or acquire characteristics of smooth muscle and transform into myofibroblasts that participate in wound contraction. The latter phenomena are regulated by the physiologic needs and/or the microenvironmental stimuli present at the wound. It appears that if the signal to down-regulate fibroblast activity is delayed beyond a specific time point, apoptosis is permanently impaired, ultimately leading to an imbalance between collagen synthesis and degradation[29] and the formation of excessive scar tissue.

Angiogenesis

Besides initiating the inflammatory response through interactions with leukocytes, microvascular endothelial cells play a key role in the proliferative phase of repair. The formation of new capillaries from pre-existing ones (angiogenesis) is necessary to restore oxygenation and to provide required nutrients to the granulation tissue newly formed within the wound. Angiogenesis, which occurs in response to tissue injury and hypoxia, is a complex and dynamic process mediated by diverse soluble factors provided by the serum and the surrounding ECM. These factors are, in particular, angiogenic inducers, including growth factors [most notably vascular endothelial growth factor (VEGF), fibroblast growth factor (FGF)-2, platelet-derived growth factor (PDGF), and members of the transforming growth factor (TGF)-β family],[30] chemokines and angiogenic enzymes (notably the serine proteinase thrombin), endothelial-specific receptors, and adhesion molecules, such as integrins,[31] many of which are released during the inflammatory phase of repair.

Construction of a vascular network requires sequential steps that include augmented microvascular permeability, the release of proteinases from activated endothelial cells with subsequent local degradation of the basement membrane surrounding the existing vessel, migration and sprouting of endothelial cells into the interstitial space, endothelial cellular proliferation and differentiation into mature blood vessels (i.e., arterioles and venules), eventually followed by regression and involution of the newly formed vasculature as tissue remodels.[32] Angiogenesis depends not only on the cells and cytokines present, but also on the production and organization of components of the ECM that provide a scaffold through which endothelial cells can migrate and a reservoir and modulator for growth factors. Thus, endothelial cells at the tip of capillaries begin their migration into the wound in response to angiogenic stimuli and the absence of neighboring cells on the second day after injury. Cytoplasmic pseudopodia extend through fragmented basement membranes; subsequently, the entire endothelial cell migrates into the perivascular space. Cells remaining in the parent vessel near the tip of the angiogenic sprouts begin to proliferate, providing a continuous source of microvascular endothelial cells for angiogenesis. A new capillary sprout has no lumen when it first develops; after it fuses with a neighboring sprout to form an arcade, it canalizes, allowing erythrocytes to pass into and through it. Formation of a lumen probably involves the joining of plasma membranes of individual and/or adjacent cells, as well as extensive intracellular vacuolization followed by fusion of the vacuoles to form "ring cells," which ultimately fuse to form seamless capillaries. Capillaries then become stable as endothelial cells interact with the new basement membrane within 24 hours of new vessel formation and via the recruitment of pericytes and smooth muscle cells. In healing wounds, this vigorous angiogenic response results in a density of vessels that far exceeds that of capillaries in normal, uninjured tissue[33] and provides the granulation tissue with its red, granular appearance.

After the stroma has been completely reconstituted, a rich vascular supply to the wound is no longer needed. Pro-angiogenic stimuli are down-regulated and/or the local concentration of anti-angiogenic factors (thrombospondin, interferon gamma-induced protein 10/CXC motif chemokine 10, and Sprouty-2)[34,35] increases, and most of the recently formed capillary network quickly involutes through the activity of matrix metalloproteinases (MMPs),[36] in particular MMP-1 and MMP-10,[37] and selective apoptosis of endothelial cells. The color of the wound pales as the rich capillary bed disappears from the granulation tissue.

Epithelialization

Epithelialization is defined as the process of covering denuded epithelial surfaces and is essential for successful closure of the wound. In addition to the aforementioned hemostatic activities that establish a temporary barrier, the residual epithelium beneath the clot moves centripetally to participate in closure of the wound. Even though epithelial migration commences 24–48 hours after wounding, the characteristic pink rim of new epithelium (Figure 1.6) is not macroscopically visible until some time later. This "lag" varies according to the species of animal and the site, size, and substrate of the wound. For example, epithelialization is accelerated in a partial-thickness wound because migrating cells arise not only from the residual epithelium at the wound's periphery but also from remaining epidermal appendages. Furthermore, the basement membrane is intact in this type of injury, precluding a lengthy regeneration. On the other hand, during second-intention healing of a full-thickness wound,

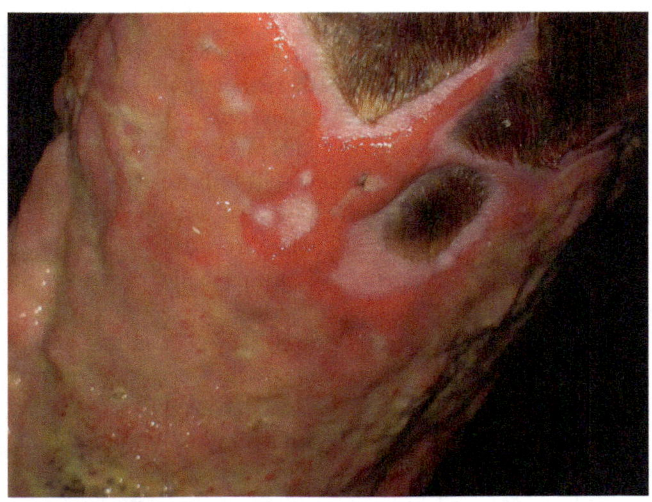

Figure 1.6 Large full-thickness metatarsal wound that healed partially by second intention and was subsequently grafted successfully. The wound showed excellent epithelialization from the healing margin of the wound. The healthy epithelial tissue is characterized by an area of hyperemia adjacent to it. Courtesy of Dr. Derek Knottenbelt.

epithelialization cannot proceed until a bed of granulation tissue has formed. In full-thickness, 7–9 cm^2 wounds created experimentally in horses and ponies and left to heal by second intention, after an initial lag phase, epithelialization progressed over the wound surface at a rate of 0.63 mm/week for metatarsal wounds in ponies, 0.48 mm/week for metatarsal wounds in horses, 0.75 mm/week for buttock wounds in ponies, and 0.62 mm/week for buttock wounds in horses between the third and the seventh week of healing.[38]

The regenerative capacity of the epidermis relies on keratinocyte stem cells (KSC) that reside within specific microenvironments referred to as stem cell niches. The following three niches have been identified: the bulge of the hair follicle (HF), the base of the sebaceous gland, and the basal layer of the interfollicular epidermis (IFE).[39] In response to epidermal injury, the HF and IFE niches participate in epithelialization of the defect.[40]

To close the defect in the epidermis, keratinocytes at the wound's edge must first loosen their adhesions to each other (desmosomes) and to the basal lamina (hemidesmosomes) and develop the flexibility required to migrate over the new matrix. Numerous regulators play a critical role in modulating the proliferation and migration of keratinocytes during epithelialization; these include chemokines, cytokines, integrins, keratins, ECM molecules, and MMPs, among others. A discussion of these is beyond the scope of the text; the reader is referred to a recent review of the subject.[41]

Additionally, various degradative enzymes necessary for the proteolysis of components of the ECM are up-regulated within cells at the leading edge of neo-epithelium, facilitating ingestion of the clot and debris found along the migratory route. This route is determined by the array of integrin receptors for various ECM proteins, expressed on the surface of migrating epithelial cells. Once the surface of the wound is covered by epithelial cells contacting one another, further migration is inhibited by the expression, within the ECM, of laminin, a major factor responsible for adhesion of epithelial cells.

Although initial cellular migration does not require an increase in cellular multiplication, basal keratinocytes at the wound's margin do begin to proliferate 1–2 days after injury to replenish the migratory front; this corresponds histologically to epithelial hyperplasia (Figure 1.7). The new cells leap-frog over those at the wound margin and adhere to the substratum, only to be replaced in turn by other cells coming from above and behind. The newly adherent monolayer subsequently restratifies to restore the original multi-layered epidermis.

In full-thickness wounds healing by second intention, such as those commonly managed in equine practice, provisional matrix is eventually replaced by a mature basement membrane. Repairing epidermis reassembles its constituents from the margin towards the center of the wound.[17] Epidermal cells then revert to a quiescent phenotype and become attached to this new basement membrane through hemidesmosomes and to the underlying neodermis through type VII collagen fibrils. This particular aspect of epithelialization is time consuming, occurring long after total coverage of the wound by epithelium is apparent, which may explain the continued fragility of neoepidermis for extended periods after repair is macroscopically complete. This is particularly evident in large wounds of the limb, where new epidermis is often thin and easily traumatized (Figure 1.8).

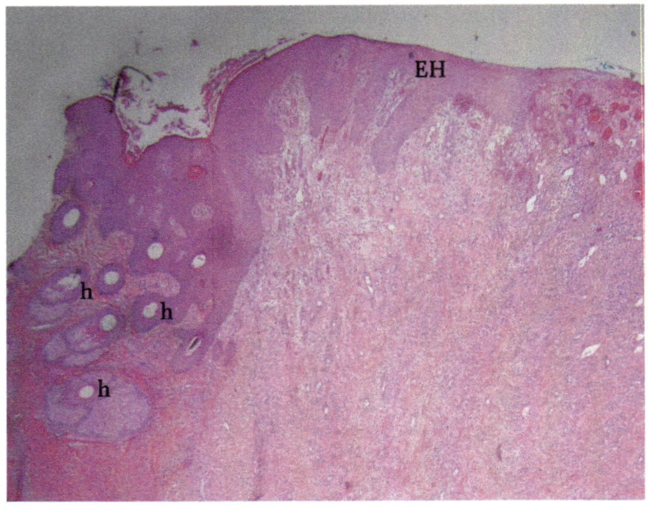

Figure 1.7 Photomicrograph of a wound edge sample of tissue. Normal unwounded skin to the left demonstrating epidermal appendages (h, hair follicles); new hyperplastic epithelium (EH) to the right, overlying granulation tissue bed. Source: Theoret 2004.[42] Reproduced with permission of Elsevier.

Matrix synthesis and remodeling (also referred to clinically as the maturation phase)

Mature ECM is a non-cellular scaffold composed of proteins, glycosaminoglycans, polysaccharides, and water, that facilitates bidirectional communication between cells and their biochemical/biophysical environment.[43] During the remodeling phase (occurring from 3 weeks to up to 1 year after injury), the components of the ECM undergo certain changes to ensure strength, integrity, and function of the replacement tissue.

In addition to epithelialization, contraction contributes to the successful closure of full-thickness wounds. Contraction is defined as a process whereby both dermis and epidermis bordering a full-thickness skin deficit are drawn from all sides centripetally over the exposed wound.[44] This usually occurs during the second week after injury. Wound contraction not only accelerates closure, it also enhances the cosmetic appearance and strength of the scar because proportionally less area of the wound must be covered by newly formed epithelium of inferior quality, which is fragile and lacks normal nervous, glandular, follicular, and vascular components (Figure 1.8b). For this reason, a high degree of contraction is a desired feature of wound repair, at least in the horse.

Wound contraction is thought to result from a combination of tractional forces generated by migrating fibroblasts and the action of a specialized fibroblast phenotype, the myofibroblast. As fibroblasts migrate into the provisional matrix of the wound under the influence of various cytokines, tension within the wound reaches the threshold required, along with the action of TGF-β1 and the ED-A splice variant of fibronectin,[45] to trigger fibroblasts to differentiate into myofibroblasts.[46] The latter are the most abundant cellular elements of healthy granulation

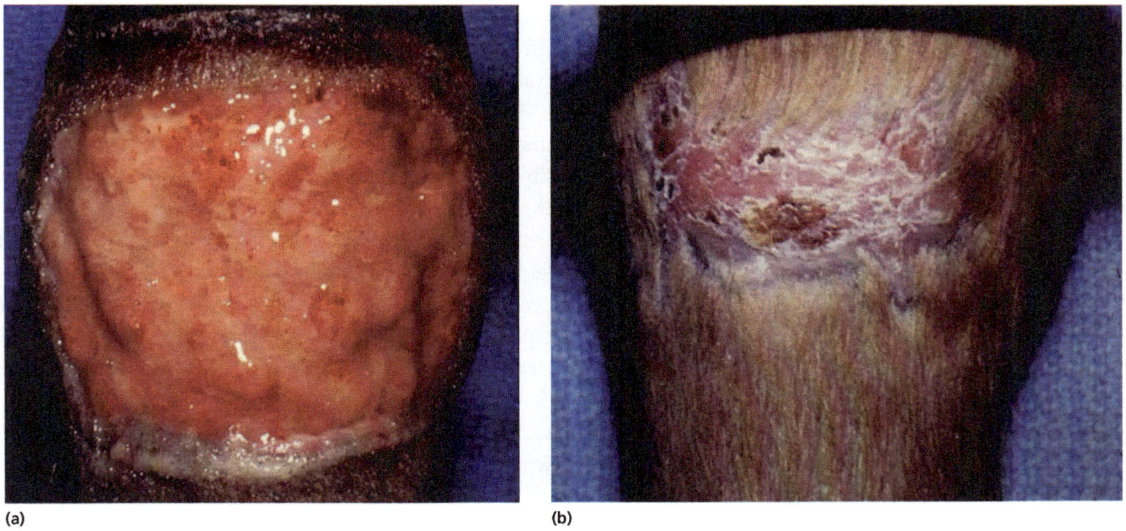

Figure 1.8 **(a)** A 5-day-old, full-thickness, experimentally created wound over the dorsal surface of the fetlock. Granulation tissue is beginning to fill the wound. **(b)** The same wound, 75 days after creation. Neoepidermis is thin, dry, and hairless, and could be easily traumatized. Courtesy of Dr. Ted Stashak.

tissue and are aligned within the wound along the lines of contraction. The most striking feature of the myofibroblast is a well-developed alpha smooth muscle actin (α-SMA) microfilamentous system, arranged parallel to the cell's long axis and in continuity with the components of the ECM via various integrins. In addition to these cell–substratum links, intercellular connections, such as gap junctions and hemidesmosomes, ensure that neighboring cells exert tension on one another.

Wound contraction is divided into three phases. An initial lag phase (wherein skin edges retract, and the area of the wound increases temporarily for 1–2 weeks, depending on its anatomic location) occurs prior to substantial fibroblastic invasion of the wound, as a prerequisite for contraction. Subsequently, a period of rapid contraction is followed by one of slow contraction as the wound approaches complete closure. The number of myofibroblasts found in a wound appears proportional to the need for contraction, and thus, as repair progresses and the rate of contraction slows, this number decreases accordingly. During wound contraction, the surrounding skin stretches by intussusceptive growth, and the wound takes on a stellate appearance.

Contraction ceases in response to one of three events: the wound's edges meet, causing contact inhibition to halt the processes of epithelialization and contraction; tension in the surrounding skin becomes equal to or greater than the contractile force generated by the α-SMA of the myofibroblasts; or, in the case of chronic wounds, a low number of myofibroblasts in the granulation tissue may result in failure of the wound to contract, despite laxity in the surrounding skin. In the latter case, the granulation tissue is pale and consists primarily of collagen and ground substance. Wound contraction is greater in regions of the body with loose skin than in regions where skin is under tension, such as the distal extremity of the equine limb. Although the shape of the wound has been speculated to influence the process of contraction, this does not appear relevant in wounds of the distal limb where skin is tightly stretched and not easily moved.[47]

Wound contraction was measured in full-thickness, 7–9 cm^2 experimental wounds left to heal by second intention on the limbs and hindquarters of horses and ponies. The wounds were bandaged for the first 3 weeks then left unbandaged. Following an initial lag phase of 1 week, wound contraction became apparent in buttock wounds of horses and ponies and in metatarsal wounds of ponies. The percentage decrease in wound surface area attributable to wound contraction between the second and the fourth week of healing was 47% for the body wounds of ponies vs. 35% for the limb wounds of ponies, and 38% for the body wounds of horses vs. 0% for the limb wounds of horses. After week 4, the rate of wound contraction slowed to less than 5% per week for these wounds, up to complete healing. The metatarsal wounds of horses showed a different pattern: the lag phase of healing lasted 4 weeks and this was followed by an average rate of contraction that did not exceed 2.5% per week.[38]

As contraction concludes, myofibroblasts disappear, either by reverting to a quiescent fibroblastic phenotype or by apoptosis,[28] primarily in response to reduced tension within the ECM.[48] The myofibroblast persists in fibrotic lesions where it may be involved in accumulation of more ECM and pathologic contracture, a condition leading to substantial morbidity, particularly when it involves joints or orifices, but rarely encountered in the horse.

The conversion of ECM from granulation to scar tissue constitutes the final phase of wound repair, also referred to as maturation, and consists of synthesis of connective tissue, lysis, and remodeling. Proteoglycans replace hyaluronan during the second week of repair, support the deposition and aggregation of collagen fibers, and make the mature matrix more resilient. Collagen macromolecules provide the tensile strength to the wound as their deposition peaks within the initial week, when healing occurs by first intention, and between 7 and 14 days, when healing occurs by second intention, in the laboratory rodent.

Although this corresponds to the period of most rapid gain in strength, only 20% of the final strength of the skin wound is achieved within the first 3 weeks of repair. At this time, collagen synthesis is balanced by collagen lysis, which normally prevents accumulation of excessive amounts of collagen and formation of a pathologic scar. The balance between synthesis and degradation determines the overall strength of a healing wound at a particular time. The first newly deposited collagen tends to be oriented randomly and, therefore, provides little tensile strength, whereas during remodeling, the fibers reform along lines of stress and, therefore, resist dehiscence more effectively. Cross-linking of the later-formed collagen is also more effective, but never occurs to the same extent as in the original tissue. The new collagen weaves into that which pre-existed and also appears to bond to the ends of old collagen fibers. These welds are points of weakness, which may rupture when stressed.

Remodeling of ECM within a wound depends on the presence of various proteolytic enzymes (proteinases) released from inflammatory and mesenchymal cells, such as MMPs and serine and cysteine proteinases (cathepsins). Those of the MMP family are collectively capable of degrading virtually all components of the ECM. Although MMPs are not constitutively expressed in skin, up-regulation occurs whenever proteolysis is required, such as during cellular migration and remodeling of the matrix. Inactive precursors of the MMPs (pro MMPs) are cleaved in the extracellular space by proteinases, such as plasmin and trypsin, left over from the inflammatory and proliferative phases, but also by other MMPs. To date, two dozen different MMPs, all distinct gene products, have been characterized.[27]

Based on domain organization and preference for substrate, MMPs may be divided into the following groups: 1 – collagenases; 2 – gelatinases; 3 – stromelysins; 4 – matrilysins; 5 – metallo-elastases; 6 – membrane-type MMPs; 7 – other MMPs.[49] Although the major function of most MMPs is probably to process bioactive molecules, such as chemokines and cytokines, as well as their respective receptors, their ability to degrade ECM proteins, as demonstrated by some members of the MMP family (MMP1, MMP3, MMP13, and MMP14 are capable of cleaving collagen; MMP7 can process syndecan-1 and elastin), suggests they have a role in remodeling during wound healing.[27] Comprehensive lists of MMPs, including their physiologic and *in vitro* substrates, can be found in proteinase databases.[50,51]

Homeostasis between collagen synthesis and degradation during the remodeling phase depends on the simultaneous presence of MMPs and non-specific inhibitors, such as α2-macroglobulin and α1-antiprotease, as well as natural specific inhibitors, the tissue inhibitors of metalloproteinases (TIMPs). TIMPs are a gene family of four structurally related members, TIMP-1 through -4, that inhibit conversion of MMPs from a zymogen to an activated state and that irreversibly bind to the catalytic site of active MMPs.[49]

Under most circumstances, an imbalance between MMPs and TIMPs leads to abnormal resolution and delayed repair. Indeed, although the presence of MMPs is essential for the wound to mature, it may also be responsible for the inability of chronic wounds to heal. For example, fluid found in chronic wounds is characterized by elevated concentrations of proteinases, particularly MMP-9 and serine proteinases, which lead to excessive degradation of proteins and the inactivation of critical growth factors. Chronic wounds also contain reduced concentrations of TIMPs, in particular TIMP-1.[52]

Wound remodeling continues for up to 2 years, during which time there is no net increase in collagen content, but instead, the collagen fibers rearrange into a more organized lattice-like structure, under the influence of local mechanical factors, progressively increasing the tensile strength of scar tissue. The majority of type III collagen fibers laid down early in healing are replaced by collagen type I, fibers become increasingly cross-linked, and the normal skin ratio of 4:1 type I to type III collagen is re-established. Glycosaminoglycans are steadily degraded until they reach concentrations found in normal dermis. The duration of the maturation phase depends on a variety of factors, including the patient's genetic makeup, age, location of the wound, type of injury, and duration of inflammation.

At maximum strength, cutaneous wounds in mice remain 15–20% weaker than the normal surrounding tissue,[53] but a study in horses showed that cutaneous wounds, fully healed by second intention, withstood a maximum breaking load equivalent to only 60% of the breaking force of normal, intact skin.[54] Importantly, skin appendages are usually not regenerated after wounding, resulting in a loss of other functions of skin.

Non-invasive methods to monitor healing

There are objective, non-invasive methods to monitor the progress and assess the quality of healing of cutaneous wounds, focusing on anatomic, mechanical, physiologic, and esthetic properties.[55] The goal of these technologies is to provide detailed information regarding skin components imperceptible to visual inspection and that enable the clinician to assess the severity of a wound and its healing potential, thereby guiding therapeutic decisions. Optical technologies that have, to date, been applied to wound assessment in humans include: near infrared imaging, thermal imaging, optical coherence tomography, orthogonal polarization spectral imaging, fluorescence imaging, laser Doppler imaging, microscopy, spatial frequency domain imaging, photoacoustic detection, and spectral/hyperspectral imaging.[56] Both infrared thermography (IRT) and near infrared spectroscopy (NIRS) have been used in the author's laboratory to study the healing of experimental wounds in horses.[57,58] Near infrared spectroscopy provides quantitative information on the structural and chemical components of cutaneous tissue, specifically oxygen saturation, hemoglobin, and water content. This tool enabled the identification of hypoxia in limb wounds relative to body wounds during the early phase of healing in horses.[57] Concomitantly, cutaneous wound temperature, as measured by IRT, and by extension skin blood flow, was found to be significantly lower in limb wounds than in body wounds.[58] Because low oxygen levels may promote a feeble yet prolonged inflammatory response to wounding, which could interfere with and retard the subsequent phases of healing, these experimental data aid our understanding of the impaired healing that commonly afflicts horses, particularly where limb wounds are concerned.

Other tools allow the measurement of wound dimensions to improve objective monitoring during healing, in view of adjusting the treatment plan, if required, and facilitating communication with the horse owner. A couple of recent studies have evaluated the accuracy and reliability of some of these methods when used in horse wounds.[59,60] Two-dimensional (2-D) measurements of the area of the scar/wound can be taken using manual planimetry, digital planimetry or digital imaging combined with computer-aided analysis. With manual planimetry, the borders of the wound/scar are traced on to sterile acetate film placed over the wound and used to approximate measurements of area by counting squares of known size within the boundaries of the tracing on a superimposed reference grid (i.e., graph paper). With digital planimetry, acetate tracings of the wound are digitized by retracing them on to a tablet, allowing automated calculations.[59] Digital imaging and computer-aided analysis are based on the concurrent viewing of a reference scale/ruler on images of the wound (placed for the purpose of calibration) and calculation of measurements of area from tracings of the image using a commercial software, such as the open-source image processing program, Image J.[61] Although 2-D planimetry provides a reproducible and inexpensive way of measuring the surface area of a scar/wound,[62] useful to quantitate epithelialization and contraction of a healing wound, it does not capture the specific characteristics of a granulation bed, nor does it allow measurements of the wound's volume. Quantitative topographic methods allowing 3-D assessments have been tested in wounds of horses, and based on these tests, investigators found that stereophotogrammetry can be applied for 3-D reconstructions and analyses of equine wounds using a self-developing camera system and commercially available software (Photomodeler Scanner).[59] A laser beam wound camera (SilhouetteStar, ARANZ Medical) was also shown to be capable of accurately determining the area and depth of experimental wounds on horse cadavers.[60]

Mediators of wound repair

Wound repair relies on a complex amalgamation of interactive processes involving formed elements of blood (e.g., erythrocytes, platelets, leukocytes), ECM, and mesenchymal cells. Although histologic and morphometric observations have lead to a detailed description of the kinetics of cellular and macromolecular components involved in repair, much remains to be learned about the regulation of such activities. Restoration of structural integrity and partial functional properties appears to rely on soluble mediators, synthesized by cells present within the wound or within the surrounding tissue, that coordinate migration, proliferation, and synthesis of proteins by the various cellular populations involved in the repair process.

Cytokines, defined as 4–60 kDa signaling glycoproteins released by most nucleated cells, are among the most important soluble mediators regulating wound repair. They act in concentrations of 10^9–10^{12} M in an autocrine (same cell), paracrine (adjacent cell), or endocrine (distant cell) fashion, via cell surface receptors. Receptors are proteins with an extracellular site to bind the cytokine and a transmembranous component to transmit the signal to the intracellular site where it must reach nuclear DNA for a specific response to occur. Cells may have different numbers of receptors for different factors; the concentration of factors in the area and the number of receptors that are bound determine the response generated. Growth factors are cytokines that exert primarily mitogenic influences. Both *in vivo* and *in vitro* studies analyzing non-healing wounds have shown deregulation of various cytokines, suggesting a potential target for therapy that has led to a robust interest in using exogenous cytokines in the clinical setting to improve outcomes of healing wounds.[63]

The cytokines that play a significant role in wound repair are summarized in Table 1.1. For more detail, the reader is referred to a comprehensive review of the topic.[64]

Table 1.1 Cytokines involved in wound repair.

Name	Abbreviation	Source	Major function
Granulocyte macrophage colony stimulating factor	GM-CSF	Macrophage, lymphocyte, fibroblast, endothelial cell	Differentiation and maturation of hematopoietic stem cells; recruitment of inflammatory cells; mediation of epidermal proliferation; promotion of myofibroblast differentiation and wound contraction
Interferon	IFN	Monocyte and macrophage, lymphocyte, mesenchymal cell	Proinflammatory; release of other cytokines; inhibits fibrosis
Interleukin	IL	All nucleated cells, in particular macrophage and lymphocyte	Proinflammatory; enhances epithelialization, angiogenesis, and remodeling
Tumor necrosis factor	TNF	Macrophage, lymphocyte, mast cell	Proinflammatory; enhances angiogenesis, epithelialization, and remodeling
Connective tissue growth factor	CTGF	Fibroblast	Mediator of TGF-β activity (cell proliferation and ECM accumulation)
Epidermal growth factor	EGF	Platelet, saliva	Epithelialization; chemotactic and mitogenic to fibroblast
Transforming growth factor-α	TGF-α	Macrophage, epithelial cell	MMP synthesis (remodeling); angiogenesis
Fibroblast growth factor (basic)	FGF-2	Inflammatory cell, fibroblast, endothelial cell, keratinocyte	Chemotactic and mitogenic to fibroblast and epithelial cell; protein synthesis; angiogenesis
Insulin-like growth factor	IGF	Liver, platelet	Chemotatic and mitogenic to endothelial cell; migration of epithelial cell; fibroblast proliferation; protein and GAG synthesis
Keratinocyte growth factor	KGF (FGF-7)	Fibroblast	Chemotactic and mitogenic to epithelial cell; mitogenic to endothelial cell
Platelet-derived growth factor	PDGF	Platelet	Chemotactic to inflammatory cell and smooth muscle cell; increases keratinocyte motility; mitogenic to fibroblasts; enhances protein synthesis; induction of myofibroblast phenotype
Transforming growth factor-β	TGF-β	Platelet, lymphocyte, mast cell, monocyte and macrophage, endothelial cell, epithelial cell, fibroblast	Chemotactic to inflammatory and mesenchymal cell; fibroblast proliferation; protein synthesis; ECM deposition (inhibition of MMP; induction of TIMP); wound contraction
Vascular endothelial growth factor	VEGF	Macrophage; fibroblast; endothelial cell; epithelial cell	Angiogenesis

Conclusion

The equine practitioner, when presented with a wounded horse, should fully understand the physiologic mechanisms underlying repair to enable design of an appropriate treatment plan. In the following chapters of this book, experienced authors share their opinion on how to best manage specific injuries. The reader benefits from a detailed understanding of the different phases of healing, as well as thorough knowledge of the mediators governing them, because these dictate the approach to follow, particularly when the wound is complicated by chronic inflammation and/or an excessive proliferative response.

References

1. Theoret CL. Wound repair and specific reaction to injury. In: Auer JA, Stick JA (eds). *Equine Surgery*, 3rd edn. WB Saunders: Philadelphia, 2005: 44.
2. United States Department of Agriculture. *National Animal Health Monitoring System Part I: Baseline reference of equine health and management, 2005. #N451.1006*. www.aphis.usda.gov/animal_health/nahms/equine/downloads/ equine05/Equine05_dr_PartI.pdf (accessed June 3, 2016).
3. Sánchez-Casanova RE, Masri-Daba M, Alonso-Díaz MÁ, *et al.* Prevalence of cutaneous pathological conditions and factors associated with the presence of skin wounds in working equids in tropical regions of Veracruz, Mexico. *Trop Anim Health Prod* 2014; **46**: 555.
4. Owen KR, Singer ER, Clegg PD, *et al.* Identification of risk factors for traumatic injury in the general horse population of north-west England, Midlands and north Wales. *Equine Vet J* 2012; **44**: 143.
5. Inness CM, Morgan KL. Polo pony injuries: player-owner reported risk, perception, mitigation and risk factors. *Equine Vet J* 2015; **47**: 422.
6. Theoret CL, Bolwell CF, Riley CB. A cross-sectional survey on wounds in horses in New Zealand. *N Z Vet J* 2016; 64: 90.
7. Sole A, Bolwell CF, Dart A, *et al.* A cross-sectional survey of wounds in horses in Australia. *Aust Eq Vet* 2015; **34**: 68.
8. Perkins NR, Reid SW, Morris RS. Profiling the New Zealand Thoroughbred racing industry. 2. Conditions interfering with training and racing. *N Z Vet J* 2005; **53**: 69.
9. Stashak TS, Theoret CL. Integumentary system: wound healing, management, and reconstruction. In: Orsini JA, Divers TJ (eds). *Equine Emergencies: Treatment and Procedures*, 4th edn. Elsevier: St-Louis, MO, 2014: 239.
10. Wulff BC and Wilgus TA. Mast cell activity in the healing wound: more than meets the eye? *Exp Dermatol* 2013; **22**: 507.
11. *Precepts*, Ch. 1, as translated by W. H. S. Jones (1923).
12. Proksch E, Brandner JM, Jensen J-M. The skin: an indispensable barrier. *Exp Dermatol* 2008; **17**: 1063.
13. McLafferty E, Hendry C, Alistair F. The integumentary system: anatomy, physiology and function of skin. *Nursing Standard* 2012; **27**: 35.
14. Wilmink J. Unpublished data on skin thickness in the horse.
15. de Groot PG, Urbanus RT, Roest M. Platelet interaction with the vessel wall. *Handb Exp Pharmacol* 2012; **210**: 87.
16. Herter JM, Rossaint J, Zarbock A. Platelets in inflammation and immunity. *J Throm Haemost* 2014; **12**: 1764.
17. Singer AJ, Clark RAF. Cutaneous wound healing. *New Engl J Med* 1999; **341**: 738.
18. Simpson DM, Ross R. The neutrophilic leukocyte in wound repair – a study with antineutrophil serum. *J Clin Invest* 1972; **51**: 2009.
19. Dovi JV, He LK, DiPietro LA. Accelerated wound closure in neutrophil-depleted mice. *J Leukoc Biol* 2003; **73**: 448.
20. Delavary BM, van der Veer WM, Van Egmond M, *et al.* Macrophages in skin injury and repair. *Immunobiol* 2011; **216**: 753.
21. Novak ML, Koh TJ. Phenotypic transitions of macrophages orchestrate tissue repair. *Am J Pathol* 2013; **183**: 1352.
22. Martin P, D'Souza D, Martin J, *et al.* Wound healing in the PU.1 null mouse – tissue repair is not dependent on inflammatory cells. *Curr Biol* 2003; **13**: 1122.
23. Duffield JS, Forbes SJ, Constandinou CM, *et al.* Selective depletion of macrophages reveals distinct, opposing roles during liver injury and repair. *J Clin Invest* 2005; **115**: 56.
24. Wynn TA. Fibrotic disease and the T(H)1/T(H)2 paradigm. *Nat Rev Immunol* 2004; **4**: 583.
25. Greenhalgh DG. The role of apoptosis in wound healing. *Int J Biochem Cell Biol* 1998; **30**: 1019.
26. Martins-Green M. The Yin and Yang of integrin function in re-epithelialization during wound healing. *Adv Wound Care* 2013; **2**: 75.
27. Gill SE, Parks WC. Metalloproteinases and their inhibitors: regulators of wound healing. *Int J Biochem Cell Biol* 2008; **40**: 1334.
28. Desmoulière A, Redard M, Darby I, *et al.* Apoptosis mediates the decrease in cellularity during the transition between granulation tissue and scar. *Am J Pathol* 1995; **146**: 56.
29. Luo S, Benathan M, Raffoul W, *et al.* Abnormal balance between proliferation and apoptotic cell death in fibroblasts derived from keloid lesions. *Plast Reconstr Surg* 2001; **107**: 87.
30. Pardali E, Goumans MJ, ten Dijke P. Signaling by members of the TGF-beta family in vascular morphogenesis and disease. *Trends Cell Biol* 2010; **20**: 556.
31. Liekens S, De Clerq E, Neyts J. Angiogenesis: regulators and clinical applications. *Biochem Pharmacol* 2001; **61**: 253.
32. Li J, Zhang Y-P, Kirsner RS. Angiogenesis in wound repair: angiogenic growth factors and the extracellular matrix. *Microsc Res Tech* 2003; **60**: 107.
33. DiPietro LA. Angiogenesis and scar formation in healing wounds. *Curr Opin Rheumatol* 2013; **25**: 87.
34. Bodnar RJ, Yates CC, Rodgers ME, *et al.* IP-10 induces dissociation of newly formed blood vessels. *J Cell Sci* 2009; **122**: 2064.
35. Wietecha MS, Chen L, Ranzer MJ, *et al.* Sprouty2 downregulates angiogenesis during mouse skin wound healing. *Am J Physiol Heart Circ Physiol* 2011; **300**: H459–H467.
36. Zhu WH, Guo X, Villaschi S, *et al.* Regulation of vascular growth and regression by matrix metalloproteinases in the rat aorta model of angiogenesis. *Lab Invest* 2000; **80**: 545.
37. Davis GE, Senger DR. Endothelial extracellular matrix. Biosynthesis, remodeling, and functions during vascular morphogenesis and neovessel stabilization. *Circ Res* 2005; **97**: 1093.
38. Wilmink J. Unpublished data on the rates of wound contraction and epithelialization in equids.

39. Boehnke K, Falkowska-Hansen B, Stark HJ, *et al.* Stem cells of the human epidermis and their niche: composition and function in epidermal regeneration and carcinogenesis. *Carcinogenesis* 2012; **33**: 1247.
40. Lau K, Paus R, Tiede S, *et al.* Exploring the role of stem cells in cutaneous wound healing. *Exp Dermatol* 2009; **18**: 921.
41. Pastar I, Stojadinovic O, Yin NC, *et al.* Epithelialization in wound healing: a comprehensive review. *Adv Wound Care* 2014; **3**: 445.
42. Theoret CL. Update on wound repair. *Clin Tech Equine Pract* 2004; **3**: 110.
43. Wong VW, Gurtner GC, Longaker MT. Wound healing: a paradigm for regeneration. *Mayo Clin Proc* 2013; **88**: 1022.
44. Desmoulière A, Gabbiani G. The role of the myofibroblast in wound healing and fibrocontractive diseases. In: Clark RAF (ed). *The Molecular and Cellular Biology of Wound Repair*, 2nd edn. Plenum Press: New York, 1996: 391.
45. Serini G, Bochaton-Piallat ML, Ropraz R, *et al.* The fibronectin domain ED-A is crucial for myofibroblastic phenotype induction by transforming growth factor-beta1. *J Cell Biol* 1998; **142**: 873.
46. Hinz B. Masters and servants of the force: the role of matrix adhesions in myofibroblast force perception and transmission. *Eur J Cell Biol* 2006; **85**: 175.
47. Madison JB, Gronwall RR. Influence of wound shape on wound contraction in horses. *Am J Vet Res* 1992; **53**: 1575.
48. Grinnell F, Zhu M, Carlson MA, *et al.* Release of mechanical tension triggers apoptosis of human fibroblasts in a model of regressing granulation tissue. *Exp Cell Res* 1999; **248**: 608.
49. Martins VL, Caley M, O'Toole EA. Matrix metalloproteinases and epidermal wound repair. *Cell Tissue Res* 2013; **351**: 255.
50. PMAP-CutDB Proteolytic Event Database. http://cutdb.burnham.org (accessed June 6, 2016).
51. MEROPS the Peptidase Database. http://merops.sanger.ac.uk (accessed June 6, 2016).
52. Yager DR, Chen SM, Ward SI, *et al.* Ability of chronic wound fluids to degrade peptide growth factors is associated with increased levels of elastase activity and diminished levels of proteinase inhibitors. *Wound Repair Regen* 1997; **5**: 23.
53. Levenson SM, Geever EF, Crowley LV, *et al.* The healing of rat skin wounds. *Ann Surg* 1965; **161**: 293.
54. Monteiro SO, Lepage OM, Theoret CL. Effects of platelet-rich plasma on the repair of wounds on the distal aspect of the forelimb in horses. *Am J Vet Res* 2009; **70**: 277.
55. Junker JPE, Philip J, Kiwanuka E, *et al.* Assessing quality of healing in skin: review of available methods and devices. *Wound Repair Regen* 2014; **22**: 2.
56. Paul DW, Ghassemi P, Ramella-Roman JC, *et al.* Noninvasive imaging technologies for cutaneous wound assessment: a review. *Wound Repair Regen* 2015; **23**: 149.
57. Celeste CJ, Deschene K, Riley CB, Theoret CL. Regional differences in wound oxygenation during normal healing in an equine model of cutaneous fibroproliferative disorder. *Wound Repair Regen* 2011; **19**: 89.
58. Celeste CJ, Deschesne K, Riley CB, Theoret CL. Skin temperature during cutaneous wound healing in an equine model of cutaneous fibroproliferative disorder: kinetics and anatomic-site differences. *Vet Surg* 2013; **42**: 147.
59. Labens R, Blikslager A. Precision of a photogrammetric method to perform 3D wound measurements compared to standard 2D photographic techniques in the horse. *Equine Vet J* 2013; **45**: 41.
60. Van Hecke LL, De Mil TA, Haspeslagh M, *et al.* Comparison of a new laser beam wound camera and a digital photoplanimetry-based method for wound measurement in horses. *Vet J* 2015; **203**: 309.
61. ImageJ Image Processing and Analysis in Java. http://imagej.nih.gov/ij (accessed June 6, 2016).
62. Perry DM, McGrouther DA, Bayat A. Current tools for noninvasive objective assessment of skin scars. *Plast Reconstr Surg* 2010; **126**: 912.
63. Barrientos S, Brem H, Stojadinovic O, *et al.* Clinical application of growth factors and cytokines in wound healing. *Wound Repair Regen* 2014; **22**: 569.
64. Kiwanuka E, Junker J, Eriksson E. Harnessing growth factors to influence wound healing. *Clin Plast Surg* 2012; **39**: 239.

CHAPTER 2

Differences in Wound Healing between Horses and Ponies

Jacintha M. Wilmink, DVM, PhD

Chapter Contents

Summary

Observing differences in wound healing between horses and ponies has provided valuable information about the intrinsic process of wound healing and the common complications encountered when managing traumatic wounds in the equid. Ponies heal faster and with fewer complications than do horses. To a large extent, these differences can be explained by disparity in the local inflammatory response, which, in turn, relates to differences in the functional capacity of leukocytes. Research data indicate that a maximal effect of treatment will be obtained in clinical practice if a differential approach is used, optimizing conditions for each successive phase of wound healing. In particular, the effect of treatment on the inflammatory response is of paramount importance to the other phases of healing and should, therefore, always be considered when managing a wound. When treating wounds healing by second intention, inflammation should be stimulated until the wound has filled with granulation tissue, and thereafter it should be inhibited.

Horses and ponies: same species, different healing characteristics

The horse evolved over the course of millions of years from a small forest dweller to a large ungulate that inhabited the vast open plains of the temperate zone. It became a "flight" animal whose instinctive reaction to danger is to run.[1] Evolution took place as a response to various environmental and climatic challenges, and the development of special features resulted from selection by mankind. Both evolution and selection led to the large variety of breeds known today.

The equine species can be roughly subdivided into horses and ponies, and this division is determined by the height of an adult at the withers (ponies are <1.48 m). Whether ponies are just small horses has been debated for decades. The discussion of this topic, with respect to wound healing, started in the 1980s when Bertone *et al.*[2] found, in a study examining second-intention healing, that wounds of ponies heal faster than those of horses and without the formation of exuberant granulation tissue (EGT). Other authors, however, reported that wounds of ponies do develop EGT,[3,4] and the faster healing of wounds in ponies could not be confirmed.[4] Because a difference in wound healing between horses and ponies might provide information about the basic biology of equine wound healing and about the complications commonly associated with wound repair in this species, Wilmink *et al.* performed a series of experiments to investigate differences in wound healing between horses and ponies.[5–7] They proved that skin wounds in ponies heal faster and with fewer complications than do similar wounds in horses and demonstrated that these differences were based on the

Equine Wound Management, Third Edition. Edited by Christine Theoret and Jim Schumacher.

Companion website: www.wiley.com/go/theoret/wound

efficiency and capacity of the leukocyte to produce various mediators.[8,9] Differences in healing are, however, apparently not related to body size. This is confirmed by a study in donkeys and Caspian miniature horses, equine subspecies of similar size, which showed that wound healing in donkeys is faster than healing in Caspian miniature horses.[10]

What remains to be elucidated is the cause of the observed differences in healing between horses and ponies. The longer period of domestication of the horse may have precluded natural selection against poor healing, because the wounded horse was/is tended to by man. Additionally, the artificial selection of various features, such as height, athletic capacity, and appearance, might have favored the development of some diseases and undesirable characteristics, including the reduced efficiency of leukocytes. Moreover, horses with wounds so poorly healed that athletic ability is impaired are often used for breeding, thus perpetuating a hereditary tendency toward poor healing. In contrast, ponies have been domesticated for a much shorter time, and, consequently, a poor capacity for healing may have been eliminated by natural selection. Moreover, artificial selection within pony breeds has been less intense, and many pony breeds maintain subpopulations (and genetic reserves) in the wild. The hypothesis that natural and artificial selection have an influence on wound healing is supported by the faster healing of donkeys compared to Caspian miniature horses,[10] the latter being selected based on a special feature, namely their speed.

The physiologic and pathophysiologic differences in healing observed between horses and ponies with experimentally induced wounds have since been corroborated by other research[7–9,11,12] and by clinical observation. These observations have resulted in improvements in guiding the management of wounds of equids and led to faster healing and the prevention of complications.

First-intention healing (primary wound closure)

Primary closure of traumatic wounds of horses is preferred over healing by second intention because healing by primary intention is usually faster, and the cosmetic and functional results are better. Unfortunately, either partial or complete wound dehiscence may ensue after primary closure. Whether or not a wound dehisces depends on many factors, including those relating to the wound itself, to the horse, to the treatment, and to the environment.[13,14]

The success of primary closure of traumatic wounds was evaluated retrospectively by Wilmink *et al.* in more than 500 equine patients admitted to a referral clinic.[7] The study revealed that primary closure is significantly more often successful in ponies than in horses (Figure 2.1), and that bone sequestra form significantly less often in ponies when bone is exposed during

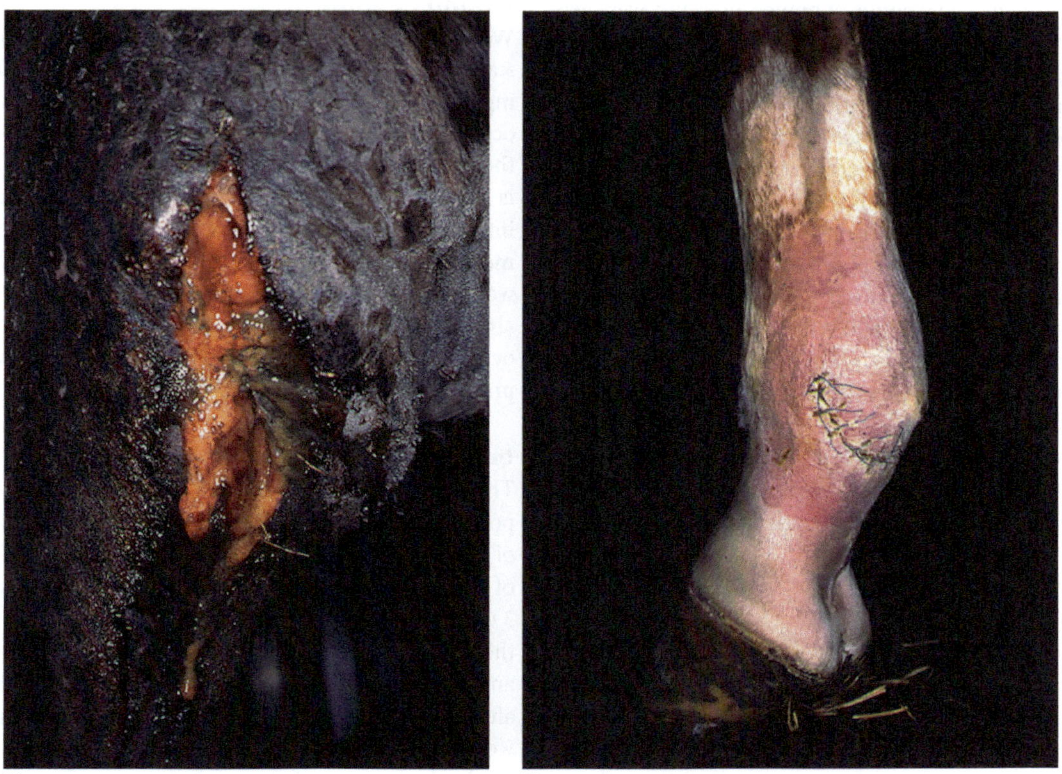

(a) (b)

Figure 2.1 **(a)** Wound on the elbow of a horse, which suffered dehiscence following primary closure, as a result of infection. **(b)** Wound on the distal aspect of the limb of a 4-year-old pony with an open fetlock joint and damage to the lateral collateral ligament. The wound was sutured approximately 8 hours after it occurred and it healed successfully, without dehiscence. Source: (b) Wilmink 2004.[15] Reproduced with permission of Elsevier.

injury. The predominant cause of wound dehiscence and of sequestration of bone is infection.[7,16,17] Other factors contributing to dehiscence are tension on the wound's margins, excessive movement of the sutured region, and involvement of certain structures, such as tendons, ligaments, and synovial cavities. Other factors besides infection contributing to formation of a sequestrum include exposure of cortical bone and extensive trauma.[18] The risk of infection is influenced by many factors, including the time elapsed since injury, the degree of contamination, the degree of tissue damage, and the thoroughness of debridement and irrigation. Wound debridement determines the concentration of bacteria left in the wound and is one factor that can be controlled clinically.[13,14,17] The concentration of bacteria, in combination with factors at the wound that facilitate bacterial colonization, such as the presence of dead space, a hematoma, and devitalized tissue, is critical to whether or not a wound becomes infected (the reader is referred to Chapter 4 for more information about factors involved in the development of infection). Although bacterial colonization and development of infection are greatly influenced by the administration of antibiotics, the effectiveness of the patient's own local defense, its acute inflammatory response, is as least as important to the prevention of infection.[19]

In the aforementioned retrospective study by Wilmink *et al.*, all these factors relating to wound infection were evaluated and compared between horses and ponies.[7] Ponies and horses did not differ with respect to age and gender, nor with respect to wound characteristics, such as location, duration, contamination, and treatment. The wounds of ponies, however, were generally deeper, and ponies were more apt to suffer laceration of an extensor tendon, to incur damage to the periosteum, to have exposed bone, and to have their wound closed while standing, rather than while anesthetized. Additionally, ponies were significantly less likely to receive antimicrobial therapy and to be administered a non-steroidal anti-inflammatory drug (NSAID). Ponies were, therefore, at greater risk of bacterial challenge than were horses because their wounds were deeper and debridement was less complete since it was performed with the ponies standing, and because they were less likely to receive antimicrobial therapy. In spite of this greater risk, wound infection occurred less often, implying that the acute inflammatory response in ponies is more effective than that of horses at reducing bacterial contamination. The more frequent use of NSAIDs in horses, however, may have contributed to a reduced effectiveness of the inflammatory response.

Second-intention healing

Wounds are allowed to heal by second intention when closure is not feasible or affordable, or when a wound dehisces after being closed primarily. Second-intention healing was investigated in horses and ponies by creating excisional wounds on the metatarsi and buttocks that extended through the periosteum of the metatarsal bone or 18 mm into the muscle on the buttocks, in imitation

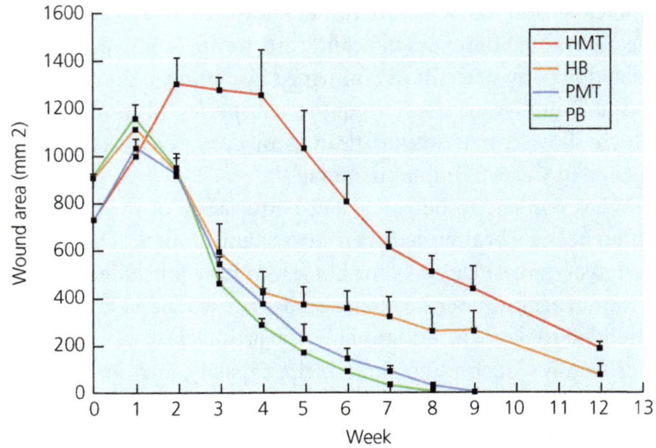

Figure 2.2 Wound area as a function of time (mean + s.e.m.). HMT, metatarsal wounds of horses; HB, body wounds of horses; PMT, metatarsal wounds of ponies; PB, body wounds of ponies. Source: Wilmink 1999.[5] Reproduced with permission of John Wiley & Sons.

of clinical wounds.[5,6] This investigation found that wounds of ponies heal significantly faster than do wounds of horses (Figure 2.2) and that the speed and efficiency of healing seem related to remarkable differences between horses and ponies in the phases of healing.[5,6] Subsequent studies showed that these differences can be attributed to variations in the function of leukocytes.[8,9,11]

Clinically apparent phases during wound healing

Wound healing is often divided into general phases of hemostasis, inflammation, proliferation, and synthesis and remodeling of matrix (see Chapter 1). Because these phases overlap and occur simultaneously in all tissue components, distinguishing them from one another is difficult. Consequently, this division is somewhat academic. In a clinical setting, dividing healing into the following macroscopically apparent events may be more practical: inflammation, formation of granulation tissue, wound contraction, and epithelialization. Although these events also overlap, they largely succeed one another and occur more or less chronologically. Moreover, they are clearly visible to the practitioner observing second-intention healing.

Inflammation

The inflammatory response to wounding is more prompt in ponies, as demonstrated by comparing the leukocytic infiltration of experimental wounds of ponies and horses.[6] High numbers of polymorphonuclear cells (PMNs) are found during the first 3 weeks of healing, after which the PMNs disappear rapidly from the wounds of ponies. In contrast, the influx of PMNs is sluggish and weak in horses, but PMNs persist so that, beginning 4 weeks after wounding, the number of PMNs exceeds those in the wounds of ponies.[6]

The leukocytes of ponies are more efficient than those of horses. An *in vitro* study showed that the leukocytes of ponies produce more reactive oxygen species, such as H_2O_2

or O^- radicals, necessary for bacterial killing after phagocytosis.[9] Within tissue cages implanted subcutaneously and in newly formed granulation tissue, the leukocytes of ponies also produce higher concentrations of other inflammatory mediators, including tumor necrosis factor (TNF)-α, interleukin (IL)-1, and transforming growth factor (TGF)-β, essential to the reinforcement of the inflammatory response, to the induction of fibroplasia, and to wound contraction.[8,9] The superior production of these mediators can thus explain the higher initial influx of leukocytes into wounds of ponies.

Migrated leukocytes, in turn, release more biologically active substances, thus creating a positive feedback that enhances the inflammatory response.[19,20] This feedback may account for the faster debridement of non-viable tissue and fibrin in wounds of ponies, leading to the faster development of a healthy bed of granulation tissue. In contrast, granulation tissue in the wounds of horses retains an irregular and purulent appearance, along with persistent deposits of fibrin.[5,6] An enhanced inflammatory response observed in ponies can, likewise, translate into a more efficient local defense against contaminating bacteria, leading to a superior control of wound infection.[7] A stronger acute inflammatory response, thus, averts the development of chronic, low-grade inflammation and leads to a faster and more thorough preparation of the wound for repair. Indeed, chronic inflammation, such as that seen in horses,[6] perpetuates the release of tissue-damaging lysosomal enzymes, as well as mediators, such as TGF-β, which in turn, over-stimulate fibroplasia and lead to the formation of EGT, which inhibits contraction.[19,21–23]

In summary, the inflammatory response to wounding in ponies is stronger and more succinct; this response appears to be more efficient for healing. In contrast, the inflammatory response in horses is weak in onset but persists over time, and this poor but persistent response may be due to the lower initial production of inflammatory mediators.

Formation of granulation tissue

In a study by Wilmink *et al.*, granulation tissue formed faster in experimental wounds of horses than in those of ponies.[5] The abundant granulation tissue in the wounds of the limbs of horses was observed to push the edges of the wound apart, which may explain why experimental wounds on the limbs of horses enlarged so dramatically during the first 2 weeks after they were created (Figure 2.2). Between weeks 2 and 3 of healing, the granulation tissue of all wounds on the limbs and buttocks of horses and ponies protruded above the level of the surrounding skin and was characterized as excessive (clinically referred to as EGT or "proud flesh"); protrusion of granulation tissue was most prominent in wounds on the limbs of horses (Figure 2.3). The wounds were left unbandaged after week 3, and during week 4 EGT disappeared spontaneously from wounds, except those on the limbs of horses, where the excess tissue had to be trimmed to promote healing.[5] The granulation tissue in horses was traversed by grooves and clefts for a much longer period, and presented a yellowish purulent surface up to week 5 after wounding. The appearance of the granulation tissue on the limbs may have been due to the weak and delayed onset followed by prolongation of the inflammatory phase. In contrast, the granulation tissue in the wounds of the ponies was smooth, regular, and achieved a healthy pink color significantly sooner (Figure 2.4).[5] It was microscopically apparent that fibroblasts continued to proliferate in horse wounds even after granulation tissue filled the wound bed, whereas fibroblasts in pony wounds ceased proliferating at this time. Granulation tissue in wounds of horses presented a chaotic cellular pattern and appeared persistently inflamed, whereas it was organized regularly in pony wounds (Figure 2.5).[6]

There may be a causal relationship between persistent inflammation and the continuous proliferation of fibroblasts and the synthesis of granulation tissue, via the activity of mediators, such as TNFα, IL-1, IL-6, platelet-derived growth factor (PDGF), TGF-β, and basic fibroblast growth factor (bFGF), which are known to induce fibrosis.[22–24] However, the formation of granulation tissue was less extensive in the wounds of ponies than in those of horses, particularly those located on the limb, even though the granulation tissue of ponies initially contained higher concentrations of TNFα, IL-1, and TGF-β,[5,8,9] which mediate the migration and proliferation of fibroblasts and endothelial cells.[22] Furthermore, fibroblasts from limbs of ponies are known to proliferate faster *in vitro* than those of horses,[11,25] even though fibroplasia seems more rapid, *in vivo*, in horses. Apparently, the balance of mediators, the interaction of mediators with other factors, and time-scale of the presence of mediators *in vivo* are more important than the absolute concentration of mediators in determining the rate of cellular growth, stressing once more the significance of the overall course of the inflammatory response.

The formation of granulation tissue in horses is excessively fast, compared to that of other species[26] and to what is observed in ponies.[5] The fast formation and persistent proliferation of granulation tissue, caused by an unrelenting inflammatory response, clearly contribute to the formation of EGT.[5,6]

Wound contraction

Contraction of wounds of ponies is faster and significantly more pronounced than is contraction of wounds of horses, and contraction of wounds on the body is faster and significantly more pronounced than is contraction of wounds on the limb (Figure 2.6).[5] As a result, second-intention healing is significantly faster in ponies than in horses and significantly faster in wounds on the body than in wounds on the limb (Figure 2.2).[5]

Histologic examination of wounds showed that the myofibroblasts in newly formed granulation tissue of wounds of ponies are organized into a regular pattern within 2 weeks after wounding; the cells are oriented perpendicular to the vessels and parallel to the wound's surface. This pattern is thought to enhance contraction because a good bond between fibroblasts and the surrounding ECM is required for the contractile forces exerted by smooth muscle actin filaments within the fibroblasts

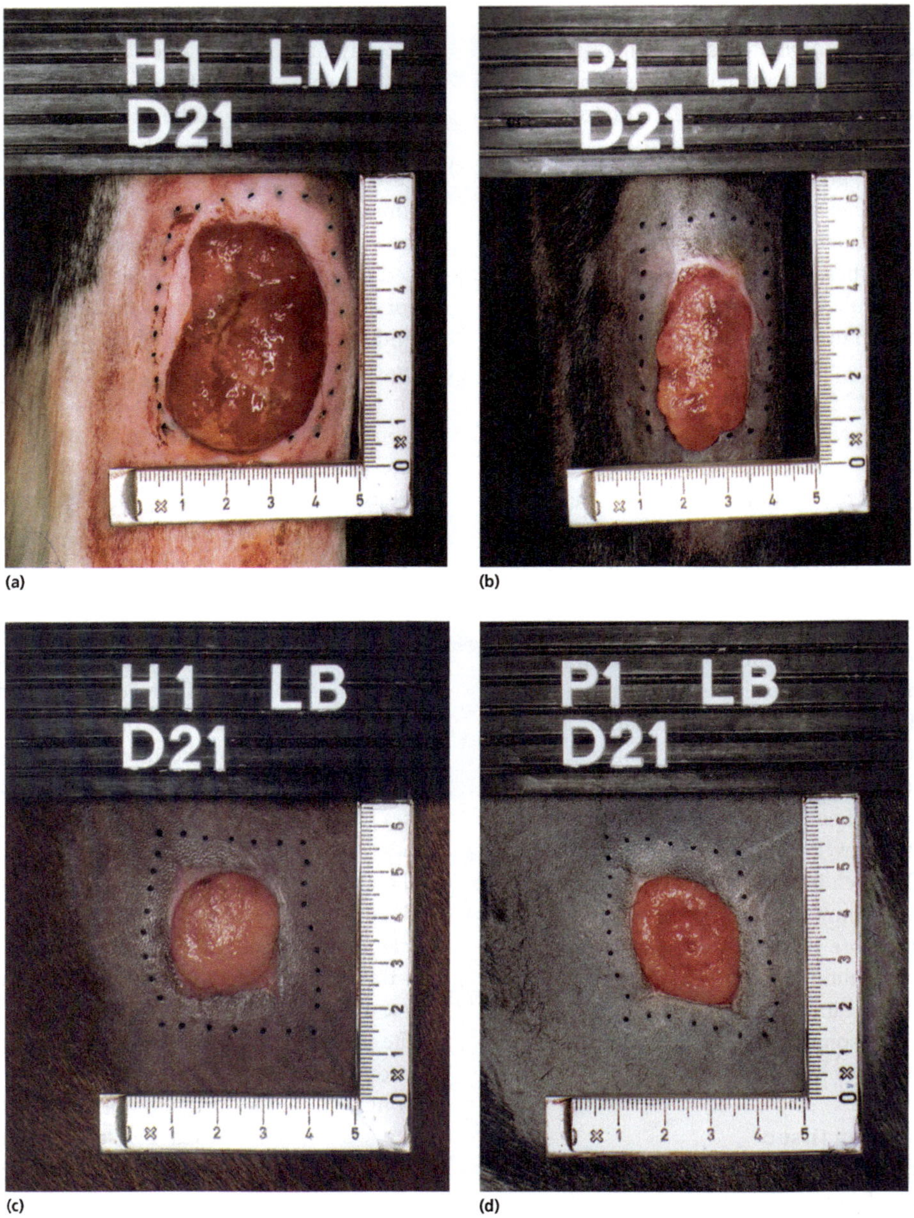

Figure 2.3 After 3 weeks, the limb wounds of horses **(a)** contained more exuberant granulation tissue than the limb wounds of ponies **(b)**. In the same timeframe, the wounds on the buttocks of horses **(c)** and ponies **(d)** had formed some exuberant granulation tissue protruding above all wound margins. Source: (a and b) Wilmink 2004.[15] Reproduced with permission of Elsevier.

to pull the margin of the wound centripetally (i.e., towards the center of the wound).[27,28] Although the number of fibroblasts and the amounts of smooth muscle actin and collagen do not differ between wounds of horses and those of ponies, the alignment of myofibroblasts of horses is delayed (Figure 2.5).[6]

Wound contraction occurs when the forces exerted by myofibroblasts exceed centrifugal (i.e., outward) forces and the local resistance to displacement. Centrifugal forces present in the skin of horses and ponies are similar, as evidenced by the identical enlargement that occurs immediately after the creation of experimental wounds (Figure 2.2). Moreover, there is no reason to believe that the local resistance to contraction in horses and ponies should differ. Variations in wound contraction are, therefore, most likely related to differences in the contractile force generated by myofibroblasts within the granulation tissue.

Surprisingly, the inherent capacity of fibroblasts of ponies to contract, *in vitro*, is similar to that of horses,[11] suggesting that factors in the wound, such as the presence of inflammatory mediators, determine the contractile forces exerted by myofibroblasts and hence the extent of contraction. Indeed, inflammatory mediators, in particular TGF-β, wield major effects on contraction. Interestingly, the concentration of TGF-β

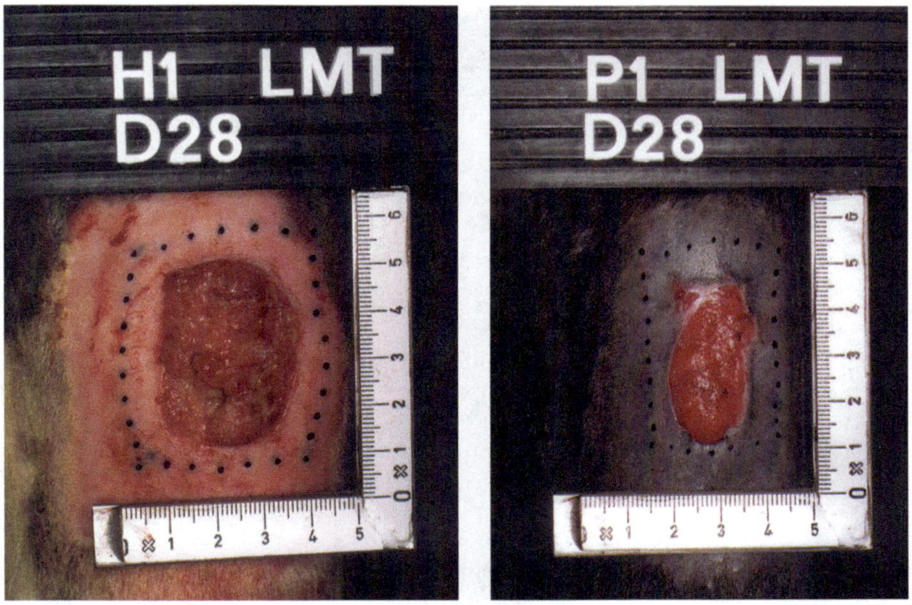

(a) (b)

Figure 2.4 **(a)** By 4 weeks after wounding, the granulation tissue of the limb wounds of horses was traversed by grooves and clefts, and on its surface was a purulent exudate. **(b)** The granulation tissue of pony wounds, on the other hand, was smooth, regular, and had a healthy pink color. Source: Wilmink 2004.[15] Reproduced with permission of Elsevier.

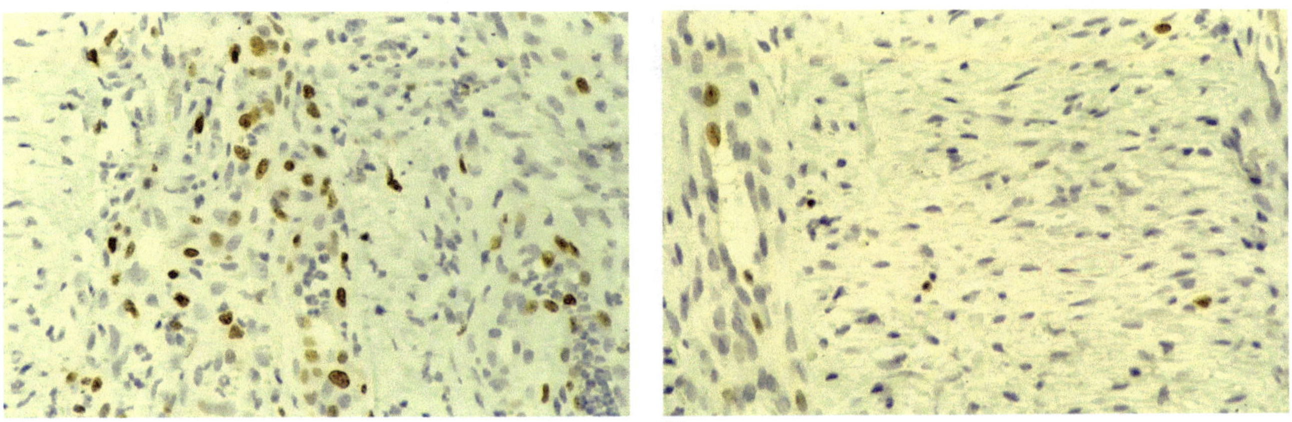

(a) (b)

Figure 2.5 Typical microscopic appearance of the granulation tissue of metatarsal wounds 6 weeks after wounding (DAP-filter, MIB). **(a)** In horses, many brown-colored cells, actively synthesizing DNA and preparing for mitosis, were present. Note the irregular arrangement of the fibroblasts in the tissue and the presence of polymorphonuclear leukocytes. **(b)** In ponies, only a few brown-stained cells are seen in the regularly organized granulation tissue. Source: Wilmink 1999.[6] Reproduced with permission of John Wiley & Sons.

is significantly higher in the newly formed granulation tissue of experimental wounds of ponies.[8] This may explain the faster organization of myofibroblasts and the more extensive contraction observed in wounds of ponies because TGF-β stimulates the differentiation of fibroblasts into myofibroblasts;[29] induces α-smooth muscle actin, α1β1 and α1β2 integrins, collagen, and fibronectin, all factors necessary to wound contraction;[30] and enhances contractile forces.[31] Furthermore, because other inflammatory mediators, such as prostaglandin (PG)E_1, PGE_2, TNFα, IL-1, IL-6, and interferon (IFN)-γ inhibit contractility,[32] a chronic inflammatory response, characteristic of wounds of horses, may exacerbate the deficiency of contraction noted in wounds of horses.

In summary, wounds of ponies heal faster by second intention than do wounds of horses because contraction contributes more to closure of wounds of ponies than to wounds of horses (Figures 2.2 and 2.6). The differences in contraction are not caused by disparity in the innate contractile capacity of the fibroblasts but by the balance of mediators in the wound's environment. The poorer contribution of contraction to closure of wounds on the limb of horses can be attributed to the initial low production of TGF-β and the frequent occurrence of chronic inflammation.[5,6,8]

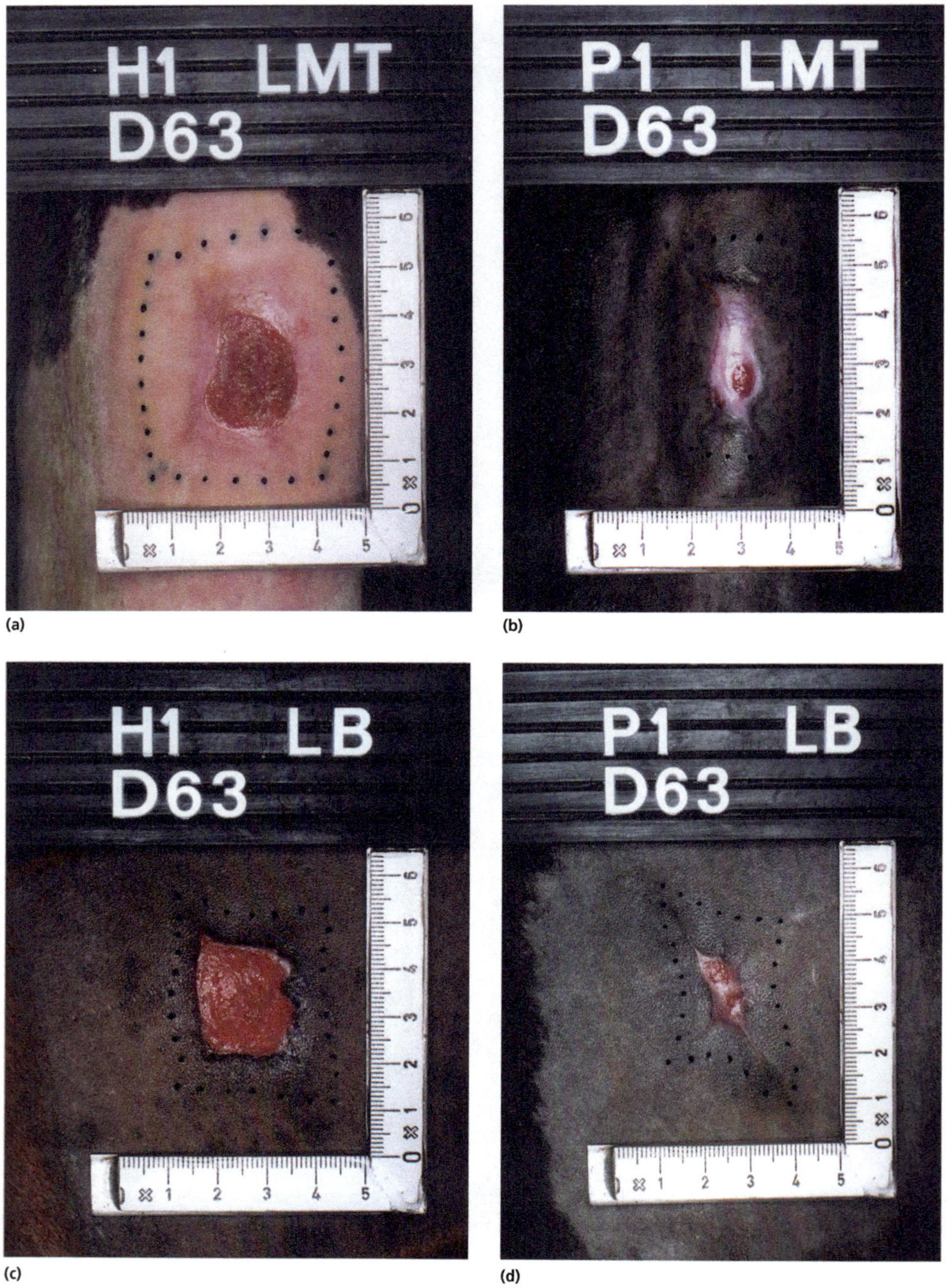

Figure 2.6 After 9 weeks of healing, the contribution of contraction to wound closure can be appreciated by observing the tattoo patterns close to the original margin of the wound. **(a)** The metatarsal wounds of horses have decreased in size. The tattoos show that the wounds have contracted minimally, whereas pronounced epithelialization is visible. **(b)** Closure of the metatarsal wounds of ponies was, to a large extent, the result of contraction and some epithelialization. **(c)** The buttock wounds of horses also healed mainly by contraction, with a small amount of epithelialization. **(d)** The buttock wounds of ponies healed, mainly by contraction, with very little epithelialization. The scar of this pony was unfortunately superficially damaged while shaving the hairs around the scar for the photographs. Source: (a and b) Wilmink 2004.[15] Reproduced with permission of Elsevier.

Epithelialization

Proliferation of epithelial cells in experimental wounds of horses was similar to that of epithelial cells in experimental wound of ponies during the first weeks of healing. Cellular proliferation was temporarily reduced when EGT developed at 3 weeks in wounds on the limbs and the buttocks of horses and ponies.[6] After the third week of healing, an inverse correlation developed between the area of epithelialization and wound contraction, so that wounds contracting the most epithelialized the least (pony versus horse wounds, buttock versus limb wounds) (Figure 2.6, Figure 2.7).[5] This inverse correlation likely developed because the circumference of the wound margin

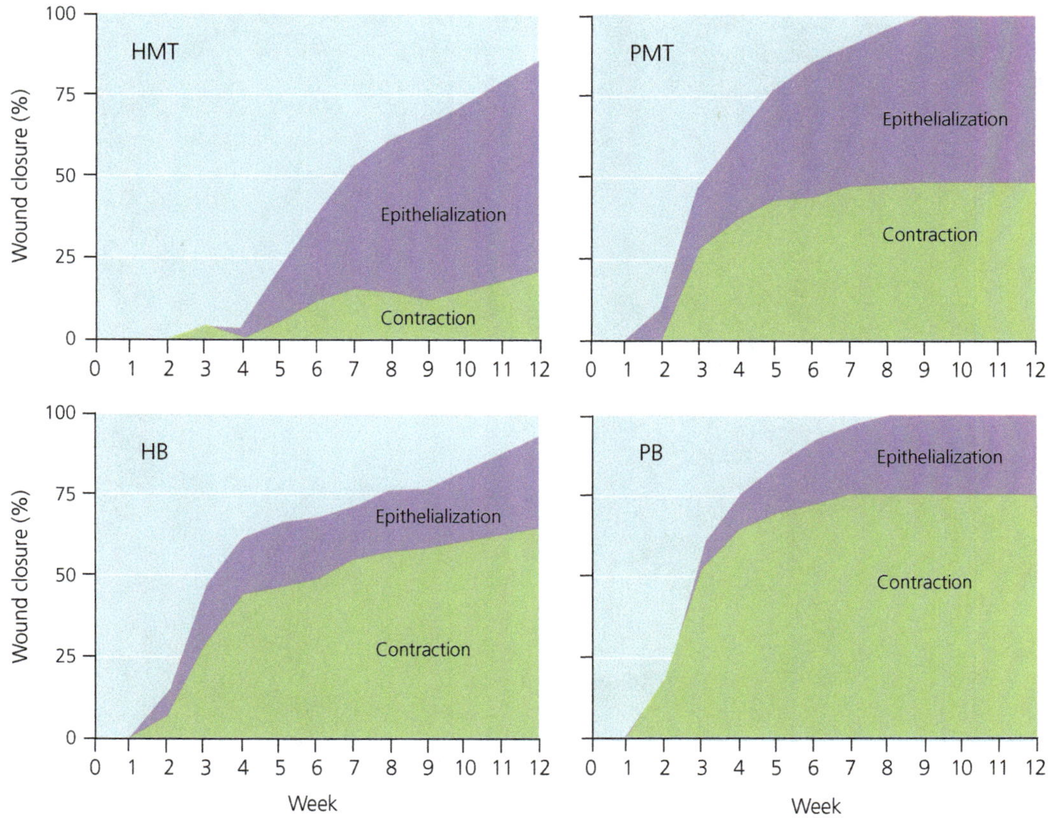

Figure 2.7 Relative contribution of contraction and epithelialization to wound closure. For abbreviations see Figure 2.2. The correlation between the epithelialized area and wound contraction is inversed, so that wounds demonstrating the most contraction show the least amount of epithelialization (pony versus horse wounds, body versus limb wounds). Source: Wilmink 1999.[5] Reproduced with permission of John Wiley & Sons.

furnishing migrating and proliferating epithelial cells decreased. Thus, more epithelialization was seen when wound contraction was poor, such as occurred in wounds on the limb of horses (Figure 2.6).[5] Epithelialization of these poorly contracting wounds was significantly faster than was epithelialization of rapidly contracting wounds from 6 weeks onward, resulting in the largest area of newly formed, inferior-quality epithelium and the most pronounced scars (Figure 2.8).[5]

Epithelialization is also hindered by persistent inflammation, which promotes release of toxic products and lysosomal enzymes from leukocytes. These toxic products not only damage tissue but also inhibit epithelial mitosis by altering the critical balance of cytokines and growth factors upon which epithelial cells depend.[33] Additionally, epithelial mitosis appears to be negatively influenced by the presence of EGT and/or factors inducing EGT,[34] as suggested by the finding that the mitotic activity of epithelial cells in all wounds temporarily diminishes when EGT is present.[6]

In other words, epithelialization slows when contraction is rapid, as seen in ponies. An increased rate of epithelialization, as seen in wounds on the limb of horses, however, has little effect on the speed of healing because epithelialization is inherently slow. A more extensive scar, characterized by fragility, poor attachment to the underlying basement membrane, and the absence of skin appendages, is formed when epithelialization is the primary mode of wound closure (Figure 2.8).[35]

Clinical application of the results of research

Traumatic wounds of ponies are more apt to heal with a favorable cosmetic and functional outcome than are similar wounds of horses. This usually translates into lower costs of treatment for ponies than for horses. A pony's better prognosis for favorable healing may justify treatment even when a wounded pony has such a low economic value that the owner is reluctant to treat the pony.

First-intention healing (primary wound closure)

The results of the study by Wilmink *et al.* examining primary-intention healing and formation of sequestra in horses and ponies[7] illustrate the detrimental effect of infection in the process of healing and the substantial role of the inflammatory response in local defense. As yet, there are no proven ways to stimulate the inflammatory response in sutured wounds to improve local defense mechanisms, signifying that preventing infection is of paramount importance, particularly for horses.

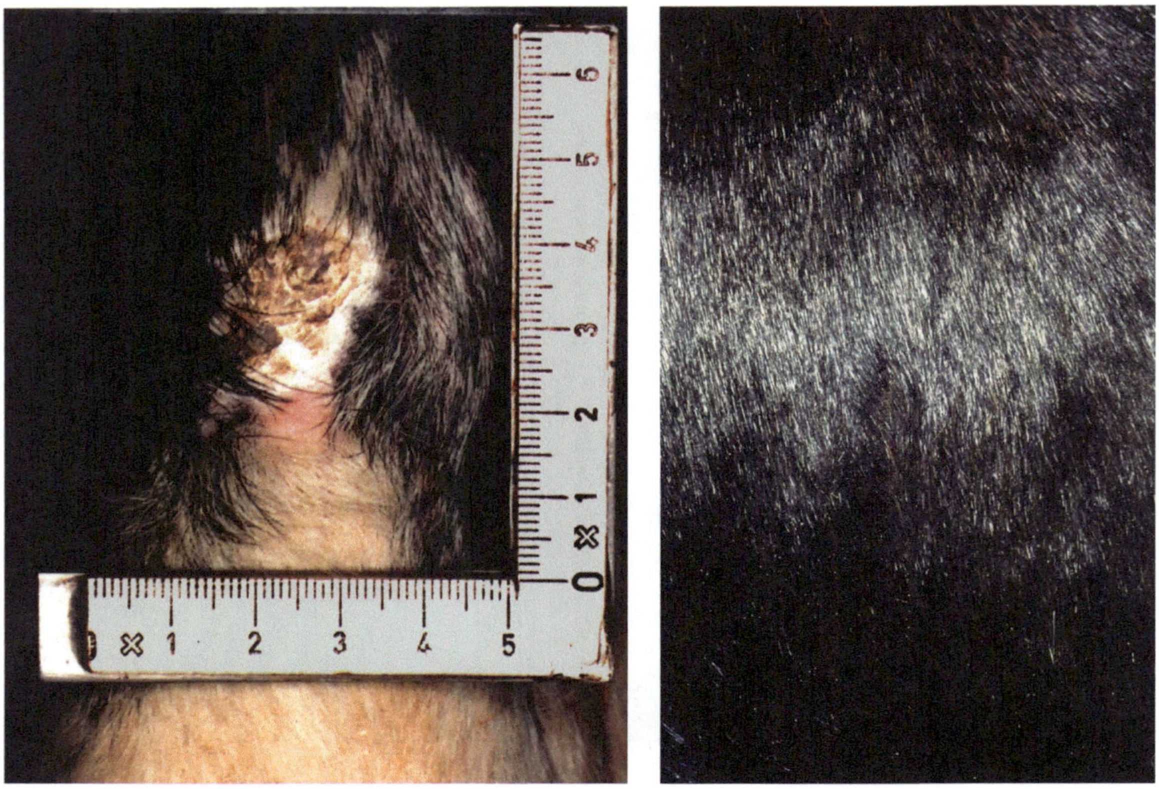

(a) (b)

Figure 2.8 Scar of a metatarsal wound of a horse **(a)** and a buttock wound of a pony **(b)** 1.5 years after healing. The limb wound in the horse healed mainly by epithelialization, leaving an unsightly scar. The buttock wound of the pony closed mainly by wound contraction, leaving no visible scar. Source: Wilmink 2004.[15] Reproduced with permission of Elsevier.

To prevent infection, as many bacteria as possible should be removed by debridement and irrigation, and, therefore, because surgical debridement is more difficult when the patient is standing, general anesthesia should be the preferred method of restraint, especially when the wound to be debrided is extensive. Debridement of exposed cortical bone appears to protect the bone from infection and subsequent formation of a bone sequestrum. Proliferation and invasion of bacteria remaining after debridement can be prevented by appropriate antimicrobial prophylaxis. Equids suffering from an acute extensive traumatic wound should be administered a broad-spectrum antibiotic as soon as possible after wounding, even if the patient is to be referred to a hospital better equipped to treat it. Antimicrobial therapy should be administered intravenously to ensure an immediate and adequate concentration of the antimicrobial drug within the wounded tissue (the reader is referred to Chapter 19 for more information about antibiotic therapy).

Sutured wounds on a limb should be protected with a bandage or cast to reduce edema and to increase the local temperature, thereby facilitating perfusion of the wound with an adequate supply of leukocytes and oxygen. Bandaging also stimulates biologic processes, such as the production of endothelial and epithelial cells and fibroblasts as well as the synthesis of components of the extracellular matrix (the reader is referred to Chapter 6 for more information about the products used to dress and bandage wounds and Chapter 7 for information about the techniques of bandaging, splinting, and casting).

The fact that the inflammatory response should initially be stimulated, rather than inhibited, implies that the wounded equid should not be administered a corticosteroid, topically or systemically. Furthermore, the routine use of NSAIDs should be avoided, because NSAIDs have been reported to exert adverse effects on wound healing.[36–40] High doses and prolonged use of a NSAID have been shown to reduce inflammation in surgical wounds of horses and ponies;[36,37] consequently, administration of a NSAID may increase the likelihood of infection in a traumatic wound. Additionally, certain NSAIDs have been shown to exert an adverse effect on skin flap survival.[39] Administration of a NSAID may be warranted, however, if the equid is severely lame or if the wounded region is so swollen that local circulation could be compromised. In these instances, a NSAID should be administered, but at the lowest effective dose and for as short a duration as possible. Topical use of disinfectants and antibiotics should also be avoided as many products are toxic to wound cells or inhibit leukocyte function.[41] Similarly, local anesthetics should not be infiltrated close to the wound, as these agents are also toxic for leukocytes and reduce their mobility and metabolism.[42–44] Consequently, regional (perineural) anesthesia or a line block performed distant to the wound is preferred.[13]

In conclusion, measures should be taken to reduce contamination and to minimize the detrimental effects of treatment on the normal inflammatory response, particularly when the wounded equid is a horse.

> **What to do**
>
> - Consider using general anesthesia, rather than sedation and regional or local anesthesia, to debride and suture wounds on the limbs of horses. Debridement is usually more thorough when the horse is anesthetized.
> - Limit the use of NSAID therapy when treating a horse for an acute wound to avoid hindering the natural inflammatory response to injury. NSAID therapy may increase the risk of dehiscence after primary closure.
>
> **What to avoid**
>
> - Avoid infiltrating a local anesthetic agent near a wound or applying a disinfectant to a wound because local anesthetic agents and disinfectants weaken the inflammatory response by harming leukocytes.

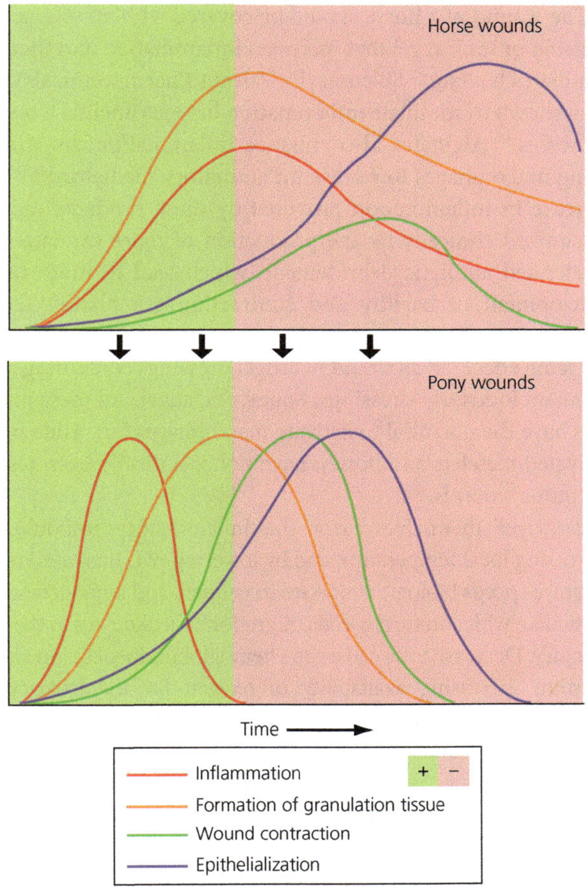

Figure 2.9 Schematic representation of the healing phases of wounds of equids. Inflammation should initially be stimulated (green shaded area) until the wound has filled with granulation tissue, and, thereafter, it should be arrested (pink shaded area) to reduce the formation of Exuberant Granulation Tissue and facilitate contraction and epithelialization. In fact, horse wounds should be treated so that the pattern of healing resembles that of ponies.

Second-intention healing

Modulating the inflammatory response

The inflammatory response orchestrates the entire healing process. The acute inflammatory response is a requisite for launching healing,[27] whereas chronic or persistent inflammation hinders wound contraction and epithelialization.[45] The inflammatory response in wounds of horses is weak initially and fails to resolve appropriately, and therefore, inflammation initially should be stimulated and later inhibited.[15,46] The primary aim of initial treatment of a wound on a horse is to modulate the inflammatory response so that it more closely resembles that of wounds of ponies (Figure 2.9). This means that inflammation should be encouraged until the wound has filled with granulation tissue and that it should be inhibited from that point onward to reduce the formation of EGT and facilitate contraction and epithelialization.[15,46] The inflammatory response can be controlled during second-intention healing, because the wounded tissues are accessible, whereas it is difficult to control during primary-intention healing. When the inflammatory phase of healing is modulated, the successive phases of the healing process are simultaneously influenced. Thus, the initial enhancement of inflammation boosts the formation of granulation tissue, which in turn hastens wound contraction; precluding chronic inflammation benefits both wound contraction and epithelialization. Treatment of equine wounds healing by second intention, therefore, can be improved by modulating the inflammatory phase, which can be either stimulated or inhibited.

> **What to do**
>
> - Stimulate inflammation until the wound has filled with granulation tissue.
> - Inhibit inflammation after the wound has filled with granulation tissue.

Stimulating the acute inflammatory response

The initial inflammatory response in wounds of horses should be encouraged, and in no manner limited, until the cavity of the wound has filled with granulation tissue. The inflammatory response can be facilitated, and the risk of infection reduced by surgical debridement, regardless of whether or not a wound is to be sutured. Although surgical debridement is necessary when contamination, necrosis, exposed bone or a frayed tendon are present within the wound of an equid, surgical debridement is especially important when the wound is that of a horse because cellular debridement of wounds of horses by the inflammatory response is slow.

The wound of a horse should be covered with an interactive dressing or topical gel that increases inflammation and thereby stimulates healing.[47] Solcoseryl® (Valeant Pharmaceuticals) has been shown to stimulate inflammation in experimental wounds of horses.[12] Alginates also enhance inflammation, by stimulating macrophages to release inflammatory mediators;[48,49] the increase in inflammation provided by these products can be recognized clinically by the production of more exudate and accelerated autolytic debridement, which lead to more rapid development of healthy and contracting granulation tissue (Figure 2.10). Products containing activated platelets also have the same effect,[50,51] as would hydrogel dressings containing acemannan, Iodosorb® dressings, honey, and sugar. All these products have the potential to activate macrophages but, aside from activated platelets and honey, have not specifically been tested in equine wounds.[51,52]

Bandages themselves favor the inflammatory response by increasing local temperature and by lowering pH. Increased temperature speeds biologic processes in general, and angiogenesis in particular, which in turn speeds migration of leukocytes to the site of injury. Decreased pH causes the hemoglobin dissociation curve to shift, increasing availability of oxygen for the leukocytes, required for the oxidative burst used to kill bacteria after phagocytosis. Bandages consequently enhance the formation of granulation tissue, most importantly by increasing the oxygen gradient between the granulation tissue and the wound's surface.[3]

Stimulating the initial inflammatory response in wounds of horses to a greater degree and in a more specific way is not yet possible, although this might be beneficial to the progression of healing. Interestingly, Solcoseryl® (Valeant Pharmaceuticals), a topical gel found to stimulate the acute inflammatory response in horses, did not exert comparable effects in ponies.[12] Apparently, the suboptimal, initial inflammatory response in horses can be stimulated more effectively than the already adequate one in ponies. Although this might suggest that the choice for special dressings and topical products that enhance the initial inflammatory response is less critical for ponies than for horses, the benefits are certainly seen in clinical practice when using interactive dressings for extensive wounds on the limbs of ponies (Figure 2.11).

Inhibition of the early inflammatory response should also be avoided when healing is occurring by second intention. The use of corticosteroids is, therefore, contraindicated, and the prolonged administration of a NSAID, including a selective cyclooxygenase-2 (COX-2) inhibitor, is questionable.[36–40] Agents toxic to leukocytes, such as many antiseptics, caustics, and astringents, should be avoided. Antiseptics, even when sufficiently diluted, should not be used routinely but only in cases of a bacterial threat and only for a short time. Additionally, wet bandages and hydrotherapy using cold water can be detrimental because they transiently decrease the temperature in local tissue, causing vasoconstriction. A decrease in temperature slows biologic processes, and vasoconstriction limits the influx of leukocytes, nutrients, and oxygen to the wound. For optimal healing, the wetting agent for a dressing and the fluid used for irrigation should be warm (~38 °C) to avoid transient vasoconstriction.[53]

What to do

- Surgically debride the wound, when necessary, even if a wound is not to be sutured, because autolytic debridement of wounds of horses is slow.
- Bandage a wound and apply interactive dressings that stimulate inflammation until the wound has filled with granulation tissue.

What to avoid

- Do not use any product that reduces inflammation, such as a NSAID or a corticosteroid, or that is toxic to inflammatory cells or fibroblasts, such as an antiseptic.

Inhibiting the inflammatory response

As soon as the cavity of a wound has filled in with granulation tissue, the inflammatory response should no longer be encouraged but instead inhibited. Chronic inflammation, inherent to wounds on limbs of horses, enhances the formation of EGT and delays contraction, through persistently elevated concentrations of several mediators (see Chapter 15), and inhibits epithelialization. A direct link between persistent inflammation and delayed wound healing has also been demonstrated in experimental wounds of rabbits.[45]

First, stimuli causing a chronic inflammatory response, such as bone sequestra, foreign bodies or necrotic tissue, should be identified and eliminated from the wound. Additionally, the wound must be protected from environmental microorganisms and foreign material, which can be achieved by covering the wound's surface with inert semi-occlusive absorbing dressings (e.g., Tegaderm foam adhesive, 3M). The number of bacteria on the wound's surface must be controlled because bacteria are strongly chemoattractive to leukocytes, the presence of which perpetuates inflammation. Reduction of surface contamination can be achieved by excising the superficial layer of granulation tissue, thereby removing clefts in which bacteria reside and eliminating many leukocytes and mediators of inflammation, which accumulate in the superficial layers of the granulation tissue. Surface contamination may be further decreased by dressing the wound for 1 or 2 weeks with an antiseptic wound dressing that absorbs exudate (the reader is referred to Chapter 6 for more information about dressings). Systemic antimicrobial therapy is ineffective in reducing the concentration of bacteria on a wound because antibiotics administered systemically often fail to reach a therapeutic concentration within granulation tissue and at its surface.[54] This failure occurs because, in spite of the good blood supply to granulation tissue, fibrin accumulation at the base of granulation tissue prevents adequate penetration of drugs.[54]

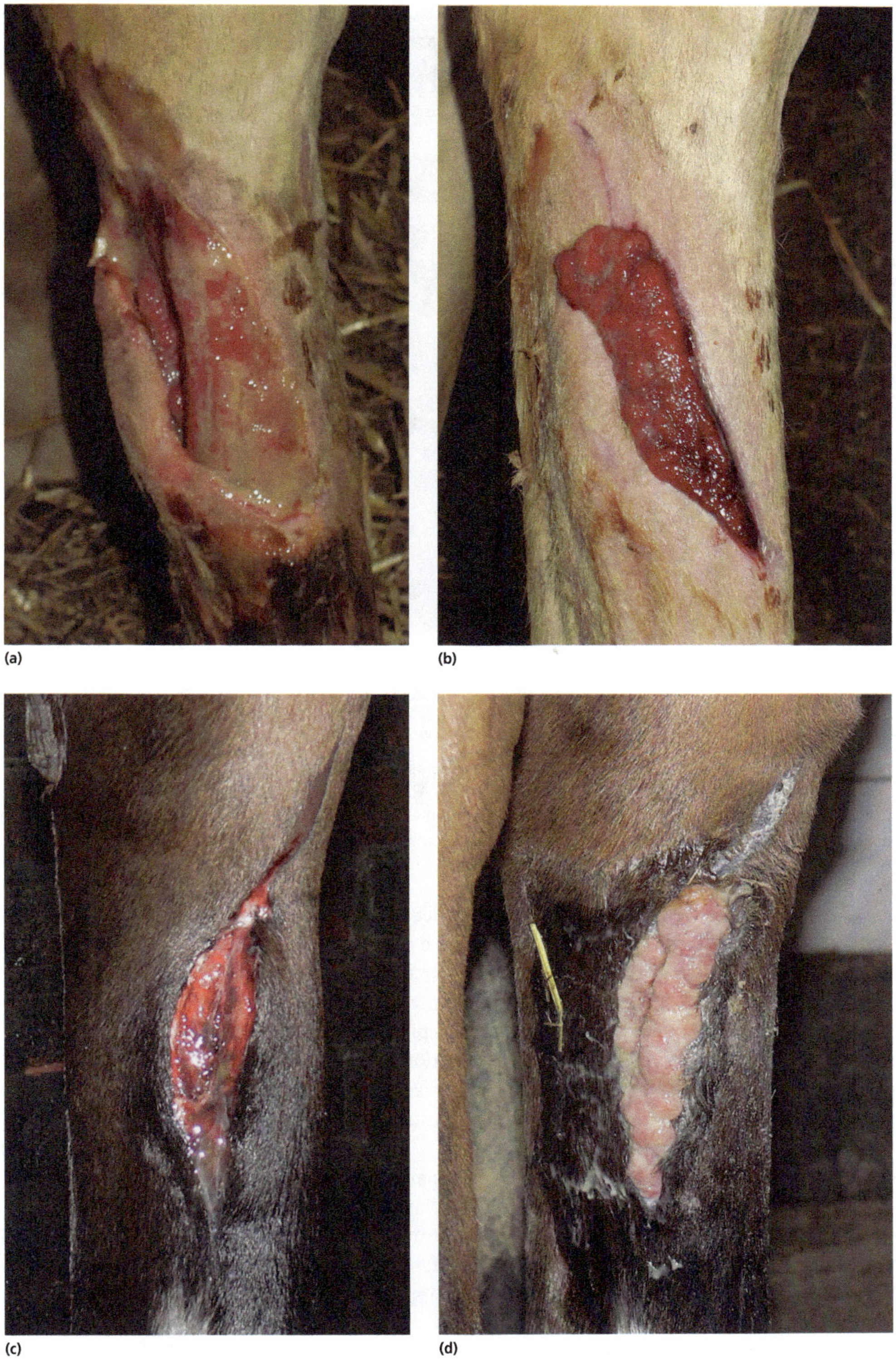

Figure 2.10 (**a**) This traumatic wound on the dorsal surface of the metatarsus of a horse, with extensive undermining, was treated with alginate dressings to stimulate the acute inflammatory response. (**b**) After 13 days, the wound was filled with healthy and contracting granulation tissue. (**c**) A different traumatic wound at a similar location in a horse, but with less undermining and no involvement of the metatarsal bone. The wound was treated with several types of silver foam dressing that do not modulate inflammation. (**d**) After 20 days, the wound was filled with EGT characterized by an irregular surface, riddled by a deep cleft. This wound failed to contract.

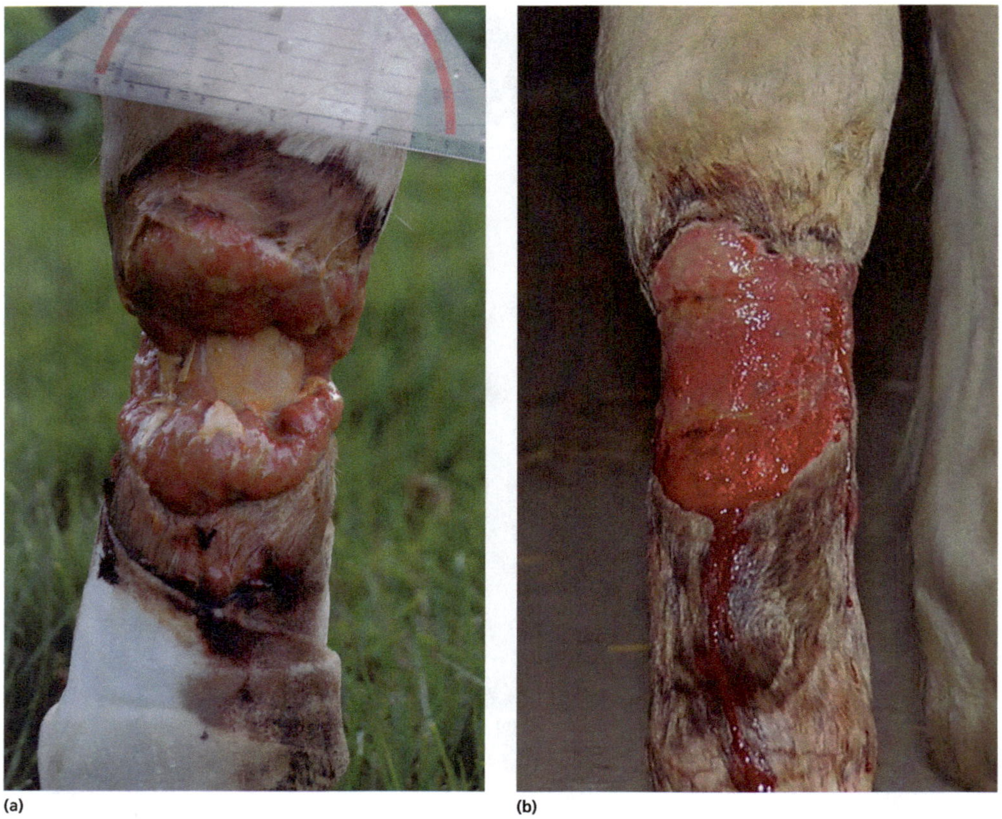

Figure 2.11 **(a)** A large degloving injury on the dorsal surface of the metacarpus of a pony, with exposed bone and lacerated extensor tendons. The wound was debrided and treated with alginate dressings to stimulate inflammation. **(b)** After 15 days, the exposed bone was covered and the wound was filled by granulation tissue. Treatment was continued with a foam dressing. A wound of these dimensions and depth may require at least twice the time to achieve a similar outcome when treated with a non-adherent dressing that is not interactive.

Chronic inflammation can be directly controlled by the topical application of a corticosteroid. A corticosteroid should be applied infrequently, and preferably only once, however, because its effects are not limited to just the inflammatory phase of healing. Theoretically, a similar inflammation-reducing effect could be expected from administering a NSAID, but such an effect has only been shown when parenteral administration is long-term, the dose is high, and the wound is acute.[36,37] Whether or not a clinically apparent effect could be achieved if the wound is chronic is questionable because, as is the case for antimicrobials, fibrin deposits may prevent the NSAID from penetrating the granulation tissue.[54] The effect of a topically applied NSAID on chronic equine wounds is unknown, but topical application of a non-steroidal, non-selective cyclooxygenase (COX) 1-2 inhibitor to experimental wounds of rabbits suffering chronic inflammation did not affect the number of leukocytes in the wounds and the NSAID delayed wound closure.[45] In conclusion, chronic inflammation is most effectively reduced by topical application of a corticosteroid.

Treatments that focus on reducing surface contamination and chronic inflammation concomitantly favor contraction and epithelialization. First, such treatments decrease the concentration of leukocytes on the wound, which in turn reduces the toxic effect of leukocytes on epithelialization, and they reduce the concentration of contraction-inhibiting inflammatory mediators. Second, such treatments decrease the risk of the wound developing EGT, the presence of which has a detrimental influence on contraction and epithelialization. Specific therapies to directly stimulate contraction and epithelialization are not yet available; consequently, contraction and epithelialization can be stimulated only indirectly, by modulating the inflammatory response.

That there is a need to specifically target wound contraction, particularly that of horses, is clear because the rate of contraction determines the speed of second-intention healing and the final cosmetic outcome (Figures 2.6 and 2.8).[5] Because the differences in wound contraction between horses and ponies appear to be caused by local tissue factors, rather than by the innate contractile capacity of fibroblasts, influencing the process may indeed be feasible.[11] Wound contraction is stimulated by TGF-β[31] but inhibited by many other inflammatory mediators abundant in a chronic inflammatory milieu.[32] It might be expected that TGF-β applied to wounds of horses would stimulate contraction, but this was not found in an experimental study,[55] possibly because the formulation of TGF-β or the timing of application was suboptimal. Interestingly, the rate of wound contraction is increased when partial-thickness skin grafts are applied (i.e., Meek micrografts).[56] Certain dermal factors present in the grafts likely stimulate contraction, but covering the wound surface with grafts also reduces inflammation, which indirectly stimulates contraction (the reader is referred to Chapter 18 for more information about skin grafting).

Epithelialization requires a smooth, healthy bed of granulation tissue that does not protrude above the level of the adjacent skin, along with a moist environment. Epithelialization benefits, therefore, from the measures taken to reduce surface contamination and chronic inflammation because it is inhibited by EGT and by toxic products produced by leukocytes.[19] The environment can be made moist by applying a semi-occlusive dressing; fully occlusive dressings, with the exception of silicone gel dressings,[57] should be avoided in the management of equine wounds because they prolong healing time by providing an environment that encourages bacterial growth, which in turn stimulates chronic inflammation, resulting in excess exudate and EGT.[58] Semi-occlusive foam dressings have the capacity to absorb exudate and bacteria and limit the influence of toxic products released from degenerated leukocytes within exudate. Epithelialization of large wounds is dramatically enhanced by skin grafting, which increases the margins from which epithelial cells proliferate and migrate. Measures to optimize the conditions for epithelialization are more critical in horses than in ponies because epithelialization is the predominant mechanism of closure of wounds on the limbs of horses, whereas epithelialization and contraction contribute equally to closure of wounds on the limbs of ponies.

What to do

- Limit the number of bacteria at the wound's surface, and protect the wound from contamination by bandaging.
- Be gentle with the tissues by avoiding application of irritating substances because these sustain chronic inflammation.
- Debride the wound when its surface has an unhealthy appearance or when healing is delayed, to reduce the number of bacteria and inflammatory cells.
- Cover the wound with an inert semi-occlusive dressing that efficiently absorbs exudate, including bacteria and toxic products released from degenerated leukocytes.
- Apply a corticosteroid topically but only when chronic inflammation delays healing and only to the frequency necessary to keep granulation tissue from becoming exuberant.
- Use skin grafts on extensive wounds of the limb to promote contraction and epithelialization.

Conclusion

Observing the differences in wound healing between horses and ponies has provided valuable information about the intrinsic process of wound healing and the common complications encountered when managing traumatic wounds of equids. Ponies heal faster and with fewer complications than do horses. These differences can, to a large extent, be explained by the disparity in the local inflammatory response, which, in turn, relates to differences in the functional capacity of leukocytes. Research data indicate that, in clinical practice, a maximal effect of treatment can be obtained by using a differential approach to wound healing that optimizes conditions for each successive phase of wound healing. The effect of treatment on the inflammatory response is of paramount importance to the other phases of healing and, therefore, modulation of the inflammatory phase of healing should always be considered when managing a wound. During treatment of wounds healing by second intention, inflammation should be stimulated until the wound has filled with granulation tissue, and thereafter it should be retarded.

References

1. Simpson GG. *Horses: the Story of the Horse Family in the Modern World and Through Sixty Million Years of History.* New York: Oxford University Press, 1951.
2. Bertone AL, Sullins KE, Stashak TS, *et al.* Effect of wound location and the use of topical collagen gel on exuberant granulation tissue formation and wound healing in the horse and pony. *Am J Vet Res* 1985; **46**: 1438.
3. Fretz PB, Martin GS, Jacobs KA, *et al.* Treatment of exuberant granulation tissue in the horse: evaluation of four methods. *Vet Surg* 1983; **12**: 137.
4. Barber SM. Second intention wound healing in the horse: the effect of bandages and topical corticosteroids. *Proc Am Assn Equine Practnrs* 1990; **35**: 107.
5. Wilmink JM, Stolk PWT, van Weeren PR, *et al.* Differences in second-intention wound healing between horses and ponies: macroscopical aspects. *Equine Vet J* 1999; **31**: 53.
6. Wilmink JM, van Weeren PR, Stolk PWT, *et al.* Differences in second-intention wound healing between horses and ponies: histological aspects. *Equine Vet J* 1999; **31**: 61.
7. Wilmink JM, van Herten J, van Weeren PR, *et al.* Study of primary-intention healing and sequester formation in horses compared to ponies. *Equine Vet J* 2002; **34**: 270.
8. Van Den Boom R, Wilmink JM, O'Kane S, *et al.* Transforming growth factor-β levels during second intention healing are related to the different course of wound contraction in horses and ponies. *Wound Repair Regen* 2002; **10**: 188.
9. Wilmink JM, Veenman JN, van den Boom R, *et al.* Differences in polymorphonucleocyte function and local inflammatory response between horses and ponies. *Equine Vet J* 2003; **35**: 561.
10. Azari O, Molaei MM, Hojabri R. Differences in second-intention wound healing of distal aspect of the limb between Caspian miniature horses and donkeys: macroscopical aspects. *Comp Clin Pathol* 2012; **21**: 731.
11. Wilmink JM, Nederbragt H, van Weeren PR, *et al.* Differences in wound contraction between horses and ponies: the in vitro contraction capacity of fibroblasts. *Equine Vet J* 2001; **33**: 499.
12. Wilmink JM, Stolk PTW, van Weeren PR, *et al.* The effectiveness of the haemodialysate Solcoseryl® for second-intention healing in horses and ponies. *J Vet Med* 2000; **47**: 311.

13. Caron JP. Management of superficial wounds. In: Auer JA, Stick JA (eds). *Equine surgery*, 2nd edn. WB Saunders: Philadelphia, 1999: 232.
14. Stashak TS. Selection of approaches to wound closure. In: Stashak TS, Theoret CL (eds). *Equine Wound Management*, 2nd edn. Wiley Blackwell: Iowa, 2008: 177.
15. Wilmink JM, van Weeren PR. Differences in wound healing between horses and ponies: application of research results to the clinical approach of equine wounds. *Clin Techn Equine Pract* 2004; **3**: 123.
16. Moens Y, Verschooten F, De Moor A, *et al.* Bone sequestration as a consequence of limb wounds in the horse. *Vet Radiol* 1980; **21**: 40.
17. Stashak TS. Management practices that influence wound infection and healing. In: Stashak TS, Theoret CL (eds). *Equine Wound Management*, 2nd edn. Wiley Blackwell: Iowa, 2008: 85.
18. Hanson RR. Management of avulsion wounds with exposed bone. *Clin Tech Equine Pract* 2004; **3**: 188.
19. Cotran SC, Kumar V, Robbins SL. Cellular growth and differentiation: normal regulation and adaptations; inflammation and repair. In: Schoen FJ (ed). *Robins Pathologic Basis of Disease, vol 1*, 5th edn. WB Saunders: Philadelphia, 1994: 35.
20. Rook G, Balkwil F. Cell-mediated immune reactions. In: Crowe L (ed.) *Immunology*, 5th edn. Mosby International Ltd: London, 1998: 121.
21. Wahl SM. The role of lymphokines and monokines in fibrosis. *Ann N Y Acad Sci* 1985; **460**: 224.
22. Turck C, Dohlman JG, Goetzl E. Immunological mediators of wound healing and fibrosis. *J Cell Physiol* 1987; **5**: 89.
23. Roberts AB, Sporn MB, Assoian RK, *et al.* Transforming growth factor type β: rapid induction of fibrosis and angiogenesis *in vivo* and stimulation of collagen formation in vitro. *Proc Nat Acad Sci USA* 1986; **83**: 4167.
24. Kovacs EJ. Fibrogenic cytokines: the role of immune mediators in the development of scar tissue. *Immunol Today* 1991; **12**: 17.
25. Miller C, Wilson DA, Keegan KG, *et al.* Growth characteristics of fibroblasts isolated from the trunk and distal aspect of the limb of horses and ponies. *Vet Surg* 2000; **29**: 1.
26. Chvapil M, Pfister T, Escalada S, *et al.* Dynamics of the healing of skin wounds in the horse as compared with the rat. *Exp Mol Pathol* 1979; **30**: 349.
27. Clark RAF. Basics of cutaneous wound repair. *J Dermatol Surg Oncol* 1993; **19**: 693.
28. Darby I, Skalli O, Gabbiani G. α-smooth muscle actin is transiently expressed by myofibroblasts during experimental wound healing. *Lab Invest* 1990; **63**: 21.
29. Desmoulière A, Geinoz A, Gabbiani F, *et al.* Transforming growth factor-β1 induces α-smooth muscle actin expression in granulation tissue myofibroblasts and in quiescent and growing cultured fibroblasts. *J Cell Biol* 1993; **122**: 103.
30. Ignotz RA, Heino J, Massague J. Regulation of cell adhesion receptors by transforming growth factor-β. *J Biol Chem* 1989; **264**: 389.
31. Montesano R, Orci L. Transforming growth factor β stimulates collagen-matrix contraction by fibroblasts: implications for wound healing. *Proc Natl Acad Sci USA* 1988; **85**: 4894.
32. Ehrlich HP, Wyler DJ. Fibroblast contraction of collagen lattices *in vitro*: inhibition by chronic inflammatory cell mediators. *J Cell Physiol* 1983; **116**: 345.
33. Stadelmann WK, Digenis AG, Tobin GR. Physiology and healing dynamics of chronic cutaneous wounds. *Am J Surg* 1998; **176**: 26.
34. Van Ruissen F, van Erp PE, de Jongh GJ, *et al.* Cell kinetic characterization of growth arrest in cultured human keratinocytes. *J Cell Sci* 1994; **107**: 2219.
35. Jacobs KA, Leach DH, Fretz PB *et al.* Comparative aspects of the healing of excisional wounds on the leg and body of horses. *Vet Surg* 1984; **13**: 83.
36. Gorman HA, Wolff WA, Frost WW, *et al.* The effect of oxyphenylbutazone on surgical wounds of horses. *J Am Vet Med Assoc* 1968; **152**: 487.
37. Busti AJ, Hooper JS, Amaya CJ, *et al.* Effects of perioperative antiinflammatory and immunomodulating therapy on surgical wound healing. *Pharmacother* 2005; **25**: 1566.
38. Su WH, Cheng MH, Lee WL, *et al.* Nonsteroidal anti-inflammatory drugs for wounds: pain relief or excessive scar formation? *Mediators Inflamm* 2010; **2010**: 413238.
39. Ren H, Lin D, Mou Z, *et al.* The adverse effect of selective cyclooxygenase-2 inhibitor on random skin flap survival in rats. *PLoS One* 2013; **8**: e82802.
40. Kahn LH, Styrt BA. Necrotizing soft tissue infections reported with nonsteroidal antiinflammatory drugs. *Ann Pharmacother* 1997; **31**: 1034.
41. Agarwal S, Piesco NP, Peterson DE, *et al.* Effects of sanguinarium, chlorhexidine and tetracycline on neutrophil viability and functions in vitro. *J Periodontal Res* 1997; **32:** 335.
42. Maeda K, Sakonju I, Kumakura A, *et al.* Effects of lidocaine hydrochloride on canine granulocytes, granulocyte CD11b expression and reactive oxygen species production. *J Vet Med Sci* 2010; **72**: 141.
43. Eriksson AS, Sinclair R, Cassuto J, *et al.* Influence of lidocaine on leukocyte function in the surgical wound. *Anesthesiol* 1992; **77:** 74.
44. Smith CJ, Edwards AE, Gower DE, *et al.* Leucocyte migration: effects of in vitro exposure to anaesthetic agents: possible potentiation of effects by adrenaline. *Eur J Anaesthesiol* 1992; **9:** 463.
45. Qian LW, Fourcaudot AB, Yamane K, *et al.* Exacerbated and prolonged inflammation impairs wound healing and increases scarring. *Wound Repair Regen* 2016; **24**: 26.
46. Wilmink JM, van Weeren PR. Second intention repair in the horse and pony and management of exuberant granulation tissue. *Vet Clin North Am Equine Pract* 2005; **21**: 15.
47. Chvapil M, Holubec H, Chvapil T. Inert wound dressing is not desirable. *J Surg Res* 1991; **51**: 245.
48. Turner TD. The development of wound management products. In: Krasner DL, Rodeheaver GT, Sibbald RG (eds). *Chronic Wound Care: A Clinical Source Book for Healthcare Professionals*, 3rd edn. Wayne PA: HMP Communications, 2001: 293.
49. Thomas A, Harding KG, Moore K. Alginates from wound dressings activate human macrophages to secrete tumour necrosis factor-alpha. *Biomaterials* 2000; **21**: 1797.
50. Carter CA, Jolly DG, Worden CE, *et al.* Platelet-rich plasma gel promotes differentiation and regeneration during equine wound healing. *Exp Mol Path* 2003; **74**: 244.
51. Monteiro S, Lepage OM, Theoret CL. Effects of platelet-rich plasma on the repair of wounds on the distal aspect of the forelimb in horses. *Am J Vet Res* 2009; **70**: 277.

52. Dart CM, Perkins NR, Kelly A, *et al.* The effect of short- and long-term treatment with Manuka honey on second intention healing of contaminated wounds on the distal aspect of the forelimbs in horses. *Vet Surg* 2013; **42**: 154.
53. Niemzura RT, DePalma RG. Optimum compress temperature for wound hemostasis. *J Surg Res* 1979; **26**: 570.
54. Robson MC, Edstom LE, Krizek TJ. The efficacy of systemic antibiotics in the treatment of granulating wounds. *J Surg Res* 1974; **16**: 299.
55. Steel CM, Robertson ID, Thomas J, *et al.* Effect of topical rh-TGF-β1 on second intention wound healing in horses. *Aust Vet J* 1999; **77**: 734.
56. Wilmink JM, Van Den Boom R, Van Weeren PR, *et al.* The modified Meek technique as a novel method for skin grafting in horses: evaluation of acceptance, wound contraction and closure in chronic wounds. *Equine Vet J* 2006; **38**: 324.
57. Ducharme-Desjarlais M, Lepault E, Celeste C, *et al.* Determination of the effect of a silicone dressing (CicaCare®) on second intention healing of full-thickness wounds of the distal limb of horses. *Am J Vet Res* 2005; **66**: 1133.
58. Howard RD, Stashak TS, Baxter GM. Evaluation of occlusive dressings for management of full-thickness excisional wounds on the distal portion of the limbs of horses. *Am J Vet Res* 1993; **54**: 2150.

CHAPTER 3

Selected Factors that Negatively Impact Healing

Andrew J. Dart, BVSc, PhD, Diplomate ACVS, Diplomate ECVS, **Albert Sole-Guitart**, DVM, Diplomate ACVS, **Ted S. Stashak**, DVM, MS, Diplomate ACVS, and **Christine Theoret**, DMV, PhD, Diplomate ACVS

Chapter Contents

Summary

Wound healing is achieved through orchestrated phases that must occur in the proper sequence and time. Many factors impair normal healing by interfering with one or more of its phases. This chapter reviews the most important factors known to negatively affect healing and describes the mechanisms whereby they exert their detrimental effects. The factors discussed include patient-related factors (horse versus pony, age, nutritional status, disease, and tissue perfusion) and wound-related factors (causes and types of wounds, age and location of the wound, involvement of structures other than skin, nature of the wound, previous treatment, neoplastic transformation, and bioburden). A better understanding of the influence of these factors on repair may lead to a therapeutic approach that negates or diminishes their effects, thereby improving healing and resolving non-healing wounds.

Introduction

Wound healing is a carefully orchestrated series of events that are temporally and spatially linked in a process leading, ultimately, to repair. Many generic factors are known to influence healing, irrespective of species. Systemic and local factors can influence a wound's microenvironment and thereby influence the progression of healing. By identifying and, when possible, manipulating these factors, wounds should proceed to complete healing. Whereas some factors, such as the type and location of the injury, cannot be manipulated, their impact on healing should be considered prior to designing and implementing a plan to manage a wound and providing a prognosis.

Patient factors

Horse versus pony

To optimize wound healing in equids, the clinician should recognize that the horse's response to injury is different to that seen in other species and even to that seen in ponies. The initial inflammatory response of horses to trauma is sluggish and less intense, which, in turn, delays the development of a healthy bed of granulation tissue, resulting in slower and sometimes problematic healing.[1–5] This type of response is more commonly seen in wounds of the distal aspect of the limb (i.e., up to and including the carpus and tarsus) of horses compared to wounds

Equine Wound Management, Third Edition. Edited by Christine Theoret and Jim Schumacher.

Companion website: www.wiley.com/go/theoret/wound

of the body. One outcome is that wounds of horses, particularly those on the distal aspect of the limb, are more subject to infection, formation of exuberant granulation tissue (EGT), and delayed healing. This observation correlates with clinical studies that report that ponies are less susceptible to wound dehiscence, less likely to form a bony sequestrum, less likely to develop EGT, and less likely to suffer from delayed wound healing compared to horses.[1] For more information on the differences in healing between horses and ponies, the reader is referred to Chapter 2.

Age of the patient

Advanced age of the patient is known to influence healing in humans, and this has also been documented in experimental animal models.[6] In laboratory animal models, old animals suffer from delayed formation of granulation tissue with reduced tensile strength of the wound early in the healing process, as well as delayed epithelialization and delayed wound closure.[7] Tissue ischemia has been implicated as the cause of these delays, but studies investigating the influence of age on wound healing vary widely, and the anatomic, physiologic, and biologic processes differ substantially between species, making translation of results from one species to another inaccurate.[7] The wound-healing process in healthy, elderly humans appears to resemble that of younger patients, in terms of reaching a similar endpoint, and is usually protracted rather than impaired.[6,8] In aged human skin, the function of macrophages is impaired, proliferation of keratinocytes is decreased, and the dermis is atrophied, all of which when combined, likely lead to a reduced ability of skin wounds of aged patients to progress promptly through all phases of healing.[7] Clinical features apparent during wound healing in human patients over 60 years old include a sluggish inflammatory reaction, a less effective immune response, and a reduction in the capacity of cellular replication, leading to delayed angiogenesis, collagen synthesis, and epithelialization.[8,9]

The effect of advanced age on healing has not been investigated in horses. The impact of aging on wound healing in animals is likely to be less important than in humans because of the relatively lower proportion of geriatric patients in veterinary practice. But, as the standard of veterinary care improves and the emotional value of pets increases, domestic animals are expected to live longer, such that an effect of advanced age on healing may become apparent. The appearance of age-onset diseases probably bears a greater impact on wound healing in animals than does advanced age itself.[7,10] Because equids seem to be more resistant to age-related diseases than do smaller companion animals, advanced age is unlikely to be a significant detriment to wound healing in horses.

Nutritional status and disease

Suitable nutrition is required to sustain cellular repair during wound healing because nutrients are essential to the many biologic processes occurring in the skin. Suitable nutrition is particularly important when cellular division, movement, and differentiation are up-regulated in response to injury.[11] Consequently, in severely malnourished patients, the progression of healing is impeded, and the scar tissue that eventually fills the wound has a decreased tensile strength and is, therefore, susceptible to reinjury.[11,12] The metabolic status (positive or negative) at the time of injury is also important because the energy requirements of healing represent an additional burden to the patient. The new demands imposed by healing cannot be met when the patient is in a negative metabolic state.

Macronutrients (i.e., proteins, carbohydrates, and fats) and micronutrients (e.g., vitamins A, B complex, C, E, and K, and minerals, such as copper, iron, and zinc) are known to play important roles in wound healing.[11] Proteins provide major building blocks for cellular renewal and tissue growth after injury, and adequate protein is needed to maintain a positive nitrogen balance. Protein deficiency may affect hemostasis, inflammation, immunity, formation of granulation tissue, remodeling, and epthelialization.[11,12] Deficiencies of the amino acids cysteine, proline, arginine, tyrosine, and histidine have been shown to adversely affect wound healing by negatively affecting angiogenesis, formation of collagen, and wound remodeling.[11–13] Carbohydrates are the principal source of energy that sustains the high metabolic demands of tissue regeneration.[11] Fats provide energy and contribute to inflammation and synthesis of cell membranes and intracellular matrix.[11]

Various human and animal studies have incriminated a vitamin or mineral deficiency in situations of impaired healing.[11,14] A deficiency of vitamin A is associated with impaired synthesis and stability of collagen, impaired contraction and epithelialization of wounds, and an increase in the patient's susceptibility to infection.[11,15] Deficiency of vitamin B complex is associated with several skin disorders and anemia, each of which may affect wound healing.[11] Deficiency of vitamin C has been implicated in impaired synthesis of collagen and scarring, as well as reduced responsiveness and function of the immune system.[11] Vitamin E is important for stabilization of the cell membrane, and vitamin K plays a key role in hemostasis.[11] Iron is essential for production of red blood cells and synthesis of collagen.[16] Copper deficiency is associated with formation of defective collagen and elastic tissue, leading to reduced tensile strength of the scar.[17] Zinc is a component of key enzyme systems needed for cellular replication and synthesis of protein (e.g., the metalloproteinases that play an important role in the proteolytic remodeling of extracellular matrix during tissue repair).[18] However, a recent study found that wounds of rats treated topically with zinc gluconate healed similarly and contained equivalent bacterial loads as wounds treated with the carrier solution (isotonic saline solution or chlorhexidine) alone.[19]

Concurrent disease may affect wound healing. For example, Cushing's disease (*pars intermedia* dysfunction), which affects mainly older horses, is characterized by high serum concentrations of endogenous cortisol that might suppress inflammation to such an extent that healing could be impaired.[20] High serum concentrations of glucocorticoids may also be found in horses in response to stress. Protracted periods of hyperglucocorticoidemia may decrease the expression of pro-inflammatory cytokines, including interleukin-1, interleukin-6, and tumor necrosis factor-α, and some chemoattractants required for the inflammatory phase of wound healing and for supporting the migration of immune cells.[21,22] Whereas Cushing's disease and consistently elevated production of glucocorticoids are associated with an increased risk of infection and impaired healing of wounds of humans, their clinical impact on healing of wounds of horses is less clear. More importantly, the stress of a severe injury may decrease appetite, thereby leading to an intake of energy and nutrients insufficient to meet the demands of healing tissues.

Tissue perfusion/oxygen tension

Effective wound healing requires adequate circulation, itself dependent on sufficient hydration, to ensure optimal tissue perfusion and oxygenation. Oxygen is essential to several critical mechanisms underlying wound healing, including bacterial killing, collagen synthesis, and epithelialization. Oxygen plays a pivotal role in eliminating anaerobic bacteria and in reducing formation of biofilm and colonization by microorganisms resistant to antimicrobial drugs. The guideline of debriding a wound back to healthy bleeding tissue is based on the principle that healing progresses more quickly and efficiently under conditions where the granulation bed is well perfused and free from avascular and necrotic debris.[23]

Because most of the oxygen in blood is carried by hemoglobin, anemia might be expected to impair healing. Normovolemic anemia, with a hematocrit above 20%, however, in the presence of adequate blood flow and tissue perfusion, does not seem to be detrimental to wound healing.[24,25] Conversely, hypovolemia can compromise tissue perfusion, thereby negatively impacting healing, mostly by a decrease in activity of leukocytes and production of collagen.[26,27]

Wounding disrupts the local blood vessels, leading to acute hypoxia in the wounded tissues. Hypoxia favors angiogenesis, and the newly formed, temporary capillaries carry much needed oxygen into the wound's microenvironment. Oxygen tension of tissue near capillaries at a wound's margin is between 60 and 90 mmHg compared to oxygen tensions of 30–50 mmHg in normal, uninjured tissue. Cells consume oxygen thereby creating an oxygen gradient between the edge of the wound and the center of the wound.

In humans, the concentration of oxygen in tissue is closely correlated to the progression of wound healing.[25] Chronic, non-healing wounds are hypoxic relative to normally healing acute wounds, with tissue oxygen tensions ranging from 5–20 mmHg.[28] Studies in horses have shown that perfusion of chronic wounds of the limb is significantly inferior to perfusion of non-chronic body wounds.[29,30] Tissue perfusion is even worse in limb wounds that go on to form EGT.[29,30] Metabolic disturbances suggestive of a deficient oxygen supply have been identified in equine limb wounds that have developed EGT,[30] and a relative state of hypoxia during the inflammatory phase of repair of limb wounds, possibly due to occlusion of microvessels, secondary to endothelial hypertrophy, has also been identified.[31,32]

New blood vessels forming in an hypoxic environment are immature and bleed easily,[33] which may explain the friable and hemorrhagic nature of equine EGT observed clinically. Because the phagocytic ability of leukocytes is oxygen dependent,[34] the presence of hypoxia may explain the inefficient inflammatory response documented in limb wounds of horses thought to contribute to the development of EGT.[4,5] Furthermore, low oxygen concentrations encourage angiogenesis, the growth of fibroblasts, and the synthesis by fibroblasts of components of the extracellular matrix, such as collagen, another mechanism whereby the hypoxia present in limb wounds might favor the development of unhealthy EGT.

Tip

- Effective wound healing requires adequate circulation to ensure optimal tissue perfusion and oxygenation. Oxygen is essential for the elimination of bacteria, collagen synthesis, and epithelialization, which are all critical to healing.

What to do

- Wound healing can be optimized by debriding the wound back to healthy bleeding tissue, using appropriate dressings, addressing hydration, and providing effective analgesia. Healing progresses more quickly and efficiently under conditions where the granulation bed is well perfused and free from avascular and necrotic debris.

What to avoid

- Excessive granulation tissue is associated with poor oxygen tension within the wound and will delay healing. Once excessive granulation tissue forms it should be excised back to healthy bleeding tissue flush with the wound edges.

Wound factors

Causes and types of wounds

Surgical wound

Surgical wounds are often classified, based on their degree of intrinsic microbial contamination, into clean, clean-contaminated, contaminated, and dirty or infected (Table 3.1).

Wound healing complications develop less frequently after elective surgical procedures than they do after emergency procedures in horses.[36–38] Stabilizing or improving the physiologic status of a patient before performing an emergency procedure, as well as addressing systemic infection prior to surgery, is likely to reduce the incidence of incisional complications. Careful surgical planning and sound anatomic knowledge of the region to be exposed, combined with good surgical technique while maintaining tissue perfusion and oxygenation with appropriate fluid therapy, optimize healing. Sharp dissection with a scalpel, where possible, is preferred to blunt dissection or the use of surgical scissors. Hemostasis should be effective, tissue should be preserved and handled carefully, and closure, using appropriate suture material, should be accurate. Application of a suitable antimicrobial regimen may be warranted (the reader is referred to Chapter 4 for more detail). After surgery, the wound may require support by a bandage, after applying an appropriate dressing (the reader is referred to Chapter 6 for more information regarding dressings).

Table 3.1 National Research Council Operative Wound Classifications.[35]

Category	Description
Clean	Elective, primary closure, no drains, non-traumatic, no infection, no inflammation, aseptic technique maintained
Clean–contaminated	Gastrointestinal, respiratory, urogenital tracts entered under controlled conditions and with expected amount of contamination or minor break in aseptic technique
Contaminated	Open, fresh traumatic wound; gross contamination from gastrointestinal tract, opening of urogenital or biliary tract with infected bile or urine; incisions in which purulent material is encountered or major break in aseptic technique
Dirty or infected	Traumatic wound with retained devitalized tissue and/or foreign bodies, and/or fecal contamination or delayed treatment or from a dirty source; perforated viscus encountered or acute bacterial inflammation with purulent exudate encountered

The duration of surgery influences the likelihood of infection and subsequent complications of healing. For example, the incidence of infection in the horse after orthopedic surgery increases 3.6-fold as surgery time extends beyond 90 minutes,[36] whereas the incidence of incisional complications after abdominal surgery doubles when the procedure extends beyond 120 minutes.[37] The association between complications of healing and duration of surgery are probably multifactorial but are likely to reflect additional tissue trauma, drying of tissues, poor tissue perfusion, and increased opportunity for bacterial contamination.[39]

Accidental wound

Accidental wounds may be categorized as closed (e.g., bruise, hematoma, contusion) or open (e.g., abrasion, puncture, laceration, avulsion, degloving, burn), the latter constituting the majority of accidental wounds encountered in equine practice. The greater the inciting trauma, the more severe is the soft-tissue damage and the greater is the risk of subsequent infection. For example, sharp lacerations caused by metal or glass are unlikely to become infected because they are rarely associated with contamination, necrosis, or alteration of the skin's vascular supply.

Conversely, crush injuries and injuries characterized by avulsion and tearing of tissue are at greatest risk for infection because of extensive thrombosis of associated vessels and subsequent loss of blood supply. These types of wounds are almost 100-fold more likely to become infected than those caused by shearing forces.[40] The blood supply to the distal extremity of a horse's limb is commonly compromised, for instance, when wire encircles the limb, thereby creating a tourniquet-like effect. Wounds caused by entrapment of the limb between fixed objects (e.g., a cattle guard or a stall door and wall) or by impact from collision with a solid object or from a kick, are especially susceptible to infection because of the magnitude of soft-tissue injury (Figure 3.1).

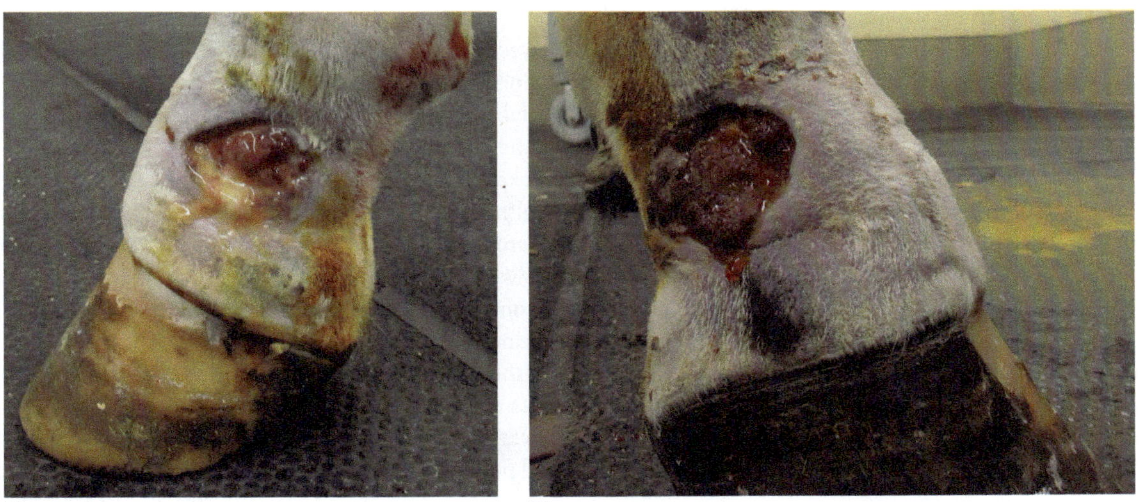

(a) (b)

Figure 3.1 Example of extensive trauma to the distal aspect of the limb. The wounds were incurred several days prior to presentation and were caused by entrapment of the foot between panels. The wounds' size and the degree of lameness had increased despite antimicrobial and anti-inflammatory therapy. Both wounds communicated with the pastern joint, and a stress radiograph confirmed rupture of the lateral collateral ligament of the proximal interphalangeal joint. (**a**) Lateral view. (**b**) Medial view.

Puncture wounds are susceptible to infection because the penetrating tract often closes, trapping bacteria deep within the tissues. Deep puncture wounds, where the point of perforation is small, may not allow sufficient drainage of contaminated fluids. Accumulation of these fluids within the wound provides an ideal environment for bacterial multiplication, particularly of anaerobic microorganisms. Opening the tract to ensure drainage, irrigating the tract, and packing it with saline-soaked sterile gauze, reduce the risk of infection becoming established.

Tip

- The contamination of a synovial structure (joint, bursa, tendon sheath), as a result of a small puncture wound, may go unnoticed unless contamination of the structure is accompanied by lameness, effusion of the synovial structure, heat over the wounded region, or signs of pain when the affected area is palpated.

What to do

- If perforation of a synovial structure is suspected, thorough physical and lameness examinations should be performed, along with ancillary diagnostic tests, which might include radiographic and/or ultrasonographic examinations and synoviocentesis to obtain fluid for cytologic analysis and bacterial culture and antimicrobial sensitivity testing. Synoviocentesis should be performed at a site remote from the wound, and after synovial fluid is collected, a sterile irrigation solution should be injected into the synovial cavity, under pressure. Egress of fluid from the wound after injection indicates that the wound communicates with the synovial structure.

What to avoid

- Synoviocentesis prior to acquiring radiographic or ultrasonographic images should be avoided to prevent introduction of air into the synovial space because air in a synovial space complicates interpretation of radiographic and ultrasonographic images.

For more information regarding the diagnosis and management of wounds involving synovial structures, the reader is referred to Chapter 16.

Age of the wound (time elapsed since injury)

A wound, either surgical or accidental, is a disruption in the integrity of the skin, which renders underlying tissues susceptible to contamination. A properly managed, clean or minimally contaminated wound should progress through the normal phases of repair. The probability that healing becomes delayed is related, at least in part, to the degree of contamination, the extent of tissue trauma, and the host's response. These factors are particularly important in accidental wounds of horses, because accidental wounds are often contaminated with foreign material and large numbers of various microorganisms.

Historically, an accidental wound, if prepared properly, was considered suitable for primary closure, with little risk of infection, if it was less than 6–8 hours old. This time, referred to as the "golden period," was based on research conducted in laboratory animals and was related to the time required for multiplying bacteria in a closed surgical wound to reach an infective concentration, considered to be more than 10^5 organisms per gram of tissue or milliliter of exudate.[41] This concept of a golden period is largely outdated.[42] Although an open wound often can tolerate a greater bioburden (e.g., 10^6 bacteria) without showing signs of deterioration,[43] the wound's outcome depends predominantly on the adequacy of the host's immune response, the virulence of contaminating bacteria, and local environmental factors (e.g., the presence of devitalized tissue or foreign material) that can potentiate the virulence of bacteria.[44]

Although the duration since injury may be given some consideration, the approach to wound management should be selected in light of other factors, such as the degree and type of contamination, the location and type of wound, including the extent of the trauma to the blood supply and to other nearby or underlying structures, the management of the wound prior to presentation, and the patient's overall physical condition and immune status. Many veterinarians become very astute at visually assessing wounds and at determining if the wound is suitable for primary closure or whether a different approach to wound management is more appropriate. The reader is referred to Chapters 4 and 8 for more information regarding the selection of appropriate methods to manage wounds.

Location of the wound

Specific healing limitations characterize different anatomic regions. For example, wounds on the distal aspect of the limb of horses, left to heal by second intention, expand during the first 2 weeks after trauma, in contrast to those on the body, which change little in size.[45] The increase in size of wounds on the distal aspect of the limb can be substantial, with the surface area of the wound almost doubling over a 2-week period. This time of expansion is referred to as the "lag phase" of healing. After a healthy bed of granulation tissue has formed, the wound starts to contract. The percentage decrease in the surface area of the wound attributable to contraction is greatest between the second and fourth weeks of healing. The capacity of body wounds to heal through contraction far exceeds that of wounds on the distal aspect of the limb. In a well-designed study, the rates of contraction and epithelialization of experimental, full-thickness wounds (7–9 cm^2) on the body and limbs of horses and ponies, left to heal by second intention, were measured. The percentage decrease in wound surface area attributable to wound contraction between the second and the fourth weeks of healing was 47% for the body wounds of ponies vs. 38% for the body wounds of horses and 35% for the limb wounds of ponies vs. 0% for the limb wounds of horses. After week 4, the rate of wound contraction slowed to less than 5% per week for the wounds of ponies and the body wounds of horses, up to complete healing. The metatarsal wounds of horses showed a different pattern: the lag phase of healing lasted 4 weeks and this was followed by an average rate of contraction that did not exceed 2.5% per week.[46] These differences in rates of contraction between wounds on the body and those on the limb have been attributed to the poorly oriented fibroblasts and myofibroblasts within the immature granulation tissue of limb wounds of horses.[47] In these same experimental limb and body wounds, epithelialization progressed over the wound's surface at a rate of 0.75 mm/week between weeks 3 and 7 of healing for body wounds of ponies, 0.62 mm/week for body wounds of horses, 0.63 mm/week for limb wounds of ponies, and 0.48 mm/week for limb wounds of horses.[46]

Moreover, wounds to the distal aspect of the limb of horses are often heavily contaminated with foreign material, including feces. Whereas short exposure to feces has been shown to improve healing of experimental wounds on the distal aspect of the limb of horses, perhaps by stimulating the acute inflammatory response,[48] wounds contaminated by feces, which may contain up to 1×10^{11} organisms/gram, are likely to become infected if not treated properly. For more information regarding the management of wounds on the distal aspect of the limb, the reader is referred to Chapters 8 and 13.

Finally, wounds on the distal aspect of the limb of horses are more susceptible to the formation of EGT than are similar wounds located elsewhere on the body.[49] The exact location of the wound on the limb further influences healing and formation of EGT; wounds over the dorsal surface of the metacarpo/metatarsophalangeal joint heal more slowly than similar wounds located over the dorsal surface of the metacarpus/metatarsus. Additionally, limb wounds located on the extensor and flexor surfaces of joints and the heel bulbs appear prone to the development of EGT. The reader is referred to Chapter 15 for more information regarding EGT.

Joints, tendons, and ligaments, all of which are vital to normal musculoskeletal function, are not protected by muscle at the distal aspect of the limb of horses. Consequently, a full-thickness skin wound in this location is likely to damage one or all of these structures, causing a substantial increase in the cost of treatment and a guarded or poor prognosis for return to function. Large wounds over bony prominences, particularly those involving the distal aspect of the limb, heal more slowly than those in other regions because they are subjected to excessive movement and high tension. Movement disrupts capillary buds, collagen deposits, and fragile new epithelium, thereby perpetuating the inflammatory response, which, in turn, favors the production of EGT. Although primary closure or delayed closure (primary or secondary) of wounds in these regions may assist healing, it can also be problematic because tension on the suture line might compromise blood supply to the skin. For this reason, many wounds over bony prominences are allowed to heal by second intention.

What to do

- External coaptation (i.e., bandages, splints, or casts) should be used to stabilize a sutured or non-sutured wound in a highly mobile region.

Tip

- If the wound is located in a region where it is subjected to pressure when the horse is recumbent (e.g., *tuber coxae*), preventing the horse from lying down (e.g., by cross-tying the horse or by attaching the horse's lead to an overhead wire) often allows the wound to heal by second intention.

Involvement of structures other than the skin

When assessing a wound in close proximity to a critical anatomic structure, the possibility of damage to that structure should be investigated. Critical structures that may be involved in a wound include synovial cavities, bone, tendon or ligament, pleural or abdominal cavities, eyes, and the paranasal sinuses. The reader is referred to Chapters 16, 14, 17, 12, and 11, respectively, for more information about the management of wounds involving one or more of these structures.

Synovial cavities (joints, tendon sheaths, or bursae) in close proximity to the wound should be examined for involvement, after cleansing the wound, by exploring the wound digitally with a gloved hand or with a sterile probe, by using radiography with a sterile metallic probe inserted in the wound or contrast material injected into the wound, or by using synovial distension. When using synovial distension to verify communication between a synovial cavity and a wound, the needle should be inserted into the synovial cavity at a site remote to the wound (Figure 3.2). The reader is referred to Chapter 4 for a more complete discussion of approaches to wound exploration and to Chapter 16 for more information regarding the diagnosis of synovial involvement and management of wounds involving a synovial structure. Timely identification of synovial involvement and the use of aseptic techniques minimize the risk of more contamination and subsequent infection, thereby optimizing the outcome of a horse with a wound involving a synovial cavity.

Injuries that expose tendons may heal with difficulty by second intention because movement of the tendon within a wound often results in the formation of two separate beds of granulation tissue, one on the tendon and the other on the tissue surrounding the tendon (Figure 3.3).

Tip

- Immobilizing the limb with a splint or a cast restricts movement of the tendon, allowing the separate granulation beds to become confluent, thereby enabling the wound to contract effectively.

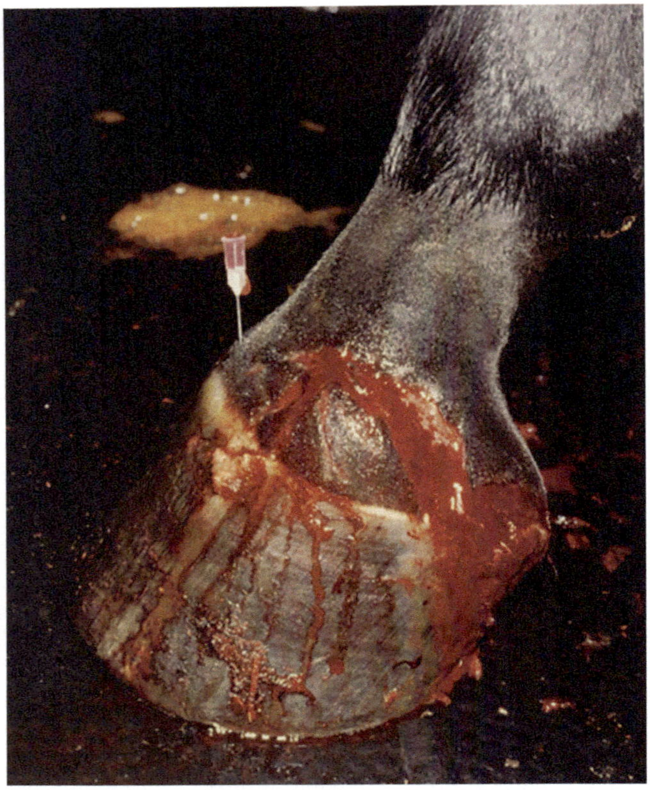

Figure 3.2 A sterile needle has been placed into the distal interphalangeal (coffin) joint at a site remote to the wound. Source: Stashak TS. Wound infection: contributing factors and selected techniques for prevention. *Proc Am Assoc Eq Pract* 2006; **52**: 270. Reproduced with permission of American Association of Equine Practitioners.

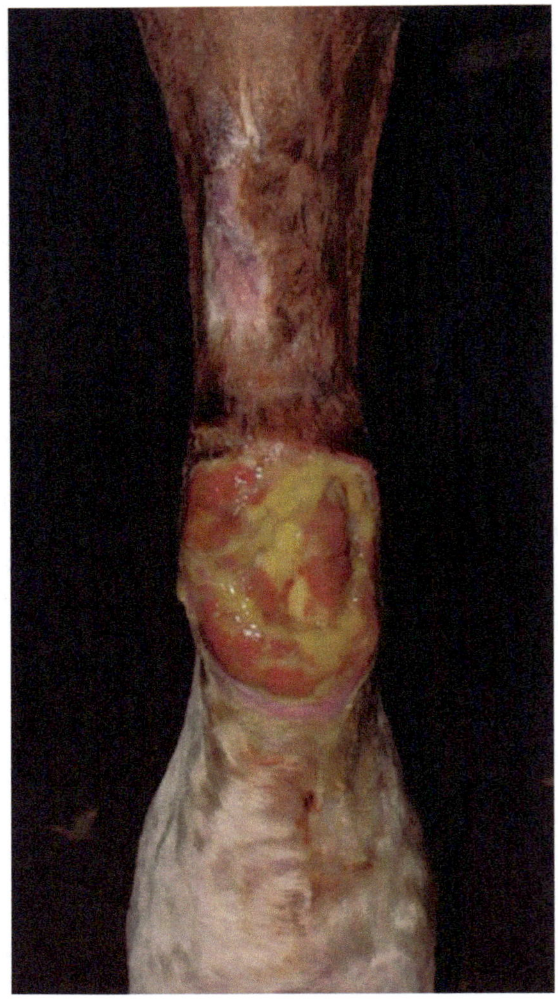

Figure 3.3 Granulating cast sore 3 weeks after the removal of a cast used to manage a laceration over the dorsal surface of the fetlock. Concentric rings of granulation tissue have formed as a result of differential movement between the skin, subcutaneous tissues, paratenon, and the underlying common digital extensor tendon. A portion of the tendon is visible distally with the proximal portion of the tendon covered by granulation tissue.

Exposure of bone in degloving wounds at the distal aspect of the limb is common, and damage to the periosteum is likely to lead to the formation of a bone sequestrum. Damage to or exposure of the periosteum and surrounding soft tissues may compromise the blood supply to the cortex of the bone. Collateral cortical blood supply may be insufficient to maintain the viability of the traumatized bone. During the first week after injury, exposed bone with adequate blood supply should start producing granulation tissue. Conversely, avascular bone, which usually appears off-white, develops no granulation tissue. Nevertheless, avascular bone may be masked by the gradual ingrowth of granulation tissue from surrounding soft tissues. Healthy cortical bone beneath a sequestrum may produce granulation tissue that may expel the sequestrum from the wound, but more commonly, granulation tissue emanating from the surrounding soft tissues traps the sequestrum within the wound (Figure 3.4). A bone sequestrum acts as a foreign body and harbors bacteria, causing chronic inflammation and, subsequently, the formation of EGT. The bone sequestrum usually makes a radiographic appearance 10–14 days after periosteal injury. A small sequestrum may be resorbed within the healing wound, but in most cases, the sequestrum must be removed surgically. The reader is referred to Chapter 14 for more information regarding the management of bone sequestra.

Wounds to the chest may involve the pleural cavity and are often associated with pneumothorax, hemothorax, or septic pleuritis. If involvement of the pleural cavity is suspected, thorough physical, radiographic, and ultrasonographic examinations are warranted. Hematologic examination can be useful in determining the extent of blood loss and/or the presence of infection. Injuries to the abdomen may be associated with septic peritonitis and damage to or herniation of viscera. Ultrasonographic examination of the viscera and cytologic examination of peritoneal fluid, obtained by paracentesis, are useful aids in diagnosing septic peritonitis. Surgical treatment may be required. Wounds that extend to body cavities may result in systemic complications such as blood loss and poor perfusion, hypoxia or sepsis that may cause chronic debilitation and negatively impact wound healing.

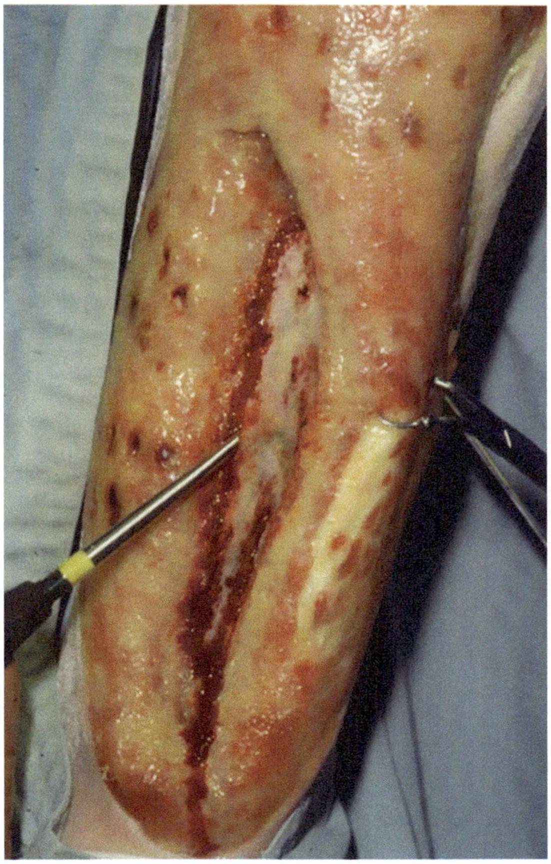

Figure 3.4 Degloving injury of 3 months duration involving the dorsal surface of the metatarsus. A linear defect in the unhealthy-looking granulation tissue was associated with wound drainage as well as stalled wound contraction, signs indicating the presence of a sequestrum. The sequestrum was removed from the sedated, standing horse using local anesthesia.

The reader is referred to Chapter 12 for more information regarding the management of wounds involving the chest or abdomen.

Nature of the wound

The shape, size, and depth of a wound can affect the rate of healing. Wounds on the extremities in which the orientation of a flap of skin is at odds with the distribution of blood vessels often experience a delay in healing and are more susceptible to infection. Arteries in the limbs run from proximad to distad so that large flaps of skin presenting as an inverted "V" suffer compromise to their blood supply (Figure 3.5). For healing to be successful, blood supply must be provided by underlying tissues, or, when the wound is sutured, from vessels that traverse the suture line to revascularize the flap. Because the flap is susceptible to avascular necrosis that inevitably leads to dehiscence after primary closure, delaying suturing this type of wound until a healthy bed of granulation tissue forms may be best. This approach is referred to as "delayed secondary closure" and is described at greater length in Chapter 8.

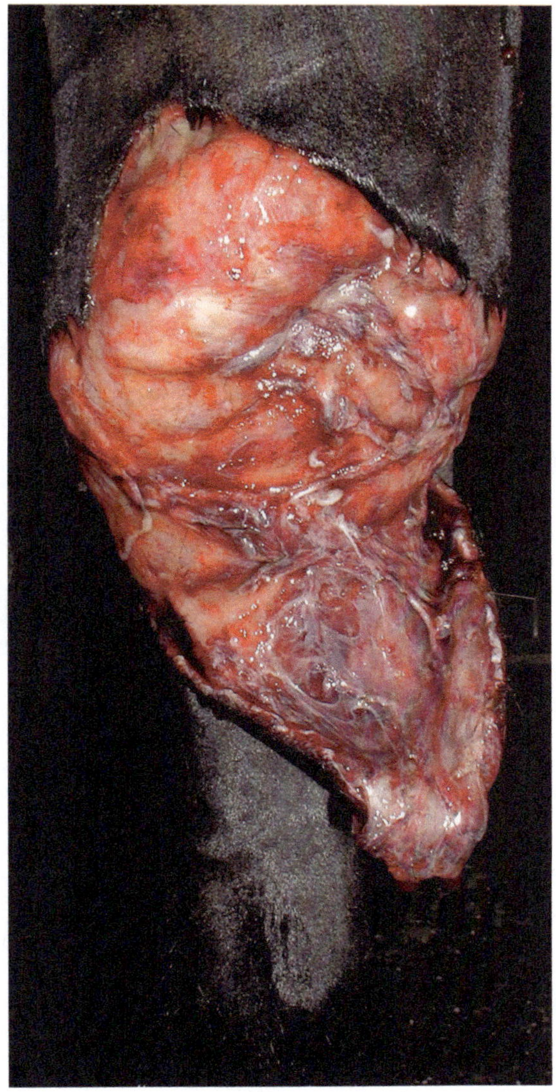

Figure 3.5 Example of an inverted "V"-shaped wound over the dorsal surface of the carpal region. This configuration compromises blood supply to the skin and subcutaneous tissues, resulting in poor wound healing. Courtesy of Dr. Christophe Celeste.

What to do

- The flap should be stabilized in a somewhat normal position with a few large tension sutures, while awaiting definitive treatment, to preserve it from recoil/retraction and to protect the underlying tissues, such as bone and/or tendon, from further injury or dessication (Figure 3.6).

Seromas, hematomas, and edema impede healing and increase the risk of infection by distracting the wound's edge and by reducing capillary perfusion from the pressure they exert on the local blood supply. Large, superficial hematomas that develop from trauma are best left for 5–7 days before being drained to allow for adequate hemostasis. Early and ineffective drainage may lead to recurrence of the hematoma. A drain may be

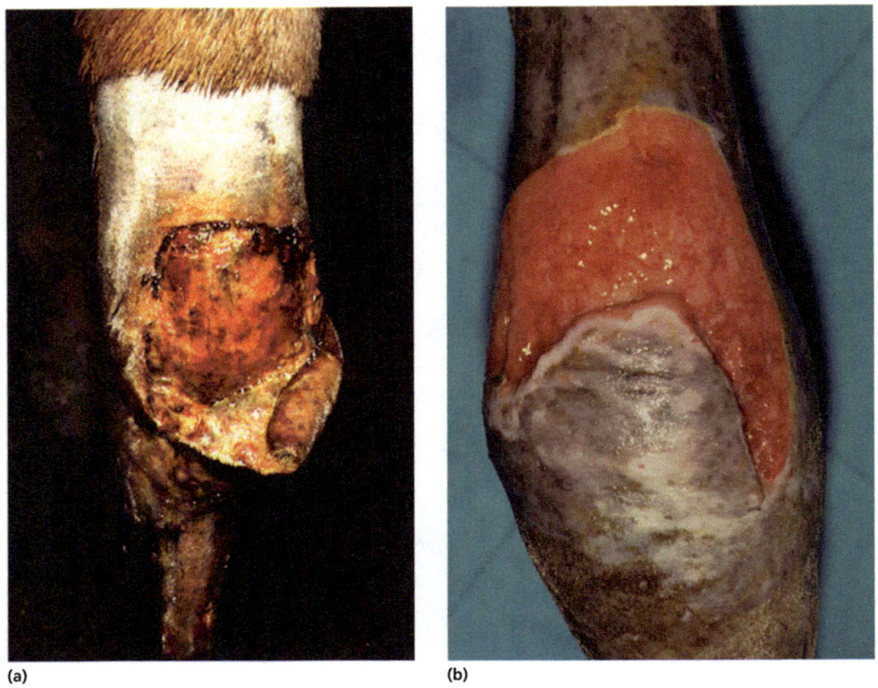

Figure 3.6 Example of a flap wound over the dorsal surface of the carpal region. The flap is positioned such that it is at odds with the limb's major distribution of blood vessels. **(a)** At presentation, ~6 hours after injury; note the absence of subcutaneous tissue at the proximal limit of the flap. The tip of the flap felt cool. After cleansing the wound, the skin flap was elevated into its normal position, after which a bandage splint was applied. **(b)** Five days after injury. The skin flap had retracted, and a healthy bed of granulation tissue had formed. This flap should have been stabilized, in as normal a position as possible, using a few large tension sutures. This would have prevented retraction of the skin flap, which complicates delayed closure of the wound.

inserted into a hematoma to ensure drainage, but to do so poses a risk of ascending infection and may be ineffective in draining large amounts of clotted blood. The reader is referred to Chapter 9 for more information about the use of drains in managing wounds.

What to do

- Edema can be controlled by applying cold therapy immediately after injury and subsequently applying a bandage and initiating exercise.

Tip

- A wounded limb that has been bandaged for an extended time often swells within a few hours after the bandage has been removed, especially if the horse is inactive or is confined. Swelling can be minimized by scheduling bandage removal to coincide with an increase in exercise brought about by moving the horse from a stall to a small paddock.

Previous treatments (used by owner)

Various topical and/or systemic treatments may negatively influence healing by slowing cellular proliferation and hindering the immune response of the patient. For more information regarding the effects of various systemically administered drugs, such as antimicrobial drugs, glucocorticosteroids, and non-steroidal anti-inflammatory drugs, the reader is referred to Chapter 4.

Many topical treatments, particularly those for which only anecdotal evidence exists, have been shown to be, at best, unreliable in promoting healing. At worst, some topical treatments, such as application of a caustic agent, may exert a negative effect. Topical agents should be applied to wounds to serve a specific purpose; this highlights the importance of understanding the properties of the active ingredients of the selected product and their proposed effects on healing tissues. For more information about topical wound-care products, the reader is referred to Chapter 5.

What to avoid

- Over-the-counter products that fail to provide a list of ingredients should not be used on wounds.

Neoplastic transformation and cutaneous habronemiasis

Neoplastic transformation at a wound site, although uncommon, should be considered when examining any non-healing, chronic, granulating wound. Transformation of a wound into sarcoid or squamous cell carcinoma has been reported in horses.[20] Apparently, the transformation can occur at a wound at any site on the body. Whereas transformation of a wound into

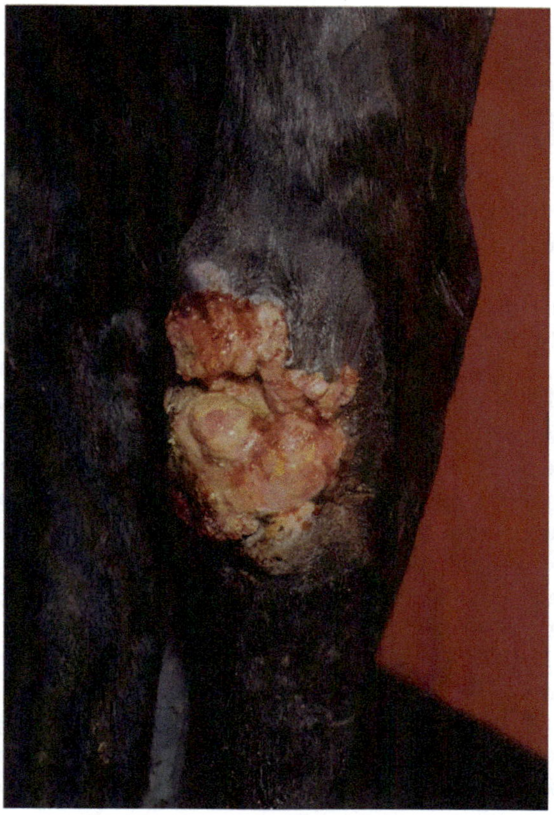

Figure 3.7 Example of a wound that would not heal after repeated attempts to excise the granulation tissue. Histologic examination of the tissue revealed a squamous cell carcinoma.

sarcoid is more likely to occur in a horse with a sarcoid at another site on its body, no such relationship has been established for transformation of a wound into a squamous cell carcinoma. A typical history for neoplastic transformation includes failure of a granulating wound to heal after repeated attempts to debride the granulation tissue or dehiscence of a sutured wound in the absence of an identifiable cause (Figure 3.7). For more information about sarcoid transformation at wound sites, the reader is referred to Chapter 21.

Cutaneous habronemiasis is a common cause of granulomas in horses in some parts of the world. It is caused, in part, by the larvae of the spirurida stomach worms, including *Habronema musca*, *Habronema majus*, and *Draschia microstoma*. Larvae feeding on pre-existing wounds cause a chronic granulomatous reaction as they migrate, halting the healing process. Lesions caused by habronemiasis are chronic and are most commonly seen around the eyes (particularly adjacent to the medial canthus), on the male genitalia, on the distal aspect of the limbs, and at the commissures of the lips (Figure 3.8).[50] The wounds typically contain yellow, calcified material the size of rice grains, and histologic examination of tissue from the wound reveals necrotic foci in a dense fibrous stroma infiltrated with eosinophils and macrophages. The incidence of yearly recurrence is high in certain individuals. Conversely, some horses are resolutely resistant.

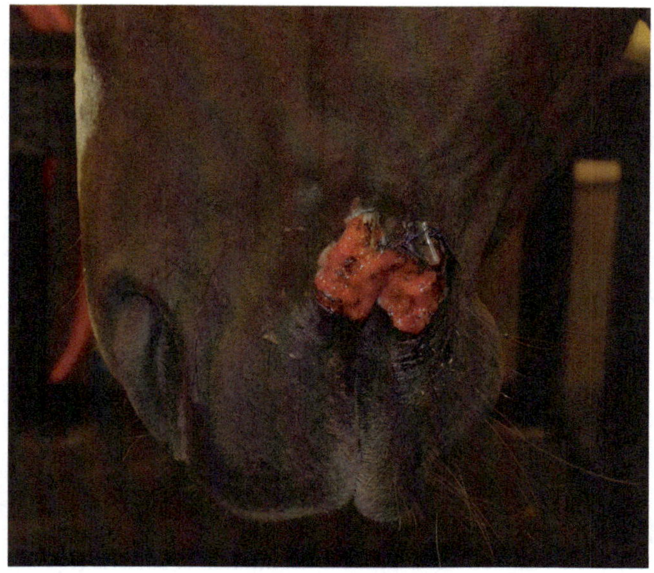

Figure 3.8 A chronic, non-healing wound at the commissure of the mouth. Despite repeated sharp debridement and excision of the granulation tissue, followed by primary closure of the defect, the wound would not heal. Histologic examination of the granulation tissue revealed habronemiasis.

Tips

- Habronemiasis can be easily confused with neoplastic and other non-neoplastic cutaneous masses in horses. Seasonality is an important issue, with the majority of cases occurring in the summer and early fall. Moreover, histologic examination of a wound sample (acquired by biopsy or by resection of the lesion) helps confirm the diagnosis, thereby enabling initiation of appropriate therapy.
- Fly control and regular deworming with ivermectin may reduce the incidence of habronemiasis.

What to do

- Treatment with ivermectin (200 μg/kg), administered intramuscularly may be effective, but extensive surgical debridement or excision of the affected wound may be required if the horse fails to respond to medical therapy.
- Where complete surgical resection of the affected area is not possible, topical application or intralesional injection of a corticosteroid, to reduce the inflammatory response associated with habronemiasis, may be used to complement surgical therapy.

Wound bioburden

Although wounds cease to heal for a number of reasons, perhaps the most common is associated with the effects of the wound's bioburden, which are influenced by the sheer quantity of colonizing microbes, the mixture of species within the wound, and the effects of microbial toxins.[51]

Contamination and infection of accidental wounds left to heal by second intention should be considered separately from surgical site infection, which has been well characterized.[52] The majority of this section addresses the effects of the bioburden on accidental wounds healing by second intention.

Wound infection can be defined as multiplication of bacteria to such an extent that the host's defenses are overwhelmed, resulting in disruption of healing and damage to the wound.[53] Infection is the endpoint of a continuum of events that reflects the microorganisms' impact on the wound and the host's reaction to this impact.

Bacterial impact continuum

Several classification systems and many definitions have been used to categorize the impact of bacteria on a wound and on the patient. The classical definition is that more than 10^5 microorganisms per gram of tissue or per milliliter of exudate constitutes infection.[41] This number serves as a reasonable threshold for infection in a closed surgical wound that tends toward predictability.[51] An open wound left to heal by second intention, however, often can tolerate a higher concentration of bacteria (e.g., up to 10^6) without showing signs of infection.[41] The outcome is predominantly dependent on the adequacy of the host's immune response and the virulence of contaminating bacteria, as well as local environmental factors (such as the presence of foreign or necrotic material) that might potentiate the virulence of bacteria.[44]

In many clinical settings, accurate determination of the concentration and types of bacteria may not be possible. Consequently, clinicians must rely on clinical signs exhibited by the patient to establish the position of the wound along the bacterial impact continuum.[52] Quantitative and qualitative microbiologic testing of tissue or fluid from the wound, when available, may be used to confirm the diagnosis and guide the selection of appropriate antimicrobial therapy.[43] Importantly, even if the results of microbiologic testing do not indicate infection, a wound should be considered infected if clinical signs of infection, such as heat, swelling, and pain caused by palpation of the wounded region, are present.

A simple classification system that can be used to assist practitioners in determining how bacteria might be impacting a wound healing by second intention is outlined in Table 3.2. This system of classification is not absolutely related to increasing concentrations of bacteria but, in many instances, larger numbers and an increasing variety of bacteria, in particular, anaerobic bacteria, will lead to greater impairment to healing and sometimes to local and/or systemic effects.[52] This progression may also be influenced by the presence of a maturing bacterial biofilm in the wound.[53]

Microorganisms do not replicate in a *contaminated* wound, and a contaminated wound shows no clinical signs of infection. All accidental wounds in horses are at least contaminated. A wound is considered *colonized* when the contaminating bacteria, often resident skin microorganisms, have adhered to the wound and proliferate, thereby competing with healing tissue for nutrients and oxygen. The microbial by-products may be deleterious to the normal physiologic processes of healing;[9] if the growth and death of microbes is kept in balance by the host's immune system, however, the wound does not become infected and heals uneventfully.

There is a point along the continuum of bacterial impact where *critical colonization* occurs. At this point, replicating microorganisms can no longer be managed by the immune system and invade the wound's surface causing a *topical infection* that delays wound healing. When contamination changes to this state of critical colonization (infection), the wound's bioburden becomes the most important factor impeding healing.[54] Many of the classical signs of infection are absent, but the wound bed may appear unhealthy.[55] Specifically, an infected wound may be dull looking and may contain a copious amount of exudate and exuberant, friable granulation tissue, which may appear to be sloughing. The size of the wound may fail to decrease and may even increase.[52]

Further along the continuum, *local infection* arises, which is characterized by bacterial invasion of the local tissues (i.e., those

Table 3.2 Clinical manifestations of the increasing bacterial impact on wound healing.[52]

Level of bacterial impairment	Bacterial activity	Degree of impairment to wound healing and clinical signs
Contamination	Bacteria are on the wound's surface. No division is occurring	No impairment to healing No obvious clinical signs of infection
Colonization	Bacteria are dividing	No impairment to healing. No obvious clinical signs of infection. (Clinical wound appearance does not usually differ from contamination)
Topical infection (critical colonization)	Bacteria are dividing. Bacteria and/or their products have invaded the wound's surface. There might be an increasing variety of bacteria present. Biofilm may be present	No obvious clinical signs of infection. (Clinical wound appearance does not usually differ from contamination)
Local infection	Bacteria and/or their products have invaded the local tissues	Impairment to healing Usually obvious clinical signs of infection localized to wound environment and immediate peri-wound tissue
Regional/spreading infection/cellulitis	Bacteria and/or their products have invaded surrounding tissues	Impairment to healing. Usually obvious clinical signs of infection. May have systemic clinical signs
Sepsis	Bacteria and/or their products have entered the bloodstream and may spread to distant sites or organs	Impairment to healing. Usually obvious systemic clinical signs: patient usually acutely unwell. Damage to organs may occur

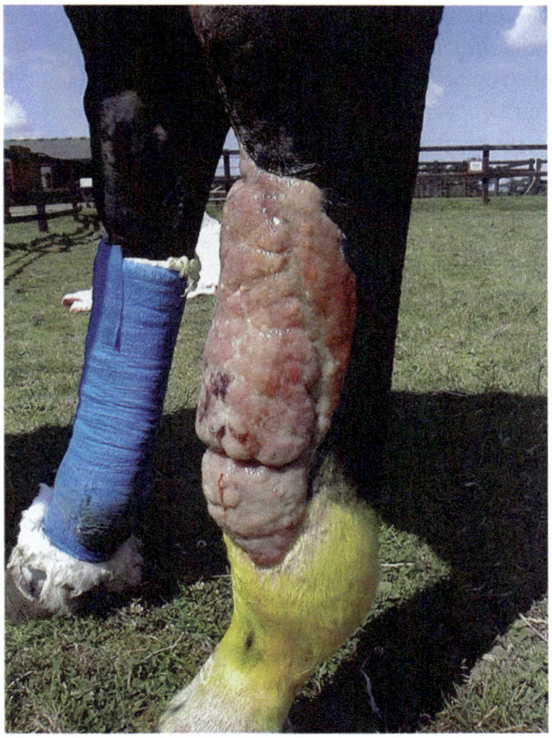

Figure 3.9 Example of a chronic wound showing local signs of infection: the granulation tissue has an irregular surface (clefts and tunnels), has become exuberant, and is covered by unhealthy exudate. Courtesy of Dr. D. Knottenbelt.

beyond the wound's surface), usually accompanied by obvious clinical signs of infection localized to the wound's immediate vicinity. At this point in the continuum, the wound usually increases in size, its granulating surface may exhibit irregularities (e.g., clefts and tunneling), and its exudate is often purulent and malodorous (Figure 3.9).

Regional or spreading infection/cellulitis occurs when the replicating microorganisms spread beyond the wound to injure surrounding tissues, thereby eliciting an immune response from the host.[56] This stage in the continuum is recognized clinically by heat, induration, signs of pain, and swelling, and sometimes by fever.

Wound infection might finally result in *sepsis*, although this is rare in horses because the immune response is usually functional and not easily overwhelmed.

Risk factors

Whether or not infection develops in a contaminated wound depends on many factors, including but not limited to: (1) dose of microorganisms; (2) virulence of microorganisms; (3) wound environment; (4) mechanism of injury; and (5) host response.

The virulence of a microorganism is related to its ability to adhere to eukaryotic cell surfaces, multiply, and evade the host's immune response. The virulence of different microorganisms varies and influences the dose of bacteria required to induce infection. The concentrations of bacteria per gram of tissue or milliliter of exudate necessary to cause infection in a closed surgical wound (10^5 bacteria) or an open wound (10^6 bacteria) have been established, but beta-hemolytic streptococci, notably *S. pyogenes*, are pathogenic at substantially lower concentrations than are many other bacterial species.[57] Moreover, polymicrobial interaction, where two or more microorganisms act synergistically, is likely to decrease the bacterial dose required for infection to result from contamination. For example, co-infection of *Staphylococcus aureus* and *Pseudomonas aeruginosa* is more virulent than infection caused by either species alone.[58] Bacteria found in open wounds are commonly considered to be aerobic, but anaerobic species are now also thought to play a role in infection because the frequency at which they can be isolated from chronically infected wounds has increased.[59]

Although chronic human and equine wounds share many pathophysiologic features,[60] the microbiologic burden of chronic wounds of equids has not been studied to the same extent as that of chronic wounds of humans. Two recent investigations, nevertheless, provide evidence for polymicrobial infection of chronic wounds of equids and show that the microbial genera found in chronic wounds of equids are very similar to those found in chronic wounds of humans, with commensal organisms acting as opportunistic pathogens when the wound's environment is favorable to their replication.[61,62] In the first study, the most common bacteria isolated and cultured from wound swabs were *P. aeruginosa*, *Staphylococcus epidermidis*, *Serratia marcescens*, *Enterococcus faecalis*, and *Providencia rettgeri*. Slight differences were found between isolates cultured from swabs of the wound's surface and those cultured from wound tissues harvested by biopsy.[61] The second study confirmed the polymicrobial community harbored in the wound environment of equids. The average number of bacterial species identified from swabs of the wound's surface was 3.02 ± 1.65 (range 0–8). The species most often isolated from chronic wounds was *P. aeruginosa*, whereas the most commonly isolated genus was *Staphylococcus*. Obligate anaerobic bacteria made up 6.8% of the total isolates.[62]

Wounds on the distal aspect of limbs of horses are often contaminated with feces and soil, making them highly susceptible to infection. This relates, at least partially, to the role of components of soil in potentiating infection. Specific infection-potentiating factors have been identified in soil, in its organic components as well as in its fractions of inorganic clay.[63,64] The ability of these factors to incite infection seems related to damage to the host's defenses, in particular to a reduction in the efficiency of leukocytes to ingest and kill bacteria and to a decrease in specific humoral factors and neutralizing antibodies, thereby eliminating the bactericidal activity of serum. Consequently, for wounds contaminated by these fractions, only 100 bacteria per gram of tissue or milliliter of exudate may be necessary to elicit infection.[63] Other components of the wound's environment that may drive the wound along the bacterial continuum include foreign material (wood, metal, gloving powder,[65] suture, orthopedic implants, drains, etc.), necrotic tissue (including bone sequestra), hematoma or seroma, or compromised vascular supply.[51] For example, a large comprehensive study reviewing the epidemiology of wound infections of human patients, found that formation of a hematoma or seroma was a leading factor in decreasing a wound's resistance to infection.[66] For information regarding approaches to the management of a hematoma or seroma, the reader is referred to Chapters 4 and 8.

A deficient response by the host is a relatively common cause of infection of wounds of humans who suffer from diseases such as diabetes, obesity, or a vascular disorder. Fortunately, equine patients usually have a functional immune system and, unless suffering from polytrauma or malnutrition, should mount an appropriate immune response to wounding.

Effects on healing

The wound offers bacteria an attractive environment in which they can flourish and, if able to overcome the host's response, cause substantial damage locally and systemically.

Infection is a major cause of delayed wound healing, reduced gain of tensile strength, and dehiscence after closure. The mechanism whereby these detrimental effects of infection occurs is probably the release of bacterial enzymes and metalloproteinases that degrade fibrin (required for migration of fibroblasts and for phagocytic activity of macrophages) and inhibit cytokines responsible for orchestrating healing. Accumulating exudate, in addition, physically forces the wound's edges apart.

Colonizing bacteria consume local oxygen required for healing, release free radicals damaging to tissues, and produce endotoxins that can activate coagulation, causing thrombosis of the microvasculature nourishing the wound,[52] or cause systemic organ or immune dysfunction. Endotoxins also favor the release of more inflammatory mediators, thereby leading to a chronic inflammatory state,[52] as is commonly seen in wounds on the limbs of horses.[1,4]

The overall effect of wound infection is increased costs, increased use of resources due to delayed healing, lost productivity, and pain.

Biofilms

In the previous sections of this chapter, bacteria were viewed from the perspective of planktonic (free-floating) pathogens proliferating and exerting their virulence, mostly as individual organisms. In the case of chronic wounds, however, microbes often exist as sessile (attached), multicellular consortiums known as biofilms.[67] The microbes in biofilms adhere to each other and/or surfaces or interfaces by a self-secreted, three-dimensional, extracellular polysaccharide (EPS) matrix.[68]

Formation of biofilm on a surface can be divided very broadly into three stages: microbial attachment, growth, and detachment.[69] Under natural conditions, planktonic bacteria reversibly adhere to a surface within minutes (stage 1).[70,71] In stage 2, biofilm-growing bacteria bind irreversibly to the surface and become sessile within 2–4 hours, then multiply and differentiate, changing patterns of gene expression in ways that promote survival (usually the result of a type of communication between bacteria known as quorum sensing). After 6–12 hours of firm attachment, the bacteria begin secreting a slimy substance (EPS) around the micro-colonies (stage 3). Once a biofilm has reached maturity (usually within 24 hours),[72] focal areas of the biofilm dissolve to shed planktonic cells, microcolonies and fragments of biofilm, which can disperse and attach to other parts of the wound bed, thereby forming metastatic daughter biofilms in the surrounding area; this occurs within 2–4 days, depending on the species and growth conditions.[71,73]

Biofilms cannot be seen with the naked eye. Rather, confocal or scanning electron microscopic evidence of microbial aggregation/EPS from wound samples is required to confirm the presence of a biofilm. Evidence of the presence of biofilms in wounds of human patients has been provided using scanning electron and confocal microscopy.[74] Biofilms tend to occur more frequently in chronic wounds (60%) than in acute wounds (6%), suggesting a possible role of biofilms in the chronicity of wounds.[74] Although less research has been done on biofilms in animals, biofilms are believed to be involved in many diseases of animals, including wound infections.[75] Two studies recently found evidence of the presence of biofilms in the wounds of horses.[61,62] One study detected polymer-embedded aggregates of bacteria using light microscopy of Gram-stained tissue harvested from the edge of chronic wounds on the limb of eight horses,[61] and the other found that tissue from eight of 13 chronic wounds of horses, examined microscopically after Gram staining, showed evidence that bacterial biofilms were present.[62] Furthermore, bacteria cultured from chronic and acute wounds and examined by microtiter plate assay showed significantly higher potential to form biofilm than did bacteria isolated from intact skin from the same horse.[62]

Single species of bacteria can make up a biofilm, but, more often, biofilms are comprised of multiple species of aerobic and anaerobic bacteria, and, occasionally, yeast, fungi, or protozoa. These organisms interact and develop stable, symbiotic relationships through complex intercellular communications, or quorum sensing, deep within the wound where they can be difficult to isolate and identify.[76,77] Traditional culturing techniques may be inadequate in establishing a comprehensive composition of a biofilm[78] but have identified *Staphylococcus*, *Pseudomonas*, and *Enterococcus* as the predominant organisms in the biofilm of chronic wounds in humans. Molecular analyses of chronic wound samples revealed diverse polymicrobial communities and the presence of bacteria, including strictly anaerobic bacteria, not revealed by culture.[74] In fact, a recent profiling study using 16S RNA sequencing demonstrated an average of 17 genera per wound, most of which were anaerobic.[79] Biofilms found in wounds of horses can be caused by environmental organisms such as *P. aeruginosa*, commonly found in infected wounds. Species of bacteria that constitute part of the normal microflora of the skin have also been incriminated in the formation of biofilms. These normally harmless commensal organisms may become pathogenic through a combination of endogenous and exogenous factors.

The presence of biofilms has important implications for the management of chronic wounds in horses because the infection resulting from biofilms is more resistant to traditional means of therapy. This is because biofilms protect microorganisms embedded within them, improving their tolerance to the host's immune system, environmental stresses, and antimicrobial therapy, whether it is administered topically (antiseptics) or systemically (antibiotics).[80] Additionally, community living allows easier transfer of genes leading to sharing of advantageous attributes, such as increased virulence.[81] For example, human leukocytes easily kill planktonic *S. aureus*, but when the same microorganism resides in a biofilm, its elimination may require a 1000-fold increase in leukocytes.[75] Likewise, *S. aureus*, when growing within a biofilm, is reported to be up to 100-fold more resistant to antimicrobial therapy when compared to its planktonic counterparts.[82] Neither phagocytes nor antimicrobial agents may be able to readily penetrate the slimy exopolymer, and if antimicrobial agents do succeed in penetrating it, they may be rendered inactive.[83,84]

Although not all wounds with biofilm exhibit typical signs of infection, biofilms may, nevertheless, impair healing by competing for metabolic resources and by interfering with the inflammatory response to wounding. Indeed, biofilms have been shown to induce a chronic non-healing inflammatory phase of healing.[85] Furthermore, biofilms have been shown to delay epithelialization, at least in a murine model.[86]

The ability of the host to control pathogenic organisms decreases as the biofilm matures.[73] Consequently, efforts to prevent or slow formation of a biofilm should be implemented as soon as possible. A biofilm-based wound-care regimen should be multifaceted, with debridement as its most essential component (the reader is referred to Chapter 4 for a thorough description of methods of wound debridement). In addition to removing devitalized tissues that serve as a fertile environment for bacteria, debridement physically disrupts the biofilm structure. The result is a period of reassembly during which organisms are more susceptible to antimicrobial therapies that may prevent bacterial reattachment and limit or prevent reinfection.[87]

The best sample for bacterial culture and antimicrobial sensitivity testing is a deep tissue biopsy specimen, or, if such a sample cannot be obtained, a swab of the deepest tissues, or both. Traditional methods of culture may not be adequate to establish the bacterial composition of biofilm in chronic wounds, complicating the selection of appropriate antimicrobial therapy.[78] In fact, biofilms of chronic wounds are characteristically polymicrobial, and sophisticated molecular techniques are required to identify the bacterial components of the biofilm. If antimicrobial drugs are administered systemically as part of the treatment, the minimum inhibitory concentrations (MIC) established by antimicrobial sensitivity testing may provide suboptimal dosing regimens and should be replaced with minimum biofilm eradication concentrations (MBEC).[75] Antiseptics, in particular the two biofilm-active antiseptics, octenidine and polyhexanide,[73] and silver-based wound dressings are used concurrently to combat biofilms in wounds of human patients.[88] The reader is referred to Chapter 5 for more information about topical wound-care products and to Chapter 6 for more information about wound dressings.

Unfortunately, a situation may arise wherein microorganisms referred to as "persisters" survive a recommended course of antimicrobial therapy because they are protected within the exopolymer matrix of the biofilm, which limits antibiotic penetration.[89] Withdrawal of the antimicrobial drug allows these "persisters" to replicate and, when conditions are appropriate, undergo a phenotypic change to become planktonic and free of the biofilm but with an increased ability to resist antimicrobial drugs and the host's immune response. Antibiotic chemotherapy is becoming increasingly ineffective in the treatment of biofilm infections because of antibiotic resistance.[80] This discovery has led to new strategies to deal with some diseases caused by biofilms. One of these consists of a pulsed dosing regimen wherein low doses of antimicrobial drugs are administered for an extended time while cycling with medication-free periods. This replaces the more classic short-term, continuous high-dose regimen. Using a low dose of antimicrobial drug, or alternatively, concurrently using low doses of two or three antimicrobial drugs targeting the biofilm, is associated with less risk of antibiotic resistance. This approach is postulated to be more effective in achieving a 100% kill and, therefore, less likely to leave behind microorganisms capable of developing antimicrobial resistance.[89] The reader is referred to Chapter 19 for more information regarding the therapeutic approach to eliminating bacterial biofilms.

It is not possible to categorically state when a wound is biofilm-free, because definitive clinical signs of a biofilm and available laboratory tests to detect a biofilm are lacking. Consequently, the most likely clinical indicator of a biofilm-free wound is progression of healing, with reduced formation of exudate and tissue slough.[88]

Conclusion

The rate and success of wound healing is determined by many factors, some of which cannot be manipulated because they already exist when the wounded horse is presented for treatment. Wound bioburden is, without a doubt, the most important impediment to healing but, fortunately, one that can be positively influenced.

Recognizing the factors that negatively impact healing and preventing or correcting these factors are key to promoting repair and returning the horse to its normal function as soon as possible, while achieving a cosmetic outcome.

References

1. Wilmink JM, van Herten J, van Weeren PR, *et al.* Retrospective study of primary intention healing and sequestrum formation in horses compared to ponies under clinical circumstances. *Equine Vet J* 2002; **34**: 270.
2. Bertone AL, Sullins KE, Stashak TS, *et al.* Effect of wound location and the use of topical collagen gel on exuberant granulation tissue formation and wound healing in the horse and pony. *Am J Vet Res* 1985; **46**: 1438.
3. Wilmink JM, Stolk PW, van Weeren PR, *et al.* Differences in second intention wound healing between horses and ponies: macroscopic aspects. *Equine Vet J* 1999; **31**: 53.
4. Wilmink JM, van Weeren PR, Stolk PW, *et al.* Differences in second intention wound healing between horses and ponies: histological aspects. *Equine Vet J* 1999; **31**: 61.
5. Wilmink JM, Veenman JN, van den Boom R, *et al.* Differences in polymorphonucleocyte function and local inflammatory response between horses and ponies. *Equine Vet J* 2003; **35**: 561.
6. Gosain A, DiPietro LA. Aging and wound healing. *World J Surg* 2004; **28**: 321.
7. Kim DJ, Mustoe T, Clark RA. Cutaneous wound healing in aging small mammals: a systematic review. *Wound Repair Regen* 2015; **23**: 318.
8. Stotts N, Wipke-Tevis D, Wopf H. Cofactors in impaired healing. In: Krasner D, Rodheaver G, Sibbald G (eds). *Chronic Wound Care: A Clinical Source Book for Healthcare Professionals*, 4th edn. HMP Communications: Malvern, PA, 2007: 215.
9. Guo S, DiPietro LA. Factors affecting wound healing. *J Dent Res* 2010; **89**: 219.
10. Wolf NS. Cell replication rates *in vivo* and *in vitro* and wound healing as affected by animal age, diet, and species. In: Wolf NS (ed). *The Comparative Biology of Aging*. Springer: The Netherlands, 2010: 97.
11. Brown KL, Phillips TJ. Nutrition and wound healing. *Clin Dermatol* 2010; **28**: 432.
12. Stechmiller JK. Understanding the role of nutrition and wound healing. *Nutr Clin Pract* 2010; **25**: 61.
13. Wild T, Rahbarnia A, Kellner M, *et al.* Basics in nutrition and wound healing. *Nutrition* 2010; **26**: 862.
14. Varani J, Warner RL, Gharaee-Kermani M, *et al.* Vitamin A antagonizes decreased cell growth and elevated collagen-degrading matrix metalloproteinases and stimulates collagen accumulation in naturally aged human skin. *J Invest Dermatol* 2000; **114**: 480.
15. Hunt TK. V: Vitamin A and healing. *J Am Acad Dermatol* 1986; **15**: 817.
16. Wright JA, Richards T, Srai SK. The role of iron in the skin and cutaneous wound healing. *Front Pharmacol* 2014; **5**: 156.
17. Gosling P, Rothe HM, Sheehan TM, *et al.* Serum copper and zinc concentrations in burns in relation to surface area. *J Burn Care Rehabil* 1995; **16**: 481.
18. Saper RB, Rash R. Zinc: an essential micronutrient. *Am Fam Physician* 2009; **79**: 768.
19. Kaufman KL, Mann FA, Kim DY, *et al.* Evaluation of the effects of topical zinc gluconate in wound healing. *Vet Surg* 2014; **43**: 972.
20. Knottenbelt DC. *Handbook of Equine Wound Management*. WB Saunders: Liverpool, 2003: 29.
21. Godbout JP, Glaser R. Stress-induced immune dysregulation: implications for wound healing, infectious disease and cancer. *J Neuroimmune Pharmacol* 2006; **1**: 421.
22. Boyapati L, Wang HL. The role of stress in periodontal disease and wound healing. *Periodontol 2000* 2006; **44**: 195.
23. Franz MG, Robson MC, Steed DL, *et al.* Guidelines to aid healing of acute wounds by decreasing impediments of healing. *Wound Repair Regen* 2008; **16**: 723.
24. Heughan C, Grislis G, Hunt T. The effect of anemia on wound healing. *Ann of Surg* 1974; **179**: 163.
25. Wutschert R, Bounameaux H. Determination of amputation level in ischemic limbs. Reappraisal of the measurement of $TcPO_2$. *Diabetes Care* 1997; **20**: 1315.
26. Jonsson K, Jensen JA, Goodson WH, *et al.* Assessment of perfusion in postoperative patients using tissue oxygen measurements. *Br J Surg* 1987; **74**: 263.
27. Hunt TK, Hopf W, Hussain Z. Physiology of wound healing. *Adv Skin Wound Care* 2000; **13**: 6.
28. Hopf HW, Rollins MD. Wounds: an overview of the role of oxygen. *Antioxid Redox Signal* 2007; **9**: 1183.
29. Celeste CJ, Deschene K, Riley CB, *et al.* Regional differences in wound oxygenation during normal healing in an equine model of cutaneous fibroproliferative disorder. *Wound Repair Regen* 2011; **19**: 89.
30. Sorensen MA, Petersen LJ, Bundgaard L, *et al.* Regional disturbances in blood flow and metabolism in equine wound healing with formation of exuberant granulation tissue. *Wound Repair Regen* 2014; **22**: 647.
31. Lepault E, Celeste C, Dore M. Comparative study on microvascular occlusion and apoptosis in body and limb wounds in the horse. *Wound Repair Regen* 2005; **13**: 520.
32. Dubuc V, Lepault E, Theoret CL. Endothelial cell hypertrophy is associated with microvascular occlusion in horse wounds. *Can J Vet Res* 2006; **70**: 206.
33. Tandara AA, Mustoe TA. Oxygen in wound healing – more than a nutrient. *World J Surg* 2004; **28**: 294.
34. McGovern NN, Cowburn AS, Porter L, *et al.* Hypoxia selectively inhibits respiratory burst activity and killing of *Staphylococcus aureus* in human neutrophils. *J Immunol* 2011; **186**: 453.
35. Centers for Disease Control and Prevention: Surgical Site Infection (SSI) Event. January 2015 (mod. April 2015): 9–26. www.cdc.gov/nhsn/PDFs/pscManual/9pscSSIcurrent.pdf
36. MacDonald D, Morley P, Bailey J, *et al.* An examination of the occurrence of surgical wound infection following equine orthopaedic surgery (1981–1990). *Equine Vet J* 1994; **26**: 323.
37. Klohnen A, Brauer T, Bischofberger A. Incisional complications following exploratory laparotomy using antibacterial coated suture material for subcutaneous closure: prospective randomised study in 100 horses. *Equine Vet J* 2010; **42**: 304.
38. Wilson D, Baker G, Boero M. Complications of celiotomy incisions in horses. *Vet Surg* 1995; **24**: 506.
39. Costa-Farre C, Prades M, Ribera T, *et al.* Does intraoperative low partial pressure of oxygen increase the risk of surgical site infection following emergency laparotomy in horses? *Vet J* 2014; **200**: 175.
40. Edlich RF, Rodeheaver GT, Morgan RF, *et al.* Principles of emergency wound management. *Ann Emerg Med* 1988; **17**: 1284.

41. Robson MC, Heggers J. Bacterial quantification of open wounds. *Mil Medicine* 1969; **134**: 19.
42. Zehtabchi S, Tan A, Yadav K, *et al.* The impact of wound age on the infection rates of simple lacerations repaired in the emergency department. *Injury* 2012; **43**: 1793.
43. Miller M. Wound infection unravelled. *J Commun Nurs* 2001; **15**: 31.
44. Bowler PG. The 10^5 bacterial growth guideline: reassessing its clinical relevance in wound healing. *Ostomy Wound Manage* 2003; **49**: 44.
45. Jacobs KA, Leach DH, Fretz PB, *et al.* Comparative aspects of the healing of excisional wounds on the leg and body of horses. *Vet Surg* 1984; **13**: 83.
46. Wilmink JM. Unpublished data on the rates of wound contraction and epithelialization in equids.
47. Wilmink JM, Nederbragt H, van Weeren PR, *et al.* Differences in wound contraction between horses and ponies: the *in vitro* contraction capacity of fibroblasts. *Equine Vet J* 2001; **33**: 499.
48. Bischofberger AS, Dart CM, Perkins NR, *et al.* The effect of short- and long-term treatment with Manuka honey on second intention healing of contaminated and noncontaminated wounds on the distal aspect of the forelimbs in horses. *Vet Surg* 2013; **42**: 154.
49. Knottenbelt DC. Equine wound management: are there significant differences in healing at different sites on the body? *Vet Dermatol* 1997; **8**: 273.
50. Pusterla N, Watson JL, Wilson D, *et al*: Cutaneous and ocular habronemiasis in horses: 63 cases (1988–2002). *J Am Vet Med Assoc* 2003; **222**: 978.
51. Kingsley A. The wound infection continuum and its application to clinical practice. *Ostomy Wound Manage* 2003; **49**: 1.
52. Position document of the Australian Wound Management Association: Bacterial impact on wound management: from contamination to infection. Australian Wound Management Association Inc. Version 1.5, October 2011; www.awma.com.au (consulted May 12th 2015).
53. Percival S, Bowler P. Biofilms in wounds. *Wound Repair Regen* 2008; **16**: 234.
54. Horrocks A. Prontosan wound irrigation and gel: management of chronic wounds. *Br J Nurs* 2006; **15**: 1222.
55. Schultz GS, Sibbald RG, Falanga V, *et al.* Wound bed preparation: a systematic approach to wound management. *Wound Repair Regen* 2003; **11**: 1.
56. Edwards R, Harding KC. Bacteria and wound healing. *Curr Opin Infect Dis* 2004; **17**: 91.
57. Robson MC. Wound infection: a failure of wound healing caused by an imbalance of bacteria. *Surg Clin North Am* 1997; **77**: 637.
58. Serra R, Grande R, Butrico L, *et al.* Chronic wound infections: the role of *Pseudomonas aeruginosa* and *Staphylococcus aureus*. *Expert Rev Anti Infect Ther* 2015; **13**: 605.
59. Bowler P, Duerden B, Armstrong D. Wound microbiology and associated approaches to wound management. *Clin Microbiol Rev* 2001; **14**: 244.
60. Theoret CL, Wilmink JM. Aberrant wound healing in the horse: naturally occurring conditions reminiscent of those observed in man. *Wound Repair Regen* 2013; **21**: 365.
61. Freeman K, Woods E, Welsby S, *et al.* Biofilm evidence and the microbial diversity of horse wounds. *Can J Microbiol* 2009; **55**: 197.
62. Westgate SJ, Percival SL, Knottenbelt DC, *et al.* Microbiology of equine wounds and evidence of bacterial biofilms. *Vet Microbiol* 2011; **15**: 152.
63. Rodeheaver G, Pettry D, Turnbull V, *et al.* Identification of the wound infection-promoting factors in soil. *Am J Surg* 1974; **128**: 8.
64. Edlich RF, Rodeheaver GT, Thacker JG, *et al.* Revolutionary advances in the management of traumatic wounds in the emergency department during the last 40 years: Part I. *J Emerg Med* 2010; **38**: 40.
65. Edlich RF, Long WB, Gubler, *et al.* Dangers of cornstarch powder on medical gloves: seeking a solution. *Ann Plast Surg* 2009; **63**: 111.
66. Cruse PJ, Foord R. The epidemiology of wound infections: a 10-year prospective study of 62 939 wounds. Symposium on surgical infections. *Surg Clin of North Am* 1980; **60**: 27.
67. Davis SC, Ricotti C, Cazzaniga A, *et al.* Microscopic and physiologic evidence for biofilm-associated wound colonization *in vivo*. *Wound Repair Regen* 2008; **16**: 23.
68. Thomson CH. Biofilms: do they affect wound healing? *Int Wound J* 2011; **8**: 63.
69. Lappin-Scott HM, Bass C. Biofilm formation: attachment, growth, and detachment of microbes from surfaces. *Am J Infect Control* 2001; **29**: 250.
70. Davies D, Chakrabarty A, Geesey G. Exopolysaccharide production in biofilms: substratum activation of alginate geen expression by *Pseudomonas aeruginosa*. *Appl Environ Microbiol* 1993; **59**: 1181.
71. Phillips PL, Wolcott RD, Fletcher J, *et al.* Biofilms made easy. *Wounds International* 2010; **1**: 1.
72. Wolcott RD, Rhoads DD, Bennett ME, *et al.* Chronic wounds and the medical biofilm paradigm. *J Wound Care* 2010; **19**: 45.
73. Daeschlein G. Antimicrobial and antiseptic strategies in wound management. *Int Wound J* 2013; **10** Suppl 1: 9.
74. James GA, Swogger E, Wolcott R, *et al.* Biofilms in chronic wounds. *Wound Repair Regen* 2008; **16**: 37.
75. Olson ME, Ceri H, Morck DW, *et al.* Biofilm bacteria: formation and comparative susceptibility to antibiotics. *Can J Vet Res* 2002; **66**: 86.
76. Hansen SK, Rainey PB, Haagensen JA, *et al.* Evolution of species interactions in a biofilm community. *Nature* 2007; **445:** 533.
77. Kaeberlein T, Lewis K, Epstein SS. Isolating "uncultivable" microorganism in a pure culture in simulated natural environment. *Science* 2002; **296**: 1127.
78. Kirketerp-Moller K, Jensen PO, Fazli M, *et al.* Distribution, organization and ecology of bacteria in chronic wounds. *J Clin Microbiol* 2008; **46**: 2717.
79. Han A, Zenilman JM, Melendez JH, *et al.* The importance of a multifaceted approach to characterizing the microbial flora of chronic wounds. *Wound Repair Regen* 2011; **19**: 532.
80. Clutterbuck AL, Woods EJ, Knottenbelt, *et al.* Biofilms and their relevance to veterinary medicine. *Vet Microbiol* 2007; **121**: 1.
81. Percival S, Bowler P. Biofilms and their potential role in wound healing. *Wounds* 2004; **16**: 234.
82. Leid JG, Shirtliff ME, Costerton JW, *et al.* Human leukocytes adhere to, penetrate, and respond to *Staphylococcus aureus* biofilms. *Infect Immun* 2000; **70**: 6339.

83. Hoyle BD, Jass J, Colsterton JW. The biofilm glycocalyx as a resistance factor. *J Antimicrob Chemother* 1990; **26**: 1.
84. Xavier JB, Forster KR. Cooperation and conflict in microbial biofilms. *Proc Natl Acad Sci USA* 2007; **104**: 876.
85. Wolcott R, Rhoads D, Dowd S. Biofilms and chronic wound inflammation. *J Wound Care* 2008; **17**: 333.
86. Schierle CF, de la Garza M, Mustoe TA, *et al.* Staphylococcal biofilms impair wound healing by delaying reepithelialization in a murine cutaneous wound model. *Wound Repair Regen* 2009; **17**: 354.
87. Wolcott RD, Rumbaugh KP, James G, *et al.* Biofilm maturity studies indicate sharp debridement opens a time-dependent therapeutic window. *J Wound Care* 2010; **19**: 320.
88. Leaper DJ, Schultz G, Carville K, *et al.* Extending the TIME concept: what have we learned in the past 10 years? *Int Wound J* 2012; **9**: 1.
89. Lewis K. Riddle of biofilm resistance. *Antimicrob Agents Chemother* 2001; **45**: 999.

CHAPTER 4

Management Practices that Influence Wound Infection and Healing

Andrew J. Dart, BVSc, PhD, Diplomate ACVS, Diplomate ECVS, **Albert Sole-Guitart**, DVM, Diplomate ACVS, **Ted S. Stashak**, DVM, MS, Diplomate ACVS, and **Christine Theoret**, DMV, PhD, Diplomate ACVS

Chapter Contents

Summary

The aim of wound management is to optimize healing in an effort to return the horse to its previous function as rapidly as possible, while respecting the financial constraints of the owner. Infection, with its associated excessive or inappropriate inflammation, is the single most likely cause of delayed healing of wounds healing by second intention. Effective wound preparation, exploration, cleansing via irrigation, and debridement are central to reducing the incidence of infection and promoting uncomplicated healing of accidental wounds. Antimicrobial drugs should be used only when there is clinical evidence of infection or when development of an infection would be life-threatening or career-ending for the patient. Although empiric broad-spectrum antimicrobial therapy may be used initially, definitive selection of antimicrobial drugs should be based on the results of bacterial culture and sensitivity testing of isolates. The use of antimicrobial drugs in surgical wounds should never replace aseptic and atraumatic surgical technique. Where there is evidence of formation of biofilm, repeat debridement and topical administration of antimicrobial drugs should be central to any treatment plan.

Introduction

The aim of wound management is to optimize healing in an effort to return the horse to its previous function, as rapidly as possible, while respecting the financial constraints of the owner. Infection, with its associated excessive or inappropriate inflammation, is

Equine Wound Management, Third Edition. Edited by Christine Theoret and Jim Schumacher.

Companion website: www.wiley.com/go/theoret/wound

the single most likely cause of delayed healing of wounds healing by second intention.

This chapter reviews selected management practices that influence wound infection and healing. The subject is approached in the order in which a wounded horse would be evaluated and managed.

Initial assessment

When attending a horse that has suffered an accidental wound, excessive hemorrhage should be addressed immediately. Thereafter, a thorough history is obtained, and a general physical examination is performed to identify any important systemic problems prior to addressing the wound. Shock, injury to the central nervous system, peripheral nerve damage, fracture, systemic disease, or malnutrition may all negatively affect healing.

If a tetanus toxoid booster has not been administered to the horse within the past year, it should be given at this time, even if the wound shows no signs of infection. The time between the occurrence of a wound and the onset of signs of tetanus can range from 2 days to 2 months.[1] Tetanus antitoxin should be administered only if the horse has no history of receiving tetanus vaccination or if it exhibits clinical signs of tetanus. In these cases, tetanus toxoid should be administered concurrently, but at a site remote from where the antitoxin was injected.

Visual appraisal of the wound

The horse usually should be tranquilized or sedated before the wound is examined, to diminish the horse's pain and anxiety and thereby facilitate a careful examination. Nevertheless, substantial blood loss caused by wounding should be considered when selecting the drug. Some tranquilizers, such as acepromazine maleate, may cause vasodilation, which in turn causes hypotension by blocking alpha-adrenergic receptors,[2] thereby exacerbating pre-existing low blood pressure. Furthermore, acepromazine has been shown to neutralize reactive oxygen species produced by stimulated equine neutrophils, at least *in vitro*.[3] This may have important implications on the acute inflammatory response to wounding in horses, which is known to be deficient relative to that of ponies and other species.[4]

Special attention should be paid to the manner in which the wound was incurred, the time elapsed since wounding, the location, shape and depth of the wound, the extent of tissue damage, especially the state of the local vascular supply, potential involvement of underlying structures, such as synovial or body cavities, bone or tendon, and the extent of gross contamination of the wound. The reader is referred to Chapter 3 for more information about the factors that impair wound healing. In particular, the clinician must take special care to identify signs of inflammation and/or acute infection, such as swelling, heat, and pain. The cause of the infection can be confirmed later by the results of microbiologic testing.

The overall aim of visually inspecting the wound is to make informed decisions on the subsequent steps required to manage factors that negatively influence healing. Of particular importance is the management of contamination by using appropriate measures, such as wound irrigation and debridement and the institution of antimicrobial therapy, when indicated.

Local anesthesia

Local or regional anesthesia to desensitize the wound may be used, often in conjunction with tranquilization or sedation, to facilitate examination, exploration, and treatment of a wound while the horse is standing. It can also be used to provide pain relief of variable duration. Local anesthetic solutions have been shown, in humans, to exhibit antimicrobial effects against a wide spectrum of pathogens.[5]

Studies in laboratory animals have inconsistently found that common anesthetic solutions, including 2% lidocaine and 0.5% bupivacaine, may increase edema and inflammation, and inhibit synthesis of collagen. Local anesthetic solutions, however, have no long-term effects on the rate or quality of healing, when infiltrated postoperatively into surgically created cutaneous wounds to manage pain.[6,7] Until recently, it was thought that local anesthetic solutions containing epinephrine/adrenaline should be avoided because of their vasoconstrictive effect, but it appears that the effects of local anesthetic solutions on wound healing are not influenced by the presence of epinephrine/adrenaline in the solution.[8] Some older studies do suggest, however, that local anesthetic solutions may be toxic to leukocytes,[9] which might further hamper the already weak inflammatory response to wounding when administered intralesionally on the limbs of horses.

Instilling local anesthetic solution perineurally (i.e., using regional anesthesia) reduces the volume of local anesthetic solution required to desensitize the wound. The solution is deposited around the nerve or nerves innervating the site of the wound but remote from it. This technique can be used to desensitize wounds to the head or to the distal aspect of the limb, in particular, those wounds located in the foot or pastern. In these areas, because the nerves are easily palpated, the technique provides a simple, precise, and reliable approach to desensitizing the wound. Alternatively, regional anesthesia, in the form of a "U" or an "L" block can achieve the desired desensitization, while avoiding the potential side-effects associated with intralesional anesthesia. Intralesional anesthesia, although more invasive, is effective and provides good compliance by the patient, and is, therefore, commonly used in practice, especially for wounds in regions that are difficult to desensitize by using perineural anesthesia.

Ideally, the anesthetic solution should be infiltrated intralesionally after cleansing the wound and clipping the surrounding hair to minimize seeding contaminants into deeper tissues. The anesthetic agent should be distributed evenly along the wound's edge to minimize the total dose administered. To facilitate this, the entire length of the needle (20–22 gauge; 1–1.5 in) can be inserted subcutaneously from within the wound, parallel to the wound's edge, to the needle's hub. A small volume of local anesthetic solution is injected as the needle is withdrawn; the volume of anesthetic solution injected should be less than that that would markedly deform the wound's edge. This technique is usually well tolerated by the horse. Generally, 2% lidocaine or mepivacaine hydrochloride is used, and either provides approximately 2 hours of clinically effective and safe anesthesia.[10] Bupivacaine hydrochloride is longer acting, providing 4–8 hours of anesthesia, and therefore, may contribute to postoperative analgesia.[10]

Some horses may experience postanesthetic pain as a consequence of either the anesthetic solution used or the anesthetic technique. Lidocaine has been reported to produce a less intense inflammatory reaction than mepivacaine or bupivacaine when injected subcutaneously in rats,[11] but no studies have specifically compared the horse's inflammatory response to various local anesthetic solutions injected subcutaneously. The intensity of the inflammatory response does not appear to be related to the concentration of the drug.[11] Although subcutaneous infiltration of a local anesthetic solution is the most common approach to desensitizing a wound, evidence suggests that a topical anesthetic cream (e.g., lidocaine/prilocaine) provides sufficient analgesia to allow debridement of an open surgical wound, at least in human patients.[12] In a recent study, applying an anesthetic cream to the labia of mares was as effective as subcutaneous infiltration of a solution of lidocaine in providing local anesthesia when performing episioplasty.[13] If a topical anesthetic cream/gel is used to provide analgesia, the veterinarian should keep in mind that the onset of blockade may take 45–60 minutes, which is much slower than that achieved by subcutaneous infiltration of local anesthetic solution.[12,13]

What to do

- Local anesthesia can facilitate examination, exploration, and treatment of wounds without affecting healing. Perineural anesthesia of regional nerves, remote to the wound, when possible, is preferred over local infiltration of the wound because anesthesia provided in this manner minimizes the volume and the local effects of the drug.

Tip

- Inserting the needle from within the wound, to the hub of the needle, parallel to the wound's edge and depositing the anesthetic solution as the needle is withdrawn helps distribute the anesthetic solution evenly.

General anesthesia and duration of surgery

Rarely must the horse be anesthetized to initially examine and cleanse the wound, but for foals or horses unaccustomed to being handled, general anesthesia may be necessary to ensure the safety of the patient and the attending veterinarian. Similarly, examination, cleansing, and initial treatment of the wound may be easier with the horse anesthetized if the wound is large and/or heavily contaminated or if it involves a structure other than skin, such as a bone, synovial cavity, tendon, or body cavity.

The depth and duration of anesthesia and the duration of surgery[14] have been shown to independently increase the risk of postoperative infection in clean and clean-contaminated wounds of dogs.[15–17] The rates of wound infection were shown to increase by 0.5% per minute after 60 minutes of anesthesia.[17] This translates to a 30% greater risk of postoperative infection for each additional hour of anesthesia. The rate of infection was shown to double after 90 minutes of surgery and nearly triple when surgery exceeded 120 minutes.[15] Incisional complications of horses undergoing ventral midline celiotomy were twice as likely when surgery took longer than 2 hours,[18] and patients undergoing orthopedic procedures were 3.6 times more likely to develop a surgical site infection (SSI) when the time of surgery exceeded 90 minutes.[19]

Excessive depth of anesthesia reduces perfusion and oxygenation of tissue, whereas prolonged anesthesia impairs the function of alveolar macrophages and depresses systemic migration and function of leukocytes.[20,21] Decreased tissue oxygenation, associated with excessive depth of anesthesia, is a critical factor in the development of SSI because it hinders neutrophil-mediated oxidative killing, a mechanism essential to defense against surgical pathogens.[22] Human patients who suffer from decreased tissue oxygenation in the perioperative period are at risk of SSI.[23] A low intraoperative arterial partial pressure of oxygen has been shown to contribute to the development of SSI following colic surgery in horses.[24] In this latter study, a nine-fold increase in the risk of SSI was observed when the period of general anesthesia exceeded 2 hours and the PaO_2 was <80 mmHg, indicating an additive effect of these two factors.

Although anesthetic agents and monitoring of anesthetized horses to optimize oxygenation and tissue perfusion continue to improve, surgeons must nevertheless carefully plan and execute surgical procedures to minimize the time a patient is anesthetized. The benefits of using general anesthesia in a well-equipped hospital environment to allow for a systematic and controlled surgical approach to manage complex wounds should not be underestimated. The advantages of treating wounds with the horse anesthetized are often lost, however, if the procedure is performed in the field.

What to do

- Reduce the depth and duration of anesthesia, and ensure that the anesthetized patient is properly hydrated. Consider insufflating the horse with oxygen postoperatively.

What to avoid

- Avoid undertaking prolonged surgical procedures with the horse anesthetized, in a field situation.

Wound preparation

Hair removal

The objective of wound preparation is to reduce contamination and produce a clean surgical site. A clear benefit of removing hair preoperatively from human patients on reducing the rates of SSI has not been established.[25] One study showed that effective aseptic preparation of the carpal and distal interphalangeal joints of horses (for arthrocentesis) can be achieved without removing hair.[26] Nevertheless, in veterinary patients, hair is usually removed from the surgical site and from the periphery of an accidental wound because it can interfere with the surgeon's ability to clean and suture the edges of the wound.

Methods of removing hair include clipping, shaving, and chemical depilation, though the latter is seldom used in veterinary medicine and contraindicated in the case of an open (accidental) wound. If the area around the wound on a horse is to be shaved, the hair is usually clipped before shaving commences. Clipping or shaving may "nip" the skin at its creases thereby causing abrasions and microscopic cuts that may subsequently become contaminated by opportunistic pathogens.[27] Of these two approaches, clipping appears to be the less traumatic and was shown, in humans, to be associated with a lower incidence of SSI.[25] Good-quality, sharp, clean equipment suited to the purpose reduces the risk of damaging and contaminating skin. Using a guarded razor (i.e., a safety or disposable razor) instead of an open-bladed system (e.g., a scalpel or Wick blade) may reduce injury to the skin. The clipper head should be disinfected between patients to minimize the risk of cross-contamination.

Removing the hair surrounding an accidental wound may contaminate the open wound with hair clippings and dander. To ensure against this risk, a sterile, water-based lubricating gel should be placed onto the wound prior to clipping. The gel prevents tiny hairs from accumulating on the wound and can be easily rinsed from the wound after clipping. Alternatively, sterile gauze sponges soaked in sterile isotonic fluid or a water-based lubricating gel can be packed into the wound prior to clipping. Sponges are removed after each stage of the preparation, the wound rinsed, and packing replaced. A wide margin of hair should be removed at the wound's periphery, and the loose hair vacuumed away from the clipped site. Scissors often work better than clippers for removing long hair at the wound's edge.

> **Tip**
>
> - Place sterile gauze swabs soaked in a water-based lubricating gel or isotonic saline solution onto the wound prior to clipping, to prevent hair entering the wound.

Skin preparation

Patient

In the case of an accidental wound, the skin adjacent to the open wound should be prepared as if for aseptic surgery. It is common practice to don sterile gloves for the final stage of skin preparation. Skin is usually prepared immediately prior to irrigating and debriding the wound. If the wound is heavily contaminated or infected, it may be necessary to perform skin preparation again after surface debridement of the wound is complete and before further surgical manipulation. The skin surrounding the wound is prepared by scrubbing it with an antiseptic detergent to remove oils, dirt, and debris and then rinsing it with sterile isotonic saline solution or 70% isopropyl alcohol. Antiseptic scrubs and isopropyl alcohol are cytotoxic and should not contact the wound itself.[28]

Povidone–iodine (PI) and chlorhexidine (CH) are the two most commonly used surgical detergents. A common PI-based detergent is Betadine®, which is a complex of iodine and polyvinylpyrrolidone (povidone), a synthetic polymer. Betadine is available as a 7.5% w/w surgical detergent equivalent to 0.75% available iodine. A study showed that the skin of horses can be prepared for aseptic surgery using a 10-minute scrub with PI, a 5-minute scrub with PI, three 30-second scrubs with PI, or by blotting the surgical site with a commercial, one-step iodophor surgical solution.[29] Chlorhexidine is available as a 4% CH gluconate detergent (Hibiclens, Mölnlycke Health Care). A recent study in horses showed that skin preparation using a 4% CH gluconate detergent without repeated mechanical scrubbing (i.e., back and forth motion of CH gluconate-soaked gauze sponges for less than 15 seconds, just long enough to produce a lather, then leaving the detergent in contact with the skin for 255 seconds) was as effective in reducing bacterial counts on the skin as the standard 5-minute mechanical preparation.[30]

Both PI and CH have broad-spectrum antimicrobial activity, but PI is reported by the manufacturer to be active against viruses, fungi, protozoa, and yeast. As an antiseptic skin detergent, CH is suggested to have superior antibacterial activity and a greater residual effect due to its ability to bind to the *stratum corneum*. Clinically, however, PI and CH appear to be equally effective as surgical scrub detergents.[31,32] One disadvantage of CH detergent is that short exposure of the detergent to the eye, even in small concentrations, can lead to conjunctivitis and corneal opacification.[33,34]

Either 70% isopropyl alcohol or sterile, 0.9% saline solution are commonly used to rinse between applications of antiseptic detergents. Rinsing with 70% isopropyl alcohol has been reported to decrease the residual antimicrobial activity of 4% CH gluconate detergent.[35] The authors of that study were unable to provide a basis for this finding, and clinically, this loss of antimicrobial activity may not translate into an increased risk of infection, particularly if the procedure is short. With this in mind, however, rinsing with sterile isotonic saline solution may be more appropriate than rinsing with isopropyl alcohol when using a CH-based detergent. In contrast, 70% isopropyl alcohol potentiates the antimicrobial activity of PI by increasing the release of free iodine.[31,36] Isopropyl alcohol also has considerable antibacterial activity when used alone at 70% or 99%.[36] Consequently, the combination of PI surgical detergent and 70% isopropyl alcohol rinse, used commonly in equine practice, is effective for preparing skin for surgery. Systematic reviews of the literature in human medicine suggest there is little evidence to favor one skin antiseptic detergent over another, at least for clean surgery. Extrapolating the findings of these studies to animals must nevertheless be done with caution because cleansing the skin of animals may be more difficult than cleansing the skin of people. Moreover, the reader should be aware that PI, as a 10% solution, can occasionally cause a transient, acute contact dermatitis in people;[37] in the authors' experience, it can also cause the same in horses, particularly when applied to the throatlatch or inguinal regions.

Wounds to the hoof require special preparation that involves removing the superficial layer of hoof wall and exfoliating the sole with a rasp and hoof knife before scrubbing with PI detergent. This approach was shown to be more effective in reducing bacterial concentration than a 6-minute scrub with PI followed by 24-hour submersion in PI solution-soaked cotton.[38] Moreover, a recent study found that a prolonged soak (12 hours) with either iodine tincture or PI damages the skin and favors bacterial recolonization.[39] Nevertheless, although bacterial concentration is significantly reduced by removal of the superficial layer of the hoof, prior to scrubbing, final bacterial counts were shown to exceed 10^5 bacteria per gram of tissue, sufficient to induce infection if the local environment and the host's immune response are compromised.

What to do

- Both CH and PI are suitable antiseptic skin detergents. Scrubs with CH detergent may be best alternated with rinses of sterile 0.9% saline solution when preparing the skin, whereas scrubs with PI detergent may be better alternated with rinses of 70% isopropyl alcohol.

What to avoid

- Avoid direct contact of an antiseptic skin detergent or alcohol with an open wound.

Surgeon

The inadvertent transfer of microorganisms from the surgeon to the patient can result in SSI. Surgeons usually wear sterile gloves to prevent transferring bacteria from their hands to the patient, but gloves may be perforated during surgery.[40] Hands, therefore, should be as bacteria-free as possible prior to gloving, and to achieve this, surgical hand antisepsis should be performed immediately before donning sterile gloves when preparing for a surgical procedure.[41] The following three types of antiseptic solutions are available for surgical hand antisepsis: aqueous scrubs, alcohol rubs, and alcohol rubs containing additional active ingredients.

The most commonly used products for surgical hand antisepsis in the human healthcare field are aqueous scrubs containing CH or PI. According to a recent survey, this also seems to be the case for veterinary surgeons, 80% of whom used water-based hand scrubbing with CH gluconate or PI detergents for hand antisepsis in 2011.[42] Scrubbing the dirty hands of large-animal veterinarians with CH or PI detergent prior to gloving initially reduces colony forming units (CFU) by ~80% on those hands for up to 120 minutes.[43] However, prolonged residual effect is an important feature of presurgical hand antisepsis because hair follicles, as well as sebaceous and sweat glands, are sources of recolonization of the surgeon's skin by bacteria, which may be a problem in the case of a perforated glove. Bacterial regrowth occurs faster after scrubbing with PI than with CH.[44]

Several alcohol-based handrubs have been licensed for the commercial market and include long-acting compounds (e.g., CH gluconate and quaternary ammonium compounds) that limit regrowth of bacteria on the gloved hand. According to the World Health Organization, the antimicrobial efficacy of alcohol-based formulations, when applied a minimum of three times, for a period of 3–5 minutes, is superior to that of all other currently available methods of preoperative surgical hand preparation in the human healthcare field.[44] These alcohol-based rubs offer the advantage of rapid and immediate action, as well as reduced skin damage after repeated use, thereby improving compliance to the protocol for surgical hygiene, and their use saves large quantities of water. Not every alcohol rub solution sold over the counter, however, is appropriate for use in surgical hand preparation, because some may contain an ineffective concentration of alcohol. The alcohol-based rub used for preoperative surgical hand preparation should meet the standards required by the American or European regulatory agencies.

The body surface of veterinary patients is likely to have higher bacterial counts than that of human patients, potentially resulting in greater contamination on the hands of veterinary surgeons. Consequently, products for surgical hand antisepsis of veterinary surgeons, specifically, should be tested to verify their effectiveness. One study compared the efficacy of a commercial alcohol-based handrub containing 45% 2-propanol, 30% 1-propanol, and 0.2% mecetronium ethylsulfate (Sterillium, Bode-Chemie) with that of two common detergent scrubs, 4% CH digluconate (Hibiscrub, Regent Medical) and 7.5% PI (Vetclean, Ecuphar), in reducing the number of CFU found on hands of equine and small-animal surgeons.[45] The alcohol-based rub and CH digluconate detergent scrub had a similar immediate effect, although the sustained effect was significantly better for the alcohol rub.[45] The PI detergent scrub had a significantly lower immediate and sustained effect.[45] A recent study comparing the efficacy of a 5-minute scrub with 4% CH gluconate water-based detergent scrub to that of a 90-second application of a commercial alcohol-based hand rub containing 1% CH gluconate and 61% ethyl alcohol in an emollient (Avagard™, 3M Healthcare), for hand antisepsis for sterile, equine elective surgical procedures, found no statistically significant difference in mean bacterial CFUs between the two techniques immediately after hand antisepsis or after surgery.[46] A similar study conducted at Massey University likewise showed no difference in the mean bacterial CFUs either immediately or 120 minutes after preparation with either CH scrub or with Avagard™, for clean, contaminated hands or for dirty hands (simulated by soaking hands for 5 minutes in a 20% w/v solution of horse feces).[47]

Nevertheless, more studies are needed to verify the impact of hand antisepsis on rates of SSI rather than on CFU. The only such study performed in the human healthcare field found that hand rubbing with an alcohol solution was as effective as hand scrubbing with an antiseptic soap, either PI or CH, for preventing SSI.[48]

> **Tip**
>
> - The commonly used 4% CH and 7.5% PI aqueous hand scrubs are suitable for surgical hand preparation in veterinary surgery. There is evidence that scrubbing with 4% CH gluconate provides longer residual activity. Scrubs are usually applied and rinsed, three times, within a 3–5-minute period. New data on alcohol-based hand rubs are promising.

Irrigation/cleansing of accidental wounds

Wound irrigation/cleansing remains an important component in managing accidental wounds. The objective of irrigation is to gently remove loosely adhered contaminants, bacteria, and devitalized tissue from the wound's surface, using a continuous or pulsatile flow of fluid. More specific techniques of cleansing and debriding should be used if contaminants cannot be removed by using gentle irrigation.

Although irrigation with tap water or a sterile isotonic saline solution may be all that is needed to adequately cleanse a lightly contaminated, acute wound (<3 hours' duration) in preparation for primary closure, more chronically contaminated wounds (>3 hours' duration), particularly those involving the distal aspect of the limb, often require debridement, in addition to irrigation, before they can be sutured. Wounds healing by second intention require repeat irrigation as long as they contain superficial slough, excess exudate, visible debris, or any residue from topically applied wound-care products or from dressings, that might delay healing.

Irrigation may be used before, after, or as an alternative to debridement, depending on the amount of contamination or tissue damage.[49] For example, briefly soaking the desiccated surface of a wound or the surface of a wound containing dry, imbedded debris with moist gauze (a form of dressing debridement) hydrates the wound, softening the underlying tissue, and thereby enhancing irrigation.

In equine practice, the delay between the time of wounding and the time the patient is presented is often substantial. Unfortunately, the effectiveness of irrigation decreases as the wound ages. For example, one study using a complex musculoskeletal wound model in goats found that irrigation resulted in a 70%, 52%, and 37% reduction in bacterial counts at 3, 6, and 12 hours, respectively, after the wounds were inoculated with *Pseudomonas aeruginosa*.[50] This is because bacteria invade tissue and aggregate to form a biofilm that becomes more resistant to irrigation over time. A biofilm-based wound-care management plan, with debridement as its central component, should be instituted after a biofilm forms (more information on the management of biofilms is available later in this chapter and also in Chapter 19).

The three major variables of irrigation are method of delivery, volume delivered, and solution delivered.

Irrigation technique/delivery method

Pressurized wound irrigation is more effective in cleansing the wound than is swabbing, and consequently more cost effective because it shortens the time required for wounds to heal by second intention and is better tolerated by the patient (Figure 4.1).[51] The overall conclusion of a critical review conducted on wound

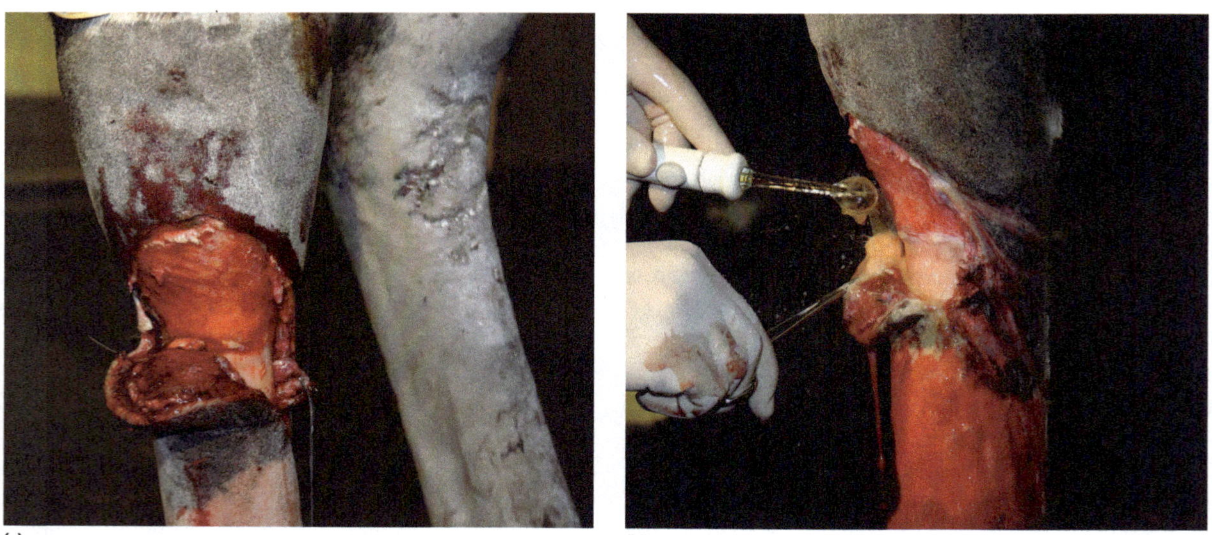

(a) (b)

Figure 4.1 **(a)** Example of a wound on the dorsal surface of the proximal metatarsus, close to the hock. The tarsometatarsal and distal intertarsal joints were injected with sterile isotonic saline solution to investigate a potential communication with the wound. These tarsal joints were not affected, however, exposure of the third metatarsal bone created a risk for sequestrum formation. **(b)** A Waterpik® Water Flosser was used for wound cleansing and irrigation and the limb was radiographed 7 days later to determine whether a sequestrum had developed.

irrigation is that optimal irrigation pressures have yet to be determined for different degrees of wound contamination in humans.[52] Likewise, the relationship between irrigation pressure and the ability to reduce bacterial counts and eliminate debris from contaminated wounds of horses has not been studied. Nevertheless, in the authors' experience, pressures ranging from 8 to 15 psi are beneficial in achieving the objectives of irrigation when managing wounds in horses. Our recommendations to use irrigation pressures between 8 and 15 psi echo those recently made by wound-care experts in the field of human healthcare who claim that this range of pressure is strong enough to overcome adhesive forces of bacteria.[53] Although higher pressures are more effective in removing necrotic tissue and foreign particles, high pressures have been shown to drive contaminants deeper into the wound or surrounding tissues, including into cancellous bone.[54] High irrigation pressures may also damage granulation or epithelial tissues,[55,56] thereby increasing the rate of wound infection and delaying healing. Furthermore, the likelihood of causing aerosolization of bacterial particles and subsequent environmental dispersal of airborne microorganisms, may increase as irrigation pressure increases.[57] In summary, the benefits of higher pressures in reducing bacterial count, dirt, and tissue debris in heavily contaminated wounds may outweigh the risk of tissue injury. Conversely, in relatively clean wounds, the potential damage of tissue resulting from high-pressure irrigation may outweigh the benefits.[52]

Pressures of 8–15 psi cannot be attained with gravity flow but can be obtained by using a 35- or 60-mL syringe and an 18- or 19-gauge needle,[58] a spray bottle, or some of the commercially available irrigation devices. A syringe with an attached 19-gauge needle typically delivers an output pressure range of 11–31 psi; however, the end pressure that reaches the wound could be as low as 8 psi.[58] Although no studies have documented the ranges of psi delivered by a spray bottle with an adjustable nozzle, the experience of the third author supports the effectiveness of this method of delivery. Commercially available, battery-powered, irrigation devices (e.g., Stryker Interpulse System; Equine Hydro-T, info@hydrot.com) are capable of delivering very high pressures (70 psi), but their pressure output can be adjusted to deliver fluid at 10–15 psi.

Fluid volume is another important component of wound irrigation; as volume increases, so does cleansing, up to a point, but the optimal volume with which to irrigate is unknown.[59] The volume of fluid should reflect the degree of contamination and the size of the wound. At minimum, the gross contaminants should be removed, and irrigation should be discontinued before tissues become waterlogged.

What to do

- Use 10–15 psi to irrigate most tissues, including bone, exposed by wounding. This can usually be achieved using a 35- or 60-mL syringe and an 18- or 19-gauge needle.

What to avoid

- Avoid using excessive pressure (>20 psi) and a greater volume of irrigation solution than that needed to cleanse the wound because either may damage healthy tissues, thereby potentiating infection and delaying healing.

Tip

- Contaminated wounds of horses may be cleansed by repeat irrigation combined with debridement.

Irrigation solutions

The ideal irrigant is sterile, isotonic, normothermic, non-toxic, hypoallergenic, and compatible with any additives (antibiotics or antiseptics). Furthermore, it should be readily available, and its use cost effective.

Several different products can be used for irrigating wounds, such as potable tap water, isotonic saline solution, Ringer's solution, and solutions containing active ingredients, such as antimicrobial agents.

Isotonic crystalloids, such as sterile isotonic saline solution or lactated Ringer's solution, are commonly used but are expensive when large volumes are used on multiple occasions. A systematic review of the effects of irrigating wounds in human patients with isotonic saline solution or potable tap water concluded that using tap water is more economical and as effective as using isotonic saline solution in cleansing acute and chronic wounds, and that using tap water does not seem to increase the risk of infection or delay healing over that which occur when the irrigant is isotonic saline solution.[60] Where potable tap water is not available, boiled and cooled water or distilled water are acceptable alternatives.

Additives

Although irrigation with potable tap water, isotonic saline solution or Ringer's solution may be sufficient to cleanse a fresh accidental wound, many wounds encountered in equine practice are not fresh and/or are heavily contaminated. No diagnostic test exists to allow practitioners to identify whether the bacterial load in the wound is capable of causing infection. For this reason, chronic accidental wounds and those exhibiting signs of infection or in which a biofilm is suspected, might benefit from irrigation with a solution containing an additive intended to decrease the bacterial inoculum in the wound to a concentraton that can be managed by the host's defences.

Antiseptics Antiseptics, defined as "agents that destroy or hinder the growth of microorganisms in or on living tissue,"[61] are often added to irrigants. In the absence of evidence-based guidelines for clinical practice, the use of antiseptics continues to provoke a great deal of debate among clinicians. Past *in vitro* experiments demonstrated that some antiseptics caused a variable amount of disruption to collagen synthesis, were toxic to fibroblasts, impaired migration of epithelial cells and/or inhibited the microcirculation.[62] Other studies demonstrated the toxic effects of antiseptics on keratinocytes and leukocytes.[63,64] Although possibly not a true reflection of the *in vivo* situation, these *in vitro* studies are at the source of the debate about whether antiseptics used for wound management do more harm than good.[65,66]

A definite advantage of antiseptics over antibiotics, if either is to be added to the irrigant, is that antiseptics have a broad antimicrobial spectrum coupled with a reduced propensity for inducing bacterial resistance. With the emergence of multi-resistant strains of organisms, there is a renewed interest in using antiseptics in wound management. The cytotoxicity of antiseptics appears to be concentration dependent, with some antiseptics (e.g., PI and CH) maintaining antimicrobial efficacy at a low, non-cytotoxic concentration.[28]

An "all or none" approach to using an antiseptic for irrigation would simplify decision making, but this approach fails to address the complexities of wounds encountered in clinical practice. Some wounds are seen early and are minimally contaminated, whereas others may be hours old and heavily contaminated, colonized, or infected (the reader is referred to Chapter 3 for more information about the bacterial impact continuum). Consequently, practitioners should be familiar with the properties of the commonly used commercial antiseptics to make the most informed choice of which antiseptic to use on a particular wound. Iodine and CH are discussed here because they are the two antiseptics most commonly added to irrigants by veterinary practitioners. The reader is referred to Chapter 5 for a comprehensive coverage of commercial wound cleansers and antiseptics.

Iodine has a broad antimicrobial spectrum and is reported to be effective against Gram-positive and Gram-negative bacteria, viruses, fungi, yeasts, molds, and protozoans.[67] None of these organisms are known to resist it, but iodine can be inactivated by blood, serum proteins, and other organic matter.[67] Active, "free" iodine is usually coupled to a carrier (an iodophor) that acts as a slow-releasing reservoir. This serves to reduce the toxicity of iodine (characteristic of aqueous solutions) and to overcome its inactivation by organic material. Two iodophor-formulations of iodine are available: povidone–iodine (PI) and cadexomer–iodine (CI). Because CI is supplied as a hydrophilic modified-starch polymer bead that gradually releases incorporated iodine into the wound, it is best used as dressing and not for irrigating wounds.

PI or polyvinylpyrrolidone–iodine complex (Betadine®) is a combination of elemental iodine bound to the synthetic, water-soluble polymer, polyvinylpyrrolidone surfactant. Betadine is available as a 10% solution in water.[68] The bactericidal component of Betadine is free iodine, approximately one part per million (1 ppm).[68] Diluting the PI solution actually increases the liberation of free iodine, and consequently increases the bactericidal effects of the solution.[69]

The existing evidence regarding the efficacy of PI as an antiseptic is complicated by conflicting results from laboratory, human, and animal studies using different experimental designs.[67] Iodine does appear to have a place in wound management, however, and may be particularly useful when irrigating heavily contaminated or infected wounds. There are no studies to support the use of PI in non-infected wounds of either humans[67] or horses, but open wounds, of dogs, at risk of infection, were found to heal more rapidly when irrigated with diluted PI than were similar wounds irrigated with isotonic saline solution.[70] More studies using horses are needed to determine the bactericidal concentration and the cytotoxic effects of different concentrations of PI, particularly on neutrophils and macrophages, which are important to the initial inflammatory phase of wound healing. The degree of contamination and the stage of bacterial colonization likely affect the efficacy of PI. On the balance of evidence, PI solutions for irrigation are probably safe and effective at reducing the likelihood of infection developing in heavily contaminated wounds of horses when delivered at concentrations of 0.1–0.2% (10–20 mL/L).

What to do

- Addition of 10–20 mL/L of 10% PI solution to the irrigant should be reserved for heavily contaminated wounds at risk of infection or those exhibiting clinical signs of infection.

Tip

- Iodine solution is inactivated in the presence of organic matter, including blood and serum and, therefore, should not be used as a wound dressing (i.e., gauze soaked with dilute PI). Conversely, gauze soaked in a dilute solution of chlorhexidine diacetate may be used to dress wounds contaminated with organic matter.

Both **chlorhexidine digluconate** and **chlorhexidine diacetate** (2%) are also commonly used as additives for wound irrigation. CH exerts rapid antimicrobial activity against a wide spectrum of non-sporing bacteria, including *Staphylococcus aureus*, *Pseudomonas aeruginosa*, and a wide range of clinical isolates,[36] but resistance of methicillin-resistant *S. aureus* (MRSA) to CH diacetate has been observed.[71] *Proteus* spp. and *Pseudomonas*

What to do

- Addition of antiseptics to wound irrigation solutions may be best reserved for wounds that are heavily contaminated and at risk of infection or those exhibiting clinical signs of infection.

What to avoid

- Avoid liberally pouring antiseptics (e.g., PI or CH) into a bucket of water or a bottle of isotonic saline solution to use as an irrigant. Using the correct concentration of an antiseptic optimizes the antiseptic's antibacterial effects and minimizes the antiseptic's cytotoxic effects on healing tissues.

Tip

- CH diluted to a 0.05% solution is safe and effective for use as a wound irrigation solution.

spp. appear to also have developed or possess a resistance to this antiseptic. CH diacetate has no effect against fungi or *Candida*,[72] and a recent study showed that microorganisms in biofilms have greater resistance to CH than do bacteria not contained within a biofilm.[73] Irrigation with a dilute solution of CH diacetate may improve healing of open wounds at risk of infection.[74–76] CH should be diluted to a 0.05% solution (1:40 = 25 mL of the 2% concentrate diluted with 975 mL of sterile isotonic crystalloid solution) for use as an antiseptic for irrigating wounds of horses, as is recommended in humans.[53]

Antibiotics The emergence of antimicrobial-resistant strains of bacteria commonly found on the skin has become a concern, even in equine practice.[77–79] Consequently, the indiscriminate addition of an antibiotic to a wound irrigant is not in line with current knowledge of antibiotic stewardship.

More information regarding topically administered antibiotics is available later in this chapter and in Chapter 5.

Commercial wound cleansers

A commercial wound cleanser may be used when enhanced cleansing is required. Most ionic and many non-ionic surfactants present in wound cleansers, however, have been shown to be toxic to cells, to delay healing, and to inhibit the wound's defense against infection.[28] For a more complete discussion of wound cleansers, the reader is referred to Chapter 5.

To cleanse a heavily contaminated wound, the wound can be sprayed with a wound cleanser, gently scrubbed with sterile gauze sponges, and then thoroughly irrigated with sterile isotonic saline solution. The coarseness of the scrubbing device should be minimal because wounds scrubbed with coarse sponges have been shown to be significantly more susceptible to infection.[80] An advantage of commercial wound cleansers is that they contain a surfactant that substantially reduces the coefficient of friction between the scrubbing device and the wound.[80]

What to do

- Select wound cleansers with little cytotoxicity (e.g., Kendall Constant-Clens® Wound Cleanser, Briggs Healthcare; Shur-Clens® Wound Cleanser, Convatec; EquineVet™ Acemannan Wound Cleanser, Carrington Labs, or Vetericyn® Wound Wash, Innovacyn). For a complete list of wound cleansers, see Table 5.1 in Chapter 5.

Wound exploration

After the wound has been cleansed, it should be explored digitally to determine its boundaries, to identify involvement of structures deep to the skin, including bone, tendon, ligament, and synovial structures, or to confirm the presence of a foreign body. The examiner should wear sterile gloves, from which talcum powder has been rinsed away with sterile isotonic saline solution, prior to touching the wound. Talcum powder may act as a foreign body and has been shown to elicit signs of toxicity by every tissue in the body.[81] If digital exploration is inhibited by the size of the wound, a sterile probe or surgical instrument can be used to measure the depth of the wound, to determine if a foreign body is present, or to verify if bone has been contacted.

If the wound is deep or involves bone, the wounded region may be examined radiographically, using plain and contrast radiographs obtained with and without a probe, to identify a fracture, a foreign body, or the relationship of the wound to bone or to a synovial cavity (Figure 4.2). One must keep in mind that some foreign bodies may not appear on radiographs and that contrast dyes do not always define the limits of the wound accurately. The effectiveness of the contrast study can be improved by slowly moving the affected body part through a range of motion while the contrast medium is being injected, thereby ensuring better distribution of the contrast medium to all areas involved in the wound (Figure 4.3).

Particular attention should be paid to the presence of fluid discharging from a wound located near a synovial structure (joint, tendon sheath, bursa), especially if the wound is located at the distal aspect of the limb, because fluid discharging from a wound is suggestive of synovial penetration. Normal synovial fluid, because of its high viscosity, forms a "string" between the thumb and forefinger. This sign of normality is eliminated by the activity of degradative enzymes produced during inflammation. Unless the wound is fresh or unless the synovial cavity is able to drain freely, communication of the wound with a synovial structure usually causes a moderate to severe lameness due to the pressure exerted by the increased volume of fluid within the closed synovial space, and trapping of inflammatory mediators. If the limb is flexed and extended, the accumulated fluid is often forced to exit the wound, under pressure, in a stream.

Obtaining synovial fluid for gross and cytologic examinations and perhaps for microbial culture and antimicrobial sensitivity testing of isolates, is one of the first steps taken to determine if a synovial structure is infected. If synovial penetration is suspected, but no synovial fluid is present at the site of the wound, an area overlying the synovial structure, remote from the wound, should be aseptically prepared for sampling (Figure 4.4).

After collecting a sample, sterile, isotonic saline solution should be injected, under pressure, into the synovial structure; this solution flows from the wound if the synovial capsule has been breached. If breached, the synovial structure should be lavaged with 3–5 L of a sterile isotonic solution. Intrasynovial damage is best determined by endoscopic examination of the synovial structure. The synovial structure is lavaged most effectively by using endoscopic instrumentation. For more information regarding the management of wounds involving synovial structures, see Chapter 16.

Radiography (with or without the use of a positive contrast medium) may be useful in documenting a fracture, joint subluxation or luxation, and the presence of a radiodense foreign body (Figure 4.2). Ultrasound may be useful in defining the

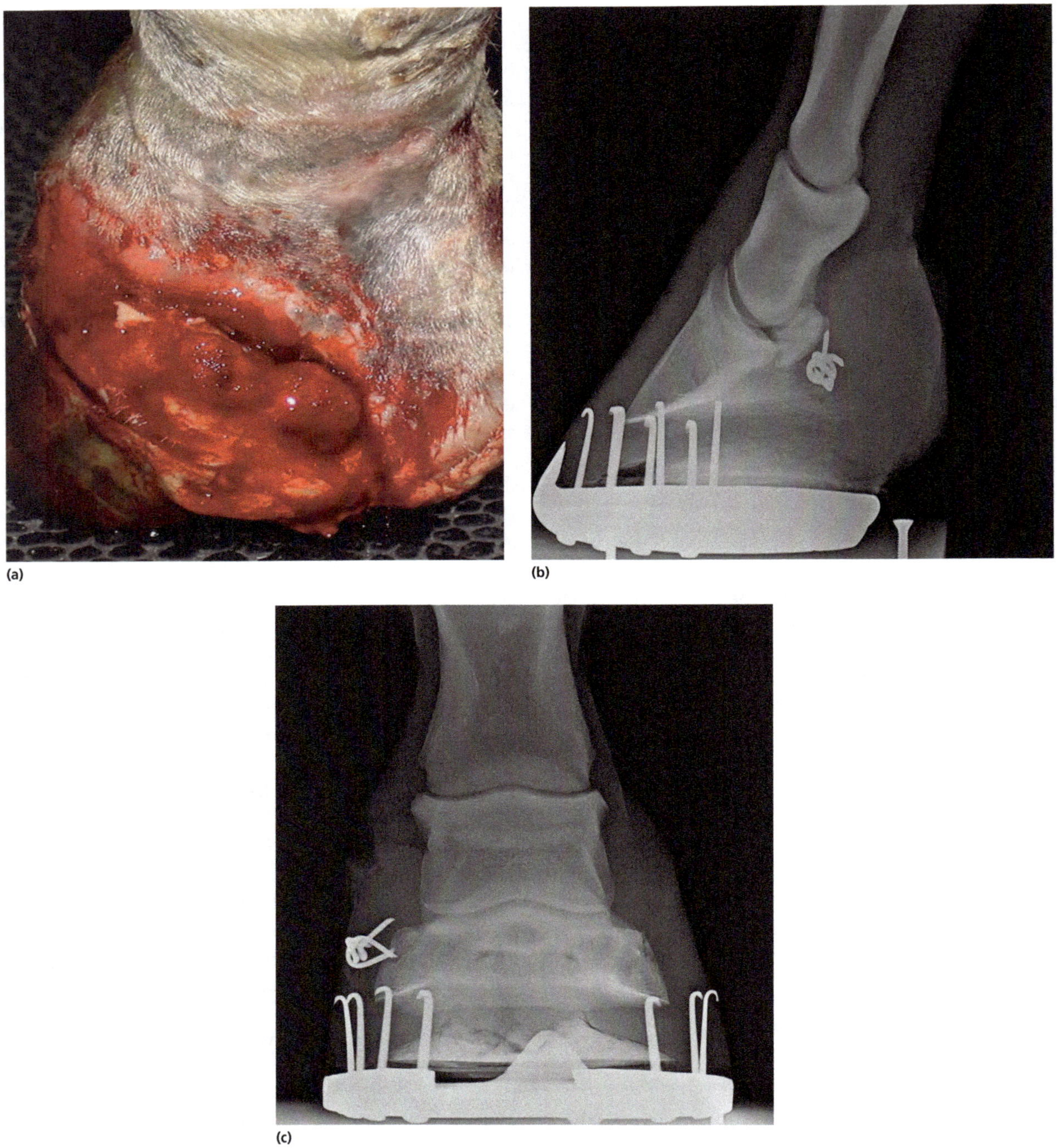

Figure 4.2 Example of a heel bulb laceration **(a)** where the foreign body (barbed wire) was not identified during visual appraisal and digital exploration of the wound. However, it was clearly identified on radiographs of the hoof **(b, c)**. None of the adjacent synovial cavities (navicular bursa, coffin joint, digital flexor tendon sheath) had been breached by the wound. The barbed wire was localized and removed under general anesthesia.

extent of soft-tissue injury, in identifying the presence of gas, fluid, or a foreign body not visible radiographically, and in identifying synovial involvement. Ultrasound can be useful in determining if a wound to the chest or abdomen has penetrated the pleural or peritoneal cavity and can assist in retrieving pleural or peritoneal fluid samples for cytologic examination and microbial culture and antimicrobial sensitivity testing of bacterial isolates.

What to do

- Wounds should be thoroughly explored to determine the extent and involvement of associated or underlying structures or the presence of a foreign body. Foreign bodies are not always obvious during radiographic or ultrasonographic examination but sometimes can be digitally palpated.

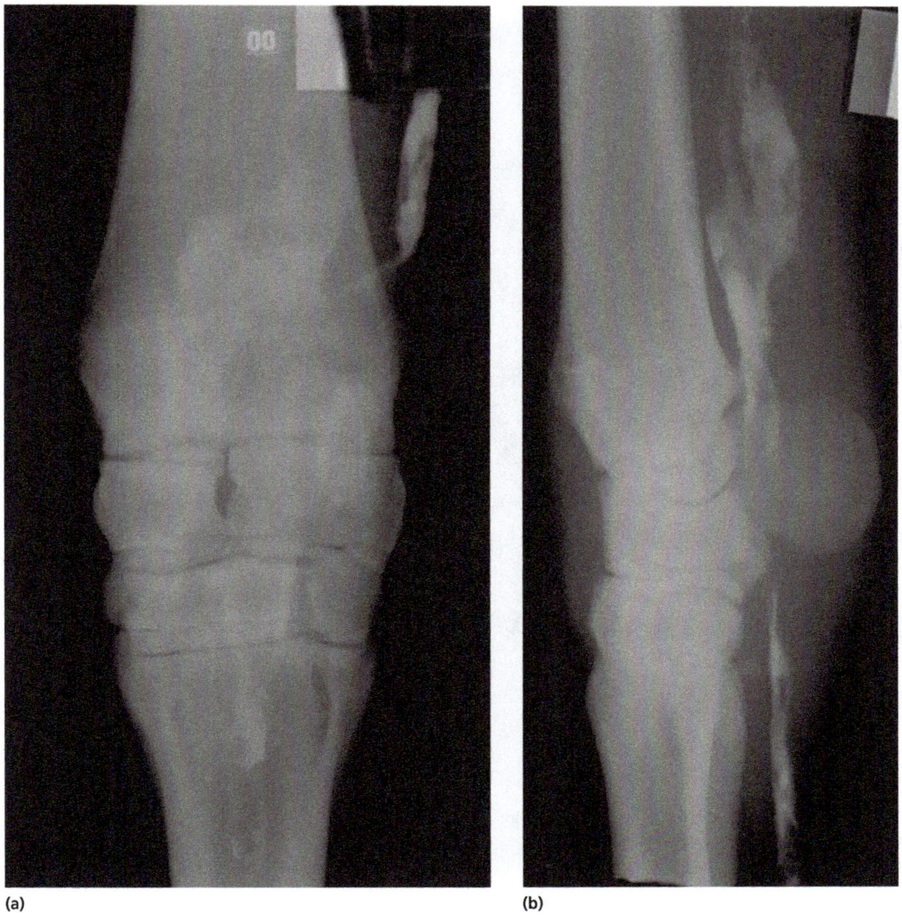

Figure 4.3 This horse suffered a penetrating wound to the lateral surface of the distal antebrachium 3 weeks earlier. Initial exploration revealed several pieces of wood in the wound, which were subsequently removed. Following debridement and irrigation, the wound was sutured and the horse received antimicrobial therapy. The horse became non-weight-bearing within 7 days and the wound broke open and began to drain 10 days postoperatively. **(a)** Craniocaudal contrast radiographic study revealing multiple filling defects (a result of pieces of wood) in the carpal canal. **(b)** Lateral radiographic view identifying multiple filling defects in the carpal canal.

What to avoid

- Do not assume that a wound has not penetrated a synovial capsule just because the wound does not directly overlie a synovial structure. Wounds may extend some distance from the point at which they penetrate the skin.

Tip

- Injection of sterile isotonic saline solution into a synovial cavity, under pressure, at a site remote from the wound, is useful to test the integrity of the synovial capsule. If the synovial capsule has been breached by the trauma, the injected fluid flows from the wound.

Wound debridement

Devitalized tissue is tissue that has no blood supply and that has no chance of becoming viable with treatment or time.[83] Accidental wounds of horses commonly contain devitalized tissue, excessively colonized, multiple organism-related biofilm or slough, exudate, and debris, including foreign material. All of these delay healing by providing a focus for infection and by exacerbating the inflammatory response.[84] Removing non-viable or foreign material through debridement reduces the bacterial load on the surface of the wound, which enhances healing. However, for healing to proceed rapidly, as much viable tissue as possible must be preserved. The wound should be debrided when it is first examined, but debridement may need to be repeated throughout healing (i.e., “maintenance” debridement) to address ongoing necrosis and infection.

Although dirt and loose debris may be rinsed away by using copious sterile irrigation, wound debridement is often used in combination with irrigation to ensure adequate preparation of the wound for healing. Various techniques of debridement available in clinical practice include autolytic, enzymatic, surgical, and mechanical debridement. Larval or maggot debridement therapy, also referred to as biodebridement, is also used in horses. The method chosen depends on various factors, such as the type, size, location, and age of the wound, the extent of tissue damage and contamination, patient tolerance, cost, expertise,

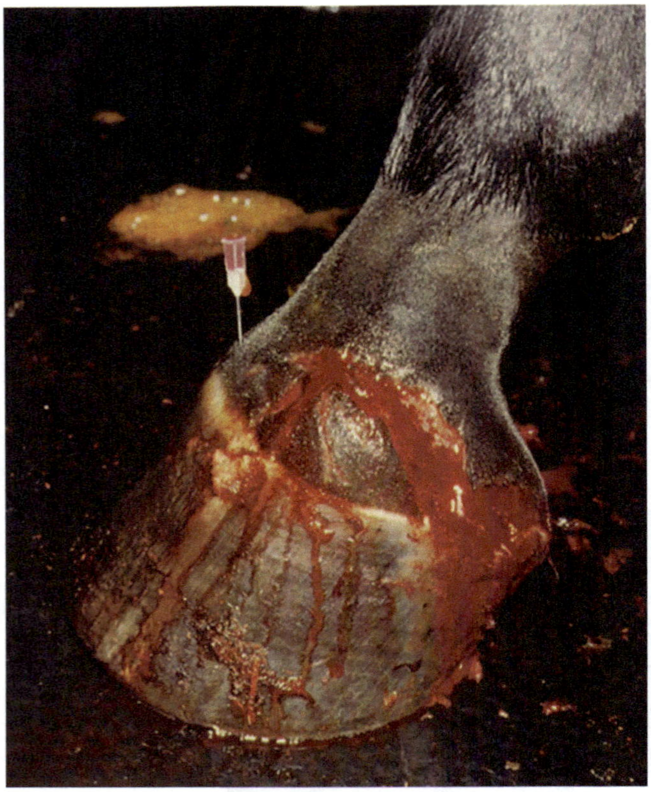

Figure 4.4 A sterile needle has been placed in the distal interphalangeal (coffin) joint at a site remote from the wound. Source: Stashak 2006.[82] Reproduced with permission of American Association of Equine Practitioners.

and available equipment. More than one type of debridement is often required to optimally prepare the wound for healing. The following sub-sections address the more common techniques of debridement available to the equine practitioner, with the aim to provide an overview of the indications, cautions, and contraindications of each.

Autolytic debridement

Debridement occurs naturally within wounds by autolysis, a process whereby devitalized tissue is softened or liquefied by the body's own enzymes, released by macrophages, mast cells, endothelial cells, keratinocytes, and fibroblasts. Autolytic debridement is selective (i.e., only devitalized tissue is liquefied) and virtually painless for the patient. If the wound is heavily contaminated or chronic, however, the autolytic process becomes overwhelmed by the sheer number of microbes or by the amount of endotoxins released from devitalized tissue.[85]

Dressing-enhanced autolytic debridement

Natural, autolytic debridement can be enhanced by applying dressings to the wound to maintain a moist environment, thereby ensuring maximum activity of the host's enzymes. Although this is perhaps the safest form of debridement, due to its selectivity, it is slow, expensive (according to the cost of the selected dressing materials), and, in the case of wounds of horses, may achieve only partial results due to its inadequate activity in the presence of necrotic tissue and debris. Consequently, another type of debridement (e.g., surgical) may be required to prepare the wound before dressing-enhanced autolytic debridement is used.

Dressings composed of honey or hypertonic saline solution promote debridement by osmosis (Figure 4.5); alginate, hydrogel, and hydrocolloid dressings support moist wound healing. The reader is referred to Chapter 6 for more information about wound dressings and to Chapter 22 for more information about the use of honey for wound management. Of note, an *in vitro* study comparing the effectiveness of various fluid-donating dressings (gauze, hydrofiber, hydrocolloid, and alginate) for debriding fibrin from blood clots of horses (using an *in vitro* model of proteinaceous coagulum or eschar) found that dressings hydrated with isotonic saline solution were better at debriding than were those hydrated with water because of their greater osmolarity.[86]

What to do

- Debridement of wounds, particularly wounds that are chronic or heavily contaminated, is an important aspect of wound management and can be combined with irrigation to prepare the wound for healing.

What to avoid

- Do not delay! Debridement should be initiated when the wound is first examined.

Tip

- Debridement may need to be repeated multiple times to address areas of ongoing necrosis.

Enzymatic debridement

Proteolytic enzymes dissolve collagenous tissue and cause superficial debris and devitalized tissue to slough.[87] These agents may be used to speed the process of autolytic debridement in areas where surgical debridement is not possible or carries risk, such as in wounds that closely approximate nerves and/or vessels.[88]

Factors that optimize debridement include a good delivery system that facilitates contact between the enzyme and the area requiring debridement, a sustained period of enzymatic activity, and an optimal wound environment.[89] Frequently, proteolytic enzymes are applied along with other topical agents to address several objectives, including balancing moisture, managing exudate, controlling the bioburden, and enhancing tissue regeneration.[90] Caution is advised when using enzymatic debridement in combination with other therapies because various wound dressings, for example iodine dressings and silver dressings, have been shown to inhibit the activity of collagenase, resulting in ineffectual debridement.[90] Little information is available about the clinical use of enzymatic debriding agents in horses.

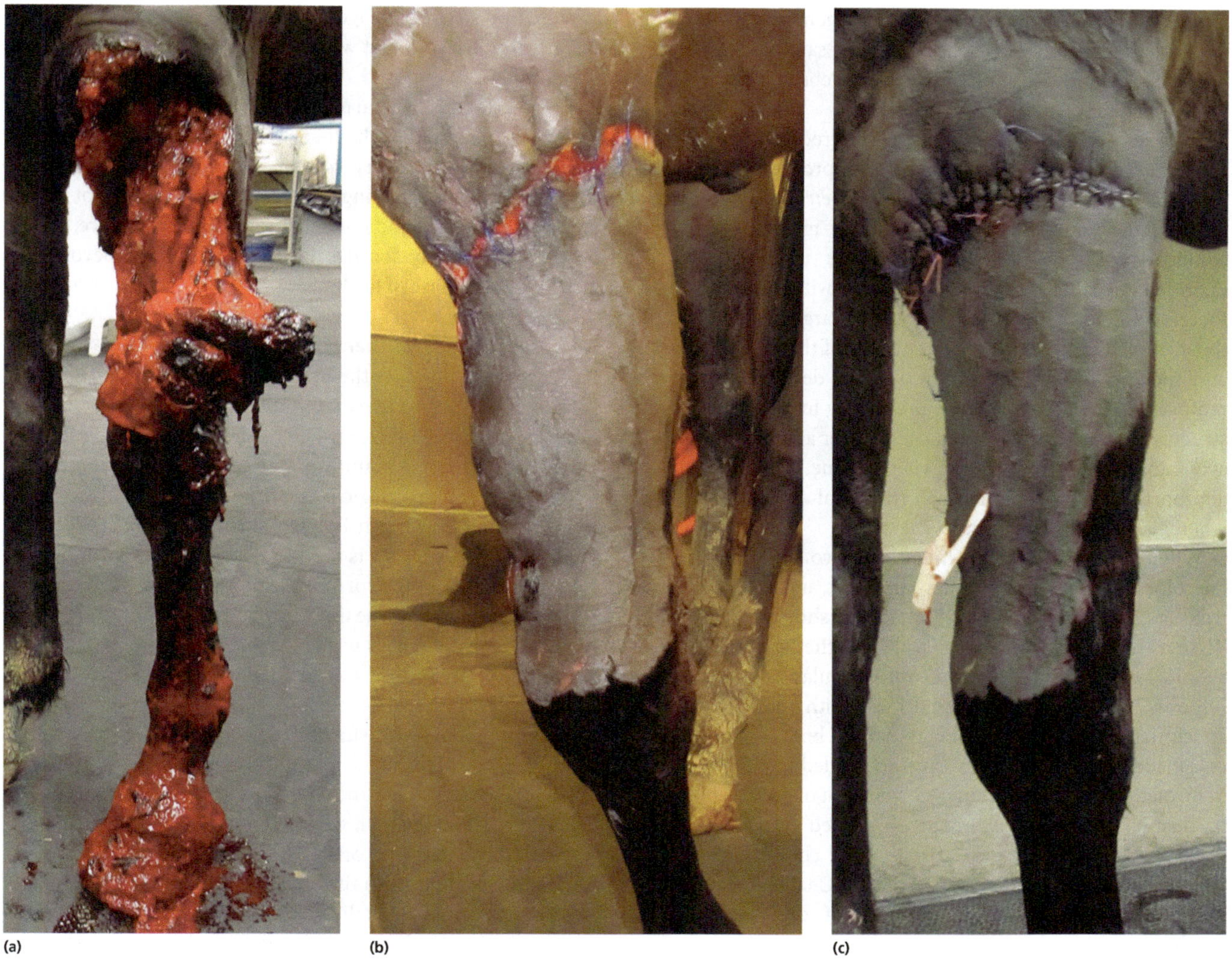

Figure 4.5 (**a**) Example of a severe wound on the dorsal surface of the antebrachium where, due to excessive contamination and the presence of non-viable tissue, closure was delayed until a bed of healthy granulation tissue had formed. (**b**) Initially, the wound was packed with hypertonic saline-soaked gauze (Curasalt™ Covidien Animal Health/Kendall) to assist autolytic debridement and the flap was temporarily replaced into a normal position and secured using several large tension sutures placed in a near–far–far–near pattern, to reduce tension and to prevent skin flap retraction. (**c**) Once a healthy bed of granulation tissue was present, the wound underwent delayed secondary closure using a combination of near–far–far–near and simple interrupted suture patterns.

A single study in horses has evaluated the debriding ability of enzymatic formulations. That study, using an *in vitro* model to simulate a dry, fibrinous chronic wound eschar, showed that traditional gauze dressings hydrated with isotonic saline solution and various forms of hydrofiber, hydrocolloid, and alginate dressing (fluid-donating dressings) were more effective in removing fibrin from blood clots than were enzymatic formulations (collagenase, papain/urea, and streptokinase/streptodornase).[86] These results suggest that proteolytic enzymes cannot penetrate thick, hard, fibrinous eschar. They may be more effective when the necrotic tissue is softer.

Although enzymatic wound debridement shows promise for eliminating necrotic debris and bacteria, this type of debridement has limitations when treating accidental wounds of equids, which are often heavily contaminated and include large areas of necrotic tissue. Until more information is available regarding the use of enzymatic debridement in the wounds of horses, other forms of debridement may be preferred.

For more information about agents used for enzymatic debridement, the reader is referred to Chapter 5.

Surgical debridement

Sharp surgical debridement using a scalpel is the optimal method for rapidly cleansing wounds containing a large amount of devitalized tissue and/or bioburden. This method of debridement is very selective because the surgeon has complete control over what tissue is removed and what tissue is left behind. The intent of debridement is to create a well-vascularized wound to support healing or skin grafting. The ability to correctly identify tissue types and anatomic structures is required to avoid further injury. Aseptic technique prevents iatrogenic contamination. Repeat surgical debridement may be necessary or, alternatively, may be followed by another form of debridement, such as dressing-enhanced autolytic debridement.

Excisional debridement may be layered, which involves sequential removal of devitalized tissue, progressing from the wound's surface to the wound's depths, or *en bloc*, which entails excising the entire wound including its margin, so that all wounded and contaminated tissues are removed. *En bloc* debridement is often used for wounds with draining tracts. Piecemeal debridement is used for very large wounds, usually those of the body. Beginning at one side of the wound's margin and moving toward the other side, all devitalized tissue is removed a little at a time while preserving important anatomic structures. Staged debridement occurs over a number of days to avoid inadvertent removal of viable tissue. This approach is appropriate for most wounds on the distal aspect of the limb, where tissue is at a premium.

When performing debridement, the two governing criteria are color and attachment. White, tan, black, and green tissues, as well as those that are poorly attached, should be debrided. Tissues that are pink to dark purple and that are well attached should be spared. Devitalized, non-articular bone should be removed, whereas well perfused bone with robust soft-tissue attachments should be left. Fragments of bone with questionable viability should be aggressively debrided to reduce the risk of formation of a sequestrum. Debridement of cortical bone that has lost its periosteum is best accomplished with a hip arthroplasty rasp, but a bone rasp, curette, bone chisel, or osteotome can be used. The reader is referred to Chapter 14 for more information about the management of degloving injuries involving denuded bone.

What to do

- The aim of sharp debridement is to remove all contaminated and devitalized tissue.

What to avoid

- Avoid damaging healthy tissue during debridement.

Tip

- Surgical debridement is highly effective and under the control of the surgeon. Where possible, debride the wound to bleeding, healthy-appearing tissues. Begin debriding at the most distal/ventral portion of the wound to prevent blood from obstructing the view of the area still to be debrided. Have a thorough understanding of the anatomy and tissue types involved in the wound.

Mechanical debridement

Wet-to-dry dressings

Open mesh gauze may be applied to the wound, either dry, as in the case of an exudative wound, or wetted, generally with sterile saline solution, as in the case of a dry wound. This dressing is covered by a sterile bandage. The dressing clings to the wound's surface as it dries, so that when it is removed, tissue adhered to the gauze is also removed.

This type of mechanical debridement is non-selective because both healthy and unhealthy tissue are removed, indiscriminately. Consequently, wet-to-dry bandages should not be confused with moist wound healing. The dressing may disrupt angiogenesis, fibroplasia, and epithelialization and, therefore, should be used exclusively for debridement and never beyond the inflammatory phase of healing.

Hydrosurgical debridement

Hydrosurgery involves the use of pressurized water or saline solution as a cutting/cleansing tool. It provides a rapid and selective method of wound debridement. It can often be used with the horse standing, but sedation may sometimes be required. Hydrosurgical debridement is reported to be well tolerated because it is less painful than sharp debridement.[91] If hydrosurgery is used to debride a fresh wound that is to be sutured, some form of local anesthesia is necessary; conversely, local anesthesia is not usually required if hydrosurgical debridement is used to debride a wound covered by granulation tissue that has been left unsutured to heal by second intention.

A commercial hydrosurgical device (Versajet™, Smith & Nephew) is widely used in the human healthcare field to manage a variety of wounds.[92,93] This system generates a high pressure (≤15 000 psi) jet of fluid (sterile saline solution) that emerges through a tiny orifice (0.127 mm) of the handpiece. Emergence of fluid from the orifice produces suction (Venturi effect) that draws devitalized tissue into a cutting chamber where it is shredded and evacuated. This device consists of an electrically powered console and single-use, disposable handpieces. The closer to 90° that the aperture is held to the tissue, the more it excises, whereas the primary effects obtained when the aperture is held at an oblique angle are irrigation and aspiration. The system has 10 power settings, the lower of which gently cleanse and debride and the higher of which allow more resilient tissue to be excised. The Versajet Plus™ has a higher-performance handpiece that provides more rapid and aggressive surgical cutting than the standard Versajet™.[94] In contrast to the standard Versajet™ this device has been shown to be effective for debriding cortical bone.[94] A number of benefits have been claimed for this hydrosurgical device, including simultaneous dissection and aspiration of debris, sparing of viable tissues, high precision and ease of use, little bleeding, the ability to safely debride small wounds located near vital structures, and fewer debridement procedures, leading to substantial savings in cost compared to other forms of debridement.[94,95] The Versajet™ has been shown to facilitate more precise debridement and preservation of dermal tissue but with no effect on scarring or time to healing in burn wounds, when compared with scalpel debridement.[96] A recent *ex vivo* study comparing the efficacy of different methods of debridement in reducing the load of *S. aureus* from contaminated equine muscle showed that hydrosurgical debridement, using the Versajet™, was more effective than irrigation with isotonic saline solution, scraping with a scalpel blade, or a combination of irrigation and scraping.[91] It remains to be proven, however, if the tool is useful for debriding clinically encountered wounds, which are usually highly contaminated with various bacterial species and foreign organic material. Moreover, the likelihood of causing aerosolization of bacterial particles and subsequent environmental dispersal of airborne microorganisms requires more investigation.[97,98]

Ultrasound-assisted debridement

Low-frequency, ultrasound-assisted debridement (Sonaca-185, Sorling GmBH) is a relatively new technique of debridement that uses low-frequency ultrasonic waves (20–60 Hz), emitted in contact or non-contact mode, produced by streaming saline solution through tubing into a sonotrobe head.[99,100] Microcavitation, resulting from oscillation of saline gas bubbles, cleaves necrotic tissue from healthy tissue, thereby debriding the wound and disrupting the biofilm; the necrotic tissue is suctioned or washed away.[99] Healthy, more elastic tissue is preserved and stimulated to epithelialize.[100,101] Although most studies examining the efficacy of ultrasound-assisted debridement have been performed on human patients with diabetic foot ulcers,[100] the technique is suggested to be suitable for a variety of wounds.[101] Because the recommended time of treatment is 20–30 sec/cm^2 of surface area,[101] ultrasound-assisted debridement is likely less applicable to the large wounds commonly found in horses.

> **Tip**
>
> - Newer forms of mechanical debridement, using commercially available devices, such as the Versajet™ or low-frequency ultrasound devices, are effective in debriding some wounds of humans. Studies to document the efficacy and safety of such methods in debriding wounds of horses are pending.
>
> **What to avoid**
>
> - Commercial devices intended for human patients should be used with caution in horses until their efficacy and safety in debriding wounds of horses can be demonstrated.

Larval/biosurgical debridement (maggot debridement therapy)

Biosurgical debridement has recently gained in popularity, both in human[102] and in equine medicine.[103] The larvae of *Lucilia sericata* provide rapid and selective debridement, by liquefaction and digestion, of devitalized tissue. Moreover, the larvae have an antiseptic effect,[104] including against MRSA,[105] and an inhibitory effect on the formation of biofilm.[106] For more information about maggot debridement therapy, the reader is referred to Chapter 22.

Negative-pressure wound therapy/vacuum-assisted closure

Negative-pressure wound therapy (NPWT), also known as vacuum-assisted closure (VAC), is one of the newest practices used to control wound infection and positively influence wound healing. The reader is referred to Chapter 22 for more information about this modality.

A recent development in NPWT allows controlled delivery of user-selected solutions for irrigating the wound by alternating instillation and soak periods with negative pressure therapy (known as NPWT instillation or NPWTi). This therapy is designed to be used for irrigating severely contaminated wounds and thus may be of interest to the equine practitioner. Recent *in vitro* and *in vivo* (porcine) studies have demonstrated the effective wound cleansing capabilities of NPWTi without the tissue damage and environmental contamination associated with traditional wound irrigation (at low and high pressures).[107]

Antimicrobial drugs

All wounds contain microorganisms, yet the majority of wounds are not infected. Nevertheless, the spectrum of interactions between the microbial community and the host may gradually reach a point at which healing is impaired. When this transition occurs, intervention to address infection is indicated.[108] Successful antimicrobial therapy relies on the administration of an appropriate drug so that pathogens are either killed or suppressed to the extent that they are eliminated by the host's immune system and no longer interfere with healing. The appropriate drug is determined by identifying the principal pathogen(s) on the wound and its (their) antibiotic sensitivities. More information about bacterial culture and antibiotic sensitivity testing can be found in Chapter 19.

Inappropriate use of antibiotics is likely a major cause for the widespread emergence of resistant organisms, such as methicillin-resistant *Staphylococcus aureus*.[109] In addition to the worry about antimicrobial resistance, the veterinary clinician must also be concerned about the cost of wound therapy, as well as the potential for serious side effects related to some antibiotics. For example, antibiotic-associated colitis or diarrhea can be rapidly fatal, with rates of mortality ranging between 20 and 50%.[110,111] Fortunately, colitis is reported to occur in <1% of horses receiving a systemically administered antibiotic.[110]

Surgical wounds

Perioperative antibiotic therapy is not usually instituted in human patients undergoing an elective surgery falling in the category of a clean procedure (see Table 3.1 in Chapter 3), in the absence of co-morbidity or placement of an implant.[112,113] One retrospective study found that antibiotics were used in 98%

of clean, elective arthroscopic procedures of horses.[114] In this study, antibiotics were found to be primarily administered perioperatively, but the dosing regimen commonly deviated from standard antimicrobial practice recommendations for prophylactic use of antibiotics.[115]

There are few objective studies analyzing what constitutes optimal perioperative antibiotic prophylaxis for horses undergoing surgery. One study revealed a 0.5% incidence of septic arthritis in horses that had undergone elective arthroscopy (a "clean" procedure) without receiving perioperative prophylactic antibiotics.[115] This compared favorably to a 0.9% incidence of septic arthritis in horses undergoing arthroscopy that had received antibiotics preoperatively.[116] Although many factors contribute to SSI, these studies suggest that the incidence of infection in horses after clean surgical procedures is very low. Consequently, administration of prophylactic antibiotics to equine patients undergoing a clean surgical procedure of short duration, when no implant is used, is not indicated, except when the development of a SSI would be performance limiting or life threatening.[117] The use of antimicrobial drugs should never replace meticulous aseptic and atraumatic surgical technique. Halsted's principles of surgery should be strictly respected. These include: gentle handling of tissue (including keeping the tissues moist and using the correct surgical instruments); meticulous hemostasis; preservation of blood supply; strict aseptic technique; minimum tension on tissues; accurate apposition of tissue (with appropriately sized suture material); and obliteration of dead space.

Conversely, antimicrobial prophylaxis is indicated if the equine surgical patient is at high risk of infection (i.e., when the likelihood of occurrence of infection exceeds 5% without prophylactic antimicrobial use). Risk factors for infection include procedures considered clean–contaminated or contaminated (see Table 3.1 in Chapter 3), surgery times that exceed 60 minutes,[15,17–19] a deep plane of anesthesia that may affect perfusion and oxygenation of tissue,[20,21,24] and the presence of orthopedic implants.

Appropriate use of prophylactic antimicrobial drugs relies on accurate selection of drug(s), dosing regimen, and duration of use. The goal is to select an antibiotic with a narrow spectrum of activity in order to preserve the patient's normal flora and decrease the risk for the development of antimicrobial resistance. Prophylactic antimicrobial therapy should begin preoperatively so that the concentrations of the drug in serum and tissue last for the duration of surgery and exceed the minimum inhibitory concentration (MIC) for the organisms likely to be encountered.[113,118] The current recommendation in human medicine is for the preoperative dose to be administered within 60 minutes of skin incision and for redosing during surgery if the procedure extends beyond two half-lives of the antibiotic.[118] The most common antibiotics used prophylactically in equine medicine, penicillin and gentamicin, reach peak concentrations at the surgical site between 15 and 30 minutes after intravenous (IV) administration, with concentrations declining rapidly thereafter.[120–122] The half-life of potassium penicillin G (20 000 IU/kg, IV) in horses is reported to be approximately 40 minutes while that of gentamicin sulfate (6.6 mg/kg, IV) is approximately 90 minutes.[120–122]

In human patients, it is recommended that antibiotic therapy be continued for 24 hours or less, postoperatively, regardless of whether the surgery was clean, clean–contaminated, or contaminated.[123–125] Prolonged administration has been shown to result in increased morbidity, including a higher rate of hospital infection (33% higher) and of surgical wound infection (15% higher)[123] and may contribute to antimicrobial resistance.[124,125] Likewise, small-animal patients receiving postoperative antibiotics had a higher rate of wound infection (8.2%) than patients receiving no antimicrobial drugs (4.3%).[126] Two studies in horses support a short duration of prophylactic antimicrobial therapy over a longer duration of prophylactic antimicrobial therapy. The first found no benefit in administering antibiotics for 120 hours, rather than for 72 hours, to prevent incisional infections after surgery for an acute abdominal crisis.[127] The second study showed no difference in the rate of SSI between horses that received antibiotics for less than 36 hours after exploratory celiotomy and those that received antibiotics for more than 36 hours.[128]

What to do

- Decide if surgical antibiotic prophylaxis is appropriate/required.
- Determine the bacterial flora most likely to cause postoperative infection (not every species of bacteria needs to be treated for prophylactically). See Table 19.1 in Chapter 19.
- Choose an antibiotic, based on the recommendation above, with the narrowest antibacterial spectrum required. See Table 19.3 in Chapter 19.
- Choose the less expensive drug if two drugs are otherwise of equal antibacterial spectrum, efficacy, toxicity, and ease of administration.
- Administer as a single dose, based on weight, preferably IV, 60 minutes before surgery.
- Top up if surgery time exceeds more than two half-lives of the drug.
- Administer for no more than 24 hours.
- Do not substitute antibiotic prophylaxis for good surgical technique.

What to avoid

- Avoid using antibiotics in routine, clean surgical procedures.

Tip

- Minimize surgical time, adhere to sound surgical principles, and have a plan for anesthesia that minimizes time and optimizes perfusion and oxygenation of tissue.

Accidental wounds

Accidental wounds of horses are often contaminated and contain considerably damaged tissue, which may include the local blood supply. Additional factors, such as the presence of foreign bodies, the involvement of structures underlying the skin, and a long delay between the onset of injury and treatment, increase the risk that contamination will progress to colonization and infection (the reader is referred to Chapter 3 for more information about the bacterial continuum), which might ultimately exert a negative impact on healing. Consequently, antimicrobial therapy is commonly included in the wound-management regimen, particularly when the wound is at high risk of becoming infected, such as a puncture wound, a wound with devitalized tissue, a wound associated with an open fracture, or a wound that has entered a body cavity or a synovial structure. Nevertheless, antimicrobial therapy should be viewed as only one component of a multifaceted strategy, addressing both wound biology (repair) and microbial pathogenicity, which also includes appropriate irrigation and debridement. In fact, focusing primarily on the pharmacologic aspect of wound management is likely to yield unsatisfactory results.

Systemic administration

The indication for systemic antibiotic therapy is not always clear. Consequently, antimicrobial drugs are often administered empirically, as a routine adjunct to the management of open wounds. A study conducted by the United States Department of Agriculture revealed that traumatic injuries or wounds were the most common reason for the administration of antimicrobials to horses, with 3.9% of equids aged 6 months or older receiving antimicrobials for traumatic injuries over a 12-month period.[129] In the UK, 96.8% of veterinary surgeons surveyed indicated that they would prescribe antimicrobials for a contaminated wound on a limb.[130] A recent study in the UK investigating the prescribing habits of equine practitioners attending limb wounds in horses revealed that systemic antimicrobials were administered prior to referral in 83.2% (94/113) of horses, 8.5% of which received the protected third- or fourth-generation cephalosporins or fluoroquinolones.[131] Of equal concern, over half of the horses did not receive a sufficient dose; this was especially true of heavier patients, who were more likely to be under-dosed.

Inappropriate use of antibiotics should be avoided to minimize the risk of developing antibiotic resistance.[132] Systemic administration of antibiotics is warranted when the degree of infection exceeds the efforts of local control of the bioburden and when local soft-tissue infection or sepsis are apparent.[133] Suspicion that the wound contains a biofilm is also an indication for systemic antibiotic therapy, but debridement, irrigation, and topical therapies are fundamental to reducing the bacterial burden and disrupting biofilms (more on biofilms later in this chapter).

When systemic antibiotic therapy is indicated, a wound sample, for bacterial culture and antibiotic sensitivity testing of isolates, should ideally be collected before instituting therapy. The sample should be harvested from the depth of the wound rather than from its contaminated surface. This enables targeting the microorganisms with a narrow-spectrum antimicrobial drug. One should bear in mind, however, that routine culture is a poor clinical indication of the bacterial population found in biofilms, which are common in chronic wounds.[134] Broad-spectrum antibiotics are selected empirically, based on expected pathogens, and used initially while awaiting the results of culture and sensitivity testing. Table 19.1 lists the common bacteria isolated from various types of wounds in horses, and Table 19.3 lists the likely antibiotic sensitivities for each pathogen, as a basis for empiric antibiotic choices that are most likely to be useful. If clinical signs of infection evolve, final selection of the antibiotic is based on the results of culture and sensitivity tests. The goal of antimicrobial therapy is to eradicate infection using a narrow-spectrum, cost-effective, safe drug.

Acute or superficial wound infections of horses are usually the result of one dominating microorganism, whereas chronic or deep wound infections of horses are often polymicrobial.[128,135] Antibiotics selected for use should reflect this microbial epidemiology,[132,135] bearing in mind the prevalence of antimicrobial resistance and the importance of using a narrow-spectrum antibiotic based on antibiotic sensitivity testing of bacterial isolates.[136] While awaiting the test results, penicillin or trimethoprim–sulfonamide, or a combination of both, are often used empirically to treat acute or superficial wound infections. Deep wounds, including those involving synovial cavities, are usually best treated with a β-lactam antibiotic along with an aminoglycoside, such as gentamicin sulfate or amikacin sulfate, because infections are often polymicrobial.[128,137] Ceftiofur sodium or enrofloxacin are generally reserved for infections where bacteria have been shown, by culture and sensitivity testing, to be resistant to penicillin or aminoglycosides.[128,137] Enrofloxacin is not recommended for use in young horses because it can lead rapidly to non-inflammatory arthropathy in immature animals.[138] High doses of penicillin and metronidazole are recommended for treating deep fascial cellulitis, septic myositis, or pyonecrotic processes associated with *Clostridia* spp.[128,136]

If the antibiotic is administered systemically, the intravenous route should be used initially because the concentration of a drug is more predictable when the drug is administered by that route than when it is administered by other routes. Oral or intramuscular administration is often used after an adequate concentration of the drug in the blood has been achieved. Regional intravenous perfusion provides a high concentration of the antimicrobial drug at the target and is particularly useful in the management of infected wounds on the distal aspect of the limb of horses. More information about regional limb perfusion can be found in Chapters 16 and 19. The duration of treatment is primarily dictated by the patient's response to therapy, with a positive response characterized by the resolution of infection and the normal progression of healing. The reader is referred to Chapter 16 for more information about the management of wounds involving synovial structures and to Chapter 19 for more information about the management of severely infected wounds.

What to do

- Where antibiotic therapy is indicated, a wound sample should be collected, ideally before instituting therapy, for bacterial culture and antibiotic sensitivity testing of isolates. This enables selection of the most appropriate drug with the narrowest spectrum of activity.
- Use validated weigh tapes or portable weighbridges to obtain an accurate estimate of the horse's weight, in an effort to prevent under-dosing of antimicrobials when these are required.

What to avoid

- Avoid the empiric use of antibiotics for the management of open wounds without evidence of infection.

Tip

- While awaiting the results of culture and sensitivity testing, base the choice of antimicrobial drug on the pathogens most likely present in the wound (see Tables 19.1 and 19.3).

Topical administration

> Perhaps the most deceptively simple of all therapeutic procedures is the treatment of cutaneous infection with topical medication. Despite the unique accessibility of the skin to scientific investigation, it has for too long been the playground of crude empiricism.
>
> (Professor Sydney Selwyn)[139]

Systemic antibiotic therapy is indicated in cases of severe wound infection that is detrimental to healing. If, however, the infected wound is poorly perfused or contains a biofilm, topically applied antimicrobial therapy may have an advantage over the same antimicrobial drug administered systemically because topical application delivers a higher concentration of medication directly to the desired area and is less likely to cause bacterial resistance. Two categories of topical antimicrobial drugs may be used in the management of open wounds: antiseptics and antibiotics.

Antiseptics

Antiseptics are agents that destroy or inhibit the growth of microorganisms in or on living tissue. Unlike antibiotics that act selectively on a specific target, antiseptics have a broader spectrum of activity and target bacteria, fungi, viruses, protozoa, and even prions. Resistance towards antiseptics has been reported but is substantially less common than that towards antibiotics.[140] Furthermore, contact sensitization to antiseptics is seen less often than with topically applied antibiotic drugs.[141]

The antiseptics most commonly used in wound management include PI, chlorhexidine, polyhexamethylene biguanide, hydrogen peroxide, hypochlorous acid, silver nitrate, and honey, among others (the reader is referred to Chapter 5 for more information about topical wound-care products and to Chapter 22 for more information about honey). The usefulness of antiseptics on intact skin (that of the surgeon or of the patient) is well established. The usefulness of antiseptics is discussed in the sections on wound preparation and cleansing/irrigation, earlier in this chapter. Conversely, the usefulness of antiseptics as anti-infective agents for open wounds remains an area of debate.[74] Evidence regarding the "biocompatibility index", which is the ratio between the antimicrobial effectiveness and the tissue's tolerance of a given product is conflicting.[142] Although the evidence is based primarily on studies performed *in vitro*, the prevailing consensus is that the judicious use of dressings containing an antiseptic agent can be a valuable option for controlling infection and promoting healing.[143]

What to do

- When appropriate, select an antiseptic over an antibiotic for topical application, because the former is less likely to be associated with the development of resistance.

What to avoid

- More is not always better, and high concentrations of many antiseptics are cytotoxic to healthy tissues.

Tip

- Use recommended concentrations of antiseptics that optimize reductions in bacterial concentrations while minimizing deleterious effects on healthy tissues. Dilute PI solution-soaked dressings are not recommended for use on wounds because they are inactivated by organic material, but cadexomer–iodine dressings are effective in reducing the bacterial concentration on wounds.

Antibiotics

Antibiotics to be administered topically to open wounds are usually in an ointment-based vehicle that supports moist wound healing.[144] The most common commercial formulations contain silver sulfadiazine, gentamicin, nitrofurazone, a cephalosporin, fusidic acid, or a combination of bacitracin, polymyxin B, and neomycin (the reader is referred to Chapter 5 for more information about topical wound-care products). The theoretical advantages of topical over systemic administration of an antibiotic include the ability of topical administration to achieve higher local concentrations of the drug, a lower incidence of antimicrobial resistance, and reduced systemic side-effects.[145] Recent meta-analyses and systematic reviews, however, suggest there are few proven indications for topically applied antibiotics in the realm of wound management, except for wounds suffering ischemia or for wounds plagued with biofilm.[146] That said, these reviews pertain to the human medical literature and concern primarily burn wounds and chronic wounds (e.g., diabetic foot ulcers, pressure ulcers, chronic leg ulcers), where the underlying pathophysiology may differ considerably from the type of wound commonly encountered in equine practice. Unfortunately, little to no evidence is available in the veterinary literature to help design an evidence-based approach for the use of topical antibiotics to manage wound infection in horses.

What to do

- There is little evidence to suggest a place for topical application of antibiotics in the management of wounds of horses. If topical antibiotics are to be used, the wound must be debrided before application.

What to avoid

- Antibiotics administered topically are less likely to lead to resistance than are antibiotics administered systemically. Nevertheless, empiric use of topically applied antibiotics, where there is no clear indication to support it, should be proscribed.

Tip

- Manuka honey (UMF >10) may provide an alternative topical wound-care product when topical antimicrobial treatment is warranted.

Biofilms

Standard techniques of bacterial culture are inappropriate to phenotype bacteria in biofilms. Similarly priced diagnostic tests based on such technologies as polymerase chain reaction (PCR), sequencing technologies, and PCR/mass spectrometry, however, can characterize the phenotype of bacterial populations within biofilms and are particularly useful for characterizing polymicrobial communities.

Nevertheless, even when antibiotic therapy is based on a precise identification of the microbial pathogens and their antibiotic sensitivities, chronic biofilm infections may be resistant to antibiotic therapy because the microorganisms composing biofilm are protected from antibiotics by a self-produced, extracellular, polymeric matrix. Consequently, biofilm infections often recur after the course of antibiotic therapy is finished. Immature biofilms are more vulnerable to antibiotics, so frequent debridement to remove the biofilm is a mainstay of therapy.[147] An antiseptic or antibiotic may be applied topically to treat biofilm-infected wounds; the treatment should be applied within 4 hours of debriding, before the biofilm reforms.[148,149]

For more information about the therapeutic approach to bacterial biofilms, the reader is referred to Chapter 19.

Antimicrobial resistance

Antimicrobial resistance is described as the acquired ability of a microorganism (including bacteria, fungi, viruses, and parasites) to survive in the presence of concentrations of a chemical that are normally lethal to the microorganism of that species.[150] The evolution of resistant strains is a natural phenomenon that occurs when microorganisms replicate themselves erroneously or when resistant traits are exchanged between them. The inappropriate use of antimicrobial drugs, including use in animal husbandry, also accelerates the emergence and spread of drug-resistant strains.[151]

Resistance causes diseases to become more difficult to cure, thereby leading to increased costs associated with more doctor/veterinarian visits and the use of stronger and more expensive drugs. This may lead to serious welfare implications characterized by longer and more complicated illnesses and more deaths caused by infection. In fact, the increase in multi-drug-resistant bacteria has led the European Centre for Disease Prevention and Control to rate antimicrobial resistance as one of the most important infectious disease threats in Europe.[152] The 2014 World Health Organization (WHO) report on global surveillance of antimicrobial resistance stated that "without urgent, coordinated action, the world is heading towards a post-antibiotic era in which common infections and minor injuries, which have been treatable for decades, can once again kill."[151]

Staphylococcus aureus is an important cause of wound infection in companion animals, and infections with methicillin-resistant *S. aureus* (MRSA) are of particular concern due to limited options for treatment and the zoonotic potential of infection.[77] Resistance is the result of staphylococcal production of an altered penicillin-binding protein, which is the target molecule for β-lactam antibiotics, including penicillins and cephalosporins. In addition to being resistant to β-lactam antibiotics, MRSA is frequently resistant to other antimicrobial classes, such as the fluoroquinolones, tetracyclines, aminoglycosides, and potentiated sulfonamides.[153] Furthermore, many equine MRSA strains have a wider resistance profile than generally seen in human and small animal isolates.[153]

Sampling of the nasal passages of horses in hospitals and/or farms, internationally, has revealed a prevalence of 0–12% of carriers of MRSA.[154–158] The prevalence is even higher (40%) for horses requiring long-term hospitalization (≥6 months).[158] A recent study identified MRSA, predominantly from the CC398 lineage, in the wounds of an alarming proportion (138/604; 22.8%) of horses from which samples were obtained.[77] As with non-resistant varieties of microorganisms, however, carriage of or colonization with MRSA must be distinguished from MRSA infection.

The first documentation of an equine case of MRSA infection occurred in 1996,[159] and the number of reported infections since then has steadily risen. MRSA infections can involve a variety of sites in horses, but sites most commonly encountered are surgical or accidental wounds. Recovering MRSA from standard swabs taken from infected wounds is not difficult and is usually achieved by routine methods of culture. Methicillin resistance is identified during routine susceptibility testing of *S. aureus* isolates when methicillin, oxacillin, or cefoxitin antimicrobial discs are used.[153]

Although comprehensive guidelines have been produced for the treatment of MRSA in humans, detailed evidence-based guidelines are not widely available for equine practitioners. Nevertheless, broad principles for treatment and control of MRSA in horses have been established (Box 4.1).[160,161]

The WHO has prioritized critically important antimicrobial drugs for use in human medicine (http://apps.who.int/iris/bitstream/10665/77376/1/9789241504485_eng.pdf). This document is intended for public health and animal health authorities, practicing physicians and veterinarians, and other interested stakeholders involved in managing antimicrobial

Box 4.1 Principles for treatment and control of MRSA in horses. Adapted from Maddox *et al.*[153]

- Select antimicrobial drugs based on culture and sensitivity testing.
- Remove foreign material and implants where possible.
- Identify and treat concurrent conditions.
- Treat superficial infections topically with antibacterial drugs.
- Confine treatment of infection to the infected area, such as by regional limb perfusion.
- Use basic techniques of hygiene and isolation, such as: isolating MRSA-infected patients; using hand hygiene with alcohol-based sanitizers; using disposable protective clothing, gloves, and masks; and disposing of clinical waste immediately and safely.
- Identify animals at risk.
- Eliminate inappropriate antimicrobial use.

resistance, to ensure that critically important antimicrobial drugs are used prudently in human and veterinary medicine. The two determining criteria for this classification are that the drug is the sole therapy or one of few options to treat serious human disease and that the organism causing this disease or its resistance genes can be acquired from non-human sources.

The fluoroquinolones, third- and fourth-generation cephalosporins, macrolides, and glycopeptides have been categorized as being of highest priority for risk management. The most recent list has, for the first time, also included veterinary drugs exclusively used in animals (e.g., ceftiofur, cefquinome, enrofloxacin, and marbofloxacin) to highlight their potential impact on development of resistance.

Carbapenems, lipopeptides, and oxazolidinones currently have no veterinary equivalent. These classes, as well as any new class of antimicrobial drug developed for human therapy, should not be used in animals, plants, or in aquaculture.

The World Organization of Animal Health (OIE) has produced a corresponding list of antimicrobial drugs critically important in veterinary medicine to complement the identification of such antimicrobials used in human medicine. The aim is to identify overlapping requirements and find a balance between public health considerations and animal health needs (http://www.oie.int/fileadmin/Home/eng/Our_scientific_expertise/docs/pdf/Eng_OIE_List_antimicrobials_May2015.pEdf).

What to do

- Select the correct antibiotic (based on culture and sensitivity testing of bacterial isolates), not only initially but also periodically during the course of treatment, to ensure that treatment does not select for resistant mutants.
- Counsel horse owners about the proper use of such drugs and the importance of administering them as directed (e.g., do not skip doses; do not save antibiotics/never use leftover medication).
- For personnel working in equine clinics, strict adherence to hand-hygiene guidelines are central to the control of nosocomial infections.

Anti-inflammatory drugs

The inflammatory phase of the wound healing cascade serves to purge the wound of alien substances and disposes of dead tissue through autolytic debridement. Simultaneously, the inflammatory cells liberate mediators, including cytokines, growth factors, and prostaglandins (PGs), that amplify and sustain the events to follow, including formation of granulation tissue, epithelialization, contraction, and remodeling. The intensity of the inflammatory response is strongly correlated to the severity of trauma and is generally thought to determine the extent of scarring. PGE_2 specifically, however, is credited with decreasing proliferation of fibroblasts, inhibiting synthesis of collagen, and enhancing the expression of matrix metalloproteinases, thereby decreasing the excessive accumulation of scar tissue.[162]

Although knockout experiments suggest that wound repair is improved in mice depleted of inflammatory cells,[163,164] this improvement holds true only when conditions are sterile – conditions that are very different from those encountered clinically in equine practice. In fact, a deficient acute inflammatory response appears to be an important contributor to the delayed healing regularly encountered in wounds on the distal aspect of limbs of horses.[4] Consequently, although studies in other species may show advantages to inhibiting the inflammatory response to wounding, extrapolating these data to the horse must be done with caution since a robust inflammatory response to wounding is required for healing to proceed normally and promptly through its phases.

Non-steroidal anti-Inflammatory drugs

Non-steroidal anti-inflammatory drugs (NSAIDs) are a class of drugs that provide analgesic and antipyretic effects, and in higher doses, anti-inflammatory effects. They inhibit the activity of cyclooxygenase-1 (COX-1) and cyclooxygenase-2 (COX-2) enzymes, and thereby, the synthesis of eicosanoids, such as PGs, thromboxanes, and leukotrienes. The NSAIDs most commonly used in horses are phenylbutazone, flunixin meglumine, and more recently, the selective COX-2 inhibitors carprofen, meloxicam, and firocoxib (Table 4.1).[165] Inhibition of COX-2 enzyme in the horse may provide anti-inflammatory,

Table 4.1 Doses for non-steroidal anti-inflammatory drugs commonly used in horses.[165]

Drug	Dose	Route
Phenylbutazone	2.2–4.4 mg/kg, q12hr	Intravenous, oral
Flunixin meglumine	0.25–1 mg/kg, q8–24 hr	Intravenous, intramuscular, oral
Carprofen	0.7 mg/kg, q24hr	Intravenous, oral
Ketoprofen	2.2 mg/kg, q24hr	Intravenous
Meloxicam	0.6 mg/kg, q24hr	Oral
Firocoxib	0.1 mg/kg, q24hr	Oral

analgesic, and antipyretic effects without causing the common adverse effects on the gastrointestinal system, including right dorsal colitis, attributed to COX-1 enzyme inhibitors.[166]

There is good evidence that pain and the stress responses to pain may act to promote wound healing in the short term. The protracted release of pain mediators, however, can create an imbalance in cellular activity, starting with exacerbated inflammation and progressing to excessive fibrosis, which may be particularly evident in burn patients, whose scarring often becomes hypertrophic.[167–170] Consequently, NSAIDs are often prescribed and used postoperatively to control pain in humans. In hairless mice, neither selective inhibition of COX-2, nor non-selective inhibition of COX-1 and COX-2, significantly affected the healing of surgical skin wounds up to 28 days post-incision,[171] although, in rats, non-selective NSAIDs have been shown to significantly decrease deposition of collagen at the wound.[172]

The effects of administering a NSAID to equine patients during the early phase of wound healing have not been investigated extensively. One study examining incisional healing found that oxyphenbutazone administered to horses at a loading dose of 12 mg/kg (for 2 days) and a maintenance dose of 6 mg/kg (for 5 days) significantly reduced inflammation and formation of granulation tissue.[173] Another study of incisional complications after celiotomy in horses found no association between administration of a NSAID and wound complications.[174] Pain management is mandatory where signs of discomfort (e.g., pain on palpation, lameness, swelling) are present after injury, and there is evidence in humans that early intervention and effective management of pain are likely to be associated with a lower cumulative dose of analgesics required during treatment.[175] The COX-2 selective inhibitors, although substantially more expensive, reduce the risk of side-effects attributed to COX-1 inhibitors.

What to do

- Where indicated, NSAIDs (ideally COX-2 inhibitors) should be used in horses to manage pain. Adjust to effect and administer for the shortest duration possible.

What to avoid

- NSAIDs should be used at the correct therapeutic dose rates and intervals to optimize the anti-inflammatory effects and reduce the potential side-effects of overdosing. Using higher doses to enable less frequent administration should be avoided.

Tip

- Using a dosing regimen at the higher end of the therapeutic recommendation initially to establish effective pain management, then decreasing the dose in relation to response may lead to a lower cumulative dose and improve the overall demeanor, appetite, and systemic state of the patient, which may contribute to healing.

Corticosteroids

The general consensus is that use of corticosteroids, either systemically or topically, should be avoided unless their use is indicated to treat co-morbidities, because they slow repair.[176–178]

Corticosteroids are administered systemically to treat various inflammatory conditions in humans, including rheumatoid arthritis, gout, and inflammatory bowel disease. Consequently, the dosing, duration, and timing of perioperative administration of corticosteroids has been studied in laboratory animals and by retrospective studies of human patients to determine whether systemically administered corticosteroids impair wound healing. A recent, comprehensive literature review found that complications of wound healing, such as infection and dehiscence, increase 2–5-fold in patients receiving a systemically administered corticosteroid for at least 30 days before surgery.[177] The negative impact of corticosteroids on wound healing, however, seems to be related mostly to duration.[179] Indeed, even a high systemic dose of a corticosteroid had no clinical effect on wound healing if administered for less than 10 days prior to surgery.[177]

Equine patients rarely suffer from medical conditions that would benefit from an extended course of a systemically administered corticosteroid, and the doses usually recommended for these medical conditions are relatively low. No information exists as to the negative effects on healing that such a therapy might exert in a horse suffering concomitantly from a skin wound. Topical administration of a corticosteroid has been advocated for the management of EGT, to reduce the chronic inflammation associated with this condition.[180] The probable benefits of topical corticosteroid therapy in reducing the excessive fibroblastic response to chronic inflammation outweigh the negative effects on wound healing, such as reduced tensile strength.[181] The authors recommend applying a corticosteroid ointment or cream on one or two occasions, at the first sign of excessive fibroplasia, after all possible causes of chronic inflammation, such as the presence of non-viable tissue, foreign material, and contamination, have been eliminated. The reader is referred to Chapter 15 for more information about the management of EGT.

What to do

- A corticosteroid ointment or cream may be applied to a wound to reduce EGT. Apply topically to the wound on one or two occasions when EGT first appears.

What to avoid

- Do not apply a corticosteroid to treat chronic inflammation in a wound before first ensuring there are no underlying causes of inflammation, such as contamination or the presence of foreign material or necrotic tissue.

Suture material and pattern

Inappropriate suture material and improper suturing technique may exert a negative impact on healing. Surgeons must carefully assess each wound and choose a suture material that minimizes the likelihood of inflammation, thereby maximizing the opportunity for healing. Carefully debriding devitalized tissue to healthy bleeding tissue that can be comfortably apposed without causing excessive tension, after hemostasis has been achieved, optimizes healing. A suitable suture material and pattern allows the surgeon to approximate tissue and minimize or eliminate dead space where exudate, serum, or air could accumulate, thereby predisposing the wound to infection. When dead space cannot be eliminated with sutures, a drain may provide a suitable exit for the fluid, or a pressure bandage may diminish the dead space (Figure 4.6).

Sutures are foreign material and, therefore, cause variable tissue reaction that may be exacerbated in the presence of tissue trauma and infection. Moreover, suture material itself may act as a nidus for infection and may contribute to the formation of biofilm.[182] Generally, synthetic absorbable and non-absorbable suture materials cause less reaction than do sutures composed of a natural substance. Monofilament suture causes less tissue drag and tissue reaction than do twisted or braided sutures. The suture pattern used to close a wound may damage tissue and, therefore, must be carefully selected according to the wound's characteristics. The reader is referred to Chapter 9 for more information about suture materials, suturing techniques, and drains.

Dressings and bandages

Bandages are usually comprised of a primary layer (the dressing), a secondary layer that absorbs exudate not absorbed by the dressing and provides protection and some support, and a tertiary layer that compresses and holds the other layers in place. The reader is referred to Chapter 6 for more information about wound dressings.

Bandages that are applied too tightly may restrict blood flow and delay healing, whereas bandages applied too loosely may insufficiently restrict movement where stabilization is required or may slip and irritate the wound or damage adjacent structures, such as tendons. Changing bandages too frequently not only inflates the cost of wound management but may also damage fragile migrating epithelial cells that have not yet firmly attached to the underlying wound. The reader is referred to Chapter 7 for more information about techniques of bandaging and casting.

Full-thickness wounds on the distal aspect of the limb of horses are more likely to develop EGT when covered with a bandage or cast than are similar wounds left unbandaged.[183–188] EGT develops because bandaging or casting induces the following: 1) the oxygen gradient between the deeper tissues and the surface of the wound is increased, stimulating angiogenesis; 2) oxygen tension in the wound's tissues is reduced, enhancing proliferation of fibroblasts; and 3) a moist, warm, and acidic environment is created, favoring cellular migration and proliferation. Furthermore, some dressings may irritate the wound, evoking more inflammation, or cause exudate to accumulate at the

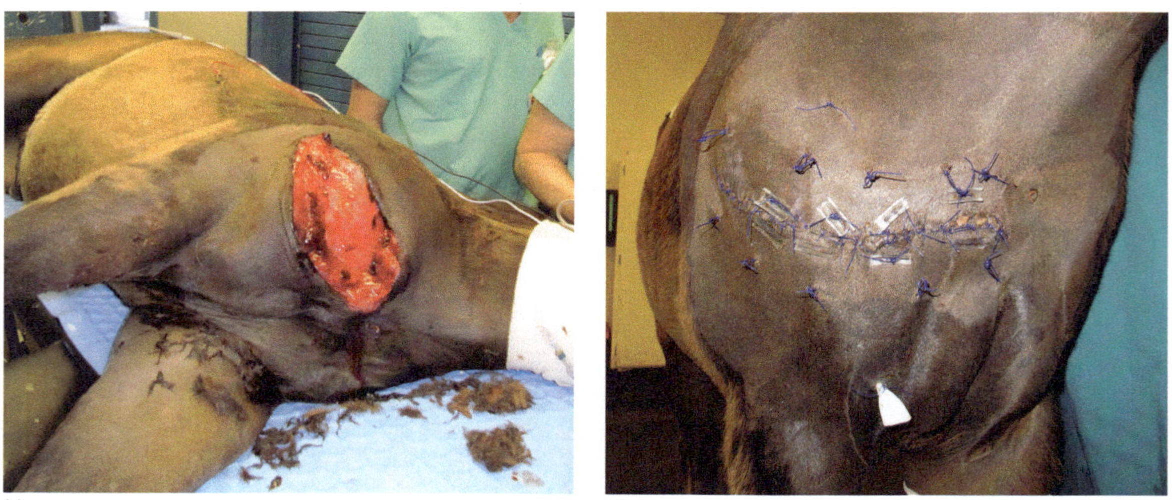

(a) (b)

Figure 4.6 **(a)** Example of an acute and mildly contaminated wound. After sharp debridement the wound was closed primarily. Due to the location over the point of the shoulder the wound was under tension. **(b)** A combination of tension-relieving sutures (near–far–far–near and vertical mattress), in addition to four horizontal mattress sutures with rubber stents, were used to reduce the risk of dehiscence. Suture loops were placed 10 cm above and below the suture line in order to secure a stent bandage to prevent contamination and to reduce edema (stent bandage not shown). A drain was used and made to exit ventral to the wound and away from the suture line, to achieve effective drainage of the dead space. The drain was sutured in place (topmost suture and ventral suture at the exit point of the Penrose drain).

wound's surface. In this respect, management practices can explain, at least partially, why EGT is more often seen in limb wounds, which are usually bandaged, than in body wounds, which are not commonly bandaged. Readers are referred to Chapter 15 for more information about EGT.

Although bandages and casts promote the formation of EGT, this does not preclude their use in managing wounds. To the contrary, bandages exert many positive influences on healing. They keep the wound clean and prevent contamination and irritation by environmental factors, such as dirt and straw, all of which induce inflammation. They facilitate administration of local wound therapies, stimulate more rapid formation of granulation tissue, which is required for healing, accelerate epithelialization by creating a moist environment, encourage the development of a more cosmetic scar, reduce the risk for sarcoid transformation of the wound, and protect the wound from trauma. Moreover, when the EGT is trimmed regularly, overall wound healing does not appear delayed, at least in small wounds created experimentally in horses.[188–190] Larger clinical wounds should be bandaged when appropriate, but bandages should be removed as soon as practical after a healthy bed of infection-resistant granulation tissue forms, to avoid the development of EGT.

Conclusion

Normal wound healing is comprised of a well-orchestrated series of events that ultimately lead to repair of injured tissues. The healing of wounds of horses, particularly those wounds on the distal aspect of the limb, can be problematic because horses have a weak acute inflammatory response that negatively impacts the subsequent phases of healing. Moreover, wounds in this location are characterized by a relatively poor blood supply, are often heavily contaminated, and often characterized by substantial damage, all of which may complicate normal healing.

Infection is the single most likely cause of delayed healing of open wounds. Infection-related delays are further complicated by the difficulty in eradicating biofilms and by the increasingly prevalent phenomenon of antibiotic resistance. By using an appropriate and careful approach to wound management, the veterinarian can influence the outcome of healing; specifically, by properly preparing, exploring, irrigating, and debriding the wound, the risk of wound infection and the likelihood of development of biofilm can be reduced substantially.

References

1. van Galen G, Delguste C, Sandersen C, *et al.* Tetanus in the equine species: a retrospective study of 31 cases. *Tijdschr Diergeneeskd* 2008; **133**: 512.
2. Pesquito M, Amory H, de Moffarts B, *et al.* Evaluation of acepromazine-induced hemodynamic alterations and reversal with norepinephrine infusion in standing horses. *Can Vet J* 2013; **54**: 150.
3. Sandersen C, Mouithys-Mickalad A, de la Rebiere G, *et al.* Modulating effects of acepromazine on the reactive oxygen species production by stimulated equine neutrophils. *Vet Anesth Analg* 2011; **38**: 83.
4. Wilmink JM, Veenman JN, van den Boom R *et al.* Differences in polymorphonucleocyte function and local inflammatory response between horses and ponies. *Equine Vet J* 2003; **35**: 561.
5. Johnson SM, Saint John BE, Dine AP. Local anesthetics as antimicrobial agents. *Surg Infect (Larchmt)* 2008; **9**: 205.
6. Hanci V, Hakimogiu S, Ozacmak H, *et al.* Comparison of bupivacaine, lidocaine and tramadol infiltration on wound healing in rats. *Rev Bras Anesthesiol* 2012; **62**: 799.
7. Waite A, Gillver SC, Masterson GR, *et al.* Clinically relevant doses of lidocaine do not impair cutaneous healing on mice. *Br J Anaesth* 2010; **104**: 768.
8. Rodrigues FV, Hochman B, Wood VT, *et al.* Effects of lidocaine with epinephrine or with buffer on wound healing in rat skin. *Wound Repair Regen* 2011; **19**: 223.
9. Eriksson AS, Sinclair R, Cassuto J, *et al.* Influence of lidocaine on leukocyte function in the surgical wound. *Anesthesiol* 1992; **77**: 74.
10. University of British Columbia. Bupivicaine versus lidocaine anaesthesia. *Clin Trials US Nat Inst Health.* https://clinicaltrials.gov/ct2/show/NCT01751347 (accessed April 2015).
11. Ribeiro PD Jr, Sanches MG, Okamoto T. Comparative analysis of tissue reactions to anesthetic solutions: histological analysis in subcutaneous tissue of rats. *Anesth Prog* 2003; **50**: 169.
12. Blanke W, Hallern BV. Sharp wound debridement in local anaesthesia using EMLA cream: 6 years' experience in 1084 patients. *Eur J Emerg Med* 2003; **10**: 229.
13. Erkert RS, Macallister CG, Campbell G, *et al.* Comparison of topical lidocaine/prilocaine anesthetic cream for local infiltration of 2% lidocaine for episioplasty in mares. *J Vet Pharmacol Ther* 2005; **28**: 299.
14. Eugster S, Schawalder P, Gasche F, Boerlin P. A prospective study of postoperative surgical site infections in dogs and cats. *Vet Surg* 2004; **33**: 542.
15. Brown DC, Conzemius MG, Shofer FS, *et al.* Epidemiologic evaluation of postoperative wound infections in dogs and cats. *J Am Vet Med Assoc* 1997; **210**: 1302.
16. Nicholson M, Beal M, Shofer F, *et al.* Epidemiologic evaluation of postoperative wound infection in clean contaminated wounds: a retrospective study of 239 dogs and cats. *Vet Surg* 2002; **31**: 577.
17. Beal MW, Brown DC, Shofer FS. The effects of perioperative hypothermia and the duration of anesthesia on postoperative wound infection rate in clean wounds: a retrospective study. *Vet Surg* 2000; **29**: 123.
18. Wilson DA, Baker GJ, Boero MJ. Complications of celiotomy incisions in horses. *Vet Surg* 1995; **24**: 506.
19. MacDonald DG, Morley PS, Bailey JV, *et al.* An examination of occurrence of surgical wound infection following orthopaedic surgery. *Equine Vet J* 1994; **26**: 323.
20. Kotani N, Hashimoto H, Sessler DI, *et al.* Intraoperative modulation of alveolar macrophage function during isoflurane and propofol anesthesia. *Anesthesiol* 1998; **89**: 1125.
21. Ciepichal J, Kubler A. Effect of general and regional anesthesia on some neutrophil functions. *Arch Immunol Ther Exp* 1998; **46**: 183.

22. Allen DB, Maguire JJ, Madhavian M, *et al.* Wound hypoxia and acidosis limit neutrophil bacterial killing mechanisms. *Arch Surg* 1997; **132**: 991.
23. Koutsoumbelis S, Hughes AP, Giarardi FP, *et al.* Risk factors for post-operative infection following posterior lumbar instrumented arthrodesis. *J Bone Joint Surg* 2011; **93**: 1627.
24. Costa-Farre C, Prades M, Ribera T, *et al.* Does intraoperative low partial pressure of oxygen increased the risk of surgical site infection following exploratory laparotomy in horses? *Vet J* 2014; **200**: 175.
25. Tanner J, Norrie P, Melen K. Preoperative hair removal to reduce surgical site infection. *Cochrane Database Syst Rev* 2011; Nov 9: CD004122 doi: 10. 1002/4651858.CD004122.pub4.
26. Hague BA, Honnas CM, Simpson RB, Peloso JG. Evaluation of skin bacterial flora before and after aseptic preparation of clipped and non-clipped arthrocentesis sites in horses. *Vet Surg* 1997; **26**: 121.
27. Hamilton HW, Hamilton KR, Lone FH. Preoperative hair removal. *Can J Surg* 1977; **20**: 269.
28. Rani SA, Hoon R, Najafi RR, *et al.* The *in vitro* antimicrobial activity of wound and skin cleansers at nontoxic concentrations. *Adv Skin Wound Care* 2014; **27**: 65.
29. Zubrod CJ, Farnsworth KD, Oaks JL. Evaluation of arthrocentesis site bacterial flora before and after 4 methods of preparation in horses with and without skin contamination. *Vet Surg* 2004; **33**: 525.
30. Davids BI, Davidson MJ, TenBroeck SH, *et al.* Efficacy of mechanical versus non-mechanical sterile preoperative skin preparation with chlorhexidine gluconate 4% solution. *Vet Surg* 2015; **44**: 648.
31. Lemarie RJ, Hosgood G. Antiseptics and disinfectants in small animal practice. *Comp Contin Educ Pract Vet* 1995; **17**: 1339.
32. Dumville JC, McFarlane E, Edwards P, *et al.* Preoperative skin antiseptics for preventing surgical wound infections after clean surgery. *Cochrane Database Syst Review* 2015; **21**:CD003949. doi:10.1002/14651858.CD003949.pub4.
33. Phinney RB, Mondino BJ, Hofbauer JD, *et al.* Corneal edema related to accidental hibiclens exposure. *Am J Opthalmol* 1988; **106**: 210.
34. Nasser RE. The ocular danger of hibiclens (chlorhexidine). *Plast Reconstr Surg* 1992; **89**: 164.
35. Osuna DJ, De Young DJ, Walker RL. Comparison of 3 skin preparation techniques in the dog, Part 2: Clinical trial in 100 dogs. *Vet Surg* 1990; **19**: 20.
36. McDonnell G, Russell AD. Antiseptics and disinfectants: activity, action and resistance. *Clin Microbiol Rev* 1999; **12**: 147.
37. de la Cuadra-Oyanguran J, Zaragoza-Ninet V, Sierra-Talamantes C, Alegre de Miguel V. Post-surgical contact dermatitis due to povidone iodine: a diagnostic dilemma. *Actas Dermosifiliograficas* 2014; **105**: 300.
38. Hennig GE, Kraus BH, Fister R, *et al.* Comparison of two methods for presurgical disinfection of the equine hoof. *Vet Surg* 2001; **30**: 366.
39. Johnson J, Messier S, Meulyzer M, *et al.* Effect of presurgical iodine-based disinfection on bacterial colonization of the equine peripodal region. *Vet Surg* 2015; **44**: 756.
40. Hayes GM, Reynolds D, Moens NH, *et al.* Investigation of incidence and risk factors for surgical glove perforation in small animal surgery. *Vet Surg* 2014; **43**: 400.
41. Tanner J, Swarbrook S, Stuart J. Surgical hand antisepsis to reduce surgical site infection. *Cochrane Database Syst Rev* 2008 Jan 23;(**1**):CD004288. doi: 10.1002/14651858.CD004288.pub2.
42. Verwilghen D, Grulke S, Kaempf G. Presurgical hand antisepsis. Concepts and current habits of veterinary surgeons. *Concepts and current habits of veterinary surgeons. Vet Surg* 2011; **40**: 515.
43. Wan PY, Blackford JT, Bemis DA, *et al.* Evaluation of surgical scrub methods for large animal surgeons. *Vet Surg* 1997; **26**: 382.
44. WHO guidelines on hand hygiene in health care. First global patient safety challenge clean care is safer care. *World Health Org* 2009. http://www.ncbi.nim.nih.gov/books/NBK144036/ (accessed June 2, 2015).
45. Verwilghen DR, Mainil J, Mastrococco E, *et al.* Surgical hand antisepsis in veterinary practice: evaluation of soap scrub and alcohol rub techniques. *Vet J* 2011; **190**: 372.
46. Almeida da Silveira E, Bubeck KA, Batista ER, *et al.* Comparison of an alcohol-based hand rub and water-based chlorhexidine gluconate scrub technique for hand antisepsis prior to elective surgery in horses. *Can Vet J* 2016; **57**: 164.
47. Edwards RA, Howe L, Frellstedt L, *et al.* Comparison of a waterless hand sanitation product (Avagard™) with a traditional chlorhexidine technique for pre-surgical hand preparation for equine surgery. In preparation 2015.
48. Parienti JJ, Thibon P, Heller R, *et al.* Hand-rubbing with an aqueous alcoholic solution vs traditional surgical hand-scrubbing and 30-day surgical site infection rates: a randomized equivalence study. *J Am Med Assoc* 2002; **288**: 722.
49. Rodeheaver GT. Wound cleansing, wound irrigation, wound disinfection. In: Krasner D, Rodeheaver G, Sibbald G (eds). *Chronic Wound Care*, 3rd edn. HMP Communications: Wayne, 2001: 389.
50. Owens BD, Wenck JC. Early wound irrigation improves the ability to remove bacteria. *J Bone Joint Surg* 2007; **89**: 1723.
51. Mak SS, Lee MY, Cheung JS, *et al.* Pressured irrigation versus swabbing method in cleansing wounds healed by secondary intention: a randomised controlled trial with cost effectiveness analysis. *Int J Nurs Stud* 2015; **52**: 88.
52. Chatterjee JS. A critical review of irrigation techniques in acute wounds. *Int Wound J* 2005; **2**: 258.
53. Barnes S, Spencer M, Graham D, Boehm-Johnson H. Surgical wound irrigation: a call for evidence-based standardization of practice. *Am J Infect Control* 2014; **42**: 525.
54. Kalteis T, Lehn N, Schroder H-J, *et al.* Contaminant seeding in bone by different irrigation methods: an experimental study. *J Orthop Trauma* 2005; **19**: 591.
55. Hassinger SM, Harding G, Wongworawat MD. High pressure pulsatile lavage propagates bacteria into soft tissue. *Clin Orthop Relat Res* 2005; **439**: 27.
56. Boyd JI, Wongawarowat MD. High pressure pulsatile lavage causes soft tissue damage. *Clin Orthop Relat Res* 2004; **427**: 13.
57. Allen D, LaBarbera LA, Bondre IL, *et al.* Comparison of tissue damage, cleansing and cross contamination potential during wound cleansing via two methods: lavage and negative pressure would therapy with instillation. *Int Wound J* 2014; **11**: 198.
58. Singer A, Hollander J, Subramanian S, *et al.* Pressure dynamics of various irrigation techniques commonly used in the emergency department. *Ann Emerg Med* 1994; **1**: 36.
59. Anglien JO. Wound irrigation in musculoskeletal injury. *J Am Acad Orthop Surg* 2001; **9**: 219.

60. Fernandez R, Griffiths R. Tap water for wound cleansing. *Cochrane Database Syst Rev.* 2012 Feb 15;**2**:CD003861. doi: 10.1002/14651858.CD003861.pub3
61. White RJ, Cutting K, Kingsley A. Topical antimicrobials in the control of wound bioburden: part 1. *Ostomy Wound Manage* 2006; **52**: 26.
62. Brennan SS, Leaper DJ. The effect of antiseptics on the healing wound: a study using the rabbit ear model. *Br J Surg* 1985; **72**: 780.
63. Lineaweaver WL, McMorris S, Soucy D, *et al.* Cellular and bacterial toxicities of topical antimicrobials. *Plast Reconst Surg* 1985; **75**: 394.
64. Teepe RGC, Koebrugge ES, Lowick CW, *et al.* Cytotoxic effects of topical antimicrobial and antiseptic agents on human keratinocytes *in vitro*. *J Trauma* 1993; **35**: 8.
65. Thomas GW, Rael LT, Bar-Or R, *et al.* Mechanisms of delayed wound healing by commonly used antiseptics. *J Trauma* 2009; **66**: 82.
66. Wilkins RG, Unversorben M. Wound cleaning and wound healing: a concise review. *Adv Skin Wound Care* 2013; **26**: 160.
67. Angel DE, Morey P, Storer JG, Mwipatayi BP. The great debate over iodine in wound care continues: a review of the literature. *Wound Pract Res* 2008; **16**: 6.
68. Khan NM. Antiseptics, iodine, povidone iodine and traumatic wound cleansing. *J Tiss Viabil* 2006; **16**: 6.
69. Welch J. Efficacy and safety of povidone-iodine underscored [Letter]. *J Emerg Nurs* 1992; **18**: 191.
70. Sanchez IR, Swaim SF, Nusbaum KE, *et al.* Effects of chlorhexidine diacetate and povidone–iodine on wound healing in dogs. *Vet Surg* 1988; **17**: 291.
71. Cookson BD, Bolton MC, Platt JH. Chlorhexidine resistance in methicillin-resistant *Staphylococcus aureus* or just an elevated MIC? An *in vitro* and *in vivo* assessment. *Antimicrob Agents Chemother* 1991; **35**: 1997.
72. Prince HN, Nonemaker WS, Norgard RC. Drug resistance studies with topical antiseptics. *J Pharm Sci* 1978; **67**: 1629.
73. Bonez PC, Dos Santos Alves CR, Dalmolin TV, *et al.* Chlorhexidine activity against bacterial biofilms. *Am J Infect Control* 2013; **41**: e119.
74. Drosou A, Falabella A, Kirsner RS. Antiseptics on wounds: an area of controversy. *Wounds* 2003; **15**: 149.
75. Lozier S, Pope E, Berg J. Effects of four preparations of 0.05% chlorhexidine diacetate on wound healing in dogs. *Vet Surg* 1992; **21**: 107.
76. Amber EI, Hendersen RA, Swaim SF, *et al.* A comparison of antimicrobial efficacy and tissue reaction of four antiseptics on canine wounds. *Vet Surg* 1983; **12**: 63.
77. Vincze S, Stamm I, Kopp PA, *et al.* Alarming proportions of methicillin-resistant *Staphylococcus aureus* (MRSA) in wound samples from companion animals. Germany 2010–2012. *PLoS One* 2014; **9**: e85656.
78. Bergstrom K, Bengtsson B, Nyman A, *et al.* Longitudinal study of horses for carriage of methicillin-resistant *Staphylococcus aureus* following wound infection. *Vet Microbiol* 2013; **163**: 388.
79. Woods EJ, Cochrane CA, Percival SL. Prevalence of silver resistance genes in bacteria isolated from human and horse wounds. *Vet Microbiol* 2009; **138**: 325.
80. Rodeheaver GT, Smith SL, Thacker JG, *et al.* Mechanical cleansing of contaminated wounds with a surfactant. *Am J Surg* 1975; **129**: 341.
81. Edlich RF, Woodard CR, Pine SA, Lin KY. Hazards of powder on surgical and examination gloves: a collective review. *J Long Term Eff Med Implants* 2001; **11**: 15.
82. Stashak TS. Wound infection: contributing factors and selected techniques for prevention. *Proc Am Assoc Eq Pract* 2006; **52**: 270.
83. Wounds UK. Effective debridement in a changing NHS: a UK consensus. http://www.wounds-uk.com/pdf/content_10761.pdf (accessed May 25, 2015).
84. Leaper DJ, Schultz G, Carville K, *et al.* Extending the TIME concept: what have we learned in the past 12 years. *Int Wound J* 2012; **9** Suppl 2: 1.
85. Broadus C. Debridement options: BEAMS made easy. *Wound Care Advisor* 2013; **2**: 15.
86. Pain R, Sneddon JC, Cochrane CA. *In vitro* study of the effectiveness of different dressings for debriding fibrin in blood clots from horses. *Vet Record* 2006; **159**: 712.
87. Ramundo J, Gray M. Enzymatic wound debridement. *J Wound Ostomy Contin Nurs* 2008; **35**: 273.
88. Kirshen C, Woo K, Ayello EA, *et al.* Debridement: a vital component of wound bed preparation. *Adv Skin Wound Care* 2006; **19**: 506.
89. Smith RG. Enzymatic debriding agents: an evaluation of the medical literature. *Ostomy Wound Manage* 2008; **54**: 16.
90. Shi L, Ermis R, Kiedaisch B, Carson D. The effects of various wound dressings on the activity of debriding enzymes. *Adv Skin Wound Care* 2010; **23**: 456.
91. Skärlina EM, Wilmink JM, Fall N, *et al.* Effectiveness of conventional and hydrosurgical debridement methods in reducing *Staphylococcus aureus* inoculation of equine muscle *in vitro*. *Equine Vet J* 2015; **47**: 218.
92. Rennekampff HO, Schaller HE, Wisser D, Tenenhaus M. Debridement of burn wounds with a water jet surgical tool. *Burns* 2006; **32**: 64.
93. Mosti G, Iabichella ML, Picerni P, *et al.* The debridement of hard to heal leg ulcers by means of a new device based on Fluidjet technology. *Int Wound* 2005; **2**: 307.
94. Oosthuizen B, Mole T, Martin R, *et al.* Comparison of standard surgical debridement versus the Versajet Plus™ hydrosurgery system in the treatment of open tibia fractures: a prospective open label randomized controlled trial. *Int J Burns Trauma* 2014; **4**: 53.
95. Granick MS, Postnett J, Jacoby M, *et al.* Efficacy and cost effectiveness of a high powered parallel waterjet for wound debridement. *Wound Repair Regen* 2006; **14**: 394.
96. Hyland EJ, D'Cruz R, Menon S, *et al.* Prospective, randomised controlled trial comparing Versajet™ hydrosurgery and conventional debridement of partial thickness paediatric burns. *Burns* 2015; **41**: 700.
97. Bowling FL, Stockings DS, Edwards-Jones V, *et al.* Hydrodebridement of wounds: effectiveness in reducing wound bacterial contamination and potential for air bacterial contamination. *Foot Ankle Surg* 2009; **2**: 13.
98. Sonnegren HH, Strombeck L, Aldenborg F, Faergemann J. Aerolized spread of bacteria and reduction in bacterial wound contamination with three different methods of surgical wound debridement: a pilot study. *J Hosp Infect* 2013; **85**; 112.
99. Shannon MK, Williams A, Bloomer M. Low-frequency ultrasound debridement (Sonica-185) in acute wound management: a case study. *Wound Pract Res* 2012; **20**: 200.

100. Amini S, ShoajeeFard A, Annabestani Z, *et al.* Low-frequency ultrasound debridement in patients with diabetic foot ulcers and osteomyelitis. *Wounds* 2013; **25**: 193.
101. Butcher G. Pinnuck L. Wound bed preparation: ultrasonic-assisted debridement. *Br J Nurs* 2013; **22**: S37–S43.
102. Sun X, Jiang K, Chen J, *et al.* Systematic review of maggot debridement therapy for chronically infected wounds and ulcers. *Int J Inf Dis* 2014; **25**: 32.
103. Lepage OM, Doumbia A, Perron Lepage MF, *et al.* The use of maggot debridement therapy in 41 equids. *Equine Vet J* 2012; **43**: 120.
104. Daeschlein G, Mumcouglu KY, Asadian O, *et al. In vitro* antibacterial activity of *Lucilia sericata* maggot secretions. *Skin Pharmacol Physiol* 2007; **20**: 112.
105. Bexfield A, Nigam Y, Thomas S, Ratcliffe NA. Detection and partial characterization of two antibacterial factors from the excretions/secretions of the medicinal maggot *Lucilia sericata* and their activity against methicillin-resistant *Staphylococcus aureus* (MRSA). *Microbes Infect* 2004; **6**: 1297.
106. Cazander G, van de Veerdonk M, Vandenbroucke-Grauls C, *et al.* Maggot excretions inhibit biofilm formation on biomaterials. *Clin Orthop Relat Res* 2010; **468**: 2789.
107. Allen D, LaBarbera LA, Bondre IL, *et al.* Comparison of tissue damage cleansing and cross-contamination potential during wound cleansing via two methods: lavage and negative pressure wound therapy with instillation. *Int Wound J* 2014; **11**: 198.
108. European Wound Management Association Position Document. *Management of Wound Infection*. MEP Ltd: London, 2006.
109. Weese JS, Lefebvre SL. Risk factors for methicillin-resistant *Staphylococcus aureus* colonization in horses admitted to a veterinary teaching hospital. *Can Vet J.* 2007; **48**: 921.
110. Barr BS, Waldridge BM, Morresy PR, *et al.* Antimicrobial-associated diarrhoea in three equine referral practices. *Equine Vet J* 2013; **45**: 154.
111. Baverud V, Gustafsson A, Franklin A, *et al. Clostridium difficile* associated with acute colitis in mature horses treated with antibiotics. *Equine Vet J* 1997; **29**: 279.
112. American Society of Health-System Pharmacists therapeutic guidelines on antimicrobial prophylaxis in surgery. *Am J Health-Syst Pharm* 1999; **56**: 1839.
113. Bratzler DW, Houck PM. Antimicrobial prophylaxis for surgery: an advisory statement from the National Surgical Infection Prevention Project. *Am J Surg* 2005; **189**: 395.
114. Weese JS, Cruz A. Retrospective study of perioperative antimicrobial use practices in horses undergoing elective arthroscopic surgery at a veterinary teaching hospital. *Can Vet J* 2009; **50**: 185.
115. Borg H, Carmalt JL. Postoperative septic arthritis after elective equine arthroscopy without antimicrobial prophylaxis. *Vet Surg* 2013; **42**: 262.
116. Olds AM, Stewart AA, Freeman DE, Schaeffer DJ. Evaluation of the rate of development of septic arthritis after elective arthroscopy in horses: 7 cases (1994–2003). *J Am Vet Med Assoc* 2006; **229**: 1949.
117. Southwood LL. Perioperative antimicrobials: should we be concerned about antimicrobial drug use in equine surgical patients. *Equine Vet J* 2014; **46**: 267.
118. Bratzler DW, Houck PM. Antimicrobial prophylaxis for surgery: an advisory statement from the National Surgical Infection Prevention Project. *Clin Infect Dis* 2004; **38**: 1706.
119. Bratzler DW, Dellinger EP, Olsen KM, *et al.* Clinical practice guidelines for antimicrobial practice in surgery. *Am J Health Syst Pharm* 2013; **70**: 195.
120. Horspool LJ, McKellar QA. Disposition of penicillin G sodium following intravenous and oral administration to *Equidae*. *Br Vet J* 1995; **151**: 401.
121. Love DN, Rose RJ, Martin CA, Bailey M. Serum concentrations of penicillin in the horse after administration of a variety of penicillin preparations. *Equine Vet J* 1983; **15**: 43.
122. Magdesian KG, Hogan P, Cohen ND, *et al.* Pharmacokinetics of a high dose of gentamicin administered intravenously or intramuscularly to horses. *J Am Vet Med Assoc* 1998; **213**: 1007.
123. Fernandez AH, Monge V, Garcinuno MA. Surgical antibiotic prophylaxis: effect in postoperative infections. *Eur J Epidemiol* 2001; **17**: 369.
124. Walter WP, Weber WR, Marti M, *et al.* The timing of surgical antimicrobial prophylaxis. *Ann of Surg* 2008; **247**: 918.
125. Bratzler DW, Houck PM, Richards C, *et al.* Use of antimicrobial prophylaxis for major surgery: baseline results from the National Surgical Infection Prevention Project. *Arch Surg* 2005; **140**: 174.
126. Brown DC, Conzemius MG, Shofer F, Swann H. Epidemioloic evaluation of postoperative wound infections in dogs and cats. *J Am Vet Med Assoc* 1997; **210**: 1302.
127. Durward-Akhurst SA, Mair TS, Boston R, *et al.* Comparison of two antimicrobial regimens on the prevalence of incisional infections after colic surgery. *Vet Rec* 2013; **172**: 287.
128. Freeman KD, Southwood LL, Lane J, *et al.* Post-operative infection, pyrexia and perioperative antimicrobial drug use in surgical colic patients. *Equine Vet J* 2012; **44**: 476.
129. United States Department of Agriculture Report: Equine 2005, Part I: Baseline Reference of Equine Health and Management, 2005. http://www.aphis.usda.gov/animal_health/nahms/equine/downloads/equine05/Equine05_dr_PartI.pdf. Accessed January 2016.
130. Hughes LA, Pinchbeck G, Callaby R, *et al.* Antimicrobial prescribing practice in UK equine veterinary practice. *Equine Vet J* 2013; **45**: 141.
131. Ross SE, Duz M, Rendle DI. Antimicrobial selection and dosing in the treatment of wounds in the United Kingdom. *Equine Vet J* 2015 Dec 25. doi: 10.1111/evj.12535. [Epub ahead of print]
132. Leaper D, Assadian O, Edmiston CE. Approach to chronic wound infections. *Br J Dermatol* 2015; **173**: 351.
133. Siddiqui AR, Bernstein JM. Chronic wound infection: facts and controversies. *Clin Dermatol* 2010; **28**: 519.
134. Fernandes A, Dias M. The microbiological profile of infected prosthetic implants with emphasis on which organisms form biofilms. *J Clin Diagn Res* 2013; **7**: 219.
135. Westgate SJ, Percival SL, Knottenbelt DR, *et al.* Microbiology of equine wounds and evidence of bacterial biofilms. *Vet Microbiol* 2011; **150**: 152.
136. Weese JS, Baptiste KE, Baverud V, Toutain PL. *Guidelines for Antimicrobial Use in Horses*. Blackwell Publishing: Oxford, 2008: 161.
137. Wilson WD. Rational selection of antimicrobials for use in horses. *Proc Am Assoc Equine Pract Ann Conv* 2001; **47**: 75.
138. Specht TE, Frederick G. Quinolone-induced arthropathy in immature *Equidae*. *J Am Vet Assoc* 1991; **198**: 516.

139. Selwyn S. Microbial interactions and antibiosis. In: Maibach H, Aly R (eds). *Skin Microbiology: Relevance to Clinical Infection.* Springer-Verlag: New York, 1981: 63.
140. Eriksson G, Ekland A, Kallings L. The clinical significance of bacterial growth in venous leg ulcers. *Scand J Infect Dis* 1984; **16**: 175.
141. Niedner R. Cytotoxicity and sensitization of povidone iodine and other frequently used anti-infective agents. *Dermatol* 1997; **195**: 89.
142. Muller G, Kramer A. Biocompatibility index of antiseptic agents by parallel assessment of antimicrobial activity and cellular cytotoxicity. *J Antimicrob Chemother* 2008; **61**: 1281.
143. White RJ, Cutting K, Kingsley A. Topical antimicrobials in the control of wound bioburden. *Ostomy Wound Manage* 2006; **52**: 26.
144. Spann CT, Taylor SC, Weinberg JM. Topical antimicrobial agents in dermatology. *Dis Mon* 2004; **50**: 407
145. Neely AN, Gardiner J, Durkee P, *et al.* Are topical antimicrobials effective against bacteria that are highly resistant to systemic antibiotics? *J Burn Care Res* 2009; **30**: 19.
146. Lipsky BA, Hoey C. Topical antimicrobial therapy for treating chronic wounds. *Clin Infect Dis* 2009; **49**: 1541.
147. Wolcott RD, Rumbaugh KP, James G, *et al.* Biofilm maturity studies indicate sharp debridement opens a time-dependent therapeutic window. *J Wound Care* 2010; **19**: 320.
148. Roche ED, Renick PJ, Tetens SP, Carson DL. A model for evaluating topical antimicrobial efficacy against methicillin-resistant *Staphylococcus aureus* biofilms in superficial murine wounds. *Antimicrob Agents Chemother* 2012; **56**: 4508.
149. Hajska M, Slobodnikova L, Hupkova H, Koller J. *In vitro* efficacy of various topical antimicrobial agents in different time periods from contamination to application against 6 multi-drug resistant bacterial strains isolated from burn patients. *Burns* 2014; **40**: 713.
150. Blood DC, Studdert VP. *Comprehensive Veterinary Dictionary,* 4th edn. *WB Saunders Co: London* 2011; **1–1334**.
151. World Health Organization. *Antimicrobial Fact Sheet 194 (updated April 2015).* http://www.who.int/mediacentre/fact sheets/fs194/en/ (accessed June 1, 2015).
152. Amato-Gauci A, Ammon A. Antimicrobial resistance. *The First European Communicable Disease Epidemiological Report.* European Centre for Disease Prevention and Control: Stockholm 2007: 49.
153. Maddox TW, Scantlebury CE, Clegg PD, *et al.* A review of the characteristics and treatment of methicillin-resistant *Staphylococcus aureus* (MRSA) in the horse and a case series of MRSA infection in 4 horses. *Equine Vet Educ* 2010; **22**: 91.
154. Bergström K, Bengtsson B, Nyman A, Grönlund Andersson U. Longitudinal study of horses for carriage of methicillin-resistant *Staphylococcus aureus* following wound infections. *Vet Microbiol* 2013; **163**: 388.
155. Axon JE, Carrick JB, Barton MD, *et al.* Methicillin resistant *Staphylococcus aureus* in a population of horses in Australia. *Aust Vet J* 2011; **89**: 211.
156. Bagcigil FA, Moodley A, Baptiste KE, *et al.* Occurrence, species distribution, antimicrobial resistance and clonality of methicillin and erythromycin resistant staphylococci in the nasal cavity of domestic animals. *Vet Microbiol* 2007; **121**: 307.
157. Tokataloff N, Manning ST, Weese JS, *et al.* Prevalence of methicillin-resistant *Staphylococcus aureus* colonization in horses in Saskatchewan, Alberta, and British Columbia. *Can Vet J* 2009; **50**: 1177.
158. Van den Eede A, Hermans K, Van den Abeele A, *et al.* Prevalence of methicillin-resistant *Staphylococcus aureus* (MRSA) on the skin of long-term hospitalized horses. *Vet J* 2012; **193**: 408.
159. Anzai T, Kamada M, Kanemaru T, *et al.* Isolation of methicillin-resistant *Staphylococcus aureus* (MRSA) from mares with metritis and its zooepidemiology. *J Equine Vet Sci* 1996; **7**: 7.
160. Weese JS. Methicillin-resistant *Staphylococcus aureus* in horses and horse personnel. *Vet Clin North Am* 2004; **20**: 601.
161. Hollis AR, Wilkins PA. Current controversies in equine antimicrobial therapy. *Equine Vet Educ* 2009; **21**: 216.
162. Sandulache VC, Parekh A, Li-Korotky JE, *et al.* Prostaglandin E2 inhibition of keloid fibroblast migration, contraction, and transforming growth factor (TGF)-β-1-induced collagen synthesis. *Wound Repair Regen* 2007; **15**: 122.
163. Dovi JV, He LK, DiPietro LA. Accelerated wound closure in neutrophil depleted mice. *J Leukoc Biol* 2003; **73**: 448.
164. Martin P, D'Sousa D, Martin J, *et al.* Wound healing in the PU.1 mouse – tissue repair is not dependant on inflammatory cells. *Curr Biol* 2003; **13**: 1122.
165. Robinson NE. Table of common drugs and approximate dosages. In: Sprayberry KA, Robinson NE (eds). *Current Therapy in Equine Medicine*, 7th edn. Elsevier: St Louis 2015: 933.
166. Marshall JF, Blikslager AT. The effect of non-steroidal anti-inflammatory drugs on the equine intestine. *Equine Vet J Suppl* 2011; **39**: 140.
167. Widgerow AD, Kalaria S. Pain mediators and wound healing – establishing the connection. *Burns* 2012; **38**: 951.
168. Broadbent E, Petrie KJ, Alley PG, *et al.* Psychological stress impairs early wound repair following surgery. *Psychosom Med* 2003; **65**: 865.
169. Ebrecht M, Hextall J, Kirtley LG, *et al.* Perceived stress and cortisol levels predict speed of wound healing in healthy male adults. *Psychoneuroendocrinol* 2004; **29**: 798.
170. Woo KY, Sibbald RG. Chronic wound pain: a conceptual model. *Adv Skin Wound Care* 2008; **21**: 175.
171. Blomme EA, Chinn KS, Hardy MN, *et al.* Selective cyclooxygenase inhibition does not affect the healing of cutaneous full-thickness incisional wounds in SKH-1 mice. *Br J Dermatol* 2003; **148**: 211.
172. Muscara MN, McKnight W, Asfaha S, Wallace JL. Wound collagen deposition in rats effects of an NO-NSAID and a selective COX-2 inhibitor. *Br J Pharmacol* 2000: **12**: 681.
173. Gorman HA, Wolf WA, Frost WW, *et al.* The effects of oxyphenybutazone on surgical wounds of the horse. *J Am Vet Med Assoc* 1968; **152**: 487.
174. Wilson DA, Baker GJ, Boero MJ. Complications of celiotomy incision in horses. *Vet Surg* 1995; **24**: 506.
175. Ong CKS, Lirk P, Seymour RA, *et al.* The efficacy of pre-emptive analgesia for acute postoperative pain management: a meta-analysis. *Anesth Analg* 2005; **100**: 757.
176. Hashimoto I, Nakanishi H, Shono Y, *et al.* Angiostatic effects of corticosteroid on wound healing of the rabbit ear. *J Med Invest* 2002; **49**: 61.

177. Wang AS, Armstrong EJ, Armstrong AW. Corticosteroids and wound healing: clinical considerations in the perioperative period. *Am J Surg* 2013; **206**: 410.
178. Kaufman KL, Mann FA, Kim DY, *et al.* Evaluation of the effects of topical zinc gluconate in wound healing. *Vet Surg* 2014; **43**: 972.
179. Mustoe TA, Cooter RD, Gold MH, *et al.* International Advisory Panel on Scar Management. International clinical recommendations on scar management. *Plast Reconstr Surg* 2002; **110**: 560.
180. Wilmink JM, Van Weeren PR. Treatment of exuberant granulation tissue. *Clin Tech Equine Pract* 2004; **3**: 141.
181. Alberti LR, Vasconcellos L de S, Petroianu A. Influence of local or systemic corticosteroids on skin wound healing resistance. *Acta Cir Bras* 2012; **27**: 295.
182. Konig L, Klopfleisch R, Kershaw O, Gruber AD. Prevalence of biofilms on surgical suture segments in wounds of dogs, cats and horses. *Vet Pathol* 2015; **215**: 295.
183. Fretz PB, Martin GS, Jacobs KA, *et al.* Treatment of exuberant granulation tissue in the horse evaluation of four methods. *Vet Surg* 1983; **12**: 137.
184. Bertone AL, Sulllins KE, Stashak TS, *et al.* Effect of wound location and use of topical collagen gel on exuberant granulation tissue formation and wound healing in the horse and pony. *Am J Vet Res* 1985; **46**: 1438.
185. Yvorchuk-ST Jean K, Gaughan E, St Jean G, *et al.* Evaluation of a porous bovine collagen membrane bandage for management of wounds in horses. *Am J Vet Res* 1995; **56**: 1663.
186. Theoret CL, Barber SM, Moyana TN, Gordon JR. Preliminary observations on expression of transforming growth factors beta1 and beta3 in equine full-thickness skin wounds healing normally or with exuberant granulation tissue. *Vet Surg* 2002; **31**: 266.
187. Berry DB, Sullins KE. Effects of topical application of antimicrobials on healing and granulation tissue formation in wounds of the distal aspect of the limbs in horses. *Am J Vet Res* 2003; **64**: 88.
188. Dart AJ, Perkins NR,Dart CM, *et al.* Effect of bandaging on second intention healing of wounds of the distal limb in horses. *Aust Vet J* 2009; **87**: 215.
189. Bischofberger AS, Dart CM, Perkins NR, *et al.* The effect of shorter and longer term treatment with manuka honey on second intention healing of contaminated and uncontaminated wounds on the distal aspect of the forelimbs in horses. *Vet Surg* 2013; **42**: 154.
190. Bischofberger AS, Dart CM, Horadagoda N, *et al.* The effect of manuka honey gel on the transforming growth factor β1 and β3 concentration, bacterial counts and histomorphology of contaminated full thickness wounds skin wounds in equine distal limbs. *Aust Vet J* 2016; **94**: 27.

CHAPTER 5

Topical Wound Treatments and Wound-Care Products

Stine Jacobsen, DVM, PhD, Diplomate ECVS

Chapter Contents

Equine Wound Management, Third Edition. Edited by Christine Theoret and Jim Schumacher.

Companion website: www.wiley.com/go/theoret/wound

Summary

Topical treatments have been used in wound care for centuries. Many of the treatments, however, have not – or only to a very limited degree – undergone scientific scrutiny. This is especially true for many of the products that are available over the counter. Determining the contents of many of these products can be difficult, and *as a rule of thumb, products without a list of ingredients should not be used on wounds.*

In contrast, effects of wound cleansers and solutions used for irrigation have been investigated in several studies. Although cleansers and antiseptics had, for some years, fallen out of favor due to their detrimental effects on cells cultured *in vitro*, current best evidence suggests that they may be of benefit if used judiciously. The negative impact on cell cultures has, in many studies, not been replicated when the products were used *in vivo*. Use of antiseptics on heavily contaminated or infected wounds seems to enhance healing through a reduction of the wound's bioburden.

Introduction

Products intended for topical application to wounds with the purpose of supporting and enhancing healing are plentiful in the wound-care market. Although effects of some products (e.g., wound cleansers and antiseptics) are well characterized and have been investigated *in vitro* and *in vivo* in numerous studies, the suggested benefits of other products are based on a much smaller body of evidence. Among the latter are many of the products of herbal origin and products whose purported effects rest on their content of vitamins and minerals, for which the manufacturers' claims to the efficacy of the products are based on limited scientific data. The same is true for several over-the-counter products sold through tack shops, for example the aerosol sprays used extensively by non-veterinarians for treatment of wounds that are perceived not to need veterinary attention. Using sound judgment and seeking out the best available evidence are, therefore, very important when choosing between the numerous topical wound-care products available. Topical agents should be applied to wounds to serve a specific purpose; this highlights the importance of a sound knowledge of the properties of the selected product and its proposed effects on the healing tissues. One very common approach is to apply antiseptics to any wound under the "better-safe-than-sorry" principle. This tactic is, however, inadvisable, as antiseptics may exert a negative influence on healing tissues. Antiseptics should thus be used only where necessary, i.e. in high-risk wounds and in contaminated or infected wounds, where the benefit of reducing wound bioburden outweighs potential negative side-effects on healing.

For technical reasons, it may be impossible to bandage wounds on the body or on the proximal limb of the horse. Consequently, topical wound-care products may be the only useful means to stimulate healing of wounds in these locations (Figure 5.1).

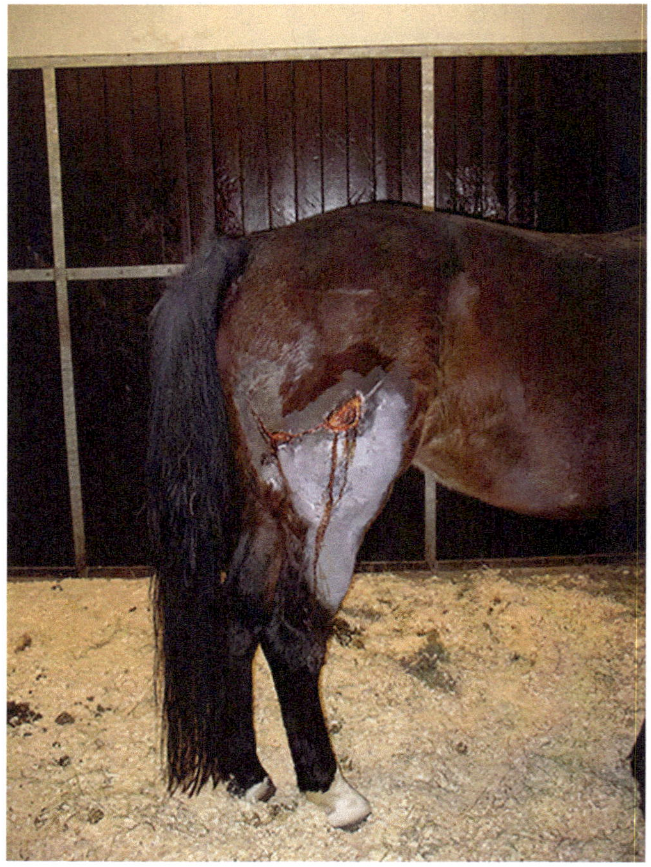

Figure 5.1 Wound on the thigh of a pony. The wound had dehisced partially after suturing. The location of this wound makes bandaging difficult. The simplest means of stimulating healing for such wounds is to apply topical products.

The purpose of this chapter is not to provide an exhaustive overview of all available products, as the sheer size of the market precludes such an endeavor. Rather, a selection of the most common products and those whose effects have been investigated in horses is presented, along with the available evidence for the effects of these selected products on healing tissues.

Wound cleansers and irrigation solutions

Foreign material, necrotic tissue, and microorganisms in the wound impede healing. The actions taken to remove these impediments are cleansing and debridement. *Cleansing*, also referred to as *wound irrigation*, involves the use of a fluid to remove loosely attached cellular debris and surface pathogens contained in wound exudate or residue from topically applied wound-care products, and *debridement* refers to the use of mechanical or chemical means to remove adherent material from the wound.

Every major supplier on the wound-care market sells a wound cleanser. In addition, a veritable myriad of products, also many over-the-counter products, are available from smaller companies. Obtaining information about the contents of different products to ascertain if the beneficial properties declared by the manufacturer hold true may be difficult.

Tip

- Only products that have been validated in scientific studies or products with known contents shown to enhance healing should be used on wounds.

Not all wounds need cleansing, and for some wounds, cleansing may traumatize fragile new tissue in the wound and the surrounding skin. For example, cleansing a clean granulating wound unnecessarily traumatizes the fragile granulation tissue. In human medicine, indications for wound cleansing have been described as:[1]

- removal of contaminants in the wound;
- removal of debris and foreign bodies after trauma;
- removal of debris and microorganisms in infected wounds;
- removal of superficial slough;
- removal of residues from dressing materials;
- removal of crusting and hyperkeratosis from the wound's edge and surrounding skin;
- removal of excess exudate and malodor;
- improvement of personal hygiene and patient comfort.

In wounds that need cleansing, wound cleansers serve important functions, and they thus deserve attention similar to that given dressings and other wound-care products. Cleansing a wound serves multiple purposes: it removes loose debris and bacteria, provides an optimal environment for healing, and facilitates assessment of the wound by optimizing its inspection. The ideal wound cleanser should be:

- hypoallergenic and non-toxic to viable tissue;
- readily available and cost effective;
- stable;
- effective in the presence of organic material, such as blood, slough, or necrotic tissue;
- capable of reducing the number of microorganisms in the wound;
- effective in removing debris, such as necrotic material and exudate.

The selected cleanser should be at body temperature prior to applying it to the wound. Wound temperature influences healing, with optimal healing occurring (in humans) at a temperature between 36 and 38 °C. Delayed healing may occur when the temperature of the wound falls below core body temperature or rises above 42 °C. Using cleansers and other solutions at temperatures lower than the core temperature can cause the temperature in the wound to be below body temperature for up to 40 minutes, and cellular division may take up to 3 hours to recommence.[2,3]

Cleansers can be applied either manually or by spraying/irrigating the wound (Figure 5.2). Using the former technique, wounds are gently wiped with swabs soaked in the cleanser; with the latter technique, the cleanser is delivered from a spray bottle, a syringe with needle, or another delivery device. When using the latter technique, the cleanser should be delivered with a pressure of no more than 15 pounds per square inch (psi), because a higher pressure tends to drive microorganisms into the wound. Appropriate pressure may be obtained with wound irrigation devices delivering specified pressures (Figure 5.3) or by attaching a 19-gauge needle to a 60-mL syringe (Figure 5.2). For more information about wound irrigation techniques, the reader is referred to Chapter 4. A study comparing cleansing of wounds, of humans, healing by second intention, by pressurized irrigation or by swabbing found that wounds cleaned by pressurized irrigation healed faster and that irrigation caused less pain and greater patient satisfaction than did swabbing. The incidence of wound infection in the two groups was similar.[4] When using the swabbing technique, the gauze swabs should be non-woven because woven gauze sheds more fibers into the wound.

Several different solutions can be used for cleansing wounds, such as isotonic saline solution, tap water, Ringer's solution, or solutions containing active ingredients. Wounds can also be cleansed with solutions containing antimicrobial agents, such as

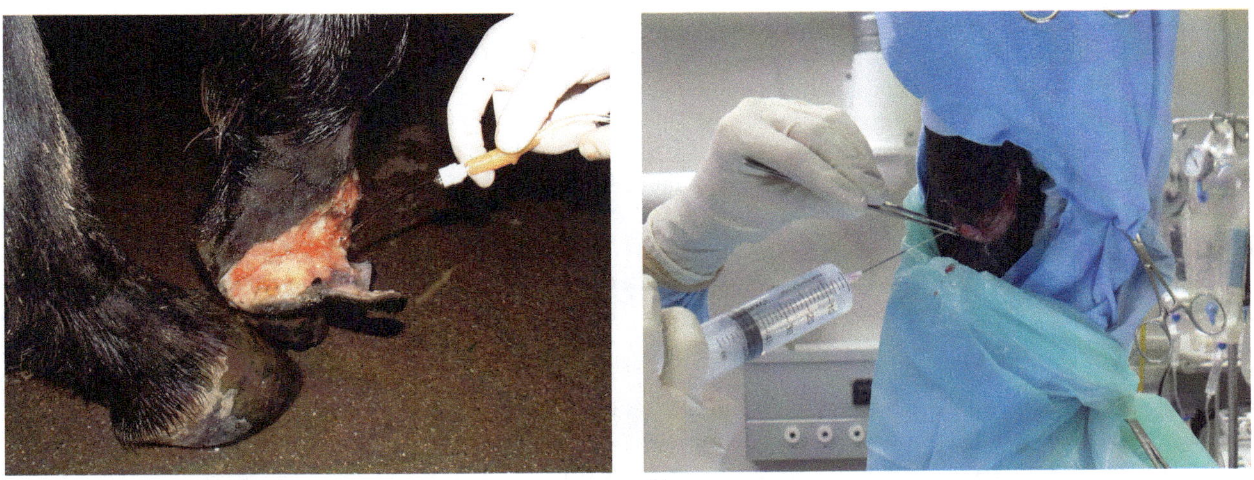

(a) (b)

Figure 5.2 **(a)** Irrigation of an acute wound using sterile isotonic saline solution. This type of passive gravity fluid flow does not provide sufficient pressure to remove contaminants or overcome the forces with which bacteria adhere to the wound. Photo courtesy of Denis Verwilghen. **(b)** To achieve an appropriate pressure (10–14 psi) fluid should be firmly expressed from a 60-mL syringe with a 19-gauge needle or through devices or spray bottles constructed to deliver the appropriate pressure. (See also Figure 5.3 and Table 5.1.)

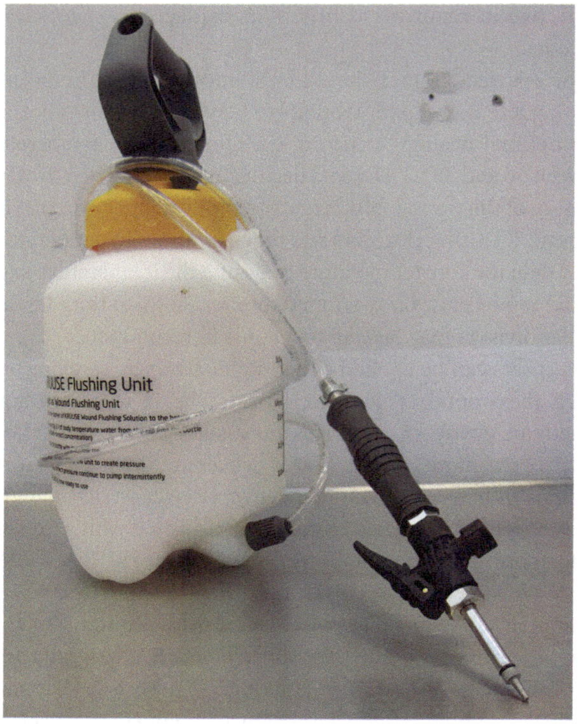

Figure 5.3 Wound irrigation device (Wound flushing unit, Kruuse) constructed to achieve appropriate pressure (10–14 psi) during wound irrigation. Moderate fluid pressure is needed to overcome the adhesion of contaminants and bacteria to the wound. High fluid pressure should be avoided because it may drive bacteria deeper into the wound.

iodine, chlorhexidine, polyhexamethylene biguanide (PHMB), ionized silver, hydrogen peroxide, sodium hypochlorite, acetic acid, alcohol, and octenidine dihydrochloride.

Isotonic saline solution

Sterile isotonic saline solution is the most appropriate and preferred cleansing solution because it is a widely available, non-toxic, isotonic solution that does not damage healing tissues. Other isotonic solutions, such as Normosol-R or lactated Ringer's solution, are equally well suited for wound cleansing. A systematic review of the effects of cleansing wounds with isotonic saline solution or tap water concluded that the current evidence suggests that irrigation using isotonic saline solution or tap water is ineffective in reducing the bioburden associated with wounds in human patients, and that the use of isotonic saline solution or tap water is not associated with improved wound healing.[5] In spite of this, many clinicians still opt to irrigate wounds with isotonic saline solution, for example after surgical debridement.

Tap water

Several studies have been performed to evaluate whether tap water is acceptable for wound cleansing. A systematic review concluded that tap water is acceptable for cleansing acute and chronic wounds, and that using tap water does not seem to increase the risk of infection or cause delayed healing of acute wounds in adult human patients.[5] Using either isotonic saline solution, distilled water, or boiled tap water to cleanse open fractures did not produce a statistically significant difference in the number of fractures developing infection.[6] Based on these studies, the hypotonicity of tap water or boiled water does not seem to cause injury to the cells in the wound – at least not to a clinically relevant extent. Tap water should not be used as a cleanser in areas where a constant supply of potable drinking water is not available. Under such circumstances, however, distilled or boiled water may be used for wound cleansing.[5]

One major advantage of using tap water as a cleanser is that it is very cheap, and thus the clinician may be more inclined to use large volumes of tap water compared to the volumes used with other cleansing fluids.

> **Tip**
>
> - Available evidence suggests that tap water may be safe for wound cleansing in areas where there is a constant supply of potable drinking water.

Commercial wound cleansers

In infected wounds, especially those where biofilm has formed, isotonic saline solution and water may not be effective cleansing solutions, because bacteria in biofilms are more resistant to irrigation than are planktonic (free-floating) bacteria. Biofilms are polymicrobial colonies protected by a matrix, which frequently form in wounds and are characterized by rapid development of resistance to mechanical disruption.

The cleansing activity of many commercial wound cleansers relies on a surfactant that breaks the bond between foreign bodies/microbes and the wound's surface, to improve efficacy. The composition of commercially available cleansers can be found in Table 5.1. *In vitro* studies have shown that many cleansers may be toxic for fibroblasts and keratinocytes.[7,8] In particular, cleansers marketed for cleaning intact skin (i.e., shampoos, body wash, and soaps) exhibit toxicity, but many products marketed for use in wounds also exert some negative effect on fibroblasts and keratinocytes *in vitro* (Table 5.1).[7,8] In comparison, wound cleansers containing the surfactant poloxamer 188 (synonym: pluronic F-68) (Shur-Clens, SAF-Clens; both from Convatec; Primaderm Dermal Cleanser, Derma Sciences) have repeatedly been shown to have low toxicity *in vitro*,[7–9] and when SAF-Clens and Shur-Clens were applied to full-thickness skin wounds in guinea pigs, no adverse effects on healing were detected (in contrast to Betadine Surgical Scrub, which significantly slowed healing).[10] Poloxamer-based cleansers mechanically cleanse wounds, but have no antimicrobial effects, and, therefore, the use of these cleansers in wounds that are prone to developing infection should be supplemented with antimicrobial treatment (Table 5.1 and Table 5.2).[9] A study comparing the use of isotonic saline solution, povidone–iodine, or Shur-Clens for cleansing acute wounds in humans prior to suturing, however, failed to demonstrate differences in the incidence of infection among wounds.[11]

Table 5.1 Commercially available wound cleansers.

Product name	Supplier	Contents	Delivery	Fibroblast toxicity index* (Rani *et al.* 2014)[8]	Time to bacterial kill** (Rani *et al.* 2014)[8]
Shur-Clens	Convatec	Poloxamer 188 (synonym: Pluronic F-68)	Pour-on/squeeze bottle	0	>24 h
Neutrophase	Novabay Pharmaceuticals	Hypochlorous acid	Pump	10	<1 min
Vetericyn	Innovacyn Inc.	Hypochlorous acid, electrolyzed water	Pump or spray bottle	10 (the study tested Puracyn, which is the equivalent product on the human wound-care market)	30 min
3M Wound Cleanser	3M	Dextrose, sodium chloride, "nutrients" (pyridoxine, zinc). Does not contain surfactant or antimicrobial agents	Squeeze bottle (8.5 psi)	10	<24 h
EquineVet Acemannan Wound Cleanser	Carrington Labs	Acemannan hydrogel, sodium lauryl sulphate, dibasic sodium phosphate	Spray bottle	10	>24 h
Biolex	Bard Medical	*Aloe vera*, proprietary non-ionic surfactant	Spray bottle	10	>24 h
SAF-Clens AF Dermal Wound Cleanser	Convatec	Poloxamer 188 (synonym: Pluronic F-68)	Spray bottle	100	24 h
Prontosan Wound Cleanser	B. Braun	Polyhexanide, betaine	Nozzled bottle (7 psi) or 40 mL single use ampoule	100	>24 h
Dermal Wound Cleanser	Smith & Nephew	Benzethonium chloride, Polysorbate 20	Spray bottle	1000	>24 h
UltraKlenz	Carrington Labs	Glycine, sucrose, benzoic acid, imidazolium compounds, dodecanoic (lauric) acid, mannitol	Spray bottle	Not assessed	Not assessed
MicroKlenz	Carrington Labs	Benzethonium chloride 0.1%, citric acid, cocamidopropyl betaine, dibasic sodium phosphate	Spray bottle	Not assessed	Not assessed
Sea-Clens	Coloplast	Saline-based	Spray bottle (7.6 psi)	Not assessed	Not assessed

* Assessed as the dilution required to maintain viable cells. The larger the number, the more toxic the product (toxicity index of 0: no dilution required; toxicity index of 100: 100-fold dilution required)
** Assessed as time to achieve a 4-log (99.99%) reduction in colony-forming units of *Staphylococcus aureus* at non-toxic dilution of the cleanser

Table 5.2 Indications and contraindications for cleansers with and without antiseptics. MRSA, methicillin-resistant *Staphylococcus aureus*; VRE, vancomycin-resistant enterococci.

Solution	Indication	Contraindication	Comments
Saline/tap water	Acute and chronic clean or minimally contaminated wounds	Saline and tap water are not effective for cleansing contaminated, necrotic, dirty or infected wounds	
Commercial cleansers with surfactant	Effective for wounds with adherent cellular debris and wounds with necrotic tissue. The presence of a surfactant means that less fluid pressure is required to remove bacteria and cellular debris	Infected wounds, as antimicrobial activity is minimal	Cleansers based on poloxamer 188 (synonym: pluronic F-68) seem to have the least toxicity, while cleansers marketed for intact skin (soaps, body washes and shampoos) the highest. See Table 5.1 for further detail
Antiseptics: silver	Wounds infected with Gram-positive and Gram-negative wound pathogens, including anaerobes and many antibiotic-resistant bacteria (MRSA, VRE), *Pseudomonas aeruginosa*, *Serratia marcescens*, fungi and yeasts (*Aspergillus* and *Candida* spp.)	Wounds that are not high risk, wounds that are not critically colonized or infected	
Antiseptics: iodine	Wounds infected with Gram-positive and Gram-negative organisms, fungi, and protozoa. Iodine is active against dermatophyte fungal infections (*Microsporum* and *Trichophyton* spp.) and has some sporicidal and virucidal activity, especially with increased exposure time	Wounds that are not high risk, wounds that are not critically colonized or infected	Cadexomer–iodine is more consistently beneficial than is povidone–iodine
Antiseptics: chlorhexidine	Wounds infected with Gram-positive bacteria and many Gram-negative bacteria, facultative anaerobes, and aerobes, yeasts, and fungi	Wounds that are not high risk, wounds that are not critically colonized or infected. Wounds infected with *Proteus*, *Serratia* and *Pseudomonas* spp., as these organisms are inherently resistant or very insensitive to the effects of chlorhexidine. Chlorhexidine has limited virucidal activity and no sporicidal activity	
Antiseptics: polyhexamethylene biguanide (PHMB)	Wounds infected with Gram-positive and Gram-negative wound pathogens, including many antibiotic-resistant bacteria, atypical organisms (e.g., *Chlamydia* and *Mycoplasma* spp.), and bacteria that form plaques and biofilms. PHMB is fungicidal against *Candida* and *Aspergillus* spp.	Wounds that are not high risk, wounds that are not critically colonized or infected. PHMB has little or no antiviral activity	Among the best antiseptics currently on the market. PHMB combines rapid and broad-spectrum antimicrobial activity with low cytotoxicity *in vitro*

Antiseptics: hydrogen peroxide	Hydrogen peroxide is mainly useful as a debriding agent: upon contact with organic matter hydrogen peroxide produces effervescence that mechanically cleanses wounds. It has sporicidal activity, but low bactericidal activity against vegetative forms of Gram-positive and Gram-negative bacteria	Hydrogen peroxide is cytotoxic and has limited bactericidal activity, therefore generally not indicated for wound cleansing	Antiseptic activity is reduced by the presence of blood. Hydrogen peroxide is cytotoxic at the efficacious concentrations (3%)
Antiseptics: sodium hypochlorite/ Dakin's solution	Wounds infected with a broad spectrum of aerobic and anaerobic organisms including *Staphylococcus aureus*, *Pseudomonas aeruginosa*, *Escherichia coli*, group D *Enterococcus*, and *Bacteroides fragilis*, as well as fungi. At higher concentrations (0.025%, which also has some cytotoxicity) Dakin's solution is effective against MRSA, *Staphylococcus epidermidis*, *Klebsiella pneumoniae*, *Enterobacter cloacae*, *Serratia marcescens*, and *Proteus mirabilis*	Wounds that are not high risk, wounds that are not critically colonized or infected. Dakin's solution has limited penetration and is therefore not suited for deep complex wounds	Conflicting cytotoxicity data, but 0.0125–0.00025% solutions seem safe
Antiseptics: hypochlorous acid	Wounds infected with very broad range of microorganisms, hypochlorous acid is active against all Gram-positive and Gram-negative bacterial, viral and fungal human pathogens, including drug-resistant staphylococci	Wounds that are not high risk, wounds that are not critically colonized or infected	Among the best antiseptics currently on the market. Hypochlorous acid combines rapid and broad-spectrum antimicrobial activity with low cytotoxicity *in vitro*
Antiseptics: acetic acid	Wounds infected with *Pseudomonas* spp.	Acetic acid is cytotoxic and has limited bactericidal activity, it is generally not recommended for wound cleansing	Limited studies are available on the cytotoxicity of acetic acid, but those available indicate that its cytotoxicity may surpass its bactericidal effects
Antiseptics: octenidine	Wounds infected with Gram-positive and Gram-negative bacteria, MRSA, plaque-forming organisms such as *Actinomyces* and *Streptococcus* spp., atypical organisms such as *Chlamydia* and *Mycoplasma* spp., fungi, some viruses	Wounds that are not high risk, wounds that are not critically colonized or infected. Octenidine has no activity against spores and protozoa	Among the best antiseptics currently on the market. Octenidine combines rapid and broad-spectrum antimicrobial activity with low cytotoxicity *in vitro*
Antiseptics: cetylpyridinium chloride	Wounds infected with Gram-positive bacteria and yeasts	Wounds that are not high risk, wounds that are not critically colonized or infected. Cetylpyridinium chloride is relatively ineffective against Gram-negative bacteria	
Antiseptics: tris-ethylenediamine tetra-acetic acid (tris-EDTA)	Wounds infected with Gram-negative bacteria, including *Escherichia coli*, *Pseudomonas aeruginosa*, and *Proteus vulgaris*	Wounds that are not high risk, wounds that are not critically colonized or infected. Tris-EDTA has little effect on Gram-positive bacteria and yeasts	Mainly useful in combination with other antiseptics (or antibiotics), because a main effect of tris-EDTA is to damage the bacterial cell membrane and increase its permeability to antimicrobial substances

Several cleansers, most of which are available over-the-counter, contain components proposed to promote healing, such as zinc (3 M Wound Cleanser, 3 M; Dermagran, Derma Sciences), *Aloe vera* (Biolex, Bard Medical; Eclipse Wound Cleanser, PRP Technologies), or vitamins (Dermagran, Derma Sciences). The effects of these compounds on healing are described later in the chapter.

Antiseptics

Antiseptics are substances that inhibit growth and development of microorganisms. The term is often used for products developed for topical application. Antimicrobial is the umbrella term for agents that kill or prevent the multiplication of microorganisms, e.g. bacteria or fungi. Antimicrobials may be antibiotics, antiseptics or disinfectants. While antibiotics are agents that act selectively against bacteria and usually against a narrow range of bacteria, antiseptics are relatively broad-acting agents that inhibit multiplication of, or kill, microorganisms. Disinfectants are also relatively non-selective with multiple sites of action and kill a wide range of microorganisms, but they are generally not suitable for use on body tissues because they are toxic to eukaryotic cells. While development of resistance to antibiotics is an increasing problem, development of resistance to antiseptics is literally unknown in the area of wound care.[12]

The use of antiseptics in wounds is controversial. Although multiple *in vitro* studies have shown that antiseptics exert negative effects on cells involved in wound healing, application of antiseptics may be indicated for cleansing and treating severely contaminated and infected wounds. The efficacy of topically applied antiseptics has also been questioned. Some argue that antiseptics are quickly denatured by contact with bodily fluids.[13] Sibbald *et al.* (2000) recommend the use of antiseptics, but only for non-healing wounds or where the local bacterial burden at the time of presentation is of greater concern than is healing the wound (Figure 5.4).[14] A Best Practice document from 2010 summarizes the current understanding of use of antiseptics in wound management by stating that “The use of topical antiseptic/antimicrobial agents is one of the key ways to assist in treating patients with signs of wound infection, and without judicious use of the products, patients may be at risk .... It is equally important to avoid using topical antiseptic/antimicrobial agents on wounds in situations where infection is not present, or where there is no significant clinical risk of infection.”[15]

Choosing the best cleanser or antiseptic for irrigation of a specific wound is not straightforward. The main dilemma is whether to select a product with antimicrobial effects or not, based on the criteria described above. Indications and contraindications for the different cleansers and antiseptics are shown in Table 5.2.

Silver

Silver has a broad spectrum of antimicrobial activity[16] and acts on multiple bacterial sites (it blocks respiratory enzymatic pathways and alters microbial DNA and the cell wall), which may decrease the risk of development of resistance.[17] Silver ions have antimicrobial effects against a broad range of Gram-positive and Gram-negative wound pathogens, including many antibiotic-resistant bacteria, such as *Staphylococcus aureus*, methicillin-resistant *Staphylococcus aureus* (MRSA), *Enterococcus faecalis*, vancomycin-resistant enterococci, *Pseudomonas aeruginosa*, and *Escherichia coli.*[18,19] Topical use of silver in infected wounds has been shown repeatedly to reduce bioburden. For example, in experimental burn wounds in rats infected with multi-drug-resistant *Pseudomonas aeruginosa*, 1% silver sulfadiazine and a silver-coated dressing (Acticoat, Smith & Nephew) reduced bacterial load more than did 3% citric acid and a dressing containing 0.5% chlorhexidine (Bactigras, Smith & Nephew).[20] Use of silver-containing dressings is described in further detail in Chapter 6.

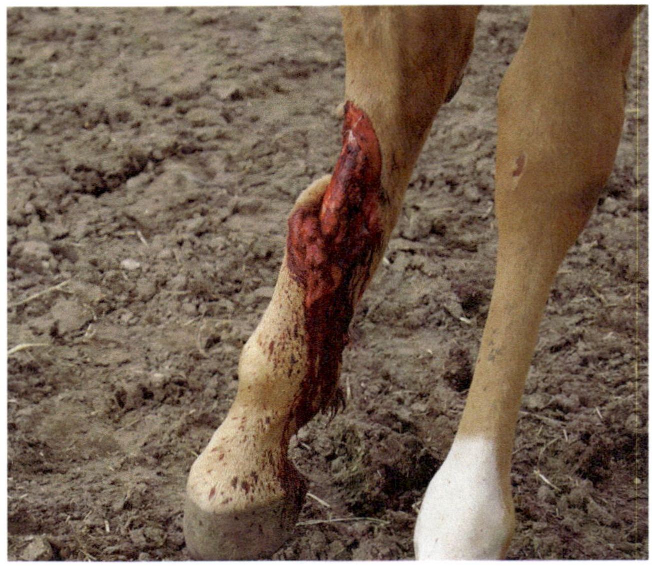

Figure 5.4 An acute, severely contaminated degloving injury. This wound is at high risk of developing infection, and will therefore benefit from being irrigated with an antiseptic solution. Photo courtesy of Tinamaria Jensen, Vinding Forlag and Tinamarias Digital Publishing.

Resistance to silver and cross-resistance between antibiotics and silver are rare.[17,21] Two studies investigating silver resistance genes in wound pathogens, including MRSA isolated from humans and horses, detected a low prevalence of silver resistance genes. Moreover, the studies showed that even those bacteria carrying the gene(s) were susceptible to the antimicrobial effects of a silver-containing hydrofiber dressing.[22,23]

A wound cleanser containing silver nitrate and menthol is commercially available (Silver-Stream, Angelini). There are no scientific studies investigating this liquid form of ionic silver, but three conference abstracts (reporting a total of eight cases of difficult-to-heal wounds in human patients) suggested that using this product to irrigate infected wounds produced positive effects.[24–26]

Another type of silver nitrate-containing product for topical application is the silver nitrate stick, where 75% silver nitrate is combined with potassium nitrate. This product has an entirely different method of action; it is used not as an antiseptic but rather as a chemical caustic agent for removing exuberant granulation tissue (EGT). When the stick/applicator is combined with water, nitric acid is produced, along with an insoluble precipitate, silver hydroxide. Nitric acid (also known as *aqua fortis* or spirit of niter) is a highly corrosive strong mineral acid, and it is the compound that initiates the biologic caustic action. It induces a chemical burn to the tissues, thereby reducing proliferation of fibroblasts. When used, it should be applied to the wound only, and a skin protectant, such as petrolatum or white paraffin, must be applied to the skin surrounding the wound to minimize harm to healthy tissues. The advancing epithelium and skin should not be touched with the silver nitrate, because to do so delays healing. In humans, silver nitrate is considered to be one of the most successful treatments for hypergranulation and has produced good results in practice.[27] Due to its harmful effects, however, cautery with strong silver nitrate should never be considered first-line therapy and should be used, with great care, for only the most stubborn areas of exuberant granulation.

Iodine compounds

Iodine is a natural element of the halogen group, is an essential nutrient in the body, and has a broad spectrum of antimicrobial activity against Gram-positive and Gram-negative organisms. Iodine exerts its antimicrobial effects by penetrating microorganisms and attacking proteins, nucleotides, and fatty acids essential for bacterial survival. Iodine is also antiviral, antifungal, and antiprotozoal. There is no known resistance to iodine.

Molecular iodine can be very toxic to tissues and cause skin pain, irritation, and inflammation. Iodophors are iodine carriers or iodine-releasing agents that act as a reservoir of the active/free iodine. By coupling iodine to these carriers, iodine is released slowly, and its toxicity is reduced. Iodine can be inactivated by blood and serum proteins and by other organic matter. The sustained release of iodine from modern wound-care products serves to overcome this issue.

Two iodophor formulations of iodine are available: povidone–iodine (PI) and cadexomer– (modified starch) iodine (CI). CI products are newer and less toxic than PI. CI is available as a powder and as an ointment (Iodosorb, Smith & Nephew). CI has been shown to accelerate healing by reducing bioburden and by directly stimulating epidermal regeneration and epithelialization.[28,29] In clinical studies in humans, the use of CI led to improved wound healing when compared with standard treatments, such as hydrocolloid dressings, paraffin gauze, wet-to-dry gauze dressings, zinc paste dressings, saline dressings, enzyme-based dressings, dextranomer dressings, and non-adherent dressings.[30] A side-effect of CI has been described as a burning or stinging sensation.

Although studies using CI have had consistently positive outcomes, evidence from studies using PI for wound management is conflicting. PI effectively reduces bacterial numbers in infected wounds. Impaired synthesis of collagen, toxic effects on fibroblasts and keratinocytes, and impaired migration of epithelial cells resulting in delayed healing have been observed in animal wound models, but there is no evidence to indicate that PI delays healing of an infected wound.[31] In a study using horses, experimental wounds treated with a 10% PI ointment under a bandage healed faster (although not statistically significantly so) than wounds treated with silver sulfadiazine cream (83 and 101 days to healing, respectively).[32]

What to do

- Prefer CI products over PI products, because studies using CI have consistently shown beneficial effects on healing, whereas studies using PI have shown more variable effects.

What to avoid

- PI should be applied with caution or not at all to wounds that are not infected; PI may be useful for wounds that are contaminated or infected.

A commonly used PI product is Betadine, which is a complex of iodine and polyvinylpyrrolidone (povidone), a synthetic polymer. The most common commercial form is a 10% solution in water yielding 1% available iodine, which is diluted to 0.1–0.2% by adding 10–20 mL of Betadine to 990–980 mL of saline. This dilution increases the availability of free iodine and minimizes cytotoxicity. PI is available as a surgical scrub, a skin cleanser with a detergent, and in other forms, and, according to its formulation, is used to disinfect hands, prepare skin for surgery, or irrigate wounds.

Chlorhexidine

Chlorhexidine is commonly used in antiseptic solutions. Chlorhexidine is a cationic biguanide that is a strong alkali virtually insoluble in water. In contrast, its salts (chlorhexidine digluconate, chlorhexidine diacetate, and chlorhexidine dihydrochloride) are soluble and used in antiseptic solutions. Chlorhexidine gluconate is the most widely used, as it is highly water soluble.

Chlorhexidine binds to the negatively charged bacterial cell wall, thereby altering the cellular osmotic equilibrium. It has activity against Gram-positive and Gram-negative bacteria, facultative anaerobes, and aerobes, yeasts including *Candida albicans*, fungi, and certain viruses. It is, however, important to keep in mind that members of the genus *Proteus* are invariably insensitive and that *Pseudomonas aeruginosa* is more resistant to chlorhexidine (and to quaternary ammonium compounds) than are other Gram-negative organisms.[33] Advantages of chlorhexidine are a prolonged residual effect due to its ability to bind to proteins in the *stratum corneum* and better activity in the presence of blood, pus, and organic debris than PI. It is well tolerated; the most frequently reported adverse reaction is contact dermatitis.

Although *in vitro* studies often suggest that chlorhexidine has adverse effects on cells, effects of topically applied chlorhexidine on *in vivo* wound healing are less clear. Topical application of two products (a skin cleanser and an aqueous solution) with 4% w/v chlorhexidine was found to have mild inhibitory effects on wound healing in guinea pigs,[34] which could have been related to chlorhexidine toxicity to newly formed keratinocytes[35] or its suppressive effects on macrophages.[36] In contrast, the use of 0.05% chlorhexidine diacetate was found to accelerate healing of full-thickness wounds on beagles.[37]

What to do

- Based on the current recommendations in humans,[38] chlorhexidine gluconate should be applied in a 0.05% concentration when used to irrigate open wounds in horses (1:40 = 25 mL of a 2% concentrate diluted with 975 mL of sterile isotonic crystalloid solution).

What to avoid

- Chlorhexidine is toxic to corneal cells[39] and joint tissues (synovial cells and chondrocytes),[40] and therefore it should be used with caution in periocular wounds and wounds communicating with synovial structures.

Polyhexamethylene biguanide

Polyhexamethylene biguanide (PHMB) (also called polyhexanide) is an antiseptic agent that exerts antimicrobial effects by adhering to and disrupting target cell membranes, causing the microorganisms to leak potassium ions and other cytosolic components, leading to cell death. PHMB has several desirable characteristics: it has very good biocompatibility,[41] low toxicity, is highly effective against susceptible and resistant strains of common Gram-positive and Gram-negative bacteria, as well as fungi found in chronic wounds, and resistance is non-existent.[42] It has been demonstrated, *in vivo*, to possess direct pro-healing effects by enhancing the proliferation of normal human keratinocytes[43] and promoting epithelialization.[44]

Tip

- PHMB seems to be among the most tissue-friendly antiseptics available and has direct pro-healing effects. This, in combination with its broad antimicrobial spectrum, makes PHMB a good choice for cleansing of contaminated and infected wounds.

In humans with chronic leg ulcers, cleansing with PHMB led to statistically significantly faster healing (time to healing 3.3 months) than cleansing with isotonic saline solution or Ringer's solution (time to healing 4.4 months) and caused 97% of problem wounds to heal within 6 months (compared to 89% of wounds in the control group),[45] a difference that was also statistically significant.

For irrigation, a solution (Prontosan, B. Braun) containing PHMB in combination with betaine, a detergent/surfactant, is available. The manufacturer describes this product as being efficient in removing biofilm. Betaine has a low surface tension, which is an important factor in the efficacy of Prontosan. Many wounds are coated with denatured proteins, lipoproteins, and lipids from cell membranes and carbohydrates. As these compounds denature, their solubility decreases. The low surface tension of betaine enhances the physical removal of debris and bacteria coating the surface of the wound.[45]

If the wound is only lightly contaminated, Prontosan should be applied to the wound's surface directly from the bottle, and the wound thoroughly cleansed. The irrigation solution should not be rinsed off after cleansing. If the wound is heavily contaminated, Prontosan should be applied by saturating a gauze compress with the solution and leaving this compress on the wound for 10–15 minutes. After the compress has been removed, the wound should be wiped lightly to remove loosened debris. The cleansing is completed by irrigating the wound again with Prontosan, which should not be rinsed off the wound.

Hydrogen peroxide

Hydrogen peroxide has been widely used to cleanse wounds. It is, therefore, paradoxical that its effects on wounds have been investigated in only a small number of studies, and, consequently, are not clear. Some studies have shown beneficial effects, but the majority of studies suggest that hydrogen peroxide may be more cytotoxic than bactericidal. There are also no definitive studies demonstrating that it has an antibacterial effect *in vivo*. Hydrogen peroxide seems ineffective in reducing the bacterial count, but has sporicidal activity.[46] One study in horses demonstrated faster healing and improved histology scores (concentrations of neutrophils and bacteria) in experimental, 2-cm diameter circular excisional wounds on the neck treated with 1% hydrogen peroxide cream (LHP cream, Bioglan Pharma AB) compared to wounds to which petrolatum or no treatment was applied. Time to complete healing in the three groups was 32, 42, and 44 days, respectively. Petrolatum did not impair wound healing in this study, but it induced the formation of EGT, perhaps because the occlusive properties of petrolatum resulted in lower oxygen tension in the wound; petrolatum-treated wounds also accumulated significantly more bacteria.[47]

Hydrogen peroxide may best serve as a chemical debriding agent. Hydrogen peroxide rapidly decomposes into water and oxygen when it combines with organic tissue or blood. During this breakdown, hydrogen peroxide produces effervescence that mechanically cleanses wounds and removes tissue debris via the release of oxygen.

What to avoid

- In view of the wide selection of commercial antiseptic wound cleansers with proven benefits to wound healing, there seems to be little justification for using hydrogen peroxide.

Dakin's solution

Dakin's solution is dilute household bleach, or sodium hypochlorite. Its antimicrobial effects were discovered by biochemist Henry Drysdale Dakin at the beginning of the 1900s, and the solution gained popularity during World War I as part of the Carrel–Dakin technique based on a concept of thorough wound cleansing (developed by the renowned French doctor Alexis Carrel) combined with irrigation with sodium hypochlorite. This technique helped save lives and mobility of numerous soldiers in the camp hospitals of World War I.[48]

Sodium hypochlorite kills bacteria and liquefies necrotic tissue by driving chlorine and oxygen into tissues. It is effective against a broad spectrum of aerobic and anaerobic organisms, as well as fungi, and it has an aggressive debriding action.[48]

Dakin's solution is available commercially in multiple dilutions ranging from "full strength" (0.5% solution, where household bleach comes as a 5% solution) and 1/40 strength (0.0125% solution). The term "full strength" refers to the highest concentration tolerable to the intact skin. Studies have shown that full-strength Dakin's solution has a negative impact on migration and viability of neutrophils, fibroblasts, and endothelial cells *in vitro*, and for this reason Dakin's solution fell out of favor for years. A recent *in vitro* study investigating the effects of antiseptics toward different fungi, however, demonstrated that in a comparison between Dakin's solution, mafenide acetate, and amphotericin B, Dakin's solution most consistently met the balance between toxicity and efficacy. A 0.00025% Dakin's solution appeared to optimize the efficacy:toxicity index,[49] thus necessitating dilution of the commercially available 0.0125% Dakin's solution 50-fold. Whether or not Dakin's solution applied to wounds at this dilution has *in vivo* antimicrobial activity towards bacteria is, however, not clear. Dakin's solution may not penetrate deep complex wounds or deeply into tissue. The original method of applying Dakin's solution therefore entailed frequent or continuous infusion into the wound through fenestrated tubes.[48,49]

> **Tip**
>
> - To make 0.5% Dakin's solution, 950 mL of tap water is boiled for 15 minutes. After the pan has been removed from the heat, ½ teaspoonful of baking soda and 95 mL unscented 5.25% household bleach is added to the boiled water. This full-strength solution should be further diluted at least 40-fold by adding 20 mL to 800 mL of boiled water before use.

Hypochlorous acid

Hypochlorous acid is produced when sodium hypochlorite is added to water and also endogenously during the respiratory burst of neutrophils. When neutrophils are activated, hydrogen peroxide is generated and converted to hypochlorous acid by the enzyme myeloperoxidase released from the granules of the neutrophils. Hypochlorous acid induces cellular death via numerous pathways, including oxidation of sulfhydryl enzymes and amino acids, ring chlorination of amino acids, oxidation of respiratory components, decreased production of adenosine triphosphate, breaks in DNA, and depressed synthesis of DNA. There are certain advantages of using hypochlorous acid over Dakin's solution. The amount of hypochlorous acid released from bleach (sodium hypochlorite) is pH dependent. Therefore electrolyzing water to make hypochlorous acid solution, as described below, ensures a product with a more consistent content of the active agent. Hypochlorous acid has been suggested to have an antimicrobial effect around 80–100 times stronger than the hypochlorite ion.[50] Hypochlorous acid solution has the added advantages of not forming the irritant chlorine gas, being more stable and not possessing the corrosive and alkaline properties of bleach.

Hypochlorous acid is highly active against all Gram-positive and Gram-negative bacterial, viral and fungal human pathogens, including drug-resistant staphylococci; a small amount of hypochlorous acid can kill spore-forming and non-spore-forming bacteria in a short time.[51,52] It may also disrupt biofilm.[8]

Several products containing hypochlorous acid are available commercially. Neutrophase (Novabay Pharmaceuticals) is a pure solution of hypochlorous acid (0.01%) in isotonic saline solution. A solution containing electrolyzed water (99.97%), sodium chloride 0.023%, sodium hypochlorite 0.004%, and hypochlorous acid 0.003% is marketed by Oculus Innovative Sciences under a number of brand names, including Dermacyn, Puracyn, Oxum, Microdacyn60, Innovacyn, and Vetricyn/Vetericyn – with the latter intended for the veterinary wound-care market. Vetericyn is made by electrochemical treatment of dilute saline solution. A pH neutral solution of hypochlorous acid, and its salt, sodium hypochlorite, is generated (Figure 5.5).

A study by Rani *et al.* (2014)[8] showed that the products based on hypochlorous acid demonstrated a very desirable combination of rapid bacterial kill and low cytotoxicity. Consequently, hypochlorous acid seems to be an ideal antiseptic.[51]

> **Tip**
>
> - Hypochlorous acid combines rapid bacterial kill with low cytotoxicity and may thus be among the most useful antiseptics currently available on the wound-care market.

A recent study showed that a homemade solution with extremely low concentration of hypochlorous acid, made by mixing 1.5 mL of "concentrated" bleach solution (8.25% sodium hypochlorite) and 1 L of distilled water (resulting in a concentration of 99.988% water and 0.012% hypochlorous acid), was as efficient as Vetericyn in inhibiting growth of *Staphylococcus aureus* and *Escherichia coli in vitro*. The homemade solution retained its antibacterial effect for at least 1 week.[53]

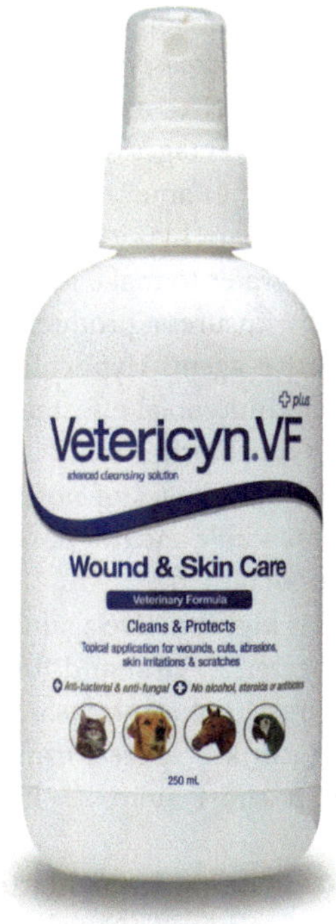

Figure 5.5 Hypochlorous acid made through electrochemical treatment of dilute saline solution, whereby a pH-neutral solution of hypochlorous acid, and its salt, sodium hypochlorite, is generated (Vetericyn, Oculus Innovative Sciences). Hypochlorous acid is highly active against all Gram-positive and Gram-negative bacterial, viral and fungal pathogens, including drug-resistant staphylococci; moreover, it combines rapid bacterial kill with low cytotoxicity *in vitro*. These desirable characteristics make hypochlorous acid very useful for wound cleansing.

Acetic acid

Dilute acetic acid is used for the treatment of chronic wounds. It has moderate bactericidal activity against many Gram-positive and Gram-negative organisms, especially *Pseudomonas aeruginosa*. Clinical antibacterial efficacy requires a concentration of at least 0.5%,[54] but solutions up to a concentration of 5% have been used for irrigation. A study evaluating the effects of a 3% solution of acetic acid on bacteria commonly found in burn wounds showed "excellent bactericidal effect of acetic acid, particularly with problematic Gram-negative bacteria, such as [....] *P. aeruginosa*."[55] Antibiotic-resistant strains of *Pseudomonas aeruginosa* are also susceptible to the effects of 3% acetic acid.[54] Effects of acetic acid on healing tissues are not entirely clear, because negative as well as positive effects on wound healing have been demonstrated. Wilson *et al.* (2005) investigated the toxicity of numerous wound cleansers towards keratinocytes and fibroblasts and found that 0.25% acetic acid had low toxicity (toxicity index of 10) compared to 3% hydrogen peroxide or 10% PI (both of which had toxicity indices of 1000).[7] Based on current best evidence, it seems that acetic acid may be indicated for cleansing wounds infected with *Pseudomonas aeruginosa*. Other acids, e.g. 3% boric acid, 2–3% citric acid, 2% ascorbic acid and 0.5–2% salicylic acid, may also be applied topically to treat *Pseudomonas aeruginosa* infections.[54]

What to do

- To make 3% acetic acid, 3 mL of acetic acid is added to 97 mL of distilled, sterile water. The acetic acid is applied as a wash/irrigation or by placing sterile gauze soaked in the solution on the wound for 15 minutes. Acetic acid should be thus applied daily or on alternate days depending on the severity of the infection. Between 2 and 15 applications have been described as necessary for resolving *Pseudomonas aeruginosa* infection in humans.[54]

Octenidine dihydrochloride

Octenidine is a bispyridinamine that exhibits a broad spectrum of antimicrobial efficacy against Gram-positive and Gram-negative bacteria and fungi. Its efficacy is not adversely affected by interfering substances, such as blood and mucus. Octenidine has strong residual activity on skin, which can still be observed 24 hours after application. When cytotoxicity of octenidine at a concentration producing a 3 $\log_{10}$ reduction of *Escherichia coli* and *Staphylococcus aureus* was compared to the cytotoxicity of other antiseptics (benzalkonium chloride, cetylpyridinium chloride, chlorhexidine digluconate, mild silver protein, PHMB, PI, silver nitrate, silver sulfadiazine, and triclosan), octenidine and PHMB were the only tested products with a biocompatibility index greater than 1, meaning that these substances were the only antiseptics more toxic to the microorganisms than to murine fibroblasts.[41] A recent review emphasized that octenidine and PHMB are the most effective, as well as best tolerated, antiseptics used in wound management today.[56]

Tip

- From the current available evidence from *in vitro* studies, octenidine, PHMB, and hypochlorous acid seem to be the best antiseptics presently on the market. All three possess the same, very desirable characteristics, as they combine rapid and broad-spectrum antimicrobial activity with low cytotoxicity, at least *in vitro*.

A study comparing the effects of octenidine and PHMB on superficial wounds in piglets showed retarded wound contraction in octenidine-treated wounds and accelerated wound contraction in PHMB-treated wounds relative to control (treatment with Ringer's solution). These effects on wound contraction resulted in significantly longer healing time in wounds treated with octenidine compared to those treated with PHMB (28 and 23 days to complete closure, respectively).[57] These findings highlight the need for well-designed *in vivo* studies to confirm results obtained with the different antiseptics *in vitro*.

Cetylpyridinium chloride

Cetylpyridinium chloride is a cationic quaternary ammonium compound with antibacterial effects. It is marketed under the name Lacerum Wound Cleanser (PRP Technologies). A study ranking several antiseptic agents according to biocompatibility index (cytotoxicity on murine fibroblast relative to microbicidal effect on *E. coli* and *S. aureus*) showed low (for *E. coli*) to moderate (for *S. aureus*) biocompatibility of cetylpyridinium chloride at the concentration needed to produce 3 $\log_{10}$ reduction of *E. coli* and *S. aureus*. The biocompatibility index of cetylpyridinium chloride was inferior to that of chlorhexidine, PHMB, and octenidine.[41]

Tris-ethylenediamine tetra-acetic acid

Tris-ethylenediamine tetra-acetic acid (tris-EDTA), when used for wound treatment, has three principal effects: it is antimicrobial, it alkalizes the wound, and it potentiates antibiotics. The antibacterial effect is achieved by lysis of the cell membrane of bacteria, especially the cell membranes of *P. aeruginosa* and other Gram-negative bacteria.[58] By lysing the membrane, tris-EDTA also increases the permeability of Gram-negative bacteria to extracellular solutes, thus making them more susceptible to antiseptics and antibiotics. Adding tris-EDTA to chlorhexidine increases the antimicrobial effectiveness of the solution. The alkalizing effect of tris-EDTA may be useful when topical application of antibiotics is planned, because activity of some antibiotics is reduced in an acidic environment. When used in combination with antibiotics, tris-EDTA has been shown to directly potentiate the antibacterial effects of multiple antibiotics, including penicillins, oxytetracycline, aminoglycosides, and fluoroquinolones.[58,59]

Use of tris-EDTA as an irrigation fluid has mainly been described for treating persistent infections in small animals, such as cystitis and otitis externa, and effects on equine wound healing are thus unknown.

Topically administered antibiotics

Applying antibiotics to the surface of a granulating wound may reduce bioburden and accelerate healing (Figure 5.6). The antibiotics more commonly used in wound management will be described here.

Triple antibiotic ointment

Triple antibiotic ointment (bacitracin, polymyxin B, and neomycin) has a wide antimicrobial spectrum, although it is usually not effective against *P. aeruginosa*. Because of its zinc content (from bacitracin) it may stimulate epithelialization. A study investigating healing, in humans, of experimental wounds infected with *S. aureus* showed that triple antibiotic ointment caused faster healing and reduced numbers of bacteria significantly better than all other antiseptics examined in the study.[60] In contrast, application of triple antibiotic ointment to equine experimental wounds resulted in delayed healing (slower rate of healing, longer time to complete closure) compared to untreated controls.[61] The reason for the delayed healing was not investigated, but it was hypothesized that the ointment's petrolatum base could be the cause of the reduced rate of healing. However, while this study showed that both the triple antibiotic ointment and petrolatum alone exerted a negative influence on healing, a previous study

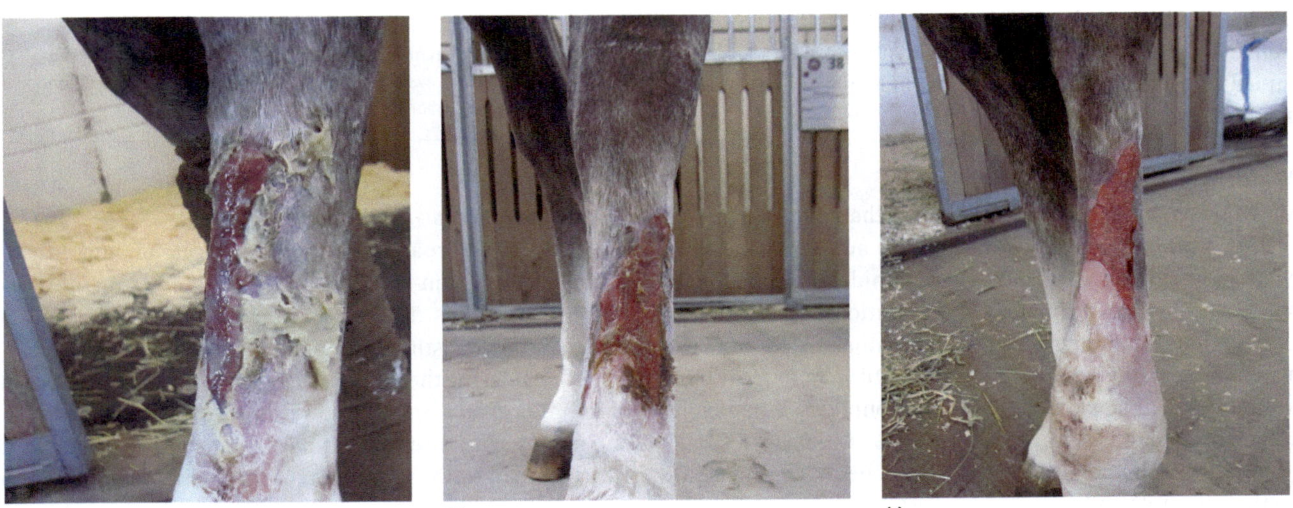

(a) (b) (c)

Figure 5.6 Granulating wound on the dorsomedial surface of the metatarsus. **(a)** The wound developed exuberant, fragile, unhealthy looking granulation tissue with signs of surface inflammation and infection. **(b)** The wound was treated by excision of exuberant granulation tissue and topical application of clindamycin under a non-adherent dressing, and 1 week later the granulation tissue was healthy with scant exudation. **(c)** The wound went on to heal without complications with no further application of antimicrobials.

did not demonstrate negative effects of cream containing petrolatum.[32]

Toxicity and development of resistance to triple antibiotic ointment are rare.

Silver sulfadiazine

Silver sulfadiazine cream contains the antibiotic sulfadiazine and silver, with the latter being responsible for the majority of the antimicrobial action of the product. Silver sulfadiazine cream is the most widely available silver product for topical application. The general merits of using silver in wound care are described under the section on Wound cleansers and irrigation solutions. Due to its effects against a broad range of Gram-positive and Gram-negative wound pathogens, including many antibiotic-resistant bacteria, the use of silver has gained popularity in wound management.

Silver sulfadiazine cream is widely used for its ability to reduce concentrations of *P. aeruginosa* and other pathogenic bacteria, in particular, in burn wounds. The effect of silver sulfadiazine is short-lived, because the silver ions quickly combine with tissue chloride to form insoluble and inactive silver compounds. The product, therefore, should be applied at least once daily. Silver sulfadiazine cream does not adhere well to the wound and, in limb wounds in horses, the cream may therefore need to be held in place by a light bandage to achieve prolonged effect.[32] After a few applications of silver sulfadiazine, a pseudo-eschar is formed on the wound surface. This "scab" provides a moist wound-healing environment, but has the disadvantage that it prohibits inspection of the wound and causes pain when it is removed. It should be gently removed on a daily basis prior to reapplying the silver sulfadiazine cream. One study in horses found that healing of experimental limb wounds treated with silver sulfadiazine was similar to that of wounds treated with PI ointment and concluded that using silver sulfadiazine had no advantage over using PI.[32]

Mafenide acetate

Mafenide is a topical sulfa antibiotic that is bacteriostatic against a wide range of Gram-positive and Gram-negative bacteria, including *P. aeruginosa*. Mafenide is available as a powder for reconstitution to make a solution for irrigation or as a cream (Sulfamylon, UDL Laboratories). In humans, mafenide is mainly used as a topical antibiotic to treat burn wounds. When applied to porcine wounds, 5% mafenide acetate compared favorably with 10% PI, 0.25% ("half-strength") Dakin's solution, 3% hydrogen peroxide, and 0.25% acetic acid in its ability to reduce bacterial concentration on the wound, and the authors of the study concluded that "Sulfamylon proved most effective in maintaining an aseptic environment while concomitantly increasing angiogenesis, proliferation of fibroblasts, and dermal thickness compared with controls."[62]

Gentamicin

Gentamicin is highly active against Gram-negative organisms, such as *Pseudomonas* spp., and some Gram-positive bacteria, including some staphylococcal strains. In a porcine wound model with wounds colonized by *S. aureus*, topical delivery of ultra-high concentrations of gentamicin (2000 μg/mL wound fluid, which is more than 1000 times the minimum inhibitory concentration) through an incubator-like wound healing platform (a polyurethane wound chamber sealed to the perimeter of the wound thus creating a protected environment), resulted in rapid decontamination of the acutely infected wounds while maintaining safe systemic concentrations of gentamicin. *In vitro*, migration and proliferation of keratinocytes were reduced at concentrations of gentamicin between 100 and 1000 μg/mL.[63]

Gentamycin cream is available at a concentration of 0.1% (1000 μg/mL), and, based on the findings in the study by Junker *et al.* (2015),[63] this concentration may exert negative effects on healing.

Nitrofurazone

Nitrofurazone has a broad antimicrobial spectrum, especially against Gram-positive organisms. It has little effect against *Pseudomonas* spp. Its primary action is bacteriostatic, but at high doses it is also bactericidal. Pus and blood reduce its antibacterial activity, and its overall potency is less than that of other antimicrobial drugs. It is hydrophilic and draws water from the wound.

What to avoid

- Nitrofurazone and other nitrofurans can cause cancer or genetic damage. For this reason, The European Union, the USA and Canada, as well as other countries, have banned the use of nitrofurans in food-producing animals, including horses. Considering this and the many alternatives available, nitrofurazone is no longer recommended for topical application to wounds.

Cephalosporins

Cefazolin has a broad Gram-positive spectrum and efficacy against some Gram-negative organisms and is mainly used to irrigate wounds. To create a solution for irrigation, 1 g of cefazolin is reconstituted in 500 mL of isotonic saline solution. Considering the much greater potential for development of antimicrobial resistance towards antibiotics than towards antiseptics, the use of antibiotic-laden irrigation fluids which spread to the environment may lead to emergence of resistant bacterial strains in hospitals or clinics and hence increase the risk of nosocomial infection that are difficult to treat.

Topically administered cefazolin has high bioavailability, and topical application results in high concentrations in wound fluid for prolonged periods and rapid systemic absorption.[64]

Fusidic acid

Fusidic acid is a bacteriostatic antibiotic with activity primarily against Gram-positive bacteria, such as *Staphylococcus* spp. and *Streptococcus* spp. It is licensed for use as its sodium salt, sodium fucidate (Fucidin 2% ointment, Leo Pharma). It is also available as a cream containing betamethasone (Fucicort, Leo Pharma). Results of studies on efficacy and effects on healing tissues are variable; the combination of fusidic acid and a glucocorticoid is more efficient than either drug alone in the treatment of infected eczema, as it combines antimicrobial action with a direct anti-inflammatory effect. In veterinary dermatology, use of fusidic acid cream is recommended for treatment of skin and wounds acutely infected with *Staphylococcus* spp.[65]

Wound-debridement agents

Autolytic debridement is the natural and highly selective process whereby endogenous proteolytic enzymes break down necrotic tissue. The endogenous enzymes are mainly produced by neutrophils invading the wound and include elastase, collagenase, myeloperoxidase, acid hydrolase, and lysosomal enzymes. In combination with moisture, these enzymes serve to rehydrate, soften, and liquefy necrotic tissue, eschar, and slough. Autolytic debridement is highly selective and virtually painless. Its main disadvantage is that it is a slow process, which may, however, be sped up by the use of dressings. Autolytic debridement can result in the production of substantial quantities of exudate, which should not be confused with exudate produced by infection (Figure 5.7). Typical practice to enhance autolytic debridement involves the use of a hydrogel to soften and break down necrotic tissue and an absorptive, occlusive or semi-occlusive dressing, which covers the hydrogel, to absorb the excess exudate. Hydrocolloid dressings are also useful for enhancing autolytic debridement.

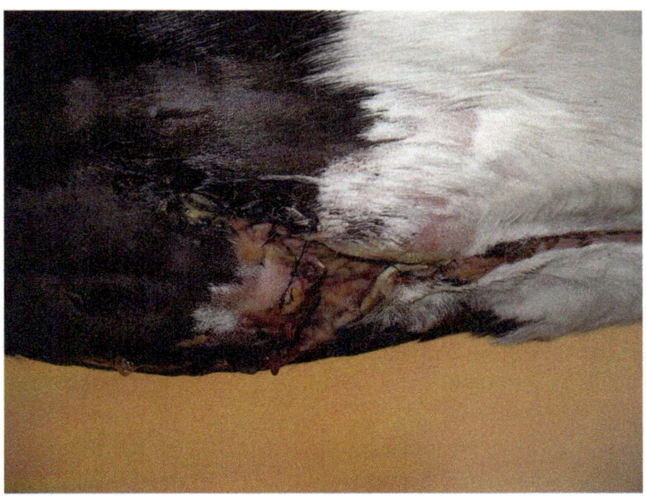

Figure 5.7 Sutured wound on the ventral abdomen. Autolytic debridement is taking place in the wound; the exudate is produced through that process and is not a sign of infection. The wound has dehisced partially, probably because sutures have been placed too close to the wound margins, which are now undergoing autolytic debridement.

In contrast to autolytic debridement, surgical debridement is fast, but also, to a certain extent, non-selective (based on the skills of the surgeon). Surgical debridement is often combined with pressurized irrigation, which also serves to debride the wound. A newer technique that combines sharp debridement and irrigation is hydrosurgery ("jet lavage"), which may, for example, be performed with the Versajet (Smith & Nephew). Hydrosurgical debridement has recently been shown to be more effective than surgical debridement with or without saline irrigation in reducing bacterial load in equine masseter muscle incubated with *S. aureus*.[66]

Other methods to achieve debridement are enzymatic, mechanical, and biosurgical (i.e., maggot debridement therapy). Numerous methods for mechanical debridement have been described, including wet-to-dry bandages (described in Chapter 6), pressurized irrigation, whirlpool therapy, and ultrasound treatment. An innovative technology for mechanical debridement, which has recently become available, is a monofilament debridement pad cut with angled tips designed to penetrate irregularly shaped areas and remove devitalized skin and wound debris (Debrisoft, Lohmann & Rauscher). Methods of debridement are described in Chapter 4.

Agents for enzymatic debridement

Enzymatic debridement is the application of exogenous enzymes to degrade necrotic tissue while preserving viable tissue. These proteolytic enzymes degrade (liquefy) the biofilm and surface coagulum of the wound, thus exposing bacteria to topically and systemically administered antimicrobial treatments. The enzymes also act to remove exudate and necrotic tissue from the wound by digesting fibrin (streptokinase) or collagen bundles (collagenase) that bind non-viable tissue to the wound surface, and by dissolving debris, thus allowing it to be absorbed into the overlying dressing or padding.[67] Excessive exudate not only hinders the effects of topically applied agents, it also breaks down extracellular matrix and impedes progression of healing. Enzymatic debridement is highly selective, leaving viable tissues intact. Major disadvantages of this technique, however, are that it has poor efficacy and is slow to achieve a clean wound. In fact, an *in vitro* study showed that autolytic debridement through the use of hydrofiber or gauze dressings hydrated in saline solution was a more efficient method of debridement (measured as protein breakdown of clotted equine blood). Autolytic debridement broke down almost 50% more protein than did dressings impregnated with proteolytic enzymes (collagenase, papain/urea or streptokinase/streptodornase).[68]

A large number of agents used for enzymatic debridement are commercially available; these are of animal, plant, or bacterial origin (Table 5.3). Enzymatic debridement is mainly useful when mechanical debridement is contraindicated, for example in patients with bleeding problems. Because alterations in blood coagulation severe enough to make sharp debridement risky or

Table 5.3 Proteolytic enzymes for wound debridement.

Origin	Enzyme	Derived from
Animal	Fibrinolysin	Bovine plasma
	Deoxyribonuclease	Bovine pancreas
	Collagenase	Red king crab *(Paralithodes camtschatica)*
	Catalase	Equine liver
Plant	Papain	Papaya
	Bromelain enzyme complex	Pineapple
Bacterial	Collagenase	*Clostridium histolyticum*
	Streptokinase	*Streptococcus* spp.
	Streptodornase	*Streptococcus haemolyticus*
	Serratiopeptidase	*Serratia* sp. E-15

Source: Modified from Strohal *et al.* 2013.[67] Reproduced with permission of EWMA.

contraindicated are rare in horses, enzymatic debridement has limited use in this species. Other indications for enzymatic debridement in horses may, however, be to avoid injury to neurovascular structures within the wound, that might be injured during surgical debridement, or when surgical debridement may result in the removal of tissue needed to reconstruct the wound at a later time. There is very limited information about clinical use of enzymatic debriding agents in horses. A pilot study using one horse concluded that the use of a product containing proteolytic enzymes derived from *Bacillus subtilis* (Travase, Flint) on an experimental wound did not confer any advantages in terms of healing rate or cosmesis.[69]

Enzymatic debriding agents are typically applied to the wound daily or twice daily. Care should be taken to avoid combining the enzymes with products containing metal, including silver dressings or products, because these diminish the biologic activity of collagenases and papain/urea. Proteolytic enzymes require moisture, and thus, enzymatic debridement agents should not be used in dry wounds.

Bacterial collagenase

Collagen is a major component of skin and thus also of non-viable tissue, and its breakdown is important in debridement. Bacterial collagenases promote healing by digesting native collagen bundles that bind non-viable tissue to the wound's surface and by dissolving collagen debris within the wound. Bacterial collagenase is unique in that it breaks the triple helical structure of both native and denatured collagens I, II, III, IV, and V at multiple points, whereby extracellular matrix- and cell surface-bound growth factors and bioactive matrix fragments are released. These fragments serve to enhance chemotaxis of macrophages and keratinocytes, fibroblasts and endothelial cells. By attracting phagocytosing macrophages and cells involved in healing, bacterial collagenase thus aids in debridement and has a direct stimulatory effect on healing. Collagenase is most efficient in the pH range 6–8, and it has no effect at pH lower than 5. The most commonly used collagenase product (Collagenase Santyl Ointment [also called Novuxol and Iruxol], Smith & Nephew) contains the collagenase clostridiopeptidase A from *Clostridium histolyticum*.[67] A major advantage of collagenase is that it is remarkably gentle on viable cells. In one study, collagenase enhanced *in vitro* proliferation and migration of keratinocytes up to 10-fold.[70] Collagenase may stimulate the formation of granulation tissue and accelerate epithelialization though the mechanisms outlined earlier.[71]

Streptokinase and streptodornase

Streptokinase is an enzyme, secreted by several species of streptococci, that serves to break down fibrin. It catalyzes the generation of plasmin from plasminogen, and plasmin degrades fibrin, fibrinogen, and certain clotting factors into peptides and amino acids. It is often used in combination with streptodornase (Varidase, Wyeth Pharmaceuticals), which is a DNAse derived from hemolytic streptococci. Streptodornase works synergistically with streptokinase to generate plasmin and also liquefies blood and nucleoproteins of dead cells and pus without exerting any effect on living cells. Streptodornase is thus particularly useful in combination with other enzymes.[67] The streptokinase–streptodornase combination was shown to be highly effective in destroying biofilms of *S. aureus in vitro*.[72]

Papain

Papain is derived from the papaya fruit. It is a meat tenderizer and liquefies fibrinous debris in a virtually pH-independent manner (i.e., papain works in the wide pH range of 3–12). It is a non-specific cysteine proteinase that denatures proteins. It is marketed as an ointment, in which papain is combined with urea (Accuzyme, Healthpoint). Urea is capable of interfering with the hydrogen bonds responsible for maintaining the tertiary structure of proteins, thus essentially causing the protein to relax. In addition, urea may disrupt some of the disulfide bonds within proteins to expose particular thiol groups, which may serve as activators of papain. The two compounds thus work synergistically to clear the wound of necrotic debris.[67] Papain has been used in wound care for many years, but relatively few studies have examined its effects. A systematic review concluded that "There is limited evidence that papain–urea-based ointment removes necrotic material from pressure ulcers more rapidly than collagenase ointment."[73] Major disadvantages of papain are the non-selective action and creation of a prominent painful inflammatory response when applied to wounds.

Fibrinolysin

Fibrinolysin of bovine origin is marketed as an ointment, in which fibrinolysin is combined with DNAse (Elase, Pfizer). The efficacy of fibrinolysin–DNAse in treatment of wounds of horses has not been investigated, and its efficacy in treatment of wounds of human patients is also not clear. When applied to chronic leg ulcers of humans, fibrinolysin–DNAse had no long-term clinical benefit in reducing purulent exudate, pain, erythema, and necrotic tissue and had no effect on the overall condition of chronic leg ulcers when compared to a placebo.[74]

Trypsin

Trypsin directly hydrolyzes a large number of naturally occurring proteins. It is available as an aerosolized spray in combination with Peru balsam and castor oil (Granulex V, Mylan Institutional Inc.). Peru balsam contains cinnamic and benzoic acids, which act as irritants and enhance blood flow by locally stimulating the capillary bed. It may also act as a mild antiseptic. Castor oil is a local protective agent that may promote epithelialization.[75] Few studies examining the effect of trypsin on wounds have been published, but trypsin seems to be less efficient than collagenase in debriding wounds.[73]

Serratiopeptidase

Serratiopeptidase is an extracellular proteolytic enzyme produced by the enterobacterium *Serratia* sp. E-15. This microorganism was originally isolated from the intestine of the silkworm caterpillar, where it is produced to allow the emerging moth to dissolve its cocoon. Serratiopeptidase hydrolyzes proteins and peptides; this hydrolysis is not restricted to specific sequences of amino acids, and the enzyme thus has a broad action. It is available coupled to pyrogenic silica in a product called SertaSil (Willingsford Limited), which is marketed specifically for veterinary wound care. In a rat model of implant-related infection with *S. epidermidis*, serratiopeptidase was successful in eradicating infection caused by biofilm-forming bacteria.[76]

Pyrogenic silica is able to bind to a wide range of molecules, including water. When SertaSil is applied topically, the silica adsorbs moisture, proteins, peptides, fragments of RNA and DNA, bacterial toxins, and other debris from the wound's surface. These effects of the silica are assisted by the serratiopeptidase bound to the silica, which, by chemical hydrolysis, breaks up the biofilm to allow more complete removal of exudate from the wound.

The manufacturer describes the product as being useful in a very wide range of acute and chronic wounds. The directions for use are to cover the wound, including its edges, with a layer of the product (1–3 mm thick) and apply a light gauze dressing. The product should initially be applied once daily until the wound is free from necrosis, pus, and infection. Thereafter, frequency of application is reduced to once every 3–5 days until the granulation phase of healing is complete. If the wound's surface appears dry (i.e., without a scab), application should be discontinued. The final layer of SertaSil should be left on the wound.

Maggot debridement therapy (biosurgery)

The use of maggots for wound debridement is described in Chapter 22.

Corticosteroids

Due to their immunosuppressive effects, corticosteroids should be expected to exert a negative influence on wound healing. Indeed, in experimental cutaneous wounds in rats, neovascularization and formation of granulation tissue were delayed in the early phases of healing, and in the later phases of healing, infiltration with neutrophil granulocytes was prolonged and there was immature fibrosis, less epithelialization and increased scab formation in wounds treated topically with 1% hydrocortisone compared to untreated controls.[77] In horses, both *in vitro* and *in vivo* studies support the negative influence of corticosteroids on wound healing. Reduction in the proliferation of isolated equine fibroblasts was reported when the cells were cultured in the presence of a corticosteroid.[78] Corticosteroids were also shown to suppress angiogenesis, inhibit epithelialization, retard wound contraction, reduce synthesis of collagen, and decrease wound tensile strength in horses.[78,79] Nevertheless, there is empirical or testimonial evidence[80] of the positive effects of topically applied corticosteroids in the management of EGT in wounds on the distal aspect of limbs of horses. In a case series including 20 horses, an ointment containing nystatin, thiostrepton, neomycin, and triamcinolone (Panalog, Novartis) applied under an occlusive hydrogel dressing was used for "maintaining granulation tissue at skin level," but results were not described any further.[80] In experimental wounds in three horses, those wounds treated with topical fluoroprednisolone applied under a non-adherent dressing healed faster than wounds treated with non-adherent dressings alone or wounds left untreated, but the cosmetic appearance of fluoroprednisolone-treated wounds was inferior to that of wounds treated with a non-adherent dressing alone.[81] In contrast to these positive findings, a study by Blackford *et al.* (1991) showed that, although experimental wounds covered by Panalog ointment decreased in size faster than control wounds dressed with a non-adherent pad and remained smaller for the first 2 weeks of healing, the time to complete healing between the two groups did not differ significantly. The size of the scar

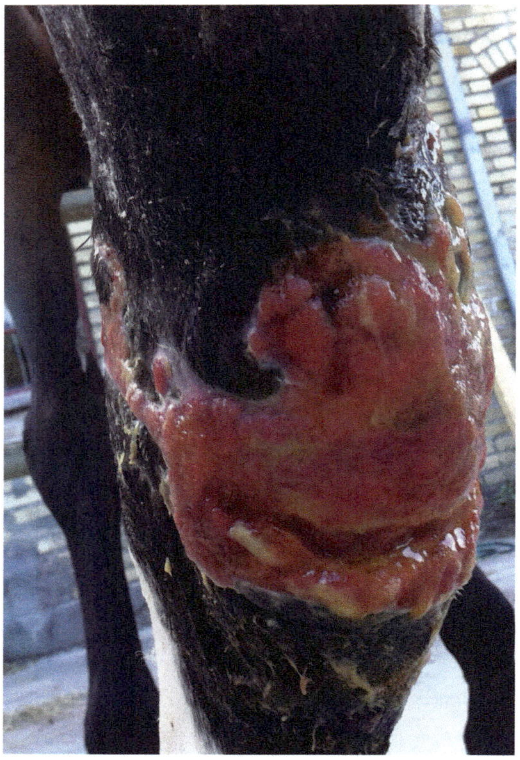

Figure 5.8 Severe, circumferential wound on the plantar surface of the left metatarsus of a mare. The wound shows signs of chronic inflammation with tenacious exudate and formation of exuberant granulation tissue. This wound will benefit from short-term topical application of a glucocorticoid cream (e.g., triamcinolone). Photo courtesy of Jørgen Didriksen.

and histologic appearance of the scar were also similar between groups.[79]

In humans, topical use of steroids has been recommended for enhancing healing of chronic, non-healing wounds characterized as being arrested in the inflammatory phase,[82] a condition that has also been described to occur frequently in horses.[83] Because chronic inflammation is a stimulus for the formation of EGT, transient suppression of the inflammatory activity of the wound bed may thus be of benefit in horses having developed EGT (the reader is referred to Chapter 15 for more information on EGT).

Wounds treated by topical application of a glucocorticoid develop a smooth and dry surface. This author advocates the transient topical use of triamcinolone ointment in granulating wounds to control excessive inflammation of the wound bed, such as in wounds coved with fibrin, wounds producing excess exudate, or wounds in which EGT recurs (Figure 5.8). It is recommended that triamcinolone be applied for a maximum of 4 consecutive days, and that treatment be alternated with antimicrobial dressings (e.g., nanocrystalline silver, fucidin ointment) to reduce the bioburden (Jacintha Wilmink, personal communication).

Sugars

Granulated sugar

Granulated sugar is a widely available and cheap product. It exerts an antimicrobial effect through its hyperosmolarity. *Pseudomonas* species seem particularly susceptible to the hyperosmolar effects of sugar.[84] Sugar moreover promotes debridement because it favors the draw of fluids through the wound. Edema is reduced due to the hygroscopic nature of sugar. Sugar is, therefore, indicated mainly for infected or sloughing wounds, in particular those with excessive exudate. Application of sugar should be discontinued when a healthy granulation bed has formed, because continued use may cause bleeding. Wounds treated with sugars often produce large amounts of transudate. Because the concentrated sugar solution causes migration of water and lymph out of the tissues and into the sugar solution, the solution becomes diluted, thereby reducing its hyperosmolar effect. Large amounts of granulated sugar should be applied, therefore, and dressings should be changed once or twice daily initially to maintain the sugar's antimicrobial effect. A large, absorptive pad should be applied over the sugar.

What to do

- A generous quantity of sugar should be used (apply to approximately 1 cm thickness). All pockets and undermined areas of the wound should be filled with sugar. Bandages should be changed once or twice daily, initially. Frequency of bandage change relates to the size of the wound and the production of exudate. Bandages should be changed if strike-through occurs. When granulated sugar is still present in the wound at the time of bandage change, the frequency of bandage changes can be reduced.[85]

Occasionally, human patients describe a burning sensation when dry granulated sugar is packed into a cavitated wound. Consequently, a paste made from 400 g caster sugar, 600 g icing sugar, 480 mL glycerin BP, and 7.5 mL hydrogen peroxide 3% BP (100 vol) has been suggested as an alternative to dry granulated sugar for abscesses and other cavities.[85] Hydrogen peroxide is combined with the glycerin and stirred; the sugars should then be added, and the ingredients mixed to a paste in a blender.

In horses, Sugardine is often used for treating hoof abscesses (Figure 5.9). Sugardine is made by adding PI to granulated sugar or icing sugar until a paste of workable consistency is produced. This hypertonic agent acts by osmotic action to draw exudate from the wound.

Honey

Honey has some of the same beneficial effects as granulated sugar and has been used in wound management for centuries. Its main antimicrobial effect is due to its hyperosmolarity and low pH. Honey, moreover, contains the enzyme glucose oxidase, which catalyzes the production of gluconic acid and hydrogen peroxide, both of which serve as mild antimicrobial agents.[86]

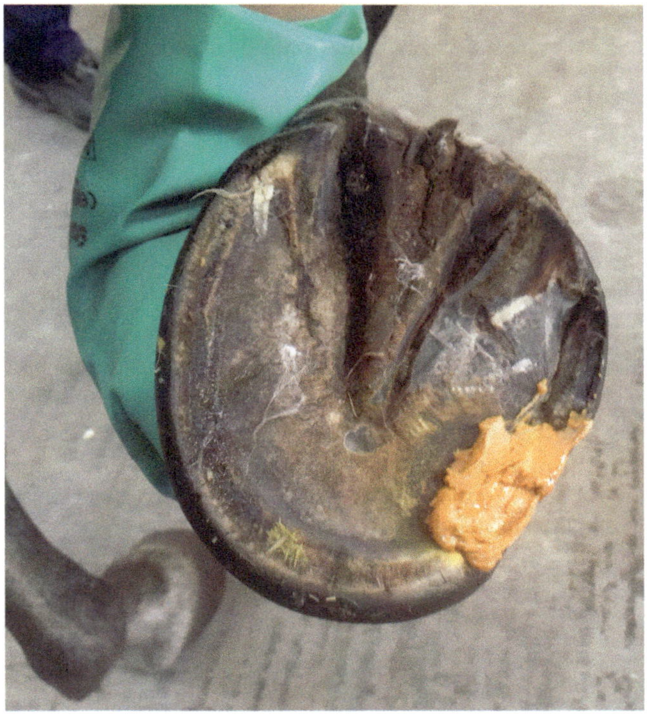

Figure 5.9 Sugardine (icing sugar mixed with iodine) applied to a hoof abscess after paring and draining of the abscess. Photo courtesy of Stine Østergaard.

Honey is also anti-inflammatory, reduces edema, stimulates fibroplasia and epithelialization, and provides nutrients required for cellular metabolism. As is the case for sugar, application of honey to the wound leads to the accumulation of moisture, thus promoting debridement and healing.

Manuka honey contains the unique antibacterial compound methylglyoxal and is, therefore, traditionally thought of as the most effective type of honey. A recent study has, however, shown that other types of honey were as efficient as or more so than Manuka honey in inhibiting the growth of bacteria obtained from equine wounds.[87] Non-sterile honey may contain *Clostridium botulinum* spores or aerobic bacteria or fungi, and consequently, only honey sterilized by gamma-irradiation should be used for treating wounds.

A study investigating the effects of Manuka honey (Summer Glow Apiaries Ltd, New Zealand) and a Manuka honey gel (Nature Vet Pty Ltd, Australia) on healing of experimental wounds on limbs of horses demonstrated that treated wounds healed faster than control wounds.[88] The two products were equally efficient, but the consistency of Manuka honey gel was superior to that of Manuka honey, preventing "run-off" when the gel was applied to wounds on the distal aspect of the limb. Consequently the need for a bandage was obviated, thereby reducing the overall cost of treatment. The beneficial effects of topical application of the Manuka honey products were most prominent during the first 3 weeks of second-intention healing. A systematic review assessing the effects of honey on the healing of acute (e.g., burns, lacerations) and/or chronic (e.g., venous ulcers) wounds in humans found evidence that honey: (1) reduced the healing time of partial-thickness burns compared to other treatments, such as polyurethane film, paraffin gauze, and leaving the burn exposed; and (2) induced faster healing of infected postoperative wounds than did antiseptics alone or gauze soaked in antiseptic solution (Eusol, i.e. lime and boric acid).[89]

Topical honey products marketed specifically for veterinary use are available from numerous sources, such as Links Medical Products, Kruuse, Aniwell, Red Horse, and Vetramil.

A more in-depth description of the use of honey in wound management is provided in Chapter 22.

Maltodextrin

Maltodextrin is a d-glucose polysaccharide. It is available as a powder and as a gel, both of which also contain 1% ascorbic acid (Multodex, DeRoyal). The powder is hydrophilic and is used in moist wounds, where the absorbed fluid turns the powder into a gel, thus providing moist wound healing.

Similar to other sugars, maltodextrin extracts fluid through the wound, thereby cleansing contaminated and infected wounds, reducing swelling, and enhancing the absorption of tenacious exudates. There is limited evidence for its effects on healing tissues, but it may positively affect chemotaxis of leukocytes, provide substrate (glucose) for cellular metabolism and healing, and induce formation of granulation tissue.[90] Based on these suggestions, maltodextrin should be used in the early phases of healing (i.e., the inflammatory and proliferative phases), especially in wounds that are contaminated or infected. Studies in humans with recalcitrant wounds or venous leg ulcers have suggested that application of maltodextrin also accelerates healing of chronic wounds.[91,92] Maltodextrin applied to experimental wounds in four horses was suggested to be more effective in reducing pain and swelling and in stimulating healing than was nitrofurazone, but the results of the study were not substantiated by statistical analyses.[93]

Maltodextrin is applied to the wound after debridement and irrigation, in a thin layer, or used to fill in cavities and undermined wounds. It should be covered by a dressing.

Vitamin- and mineral-containing wound products

Zinc

Zinc is an essential trace element in the body. Although the effects of zinc on wound healing are not entirely clear, a review on zinc in wound healing concluded that it had documented positive effects on autolytic debridement, bioburden control, and epithelialization and that the use of zinc was underappreciated in human wound care.[94] In individuals that are zinc deficient from hereditary or dietary reasons, systemically administered zinc supplements are indicated, but in otherwise normal individuals, zinc is better applied topically to the wound's surface.

Zinc can be applied as a cream/ointment or as a zinc paste bandage (a so-called Unna boot). Unna boots are composed of open-weave cotton gauze impregnated with zinc oxide paste, and they are regarded as standard treatments for leg ulcers in humans, where they promote healing and protect and soothe inflamed peri-ulcer skin.[94] In some countries, zinc oxide bandages are routinely used to dress surgical wounds in horses, but there are no scientific studies to testify to the potential beneficial effects of this practice.

On the equine wound-care market, an ointment containing 10% zinc oxide, thuja, and scarlet oil (Thuja-zinc oxide, Vedco) is available. The manufacturer describes it as a protective astringent, antiseptic, and counterirritant ointment that aids in the management of superficial wounds and abrasions in horses. Another zinc-containing wound-care product on the veterinary market is the Maxi/Guard Zn7 Derm spray (Addison Biological Laboratories, the product was previously called Maxi/Guard Zn7 Equine Wound Care Formula). The spray contains zinc gluconate, complexed with the amino acids lysine and taurine to prevent zinc precipitation in the neutral pH range, calamine lotion, vitamin C, deionized water, carboxymethylcellulose, methylparaben, and propylparaben. The product is suggested to possess healing-promoting and antipruritic functions and to dry out moist dermatitis; the manufacturer advocates the use of the spray on a wide variety of wounds, both with and without a dressing. A study involving 2 × 2 cm experimental wounds in rats did not, however, find any difference in healing between wounds treated with Zn7 Derm or with multiple controls (carrier solution alone, chlorhexidine, saline or no treatment).[77]

Tri- and tetrapeptide–copper complexes

Tri- and tetrapeptide–copper are complexes of the amino acids glycyl, histidyl, lysine, (and phenylalanine) with copper found in plasma, urine, and saliva. The tri- and tetrapeptide–copper complexes (TCC) promote several cellular and tissue activities involved in wound healing, including chemoattraction of leukocytes, angiogenesis, disposition of collagen, and growth of fibroblasts.[95] TCC are used in cosmetics as a reparative and anti-aging agent, for stimulation of hair growth, and as a wound-care product (Iamin hydrogel, Procyte). They have not been tested in horses, but in rabbits, they have been shown to stimulate formation of granulation tissue, to decrease time to healing, and to be more efficient in promoting healing of open wounds than zinc oxide.[95,96] The product should be used in the late inflammatory phase and early proliferative phase of healing to stimulate formation of granulation tissue. In dogs, TCC induced formation of EGT,[97] and therefore, equine wounds treated with TCC should be monitored closely.

Vitamins

The effects of delivering vitamins to wounds from dressings and ointments are only sparsely reported; most studies have investigated effects of oral supplementation. Vitamins can be administered to the wound's surface by oil-based liquid emulsions, creams, ointments, gauze, and silicone gel sheets.

Vitamins may serve several important functions in wound healing.[98] Vitamin A is involved in differentiation of epithelial cells and synthesis of collagen, and it has been shown to promote wound healing and to reverse corticosteroid-induced inhibition of wound healing. Vitamin C plays a central role in the synthesis of collagen and other organic components of the intracellular matrix, and the need for vitamin C is increased during the homeostatic and immune responses to accidental and surgical trauma and to infection. Vitamin E is reported to have antioxidant and anti-inflammatory functions and to promote angiogenesis and reduce scarring, but contact dermatitis has been ascribed to topical application of vitamin E.[98] Numerous vitamin-containing creams and ointments intended for skin and wound care are available over the counter, but clinical studies investigating their effects on wound healing are lacking. Consequently, recommendations for use of these products cannot currently be provided.

Herbal products

The wound-care market comprises a large number of herbal products. These preparations usually consist of small amounts of the plant combined with a delivery vehicle (e.g., an ointment). An exhaustive overview of all medicinal plants used in wound care is beyond the scope of this chapter; instead, readers may wish to consult comprehensive reviews on the topic, such as those by Pazyar *et al.* (2014),[99] Reddy *et al.* (2013),[100] or Krishnan (2006).[101] A recent review by Budovsky *et al.* (2015) gives a nice overview of the bioactive constituents responsible for the therapeutic activity of medicinal plants and their proposed targets in the body.[102] The herbal therapies mentioned below are those most widely available. It is important to note that very few of the therapies have been tested in the horse for effectiveness and/or toxicity. Examples of herbal wound-care products are shown in Table 5.4.

Aloe vera and acemannan

Aloe vera gel is extracted from the leaves of the succulent plant *Aloe vera*. The effects of *Aloe vera* have been suggested to come from multiple components of the plant, such as polysaccharides, mannans, lectins, and glycoproteins. One of these components, acemannan, stimulates macrophages to produce the cytokines, interleukin-1 and tumor necrosis factor α, which in turn, stimulate proliferation of fibroblasts, angiogenesis, epidermal growth and motility, and deposition of collagen. Acemannan may also stabilize growth factors to prolong their effects on fibroplasia.

Aloe vera has been suggested to possess numerous potentially beneficial functions, including a soothing effect, inhibition of bacterial and fungal growth, anti-inflammatory effects, synthesis and cross-linking of collagen, and increased

Table 5.4 Examples of herbal wound-care products.

Brand name	Company	Contents
Aloe Heal	Farnam	*Aloe vera*, vitamins A, D and E, safflower and sunflower seed oils
C4G ointment	Uckele	Petrolatum, beeswax, calendula, chamomile, arnica, spirit of camphor, clove oil, witch hazel, sodium copper chlorophyllin, gentian extract
Dy's Liquid Bandage	Advanced Biological Concepts	Olive oil, beeswax, pascalite clay, goldenseal, bee pollen, yarrow, chlorophyll, Oregon grape, cramp bark, shavegrass, myrrh, *Aloe vera*, cod liver oil, tea tree oil (*Melaleuca alternifolia*), propolis, calendula, honey
Equine Wound Care Oil	Feelgood Health	Linseed oil (flaxseed oil), comfrey, lavender (*Lavandula angustifolia*), St. John's Wort (*Hypericum perforatum* L.), tea tree oil
Herbal Solution	Schreiner's	*Aloe vera*, goldenseal, comfrey, myrrh, cayenne, elder
Natural Herbal Skin Cream	Botanica	Tea tree oil, comfrey, *Aloe vera*, oil of lavender
Power Dust #16 E	Silver Lining Herbs	Comfrey, capsicum, flax seed, boneset, lobelia, plantain, slippery elm, yarrow, shepherd's purse, goldenseal
Simple Relief Wound Gel	Equine Energetics	Organic essential oils of benzoin, lavender, vetiver, patchouli, geranium, immortelle, tea tree, cypress, palmarosa
Wound Heal Herbal Treatment Spray	The Equine Apothecary	*Aloe vera*, herbal tinctures in organic grain alcohol (calendula, chamomile, comfrey, echinacea, elder, goldenseal, myrrh), lavender essential oil, tea tree essential oil, vitamin E

blood flow due to dilation of capillaries. It has been used extensively in the management of burn wounds in humans. One study found that *Aloe vera* gel was more effective in increasing the rate of epithelialization of burn wounds than was silver sulfadiazine cream.[103] A recent systematic review of the use of *Aloe vera* in the management of acute and chronic wounds in humans did not, however, provide sufficient clinical evidence to support use of *Aloe vera* in wound-care management.[104]

A wide range of human and veterinary wound-care products containing acemannan are available from Carrington Labs/Medline, including wound cleansers (Carravet Acemannan Wound Cleanser, EquineVet Acemannan Wound Cleanser), amorphous hydrogels (Carrasyn, Carrasyn V, Carravet Acemannan Wound Gel, Carrasmart Gel), spray (Carrasyn spray), gauze impregnated with hydrogel (Carragauze), alginate (Carraginate with Acemannan Hydrogel), and hydrocolloid (Carrasmart Hydrocolloid with Acemannan Hydrogel). There are no studies evaluating effects of *Aloe vera*/acemannan on equine wound healing, but in dogs, acemannan hydrogel enhanced contraction and epithelialization of paw wounds and stimulated formation of granulation tissue over exposed bone.[105] *Aloe vera* and acemannan stimulate early events in wound healing and have been suggested to be most useful during the first 7 days after injury.

Chamomile

The very common medicinal chamomile plant (*Chamomilla recutita* L. Rauschert) owes its therapeutic activity to different groups of effective substances, including chamazulene, α-bisabolol, bisabolol oxides, spiroethers, and flavenoids; and chamomile has been suggested to have anti-inflammatory, antibacterial, and antifungal properties.[99] Chamomile seemed to increase healing of experimental burn wounds and ulcers in rats, better than did olive oil and corticosteroids.[106,107]

Sunflower-seed oil

Topically applied sunflower-seed oil (*Helianthus annuus*) has been shown to have positive effects on wound healing in lambs and humans.[108,109] Sunflower seeds have oleic acid and abundant unsaturated fatty acids, most prominently linoleic acid, which is a precursor of arachidonic acid. In addition, sunflower oil has been shown to have antibacterial properties.[108] Topical application of sunflower oil to experimental wounds on horses, especially those on the body, accelerated the healing process (i.e., faster reduction in the wound area and earlier ingrowth of granulation tissue). Investigators hypothesized that part of the improvement in healing was due to a more efficient inflammatory response immediately after wounding, because treated wounds had more infiltration of polymorphonuclear cells during the first 7 days after surgery than did the control wounds (saline treated). Sunflower oil was applied twice daily and all wounds (treated and control) were covered with a gauze bandage.[110]

Tea tree oil

Tea tree oil (*Melaleuca alternifolia*) has well-documented antimicrobial properties, and it may also be anti-inflammatory and may increase fibroplasia.[99] Its effects on wound healing are sparsely investigated, but authors of a small case series of 10 humans with abscesses caused by *Staphylococcus aureus* concluded that tea tree oil accelerated healing. Based on the proposed effects of tea tree oil, the product should probably be used during the inflammatory and early fibroblastic phases of healing.[111]

Comfrey

Comfrey (*Symphytum officinale*) root, described as a natural poultice, is traditionally used for the topical therapy of contusions. Allantoin, the pharmacologically active compound in comfrey, has been documented to possess numerous activities, including the removal of necrotic tissue, stimulation of mitosis, promotion of epithelialization, and proliferation of fibroblasts and their production of extracellular matrix.[99] The healing mechanism stimulated by allantoin occurs via the regulation of inflammation. Comfrey has also been demonstrated to possess antimicrobial effects.[112]

Marigold

The common garden plant marigold (*Calendula officinalis*) has been used for centuries in wound management. Similar to chamomile, aqueous extracts of marigold are used as washings or wet packs for fresh wounds. Marigold has bactericidal and anti-inflammatory, as well as free-radical scavenging properties.[113] A small study suggested that a *Calendula arensis*/*Hypericum perforatum* extract has positive effects on surgical incisions created during Cesarean section, with treated wounds reducing in size faster than control wounds treated with the carrier solution alone.[114] A systematic review of the use of marigold in wound management concluded that the plant seems to possess a number of properties, especially modification of inflammation and epithelialization and reduction of bacterial load, conducive to wound healing, and that clinical effects are observed when 2–10% marigold ointment is applied to acute and chronic wounds. The available evidence, however, was characterized as weak, and the authors concluded that investigation using more rigorous clinical methods was warranted.[115] Recommendations regarding proposed best use in horses cannot be provided.

Arnica

Arnica, most commonly *Arnica montana*, has anti-inflammatory and antipurpuric effects. Several compounds in arnica provide analgesic and anti-inflammatory activity, including sesquiterpene lactones, helenalin, and chamissonolid, which are potent inhibitors of transcription factors. Unfortunately, the plant has numerous toxic side effects, including hypertension, renal toxicity, cardiotoxicity, muscle paralysis, and even death. Only homeopathic doses are safe when the product is ingested, and topical preparations should be restricted to intact skin. This limits the usefulness of arnica in the management of wounds healing by second intention, but the plant has been used in the management of contusions, sprains, and bruises and for the treatment of joint pain. A small number of studies of arnica are available, and no uniform conclusion can be drawn from these, because both positive and negative findings are reported.[100]

Ocimum

Holy basil (*Ocimum sanctum*) has anti-inflammatory, analgesic, and immunostimulatory properties.[116,117] Flavonoids isolated from *Ocimum sanctum* scavenge free radicals *in vitro* and have antilipoperoxidant activity,[118] and these properties may serve to promote wound healing. *Ocimum sanctum* has been suggested to be beneficial in the management of abnormal healing in humans, such as in preventing keloids and hypertrophic scars.[99] Topical application of ocimum extracts to experimental wounds in rats caused healing to progress faster and resulted in increased breaking strength of the wounds.[116,118] There are no reports on use of ocimum in equine wound management.

Miscellaneous topical wound-care products

Propolis

Propolis is a compound used by bees to seal and protect their hives from bacterial and viral colonization. Propolis is made of resinous compounds and balsams (55%), beeswax (30%), aromatic oils (10%), and pollen (5%), and it contains various flavonoids, amino acids, vitamin B, and antimicrobial substances.

Propolis exhibits a significant antibacterial and antifungal activity, with stronger effects on Gram-positive bacteria than on Gram-negative bacteria.[119] In addition, propolis is a potent antioxidant that may serve to scavenge free radicals, and it has immunomodulatory and anti-inflammatory properties. The anti-inflammatory activity is mediated by several constituents, among which is a compound called caffeic acid phenyl ester (CAPE), which has been demonstrated to dampen experimentally induced inflammation (adjuvant arthritis, carrageenan edema, and pleurisy) in rats. Purified CAPE and extracts of propolis have also been shown to modulate metabolism of arachidonic acid and to suppress generation of prostaglandin and leukotrienes *in vitro* and *in vivo*.[119] A recent study showed accelerated healing, reduced activity of matrix metalloproteinases, and lower bacterial counts in chronic diabetic foot ulcers of 24 human patients treated with propolis compared to that in a cohort of recently treated historical controls that had received standard treatment.[120] The potential benefits of using propolis for the management of chronic wounds are supported by the findings of a recent report on the treatment of chronic (duration not stated in the paper) neck and shoulder wounds in 32 horses and donkeys. Wounds were managed with surgical debridement and subsequent application of propolis powder (manufacturer not specified), which was covered with gauze and a sterile bandage. Authors found that within 1 week of treatment, wounds were reduced to 70% of initial size and had good coverage with granulation tissue and no exudation; after 3 weeks of treatment, wounds in horses were reduced to 45% of initial size, while wounds in donkeys were reduced to 15% of initial size. In the same report, authors also described healing of experimental wounds (4 × 4 cm, made in the shoulder region) in five donkeys. These acute wounds treated with propolis had completely healed (100% reduction in size) by week 3, whereas wounds treated with honey were reduced by 57%, and wounds treated with isotonic saline solution were reduced by 38%.[121] Based on these findings, it seems that propolis may accelerate healing of acute as well as chronic wounds in horses.

A propolis-containing product (Corigem, Corigem Animal Wound and Infection Care) is commercially available as a spray and as a cream. The manufacturer states that the propolis was harvested from the hives of African killer bees in Brazil, and the ingredient list includes, in addition to propolis, a proprietary blend of Brazilian extracts, glycerin, mineral oil, stearic acid, propylene glycol, glyceryl stearate, PEG-100 stearate, cetyl alcohol, triethanolamine, *Aloe barbadensis* leaf juice, *Argania spinosa* kernel oil, tocopheryl acetate (vitamin E), carbomer, phenoxyethanol, and methylisothiazoline. The manufacturer recommends applying the product two to three times daily or soaking gauze with the product before applying it to the affected area.

Protein-free dialysate of calf blood

Protein-free dialysate of calf blood (Solcoseryl, ICN Pharmaceuticals [now Valeant Pharmaceuticals International]) influences proliferation and migration of fibroblasts *in vitro* in a growth factor-like fashion, perhaps via stimulation of growth factor receptors.[122] In an equine study, Solcoseryl was applied to deep wounds of the trunk and limbs.[123] Solcoseryl application was beneficial in the early stages of healing, because it provoked a greater inflammatory response, faster formation of granulation tissue, and faster contraction. With sustained use, however, it inhibited healing by causing protracted inflammation and delayed epithelialization. The perceived best use is for deep wounds during the early inflammatory phase; treatment should be discontinued at the first signs of epithelialization.

Selective serotonin reuptake inhibitor

Serotonin is a neurotransmitter with multiple functions. Apart from its effects on the central nervous system, it has many functions in peripheral tissues. Activation of serotonin receptors leads to pro-healing events such as up-regulation of growth factors, production of collagen and proliferation of fibroblasts.[124] Serotonin exerts very complex effects on immune cells such as lymphocytes and monocytes, macrophages and dendritic cells, the overall function being described as maintenance of an anti-inflammatory state.[125] Moreover, serotonin causes vascular constriction and platelet activation.[124] The effects of serotonin on healing tissues are thus very complex and may enhance as well as inhibit healing.

Ketanserin is a potent serotonergic receptor antagonist, which is commercially available as a gel (Vulketan, Elanco Animal Health). It has been proposed that its beneficial effects on healing tissues are due to: (1) improvement of the microvasculature (vasodilation, inhibition of microthrombus formation); and (2) enablement of a strong and effective inflammatory response.[124,125] In horses, the blockage of serotonin-induced fibroblast proliferation may, to some extent, counteract formation of EGT, as described below.

In humans, ketanserin was useful for the management of chronic leg ulcers,[126] but did not affect healing of fresh surgical wounds.[127] Similar conclusions can be drawn from studies of the effects of ketanserin on equine wound healing. When ketanserin gel was applied to experimental (acute) wounds on the croup of eight horses, treatment did not confer any positive or negative effects compared to control (treated with soap and water) wounds.[128] In contrast, a multicenter, randomized, controlled clinical study found that application of ketanserin gel reduced the occurrence of EGT and wound infection and resulted in better healing in accidental limb wounds of varying chronicity (average approximately 1 week old at the time of presentation).[129] In that study, ketanserin gel was compared to an antiseptic (Rivanol, ASID Veterinär Vertriebs GmbH) or a desloughing cream containing malic, benzoic, and salicylic acids (Dermaflon Crème Elevage/Dermisol cream, Pfizer Animal Health). The treatments were applied twice daily by the owner, and wounds were left unbandaged. Treatment continued until the wound healed (success), formed EGT (failure), became infected (failure), or until the end of the study at 180 days. The authors concluded that the use of ketanserin gel was two to five times more likely to lead to successful closure of the wound and that this effect was achieved through reduction of infection and of formation of EGT.

A German study involving 198 horses treated with ketanserin gel (but with no control group) concluded that the product can be used to successfully treat wounds of the body and the limbs, and that wounds treated with ketanserin gel can be covered by a dressing.[130]

The clinical studies in humans and horse suggest that ketanserin is most useful during the late inflammatory and the proliferative phases of healing.

Cyanoacrylate

Cyanoacrylate is a tissue adhesive normally used to replace sutures and staples for wound closure. While short-chain cyanoacrylates are irritating and toxic to tissues, a long-chain cyanoacrylate, octyl-2-cyanoacrylate (2-OCA), formulated for greater flexibility (Liquid Bandage) is available as an over-the-counter product intended for application to non-sutured wounds. This product forms a protective barrier on the wound's surface. Cyanoacrylate has been shown to be hemostatic and bacteriostatic,[131] and animal studies have consistently shown an absence of tissue toxicity from 2-OCA when the product is applied directly to open wounds.[132]

Studies in laboratory animals and humans have shown no adverse effects of applying 2-OCA to wounds. In a case series of horses with partial- or full-thickness lacerations, the effects of liquid cyanoacrylate (Nexaband Pump Spray, Veterinary Products Laboratory) were evaluated. The product was, in most cases, used without a bandage, and the authors concluded that cyanoacrylate had a definite function in managing second-intention healing. Cyanoacrylate was used to protect the wound from dirt, debris, and insects and to stabilize full-thickness skin lacerations, thereby allowing uninterrupted granulation and epithelialization.[80] Healing of unbandaged, experimental wounds on the distal aspect of the limb of horses treated with liquid cyanoacrylate was equivalent to that of control wounds that were covered with a hydrocolloid dressing. Applying the cyanoacrylate was faster than dressing the wounds with the hydrocolloid, and both treatments were effective in preventing the formation of EGT. In this same report, cyanoacrylate was used to treat accidental wounds to the distal extremities in 10 clinical cases; all wounds healed without the development of EGT.[133] In the inflammatory phase of healing, the cyanoacrylate dressing was difficult to manage, as wound fluid would accumulate under and disrupt/elevate the cyanoacrylate from the wound. Once the wound was covered with granulation tissue, this problem was resolved, and cyanoacrylate would stay on the wound surface for weeks. Therefore, acute wounds were initially treated with bandages or casts for 2–3 weeks to allow the wound to fill in with granulation tissue, and, before cyanoacrylate was applied, the wound received a steroid cream to minimize wound exudation.[133]

Live yeast derivative

Live yeast cell derivative (Preparation H®, Pfizer) is a water-soluble extract of yeast reported to stimulate angiogenesis, epithelialization, and formation of collagen.[134] It has been associated with improved wound healing in humans,[134] but when applied to wounds of horses, it prolonged wound healing by delaying contraction and resulted in formation of EGT.[135] Anecdotally, live yeast cell derivative has been used succesfully in the late inflammatory and early proliferative phases of healing to stimulate formation of granulation tissue in wounds with tissue loss. Application of the product should be discontinued when the wound is almost filled with granulation tissue (Christine Theoret, personal communication).

Phenytoin

Phenytoin was originally introduced in 1937 as an antiseizure medication; since that time, evidence has accumulated to show that phenytoin can also be used to promote wound healing in a variety of chronic wounds in humans, such as leg ulcers, leprosy wounds, and diabetic foot ulcers. In rabbit models of wound healing, phenytoin was shown to shorten the healing time, increase tensile strength of wounds, and improve histologic architecture of the tissue.[136,137]

Although a systematic review concluded that phenytoin may have a positive effect on wound healing in a variety of wounds in humans,[138] the effects of phenytoin on wounds of horses remain unknown.

Ozone

Ozone therapy is a form of alternative medical treatment that purports to increase the amount of oxygen in the tissues through the introduction of ozone into the body. Also, the potent oxidizing effects of ozone may be of potential benefit to wound healing, as these lead to killing of microbes. Treating bacterial cultures with 20 μg/mL of ozone in a gaseous mixture with oxygen for 5 minutes led to complete inhibition of growth of *E. coli*, *S. aureus*, *Enterococcus faecalis*, *P. aeruginosa*, and other bacterial strains.[139]

Several methods have been suggested for administering the ozone. Ozone may be mixed with various gases (often oxygen) and injected intramuscularly, intravenously, subcutaneously or administered via a method called autohemotherapy, where blood is drawn from the patient, exposed to ozone and re-injected. Although ozone is an unstable gas, it can be stabilized as an ozonide between the double bonds of a monounsaturated fatty acid such as oleic acid. In that way olive oil can be ozonated and stay thus for 2 years, if stored at 4 °C.[140] Ozone can be administered topically by: (1) placing the wounded portion of the body in a sealed, ozone-resistant bag or tent and insufflating the bag/tent with ozone; or (2) applying ozonized water or oil to the wound.[141] In humans, it is recommended that wounds be carefully cleansed before application of ozonated oil. This recommendation is derived from the observation that the bactericidal action of ozone is markedly reduced when antioxidant compounds are present; presence of 5–10% serum, for example, has been shown to block most of ozone's bactericidal effect.[142]

The methods of action of ozonated oils are not entirely clear, but it has been suggested that when the stable ozonide comes into contact with the exudate of the wound, it slowly decomposes into different peroxides, which readily dissolve in water, thereby generating hydrogen peroxide.[143] Topical application of ozone has also been suggested to directly accelerate wound repair by promoting collagen synthesis and fibroblast proliferation at the site of injury and by increasing the expression of growth factors such as platelet-derived growth factor, transforming growth factor-β, and vascular endothelial growth factor.[144]

Topical application of ozone was shown to enhance healing in experimental, critical-size bone defects in the cranium of rats[145,146] and in experimental skin wounds in guinea pigs.[144] While healing of chronic venous ulcers was accelerated by application of ozone,[147] second-degree burn wounds treated with topical ozone showed the same rate of healing as wounds treated with hyaluronic acid gel.[148] No studies have evaluated the use of ozone in the management of wounds in horses.

Long-term exposure to ozone can be deleterious to the skin because it results in depletion of antioxidants in the *stratum corneum*. In contrast, several studies and a review by Valacchi *et al.* (2005) claim that controlled, brief exposure to low ozone concentrations are beneficial in treating skin infections and wounds.[140] In 2015, however, the United States Food and Drug Administration summarized the scientific consensus and stated that ozone is a toxic gas which has, as yet, no "known useful medical application in specific, adjunctive, or preventive therapy." It is also noted that in order for ozone to be effective as a germicide, it must be present in a concentration far greater than can be safely tolerated by man or other animals.[149]

Aerosol sprays

Several of the aerosol sprays available on the wound-care market are based on the principle of using cationic biologic dyes, such as methylene blue, gentian (crystal) violet, and acriflavine in

Table 5.5 Aerosol sprays.

Product	Manufacturer	Active ingredient(s)	Use
AluShield	Neogen	Aluminum powder	Surgical sites that are not bandaged, minor lacerations
Aluspray	Vétoquinol	Aluminum powder	Surgical sites that are not bandaged, minor lacerations
Blue-Kote	Dr. Naylor	Sodium propionate, gentian violet, acriflavine, isopropyl alcohol	Minor abrasions, fungal infections
Cetrigen	Virbac	Cetrimide, di-N-propyl isocinchomeronate, diethyltoluamide	Superficial cuts, also serves as a fly repellent
Red-Kote	Dr. Naylor	Phenol, biebrich scarlet red, isopropyl alcohol	Non-drying spray that soothes and softens. For cuts, burns and slow-healing ulcers
Scarlex	Farnam	Scarlet oil, methyl salicylate, P-chloro-M-xylenol, benzyl alcohol	Superficial wounds, cuts, burns, minor skin lesions, superficial dermatitis
Scarlet Oil	First Priority	Isopropyl alcohol, methyl salicylate, benzyl alcohol, parachlorometaxylenol, biebrich scarlet red	Superficial wounds, cuts, burns, minor skin lesions, superficial dermatitis
Wound-Kote	Farnam	Isopropyl alcohol, acriflavin, methyl violet	Minor cuts and skin abrasions

local wound therapy. An overview of the ingredients of aerosol sprays commonly used in horses is shown in Table 5.5. The main active ingredients in aerosol sprays are described below.

Acriflavine

Acriflavine is a dye obtained from coal tar. It was introduced as an antiseptic in 1912 by the German medical researcher Paul Ehrlich. It is supplied in the form of an orange or brown powder. It has trypanocidal, antibacterial, and antiviral properties and is mostly used for treating vaginal trichomoniasis in women and external fungal infections in aquarium fish.[150] It has also been shown to have inhibitory effects on growth of tumors through its antiangiogenic properties.[151] Its effects on wound healing are incompletely described, and there are no reports describing the use of acriflavine in horses.

Gentian (crystal) violet

The name "gentian violet"was originally used for a mixture of methyl pararosaniline dyes (methyl violet) but is now often considered a synonym for crystal violet, which is a triarylmethane dye used as a histologic stain and in Gram staining. Crystal violet has antibacterial, antifungal, and anthelmintic properties and was formerly extensively used in human wound care. A foam bound with gentian violet and methylene blue (Hydrofera Blue, Hydrofera) showed some promise at managing stalled/chronic wounds of the lower extremity of humans, plagued with a high superficial bacterial burden, that had been unresponsive to previous treatments.[152] The possible adverse effects of gentian violet are not completely clear. A study involving 70 geriatric human patients in which gentian violet was used to treat small, open wounds and eschars of all sizes and thicknesses on an extremity showed no adverse events to the gentian violet, and 103 of 111 wounds healed completely.[153] In contrast to these findings, gentian violet has been described as having a tissue-irritating effect and adverse effects on the formation of granulation tissue, to retard gain of tensile strength, and to cause marked vascular proliferation, indicating tissue damage.[154] Several studies have revealed that gentian violet is a carcinogenic agent when used on open wounds and on mucous membranes.[155] In conclusion, it is not clear whether use of gentian violet in wound care is safe.

Scarlet oil

Although scarlet oil has been used in the treatment of wounds in horses for many years, there have been no controlled studies evaluating its effectiveness. The ingredients in scarlet oil are mineral oil, isopropyl alcohol, methyl salicylate, benzyl alcohol, pine oil, eucalyptus oil, parachlorometaxylenol, and biebrich scarlet red (Table 5.5). Pine oil is commonly used as an antiseptic in household cleaning agents. Eucalyptus has antibacterial effects against *P. aeruginosa*.[156] Scarlet oil can cause a painful contact dermatitis in some horses, causing objection to continued treatment. Most veterinarians use this agent to stimulate formation of granulation tissue, but there are no data to prove that it is of any benefit, and therefore, its use cannot be recommended.

Topical fly repellents

Although many fly repellents are commercially available, few are marketed specifically for use with wounds. Citronella oil, cedar oil, and eucalyptus oil have been used to repel insects and are contained in some wound products. Pyrethrins are a class of insecticides that are also added to some products. The author is unaware of any scientific study that examines the use of these compounds on or near wounds.

References

1. Main RC. Should chlorhexidine gluconate be used in wound cleansing? *J Wound Care* 2008; **17**: 112.
2. McGuiness W, Vella E, Harrison D. Influence of dressing changes on wound temperature. *J Wound Care* 2004; **13**: 383.

3. Magson-Roberts S. Is tap water a safe alternative to normal saline for wound cleansing? *J Community Nurs* 2006; **20**: 19.
4. Mak SS, Lee MY, Cheung JS, *et al.* Pressurised irrigation versus swabbing method in cleansing wounds healed by secondary intention: a randomised controlled trial with cost-effectiveness analysis. *Int J Nurs Stud* 2015; **52**: 88.
5. Fernandez R, Griffiths R. Water for wound cleansing. *Cochrane Database Syst Rev* 2012; **2**: CD003861.
6. Museru LM, Kumar A, Ickler P. Comparison of isotonic saline, distilled water and boiled water in irrigation of open fractures. *Int Orthop* 1989; **13**: 179.
7. Wilson JR, Mills JG, Prather ID, *et al.* A toxicity index of skin and wound cleansers used on in vitro fibroblasts and keratinocytes. *Adv Skin Wound Care* 2005; **18**: 373.
8. Rani SA, Hoon R, Najafi RR, *et al.* The in vitro antimicrobial activity of wound and skin cleansers at nontoxic concentrations. *Adv Skin Wound Care* 2014; **27**: 65.
9. Rodeheaver GT, Kurtz L, Kircher BJ, *et al.* Pluronic F-68: a promising new skin wound cleanser. *Ann Emerg Med* 1980; **9**: 572.
10. Menton DN, Brown M. The effects of commercial wound cleansers on cutaneous wound healing in guinea pigs. *Wounds* 1994; **6**: 21.
11. Dire DJ, Welsh AP. A comparison of wound irrigation solutions used in the emergency department. *Ann Emerg Med* 1990; **19**: 704.
12. International consensus. Appropriate use of silver dressings in wounds. An expert working group consensus. *Wounds Int* 2012. http://www.woundsinternational.com/other-resources/view/international-consensus-appropriate-use-of-silver-dressings-in-wounds (accessed September 1, 2015).
13. Wartret L, Armitage M. Making sense of wound cleansing. *J Comm Nurs* 2002; **16**: 27.
14. Sibbald RG, Williamson D, Orsted HL, *et al.* Preparing the wound bed – debridement, bacterial balance, and moisture balance. *Ostomy Wound Manage* 2000; **46**: 14; quiz 36–37.
15. Best Practice Statement: The use of topical antiseptic/antimicrobial agents in wound management. *Wounds UK* 2011. http://www.wounds-uk.com/pdf/content_9969.pdf (accessed September 1, 2015).
16. Jones SA, Bowler PG, Walker M, *et al.* Controlling wound bioburden with a novel silver-containing Hydrofiber((R)) dressing. *Wound Repair Regen* 2004; **12**: 288.
17. Percival SL, Bowler PG, Russell D. Bacterial resistance to silver in wound care. *J Hosp Infect* 2005; **60**: 1.
18. Parsons D, Bowler PG, Myles V, *et al.* Silver antimicrobial dressings in wound management: A comparison of antibacterial, physical, and chemical characteristics. *Wounds* 2005; **17**: 222.
19. Ip M, Lui SL, Poon VKM, *et al.* Antimicrobial activities of silver dressings: an *in vitro* comparison. *J Med Microbiol* 2006; **55**: 59.
20. Yabanoglu H, Basaran O, Aydogan C, *et al.* Assessment of the effectiveness of silver-coated dressing, chlorhexidine acetate (0.5%), citric acid (3%), and silver sulfadiazine (1%) for topical antibacterial effects against the multi-drug resistant *Pseudomonas aeruginosa* infecting full-skin thickness burn wounds on rats. *Int Surg* 2013; **98**: 416.
21. Woodward M. Silver dressings in wound healing: what is the evidence? *Primary Intention* 2005; **13**: 153.
22. Loh JV, Percival SL, Woods EJ, *et al.* Silver resistance in MRSA isolated from wound and nasal sources in humans and animals. *Int Wound J* 2009; **6**: 32.
23. Woods EJ, Cochrane CA, Percival SL. Prevalence of silver resistance genes in bacteria isolated from human and horse wounds. *Vet Microbiol* 2009; **138**: 325.
24. Kahn R. Use of a silver wound cleanse on an infected below knee amputation (BKA). *J Wound Ostomy Continence Nurs* 2011; **38**: S28.
25. Kahn R. Infected post surgical wound treated with a silver impregnated wound cleanser and NPWT. *J Wound Ostomy Continence Nurs* 2011; **38**: S28–S29.
26. Saucier D, Milne CT. Use of an ionic topical silver solution with menthol as a wound cleansing agent in venous ulcerations. *J Wound Ostomy Continence Nurs* 2012; **39**: S12.
27. Borkowski S. G tube care: managing hypergranulation tissue. *Nursing* 2005; **35**: 24.
28. Mertz PM, Davis SC, Brewer LD, *et al.* Can antimicrobials be effective without impairing wound-healing – the evaluation of a cadexomer iodine ointment. *Wounds* 1994; **6**: 184.
29. Lamme EN, Gustafsson TO, Middelkoop E. Cadexomer–iodine ointment shows stimulation of epidermal regeneration in experimental full-thickness wounds. *Arch Dermatol Res* 1998; **290**: 18.
30. Miller CN, Newall N, Kapp SE, *et al.* A randomized-controlled trial comparing cadexomer iodine and nanocrystalline silver on the healing of leg ulcers. *Wound Repair Regen* 2010; **18**: 359.
31. Angel DE, Morey P, Storer JG, *et al.* The great debate over iodine in wound care continues: a review of the literature. *Wound Pract Res* 2008; **16**: 6.
32. Berry DB, Sullins KE. Effects of topical application of antimicrobials and bandaging on healing and granulation tissue formation in wounds of the distal aspect of the limbs in horses. *Am J Vet Res* 2003; **64**: 88.
33. Russell AD. Bacterial resistance to disinfectants: present knowledge and future problems. *J Hosp Infect* 1999; **43** Suppl: S57.
34. Saatman RA, Carlton WW, Hubben K, *et al.* A wound healing study of chlorhexidine digluconate in guinea pigs. *Fundam Appl Toxicol* 1986; **6**: 1.
35. Fraser JF, Cuttle L, Kempf M, *et al.* Cytotoxicity of topical antimicrobial agents used in burn wounds in Australasia. *ANZ J Surg* 2004; **74**: 139.
36. Bonacorsi C, Raddi MSG, Carlos IZ. Cytotoxicity of chlorhexidine digluconate to murine macrophages and its effect on hydrogen peroxide and nitric oxide induction. *Braz J Med Biol Res* 2004; **37**: 207.
37. Sanchez IR, Swaim SF, Nusbaum KE, *et al.* Effects of chlorhexidine diacetate and povidone-iodine on wound healing in dogs. *Vet Surg* 1988; **17**: 291.
38. Barnes S, Spencer M, Graham D, *et al.* Surgical wound irrigation: a call for evidence-based standardization of practice. *Am J Infect Control* 2014; **42**: 525.
39. Fowler JD, Schuh JCL. Preoperative chemical preparation of the eye – a comparison of chlorhexidine diacetate, chlorhexidine gluconate, and povidone–iodine. *J Am An Hosp Assoc* 1992; **28**: 451.
40. Wilson DG, Cooley AJ, Macwilliams PS, *et al.* Effects of 0.05-percent chlorhexidine lavage on the tarsocrural joints of horses. *Vet Surg* 1994; **23**: 442.
41. Mueller G, Kramer A. Biocompatibility index of antiseptic agents by parallel assessment of antimicrobial activity and cellular cytotoxicity. *J Antimicrob Chemother* 2008; **61**: 1281.

42. Moore K, Gray D. Using PHMB antimicrobial to prevent wound infection. *Wounds UK* 2007; **3**: 96.
43. Wiegand C, Abel M, Kramer A, *et al.* Viability and proliferation of fibroblasts, keratinocytes and HaCaT-cells influenced by polihexanide. *EWMA J* 2007; **7**: 109. Poster presentation Wounds UK Conference, Harrogate, UK.
44. Daeschlein G, Assadian O, Bruck JC, *et al.* Feasibility and clinical applicability of polihexanide for treatment of second-degree burn wounds. *Skin Pharmacol Physiol* 2007; **20**: 292.
45. Andriessen AE, Eberlein T. Assessment of a wound cleansing solution in the treatment of problem wounds. *Wounds* 2008; **20**: 171.
46. Wasserbauer S, Perez-Meza D, Chao R. Hydrogen peroxide and wound healing: a theoretical and practical review for hair transplant surgeons. *Dermatol Surg* 2008; **34**: 745.
47. Toth T, Brostrom H, Baverud V, *et al.* Evaluation of LHP® (1% hydrogen peroxide) cream versus petrolatum and untreated controls in open wounds in healthy horses: a randomized, blinded control study. *Acta Vet Scand* 2011; **53**: 45.
48. Levine JM. Dakin's solution: past, present, and future. *Adv Skin Wound Care* 2013; **26**: 410.
49. Barsoumian A, Sanchez CJ, Mende K, *et al.* In vitro toxicity and activity of Dakin's solution, mafenide acetate, and amphotericin B on filamentous fungi and human cells. *J Orthop Trauma* 2013; **27**: 428.
50. Rossi-Fedele G, Guastalli AR, Dogramaci EJ, *et al.* Influence of pH changes on chlorine-containing endodontic irrigating solutions. *Int Endod J* 2011; **44**: 792.
51. Sakarya S, Gunay N, Karakulak M, *et al.* Hypochlorous acid: an ideal wound care agent with powerful microbicidal, antibiofilm, and wound healing potency. *Wounds* 2014; **26**: 342.
52. Selkon JB, Babb JR, Morris R. Evaluation of the antimicrobial activity of a new super-oxidized water, Sterilox, for the disinfection of endoscopes. *J Hosp Infect* 1999; **41**: 59.
53. Ramey DW, Kinde H. Commercial and homemade extremely dilute hypochlorous acid solutions are bactericidal against *Staphylococcus aureus* and *Escherichia coli in vitro*. *J Equine Vet Sci* 2015; **35**: 161.
54. Nagoba BS, Selkar SP, Wadher BJ, *et al.* Acetic acid treatment of pseudomonal wound infections – a review. *J Infect Public Health* 2013; **6**: 410.
55. Ryssel H, Kloeters O, Germann G, *et al.* The antimicrobial effect of acetic acid – an alternative to common local antiseptics? *Burns* 2009; **35**: 695.
56. Daeschlein G. Antimicrobial and antiseptic strategies in wound management. *Int Wound J* 2013; **10** Suppl 1: 9.
57. Kramer A, Roth B, Muller G, *et al.* Influence of the antiseptic agents polyhexanide and octenidine on FL cells and on healing of experimental superficial aseptic wounds in piglets. A double-blind, randomised, stratified, controlled, parallel-group study. *Skin Pharmacol Physiol* 2004; **17**: 141.
58. Wooley RE, Jones MS. Action of EDTA-Tris and antimicrobial agent combinations on selected pathogenic bacteria. *Vet Microbiol* 1983; **8**: 271.
59. Sparks TA, Kemp DT, Wooley RE, *et al.* Antimicrobial effect of combinations of EDTA-Tris and amikacin or neomycin on the microorganisms associated with otitis externa in dogs. *Vet Res Commun* 1994; **18**: 241.
60. Leyden JJ, Bartelt NM. Comparison of topical antibiotic ointments, a wound protectant, and antiseptics for the treatment of human blister wounds contaminated with *Staphylococcus aureus*. *J Family Pract* 1987; **24**: 601.
61. Bischofberger AS, Tsang AS, Horadagoda N, *et al.* Effect of activated protein C in second intention healing of equine distal limb wounds: a preliminary study. *Aust Vet J* 2015; **93**: 361.
62. Bennett LL, Rosenblum RS, Perlov C, *et al.* An *in vivo* comparison of topical agents on wound repair. *Plast Reconstr Surg* 2001; **108**: 675.
63. Junker JP, Lee CC, Samaan S, *et al.* Topical delivery of ultrahigh concentrations of gentamicin is highly effective in reducing bacterial levels in infected porcine full-thickness wounds. *Plast Reconstr Surg* 2015; **135**: 151.
64. Matushek KJ, Rosin E. Pharmacokinetics of cefazolin applied topically to the surgical wound. *Arch Surg* 1991; **126**: 890.
65. Werner AH, Russell AD. Mupirocin, fusidic acid and bacitracin: activity, action and clinical uses of three topical antibiotics. *Vet Dermatol* 1999; **10**: 225.
66. Skarlina EM, Wilmink JM, Fall N *et al.* Effectiveness of conventional and hydrosurgical debridement methods in reducing *Staphylococcus aureus* inoculation of equine muscle *in vitro*. *Equine Vet J* 2015; **47**: 218-222.
67. Strohal R, Apelqvist J, Dissemond J, *et al.* EWMA Document: Debridement. *J Wound Care* 2013; **22**: S1–S52.
68. Pain R, Sneddon JC, Cochrane CA. In vitro study of the effectiveness of different dressings for debriding fibrin in blood clots from horses. *Vet Rec* 2006; **159**: 712.
69. Owen R. Use of a topical enzymatic debriding agent in wounds of the equine leg (a pilot study). *Vet Med Small Anim Clin* 1975; **70**: 1101.
70. Herman IM. Stimulation of human keratinocyte migration and proliferation *in vitro*: Insights into the cellular responses to injury and wound healing. *Wounds* 1996; **8**: 33.
71. Falanga V. Wound bed preparation and the role of enzymes: a case for multiple actions of therapeutic agents. *Wounds* 2002; **14**: 47.
72. Nemoto K, Hirota K, Ono T, *et al.* Effect of Varidase (streptokinase) on biofilm formed by *Staphylococcus aureus*. *Chemotherapy* 2000; **46**: 111.
73. Ramundo J, Gray M. Enzymatic wound debridement. *J Wound Ostomy Continence Nurs* 2008; **35**: 273.
74. Falabella AF, Carson P, Eaglstein WH, *et al.* The safety and efficacy of a proteolytic ointment in the treatment of chronic ulcers of the lower extremity. *J Am Acad Dermatol* 1998; **39**: 737.
75. Noble TA, Carr DS, Gonzalez MF. Use of a trypsin, Peru balsam, and castor oil spray on the oral mucosa: case report and review of the literature. *Pharmacotherapy* 1989; **9**: 386.
76. Mecikoglu M, Saygi B, Yildirim Y, *et al.* The effect of proteolytic enzyme serratiopeptidase in the treatment of experimental implant-related infection. *J Bone Joint Surg Am* 2006; **88**: 1208.
77. Kaufman KL, Mann FA, Kim DY, *et al.* Evaluation of the effects of topical zinc gluconate in wound healing. *Vet Surg* 2014; **43**: 972.
78. Miller CB, Wilson DA, Keegan KG, *et al.* Growth characteristics of fibroblasts isolated from the trunk and distal aspect of the limb of horses and ponies. *Vet Surg* 2000; **29**: 1.
79. Blackford JT, Blackford LW, Adair HS. The use of an antimicrobial glucocorticoid oinment on granulating lower leg wounds in horses. *Proc Ann Convention Am Assoc Equine Pract* 1991; **37**: 71.

80. Bello TR. Practical treatment of body and open leg wounds of horses with bovine collagen, biosynthetic wound dressing and cyanoacrylate. *J Equine Vet Sci* 2002; **22**: 157.
81. Barber SM. Second intention wound healing in the horse: the effect of bandages and topical corticosteroids. *Proc Ann Convention Am Assoc Equine Pract* 1989; **35**: 107.
82. Bosanquet DC, Rangaraj A, Richards AJ, *et al.* Topical steroids for chronic wounds displaying abnormal inflammation. *Ann R Coll Surg Engl* 2013; **95**: 291.
83. Wilmink JM, van Weeren PR, Stolk PWT, *et al.* Differences in second-intention wound healing between horses and ponies: histological aspects. *Equine Vet J* 1999; **31**: 61.
84. Cooper R, Molan P. The use of honey as an antiseptic in managing *Pseudomonas* infection. *J Wound Care* 1999; **8**: 161.
85. Mathews KA, Binnington AG. Wound management using sugar. *Compend Contin Educ Vet* 2002; **24**: 41.
86. Mueller RS, Bergvall K, Bensignor E, *et al.* A review of topical therapy for skin infections with bacteria and yeast. *Vet Dermatol* 2012; **23**: 330, e362.
87. Carnwath R, Graham EM, Reynolds K, *et al.* The antimicrobial activity of honey against common equine wound bacterial isolates. *Vet J* 2014; **199**: 110.
88. Bischofberger AS, Dart CM, Perkins NR, *et al.* The effect of short- and long-term treatment with Manuka honey on second intention healing of contaminated and noncontaminated wounds on the distal aspect of the forelimbs in horses. *Vet Surg* 2013; **42**: 154.
89. Jull AB, Cullum N, Dumville JC, *et al.* Honey as a topical treatment for wounds. *Cochrane Database Syst Rev* 2015; **3**: CD005083.
90. Dart AJ, Dowling BA, Smith CL. Topical treatments in equine wound management. *Vet Clin North Am Equine Pract* 2005; **21**: 77.
91. Krötzsch E, Salgado RM, de la Garza AS, *et al.* A comparative evaluation of maltodextrin/ascorbic acid vs. standard care for the treatment of venous leg ulcers. *Wound Repair Regen* 2005; **13**: A17–A17.
92. Brunette G. Resolution of recalcitrant wounds with maltodextrin powder. *J Wound Ostomy Continence Nurs* 2012; **39**: S16–S16.
93. White GW. Maltodextran NF powder – a new concept in equine wound healing. *J Equine Vet Sci* 1995; **15**: 296.
94. Lansdown AB, Mirastschijski U, Stubbs N, *et al.* Zinc in wound healing: theoretical, experimental, and clinical aspects. *Wound Repair Regen* 2007; **15**: 2.
95. Gul NY, Topal A, Cangul IT, *et al.* The effects of topical tripeptide copper complex and helium-neon laser on wound healing in rabbits. *Vet Dermatol* 2008; **19**: 7.
96. Cangul IT, Gul NY, Topal A, *et al.* Evaluation of the effects of topical tripeptide–copper complex and zinc oxide on open-wound healing in rabbits. *Vet Dermatol* 2006; **17**: 417.
97. Swaim SF, Bradley DM, Spano JS, *et al.* Evaluation of multipeptide-copper complex medications on open wound healing in dogs. *J Am An Hosp Assoc* 1993; **29**: 519.
98. Boateng JS, Matthews KH, Stevens HN, *et al.* Wound healing dressings and drug delivery systems: a review. *J Pharm Sci* 2008; **97**: 2892.
99. Pazyar N, Yaghoobi R, Rafiee E, *et al.* Skin wound healing and phytomedicine: a review. *Skin Pharmacol Physiol* 2014; **27**: 303.
100. Reddy KK, Grossman L, Rogers GS. Common complementary and alternative therapies with potential use in dermatologic surgery: risks and benefits. *J Am Acad Dermatol* 2013; **68**: e127.
101. Krishnan P. The scientific study of herbal wound healing therapies: Current state of play. *Curr Anaesth Crit Care* 2006; **17**: 21.
102. Budovsky A, Yarmolinsky L, Ben-Shabat S. Effect of medicinal plants on wound healing. *Wound Repair Regen* 2015; **23**: 171.
103. Khorasani G, Hosseinimehr SJ, Azadbakht M, *et al.* Aloe versus silver sulfadiazine creams for second-degree burns: a randomized controlled study. *Surg Today* 2009; **39**: 587.
104. Dat AD, Poon F, Pham KB, *et al. Aloe vera* for treating acute and chronic wounds. *Cochrane Database Syst Rev* 2012; **2**: CD008762.
105. Swaim SF, Riddell KP, McGuire JA. Effects of topical medications in the healing of open pad wounds in dogs. *J Am An Hosp Assoc* 1992; **28**: 499.
106. Jarrahi M. An experimental study of the effects of *Matricaria chamomilla* extract on cutaneous burn wound healing in albino rats. *Nat Prod Res* 2008; **22**: 422.
107. Martins MD, Marques MM, Bussadori SK, *et al.* Comparative analysis between *Chamomilla recutita* and corticosteroids on wound healing. An *in vitro* and *in vivo* study. *Phytother Res* 2009; **23**: 274.
108. Marques SR, Peixoto CA, Messias JB, *et al.* The effects of topical application of sunflower-seed oil on open wound healing in lambs. *Acta Cir Bras* 2004; **19**: 196.
109. Vasconcelos E. The usefulness of topical application on of essential fatty acids to prevent pressure ulcers. *Ostomy Wound Manage* 1997; **43**: 48.
110. Oliveira LAT, Souza VRC, Endringer DC, *et al.* Effects of topical application of sunflower-seed oil on experimentally induced wounds in horses. *J Equine Vet Sci* 2012; **32**: 139.
111. Chin KB, Cordell B. The effect of tea tree oil (*Melaleuca alternifolia*) on wound healing using a dressing model. *J Altern Complement Med* 2013; **19**: 942.
112. Sumathi S, Kumar SS, Bharathi V, *et al.* Antibacterial activity of the plant extract of *Symphytum officinale* L. against selected pathogenic bacteria. *Int J Res Pharma Sci* 2011; **2**: 92.
113. Parente LM, Lino Junior Rde S, Tresvenzol LM, *et al.* Wound healing and anti-inflammatory effect in animal models of *Calendula officinalis* L. growing in Brazil. *J Evid Based Complementary Altern Med* 2012; **2012**: 375671.
114. Lavagna SM, Secci D, Chimenti P, *et al.* Efficacy of Hypericum and Calendula oils in the epithelial reconstruction of surgical wounds in childbirth with caesarean section. *Farmaco* 2001; **56**: 451.
115. Leach MJ. Calendula officinalis and wound healing: A systematic review. *Wounds* 2008; **20**: 236.
116. Goel A, Kumar S, Singh DK, *et al.* Wound healing potential of *Ocimum sanctum* Linn. with induction of tumor necrosis factor-alpha. *Indian J Exp Biol* 2010; **48**: 402.
117. Mequanint W, Makonnen E, Urga K. In vivo anti-inflammatory activities of leaf extracts of Ocimum lamiifolium in mice model. *J Ethnopharmacol* 2011; **134**: 32.
118. Shetty S, Udupa S, Udupa L. Evaluation of antioxidant and wound healing effects of alcoholic and aqueous extract of *Ocimum sanctum* Linn in rats. *J Evid Based Complementary Altern Med* 2008; **5**: 95.

119. Wagh VD. Propolis: a wonder bees product and its pharmacological potentials. *Adv Pharm Sci* 2013; **2013**: 308249.
120. Henshaw FR, Bolton T, Nube V, *et al.* Topical application of the bee hive protectant propolis is well tolerated and improves human diabetic foot ulcer healing in a prospective feasibility study. *J Diabetes Complications* 2014; **28**: 850.
121. Abu-Ahmed H, Abdel-Wahed RE, El-Kammar MH, *et al.* Evaluation of the effectiveness of propolis compared with honey on second intention wound healing in the equine. *Middle-East J Sci Res* 2013; **14**: 1292.
122. Schreier T, Degen E, Baschong W. Fibroblast migration and proliferation during in vitro wound healing. A quantitative comparison between various growth factors and a low molecular weight blood dialysate used in the clinic to normalize impaired wound healing. *Res Exp Med (Berl)* 1993; **193**: 195.
123. Wilmink JM, Stolk PWT, van Weeren PR, *et al.* The effectiveness of the haemodialysate Solcoseryl® for second-intention wound healing in horses and ponies. *J Vet Med, series A* 2000; **47**: 311.
124. Malinin A, Oshrine B, Serebruany V. Treatment with selective serotonin reuptake inhibitors for enhancing wound healing. *Med Hypotheses* 2004; **63**: 103.
125. de Las Casas-Engel M, Corbi AL. Serotonin modulation of macrophage polarization: inflammation and beyond. *Adv Exp Med Biol* 2014; **824**: 89.
126. Quatresooz P, Kharfi M, Paquet P, *et al.* Healing effect of ketanserin on chronic leg ulcers in patients with diabetes. *J Eur Acad Dermatol Venereol* 2006; **20**: 277.
127. Lawrence CM, Matthews JN, Cox NH. The effect of ketanserin on healing of fresh surgical wounds. *Br J Dermatol* 1995; **132**: 580.
128. Ribeiro G, Martins CB, Silva MAG, *et al.* Uso tópico de ketanserina na cicatrização de feridas cutâneas induzidas em equinos [Topical use of kentaserin on healing of experimentally-induced skin wounds in horses]. *Arq Bras Med Vet Zootec* 2009; **61**: 144.
129. Engelen M, Besche B, Lefay MP, *et al.* Effects of ketanserin on hypergranulation tissue formation, infection, and healing of equine lower limb wounds. *Can Vet J* 2004; **45**: 144.
130. van Gulik I, Vinke L, Cieslicki M. The effect of ketanserin on wound healing in horses. *Prakt Tierarzt* 2012; **93**: 802.
131. Mertz PM, Davis SC, Cazzaniga AL, *et al.* Barrier and antibacterial properties of 2-octyl cyanoacrylate-derived wound treatment films. *J Cutan Med Surg* 2003; **7**: 1.
132. Eaglstein WH, Sullivan T. Cyanoacrylates for skin closure. *Dermatol Clin* 2005; **23**: 193.
133. Blackford JT, Shires GMH, Goble DO. The use of n-butyl cyanoacrylate in the treatment of open leg wounds in the horse. *Proc Ann Convention Am Assoc Equine Pract* 1986; **32**: 349.
134. Kaplan JZ. Acceleration of wound healing by a live yeast cell derivative. *Arch Surg* 1984; **119**: 1005.
135. Bigbie RB, Schumacher J, Swaim SF, *et al.* Effects of amnion and live yeast cell derivative on second-intention healing in horses. *Am J Vet Res* 1991; **52**: 1376.
136. Dehghani S, Abrishami A. Effect of phenytoin on wound healing in rabbits. *Indian J Vet Surg* 1993; **14**: 10.
137. Naeini AT, Oryan A, Dehghani S, *et al.* Effects of topical and parenteral application of phenytoin on cutaneous wound healing in rabbits. *J Anim Vet Adv* 2008; **7**: 1537.
138. Shaw J, Hughes CM, Lagan KM, *et al.* The clinical effect of topical phenytoin on wound healing: a systematic review. *Br J Dermatol* 2007; **157**: 997.
139. Fontes B, Cattani Heimbecker AM, de Souza Brito G, *et al.* Effect of low-dose gaseous ozone on pathogenic bacteria. *BMC Infect Dis* 2012; **12**: 358.
140. Valacchi G, Fortino V, Bocci V. The dual action of ozone on the skin. *Br J Dermatol* 2005; **153**: 1096.
141. Fathi AM, Mawsouf MN, Viebahn-Hansler R. Ozone therapy in diabetic foot and chronic, nonhealing wounds. *Ozone: Science & Engineering* 2012; **34**: 438.
142. Valacchi G, Sticozzi C, Pecorelli A, *et al.* Cutaneous responses to environmental stressors. *Ann N Y Acad Sci* 2012; **1271**: 75.
143. Travagli V, Zanardi I, Valacchi G, *et al.* Ozone and ozonated oils in skin diseases: a review. *Mediators Inflamm* 2010; article ID 610418.
144. Kim HS, Noh SU, Han YW, *et al.* Therapeutic effects of topical application of ozone on acute cutaneous wound healing. *J Korean Med Sci* 2009; **24**: 368.
145. Kan B, Sencimen M, Bayar GR, *et al.* Histomorphometric and microtomographic evaluation of the effects of hyperbaric oxygen and systemic ozone, used alone and in combination, on calvarial defect healing in rats. *J Oral Maxillofac Surg* 2015; **73**: 777.
146. Ozdemir H, Toker H, Balci H, *et al.* Effect of ozone therapy on autogenous bone graft healing in calvarial defects: a histologic and histometric study in rats. *J Periodont Res* 2013; **48**: 722.
147. Solovastru LG, Stincanu A, De Ascentii A, *et al.* Randomized, controlled study of innovative spray formulation containing ozonated oil and alpha-bisabolol in the topical treatment of chronic venous leg ulcers. *Adv Skin Wound Care* 2015; **28**: 406.
148. Campanati A, De Blasio S, Giuliano A, *et al.* Topical ozonated oil versus hyaluronic gel for the treatment of partial- to full-thickness second-degree burns: a prospective, comparative, single-blind, non-randomised, controlled clinical trial. *Burns* 2013; **39**: 1178.
149. Code of Federal Regulations, Title 21, Volume 8, section 801.415, United States Food & Drug Administration, April 1, 2015. http://www.accessdata.fda.gov/scripts/cdrh/cfdocs/cfcfr/CFRSearch.cfm?fr=801.415 (accessed October 1, 2015).
150. Wainwright M. Acridine – a neglected antibacterial chromophore. *J Antimicrobial Chemother* 2001; **47**: 1.
151. Lee K, Zhang H, Qian DZ *et al.* Acriflavine inhibits HIF-1 dimerization, tumor growth, and vascularization. *Proc Natl Acad Sci U S A* 2009; **106**: 17910.
152. Coutts PM, Ryan J, Sibbald RG. Case series of lower-extremity chronic wounds managed with an antibacterial foam dressing bound with gentian violet and methylene blue. *Adv Skin Wound Care* 2014; **27**: 9.
153. Farid KJ, Kelly K, Roshin S. Gentian violet 1% solution in the treatment of wounds in the geriatric patient: a retrospective study. *Geriatr Nurs* 2011; **32**: 85.
154. Mobacken H, Zederfeldt B. Influence of a cationic triphenylmethane dye on granulation tissue growth in vivo. An experimental study in rats. *Acta Dermatol Venereol* 1973; **53**: 167.
155. Ryan TJ. Wound healing and current dermatologic dressings. *Clin Dermatol* 1990; **8**: 21.
156. Al-Saimary IE, Bakr SS, Jaffar T, *et al.* Effects of some plant extracts and antibiotics on *Pseudomonas aeruginosa* isolated from various burn cases. *Saudi Med J* 2002; **23**: 802.

CHAPTER 6

Update on Wound Dressings: Indications and Best Use

Stine Jacobsen, DVM, PhD, Diplomate ECVS

Chapter Contents

Summary

Myriads of wound-care products are on the market, and making the right choice for a specific wound can be complex, especially because the scientific literature on wound-care products in horses is sparse. To select the best possible dressing, the veterinarian must decide which material is needed to enhance healing. The clinician must then determine if antimicrobial therapy is required. Several antibacterial compounds are available for topical use and are often more effective than systemically administered antibiotics in the management of severe contamination, critical colonization, or infection. To serve the requirements of specific wounds, several combinations of antimicrobial drugs and dressings are available.

The wound milieu changes as healing progresses and so do the requirements for dressings. Continued assessment, based on a thorough clinical examination and sound knowledge of the healing process, is indicated, therefore, to maintain an optimal environment for healing.

Introduction

For many years, dressings were considered useful only for protecting the wound and removing exudate. The prevailing theory was that the wound, if kept dry, would heal uneventfully. This belief was overturned completely by the landmark study performed by George Winter and published in Nature in 1962.[1] This study showed that the moist environment under a polyethylene film increased the rate of epithelialization of experimental wounds in pigs compared to wounds that had been left exposed to air.[1] Although progress has been slow, the concept of moist wound healing is now widely accepted in wound care in humans.

Equine Wound Management, Third Edition. Edited by Christine Theoret and Jim Schumacher.

Companion website: www.wiley.com/go/theoret/wound

Another critical turning point has been the gradual realization that major pathophysiologic changes take place in the wound bed as wounds heal (the reader is referred to Chapter 1 for more information on the physiology of wound healing). Consequently, no single dressing may support the processes of wound healing in all phases. Dressing should possess more than "plug-and-seal" capabilities – they should support healing by enhancing physiologic processes within the wound. The practitioner must, therefore, recognize the different phases of healing and have good knowledge of the properties of dressing materials to be able to select the best dressing for a specific wound at a specific stage in the healing process, from amongst the enormous assortment of available dressings.

What to avoid

- Avoid using the same type of dressing throughout all phases of wound healing because the different phases have different requirements.

The evidence-based approach to choosing wound dressings in horses is hampered by the paucity of scientific evidence of how different dressings affect wound healing in this species. Today, thousands of wound-care products are marketed, but few have been investigated in the horse. In most equine studies, the dressing under investigation has been used throughout all phases of wound healing, and most studies have been performed using experimental, excisional wounds. Accepting the premise that no single material can produce the optimum microenvironment for all wounds or for all the phases of healing, it becomes evident that such study designs are suboptimal for assessing how a wound-care product would affect healing were it applied to an accidental wound in the phase of healing for which it was designed. Veterinarians are often forced to select a dressing based on studies performed in humans or laboratory rodents, or based on common sense and a pathophysiologic rationale. Extrapolating from studies performed using other species may not always be useful, because the pathophysiology of wound healing varies widely among different species. Horses are tight-skinned and thick-skinned animals,[2,3] and limb wounds in equids heal mainly by epithelialization, with contraction accounting for 15–20% of the wound closure.[4,5] In contrast, wounds of small mammals heal mainly by contraction, because small mammals are loose-skinned and have the *panniculus carnosus* muscle layer that enhances contraction.[6]

Tips

For healing to proceed at optimum speed, the wound should be:[7]

- moist with exudate, but not macerated;
- free of clinically relevant infection and excessive slough;
- free of toxic chemicals, particles, fibers, etc. released by the dressing;
- at the optimum temperature: the most appropriate temperature has not been determined in horses, but optimal healing probably occurs at core body temperature, as is the case for humans;[8]
- undisturbed by frequent or unnecessary dressing changes;
- at the correct pH: an alkaline environment has been linked to non-healing. As the wound progresses towards healing, the pH moves to neutral and then becomes acidic.[9]

Expected outcome

Even when modern dressings are used and sound principles of wound management are followed, wounds of horses, particularly those located at the distal extremity of the limb, heal slowly (the reader is referred to Chapters 3 and 15 for more information about the healing of wounds on the limbs of horses). For example, numerous experimental studies in horses have shown that even under optimal conditions, a 2.5-cm × 2.5-cm full-thickness skin defect on the distal limb takes more than 2 months (62–106 days) to heal.[10–13] Moreover, the cosmetic outcome is often unpredictable and, in some cases, less than desirable. The owner of the wounded horse should be cautioned about these facts before embarking on treatment, which, in many instances, is costly.

Desirable dressing characteristics

Important properties of dressings are listed in Table 6.1.

Minimizing heat and fluid loss is important for maintaining a warm, moist wound environment, which maximizes the rate at which healing takes place (see the following section on Moist wound healing). It is generally desirable for the dressing to be non-adherent so that pain is minimized and the healing tissues are not disrupted during dressing changes. Moreover, the dressing should be easy to use and cost effective. Although many modern dressings are more expensive than traditional materials, their use may result in more rapid response to treatment and reduced frequency of dressing change, which in turn, may considerably reduce the total cost of treatment.

Other characteristics important for dressings used in humans, such as the dressing's attractiveness and ability to reduce odor, are of lesser importance in veterinary medicine.

Moist wound healing

Moist wound healing has repeatedly been shown to promote epithelialization and reduce scarring when compared to the healing of wounds in a dry environment.[14] Use of dressings that provide moist healing not only promotes faster healing but also leads to the formation of a more cosmetic scar, which may be of great importance to some horse owners.

Providing moisture to the wound bed has the following beneficial effects on healing:

- Reduced dehydration and cellular death: wound repair requires the activity of a range of cells, such as neutrophils and

Table 6.1 Desirable characteristics of dressings and their clinical significance.

Characteristic	Clinical significance
Provide or maintain a moist wound environment	Moist wound healing has numerous advantages (see "Moist wound healing" for further details). Permeability to water vapor controls the management of exudate
Absorb wound transudates and exudates	Excess exudate, especially from chronic wounds, contains tissue-degrading enzymes that block the proliferation and activity of cells and break down extracellular matrix components and growth factors, all of which will impair wound healing. Excess exudate can also macerate surrounding skin
Modulate gaseous exchange	Reducing oxygen tension (through occlusive dressings) in the wound bed enhances angiogenesis and fibroblast proliferation, thus stimulating formation of granulation tissue
Protect the wound from bacteria and foreign material	Infection and foreign material prolong the inflammatory phase and delay collagen synthesis, inhibit keratinocyte migration and induce additional tissue damage. Foreign bodies and particles form a nidus around which bacterial growth and biofilm formation may occur
Minimize heat loss	Normal tissue temperature improves the blood flow to the wound bed and enhances the function of cells involved in healing
Provide mechanical protection of the wound and wound surroundings. Be minimally or non-adherent	Fragile new tissue will be disrupted upon removal of adherent dressings; moreover, this can be painful. Reducing tissue damage by protecting the wound and wound surroundings will provide optimal conditions for wound healing
Require infrequent changes	Temperature falls and healing tissues are disturbed during dressing change
Provide compression to minimize edema and obliterate dead space	Edema may disturb perfusion and diffusion in the wound bed and surrounding skin. In wounds with dead space, transudates and exudates may accumulate and increase the risk of wound infection and dehiscence
Be non-toxic, non-allergenic and fiber-fast (not shed foreign matter into the wound)	Toxicity, allergies and presence of particulate matter will have detrimental effects on wound healing

macrophages, fibroblasts, endothelial cell, and myofibroblasts. The function of these cells in a dry wound is much reduced.

- Increased angiogenesis: cells required for angiogenesis thrive in a moist environment.[15]
- Enhanced autolytic debridement: moisture enhances survival of neutrophils and ensures that proteolytic enzymes responsible for autolytic debridement are carried to the wound.[16]
- Increased epithelialization: blood supply to dry, crusted wounds is reduced, and the scab produces a barrier to cellular migration, thus slowing rates of epithelialization.[17]

Enhancing epithelialization is tremendously important in horses, where epithelialization plays a proportionally greater role in limb wound closure than does contraction.

- Decreased rates of infection: bacteria have been shown to pass through up to 64 layers of moist gauze. Conversely, occlusive dressings are designed to form a barrier to bacterial invasion.[18] The warm, moist environment provided by occlusive dressings seems to favor the growth of pathogenic microorganisms leading to infection, but, although occlusive dressings have been shown to encourage microbial proliferation in wounds,[19] the infection rate is actually lower under occlusive dressings than under conventional dry dressings.[20–22]
- Decreased pain and iatrogenic trauma: the moist wound bed insulates and protects nerve endings, thereby reducing pain.[23] Furthermore, when using occlusive dressings, often fewer dressing changes are required, and therefore, discomfort to the patient and damage to the advancing epithelium are reduced.

Occlusive wound healing

Moist wound healing should be distinguished from occlusive wound healing. An occlusive dressing is impermeable to water vapor, whereas semi-occlusive/semi-permeable dressings have varying degrees of permeability to water vapor and allow gaseous exchange. Both occlusive and semi-occlusive dressings cause retention of moisture in the wound bed. Semi-occlusive dressings are constructed to allow some moisture to escape from the dressing while still maintaining a moist wound-dressing interphase. They thereby provide the benefit of moist wound healing while minimizing the risk of maceration. Non-occlusive dressings are freely permeable to water vapor and gases. As a dressing absorbs exudate, the combination (dressing plus exudate) may create a partially or fully occlusive shield over the wound (Figure 6.1). For instance, a gauze or cotton wool saturated with exudate may become fully occlusive and thereby exert different effects on the healing tissues than intended. Another example is a foam dressing, which is semi-occlusive but not designed to handle the often thick exudate produced in the wounds of horses. Consequently, as the exudate accumulates in the foam, the dressing becomes occlusive and impermeable. Therefore, the frequency of dressing changes must be adapted to the clinical situation at hand rather than the theoretical fluid-handling properties of a dressing.

Occlusion results in a mildly acidic pH and a relatively low oxygen tension in the wound bed. Angiogenesis is directed towards regions of low oxygen tension,[24] and because low oxygen tension also provides optimal conditions for proliferation of fibroblasts,[25] occlusive dressings enhance cellular activities involved in the formation of granulation tissue.

While generally beneficial in other species, the use of occlusive dressings may require a more circumspect approach in horses. A study investigating the effect of applying a fully occlusive dressing to experimental wounds on the limbs of horses showed that this type of dressing caused wounds to develop more exudate, take longer to heal and require more frequent

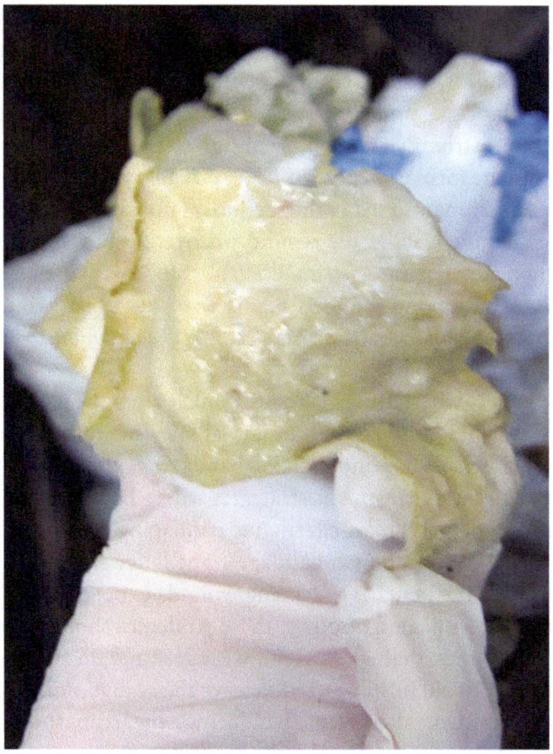

Figure 6.1 Dressing materials soaked in tenacious exudate. The exudate forms a partially or completely occlusive shield over the wound, because it is impermeable to water vapor and oxygen. The effects of the applied dressing may thus change in the presence of such thick exudate. This type of exudate may result from autolytic debridement, chronic inflammation or wound infection, i.e. from very different (patho)physiologic processes that require different treatments.

trimming of exuberant granulation tissue (EGT) (11.5 times on average until the wounds were healed at 113 days) compared to control wounds dressed with a dry, non-adherent gauze-like pad (in which EGT was trimmed on average 3.5 times until wounds were healed at 53 days).[26]

The adverse effects of occlusive dressings on the wounds of horses are, however, contested, since the authors of two case series involving six[27] and 28 horses[28] found that the use of a fully occlusive hydrocolloid dressing (Duoderm, Convatec) resulted in rapid formation of granulation tissue, which was suggested to be an advantage for horses with a severe laceration containing exposed bone or frayed tendons. Clearly, comparisons between small, superficial, experimental wounds and large, accidental wounds involving structures underlying the skin, must be made with caution.

Silicone gel sheet dressings, another form of fully occlusive dressing, have been shown to exert no negative effects on the healing of small, full-thickness skin wounds created experimentally on the limbs of horses. In fact, while the silicone gel sheet did not accelerate the overall rate of healing, treated wounds showed less propensity to form EGT and a better quality of repair than did wounds dressed with a non-adherent gauze pad.[29] Considering the divergent findings in studies using occlusive dressings for the management of wounds in horses, the effect of occluding equine wounds during the inflammatory and proliferative phases of healing appears to be poorly understood. Wounds should, therefore, be monitored closely if occlusion is anticipated, either as a result of the characteristics of the chosen dressing or the combined effect of the dressing and accumulating exudate.

To avoid the development of EGT, some authors have suggested that occlusive dressings should be used only during the inflammatory phase of healing and that their use should be discontinued at the earliest sign of formation of granulation tissue[30] or when the wound bed is covered with granulation tissue.[28] EGT developing beneath the occlusive dressing may need to be controlled by excision[26] or by other means (for more information on the management of EGT, the reader is referred to Chapter 15). Although it is occlusive, the silicone gel sheet should be considered as a unique treatment entity that differs from other types of occlusive dressings and can be used successfully throughout the proliferative phase of healing to control the development of EGT in the wounds of horses. Its mode of action and indications for use are described in more detail later in the chapter.

What to avoid

- Although beneficial in the management of wounds in humans, occlusive dressings should be used with caution in horses and only during the initial phase of healing, prior to the appearance of granulation tissue.

To bandage or not to bandage?

Bandages generally consist of three layers. The primary layer is the contact layer that lies directly against the wound, i.e. the dressings described in the following section. The secondary layer is padding that provides protection, immobilization and absorption of exudate. The tertiary layer is made of elastic and adhesive materials that serve to further immobilize, provide compression and fix the entire bandage to the limb. Bandaging techniques are described in more detail in Chapter 7.

The alternative to bandaging is to leave the wound uncovered. This causes a scab to form over the wound (Figure 6.2). Scabs are crusts of dried serum/blood containing erythrocytes, leukocytes, and platelets. They have beneficial effects in the sense that they provide a barrier against foreign material, minimize loss of fluids and proteins from the wound's surface, span the surface of the wound thereby preventing it from expanding and may facilitate wound contraction. Scabs are, however, not the ideal "dressing" because they slow epithelialization.[17] Moreover, unsightly scars may develop in wounds that are left unbandaged (Figure 6.3).[31] A study, in which experimental limb wounds in horses were either "neglected" or treated with gauzed soaked in saline, showed that moisture accelerated healing.[32] The limbs with the neglected wounds moreover

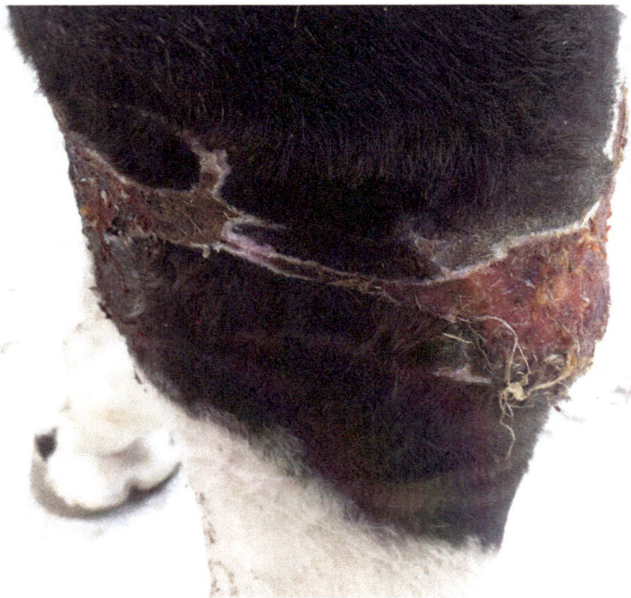

Figure 6.2 Limb wound where bandaging was discontinued. A scab has formed over the wound, and healing will continue under the scab, albeit at a slower rate and with a poorer cosmetic outcome than if appropriate dressings had been applied. The propensity for formation of EGT is reduced in wounds that are left uncovered. Contamination of the scab with bedding material or dirt rarely causes clinical problems. Photo courtesy of Jørgen Didriksen.

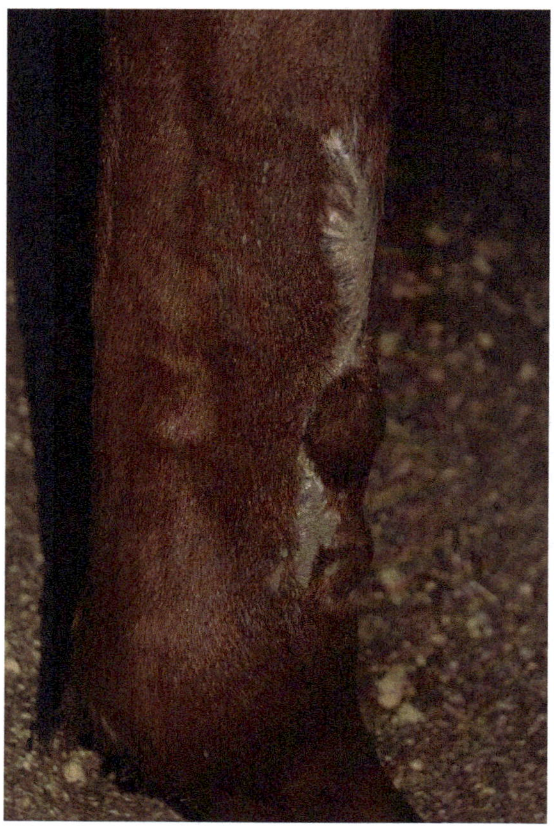

Figure 6.3 Unsightly scar that developed in a wound after bandaging was discontinued due to financial constraints. Same horse as in Figures 6.8 and 6.16. Photo courtesy of Tinamaria Jensen, Vinding Forlag and Tinamarias Digital Publishing.

became firmly and permanently swollen, and the author concluded that the lack of a support bandage had resulted in the initial cellulitis, which became organized over the course of the study.[32] Bandages and casts applied to full-thickness wounds at the distal extremity of the limb of horses have been shown to promote the formation of EGT,[31,33–35] possibly as a consequence of the effects mentioned in the section on moist wound healing. Consequently, leaving the wound uncovered may reduce the likelihood of having to trim EGT.[13,31] Moreover, it has been shown that leaving wounds exposed to air greatly reduces numbers of clostridia, *Bacteroides*, and *Pseudomonas* in the wound.[36]

In horses, where financial constraints or practicalities (e.g., temperamental horses that resent application of bandages) have dictated discontinuation of bandaging, this author has successfully used treatment strategies where bandaging is discontinued altogether, or "alternating bandaging" is used (7 days with and 7 days without a bandage). The latter strategy serves to combine the benefits of leaving wounds exposed to air and those of moist healing. Both of these strategies should only be used in wounds that are covered with granulation tissue, and the owner should be instructed to leave the scab *in situ*. If using the approach of alternating bandaging, the scab should be gently removed by irrigating the wound before applying the bandage. If bandaging is discontinued completely, this author advises horse owners to remove the scab every 7–10 days to inspect the wound that is otherwise completely covered by the scab, to ensure that granulation tissue is healthy with no crevices or necrotic areas and that epithelial ingrowth at the wound's margin is progressing as expected. Owners should be advised about the cosmetic consequences of not bandaging, and they should be warned that wounded limbs tend to swell when bandaging is discontinued, which may cause discomfort to the horse; swelling and discomfort can often be controlled by light exercise.

Selected products

Dressings are commonly classified according to the following: (1) their function in the wound (e.g., debriding, antibacterial, occlusive, absorbent, adherent); (2) the type of material used to produce the dressing (e.g., hydrocolloid, alginate, collagen, etc.); or (3) the physical form of the dressing (e.g., pad, film, foam, gel). In this chapter, dressings are classified according to their materials of composition into the following: gauze or gauze-like (i.e., "dry dressings"), alginates, hydrofibers, hydrogels, hydrocolloids, polymeric foams, polymeric films, silicone gel sheets, and biologic dressings. The indications, contraindications, and instructions for use of the different types of dressings are shown in Table 6.2, while Table 6.3 highlights the selection of dressings for specific types of wounds.

For most types of dressings, one or more antiseptic/antibacterial subtypes are available. These dressings are described at the end of the chapter.

Table 6.2 Dressings classified according to their materials of composition, their indications and contraindications, instructions for use, and examples of products.

Type of dressing	Description	Mode of action	Indications and contraindications	How to use	Examples*
Gauze and gauze-like	Traditionally made from loosely woven cotton. Non-adherent gauze-like ("dry dressings") are made from compressed cotton covered by a non-adherent thin, perforated, polyester film	Absorbs exudate and wicks it to the secondary layer of the bandage. Traditional gauze absorbs fibrin that is then removed at dressing change	Traditional gauze swabs are used to make wet-to-dry dressings for debridement of necrotic wounds Dry dressings are indicated for surgical wounds to provide sterile coverage. Contraindicated in complex wounds healing by second intention, where modern dressings with healing-enhancing properties are needed to stimulate healing	Gauze dressings should be changed often (approximately every 24 hours), in particular if used on wounds with moderate to heavy exudation (when the gauze is soaked, it no longer provides a barrier) or if used as a wet-to-dry dressing Non-adherent gauze-like pads may be left on sutured wounds for up to 1 week, depending on the status of the wound. If the non-adherent gauze-like pad is adhered to the wound at the time of dressing change, the dressing should be soaked in saline, *in situ*, for non-traumatic and pain free removal	Gauze swabs (many suppliers) Non-adherent, gauze-like: Melolin (Smith & Nephew) Telfa (Kendall) Tulle gras: Jelonet (Smith & Nephew)
Chitin and chitosan	Chitin is a polysaccharide material derived from natural sources such as fungi, yeast, and the exoskeleton of sea crustaceans. Chitosan is a derivative of chitin. Fibers from chitosan are absorbent and possess hemostatic properties	The material has a gelling and swelling action, when it comes into contact with exudate. The fibers are positively charged and will interact with the negatively charged erythrocytes to produce hemostasis. The material enhances functions of leukocytes and induces angiogenesis	Wounds with hemorrhage. Wounds in the early phases of healing, where the dressing may stimulate inflammation and ingrowth of granulation tissue	When used for hemostasis, the dressing should be handled quickly, as it becomes sticky when in contact with blood. The dressing must be pushed determinedly on to the source of the bleeding. Pressure should be applied with gauze on the chitosan and maintained for at least 2 minutes or until the chitosan adheres and the bleeding is controlled. Once used, the chitosan will not stick again, so the dressing should not be repositioned once applied. The dressing can remain in place for up to 48 hours; remove with water or saline	Chitosan: HemCon Bandage PRO (HemCon) Chitogauze PRO (HemCon) Chitoflex PRO (HemCon) Chitoderm (Trusetal Verbandstoffwerk GMBH) Kytocel (Aspen Medical Group) Chitin: Syvek (Marine Polymer Technologies) Talymed (Marine Polymer Technologies)
Alginate	Highly absorbent, biodegradable, non-woven fibers of calcium salts of alginic, mannuronic, and guluronic acids derived from seaweed. The high absorption is achieved via strong hydrophilic gel formation	Absorbs exudate (20 times the weight of the dressing) resulting in gelling and/or swelling (moist wound healing). Promotes hemostasis, inflammation (activates macrophages and mast cells), autolytic debridement and granulation tissue formation	Indicated for wounds in the inflammatory and proliferative phases, where granulation tissue coverage is needed. Suited for wounds with moderate to severe exudation, acute wounds with hemorrhage Contraindicated in wounds with minimal exudate (e.g. surgical wounds) or wounds with a dry eschar. If the alginate does not undergo gelling or swelling while on the wound, another category of dressing should be considered	Requires exudate to achieve gelling, must be pre-moistened if applied to wounds with limited exudation. The formed gel should not be confused with purulent exudate at dressing change Must be covered with a secondary layer. Should be placed on wound bed only (not on surrounding skin), and may be packed into crevices and cavities If dry, wet with saline before removal. Wound may need to be irrigated to remove fibers remaining after removal of dressing Change every 3–7 days, depending on type of dressing and amount of exudate. If used to control hemorrhage, dressing should be removed as soon as that has been achieved, otherwise dressing will dry and adhere to wound	Algisite M (Smith & Nephew) Kaltostat Calcium Sodium Alginate (Convatec) Curasorb Calcium Alginate (Kendall) Curasorb Zinc Calcium Alginate Dressing (Kendall) Biatain Alginate (Coloplast)
Hydrofiber	Fine fibers of high-purity cellulose are carboxymethylated to form sodium carboxymethylcellulose. Carboxymethylation of the cellulose alters its structure to improve its ability to absorb and retain fluid	The fibers absorb fluid and swell to form a clear, soft, cohesive gel that retains structural integrity and maintains a moist wound environment. Wound fluid and its contents, e.g. bacteria, leukocytes, and enzymes, are trapped and held within the dressing. Very little lateral wicking of fluid and thus reduced risk of periwound maceration	Indicated for wounds in the inflammatory and proliferative phases, where granulation tissue coverage is needed. Suited for wounds with moderate to severe exudation Contraindicated in wounds with minimal exudate, wounds with a dry eschar or wounds with heavy bleeding	Used in the same way as alginates – but not for bleeding wounds	Suprasorb X (Lohmann & Rauscher) Aquacell (Convatec)

(*Continued*)

Table 6.2 (*cont'd*)

Type of dressing	Description	Mode of action	Indications and contraindications	How to use	Examples*
Hydrogel	3-D network of hydrophilic polymers with a high water content (90–95%)	Donates moisture to the wound bed, promotes autolytic debridement and dissolves eschar and necrotic tissue. Has limited absorptive capacity. Has a cooling/soothing effect	Indicated for clean, acute wounds during the inflammatory phase of wound healing. Particularly suited for dry or necrotic wounds and for acute, painful wounds. May be used over exposed bone Contraindicated in infected wounds, wounds with heavy exudation or where there is skin maceration	Amorphous hydrogels are applied directly to the wound bed or may be applied to cavities, must be covered with a secondary layer May require frequent reapplication	Curafill (Kendall) Tegaderm Hydrogel Wound Filler (3M) Intrasite Gel (Smith & Nephew) Normlgel (Mölnlycke) Suprasorb G (Lohmann & Rauscher)
Hydrocolloid	Complex dressing consisting of gelatin, pectin, and carboxymethylcellulose with a polyurethane backing	Absorbed wound fluids convert components into a fully occlusive gel. Moisture is retained to a high degree in the wound bed, which facilitates autolytic debridement. May induce formation of exuberant granulation tissue in horses	Indicated during the inflammatory and early proliferation phases of healing to promote formation of granulation tissue in clean, acute wounds with minimal to moderate drainage. May be used over exposed bone. Contraindicated in infected wounds, wounds with heavy exudation, or where there is skin maceration	Dressing is self-adherent and does not require a secondary layer. Many hydrocolloids are opaque, which may make it difficult to observe the wound through the dressing. Should be removed from the wound with care, as hydrocolloids tend to adhere to the wound and may cause trauma/injury to fragile tissues upon removal. Produce odor that may be mistaken for infection Discontinue use at the earliest signs of granulation tissue formation Dressing should be changed every 4–7 days	Duoderm (Convatec) Suprasorb H (Lohmann & Rauscher) Tegaderm Hydrocolloid (3M) Replicare (Smith & Nephew)
Foam	Hydrophilic polyurethane foam, semipermeable. Some have adhesive perimeter, others a soft silicone contact layer to enhance patient comfort and decrease damage to tissues during dressing change	Large absorptive capacity, lifts excess exudate away from wound bed and stores it in its hydrocellular network, maintains appropriate moisture at dressing–wound interphase. Reduces risk of maceration	Indicated in wounds in the late proliferation phase, when completely filled with granulation tissue and requiring epithelialization and wound contraction. Useful for wounds with moderate to severe exudation. In wounds with minimal drainage a regular foam may desiccate the wound (thin/"lite" foams are available for such wounds) Contraindicated in dry wounds with a scab or eschar	Should extend over wound edges. Most manufacturers recommend dressing change every 3–7 days, but this will depend on amount of exudate and thickness of the foam. Does not require an absorptive secondary layer, as exudate is stored in the dressing	Tegaderm Foam (3M) Allevyn (Smith & Nephew) Biatain (Coloplast) Mepilex (Mölnlycke) Kendall Foam Dressing (Kendall) Tegaderm, Biatain, Mepilex and several other foams are available with soft silicone wound-contact surface
Film	Thin, transparent, polyurethane membrane coated with a layer of acrylic adhesive. Varying moisture and oxygen permeability. No absorptive capacity	Forms an impermeable barrier to microorganisms and moisture	Indicated in simple, shallow wounds (e.g. scalds and abrasions) with little or no exudation but healthy granulation tissue Can be used to cover sutures to prevent dehydration of surgical wound Contraindicated in deep, full-thickness wounds, in exudative and infected wounds	The dressing should overlap healthy skin by 3–4 cm. It may be difficult to get films to adhere to haired skin. Some films are available as sprays; these should be applied to the wound surface in several layers May be left on the wound surface for 7 days or more, depending on wound characteristics	OpSite (Smith & Nephew) Mepore Film (Mölnlycke) Suprasorb F (Lohmann & Rauscher) Tegaderm Transparent (3M) OpSite Spray (Smith & Nephew) Cavilon Spray (3M)
Silicone gel sheet	Silicone	Prevents or reduces formation of exuberant granulation tissue in horses. Mechanism of action is not completely elucidated, but may be related to hydration of the wound and surrounding skin or through occlusion of microvessels and modulation of fibroblast apoptosis	Indicated in wounds that have formed or are at risk of forming exuberant granulation tissue Contraindicated in infected or exudative wounds (has no absorptive capacity)	In wounds where exuberant granulation tissue has formed, this tissue should be excised and hemostasis achieved before applying the silicone sheet Should be reapplied every 3–5 days. The dressing may be reused several times after cleaning in mild soap and rinsing in water	Cica-care (Smith & Nephew)

* This is not an exhaustive list of product names; multiple products are available within each category of dressing. Several of the dressings are available also in one or more antibacterial subtypes; these are shown in Table 6.4.

Table 6.3 Dressing selection to promote healing in specific types of wounds. Please refer to Table 6.2 for further descriptions of the dressings and instructions for use.

Wound characteristic	Dressing	Comments
Necrotic wounds	Hydrogels Hydrocolloids Wet-to-dry gauze	Surgical, hydrosurgical, biosurgical (maggot) debridement will greatly enhance elimination of necrotic tissue
Desiccated wounds	Hydrogels Hydrocolloids	
Wounds where ingrowth of granulation tissue is required Wounds in the early proliferative phase; wounds later in the proliferative phase where crevices and cavities remain	Alginates Hydrofibers Chitosan and chitin dressings	Crevices/cavities may indicate presence of a sequestrum; wound should be thoroughly explored
Wounds with complete coverage of granulation tissue, where epithelial ingrowth is required	Foams Silicone gel sheets	If the granulation tissue is exuberant, it should first be resected surgically and hemorrhage must have abated prior to dressing the wound with a foam or a silicone gel sheet. For more information on the management of EGT, the reader is referred to Chapter 15
Wounds with excessive exudate	Alginates Hydrocolloids Foams Hypertonic saline dressings	Wounds with excessive exudation should be examined for signs of infection
Wounds in the late proliferative phase where healing is progressing normally	Films	
Sutured wounds	Gauze-like dressings (non-adherent) Films Soft silicone wound contact layer	
Small abrasions and superficial burns	Tulle gras dressings Gauze-like dressings Films Soft silicone wound contact layer	
Wounds with hemorrhage	Alginates (with zinc) Chitosan dressings	
Infected wounds	Antibacterial dressings such as silver, polyhexamethylene biguanide (polyhexanide), chlorhexidine, iodine, honey, hypertonic saline, activated charcoal, boric acid, or dialkylcarbamoylchloride	Systemic antimicrobials are only of use if there are signs of severe wound infection. In granulated wounds with superficial infection, antibacterial dressings are more efficient. For more information on the management of severely infected wounds, the reader is referred to Chapter 19

Gauze and gauze-like dressings

Gauze has been used extensively to treat the wounds of horses, especially as wet-to-dry dressings for debridement. It is inexpensive, which is one of its main attributes. Gauze sponges are either woven or non-woven. Woven sponges are traditionally made of 100% cotton fibers (threads) that are woven perpendicularly through each other, whereas non-woven sponges are a synthetic blend of melded polyester and rayon. Non-woven sponges are generally up to twice as absorbent as woven gauze and have a softer feel. Both woven and non-woven sponges are prone to linting, but non-woven sponges produce less lint. Both types of gauze are highly permeable, relatively non-occlusive, at least when dry, and have a high absorptive capacity. A wound bed dressed with gauze is thus likely to desiccate.

Wet-to-dry dressings are still widely used in equine practice to debride wounds. It is important to understand that the debridement achieved with this type of dressing is non-selective and removes healthy tissue and cells, such as epidermal cells and fibroblasts, as well as material requiring removal, such as fibrin and necrotic debris. Cross-contamination may also be an issue with this type of dressing because the saturated gauze in a wet-to-dry dressing does not provide a barrier to the environment, thus allowing microorganisms to move into and out of the wound. To create a wet-to-dry dressing, gauze soaked in isotonic saline solution is placed within a wound with exudate. As the dressing dries, exudate sticks to it. The gauze is peeled off the wound after approximately 24 hours, and adhered debris and tissue are removed along with the gauze pad. Removal can be painful.[37] One to three applications of a wet-to-dry dressing have been recommended in exudative wounds;[30] continued use is contraindicated because the non-selective nature of debridement strips away newly formed, fragile epidermis.

Using occlusive dressings (hydrogels or hydrocolloids) to assist autolytic debridement is a gentler, yet slower, approach to achieving a clean wound bed. An *in vitro* study showed that gauze, hydrofiber, hydrocolloid, and alginate dressings were the most efficient methods of debridement (measured as breakdown of protein in clotted equine blood). Hydrating the dressings in isotonic saline solution, rather than distilled water enhanced efficacy of debridement, and the authors suggested that isotonic saline solution was more efficient in donating water to the eschar.[38]

The efficient debridement achieved with a traditional gauze dressing may be attributable to the fact that the gauze's cotton fibers absorb fibrin;[39] fibrin absorbed into the gauze imbibes the saline solution, thereby increasing the surface area across which water can be donated to the eschar.

Dressing limb wounds with non-hydrated gauze swabs was shown to induce the formation of EGT.[13] Experimental, full-thickness, 2.5-cm × 2.5-cm skin wounds, on the distal extremity of limbs of horses, dressed with gauze, showed greater and more prolonged retraction than unbandaged wounds during the first weeks after wounding. In bandaged wounds, EGT required regular trimming, whereas trimming was not necessary in unbandaged wounds. There was no significant difference in the total number of days to healing or the overall rate of healing in bandaged and unbandaged wounds (75 and 66 days to healing, respectively), provided that EGT was excised regularly from the wounds dressed with gauze.[13]

Roll gauze can be used to pack cavities, such as abscesses after lancing. The packing is extracted gradually over 3–4 days. Debris, necrotic material, and bacteria are evacuated from the cavity as the gauze is extracted. Several types of medicated roll gauze are available.

When adherence of the gauze to the wound is undesirable, for example to avoid disruption of healing tissues, a tulle gras dressing (gauze impregnated with paraffin, lanolin or similar emollient e.g., Jelonet from Smith & Nephew) (Figure 6.4) may be applied. Tulle gras dressings are non-absorbent, and a secondary layer of absorbent material must be added over the dressing. Other forms of non-adherent gauze-like pads are the so-called dry dressings (e.g., Melolin from Smith & Nephew and Telfa from Kendall) (Figure 6.5). These dry dressings are typically composed of some form of gauze pad or compressed cotton covered by a non-adherent, thin, perforated polyester film (therefore sometimes also referred to as plastic film-faced dressings). These dressings allow free exchange of fluid and gas and thus do little to support moist healing. They have limited absorptive capacity and are mainly indicated for sterile coverage of sutured wounds with minimal exudation. Sterile dressings help decrease the opportunity for bacteria to enter or exit wounds, thus reducing the risks for infection and cross-contamination.

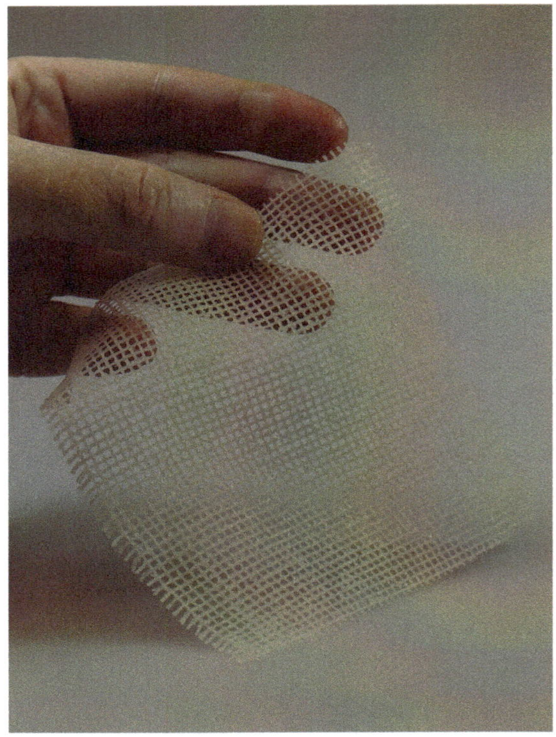

Figure 6.4 Tulle gras dressing. This dressing is indicated for use on minor burns and scalds, lacerations, abrasions, and other skin loss wounds of limited extent. Tulle gras dressings are non-absorbent, and a secondary layer of absorbent material must be placed over the dressing.

Tip

- Pouring isotonic saline solution over a dry dressing stuck to the wound eases removal of the dressing.

Dressing a sutured wound healing by primary intention

Dressing and bandaging sutured wounds healing by primary intention is generally perceived as beneficial in protecting the wound from contamination, removing exudate that escapes through the apposed wound edges, minimizing periwound edema, and providing physical support. There is, however, little evidence to support this notion.

In humans, a systematic review involving 20 randomized clinical trials with more than 3500 individuals with surgical wounds healing by primary intention concluded that there was no evidence to support that covering the wound with a dressing would reduce the prevalence of surgical site infection (SSI) compared to leaving the wound exposed. Moreover, this same review showed no difference between dressings in their ability to reduce the risk of developing an SSI.[40]

As the milieu in a recovery box and a stall is entirely different from that of a hospital bed, most equine surgeons opt to bandage surgical wounds. In support of this approach, a recent study suggests that suturing a stent over midline celiotomy wounds in horses that underwent exploratory abdominal surgery significantly reduces the occurrence of wound complications such as persistent serohemorrhagic drainage, excessive edema or purulent drainage.[41] Applying an elastic, adhesive bandage over celiotomy wounds was also shown to reduce the occurrence of postoperative incisional complications in horses.[42] For orthopedic surgeries, it is suggested that maintaining bandages for 10–14 days after arthroscopic procedures of the tibiotarsal joint is crucial for minimizing the risk of wound dehiscence and sepsis,[43] and in a study evaluating complications after arthroscopy, two out of three joints developing septic arthritis postoperatively had suffered bandage slippage.[44] Taken together, this limited evidence points to a beneficial effect of dressing and bandaging postsurgical wounds in horses. There are, however, no studies evaluating the benefits of applying dressings to accidental wounds in horses in which primary closure is the selected approach to wound management. Perceived benefits are, however, to support the apposed wound edges, immobilize, and to provide counter-pressure to minimize edema of the periwound tissues that are often also contused or inflamed.

The contact layer, also referred to as the dressing, should be chosen according to the expected amount of exudate. For smaller wounds with little exudate, a non-adhesive gauze pad or a film will suffice, whereas foam dressings are useful for surgical wounds from which moderate or heavy exudation is expected. "Lite" types of foams may be used where minimal exudation is expected, without risking wound desiccation. Adding a secondary layer of padding and an elastic/compressive tertiary layer will serve to protect the wound, keep the tissues warm and reduce edema and dead space. Where this is not possible, a stent may be sutured over the wound.

Frequency and timing of dressing changes will be based on the expected amount of exudate and the surgeon's preference. One systematic review did not find any differences in complication rates after early and late (>48 hours) dressing removal following primary closure of clean and clean-contaminated surgical wounds in humans, and one study included in the review suggested that early dressing removal resulted in shorter hospital stay and reduced treatment costs.[45]

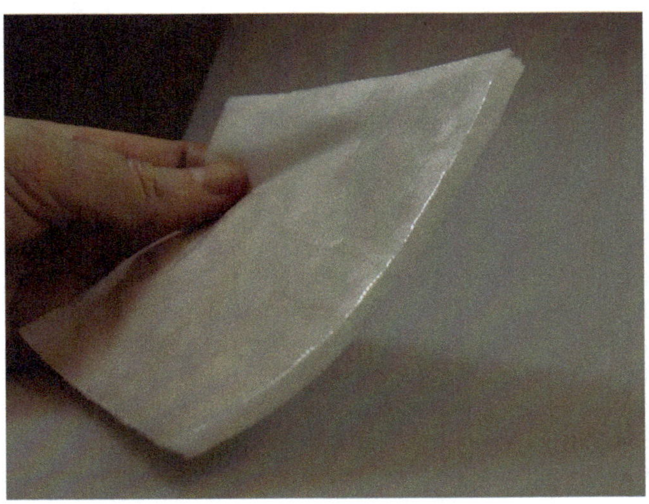

Figure 6.5 Gauze-like (also called dry or plastic film-faced) dressing. This type of dressing is made from compressed cotton and is covered by a non-adherent, thin, perforated polyester film. It is freely permeable to water vapor and oxygen. This type of dressing is mainly indicated for wounds healing by primary intention.

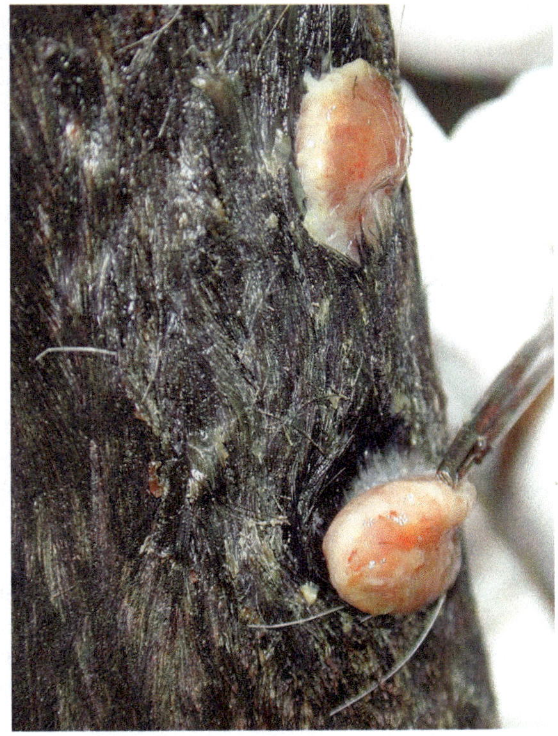

Figure 6.6 Experimental wound 28 days after the wound was created by surgical excision of 1 × 1 cm skin and periosteum. The wound was dressed with a non-adherent, gauze-like dressing during the 28 days study period. EGT mushrooming over the wound margin is apparent.

While acceptable for covering sutured wounds, dry dressings may be less ideal for wounds healing by second intention in horses. Several studies suggest that gauze-like non-adherent dressings, similar to traditional gauze,[13,26] stimulate the formation of EGT and thus may delay healing. In fact, in experimental studies on wound healing and wound management, where researchers intend to stimulate the formation of EGT, it has been demonstrated that 7–14 days of bandaging with a dry dressing is a consistent means of inducing the formation of EGT (Figure 6.6).[35,46,47]

Taken together, the available evidence thus suggests that wounds of horses healing by second intention, especially wounds at the distal extremity of the limb, benefit from dressings that promote healing better than do traditional gauze and gauze-like dressings.

Chitin and chitosan

Chitin, and its derivative chitosan, is a polysaccharide. Chitin is found in many naturally occurring organisms (e.g. fungi and yeast), and is the principal component in the exoskeleton of sea crustaceans. Chitosan, in contrast, is not found in large amounts in natural sources; therefore, the chitosan used for commercial products is derived from chitin through chemical or enzymatic treatment of shells of shrimp or crab. Chitin and chitosan are biocompatible and biodegradable agents, and they have been shown to exert positive effects on hemostasis and wound healing.

Chitosan is a hemostat; its fibers are positively charged, which enhances blood clotting by binding of the negatively charged red blood cells to the fiber. Chitosan fibers also polymerize with blood into a net-like structure, which captures red blood cells and further enhances clotting. The hemostatic properties were evaluated in combat wounds, where the main indication for use was gauze failing to achieve hemostasis. In 97% of wounds, application of the chitosan dressing (HemCon Medical Technologies Inc.) caused cessation of bleeding or greatly improved hemostasis.[48]

Tip

- Chitosan dressings may provide fast clotting in wounds with moderate to severe bleeding. This property makes chitosan dressing useful in wounds with hemorrhage after excision of EGT.

In addition to its hemostatic properties, chitosan exerts positive effects on several physiologic processes involved in the early phases of wound healing. It stimulates the initial inflammation by attracting leukocytes, and it enhances functions of polymorphonuclear leukocytes and macrophages, such as phagocytosis and synthesis of cytokines.[49] Chitosan gradually depolymerizes to release N-acetyl-β-D-glucosamine, which initiates fibroblast proliferation, helps in ordered collagen deposition and stimulates hyaluronic acid (HA) synthesis at the wound site, and it thereby may stimulate formation of granulation tissue. A chitin film was thus shown to lead to faster healing and a stronger wound than did gauze and a commercially available film (Opsite, Smith & Nephew).[50] In full-thickness cutaneous wounds in a diabetic mouse model, treatment with chitin-containing membranes resulted in an accelerated wound closure rate, probably based on an increase in angiogenesis.[51] There are no studies on effects of chitin or chitosan on healing of wounds in horses. From a pathophysiologic rationale, chitin and chitosan dressings seem to be suited for dressing wounds with hemorrhage and wounds in the early phases of healing. Chitosan dressings are available in several formats (e.g. hydrogel, powder, rope/ribbon, film and pad/sheet), from several companies (e.g. HemCom Medical Technologies Inc., Trusetal Verbandstoffwek GMBH, and Aspen Medical).

Chitin and chitosan have some intrinsic antibacterial activity, but the material is also well suited for delivering antimicrobial compounds to burns and infected wounds.[52] A proprietary dressing containing chitosan and silver nanoparticles exhibited significantly greater bactericidal activity *in vitro* than chitosan alone, and it reduced mortality from 90% to 14.3% in a *Pseudomonas aeruginosa* wound infection model in mice compared to gauze dressing.[53]

Alginates

Alginates (Figure 6.7) are made from acids obtained from seaweed. The calcium salts of alginic, mannuronic, and guluronic acids are processed into non-woven, biodegradable fibers.

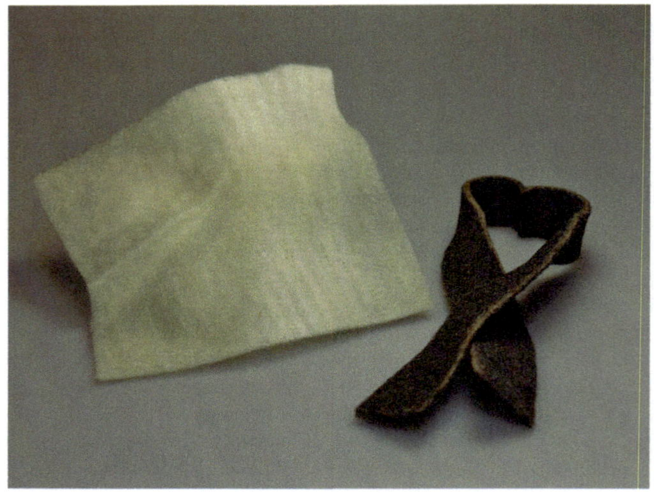

Figure 6.7 Alginate dressings. When exudate is absorbed into the dressing, alginate fibers swell, partially dissolve, and form a gel. The gel provides a moist environment in the wound and, by doing so, promotes healing. The rope form (right) contains silver, which causes the gray color. Rope dressings are useful for packing cavities.

Alginates can absorb up to 20, or more, times their weight of a wound's fluid. When an alginate dressing comes into contact with blood or exudate, ion exchange takes place between the calcium ions in the alginate and the sodium ions in blood or exudate. When sufficient calcium ions are replaced by sodium ions, the alginate fibers swell, partially dissolve, and form a gel. The gel provides a moist environment in the wound and, by doing so, promotes healing. Moreover, alginates have been shown to stimulate both inflammation and fibroplasia,[54] and from a pathophysiologic rationale they thus seem most suited to the inflammatory phase and the early proliferative phase of wound healing. A systematic review of dressings used to manage acute and chronic wounds in humans concluded that alginates were better than other modern dressing types for debriding necrotic wounds.[55] This author uses alginates until the wound bed is filled in with granulation tissue (Figure 6.8).

Due to their high absorptive capacity, alginates are useful in moderately to heavily exudative wounds. If used in wounds with little exudation, alginate dressings must be moistened with isotonic saline solution before being applied.

This author uses alginate dressing also over exposed bone, although the dressing is not marketed for that specific purpose. Formation of granulation tissue over bone denuded of periosteum is often a lengthy process because angiogenesis and fibroplasia must occur mainly from the soft tissues at the wound's margin. Applying an alginate to exposed bone, however, seems to enhance capillary ingrowth from the bone marrow (Figure 6.9). In a study involving 25 human patients with a soft-tissue defect exposing bone on the head and face, dressing the wound with an alginate compress, which was covered with a hydrocolloid dressing, provided significant advantages and resulted in good coverage of bone with high-quality granulation tissue.[56]

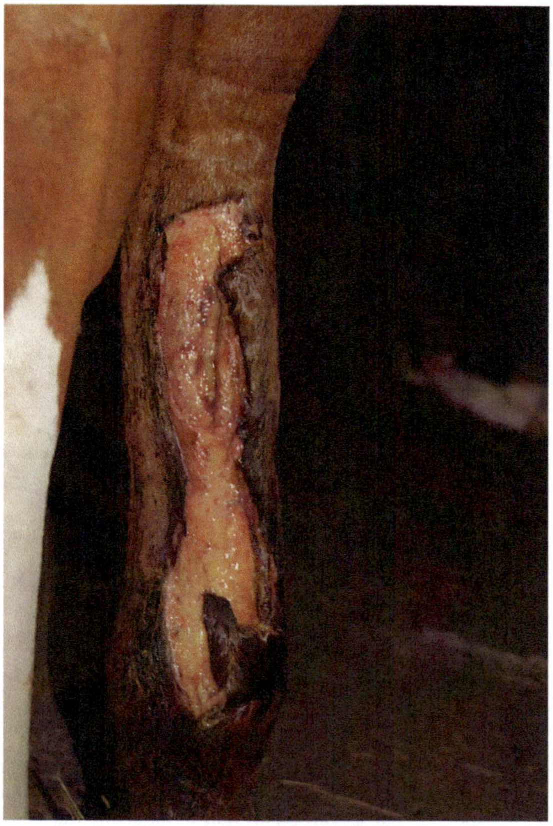

Figure 6.8 Wound requiring ingrowth of granulation tissue. Alginate dressings are useful for stimulating the formation of granulation tissue. In wounds where exudation is sparse, the alginates should be moistened with sterile saline solution before being applied to the wound. Same horse as in Figures 6.3 and 6.16. Photo courtesy of Tinamaria Jensen, Vinding Forlag and Tinamarias Digital Publishing.

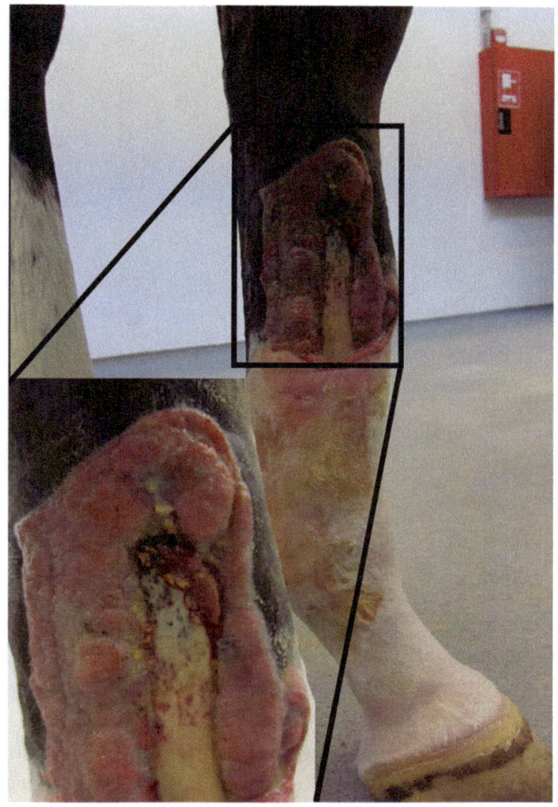

Figure 6.9 Severe degloving injury with large area of exposed bone. The wound was dressed with moistened alginates, and formation of granulation tissue is apparent at the wound edges. Moreover, capillary ingrowth, evident as pin-point red or dark spots, is evident in the cortex of the exposed third metatarsal bone (inset). Alginates are not marketed for use on exposed bone, but studies and experience have demonstrated their efficacy for stimulating ingrowth of granulation tissue over the denuded bone (see text for further details).

Alginates can also be used to achieve hemostasis. The high calcium content activates platelets and stimulates coagulation. Some alginates contain zinc, which enhances these prothrombogenic effects of the alginate.[57] Alginates have been used for hemostatic purposes after hemorrhagic surgery in humans, such as for packing the nasal cavity after trimming the nasal turbinates,[58] and to temporarily pack the alveolar socket after dental extraction.

Alginates moistened with saline solution containing 0.05% bupivacaine with adrenaline 1:200 000 have been applied to small abrasions and “road rash” in humans to temporarily relieve pain and reduce hemorrhage.[59] Although this use has not been reported in the veterinary literature, an alginate dressing used in this manner might be appropriate for treating horses with a similar injury.

Alginates are available as flat sheets suitable for covering superficial wounds and as ribbons or ropes that can be used to pack cavities (Figure 6.7). Alginate dressings are very conformable, especially when wet; and the sheet dressings can be folded and used to pack deeper wounds. The gelling action of the alginate results in varying degrees of loss of structural integrity of the alginate. The gelled dressing may resemble purulent material and should not be mistaken for that at dressing change. Because the gel does not adhere to the wound, dressing changes are pain-free, and newly formed granulation tissue is not disturbed. Moreover, the gel may trap bacteria and thus exert an antibacterial effect. A study in rats showed that in cavitated wounds experimentally infected with *Escherichia coli* and *Staphylococcus epidermidis*, packing the wound with an alginate reduced dissemination of bacteria.[60]

Hydrofibers

Hydrofiber dressings (Figure 6.10) consist of sodium carboxymethylcellulose fibers, a substance that can draw exudate away from the wound surface. Hydrofibers are very hydrophilic and, upon contact with fluid in the wound, they form a gel. Although hydrofiber dressings are very similar to alginates, they have been developed to provide superior absorbency; they absorb up to 30 times their weight in wound fluid, and retain the fluid within the interior of the dressing to reduce or eliminate lateral wicking. The dressing provides appropriate moisture at the

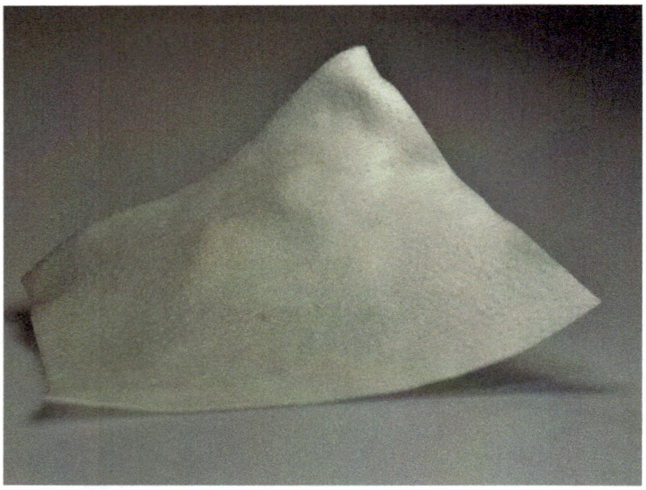

Figure 6.10 Hydrofiber dressing.

wound-dressing interphase with low risk of maceration, and therefore, an oft-cited advantage is that the dressing can be left on the wound for several days. Another important difference between alginates and hydrofibers is that the latter have no effect on hemostasis.

A study comparing alginate and hydrofiber dressings for the management of chronic leg ulcers in humans found that the dressings exerted similar effects on healing. Hydrofiber dressings were, however, more cost effective, and healthcare workers found that hydrofiber dressings had superior handling properties during application and bandage change.[61] Conversely, in a randomized study using alginates or hydrofiber dressings to cover wounds of 200 human patients after arthroplasty, skin health was better (i.e., fewer skin blisters), and patient comfort superior (i.e., less pain during removal of the dressing) in the alginate group.[62] There are no studies evaluating the use of hydrofiber dressings in horses. In humans, hydrofiber dressings are mainly indicated for use in moderately to heavily exudating wounds. A secondary layer is required to keep the hydrofiber in place.

Hydrogels

Hydrated polymers or hydrogels are dressings composed of 90–95% water and 5–10% of a polymer or co-polymer of natural gel-forming agents such as alginates, carboxymethylcellulose, polyvinylpyrrolidone and pectin. Hydrogels are able to donate moisture to dehydrated tissue. Even though hydrogels are considered to be occlusive, they can absorb some wound fluid into the polymer matrix. The high water content of hydrogel dressings cools the wound, providing pain relief.

These dressings are particularly useful for rehydrating necrotic tissue and enhancing autolytic debridement and thus are indicated for dry wounds containing necrotic tissue or an eschar (Figure 6.11). Burns, in humans, to which hydrogel dressings were applied had earlier onset of epidermal healing than did uncovered burns.[63] This earlier onset of epithelial regeneration may have been the result of a shorter debridement phase.

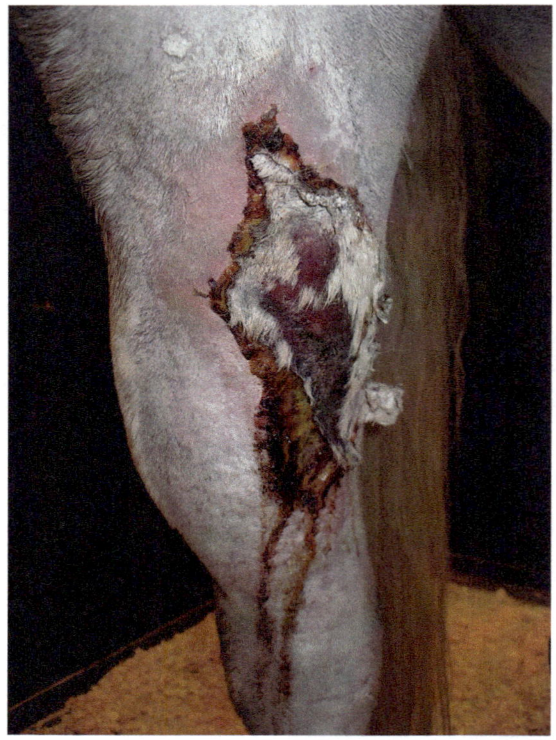

Figure 6.11 Necrotic wound sustained when the limb was caught as the horse attempted to jump over its stall door. The wound is dry and would benefit from application of a hydrogel dressing to soften the scab and stimulate autolytic debridement.

Hydrogels should be applied only to wounds that do not show signs of infection, because they may increase the risk of microorganisms spreading to surrounding tissues.[64] Hydrogels with antimicrobial properties, such as hydrogel with hypertonic saline (e.g., Hypergel from Mölnlycke), with polyhexamethyl biguanide (PHMB) (e.g., Prontosan Wound Gel from B. Braun), or hydrogel containing silver (e.g., Normlgel Ag from Mölnlycke), may be used in infected wounds. A study in horses showed that wounds dressed with a fully occlusive hydrogel sheet throughout the entire course of healing took significantly longer to heal (113 days) than did wounds dressed with a non-adherent gauze pad (53 days). The hydrogel stimulated formation of EGT, and hydrogel-dressed wounds required significantly more excisions of EGT than those dressed with the non-adherent gauze pad.[26] Consequently, such fully occlusive hydrogel sheet dressings may not be suitable for dressing the wounds of horses.

> **Tip**
>
> - Use of hydrogel dressings should be limited to the early phases of wound healing, and, to avoid formation of EGT, use of hydrogels should be discontinued at the first appearance of granulation tissue. Wounds dressed with a hydrogel should be monitored closely for development of maceration (which should prompt the clinician to change to another type of dressing with better ability to remove fluid).

Early in healing, before granulation tissue forms, hydrogel dressings are comfortable, supportive dressings; they protect the wound from additional contamination, assist in debridement, absorb some wound fluid into their polymer matrix, and reduce pain. This author often uses them over exposed bone to prevent desiccation and reduce pain.

Hydrogels are available in three forms.

- Amorphous hydrogel (Figure 6.12): free-flowing gel, packaged in tubes, foil packets, and spray bottles. These are particularly suited for dressing uneven wounds or cavities. They require a secondary dressing.
- Impregnated hydrogel: a gauze pad, rope, or strip saturated with amorphous hydrogel.
- Sheet hydrogel (Figure 6.12): a gel supported by a thin fiber mesh. The dressing can overlap intact skin without harming it. Available with and without an adhesive border and can be cut to fit the wound.

Several hydrogels containing additives that promote healing are available, for example, hydrogels containing hypertonic saline solution (e.g., Hypergel, Mölnlycke) that soften eschar and draw exudate and debris from the wound, and hydrogels containing components, such as antimicrobial drugs, HA, vitamins and microminerals, collagens, Aloe vera, or other components with suggested benefits to the healing tissues. A study investigated the effects of applying a hydrogel containing 25% propylene glycol (Solugel, Johnson & Johnson) to experimental wounds created on the limbs of horses. Propylene glycol, at this concentration, was hypothesized to enhance epithelialization, but the study did not show any advantages of using this hydrogel, because the rate of healing of wounds to which the hydrogel was applied did not differ from that of wounds covered with gauze soaked in isotonic saline solution.[12]

Hydrogels are also available as hybrid dressings, where they are combined with, for example, an alginate or a hydrocolloid.

Hydrocolloids

Hydrocolloids are complex dressings. The active surface of the dressing is coated with a cross-linked adhesive mass containing a dispersion of gelatin, pectin, and carboxymethylcellulose, together with other polymers and adhesives forming a flexible wafer (Figure 6.13). The dressing is inherently adhesive and requires no secondary layer, because it adheres well to surrounding intact skin and has a high absorptive capacity, thus enabling it to serve as a stand-alone dressing (this principle is well known in the treatment of blisters). When in contact with wound exudate, the polysaccharides and other polymers absorb water and swell, forming a gel, which is held within the structure of the adhesive matrix. Over the wound bed, moisture from the denuded tissue prevents the hydrocolloid dressing from adhering to the injured tissues. Hydrocolloid dressings are virtually impermeable to water vapor (i.e., they are fully occlusive), which conserves wound moisture to a high degree. The moist conditions produced under the dressing are intended to promote wound healing by encouraging fibrinolysis and other autolytic debridement processes, as well as angiogenesis, without causing healthy tissue to macerate and break down. Hydrocolloids are classic blister plasters, used to promote healing and reduce pain.

Occlusive dressings such as hydrocolloids have been shown to exert negative effects on wound healing in horses (EGT) and other veterinary species.[28,65,66] In spite of this bad press, the authors of a case series with six horses treated for an acute laceration of the limb concluded that, after using hydrocolloid dressings, "the healing of [the] wounds was very satisfying, fast, without development of excessive granulation tissue."[27] Similar results were obtained in a study using hydrocolloid dressings to treat severe lacerations with exposed bone, frayed tendons or ligaments, or abrasions of the fibrous joint capsule.[28] Dressings

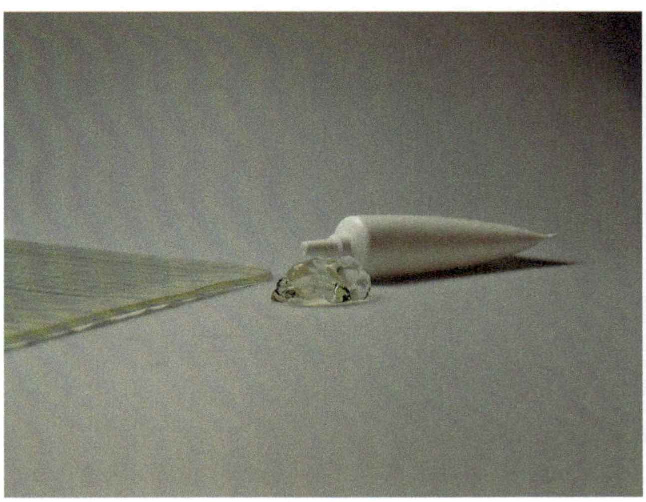

Figure 6.12 Hydrogel dressings: amorphous hydrogel to the right, sheet hydrogel to the left. Hydrogels are useful for donating moisture to dry wounds and for preventing desiccation of exposed bone or tendon.

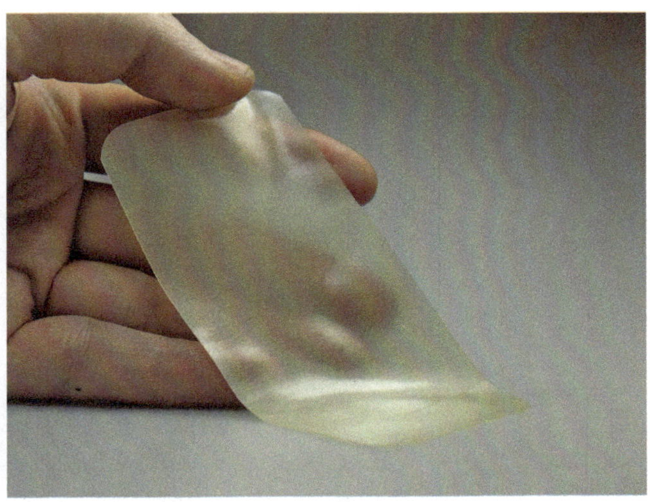

Figure 6.13 Hydrocolloid dressing. This dressing is fully occlusive, has a large absorptive capacity and provides moist wound healing. It has been implicated in the formation of EGT in horses; consequently, wounds dressed with hydrocolloids should be monitored closely.

were changed every 4–7 days, and at the first dressing change, wounds were already covered with a thin bed of granulation tissue. In wounds containing denuded bone, fibroplasia was observed to originate directly from the bone surface. Wound infection was documented in only two of the 28 horses included in the study. Based on these findings, it seems that hydrocolloid dressings can be used early in the inflammatory phase to promote the formation of granulation tissue.

Tips

- Hydrocolloids might be particularly effective when bone or connective tissue has been exposed by wounding.
- The hydrocolloid dressing should be applied only to wounds free of infection, and wounds should be monitored closely for development of infection, EGT, and maceration of the wound's margin.

Foams

Foams are non-adherent and semi-permeable, and they are designed to maintain appropriate moisture at the wound–dressing interface, which reduces the risk of maceration and promotes epithelialization. Polyurethane foam contains variably sized, small, open cells that have the ability to pull exudate from the wound by capillary action (Figure 6.14). The fluid is then held within the dressing, even when the dressing is under pressure from the bandage. Many foams have a semi-permeable polyurethane membrane backing that allows some water vapor to escape. Foams are capable of absorbing and retaining large volumes of exudate, and they are thus suitable for moderately to heavily exudative wounds. The backing reduces evaporative fluid loss and thus prevents the dressing from drying out when used in wounds with little exudation. Nevertheless, within recent years, foams suited to wounds with little exudation have become available; the names of these foams may have the suffix "lite," and whereas a regular foam may dry out the wound through its high absorptive action, "lite" foams should provide perfect conditions for healing of dry wounds. Foams thus provide a moist environment in wounds with varying degrees of exudation.

Tip

- Moisture is an important prerequisite for epithelialization, and foams are thus suitable in the proliferative phase of wound healing to ensure optimal conditions for advancing epithelium.

Additional benefits of foams are their conformability and their softness. The addition of a soft silicone layer to some products adds to the following: (1) patient comfort by reducing pain, and (2) increasing the speed of healing by minimizing stripping of newly formed epithelium when the dressing is changed. These silicone-coated foams have excellent handling properties, making them advantageous for veterinary use. They tend to stick slightly to the skin, which reduces the risk of the dressing slipping from a vertically oriented wound (i.e. on the limb) or falling off when changing the bandage of an unruly horse. Some foams come with an adhesive border to help the dressing stay in place. The adhesive borders are often of less value in horses than in humans, however, because they are not designed to adhere to the hairy skin of horses.

Different foams have very different absorptive capacities, and their permeability to water vapor also varies. Whether these differences in fluid-handling properties have any clinical impact on the healing of wounds of horses is not clear, because no studies

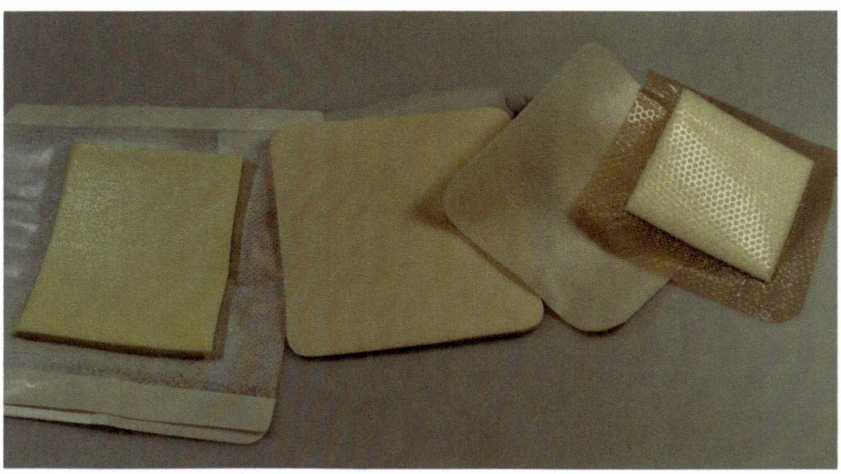

Figure 6.14 Foam dressings. Several types are shown, both with and without an adhesive border. Foams are used for wounds that have completely filled in with granulation tissue. To the right two "lite" foams are shown. These are indicated for wounds with little or no exudation, where application of a regular foam dressing might cause desiccation of the wound. The two "lite" foams shown also have a soft silicone adhesive layer on the surface. Soft silicone coating has several advantages, as it improves handling properties (by preventing slippage) of the dressing, increases patient comfort and reduces disruption of healing tissues during dressing change. Several regular foams also have a soft silicone layer (see text and Table 6.2 for details).

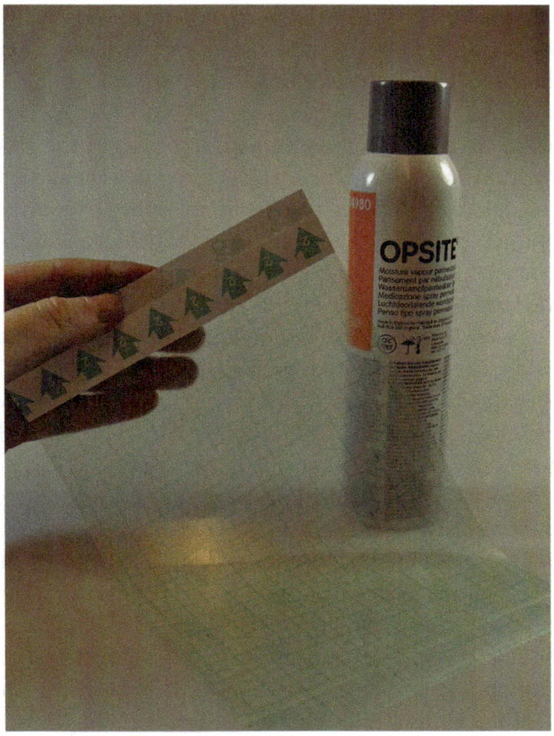

Figure 6.15 Film dressings. An example of a spray-on film dressing is shown to the right. Films are used as a "second skin" to protect the wound in the last stages of healing or to dress wounds healing by primary intention. Film dressings have very little absorptive capacity.

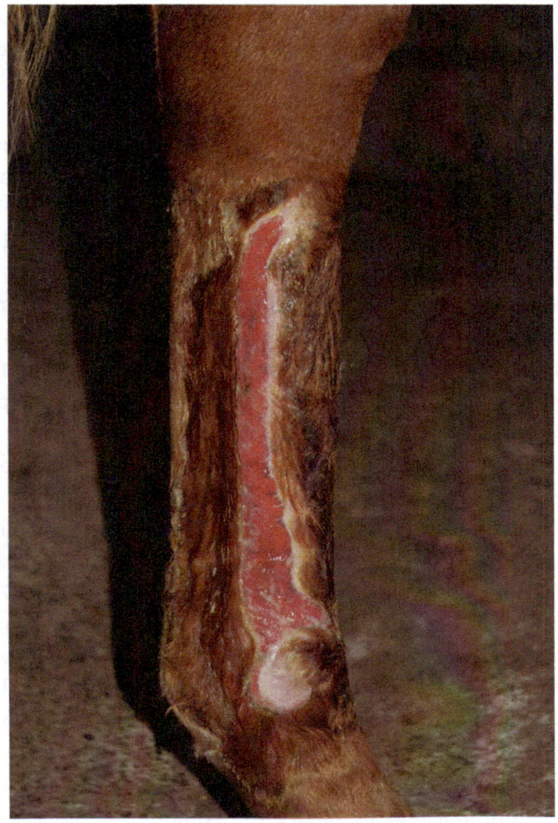

Figure 6.16 Large wound on the limb, in which healing is progressing well. The wound bed is filled with healthy granulation tissue, epithelialization is evident as the pale rim at the wound's margin. The wound may at this stage be protected by a spray-on film or dressed with a "lite" foam to limit desiccation, which would reduce the rate of epithelialization. Photo courtesy of Tinamaria Jensen, Vinding Forlag and Tinamarias Digital Publishing.

comparing the effects of different foam dressings on wound healing in the horse are available. A recent study by Kelleher *et al.* (2015)[67] showed that dressing experimental, full-thickness cutaneous wounds with a polyurethane foam (Retro-Tech Dressing, Pioneer Vet) improved the granulation tissue score (corresponding to reduced propensity for exuberance) and reduced initial wound retraction more than did dressing wounds with an absorbent, non-adherent, gauze-like pad (Curity Abdominal Pad, Covidien). Time to complete healing was similar with the two dressings. It was not clear whether the improved healing in wounds dressed with the polyurethane foam was a consequence of the foam itself or of a decreased bioburden in the wound, because the dressing was impregnated with three antimicrobial products (ionic silver, gentian violet, and methylene blue) – or a combination of both.

Films

Film dressings are usually made from a thin polyurethane membrane that is coated with adhesive (Figure 6.15). They are designed to protect the wound from friction and damage and also provide a barrier against contaminants. Film dressings are waterproof and thus protect the wound from being soaked when the horse is housed in wet conditions. They are permeable to water vapor and oxygen, to variable degrees, and they serve as a "second skin" that prevents the wound bed from dehydrating. They have no or very little absorptive capacity, making them useful only for wounds with little or no exudation. Their use in horses has not been investigated, but in humans they are used in shallow, simple wounds containing a healthy bed of granulation tissue (Figure 6.16). Because they are transparent, they are also suited for dressing surgical wounds that may then be inspected through the dressing.

Getting the sheet film to stick to the skin of horses may be difficult. This author thus prefers the spray form of films (e.g., Opsite Spray, Smith & Nephew) (Figure 6.15) that can be applied in several layers to the wound bed to protect an almost completely healed wound and provide some moisture during the last phases of healing.

Silicone dressings

Soft silicone is a particular family of silicones that is soft and exhibits "tack." Tack occurs because the silicone makes multiple points of contact with the skin surface, which results in a tight seal between the skin and the dressing. The soft silicone dressing will not adhere to the moist wound surface, but will stick slightly to the surrounding skin.

Dressings that incorporate soft silicones were developed for use in human medicine. The three main groups of soft silicone dressings possess entirely different functions targeted to suit particular clinical needs.[68]

1. Soft silicone wound contact layer in dressings that are non-absorbent and designed to allow exudate to pass through into an absorbent secondary layer. Their main purpose is to increase comfort and minimize disruption to the wound bed during dressing change.
2. Absorbent dressings with silicone adhesive. Many foam dressings incorporate a soft silicone contact layer (Figure 6.14). In these dressings the silicone is intended to form a watertight seal to prevent lateral wicking of wound fluid into the peri-wound skin, but it also serves the same purposes as the soft silicone wound contact layers (comfort, reduced slippage, protection of healing tissues).
3. Silicone gel sheets, which are self-adhesive, occlusive sheets to be used as a first line of treatment for wounds at risk of developing hypertrophic scarring or keloids (Figure 6.17).

Soft silicone wound contact layers and foams coated with soft silicone may be used to manage wounds in horses following the same indications as in humans. This author has found the silicone-coated foams very useful in horses, as the tack helps them stick to the uneven skin surface and prevents slippage.

The mode of action of silicone gel sheets is incompletely understood, but may be related to hydration, modification of oxygen tension, and/or creation of a static electric field as a result of the friction between the wound and the silicone. Several studies have demonstrated efficacy against hypertrophic scars and keloids in humans.[69] Silicone gel sheets are designed for use on closed wounds or scar tissue, and, according to the product information supplied by the manufacturer, they should not be used on open wounds (Cica-care, Smith & Nephew). Nevertheless, silicone gel sheets are recommended as the gold-standard, first-line, non-invasive option for the prevention and treatment of scars in humans[70] and are used clinically on open, surgical wounds after revising keloids.[71] A study was designed to investigate their use in horses on limb wounds predisposed to developing EGT, a fibroproliferative disorder with some of the same characteristics as keloids in humans. The silicone gel sheets prevented the formation of EGT, and the quality of healing tissues was better than that of tissues to which a non-adherent gauze pad (Melolite, Smith & Nephew) was applied.[29] This author uses silicone gel sheets on acute or chronic wounds, healing by second intention, to prevent occurrence or reduce the severity of EGT, and has not observed adverse effects (Figure 6.17).

The silicone gel sheet has no absorptive capacity and therefore, cannot be used on exudative wounds because this would result in maceration of the wound and surrounding skin. The sheet is more expensive than other dressings, but it can be reapplied (after being cleaned with mild soap and rinsed with water) several times, thus improving cost effectiveness considerably.

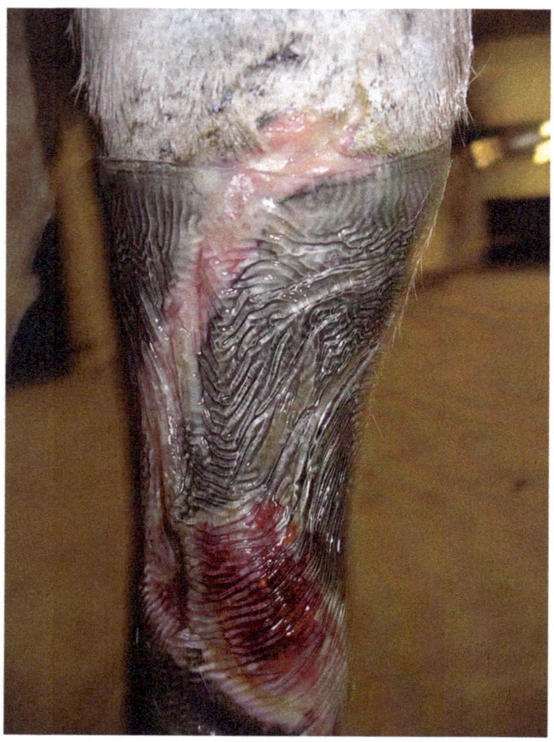

Figure 6.17 Acute wound dressed with a silicone gel sheet to prevent the formation of EGT. The wound was dressed with the silicone gel sheet until almost completely healed, and it healed without complications.

Biologic dressings

Biologic dressings purportedly promote wound healing by providing a barrier that protects the wound from infection, by maintaining a moist environment conducive to migration of epithelial cells, and by retarding the formation of EGT. Biologic dressings are designed to become incorporated into the wound, providing a scaffold that allows adhesion and migration of fibroblasts, endothelial cells, and keratinocytes, thereby enhancing fibroplasia, vascularization, and epithelialization. Tissues used in biologic dressings can be autogenous (autologous), allogeneic, or xenogeneic. Several different types of biologic dressings have been used in equine wound management, including amnion, peritoneum, skin, and processed collagen. A study evaluating the incorporation of three biologic dressings (split-thickness allogeneic skin, allogeneic peritoneum, and xenogeneic porcine small intestinal submucosa) into the wound bed, however, detected no vascularization of any of the biologic dressings. Moreover, none of them had an effect on wound infection, the inflammatory response, or the time required for wounds to heal when compared to wounds dressed with a non-adherent, synthetic pad.[72] Effects of these biologic dressings on the wounds of horses are thus not entirely clear.

Amnion

Amnion conforms well to the wound's surface, has low antigenicity, and is soft and pliable. Therefore, it causes very little abrasion, irritation, and inflammation to the wound. Fresh amnion samples contain HA and multiple cytokines and growth factors (epidermal growth factor, vascular endothelial growth factor, keratinocyte growth factor, transforming growth factor-β and others), which may also exert direct effects on wound healing.[73] The molecular mechanisms underlying the beneficial effects of amnion have, however, not been fully elucidated, as it has been shown that several of the cytokines and growth factors in amnion are removed/inactivated during processing of the membrane.[73] In horses, amnion has found the widest application in restoration of ocular surface defects, where it is described as "undeniably efficacious."[74]

In two studies, wounds of horses dressed with amnion healed faster and had a lower incidence and severity of EGT than did control wounds dressed with a non-adherent gauze pad.[75,76] The beneficial effects of using amnion were, however, less clear in a study by Howard *et al.* (1993);[26] in that study, amnion-dressed wounds did not heal faster or develop less EGT than wounds dressed with a non-adherent gauze pad.

Amnion is inexpensive, but its main drawback is that harvesting and processing of the membrane is time consuming. Several protocols for processing amnion exist, they all include washing the placenta with a balanced salt solution containing several antimicrobials (usually 50 μg/mL streptocillin, 50 μg/mL penicillin, 100 μg/mL neomycin, and 2.5 μg/mL amphotericin B) and removing the amnion from the chorion by blunt dissection. The amnion is then washed with phosphate-buffered saline containing antibiotic–antimycotic solution. The epithelium of the amnion is removed by treating it with 0.05% trypsin and 0.02% ethylene diaminetetraacetic acid in phosphate-buffered saline. The amniotic membrane is cut into manageable pieces and placed, epithelial side up, on nitrocellulose paper in a medium such as Hank's balanced salt solution with gentamicin, 10% DMSO or a mixture of glycerol and Dulbecco Eagle's medium. The membrane is stored at -80 °C until use.[74] Commercial products containing amniotic membrane (e.g. dehydrated homogenates) have recently been described.[73]

Peritoneum

Peritoneum, due to its high content of collagen, was hypothesized to enhance wound healing when used as a dressing, but when applied to experimental wounds on horses, peritoneum had no beneficial effect on infection, inflammation, or healing time when compared to a non-adherent pad. Moreover, the peritoneum proved difficult to handle.[72]

Pericardium

One study comparing a dressing of pericardium to a synthetic semi-occlusive dressing (Adaptic, Johnson & Johnson) showed that pericardium applied to experimental limb wounds in horses caused more intense inflammation (determined histologically) but resulted in subjectively better quality granulation tissue. Healing time was similar in the two groups.[77] Applying an equine pericardium biomatrix (Unite, Synovis Orthopedic and Woundcare Inc) to diabetic foot wounds in humans was considered safe and seemed to enhance healing.[78] A mesh made from bovine pericardium (Tutomesh, Tutogen Medical GmbH) proved superior to primary closure or synthetic mesh in the repair of complicated (contaminated/infected) ventral hernias in humans, where it reduced the occurrence of postoperative infection, seroma formation, and recurrence.[79]

With the advent of processed products, use of allogeneic or xenogeneic pericardium may become more widespread. There is currently insufficient evidence to suggest its proposed best use.

Processed collagen and extracellular matrix

Collagen-based matrices may be prepared from the submucosa of the small intestine, urinary bladder, or pericardium. The collagen becomes incorporated in the wound and reportedly serves as a scaffold to support adhesion and migration of fibroblasts and keratinocytes. Porcine small intestinal submucosa (PSIS) and processed collagen dressings (primarily composed of bovine collagen) have been used to treat wounds in horses.[72,80,81] Although studies in humans and laboratory animals indicate beneficial effects of collagen-based matrices on healing of chronic wounds,[82,83] none of the studies performed in horses have demonstrated advantages of applying collagen-containing dressings. Processed bovine collagen applied to wounds of horses significantly increased the degree of inflammation[80] but did not increase the rates of epithelialization or contraction, and healing time in collagen-treated wounds was similar to that of control wounds dressed with a non-adherent dressing (Release, Johnson & Johnson).[80,81] Similarly, PSIS had no beneficial effects on infection, inflammatory response, or healing time in experimental wounds in horses and dogs.[72,84]

Recently, an equine pericardium-derived biomatrix has been introduced to the market (Unite, Synovis Orthopedic and Woundcare Inc) and used for the treatment of chronic and difficult-to-heal wounds in humans. Chronic neuropathic foot wounds in humans, when implanted with the biomatrix, healed within 7 weeks.[78] There are no reports of the product being used to treat the wounds of animals.

Hyaluronic acid

Glycosaminoglycans (GAGs) are highly negatively charged molecules located primarily on the surface of cells or in the extracellular matrix. HA, or hyaluronan, is an anionic, non-sulfated GAG distributed widely throughout connective, epithelial, and neural tissues. HA, a major component of skin, has been shown to be involved in several processes important for repair of cutaneous tissue, including inflammation, angiogenesis, regulation of myofibroblast phenotype, induction of deposition of collagen, and modulation of proliferation of keratinocytes.[85]

Fetal tissue has a very high concentration of HA, and wounds of fetuses heal by regeneration, rather than by repair. High concentrations of HA are, therefore, thought to be instrumental in scarless healing. The concentration of HA in the wounds of adult people peaks at around 3 days, whereas during fetal wound healing, HA is deposited more rapidly and its concentration is sustained.[86] This has led to the hypothesis that the addition of exogenous HA to wounds might lead to scarless healing, as in the fetus. Studies so far, however, have not uniformly supported this hypothesis. While one study showed enhanced healing (rate and quality) in wounds treated with proprietary thiolated carboxymethyl-HA-based gel or film,[87] the use of HA-containing gels/dressings in dogs and horses did not accelerate healing in two other studies.[88,89] The study in dogs did, however, show beneficial effects of applying HA gel under a non-adherent dressing in the late phases of healing, where the wounds treated with cross-linked HA-based gel contracted more than did control wounds treated with the dressing alone.[88] Timing of application of HA-containing biomaterials may thus be of importance, although no firm recommendations can be made at this stage.

Several HA-containing dressings are available commercially, and a wound gel containing HA (SentrX Animal Care) is marketed specifically for veterinary application.

Current-generating bioelectric wound-care device

Electroceutical therapy is the use of electric current to stimulate impaired biologic functions. Use of microcurrents has been described in wound management, and this therapeutic modality is based on the knowledge that endogenous, direct-current electrical fields are fundamental to wound healing.[90] Electric current has been shown to accelerate migration of neutrophils, macrophages, fibroblasts, and keratinocytes ("galvanotaxis"), and to inhibit bacterial growth, including formation of *Pseudomonas aeruginosa* biofilm.[91,92] Several studies have demonstrated facilitated wound closure in wounds treated with microcurrent.[93,94] Continuous μA-level currents seemingly have better antimicrobial activity compared to pulsed currents. This principle has been exploited in a wireless electroceutical dressing (also referred to as a current-generating bioelectrical wound-care device) (Procellera Vomaris), where silver and zinc dots are printed on the surface of a polyester dressing in a matrix pattern to create multiple microbatteries with a voltage potential of 0.3–0.9 V. In the presence of a conductive fluid (wound exudate, saline solution, or hydrogel) a microcurrent of approximately 10 μA is generated, silver being the cathode, which is reduced, and zinc the anode, which is oxidized. This silver–zinc redox couple reduces molecular oxygen to a superoxide anion radical, which is the same reactive oxygen species that is the hallmark of the respiratory burst of neutrophil granulocytes.[91] The superoxide anion radical may account, at least in part, for the antimicrobial action of the dressing. More information about the technology and the different types of products available can be found at the product homepage (www.procellera.com). The dressing has the advantage that it is inherently bioelectric and thus requires no external power supply, forms an electrical field within the physiologic range, can be cut to the size of the wound, and conforms to irregular surfaces.

In a case series involving 10 horses, where the wireless electroceutical dressing was applied to acute or chronic limb wounds, the author concluded that inflammation and pain were decreased, epithelialization enhanced, and hair regrowth and cosmetic outcome improved – notwithstanding that no control group was included.[95] Although the technology is interesting and seems sound from a pathophysiologic rationale, more studies are needed, before best use of the Procellera dressing in horses can be determined.

Antimicrobial compounds

Antimicrobials are agents that kill microorganisms. The term antimicrobial is an "umbrella" term that encompasses disinfectants, antiseptics, and antibiotics. Whereas disinfectants are chemical agents, or biocides, and are used only to inhibit or kill microbes on inanimate objects, antiseptics and antibiotics may be incorporated into dressings and topical products that are applied to the wound's surface to reduce the bioburden. Microbial burden can delay wound healing but beneficial effects of bacteria have been noted under certain circumstances. For example, one author suggested that contamination may help wound healing by enhancing beneficial inflammatory processes and by increasing blood flow to the wound.[96] This is supported by the findings of a recent experimental study in horses, where excisional wounds contaminated with feces for 24 hours after wounding healed faster than non-contaminated wounds.[97]

In contrast, infection negatively affects wound healing by inducing the synthesis of pro-inflammatory cytokines that increase concentrations of matrix metalloproteinases – changes that impair wound healing. This is the rationale underlying the recommendation that bioburden in wounds be controlled. The recommendations for wound bed preparation in human patients set forth by the European Wound Management Association[98] and the guidelines to aid healing of acute wounds by decreasing impediments of healing set forth by the Wound Healing Society[99] emphasize the importance of controlling microbes in wounds. More information about wound contamination and infection can be found in Chapters 3 and 4.

In the acute phase of wound healing, systemically administered antibiotics may gain access to the wound and help control bacterial numbers. In later stages, when granulation tissue has formed in the wound, topical application of an antimicrobial agent is often more efficient than systemic administration of an antibiotic. Drug diffusion is impaired in fibrous granulation tissue, and antibiotics often do not reach a therapeutic concentration in the relatively avascular infected wound tissues.[100] Antimicrobial dressings should never replace the basic principles of wound management, and the wound and patient should always be carefully assessed. The use of antimicrobial dressings is indicated for wounds with critical colonization and superficial infection (Figure 6.18). Where clear infection extending into the deeper tissues is present, or in the presence of an established biofilm,

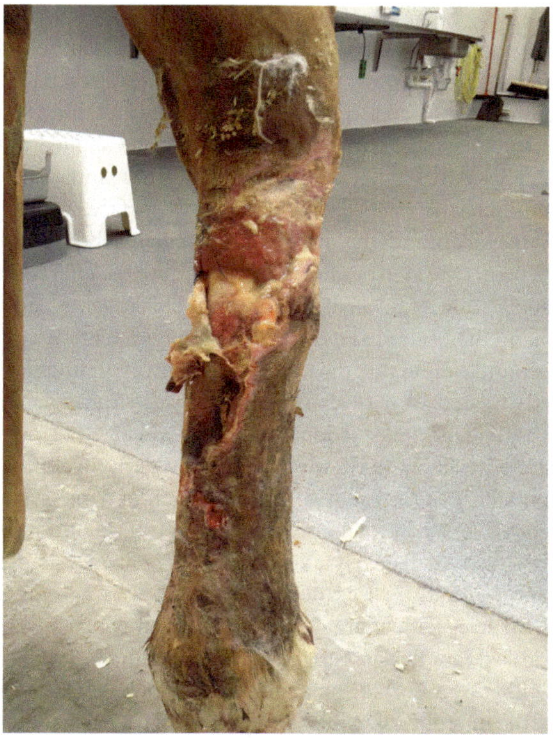

Figure 6.18 Wound on the limb, which suffered substantial dehiscence after primary closure. The remaining distal part of the skin flap is clearly necrotic (dark, dry) and will also dehisce over time. This wound should be treated with a thorough surgical or hydrosurgical debridement and covered with an alginate dressing containing silver to reduce bioburden and to stimulate the formation of granulation tissue. Although hydrocolloids may encourage autolytic debridement and the formation of granulation tissue, they are contraindicated in wounds with heavy exudation and signs of infection.

additional debridement, as well as systemically administered antimicrobial treatment, is required.

What to avoid

- Systemic administration of antibiotics should be avoided when treating infection in granulating wounds, where antimicrobial dressings are more efficacious.

A Best Practice document from 2010[101] concludes that the use of topical antiseptic/antimicrobial agents and dressings is important when treating patients with signs of wound infection, and that patients may be put at risk if such products are not used. In contrast, the document highlights that it is just as important to avoid using topical antiseptic/antimicrobial agents on wounds without infection, or where there is no significant clinical risk of infection. A 14-day trial to assess usefulness of the antimicrobial product is described, as follows.[101]

What to do

Topical antiseptic/antimicrobial agents should initially be utilized for 14 days, and the wound assessed clinically at each dressing change. If after 2 weeks:

- consistent signs of progress towards healing are observed and signs of wound infection are no longer present, antimicrobial intervention may be discontinued;
- there is improvement in the wound, but signs of infection are still present, the treatment should be continued;
- the wound shows no improvement, it is recommended that an alternative topical antiseptic/antimicrobial agent be used;
- the wound begins to show further signs of infection, the use of a systemic antibiotic should be considered, based on the results of sensitivity testing.

The antibacterial compounds that may be added to dressings are mentioned in the following sections. Antimicrobial versions of several of the types of dressing described earlier are available. Examples of combinations of dressing and antimicrobial compounds can be found in Table 6.4. Because of the variety of carrier materials and formulations available, understanding the general properties of the dressings and the advantages and disadvantages of the different antimicrobial agents is important to plan care effectively and achieve the desired outcome.

Silver

Silver has been used for its antimicrobial activity for millennia. Silver has a broad spectrum of antimicrobial activity[102] and acts in multiple ways on bacteria, including blocking respiratory enzymatic pathways and altering microbial DNA and the cell wall.[103] Laboratory studies have shown silver ions to be active against a broad range of Gram-positive and Gram-negative pathogens found in wounds, including many antibiotic-resistant bacteria, such as *S. aureus*, methicillin-resistant *S. aureus* (MRSA), *Enterococcus faecalis*, vancomycin-resistant enterococci, *P. aeruginosa*, and *E. coli*.[104,105] A silver chloride-coated nylon dressing showed *in vitro* efficacy against bacterial isolates (*E. coli*, *Klebsiella pneumoniae*, *P. aeruginosa*, *Streptococcus equi* subspecies *zooepidemicus*, and *S. aureus*) from wounds of horses.[106]

To be effective, silver must be delivered to tissues in its ionic form and in sufficient concentration. In wound-care products, silver is found in the form of elemental silver (e.g. nanocrystalline silver), an inorganic compound (e.g silver sulphadiazine, silver nitrate, silver oxide, silver phosphate, silver chloride, silver sulfate, silver–calcium–sodium phosphate, silver zirconium) or an organic complex (e.g. silver alginate, silver carboxymethylcellulose). Silver sulfadiazine cream revolutionized the management of burn wounds in the 1960s, and it is still widely used for its ability to dramatically reduce concentrations of *P. aeruginosa* and other bacteria. Silver sulfadiazine has a short duration of action, because its silver ions quickly combine with wound fluids and become inactive. Ionic silver is highly reactive and will react with chlorides and other halides, inorganic

Table 6.4 Antimicrobial dressings.

Antimicrobial compound/principle	Examples of products
Silver	Hydrogel • Normlgel Ag (Mölnlycke) Alginate • Melgisorb Ag (Mölnlycke) • Biatain Alginate Ag (Coloplast) • Suprasorb A+Ag (Lohmann & Rauscher) • Acticoat Absorbent (Smith & Nephew) Foam • Mepilex Ag (Mölnlycke) • Biatain Foam Ag (Coloplast) • Allevyn Ag (Smith & Nephew) Hydrofiber • Aquacel Ag (Convatec)
Polyhexamethyl biguanide (polyhexanide, PHMB)	Hydrogel • Kruuse HydroGel (Kruuse, 0.04% PHMB) • Prontosan Wound Gel and Prontosan Wound Gel X (B. Braun, 0.1% PHMB) Foam • Kendall AMD Antimicrobial Foam Dressing (Covidien, 0.5% PHMB) Hydrofiber • Suprasorb X+PHMB (Lohmann & Rauscher, 0.3% PHMB) Gauze • Kendall AMD Antimicrobial Gauze (Covidien, 0.2% PHMB, available as Curity packing strips, Excilon sponges, Kerlix rolls and super sponges) Non-adherent gauze-like • Telfa AMD pads (Covidien, 0.2% PHMB)
Hypertonic saline	Hydrogel • Hypergel (Mölnlycke, 20% saline) Gauze • Curity Sodium Chloride (Covidien, 20% saline, available as packing strips and pads)
Honey	Hydrogel • Manuka G (Kruuse) Superabsorbent polymer • Manuka AD (Kruuse) Gauze/tulle gras • Actilite (Advancis Medical) • Activon Tull (Advancis Medical) • Manuka ND (Kruuse) Alginate • Algivon (Advancis Medical)
Iodine	Sheet • Iodosorb dressing (Smith & Nephew, cadexomer–iodine)
Chlorhexidine	Tulle gras • Bactigras (Smith & Nephew, 0.5% chlorhexidine acetate in white soft paraffin)
Activated charcoal	Alginate Carboflex (Convatec) Fabric Actisorb Silver 220 (Johnson & Johnson, contains silver) Multicomponent • Carbonet (Smith & Nephew) • Activate (Robinson)
Boric acid	Poultice pad • Animalintex (3M)
Dialkylcarbamoylchloride (DACC)/hydrophobic interaction	Sorbact (BSN Medical, available as hydrogel sheet, gauze roll)
Octenidine (described in Chapter 5)	Hydrogel • Octenilin (Schülke)

compounds, organic acids, protein, DNA, and RNA in the wound; therefore, silver released into a wound can be rapidly consumed (in contrast, metallic silver is less reactive, thus explaining the increased efficacy of nanocrystalline silver). Silver sulfadiazine cream, therefore, should be applied at least once daily. After a few applications of silver sulfadiazine, a pseudo-eschar is formed on the wound's surface, which prohibits inspection of the wound and which, when removed, causes pain. One study in horses investigating the effects of topical application of silver-based antimicrobial agents and bandaging on the healing and development of granulation tissue in limb wounds found that the rate of healing in experimental limb wounds treated with silver sulfadiazine was similar to that of wounds treated with povidone–iodine ointment.[34]

In vitro studies have shown that more modern silver products that provide a sustained, high concentration of nanocrystalline silver are able to control microbes (including antibiotic-resistant bacteria) more effectively and rapidly than silver sulfadiazine and silver nitrate.[107,108] Nanocrystalline silver is composed of small particles with a large surface area from which silver ions are released rapidly. Dressings containing nanocrystalline silver work either by absorbing exudate and bacteria into the dressing, where the microbes are killed, or by providing a constant release of silver ions into the wound with the microbes being eliminated in the wound bed. It has been suggested that the latter type of dressing leads to a more efficient microbial killing.[109]

Bacterial resistance to silver is thought to be uncommon, and cross resistance between antibiotics and silver is rare.[96,103] In two studies investigating the presence of silver-resistance genes in wound pathogens, including MRSA, isolated from humans and horses, a low prevalence of silver-resistance genes was detected. Moreover, the studies showed that even bacteria with the gene(s) were susceptible to the antimicrobial effects of a silver-containing hydrofiber dressing.[110,111] The authors recommended, therefore, that topical use of silver be considered before using antibiotics[110] and that – considering the fact that silver-resistance genes are difficult to transfer to and be maintained by other bacteria – "the threat to wound care is small, and the positive clinical outcomes associated with silver usage far outweigh the risks of bacterial resistance."[111]

Another advantage of silver is that, in addition to its antimicrobial effects, it may affect wound healing positively by directly reducing inflammation, modulating activity of proteolytic enzymes in the wound bed, and increasing epithelialization.[96]

Despite the convincing *in vitro* results, clinical benefits of silver dressings in humans are less clear. Several systematic reviews have concluded that there is no unequivocally demonstrated benefit of using silver dressings for the management of chronically infected wounds. The lack of evidence may be due mainly to the paucity of studies with sufficient power to make firm conclusions.[112,113] A recent meta-analysis did conclude, however, that "[....] results strengthen the proposition that silver-impregnated dressings improve the short-term healing of wounds and ulcers."[112]

In horses, a study comparing the efficacy of a semi-occlusive polyurethane foam impregnated with ionic silver, gentian violet, and methylene blue (Retro-Tech Dressing, Pioneer Vet) to that of an absorbent pad (Curity Abdominal Pad, Covidien) demonstrated that, although time to wound healing was similar with the two dressings, wounds treated with the silver dressings developed granulation tissue of superior quality and healed faster in the initial phase (first 30 days).[67] Surprisingly, there were no differences in bacterial load (based on cultures of the surface of the granulation tissue) between wounds dressed with the Retro-Tech dressing and the control dressing, which may relate to the fact that the Retro-Tech dressing is designed to absorb bacteria and kill them inside the dressing, rather than to release silver to the wound.

Polyhexamethylene biguanide (polyhexanide)

PHMB (also called polyhexanide) is an antiseptic agent with a wide range of applications. It is used as a swimming pool sanitizer, a preservative in cosmetics and contact lens solutions, and can be found in wound-care products. Its mode of action is not completely understood, but it may adhere to and disrupt target cell membranes, causing them to leak potassium ions and other cytosolic components, leading to cellular death. PHMB has several desirable characteristics, such as good biocompatibility,[114] low toxicity, high effectiveness against antibiotic-susceptible and -resistant strains of common (human) Gram-positive and Gram-negative bacteria, as well as fungi found in chronic wounds, and absence of resistance.[115] PHMB has been demonstrated to possess direct pro-healing effects. For example, it enhances the *in vitro* proliferation of normal human keratinocytes[116] and promotes epithelialization *in vivo*.[117]

When the effect of a PHMB-impregnated gauze (Kerlix AMD gauze, Covidien) against bacterial isolates from small animal patients was tested, the gauze was found to be more effective than control gauze at inhibiting the growth of all Gram-positive bacteria tested, but it was effective at inhibiting only some Gram-negative bacteria (*E. coli* and *E. aerogenes*).[118] The effect of PHMB on pathogens commonly found in equine wounds has not been tested, so PHMB's antimicrobial spectrum must be inferred from results of trials using humans or species of small animals. Contraindications to the use of PHMB in humans include lavage of the peritoneal cavity and joints (cartilage toxicity), application to any part of the central nervous system and the middle or inner ear, and during the first 4 months of pregnancy.[119]

Several types of dressings containing PHMB are commercially available (Table 6.4), as is an irrigation fluid containing PHMB in combination with betadine, a detergent/surfactant (Prontosan, B. Braun). The manufacturer claims that this irrigation fluid is effective against biofilm. Because PHMB is relatively new to the wound-care market, a limited number of clinical studies has been conducted to determine the potential merits of dressing wounds with PHMB. In a multicenter, prospective, double-blind, randomized, controlled clinical trial, application of PHMB-impregnated foam to chronic foot and leg ulcers reduced wound pain and bacterial burden better than did foam free of PHMB. The size of PHMB-treated wounds decreased more than that of control wounds during the 4-week study period, though this difference was not statistically significant.[120]

Chlorhexidine

Chlorhexidine is commonly used as a disinfectant and antiseptic. Chlorhexidine is a cationic biguanide that is a strong alkali, virtually insoluble in water. In contrast, its salts (chlorhexidine digluconate, chlorhexidine diacetate, and chlorhexidine dihydrochloride) are soluble and used in antiseptic solutions. Chlorhexidine gluconate is the most widely used, as it is highly water soluble.

Chlorhexidine binds to the negatively charged bacterial cell wall, altering the cellular osmotic equilibrium. It has activity against Gram-positive and Gram-negative bacteria, facultative anaerobes and aerobes, yeasts, fungi, and certain viruses, but it is important to keep in mind that members of the genus *Proteus* are invariably insensitive and *P. aeruginosa* is more resistant to chlorhexidine (and to quarternary ammonium compounds) than other Gram-negative organisms.[121] Chlorhexidine is well tolerated; the most frequently reported adverse reaction is contact dermatitis. Chlorhexidine should be used with caution near wounds involving synovial structures, because chlorhexidine causes inflammation of the synovium. Wilson *et al.* (1994) showed that lavage of the equine tarsocrural joint with 0.05% chlorhexidine diacetate resulted in synovial ulceration, inflammation, and abundant fibrin accumulation.[122] Also, studies in dogs and humans have shown deleterious effects of chlorhexidine in the synovial compartment (severe inflammation, chondrolysis) and chlorhexidine is thus not recommended for joint lavage.[123,124]

Although some *in vitro* studies suggest that chlorhexidine has adverse effects on cells, the effects of chlorhexidine, applied topically *in vivo*, on wound healing are less clear. Topical application of chlorhexidine digluconate was found to have mild inhibitory effects on wound healing in guinea pigs,[125] which could be related to its cytotoxicity on newly formed keratinocytes,[126] or its suppressive effects on macrophages.[127] In contrast, chlorhexidine diacetate was found to accelerate healing of full-thickness skin wounds in beagles.[128] The concentration of chlorhexidine in an irrigation solution should not exceed 0.1%; solutions used for wound irrigation often contain 0.02–0.05% chlorhexidine.

Chlorhexidine is available in many types of medical products. For wound care, a tulle gras (paraffin-impregnated gauze) containing 0.5% chlorhexidine acetate (Bactigras, Smith & Nephew) is marketed for use on minor burns and scalds, lacerations, abrasions and other skin-loss wounds of limited extent, and for donor and recipient graft sites (Figure 6.4). Chlorhexidine-impregnated tulle gras dressing (Bactigras) was less effective in promoting healing and reducing pain in human patients at the donor site of a split-thickness skin graft than was a non-adherent gauze-like dressing (i.e., dry dressing) containing PHMB (Telfa AMD, Covidien).[129]

The Bactigras dressing (Smith & Nephew) has been tested in several studies using rats with burns contaminated with different microorganisms. These studies showed that the chlorhexidine-impregnated tulle gras dressing was less effective in reducing the load of multi-drug-resistant *Pseudomonas* spp. than were silver-containing products[130] but equaled silver's ability to reduce MRSA.[131] The dressing was ineffective in eliminating *Candida albicans*.[132]

Iodine

Iodine has been used in wound care since the 1800s. Because molecular iodine can be very toxic to tissues, formulations combining iodine with a carrier that decreases iodine's availability have been developed. In modern wound management, iodine is used in two forms.

- Povidone–iodine (PI): this product is a combination of molecular iodine and polyvinylpyrrolidone. Examples of dressings containing PI are Inadine (Systagenix) and Repithel (Mundipharma). PI is used most commonly in antiseptic soaps and in solutions for wound irrigation. Its use as an antiseptic is described in more detail in Chapter 5.
- Cadexomer–iodine (CI): this product consists of spherical hydrophilic beads of cadexomer-starch that contain iodine. The beads are highly absorbent and release iodine slowly into the wound. An example of a dressings containing CI is Iodosorb (Smith & Nephew).

Iodine is inactivated by blood and serum proteins and other organic matter. The sustained release of iodine from modern dressings serves to overcome this issue. The antimicrobial spectrum of iodine is the broadest of all antiseptics and includes bacteria, mycobacteria, fungi, protozoa, and viruses. Reports of iodine-resistant strains of microorganisms are exceptionally rare.

In *in vitro* studies, iodine has been shown to have cytotoxic effects on cells involved in wound healing (i.e., fibroblasts, keratinocytes), and these cytotoxic effects may cause delayed healing.[133] The cytotoxicity of iodine is concentration dependent,[134] and iodine, therefore, is used in low concentrations that are non-toxic to tissue but still retain antibacterial activity. The bactericidal activity of PI has been shown to be *highest* when the concentration of PI is *low*.[135]

It has, within recent years, become increasingly clear that the cytotoxicity of iodine demonstrated *in vitro* does not translate into clinically evident harmful effects of topical application of modern iodine-containing products to wounds. A systematic review of the beneficial and harmful effects of iodine on wounds concluded that "[....] the use of iodine in wound treatment is still defendable because the best available evidence supports neither the purported harmful effects nor a delay of the wound-healing process."[136] CI seems to accelerate healing, particularly of chronic wounds in humans. This effect can be ascribed to a reduced bioburden as well as direct stimulation of epidermal regeneration and epithelialization.[137,138]

In horses, experimental limb wounds treated with 10% PI ointment under a bandage did not heal faster than control wounds,[34] maybe because the product was applied to a non-infected wound. In humans, iodine-impregnated dressings are used for acute and chronic wounds, including burns, to prevent or eliminate critical colonization and infection. Grafted wounds dressed with a hydrogel containing 3% PI (Repithel, Mundipharma) covered by a tulle gras dressing healed faster than control wounds.[139] In a rabbit model of muscle injury severely contaminated with *S. aureus*, a PI dressing applied 3 hours after injury significantly reduced bacterial concentration. Authors suggested that the dressing is useful in heavily contaminated soft-tissue wounds, particularly acute wounds where surgical treatment must be delayed.[140]

Skin surrounding the wound to which an iodine dressing has been applied may develop contact dermatitis (as can the skin of a healthcare worker applying the dressing, if gloves are not worn). Moreover, some people describe an unpleasant burning or stinging skin sensation after application of an iodine dressing, especially a CI dressing.

Honey

Honey contains sugars (e.g., glucose, fructose, sucrose) and many other substances, such as amino acids, vitamins, minerals, and enzymes. The antibacterial properties of honey rely on its hygroscopic powers, which dehydrate bacteria. The high sugar content also inhibits microbial growth. Furthermore, honey has a low pH and contains the enzyme glucose oxidase, which oxidizes glucose to produce gluconic acid and hydrogen peroxide.[141] Honey has been shown to be active against a broad spectrum of bacteria and fungi, including *S. aureus*, coagulase-negative staphylococci, *P. aeruginosa*, and MRSA, and so far, there are no clinical reports of acquired antimicrobial resistance to honey. Manuka honey, derived from the *Leptospermum* tree that grows in New Zealand and Australia, has received particular attention, because it contains the unique antibacterial compound methylglyoxal, but a recent study showed that other types of honey were as efficient as or more so than Manuka honey in inhibiting growth of bacteria obtained from wounds of horses.[142] That study demonstrated that some of the tested honeys were contaminated with aerobic bacteria or fungi, and consequently, the authors recommended that only honey sterilized by gamma-irradiation be used for treating wounds.[142]

Two studies in horses investigated the effects of Manuka honey on healing of experimental limb wounds and demonstrated some beneficial effects, the most consistent being reduced wound retraction in the initial phases of healing.[10,97]

A more in-depth description of the use of honey in wound management is provided in Chapter 22.

Hypertonic saline solution

Hypertonic saline-impregnated dressings are infused with 20% sodium chloride, which kills bacteria by osmotic action. These dressings can be used to debride wounds and are supplied as a hydrogel (e.g., Hypergel, Mölnlycke), which facilitates autolytic debridement of dry necrotic tissue by hydrating it, and as a gauze (e.g. Curity [previously Curasalt], Kendall/Covidien), which wicks moisture away from heavily exudative wounds. Because hypertonic saline-impregnated gauze dressings depend on moisture in the wound to make them effective at debridement, they are not appropriate for minimally exudative wounds or wounds covered with dehydrated slough or eschar.

Hypertonic saline-impregnated dressings are indicated for heavily infected and necrotic wounds. These dressings should be replaced every 24 hours, and their use stopped after debridement is complete. Although used extensively in veterinary medicine, no scientific studies have investigated the effects on healing, of this type of dressing.

Activated charcoal

Activated charcoal found in some dressings adsorbs bacteria and the pro-inflammatory and tissue-damaging elements produced by them, such as endotoxin; the bacteria and these elements are then removed when the dressing is changed.[143] Activated charcoal is very efficient in controlling odor, and a study using an activated charcoal dressing containing silver (Actisorb Silver 220, Systagenix Wound Management) to treat chronic wounds in human patients suggested that this dressing has more beneficial effects on healing than does a hydrocolloid dressing.[144]

Boric acid

Boric acid is incorporated into a commercially available poultice pad (Animalintex, 3M) marketed for use in horses as a dry dressing and as a hot or cold poultice for treating such diverse conditions as abscesses, infected and dirty wounds, cracked heels, strains, sprains, sore shins, splints, bruises, capped hocks, and capped elbows. Boric acid is a mild antiseptic, and a 3% solution may exert a positive influence on wound healing in humans.[145] Boric acid is not absorbed through intact skin but is absorbed rapidly through wounds, especially through well-vascularized granulation tissue. Toxicity in horses has not been investigated, but long-term exposure in people may cause kidney damage, and, hence, only dilute solutions should be applied to wounded skin. Effects of boric acid rely on its ability to acidify the wound. Acidifying the wound aids healing by reducing bioburden, reducing toxicity of bacterial end-products, altering activity of proteases, and enhancing epithelialization and angiogenesis.

Dialkylcarbamoylchloride (DACC)

Unlike traditional antimicrobial dressings, dialkylcarbamoylchloride (DACC) contains no chemically or pharmacologically active substances. The action of DACC dressings relies on the physical principle that two hydrophobic particles bind together in the presence of moisture.[146] Common pathogenic microorganisms, such as *S. aureus*, *Streptococcus* spp., *E. coli*, *P. aeruginosa*, and *Candida albicans*, are hydrophobic and, therefore, bind to the hydrophobic DACC coating.[147] The sequestered bacteria are immobilized and removed at dressing change. Advantages of this type of dressing are that resistance does not develop, and because the dressing contains no chemicals, sensitization to and systemic absorption of harmful substances are avoided. DACC dressings should not be used with ointments and creams containing lipids because these can inhibit the hydrophobic interaction of the dressing. In addition, some antiseptics can impair the surface hydrophobicity of microorganisms, thus reducing the efficacy of the dressing.

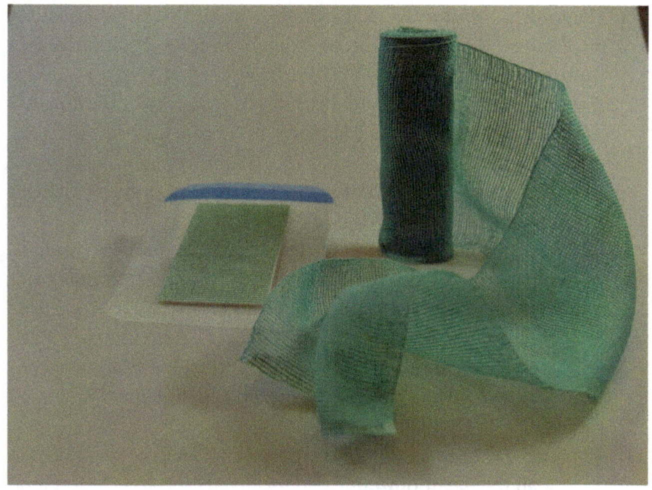

Figure 6.19 Dialkylcarbamoylchloride (DACC) dressings. These antibacterial dressings work by hydrophobic–hydrophobic interaction. Bacteria are retained in the dressing and removed at dressing change. A pad with an adhesive border (left) and a gauze suited for packing cavities (right) are shown.

In addition to its antibacterial effects, DACC may stimulate healing directly. One study showed that DACC stimulated proliferation of fibroblasts and increased the rate of healing by 100% in an *in vitro* wound model.[148]

DACC dressing are marketed by Abigo under the name Sorbact or Cutimed Sorbact. Different sizes and forms (e.g., pad, swab, ribbon, see Table 6.4) are available (Figure 6.19).

References

1. Winter GD. Formation of scab and rate of epithelialization of superficial wounds in skin of young domestic pig. *Nature* 1962; **193**: 293.
2. Davidson JM. Animal models for wound repair. *Arch Dermatol Res* 1998; **290**: S1–S11.
3. Talukdar AH, Stinson AW, Calhoun ML. Microscopic anatomy of skin of horse. *Am J Vet Res* 1972; **33**: 2365.
4. Wilmink JM, van Weeren PR, Stolk PWT, *et al.* Differences in second-intention wound healing between horses and ponies: histological aspects. *Equine Vet J* 1999; **31**: 61.
5. Sardari K, Kazemi H, Emami M, *et al.* Role of collagen cross-linking on equine wound contraction and healing. *Comp Clin Path* 2009; **18**: 239.

6. Mogford JE, Mustoe TA. Experimental models of wound healing. In: Falanga V (ed). *Cutaneous Wound Healing*, 1st edn. Martin Dunitz: London, 2001: 109.
7. Thomas S, Leigh IM. Wound dressings. In: Leaper DJ, Harding KG (eds). *Wounds: Biology and Management*, 1st edn. Oxford University Press: Oxford, 1998: 166.
8. McGuiness W, Vella E, Harrison D. Influence of dressing changes on wound temperature. *J Wound Care* 2004; **13**: 383.
9. Gethin G. The significance of surface pH in chronic wounds. *Wounds UK* 2007; **3**: 52. http://www.woundsinternational.com/media/issues/160/files/content_124.pdf (accessed August 15, 2015).
10. Bischofberger AS, Dart CM, Perkins NR, *et al.* A preliminary study on the effect of manuka honey on second-intention healing of contaminated wounds on the distal aspect of the forelimbs of horses. *Vet Surg* 2011; **40**: 898.
11. Monteiro SO, Lepage OM, Theoret CL. Effects of platelet-rich plasma on the repair of wounds on the distal aspect of the forelimb in horses. *Am J Vet Res* 2009; **70**: 277.
12. Dart AJ, Cries L, Jeffcott LB, *et al.* Effects of 25% propylene glycol hydrogel (Solugel) on second intention wound healing in horses. *Vet Surg* 2002; **31**: 309.
13. Dart AJ, Perkins NR, Dart CM, *et al.* Effect of bandaging on second intention healing of wounds of the distal limb in horses. *Austr Vet J* 2009; **87**: 215.
14. Junker JP, Kamel RA, Caterson EJ, *et al.* Clinical impact upon wound healing and inflammation in moist, wet, and dry environments. *Adv Wound Care (New Rochelle)* 2013; **2**: 348.
15. Dyson M, Young SR, Hart J, *et al.* Comparison of the effects of moist and dry conditions on the process of angiogenesis during dermal repair. *J Invest Dermatol* 1992; **99**: 729.
16. Baxter CR. Immunological reactions in chronic wounds. *Am J Surg* 1994; **167**: S12–S14.
17. Kunugiza Y, Tomita T, Moritomo H, *et al.* A hydrocellular foam dressing versus gauze: effects on the healing of rat excisional wounds. *J Wound Care* 2010; **19**: 10.
18. Mertz PM, Marshall DA, Eaglstein WH. Occlusive wound dressings to prevent bacterial invasion and wound-infection. *J Am Acad Dermatol* 1985; **12**: 662.
19. Mertz PM, Eaglstein WH. The effect of a semiocclusive dressing on the microbial population in superficial wounds. *Arch Surg* 1984; **119**: 287.
20. Hutchinson JJ, Lawrence JC. Wound-infection under occlusive dressings. *J Hosp Infect* 1991; **17**: 83.
21. Hutchinson JJ, McGuckin M. Occlusive dressings – a microbiological and clinical review. *Am J Infect Control* 1990; **18**: 257.
22. Boulton AJ, Meneses P, Ennis WJ. Diabetic foot ulcers: a framework for prevention and care. *Wound Repair Regen* 1999; **7**: 7.
23. Reddy M, Kohr R, Queen D, *et al.* Practical treatment of wound pain and trauma: a patient-centered approach. An overview. *Ostomy Wound Manage* 2003; **49**: 2.
24. Knighton DR, Silver IA, Hunt TK. Regulation of wound-healing angiogenesis – effect of oxygen gradients and inspired oxygen concentration. *Surgery* 1981; **90**: 262.
25. Alvarez OM, Mertz PM, Eaglstein WH. The effect of occlusive dressings on collagen-synthesis and re-epithelialization in superficial wounds. *J Surg Res* 1983; **35**: 142.
26. Howard RD, Stashak TS, Baxter GM. Evaluation of occlusive dressings for management of full-thickness excisional wounds on the distal portion of the limbs of horses. *Am J Vet Res* 1993; **54**: 2150.
27. Serteyn D, Mottart E. Ultilisation of an occlusive dressing, DuoDERM, on cutaneous lacerations of the legs in horses. *Ann Med Vet* 1988; **132**: 593.
28. Blackford JT, Wan PY, Latimer FG, *et al.* Treatment of distal extremity lacerations using a flexible hydroactive occlusive dressing. *Proc Ann Convention Am Assoc Equine Pract* 1993; **39**: 215.
29. Ducharme-Desjarlais M, Celeste C, Lepault E, *et al.* Effect of a silicone-containing dressing on exuberant granulation tissue formation and wound repair in horses. *Am J Vet Res* 2005; **66**: 1133.
30. Stashak TS, Farstvedt E, Othic A. Update on wound dressings: indications and best use. *Clin Techniques Eq Pract* 2004; **3**: 148.
31. Barber SM. Second intention wound healing in the horse: the effect of bandages and topical steroids. *Proc Ann Convention Am Assoc Equine Pract* 1989; **35**: 107.
32. Owen R. Use of a topical enzymatic debriding agent in wounds of the equine leg (a pilot study). *Vet Med Small An Clin* 1975; **70**: 1101.
33. Fretz PB, Martin GS, Jacobs KA, *et al.* Treatment of exuberant granulation tissue in the horse evaluation of four methods. *Vet Surg* 1983; **12**: 137.
34. Berry DB, Sullins KE. Effects of topical application of antimicrobials and bandaging on healing and granulation tissue formation in wounds of the distal aspect of the limbs in horses. *Am J Vet Res* 2003; **64**: 88.
35. Theoret CL, Barber SM, Moyana TN, *et al.* Preliminary observations on expression of transforming growth factors beta 1 and beta 3 in equine full-thickness skin wounds healing normally or with exuberant granulation tissue. *Vet Surg* 2002; **31**: 266.
36. Marshall DA, Mertz PM, Eaglstein WH. Occlusive dressings – does dressing type influence the growth of common bacterial pathogens? *Arch Surg* 1990; **125**: 1136.
37. Vermeulen H, Ubbink DT, Goossens A *et al.* Systematic review of dressings and topical agents for surgical wounds healing by secondary intention. *Br J Surg* 2005; **92**: 665.
38. Pain R, Sneddon JC, Cochrane CA. *In vitro* study of the effectiveness of different dressings for debriding fibrin in blood clots from horses. *Vet Rec* 2006; **159**: 712.
39. Hoekstra MJ, Hermans MH, Richters CD, *et al.* A histological comparison of acute inflammatory responses with a hydrofibre or tulle gauze dressing. *J Wound Care* 2002; **11**: 113.
40. Dumville JC, Gray TA, Walter CJ, *et al.* Dressings for the prevention of surgical site infection. *Cochrane Database Syst Rev* 2014; **9**: CD003091. DOI: 10.1002/14651858.CD003091.pub3.
41. Tnibar A, Grubbe Lin K, Thuroe Nielsen K, *et al.* Effect of a stent bandage on the likelihood of incisional infection following exploratory coeliotomy for colic in horses: a comparative retrospective study. *Equine Vet J* 2013; **45**: 564.
42. Smith LJ, Mellor DJ, Marr CM, *et al.* Incisional complications following exploratory celiotomy: does an abdominal bandage reduce the risk? *Equine Vet J* 2007; **39**: 277.
43. McIlwraith CW, Nixon AJ, Wright IM. Diagnostic and surgical arthroscopy of the tarsocrural (tibiotarsal) joint. In: McIlwraith CW, Nixon AJ, Wright IM (eds). *Diagnostic and Surgical Arthroscopy in the Horse*, 4th edn. Mosby Elsevier: Philadelphia, 2015: 243.
44. Borg H, Carmalt JL. Postoperative septic arthritis after elective equine arthroscopy without antimicrobial prophylaxis. *Vet Surg* 2013; **42**: 262.

45. Toon CD, Ramamoorthy R, Davidson BR, *et al.* Early versus delayed dressing removal after primary closure of clean and clean-contaminated surgical wounds. *Cochrane Database Syst Rev* 2013; **9**: CD010259. DOI: 10.1002/14651858.CD010259.pub2.
46. Sørensen MA, Petersen LJ, Bundgaard L, *et al.* Regional disturbances in blood flow and metabolism in equine limb wound healing with formation of exuberant granulation tissue. *Wound Repair Regen* 2014; **22**: 647.
47. Celeste CJ, Deschesne K, Riley CB, *et al.* Skin temperature during cutaneous wound healing in an equine model of cutaneous fibroproliferative disorder: kinetics and anatomic-site differences. *Vet Surg* 2013; **42**: 147.
48. Wedmore I, McManus JG, Pusateri AE, *et al.* A special report on the chitosan-based hemostatic dressing: experience in current combat operations. *J Trauma* 2006; **60**: 655.
49. Ueno H, Mori T, Fujinaga T. Topical formulations and wound healing applications of chitosan. *Adv Drug Deliv Rev* 2001; **52**: 105.
50. Yusof NL, Wee A, Lim LY, *et al.* Flexible chitin films as potential wound-dressing materials: wound model studies. *J Biomed Mater Res A* 2003; **66**: 224.
51. Pietramaggiori G, Yang HJ, Scherer SS, *et al.* Effects of poly-N-acetyl glucosamine (pGlcNAc) patch on wound healing in db/db mouse. *J Trauma* 2008; **64**: 803.
52. Dai T, Tanaka M, Huang Y-Y, *et al.* Chitosan preparations for wounds and burns: antimicrobial and wound-healing effects. *Expert Rev Anti Infect Ther* 2011; **9**: 857.
53. Ong SY, Wu J, Moochhala SM, *et al.* Development of a chitosan-based wound dressing with improved hemostatic and antimicrobial properties. *Biomaterials* 2008; **29**: 4323.
54. Barnett SE, Varley SJ. The effects of calcium alginate on wound-healing. *Ann R Coll Surg Engl* 1987; **69**: 153.
55. Chaby G, Senet P, Vaneau M, *et al.* Dressings for acute and chronic wounds – a systematic review. *Arch Dermatol* 2007; **143**: 1297.
56. von Lindern JJ, Niederhagen B, Appel T, *et al.* Treatment of soft tissue defects with exposed bone in the head and face region with alginates and hydrocolloid dressings. *J Oral Maxillofac Surg* 2002; **60**: 1126.
57. Segal HC, Hunt BJ, Gilding K. The effects of alginate and non-alginate wound dressings on blood coagulation and platelet activation. *J Biomater Appl* 1998; **12**: 249.
58. Sirimanna KS. Calcium alginate fiber (Kaltostat-2) for nasal packing after trimming of turbinates – a pilot study. *J Laryngol Otol* 1989; **103**: 1067.
59. La Hausse-Brown TP, Dujon DG. A dressing for 'road rash'. *Ann R Coll Surg Engl* 1997; **79**: 154.
60. Velasco JLD, Bernard MJB, Perez GT, *et al.* Clinical efficacy of sodium alginate meshes for the control of infectious dissemination by *Escherichia coli* and *Staphylococcus epidermidis* in cavitated wounds with primary healing. *Veterinaria Mexico* 2012; **43**: 285.
61. Harding KG, Price P, Robinson B, *et al.* Cost and dressing evaluation of hydrofiber and alginate dressings in the management of community-based patients with chronic leg ulceration. *Wounds* 2001; **13**: 229.
62. Ravnskog FA, Espehaug B, Indrekvam K. Randomised clinical trial comparing hydrofiber and alginate dressings post-hip replacement. *J Wound Care* 2011; **20**: 136.
63. Davis SC, Cazzaniga AL, Ovington LG, *et al.* A new hydrogel dressing accelerates 2nd-degree burn wound-healing. *J Invest Dermatol* 1991; **96**: 575.
64. Jones V, Milton T. When and how to use hydrogels. *Nursing Times* 2000; **96**: 3.
65. Morgan PW, Binnington AG, Miller CW, *et al.* The effect of occlusive and semi-occlusive dressings on the healing of acute full-thickness skin wounds on the forelimbs of dogs. *Vet Surg* 1994; **23**: 494.
66. Ramsey DT, Pope ER, Wagnermann C, *et al.* Effects of 3 occlusive dressing materials on healing of full-thickness skin wounds in dogs. *Am J Vet Res* 1995; **56**: 941.
67. Kelleher ME, Kilcoyne I, Dechant JE, *et al.* A preliminary study of silver sodium zirconium phosphate polyurethane foam wound dressing on wounds of the distal aspect of the forelimb in horses. *Vet Surg* 2015; **44**: 359.
68. Meuleneire F, Rüchnagel H. Soft silicone dressings made easy. *Wounds Int* 2013; May: 1–6. http://www.woundsinternational.com/media/issues/674/files/content_10804.pdf (accessed August 15, 2015).
69. Mustoe TA. Evolution of silicone therapy and mechanism of action in scar management. *Aesthetic Plast Surg* 2008; **32**: 82.
70. Meaume S, Le Pillouer-Prost A, Richert B *et al.* Management of scars: updated practical guidelines and use of silicones. *Eur J Dermatol* 2014; **24**: 435.
71. Gold MH, Foster TD, Adair MA, *et al.* Prevention of hypertrophic scars and keloids by the prophylactic use of topical silicone gel sheets following a surgical procedure in an office setting. *Dermatol Surg* 2001; **27**: 641.
72. Gomez JH, Schumacher J, Lauten SD, *et al.* Effects of 3 biologic dressings on healing of cutaneous wounds on the limbs of horses. *Can J Vet Res* 2004; **68**: 49.
73. Litwiniuk M, Grzela T. Amniotic membrane: New concepts for an old dressing. *Wound Repair Regen* 2014; **22**: 451.
74. Plummer CE. The use of amniotic membrane transplantation for ocular surface reconstruction: a review and series of 58 equine clinical cases (2002–2008). *Vet Ophthalmol* 2009; **12**: 17.
75. Bigbie RB, Schumacher J, Swaim SF, *et al.* Effects of amnion and live yeast-cell derivative on 2nd-intention healing in horses. *Am J Vet Res* 1991; **52**: 1376.
76. Goodrich LR, Moll D, Crisman MV, *et al.* Comparison of equine amnion and a nonadherent wound dressing material for bandaging pinch-grafted wounds in ponies. *Am J Vet Res* 2000; **61**: 326.
77. Bellenzani MCR, Matera JM, Giacóia MR. homologous pericardium as a biological dressing for treatment of distal limb wounds in horses: an experimental study. *Acta Cir Bras* 1998; **13**: 237.
78. Alexander JH, Yeager DA, Stern DS, *et al.* Equine pericardium as a biological covering for the treatment of diabetic foot wounds – a prospective study. *J Am Podiatr Med Assoc* 2012; **102**: 352.
79. Gurrado A, Franco IF, Lissidini G, *et al.* Impact of pericardium bovine patch (Tutomesh®) on incisional hernia treatment in contaminated or potentially contaminated fields: retrospective comparative study. *Hernia* 2015; **19**: 259.
80. Yvorchuk-St. Jean K, Gaughan E, St-Jean G, *et al.* Evaluation of a porous bovine collagen membrane bandage for management of wounds in horses. *Am J Vet Res* 1995; **56**: 1663.
81. Bertone AL, Sullins KE, Stashak TS, *et al.* Effect of wound location and the use of topical collagen gel on exuberant granulation tissue formation and wound healing in the horse and pony. *Am J Vet Res* 1985; **46**: 1438.
82. Elgharably H, Ganesh K, Dickerson J, *et al.* A modified collagen gel dressing promotes angiogenesis in a preclinical swine model of chronic ischemic wounds. *Wound Repair Regen* 2014; **22**: 720.

83. Elgharably H, Roy S, Khanna S, *et al.* A modified collagen gel enhances healing outcome in a preclinical swine model of excisional wounds. *Wound Repair Regen* 2013; **21**: 473.
84. Schallberger SP, Stanley BJ, Hauptman JG, *et al.* Effect of porcine small intestinal submucosa on acute full-thickness wounds in dogs. *Vet Surg* 2008; **37**: 515.
85. Aya KL, Stern R. Hyaluronan in wound healing: rediscovering a major player. *Wound Repair Regen* 2014; **22**: 579.
86. Lo DD, Zimmermann AS, Nauta A, *et al.* Scarless fetal skin wound healing update. *Birth Defects Res C Embryo Today* 2012; **96**: 237.
87. Yang G, Prestwich GD, Mann BK. Thiolated carboxymethyl-hyaluronic-acid- based biomaterials enhance wound healing in rats, dogs, and horses. *ISRN Vet Sci*; **2011**: 851593. http://www.hindawi.com/journals/isrn/2011/851593/(accessed August 15, 2015).
88. Hadley HS, Stanley BJ, Fritz MC, *et al.* Effects of a cross-linked hyaluronic acid based gel on the healing of open wounds in dogs. *Vet Surg* 2013; **42**: 161.
89. Witte SH, Olaifa AK, Lewis AJ, *et al.* Application of exogenous esterified hyaluronan to equine distal limb wounds. *J Equine Vet Sci* 2009; **29**: 197.
90. Nuccitelli R. A role for endogenous electric fields in wound healing. *Curr Top Dev Biol* 2003; **58**: 1.
91. Banerjee J, Das Ghatak P, Roy S, *et al.* Silver–zinc redox-coupled electroceutical wound dressing disrupts bacterial biofilm. *PLoS ONE* 2015; **10**: e0119531.
92. Banerjee J, Das Ghatak P, Roy S, *et al.* Improvement of human keratinocyte migration by a redox active bioelectric dressing. *PLoS ONE* 2014; **9**: e89239.
93. Huckfeldt R, Flick AB, Mikkelson D, *et al.* Wound closure after split-thickness skin grafting is accelerated with the use of continuous direct anodal microcurrent applied to silver nylon wound contact dressings. *J Burn Care Res* 2007; **28**: 703.
94. Carley PJ, Wainapel SF. Electrotherapy for acceleration of wound healing: low intensity direct current. *Arch Phys Med Rehabil* 1985; **66**: 443.
95. Varhus JD. A Novel bioelectric device enhances wound healing: an equine case series. *J Equine Vet Sci* 2014; **34**: 421.
96. Woodward M. Silver dressings in wound healing: what is the evidence? *Primary Intention* 2005; **13**: 153.
97. Bischofberger AS, Dart CM, Perkins NR, *et al.* The effect of short- and long-term treatment with manuka honey on second intention healing of contaminated and noncontaminated wounds on the distal aspect of the forelimbs in horses. *Vet Surg* 2013; **42**: 154.
98. European Wound Management Association (EWMA). *Position Document: Wound bed preparation in practice*. London: MEP Ltd, 2004. http://www.ewma.org/fileadmin/user_upload/EWMA/pdf/Position_Documents/2004/pos_doc_English_final_04.pdf (accessed August 15, 2015).
99. Franz MG, Robson MC, Steed DL, *et al.* Guidelines to aid healing of acute wounds by decreasing impediments of healing. *Wound Repair Regen* 2008; **16**: 723.
100. Robson MC, Edstrom LE, Krizek TJ, *et al.* Efficacy of systemic antibiotics in treatments of granulating wounds. *J Surg Res* 1974; **16**: 299.
101. Best Practice Statement: The use of topical antiseptic/antimicrobial agents in wound management. *Wounds UK* 2011. http://www.wounds-uk.com/pdf/content_9969.pdf (accessed August 15, 2015).
102. Jones SA, Bowler PG, Walker M, *et al.* Controlling wound bioburden with a novel silver-containing hydrofiber dressing. *Wound Repair Regen* 2004; **12**: 288.
103. Percival SL, Bowler PG, Russell D. Bacterial resistance to silver in wound care. *J Hosp Infect* 2005; **60**: 1.
104. Parsons D, Bowler PG, Myles V, *et al.* Silver antimicrobial dressings in wound management: A comparison of antibacterial, physical, and chemical characteristics. *Wounds* 2005; **17**: 222.
105. Ip M, Lui SL, Poon VKM, *et al.* Antimicrobial activities of silver dressings: an *in vitro* comparison. *J Med Microbiol* 2006; **55**: 59.
106. Adams AP, Santschi EM, Mellencamp MA. Antibacterial properties of a silver chloride-coated nylon wound dressing. *Vet Surg* 1999; **28**: 219.
107. Bowler PG, Jones SA, Walker M, *et al.* Microbicidal properties of a silver-containing hydrofiber (R) dressing against a variety of burn wound pathogens. *J Burn Care Rehabil* 2004; **25**: 192.
108. Wright JB, Lam K, Burrell RE. Wound management in an era of increasing bacterial antibiotic resistance: a role for topical silver treatment. *Am J Infect Control* 1998; **26**: 572.
109. Thomas S, McCubbin P. A comparison of the antimicrobial effects of four silver-containing dressings on three organisms. *J Wound Care* 2003; **12**: 101.
110. Loh JV, Percival SL, Woods EJ, *et al.* Silver resistance in MRSA isolated from wound and nasal sources in humans and animals. *Int Wound J* 2009; **6**: 32.
111. Woods EJ, Cochrane CA, Percival SL. Prevalence of silver resistance genes in bacteria isolated from human and horse wounds. *Vet Microbiol* 2009; **138**: 325.
112. Carter MJ, Tingley-Kelley K, Warriner RA. Silver treatments and silver-impregnated dressings for the healing of leg wounds and ulcers: a systematic review and meta-analysis. *J Am Acad Dermatol* 2010; **63**: 668.
113. Vermeulen H, Van Hattem JM, Storm-Versloot MN, *et al.* Topical silver for treating infected wounds. *Cochrane Database Syst Rev* 2007; **1**: CD005486. DOI: 10.1002/14651858.CD005486.pub2.
114. Mueller G, Kramer A. Biocompatibility index of antiseptic agents by parallel assessment of antimicrobial activity and cellular cytotoxicity. *J Antimicrob Chemother* 2008; **61**: 1281.
115. Moore K, Gray D. Using PHMB antimicrobial to prevent wound infection. *Wounds UK* 2007; **3**: 96.
116. Wiegand C, Abel M, Kramer A, *et al.* Viability and proliferation of fibroblasts, keratinocytes and HaCaT-cells influenced by polihexanide. *EWMA J* 2007; **7**: 109.
117. Daeschlein G, Assadian O, Bruck JC, *et al.* Feasibility and clinical applicability of polihexanide for treatment of second-degree burn wounds. *Skin Pharmacol Physiol* 2007; **20**: 292.
118. Lee WR, Tobias KM, Bemis DA, *et al.* In vitro efficacy of a polyhexamethylene biguanide-impregnated gauze dressing against bacteria found in veterinary patients. *Vet Surg* 2004; **33**: 404.
119. Consensus document: PHMB and its potential contribution to wound management. Wounds UK, Aberdeen, 2010. www.wounds-uk.com/pdf/content_9484.pdf (accessed August 15, 2015).
120. Sibbald RG, Coutts P, Woo KY. Reduction of bacterial burden and pain in chronic wounds using a new polyhexamethylene biguanide antimicrobial foam dressing – clinical trial results. *Adv Skin Wound Care* 2011; **24**: 78.
121. Russell AD. Bacterial resistance to disinfectants: present knowledge and future problems. *J Hosp Infect* 1999; **43 Suppl**: S57.

122. Wilson DG, Cooley AJ, Macwilliams PS, *et al.* Effects of a 0.05-percent chlorhexidine lavage on the tarsocrural joints of horses. *Vet Surg* 1994; **23**: 442.
123. Douw CM, Bulstra SK, Vandenbroucke J, *et al.* Clinical and pathological changes in the knee after accidental chlorhexidine irrigation during arthroscopy – case reports and review of the literature. *J Bone Joint Surg Br* 1998; **80B**: 437.
124. Anderson MA, Payne JT, Kreeger JM, *et al.* Effects of intraarticular chlorhexidine diacetate lavage on the stifle in healthy dogs. *Am J Vet Res* 1993; **54**: 1784.
125. Saatman RA, Carlton WW, Hubben K, *et al.* A wound-healing study of chlorhexidine digluconate in guinea pigs. *Fundam Appl Toxicol* 1986; **6**: 1.
126. Fraser JF, Cuttle L, Kempf M, *et al.* Cytotoxicity of topical antimicrobial agents used in burn wounds in Australasia. *ANZ J Surg* 2004; **74**: 139.
127. Bonacorsi C, Raddi MSG, Carlos IZ. Cytotoxicity of chlorhexidine digluconate to murine macrophages and its effect on hydrogen peroxide and nitric oxide induction. *Braz J Med Biol Res* 2004; **37**: 207.
128. Sanchez IR, Swaim SF, Nusbaum KE, *et al.* Effects of chlorhexidine diacetate and povidone iodine on wound-healing in dogs. *Vet Surg* 1988; **17**: 291.
129. Muangman P, Nitimonton S, Aramwit P. Comparative clinical study of Bactigras and Telfa AMD for skin graft donor-site dressing. *Int J Mol Sci* 2011; **12**: 5031.
130. Yabanoglu H, Basaran O, Aydogan C, *et al.* Assessment of the effectiveness of silver-coated dressing, chlorhexidine acetate (0.5%), citric acid (3%), and silver sulfadiazine (1%) for topical antibacterial effects against the multi-drug resistant *Pseudomonas aeruginosa* infecting full-skin thickness burn wounds on rats. *Int Surg* 2013; **98**: 416.
131. Ulkur E, Oncul O, Karagoz H, *et al.* Comparison of silver-coated dressing (Acticoat), chlorhexidine acetate 0.5% (Bactigrass), and silver sulfadiazine 1% (Silverdin) for topical antibacterial effect in *Pseudomonas aeruginosa*-contaminated, full-skin thickness burn wounds in rats. *J Burn Care Rehabil* 2005; **26**: 430.
132. Acar A, Uygur F, Diktas H, *et al.* Comparison of silver-coated dressing (Acticoat), chlorhexidine acetate 0.5% (Bactigrass) and nystatin for topical antifungal effect in *Candida albicans*-contaminated, full-skin-thickness rat burn wounds. *Burns* 2011; **37**: 882.
133. Thomas GW, Rael LT, Bar-Or R, *et al.* Mechanisms of delayed wound healing by commonly used antiseptics. *J Trauma* 2009; **66**: 82.
134. Fleischer W, Reimer K. Povidone–iodine in antisepsis state of the art. *Dermatol* 1997; **195**: 3.
135. Berkelman RL, Holland BW, Anderson RL. Increased bactericidal activity of dilute preparations of povidone-iodine solution. *J Clin Microbiol* 1982; **15**: 635.
136. Vermeulen H, Westerbos SJ, Ubbink DT. Benefit and harm of iodine in wound care: a systematic review. *J Hosp Infect* 2010; **76**: 191.
137. Mertz PM, Davis SC, Brewer LD, *et al.* Can antimicrobials be effective without impairing wound healing – the evaluation of a cadexomer iodine ointment. *Wounds* 1994; **6**: 184.
138. Lamme EN, Gustafsson TO, Middelkoop E. Cadexomer–iodine ointment shows stimulation of epidermal regeneration in experimental full-thickness wounds. *Arch Dermatol Res* 1998; **290**: 18.
139. Vogt PM, Reimer K, Hauser J, *et al.* PVP-iodine in hydrosomes and hydrogel – a novel concept in wound therapy leads to enhanced epithelialization and reduced loss of skin grafts. *Burns* 2006; **32**: 698.
140. Guthrie HC, Martin KR, Taylor C, *et al.* A pre-clinical evaluation of silver, iodine and Manuka honey based dressings in a model of traumatic extremity wounds contaminated with *Staphylococcus aureus*. *Injury* 2014; **45**: 1171.
141. Mueller RS, Bergvall K, Bensignor E, *et al.* A review of topical therapy for skin infections with bacteria and yeast. *Vet Dermatol* 2012; **23**: 330–E362.
142. Carnwath R, Graham EM, Reynolds K, *et al.* The antimicrobial activity of honey against common equine wound bacterial isolates. *Vet J* 2014; **199**: 110.
143. Naka K, Watarai S, Tana, *et al.* Adsorption effect of activated charcoal on enterohemorrhagic *Escherichia coli*. *J Vet Med Sci* 2001; **63**: 281.
144. Kerihuel JC. Effect of activated charcoal dressings on healing outcomes of chronic wounds. *J Wound Care* 2010; **19**: 208.
145. Borrelly J, Blech MF, Grosdidier G, *et al.* Contribution of a 3-percent boric acid solution for the treatment of deep wounds with loss of substance. *Ann Chir Plast Esthet* 1991; **36**: 65.
146. Ljungh A, Yanagisawa N, Wadström T. Using the principle of hydrophobic interaction to bind and remove wound bacteria. *J Wound Care* 2006; **15**: 175.
147. Ljungh A, Wadstrom T. Growth conditions influence expression of cell surface hydrophobicity of staphylococci and other wound infection pathogens. *Microbiol Immunol* 1995; **39**: 753.
148. Falk P, Ivarsson ML. Effect of a DACC dressing on the growth properties and proliferation rate of cultured fibroblasts. *J Wound Care* 2012; **21**: 327.

CHAPTER 7

Bandaging and Casting Techniques for Wound Management

Updated by Yvonne A. Elce, DVM, Diplomate ACVS

Chapter Contents

Summary

Bandages and splints or casts are an essential component of wound management and, when used properly, can greatly aid healing. Improper application, however, may impede healing and be detrimental to the well-being or athletic future of the horse. Many different types of bandage materials exist and are reviewed in Chapter 6. The current chapter is devoted to the principles and techniques of bandaging and casting. Splinting is discussed along with casting because either approach may be used when immobilization is required to support wound healing. Various techniques to improve the application and maintenance of bandages, splints, and casts, as well as to manage complications arising from their use, are discussed.

Introduction

Bandages, splints, and casts can be valuable aids to the healing of various wounds. Bandages protect the wound from the environment, as well as from repeated trauma. By keeping the area warm and moist, they improve cellular metabolism and migration within the wound bed. Moreover, bandages may absorb exudate and/or decrease tissue edema through mild compression. In general, bandages enhance wound healing, if properly applied and if they are adapted to the phases of wound healing. Bandages, however, may also wield some disadvantages besides the costs associated with their long-term use. Of particular concern, they may increase the risk of formation of exuberant granulation tissue (EGT) in wounds located at the distal aspect of the limb (the reader is referred to Chapter 15 for more information on equine EGT).[1–4] Wounds that produce a copious amount of discharge may suffer tissue maceration if the dressing is not adapted to this situation and if the saturated bandage is not replaced in a timely manner. Moreover, incorrectly applied bandages can damage the wound surface and/or cause inflammation in the soft tissues underlying and surrounding the wound.

Although a thick bandage decreases movement in a wounded area, a splint or cast is a more appropriate choice when immobilization

Equine Wound Management, Third Edition. Edited by Christine Theoret and Jim Schumacher.

Companion website: www.wiley.com/go/theoret/wound

would aid healing. Splints are generally applied over a well-padded bandage and decrease movement, whereas casts, applied over a bandage or not, provide the most rigid immobilization. Immobilization with a splint or cast is generally reserved for wounds over high-motion areas, such as joints (e.g., fetlock or carpus), and it should be kept in mind that even short periods of immobilization can negatively affect the health of joints and bones.[5,6]

Thus, in all cases, the benefits of bandaging and/or splinting or casting should be weighed carefully against the potential negative effects that may result from the improper use of bandages, splints, and casts.

Bandages

Materials

Bandages generally consist of three main layers.[7] The primary layer is in direct contact with the wound, the secondary layer is thicker and usually composed of cotton padding, while the tertiary layer is commonly the mechanism whereby the other layers are held in place.

The primary layer, or wound dressing, must be adapted to the nature of the wound, especially as it pertains to the phase of healing. Of the many types available, most modern dressings are considered "interactive" and are designed to either support debridement, maintain a humid wound environment, allow the passage of oxygen and/or exudate, enhance epithelialization, or exert some combination of these actions (the reader is referred to Chapter 6 for an update on the various types of wound dressings).

The secondary or intermediate layer is composed of thicker material, such as cotton or gauze, designed to absorb excess exudate not managed by the dressing, to provide padding and to limit motion somewhat.

The tertiary layer, while passive, provides some compression to decrease swelling and aids in restricting movement of the limb. Elastic, adhesive, or self-adhesive materials are commonly used for this purpose (Table 7.1).

Wound bandaging in horses usually includes these basic three layers, with some modifications according to the specific area being bandaged. Bandages applied to the head and to the foot, for example, may not comprise all three layers.

Table 7.1 Common examples of materials used for the secondary and tertiary layers of a wound bandage.

Bandage material	Purpose	Company
Kling™	Conforming gauze to support the dressing	Johnson & Johnson, Guelph, ON, Canada
Curity Synthetic undercast padding™	Conforming gauze to support the dressing	Covidien, Mansfield, MA, USA
Bandage gauze	Conforming gauze to support the dressing	Shoof International Ltd, Cambridge, New Zealand
Gamgee Highly Absorbent Padding	Secondary layer	3M, St Paul, MN, USA
Curity practical cotton roll	Secondary layer	Covidien
Curity wadding rolls	Secondary layer	Covidien
Cotton wool roll	Secondary layer	Shoof International Ltd, Cambridge, New Zealand
Vetrap™	Tertiary layer	3M
Shoof-Vet cohesive bandage	Tertiary layer	Shoof International Ltd, Cambridge, New Zealand
Kendall adhesive bandage	Tertiary layer	Covidien
Powerflex bandage	Tertiary layer	Andover, Salisbury, MA, USA
Veterinary Elastic Adhesive Tape	Tertiary layer	3M
Elastikon® Elastic Tape	Tertiary layer	Johnson & Johnson
Bandage elastic adhesive Shoof	Tertiary layer	Shoof International Ltd, Cambridge, New Zealand
Co-Ease cohesive bandage	Tertiary layer	Tempo-medical products, Scottsdale, AZ, USA

General considerations

Horses with bandages and/or splints or casts should be kept in a clean, dry area that allows for frequent visual monitoring. A clean stall or small pen with grass may be used.

Bandages should be changed regularly to avoid tissue maceration due to the excessive accumulation of exudate that is not absorbed adequately by the primary and secondary layers. The required frequency of bandage change is dictated by the nature of the underlying wound and the selected dressing.

The tertiary layer must be applied with even tension and over sufficient padding so as not to cause excessive pressure, particularly at the distal aspect of the limb where there is little soft-tissue coverage. Elasticized bandage should not be applied directly to the skin, so a small amount of the secondary layer is left uncovered proximally and distally. Adhesive tape is then applied, without tension, over those uncovered areas of the secondary layer and overlapped on to the skin. This final touch prevents foreign material from migrating under the bandage and causing skin sores or contaminating the wound.

Specific bandages

Foot and pastern bandages

Wounds to the foot are usually the result of penetrating objects or of the foot becoming caught between two surfaces. Bandages are used to cover wounds on the sole of the hoof, the coronary band or the pastern. If there is a large defect in the sole, initial bandaging used during the acute phase of healing may be followed by the long-term use of a specialized shoe, such as one with a removable plate covering the sole. If there is a defect involving the hoof wall, the hoof wall surrounding the wound is trimmed slightly shorter so that the shoe contacts the wall of the hoof, as normal, except at the affected area. A foot cast and/or a specialized shoe is necessary when a substantial portion of the hoof wall has been lost because it helps provide long-term stability to the rest of the foot during the lengthy healing and regrowth of the horn.

Wounds of the sole, hoof, or pastern first receive generic cleansing and debridement, followed by primary closure, if warranted. A dressing suitable to the state of the wound is then applied (Figure 7.1a,b), followed by a secondary layer of cotton. For wounds on the sole, a large square of cotton can be placed on the bottom of the foot and folded up over the wall of the hoof and the coronary band then attached with elastic, self-adhesive material (Figure 7.1c,d). A square patch of duct tape placed on the bottom of the foot, over the square of cotton, prevents wicking of moisture from the environment (Figure 7.1e). Finally, elastic, adhesive tape is lightly applied, circumferentially, to the top of the bandage and the surrounding skin, to prevent foreign material from migrating under the bandage (Figure 7.1f,g).

Pastern wounds involving the coronary band or heel bulb regions are bandaged in a manner similar to those on the hoof except that the bandage extends proximad to cover the wound in the pastern region. Most of these wounds are best managed with a phalangeal (foot/pastern) cast, discussed later. Lacerations of the mid and proximal pastern region may be managed by bandaging the region without including the bottom of the foot. In this case, elastic adhesive tape is used to attach the distal extremity of the bandage to the hoof wall (Figure 7.2).

What to avoid

- When applying a bandage that encompasses the hoof, the square cotton pad (secondary layer) is difficult to conform and the spaces between its corners cause some areas at the coronary band or skin over the pastern to remain unpadded; consequently, avoid placing excess pressure when applying the tertiary layer.

Tip

- Disposable baby diapers are cost effective and provide a waterproof yet absorbent secondary layer. Moreover, the diaper conforms nicely to the hoof when used for bandaging wounds of the sole.

Distal limb bandages (extending from the ground to the carpus or tarsus)

Practitioners are usually comfortable applying a bandage to the distal aspect of the limb of horses because this is a commonly traumatized area in their equine patients[8,9] and because bandages conform more readily to the metacarpus/metatarsus or fetlock than to the foot. The primary layer of the bandage (dressing) must suit the nature of the wound and is usually held in place with conforming gauze (Figure 7.3a). The thicker part of the secondary layer, consisting of cotton, is then applied (Figure 7.3b) and held in place with the tertiary layer, commonly elastic, self-adhesive wrap such as Vetrap™ (Figure 7.3c). This tertiary layer must be applied evenly, distad to proximad, leaving a small border of the secondary layer exposed at either extremity to avoid applying pressure directly to the skin. These borders are then covered loosely by an elastic, adhesive tape, such as Elastikon®, that overlaps onto the skin to prevent the entry of foreign material under the bandage (Figure 7.3d). Horsemen are commonly taught to wrap the limb in such a way that the bandage material passes from outside to inside across the palmar/plantar surface of the limb: left limbs are wrapped counter-clockwise, and right limbs are wrapped clockwise.

What to avoid

- Bunching of the bandage or uneven tension that may cause underlying tissues to swell.
- Ending the bandage at the level of the coronary band where it may rub and irritate this delicate tissue. The bandage should end a few centimeters proximal to the coronary band, on the pastern (Figure 7.3e), or more distally, over the hoof wall, where it is attached using elastic, adhesive tape (Figure 7.3d).

Carpal and tarsal bandages

Carpal and tarsal bandages resemble the bandages applied to wounds on the distal aspect of the limb, apart from two main considerations: they are more challenging to apply and maintain and they have a greater potential of causing pressure sores over areas with little soft-tissue coverage (e.g., the accessory carpal bone in the forelimb and the point of the hock in the hindlimb). Some measures can help protect against the development of cast sores related to bandages on the carpus or tarsus. For the carpal area, the conforming gauze used to secure the wound dressing can be wrapped in a figure-of-eight pattern around the carpus (Figure 7.4a), thereby relieving some pressure on the accessory carpal bone and simultaneously filling in the relative depression surrounding it. Thus, when the main part of the secondary layer (i.e., the cotton pad) is applied (Figure 7.4b), pressure is distributed evenly to the palmar surface of the carpus rather than to a focal point (accessory carpal bone). Alternatively, the layers can be applied as usual and then a small "releasing" incision can be made in the tertiary and secondary layers, directly over the accessory carpal bone, to relieve pressure at this area (Figure 7.4c–f). Another method of preventing excessive pressure on the accessory carpal bone is to create a donut of conforming gauze or rolled up stockinette and positioning it so that the hole is over the accessory carpal bone. This can be placed between the conforming gauze holding the primary layer in place and the secondary layer of cotton padding. This effectively prevents pressure on the bone when correctly positioned but, since the donut may slip, increased rather than decreased pressure may arise at a point under the bandage. Ultimately, the method used to reduce pressure on the accessory carpal bone when bandaging this area should be tailored to the materials available and the behavior of the patient.

The conformation of the hock and the combination of forces generated by the reciprocal apparatus impose some important considerations when applying a bandage to this region. Horses are reluctant to accept restricted movement of this area and frequently disrupt the bandage by hyper-flexing the hock. Placing the conforming gauze in a figure-of-eight pattern around the

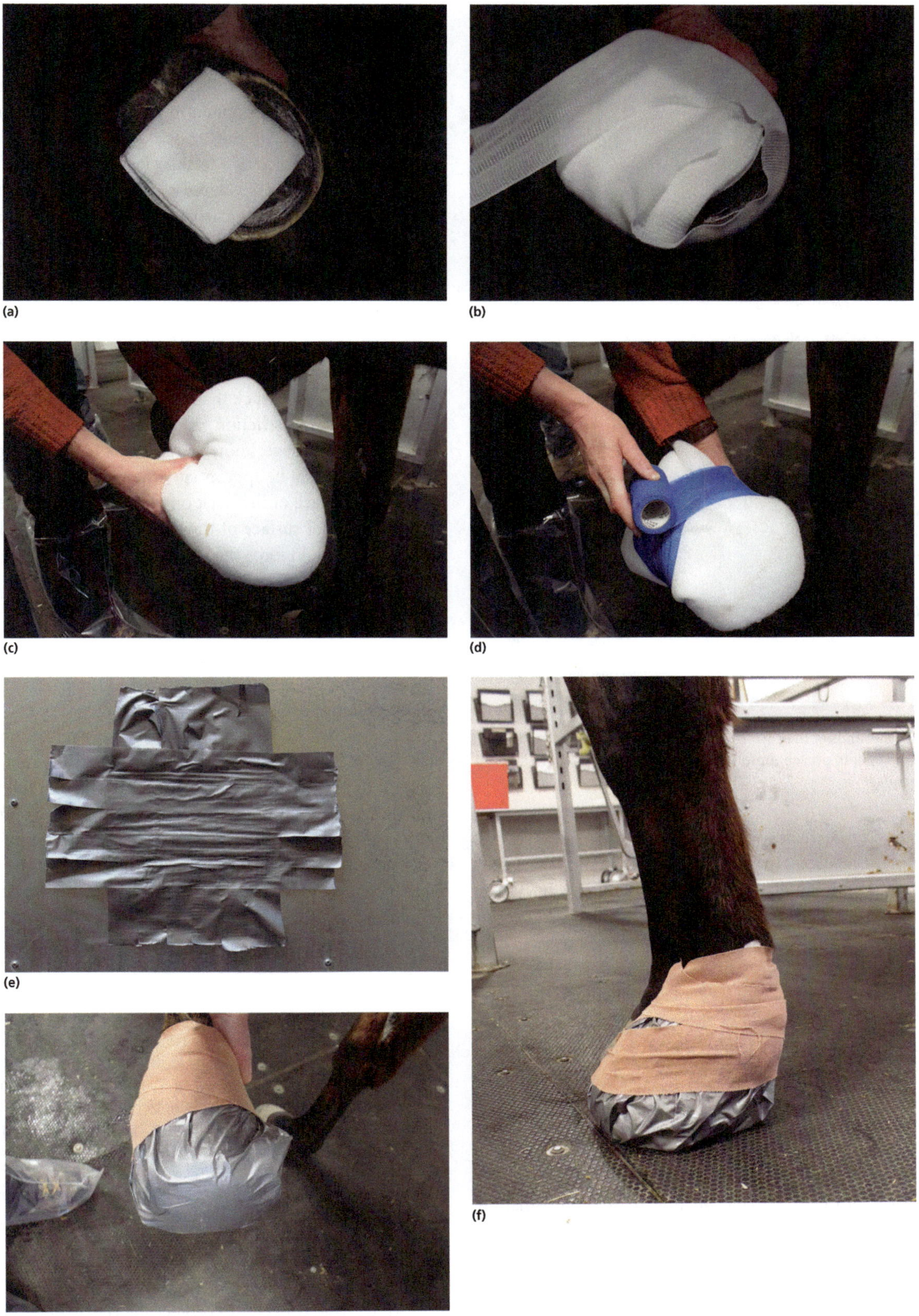

Figure 7.1 **(a)** A penetrating injury to the sole of the foot has been cleaned, irrigated, and covered with sterile gauze. **(b)** Conforming gauze (Kling™ or Conform) can be used to hold the primary layer in place on the bottom of the foot. **(c)** A cotton pad is folded into a square and then placed over the sole of the foot with the edges drawn up and over the foot and coronary band. **(d)** Elastic, self-adhesive material (Vetrap™) is used as a tertiary layer to hold the cotton in place. **(e)** Duct tape is used to make a patch in a square or a cross configuration to be placed on the bottom of the foot. It is best to do this on a clean metal surface and not a painted wall as the paint may peel off when the patch of duct tape is removed. This patch is centered over the sole of the foot with the edges coming up around the sides of the foot bandage. **(f)** To complete the foot bandage, elastic adhesive tape is applied (without tension) over the skin to prevent bedding or dirt from entering between the bandage and the skin/hoof. The final bandage provides some padding to the injured foot but also absorbs drainage and protects from further contamination. **(g)** A view of the bottom of the foot with the bandage in place. The horse should be kept in a clean and dry environment to complement the action of the protective, waterproof duct tape.

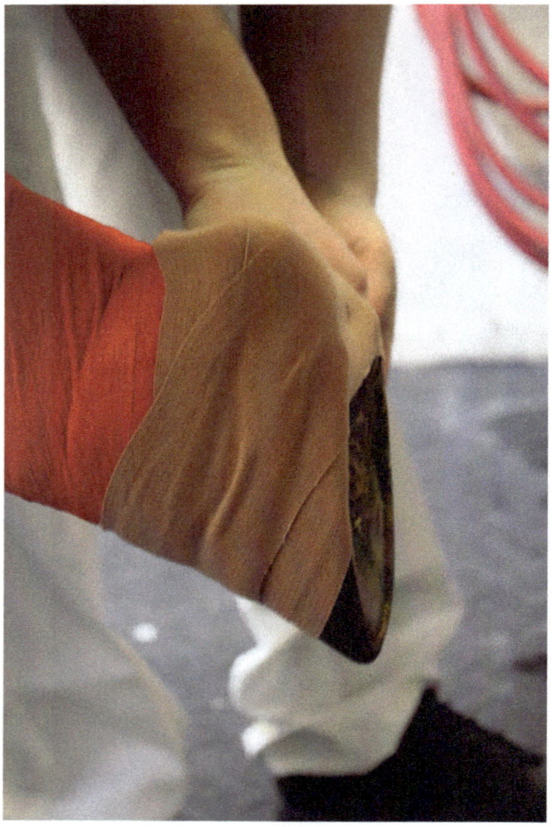

Figure 7.2 For wounds of the pastern region it is preferable to attach the bandage to the hoof to prevent upwards migration of foreign material under the bandage.

point of the hock (calcaneal tuberosity) not only relieves pressure but is also useful in preventing bandage slippage. When the tertiary layer is applied over the point of the hock, less tension should be exerted to allow unrestricted flexion of the hock. Moreover, elastic adhesive tape must be used to secure the bandage to the skin at its proximal and distal limits. Figure 7.5 shows the progression of bandage placement over the hock. Because the bandage may split over the point of the hock when the horse flexes its limb, a strip of elastic tape may be placed along the plantar surface, over the tertiary layer of the bandage, to reinforce that area without increasing pressure on the underlying skin (Figure 7.6). Placing a distal limb bandage after applying a tarsal or carpal bandage is often helpful to prevent the latter from slipping distally (Figure 7.7). Many horse owners find the hock difficult to bandage due to its conformation. Consequently, they may use various readily available materials, such as pantyhose or Velcro strips, to create an innovative bandage. The veterinarian must remain in contact with the owner and frequently verify that all is well with the horse and its bandage to ensure against constriction or rubbing.

Restricting carpal flexion by applying a full-limb bandage may be beneficial if the wound is located on the dorsal surface of the carpus. To apply a full-limb bandage, cotton padding is used to cover the entire limb (from the coronary band or fetlock to the proximal radius) once the dressing has been secured over the wound. The separate rolls of cotton used to span the entire distance should be overlapped to avoid the formation of a gap between two rolls. An elastic, self-adhesive material, such as Vetrap™ is then applied as a tertiary layer in the same fashion as for a distal limb bandage, and a relieving incision is made over the area of the accessory carpal bone. It may be easier to first apply all layers of the distal limb bandage and then add the proximal bandage, overlapping slightly at the proximal cannon bone; this avoids the need to hold the full length of cotton padding in place while applying the tertiary layer of Vetrap™. A full-limb bandage can be applied in similar fashion to the hindlimb; in that case, the tertiary layer must be applied with less tension over the point of the hock than over the rest of the limb.

When greater restriction of flexion is desired, a compact, multi-layered bandage, known as a Robert Jones bandage, can be applied. This might be appropriate when managing a wound over the plantar surface of the hock or a transversely oriented wound across the dorsal surface of the carpus; in both these instances, joint flexion would force the wound edges apart. In the case of a Robert Jones bandage, multiple secondary and tertiary layers are applied consecutively to the limb to build a uniformly compact bandage encompassing the entire limb. This thicker bandage will limit movement more than would a simple bandage.

Alternatively, a splint can be added to the palmar surface of a conventional forelimb full-limb bandage, or a full-limb cast can be used. In the case of a wound to the hindlimb, a splint made from cast material can be applied dorsally to a full-limb bandage to partially immobilize the hindlimb or a full-limb cast can be applied to support the repair of a large wound on the plantar surface of the metatarsus. The benefits provided by a full-limb cast should be carefully weighed against the potential negative consequences (discussed in the following section on splints and casts).

Tips

- Slice a rectal sleeve lengthwise and attach it as a "rain jacket" over the plantar surface of a hindlimb bandage (Figure 7.8). This is particularly useful for horses with loose manure or for mares suffering from urinary incontinence. The plastic sleeve must not completely encircle the limb because this would render the bandage occlusive and increase the likelihood of tissue maceration. A plastic rectal sleeve can also be applied to the medial surface of forelimb bandages if the horse rubs its forelimbs together.
- Smear a mixture of hot pepper and petroleum jelly over the exterior of a bandage to dissuade the horse from nibbling it.

Head bandages

A head bandage is useful to protect the repair of a head wound or a wound left open to heal by second intention, and to exert a small amount of pressure that might control the development of subcutaneous emphysema in the case of sinus penetration. Special attention to positioning and maintaining a head bandage is required to avoid ocular trauma or occlusion of the nostrils.

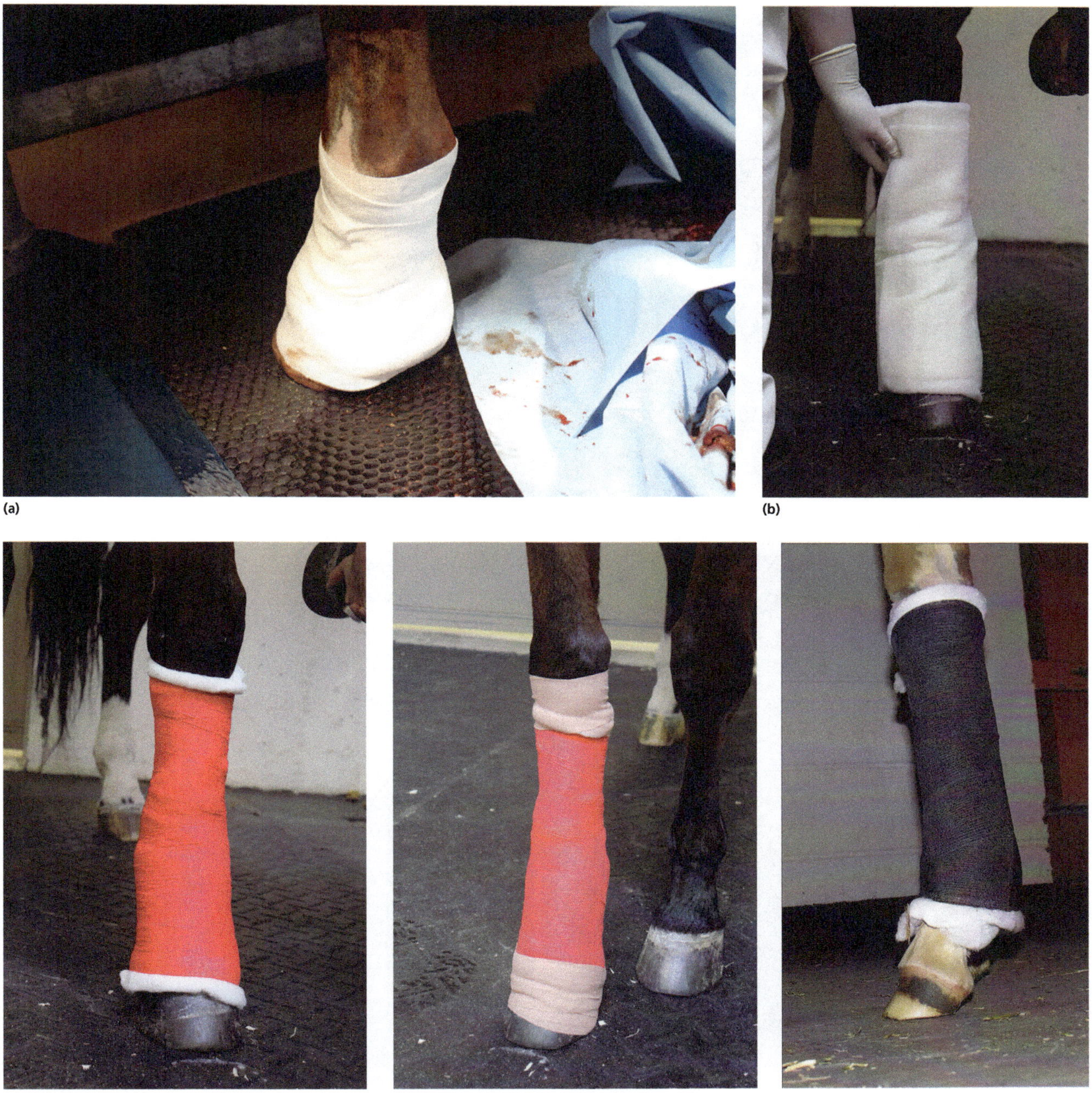

(a) (b) (c) (d) (e)

Figure 7.3 (**a**) The first step in creating a distal limb bandage is to place a dressing on the wound or suture line. This is held in place with some soft roll gauze, such as Conform. (**b**) Cotton padding is used as the secondary layer of a distal limb bandage. It must extend distally past the coronary band; it is important to avoid finishing the bandage directly over the coronary band where it may rub and cause irritation. The cotton layer protects the limb and may absorb excess exudate. (**c**) The tertiary layer, consisting of elastic, self-adhesive material, is applied using even pressure. It must cover the underlying layer of cotton except for a small border both proximally and distally, in an effort to avoid placing undue pressure on uncovered skin. (**d**) Elastic, adhesive tape is then applied, without tension, both proximally and distally to cover the extremities of the bandage and prevent bedding or dirt from migrating under the bandage. (**e**) This distal limb bandage is used to cover a wound over the cannon bone; consequently, it need not be attached to the hoof. The distal extremity rests a few centimeters above the coronary band thus sparing it from rubbing and irritation.

A simple head bandage consists of an appropriate dressing, followed by the placement of a mesh stockinette (Figure 7.9a) over the head, with holes cut out for ears and eyes (Figure 7.9b). The extremities of the stockinette can be attached to the skin with an elastic adhesive tape such as Elastikon®, placed without tension, half on the stockinette and half on the adjacent skin (Figure 7.9c). An extra length of elastic adhesive tape may span the stockinette where it covers the dressing, in an effort to secure the dressing to the surface of the wound and prevent slippage under the stockinette (Figure 7.9d). Additionally, gauze may be slipped under the

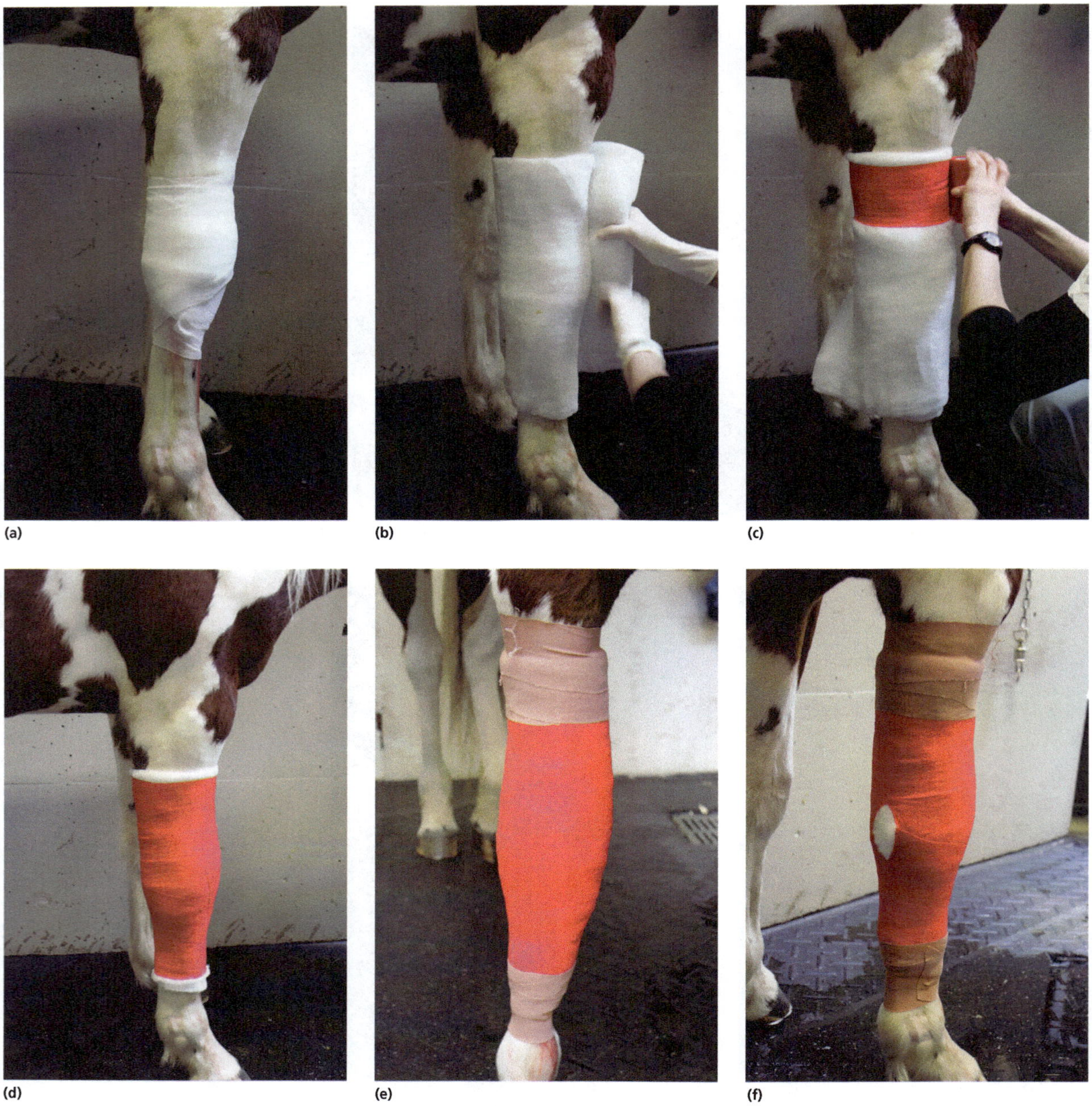

Figure 7.4 **(a)** The first step in creating a carpal bandage is to place an appropriate dressing on the wound or suture line. This is gently held in place with conforming gauze that can be placed in a figure-of-eight pattern around the carpus. **(b)** The secondary layer of cotton padding is applied as for a distal limb bandage, taking care to avoid bunching. **(c)** The tertiary layer is applied using even tension and overlapping by 50% the width of each turn of the elastic, self-adhesive material. **(d)** The bandage with the tertiary layer in place; note the snug fit required to avoid bandage slippage and bunching that would be detrimental to both the wound and the skin of the limb. **(e)** The top and bottom of the bandage can be attached to the skin using elastic, adhesive tape, applied without tension. Placement of a stall bandage distally would eliminate the need for the lowermost band of tape and may help prevent distal slippage of the carpal bandage. **(f)** To prevent the development of a pressure sore over the protuberance of the accessory carpal bone, a releasing incision is made in the bandage directly overlying this site. This protuberance can be palpated through the bandage.

stockinette over the dressing to exert gentle pressure on the wound, if required. The elastic adhesive tape can be wrapped in a figure-of-eight pattern between the eyes and around the mandible, rostral to the eyes, and then behind the ears and under the mandible, if more pressure is required to prevent emphysema or swelling from developing (Figure 7.9e). This is useful for wounds involving the sinuses. Care should be taken to avoid wrapping too tightly around the rostral extent of the bandage, which might prevent the mouth from opening, or around the throatlatch region, which could hinder swallowing or breathing. A finger should slide easily between the bandage and the skin of the throatlatch. Following enucleation, the figure-of-eight pattern with one length of the elastic adhesive tape passing over the incision is used to apply gentle pressure to the wound and to prevent the horse from rubbing the sutures. This figure-of-eight bandage is also used following repair of fractured frontal bones.

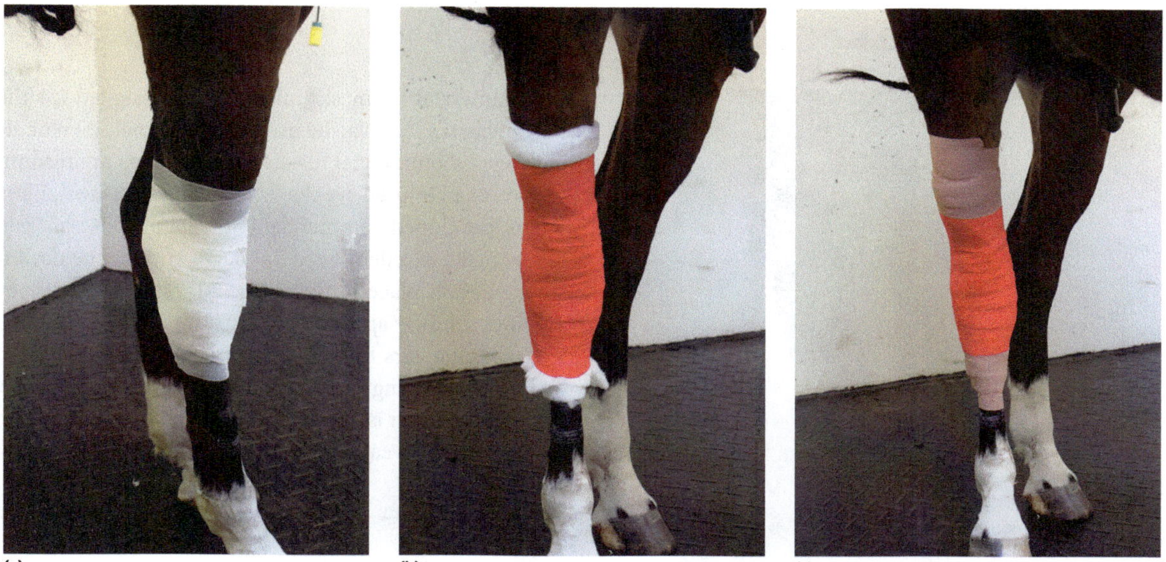

(a) (b) (c)

Figure 7.5 **(a)** A hock bandage is fashioned similarly to a carpal bandage. The selected dressing is applied to the wound and held in place using conforming gauze that is applied, in a figure-of-eight pattern, above and below the point of the hock. **(b)** The secondary layer is placed by conforming the cotton pad around the tibia and then slightly bunching it around the cannon bone when the tertiary layer is applied. As is the case with a forelimb bandage, the tertiary layer must be applied using snug, even tension and making sure to leave some cotton distally and proximally so as to avoid exerting pressure on unprotected skin. Moreover, less tension must be used when running over the point of the hock, to allow this joint to flex in spite of the bandage. **(c)** The proximal and distal extremities of the bandage can be sealed with loose turns of elastic, adhesive tape. More can be used proximally to help prevent distal slippage of the bandage.

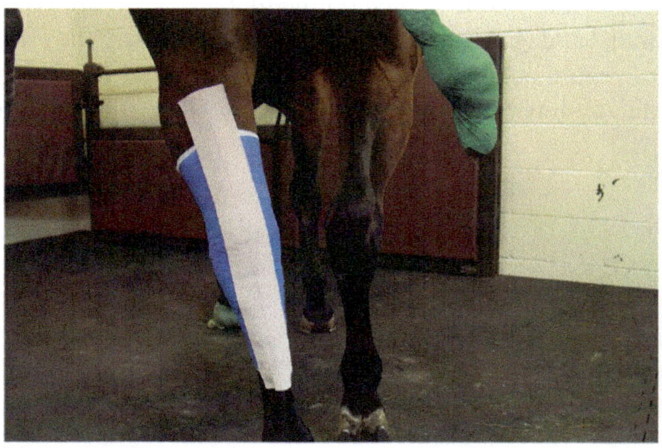

(a)

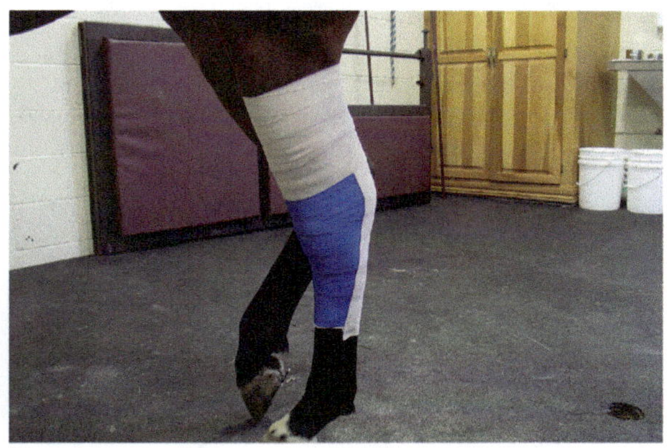

(b)

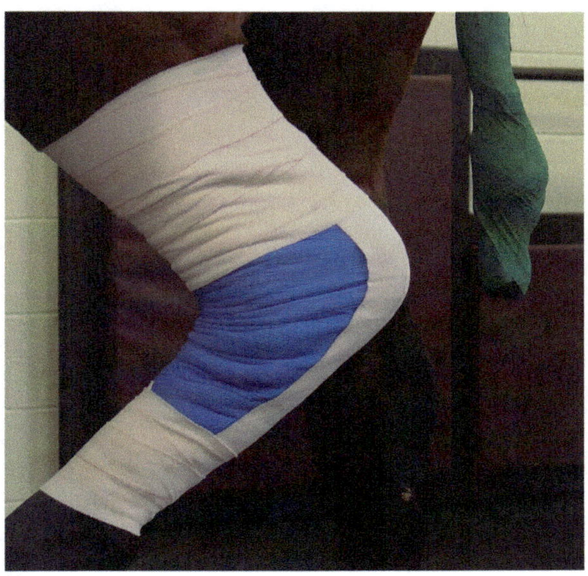

(c)

Figure 7.6 **(a)** Alternative hock bandage. A strip of elastic adhesive tape (e.g. Elastikon®) is placed longitudinally over the plantar surface of the hock region. **(b)** The strip of Elastikon® is held in place at its proximal limit by circumferential rolls of the same tape. **(c)** Bandage complete; both the proximal and distal limits of the strip of Elastikon® are secured with the same tape. The strip of Elastikon® helps limit disruption of the bandage during hock flexion. Courtesy of Dr. D. Peters.

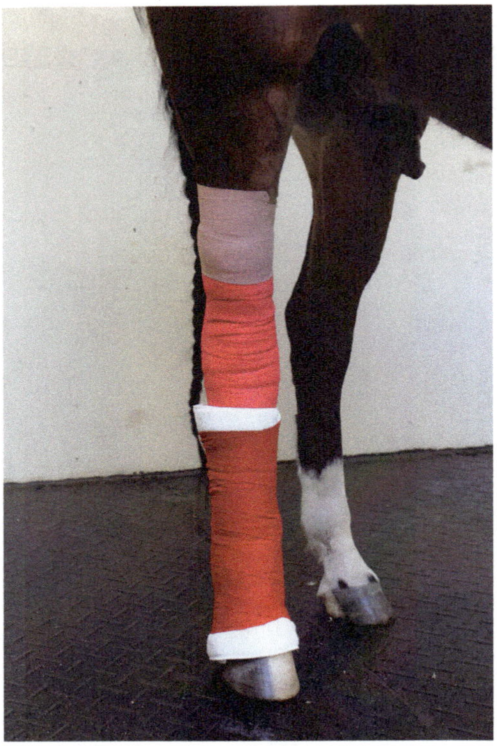

Figure 7.7 The addition of a distal limb bandage may help hold the carpal or tarsal bandage in place. Moreover, in the acute phase of wound healing, this bandage may aid in controlling the development of edema distal to the wound.

Commercial fly masks and helmets designed for the transport of horses may also be used either on their own or alongside bandages. Commercial masks with eye cups are recommended to protect an injured eye that is receiving treatment. Elastic head wraps, developed commercially for the purpose of "calming" a horse, make excellent head bandages and can be used over the stockinette in place of the elastic adhesive tape, although they are not useful for applying pressure, if that is required.

Bandaging ears that have been lacerated or partially amputated is challenging; care should be taken to avoid wrapping too tightly (the reader is referred to Chapter 11 for more information on bandaging an ear).

> **Tip**
>
> - A successful method of creating an ear bandage is to place a roll of conforming gauze in the pinna and to wrap around the ear with an elastic adhesive tape that is then looped around the mandible to stabilize the bandage.

Thoracic and abdominal bandages

When a wound is located on the thoracic or on the abdominal wall, bandaging is sometimes required to prevent the formation of ventral edema or the accumulation of fluid in dead spaces, due to gravity. Conversely, bandaging is usually not indicated

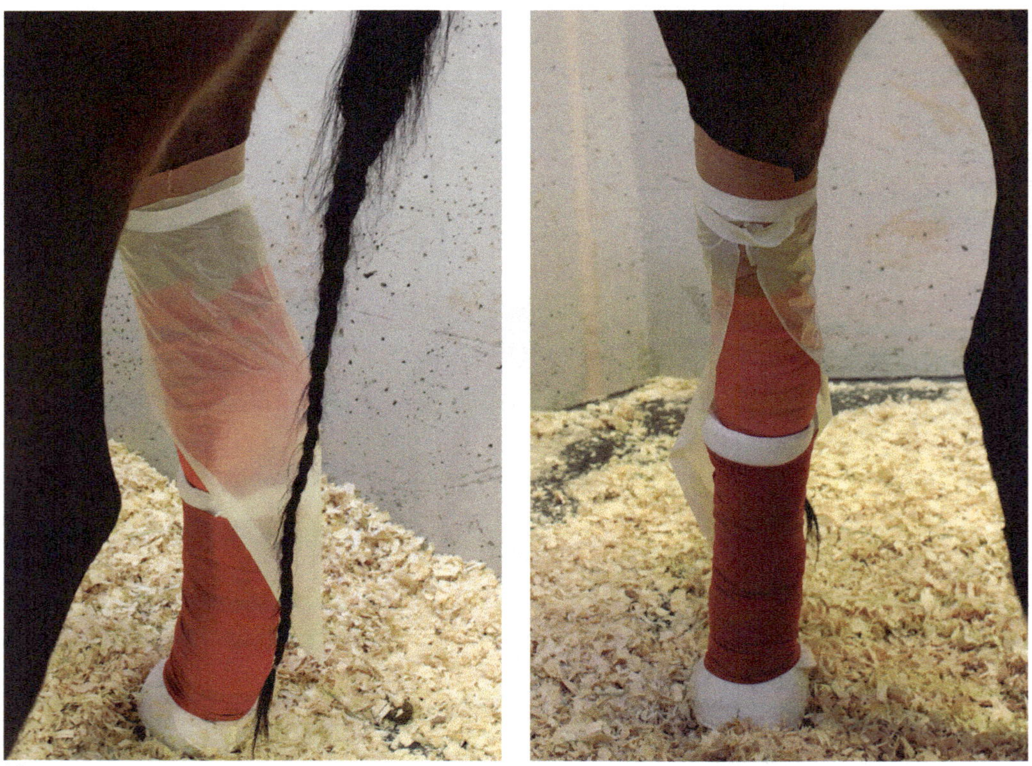

(a) (b)

Figure 7.8 **(a)** A rectal sleeve can be sliced lengthwise and attached over the plantar surface of the bandage. This should help protect it from becoming wet and may also reduce the ability of the horse to rub the two limbs together in an effort to dislodge the bandage. **(b)** Cranial view of the rectal sleeve acting as a "rain jacket."

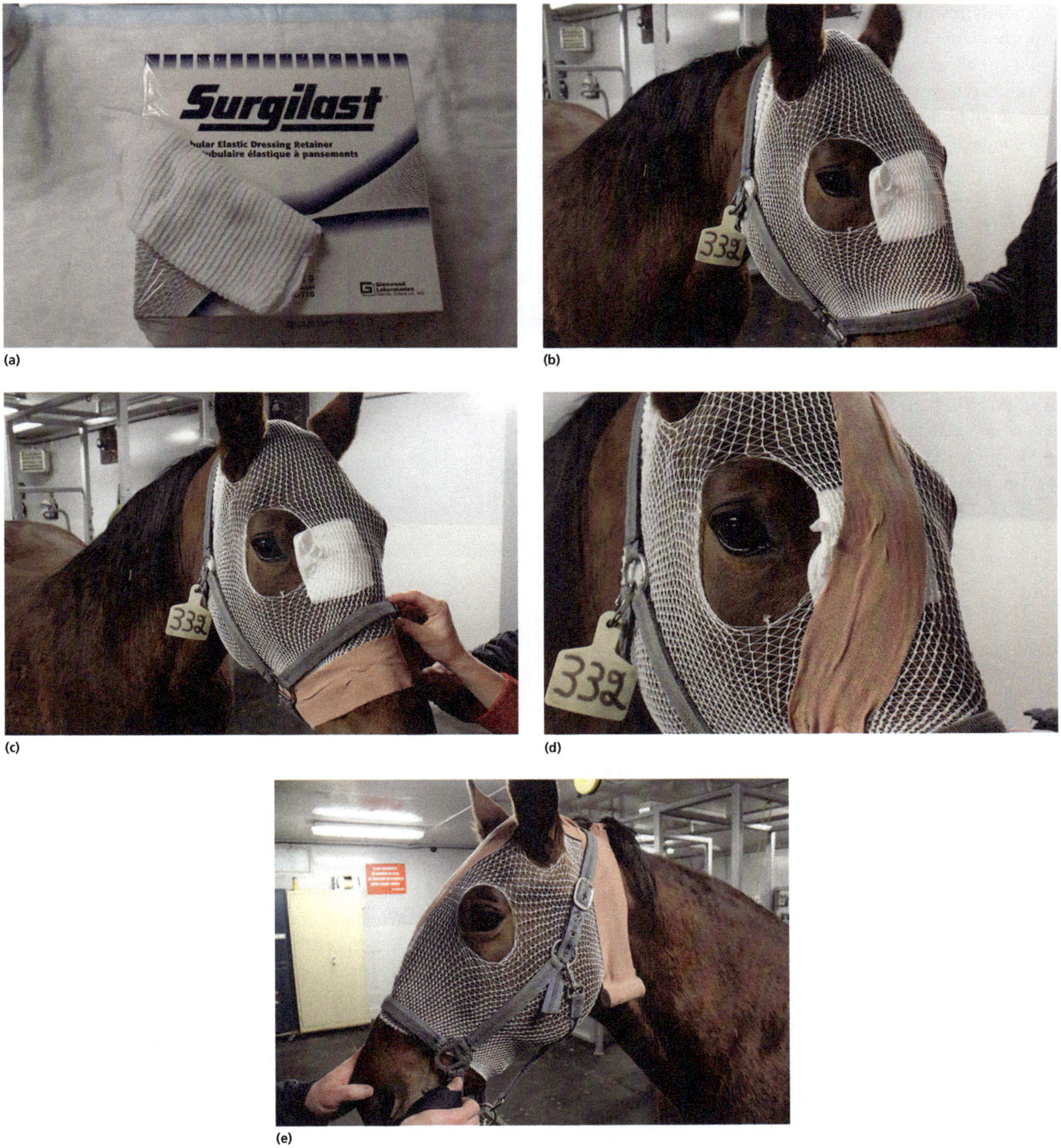

Figure 7.9 **(a)** Mesh stockinette is very useful when making a head bandage, due to its natural elasticity and the ease with which it can be torn to form eye and ear holes. **(b)** The mesh stockinette is drawn up over the head, tearing or cutting generous holes for the eyes and ears. Care must be taken to avoid occluding the nostrils or rubbing the eyes. **(c)** The two extremities of the mesh have a tendency to roll up thus uncovering the wound or interfering with the eyes. An elastic, adhesive tape (such as Elastikon®) can be applied, with light tension, to fix the two extremities to the skin. **(d)** The elastic, adhesive tape can be placed over the frontal sinus area and then looped around the face, rostrally, and behind the ears, caudally. The loops must be placed without tension but the tape may exert a small amount of compression on the dressing over the wound. **(e)** Elastic, adhesive tape has been looped behind the ears. Where the bandage passes under the throatlatch area, care must be taken to ensure it is not too tight; a finger should be easily inserted between the bandage and the underlying skin.

for wounds involving the axillary or inguinal areas. In these cases, the wound opening should remain as unobstructed as possible to allow ventral drainage and to avoid the trapping of air within the wound and surrounding subcutaneous tissues, which could lead to the development of emphysema.

To bandage a wound in the thoracic or abdominal area, the dressing is placed against the wound and overlaid by a secondary layer of cotton padding. The tertiary layer is then applied to hold everything in place and to mildly compress the wound. The best way to hold the bandage in place is to wrap the tertiary layer, often an elastic adhesive tape such as Elastikon®, around the circumference of the trunk. To ensure appropriate tension without restricting breathing, there should be room for a finger to slide easily under the bandage. Body bandages require a large amount of material and, consequently, they can be costly. An alternative to the classical tertiary layer is an adaptable commercial abdominal bandage (Figure 7.10). Because it can be laundered, it is especially useful for exudative wounds that require frequent bandage changes.

Tip

- Prior to shipping a horse with a penetrating thoracic injury to a referral hospital, plastic food wrap/cling film can be wrapped around the thorax after the wound has been dressed, and held in place with elastic adhesive tape. This may help prevent the development of a pneumothorax during transport.

Tie-over (stent) bandages

Some wounds that have either been sutured or left to heal by second intention might benefit from added protection but are located in an area that is difficult to bandage. Examples are incisions or wounds over the point of the elbow, ventral abdominal incisions after colic surgery or herniorrhaphy, wounds at the proximal extent of the fore- or hindlimb, and wounds over

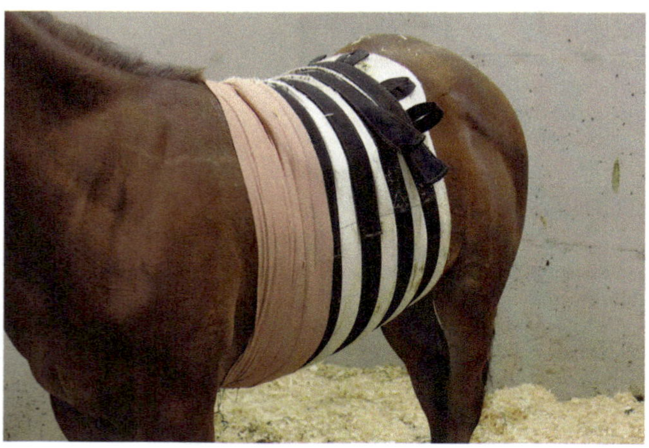

Figure 7.10 A commercial abdominal bandage has been placed over the primary and secondary layers of a bandage. Elastic, adhesive tape is used cranially to attach the bandage to the skin and thereby prevent caudal slippage.

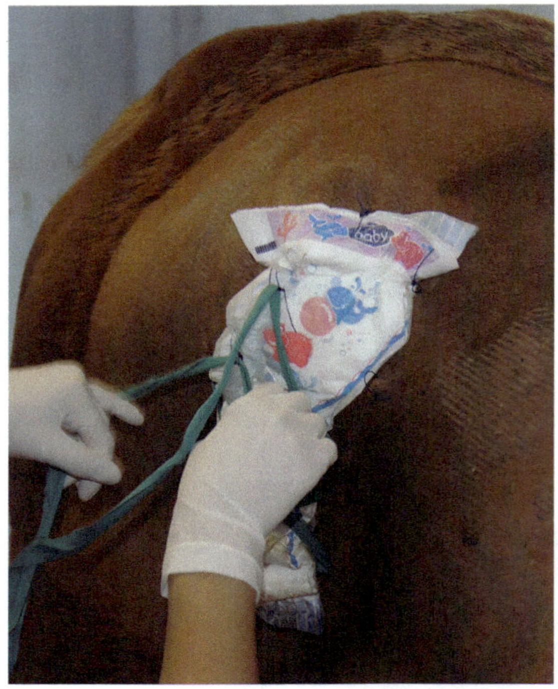

Figure 7.11 A stent bandage, made from a baby diaper, has been sutured over a wound dressing to treat a chronic abscess, which developed over the *tuber coxae* following a fracture leading to bony sequestration. Courtesy of Dr. O.M. Lepage.

the *tuber coxae*. A stent or "tie-over" bandage is fashioned by placing loops of a heavy non-absorbable suture (size 1 or 2) through the healthy skin on either side of the wound, at regular intervals (~3 cm apart). A dressing is then placed over the wound and the secondary layer might consist of a folded surgical towel, cotton padding or baby diaper. This bandage is held in place by lacing umbilical tape or string through the previously placed suture loops rather than by using a classical tertiary layer (Figure 7.11). When the general guidelines for bandage care are followed, such as keeping the bandage clean and dry, the stent is a useful protective measure for wounds located in areas difficult to bandage. For example, the use of stent bandages following exploratory celiotomy for colic was shown, in a retrospective study, to reduce the likelihood of incisional infection.[10]

Tips

- Use large, colored suture material to create the loops on either side of the wound to facilitate recognition for both placement of the laced umbilical tape (possibly under suboptimal lighting conditions) and to distinguish from incisional sutures, for accurate removal.
- Leave a fairly large space within the suture loops to facilitate threading the umbilical tape or string through them.

Special considerations of bandages for foals

Although the general bandaging techniques for foals resemble those described for adult horses, one should bear in mind the

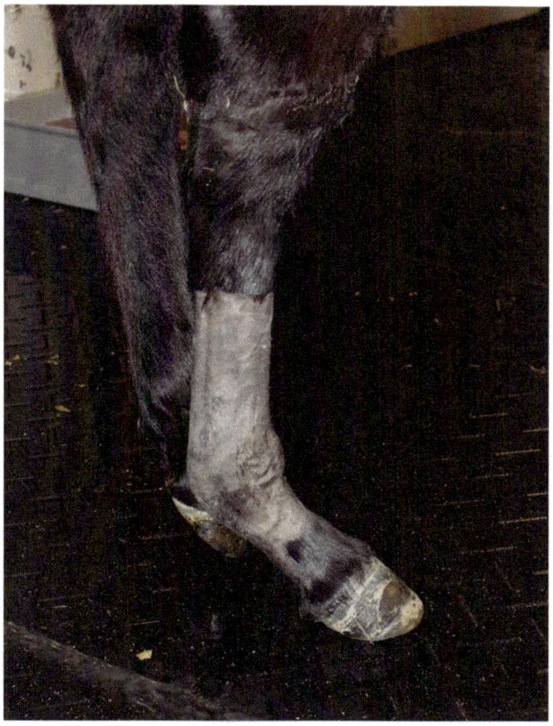

Figure 7.12 A dropped fetlock is a sign of flexor tendon laxity in this foal. It developed in response to a 2-week period of distal limb bandaging to treat a skin laceration over the medial metacarpal area. A gradual increase in exercise should help resolve the laxity; a special orthopedic shoe with a heel extension may also be required.

fragility and thinness of the skin and the relative paucity of soft-tissue coverage of deeper structures on the distal aspect of the limbs of foals. Consequently, in a foal, care should be taken to reduce the amount of pressure exerted by the tertiary layer over the cotton padding, so as not to interfere with blood supply to the skin of the limb. After a bandage has been applied to the distal aspect of the limb, the coronary band and pastern should be palpated regularly, by inserting a finger under the bandage, to monitor for swelling or a decrease in skin temperature, both of which result from excessive pressure caused by the bandaging. Moreover, bandages in foals should be changed at least once daily. Bandages applied to the limbs of neonatal foals will quickly induce laxity of the soft tissues; this may be desirable for the management of flexural deformities but not for regular wound management (Figure 7.12). Omitting the thick secondary layer may help prevent this particular complication (but will increase the likelihood of exerting undue pressure on soft tissues).

Complications relating to the use of bandages

The overall benefits of using bandages in the management of wounds in horses surpass any negative effects. Nevertheless, when bandages are incorrectly applied they may impede healing or be deleterious to the animal's health. This is particularly true of bandages used to manage wounds on the limb. If the pressure exerted by the tertiary layer is unevenly distributed or if the secondary layer slips or bunches up, zones of pressure will develop underneath. This may lead to swelling of the skin and subcutaneous tissues. Swelling may interfere with circulation and cause focal inflammation within the skin and deeper structures, in particular the flexor tendons. Swelling of the tendons, as a result of the pressure exerted by bandages, is commonly referred to as a "bandage-bow." Focal swellings are generally self-limiting and can be treated symptomatically with cold water hosing and the administration of systemic anti-inflammatory drugs if they cause lameness. If the tendon appears swollen, the extent of injury should be evaluated using ultrasound in order to determine the best management approach, which may include rest and rehabilitation.

When bandages are placed over bony prominences, such as the accessory carpal bone or the point of the hock, the pressure normally used to apply a bandage can create a pressure point given the relative absence of soft-tissue coverage in these areas. If bandaging is maintained for a prolonged period, a sore may develop as a result of pressure necrosis of the skin overlying the prominence. As a means to prevent this complication, special care should be taken when applying a bandage over bony prominences. Specifically, as outlined in the section on carpal and tarsal bandages, the tension of the tertiary layer should be diminished when passing over the bony prominence (hock) or, alternatively, a small releasing incision should be made (over the area of the accessory carpal bone). In the absence of skin necrosis, prolonged pressure exerted by a bandage can nevertheless cause bleaching of the hair, which may be perceived by some owners as a cosmetic blemish. If prolonged periods of bandaging are required for wound management, the appearance of the skin under the bandage should be carefully inspected at each bandage change and the owner warned of the possibility of the hair turning white.

If a wound is producing copious discharge, the bandage should be changed frequently to avoid skin maceration. Most importantly, an appropriate dressing, capable of managing high volumes of exudate, must be selected (the reader is referred to Chapter 6 for more information on wound dressings). Alternatively, negative-pressure wound therapy might be used (the reader is referred to Chapter 22 for more information on NPWT).

Splints and casts

In some cases it may be helpful to restrict movement of a wounded limb to prevent disruption of the healing process. This can be done by providing greater rigidity in the form of either a splint or a cast. Splints can be applied with relative ease, and removed and reapplied repeatedly, allowing for regular inspection of the injured site. Moreover, because they are non-circumferential, splints allow for natural swelling that occurs during the initial inflammatory phase following injury and are thus less likely to cause pressure-related complications. However, splints commonly shift and become displaced, leading to potentially negative consequences. Casts provide more rigidity than do splints but may lead to complications such as the development of pressure sores and orthopedic damage due to immobilization of the joints and bones. Recently, bandage casts (wherein a cast is applied over a thin bandage) were shown to have a lower risk of inducing the development of pressure sores and may thus be a better choice than more rigid traditional casts, used for orthopedic conditions, for horses requiring immobilization to assist wound healing.[11] The choice between a bandage, a splint, a bandage cast, and a cast depends on many variables and must be made on a case-by-case basis. Some variables to consider include the patient's behavior/compliance, the level and quality of monitoring present at the farm, the experience of the personnel at the farm, as well as the benefits to the wound healing vs. the potential negative effects.

Splints

Materials

Splints may be constructed from several readily available materials including polyvinyl chloride (PVC) pipe or cast material (Table 7.2). Figure 7.13 shows common materials that may be used to create a splint. Splints are applied over a standard bandage and attached to it using duct tape (3M, St Paul, MN, USA) or white tape (3M). The white tape is preferred because its porosity allows for evaporation of humidity from the bandage, thus decreasing the likelihood of maceration at the underlying wound. The splint can also be attached with elastic, adhesive tape. A splint must be closely monitored and reset immediately if it has shifted, to avoid additional injury to the limb; of course it must also be reset whenever the underlying bandage is changed.

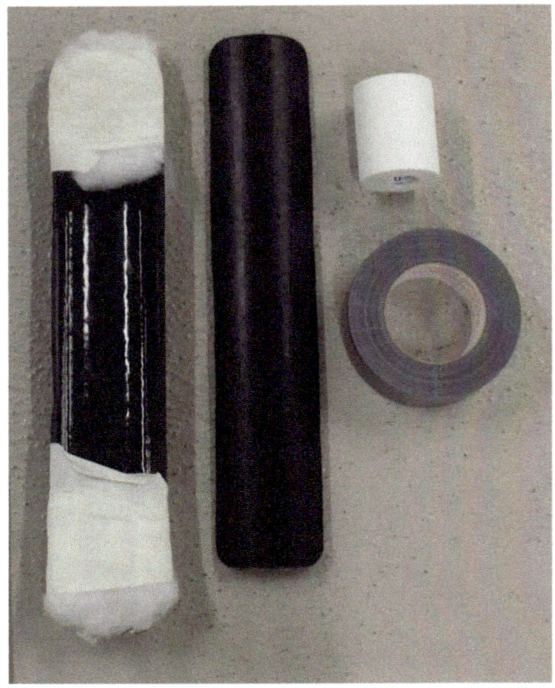

Figure 7.13 Examples of materials commonly used to build a splint: PVC pipe (that can be padded at both ends), duct tape, and white tape. The duct tape may be used temporarily (for transportation to a referral center) but the permeable white tape is preferred for chronic use as it is less likely to cause sweating under the bandage and subsequent skin maceration. Cast material can also be used to form a splint.

Table 7.2 Examples of common casting materials and how they are used in the making of a cast. Note that the time to initially dry (set) and then harden to full strength (cure) depends on the temperature of the water in which the cast material is soaked: aim for room-temperature water.

Cast material	Use	Company
Felt	At the top of the cast, or can be used to form donuts around bony protuberances	Any craft store or orthopedic felt from medical suppliers
Synthetic cast stockinette	Over dressing, beneath cast padding	3M, St Paul, MN, USA
Delta-Dry stockinette	Over dressing, beneath cast padding	BSN Medical, Hamburg, Germany
Delta-Dry cast padding	Padding that is placed over the stockinette to protect the soft tissues	BSN Medical
Vetcast Plus casting tape	Various widths of fiberglass cast material (sets in ~5 mins, supports weight bearing in 20 mins)	3M
Delta-Lite Plus casting tape	Various widths of fiberglass cast material (sets in 7 mins, supports weight bearing in 20 mins)	BSN Medical
Duct tape	Under the foot to prevent strike-through	3M
Soft-Ride boot	Velcro strap boot placed on the opposite limb to match the length of the cast limb	Soft-Ride Inc, Vermilion, OH, USA

Polyvinyl chloride pipe

Splints constructed of PVC pipe often shift around the limb when applied over a bandage. For this reason, it is helpful to secure the conforming gauze (first portion of the secondary layer of the bandage) with an elastic, adhesive tape (e.g., Elastikon®) prior to applying the rest of the secondary layer, consisting of cotton padding. This ensures better adhesion between the components of the secondary layer of the bandage, thereby preventing a cleavage plane that could facilitate displacement of the overlying splint. The cotton padding is secured to the limb with conforming gauze and elastic, self-adhesive material. Additional cotton padding is usually applied to the proximal and distal edges of the splint, before it is affixed to the bandage, to protect the limb from the PVC pipe splint.

PVC pipe, commonly 8 cm in diameter, is cut in thirds or halves, longitudinally, and the sharp edges are smoothed while the ends are rounded. For heavier horses (i.e. draft breeds or Warmbloods), two pieces of PVC pipe can be taped together one on top of the other to increase the strength of the splint, thereby preventing it from bending. PVC pipe can be heated and slightly bent according to the angulation of the limb to which it will be applied.

Cast material

The extent to which PVC piping may be intentionally bent and shaped to the limb is limited. For this reason, cast material is more often used to construct a full-limb splint for a wound on the hindlimb where prevention of hock flexion would be beneficial to healing.

A splint can be made from cast material by unrolling four to five rolls of 12–15-cm fiberglass cast tape, then folding them to the appropriate length and affixing the resulting "band" to the bandage, longitudinally, over the back of the limb. The technique for making a full, hindlimb splint from fiberglass casting tape is as follows.

1. A full, hindlimb bandage is applied.
2. The area of the bandage corresponding to where the splint is to be affixed is covered with a water-impervious shield (e.g., disposable plastic OB sleeve or plastic food wrap).
3. The first roll of fiberglass cast tape is unrolled on the plantar/caudal surface of the hindlimb to the desired length (the full-limb splint should extend from the distal metatarsus to the mid or proximal crus), then folded back on itself repeatedly with a slight side-to-side overlap (Figure 7.14 shows the folding of cast material but in this particular case, it was for application to the sole of the foot and is thus much shorter than it would be when creating a splint for the full hindlimb).
4. Additional rolls of fiberglass cast tape are then unrolled in a similar fashion over the first roll, until the desired thickness is reached; four to five rolls are commonly required. The rolls are not dipped in water until all the cast material is unrolled to the desired length and thickness.
5. The "band" of cast material is then dipped, as a whole, into water, stripped of excess moisture, and replaced on the caudal surface of the limb. It is manually molded to the limb; rubbing the cast material with a gloved hand, lubricated with water or cream, helps laminate the cast tape layers.

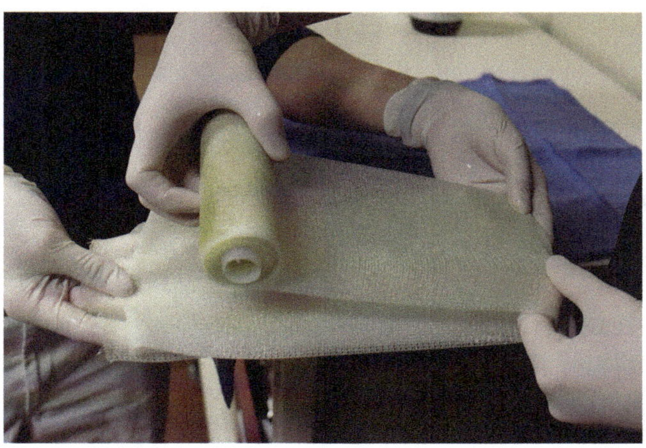

Figure 7.14 A roll of fiberglass cast tape is unrolled then folded back on itself repeatedly with a slight side-to-side overlap. In this particular case, it was for application to the sole of the foot and is thus much shorter than it would be for creating a distal or full-limb splint.

6. The splint is then held in place with conforming gauze while the cast material sets completely (until dry and hard to the touch); this should take 2–3 minutes. Thereafter, the splint is removed by cutting the plastic shield (OB sleeve or plastic food wrap) and the conforming gauze, using scissors.
7. The splint should be allowed to cure (completely harden) for at least 20–30 minutes before affixing it to the bandage on the limb (Figure 7.15).

To construct a bi-valved cast that can be used as a splint, a half-limb or full-limb bandage (not including the foot) is applied, according to the need, as previously described. Several rolls (four to five) of fiberglass cast tape are then applied over the bandage, in a manner similar to the Vetrap™, (each turn overlapping the previous by 50% and using only light tension) to increase its rigidity, thereby immobilizing the area. When the cast material is applied, a small amount of the bandage is left uncovered proximad and distad; this ensures that once it is used as a splint it does not touch unbandaged areas. Once the cast material has cured, usually within 20–30 minutes, it is cut laterally and medially into two longitudinal halves (bi-valved) to allow removal for dressing changes and wound treatment. After re-bandaging the wound, the two half casts are reapplied and secured with elastic, self-adhesive material; alternatively, just the caudal half can be used as a splint.

General considerations

Splints are most commonly used on the palmar or plantar surface of the limb to prevent flexion, when treating wounds over a joint, and to limit movement or to support the limb when a flexor or extensor tendon has been lacerated.

What to do

- Frequently monitor the splint to ensure that it has not slipped; if this occurs, the splint must immediately be repositioned.

What to avoid

- Avoid ending the splint in the middle of a long bone because this may create a fulcrum over which the bone could fracture.

Specific splints

Distal limb splints

A standard bandage is first applied to the limb. When using a straight piece of PVC pipe, cotton should be used to fill the space between the splint and the palmar/plantar surface of the pastern to help further immobilize the fetlock (Figure 7.16a); better yet, the splint can be angled dorsally at the fetlock to conform to the angulation of the limb (Figure 7.16b). The splint is attached to the bandage with white tape, duct tape or elastic adhesive tape (Figure 7.16c,d).

When a bandage cast is made with the intention of splitting it in half to be used as a splint, it can be applied with the horse standing or under general anesthesia. In the standing horse, the

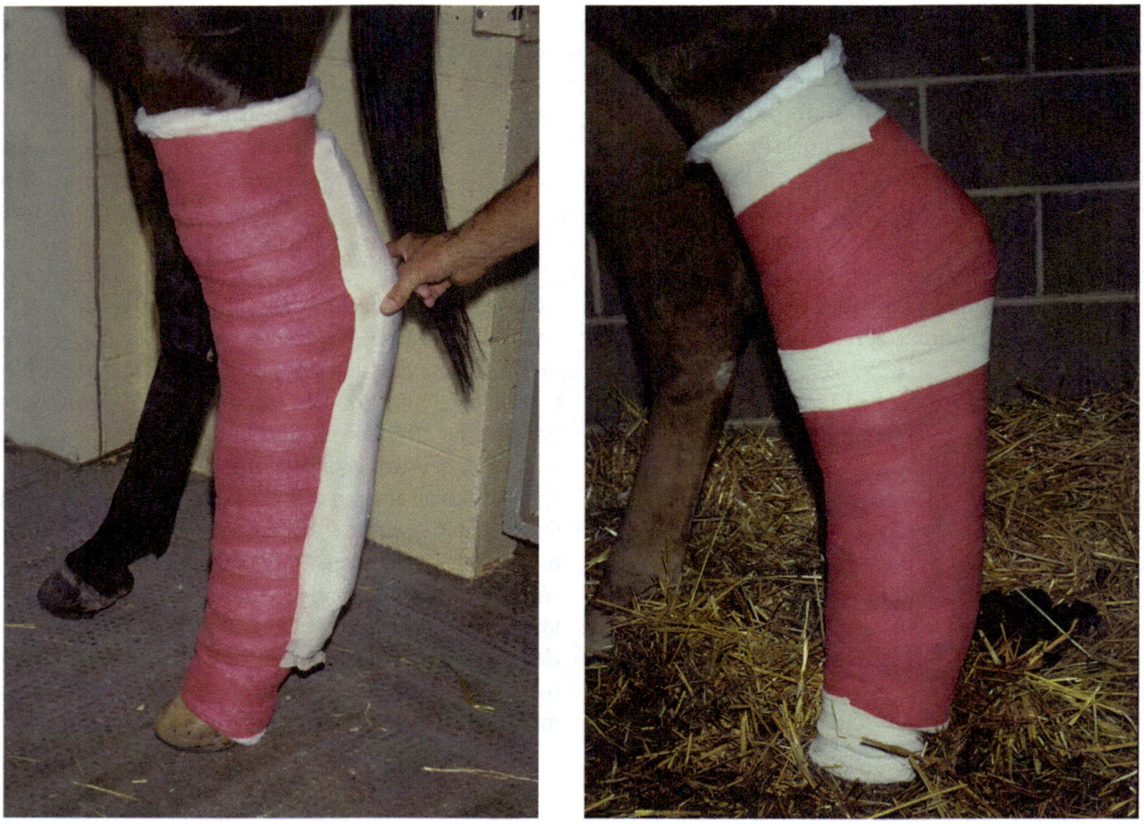

(a) (b)

Figure 7.15 (a) Cast splint for the hindlimb. The cast splint has cured and is ready to be applied to the hindlimb. (b) Vetrap™ is used to affix the cast splint to the bandage. Elastikon® is used to prevent the end of the self-adherent tape from unraveling (center) and to further secure the splint proximally and distally.

cast can be applied over the bandage without including the foot, and then cut into two halves when dry, as previously described.

Full-limb splints

Full-limb splints, in either the fore- or hindlimb, can extend from the ground or from just proximal to the fetlock up to the level of the proximal radius/tibia. A palmar splint can easily be added to a conventional forelimb full-limb bandage, or a full-limb cast can be used. Conversely, in the case of a wound to the hindlimb, a splint made from cast material is easier to conform and apply to the dorsal or the plantar surface of a full-limb bandage.

A PVC splint is relatively easy to place over a full-limb bandage in the forelimb, however the underlying bandage must not be excessively thick because this could predispose the splint to slipping around the limb. Because the splint is applied to the palmar surface of the limb, a releasing incision over the point of the accessory carpal bone fails to relieve pressure in this area; as an alternative, a donut of felt or gauze is positioned to encircle this pressure point prior to applying the cotton padding of the secondary layer of the bandage. The splint is then attached to the bandage with white tape, elastic adhesive tape, or duct tape.

The main advantage of using a full-limb splint is that it can be placed without general anesthesia, as opposed to the placement of a full-limb cast, which usually requires the horse to be recumbent, thus anesthetized.

What to do

- The donut used to protect the accessory carpal bone under a splint should be held in place with self-adhesive material to ensure that it does not migrate distally where it might create a new pressure point.

Casts

Casts may be applied immediately over a thin layer of protection intended to preserve the integrity of underlying soft tissues (traditional cast), or over a bandage (the latter referred to as "bandage–cast"). A traditional cast is most appropriate if, in addition to the skin wound, the horse also suffered significant orthopedic injury, whereas a bandage–cast is more appropriate if the therapeutic aim is to limit movement of the limb in order to support the healing of a more superficial wound. If using a traditional cast, a stockinette, a strip of felt proximally, and a layer of cast padding (either a foam-based or conforming gauze) are placed over the wound dressing prior to applying the cast material. When applying a bandage–cast, an appropriate primary layer (dressing) is first placed over the wound, followed

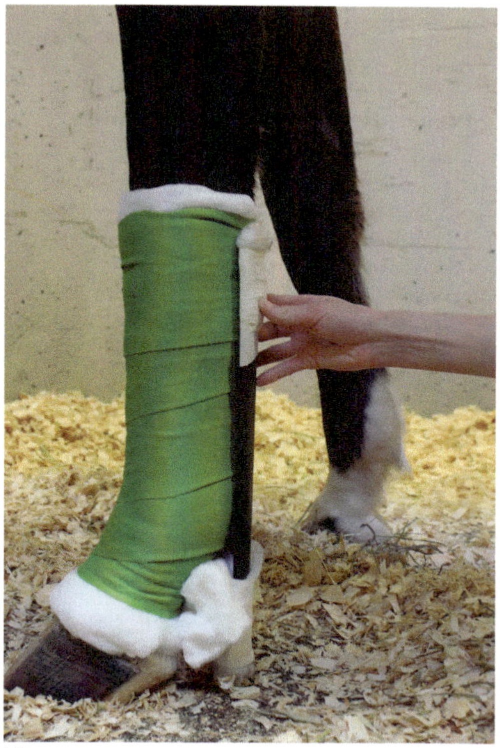

(a)

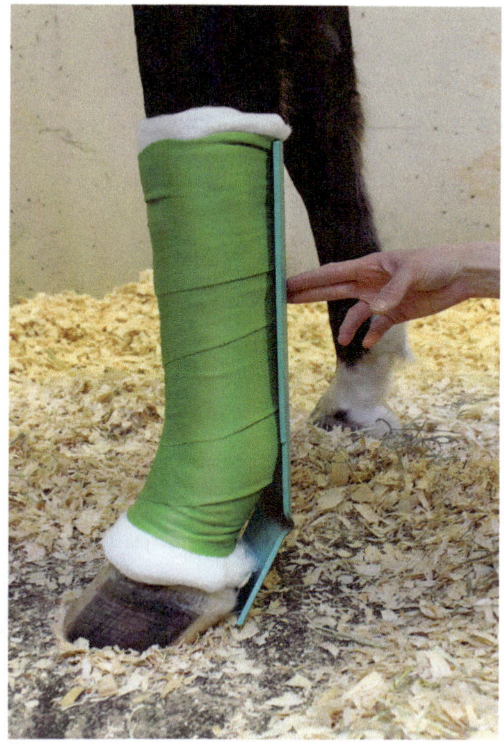

(b)

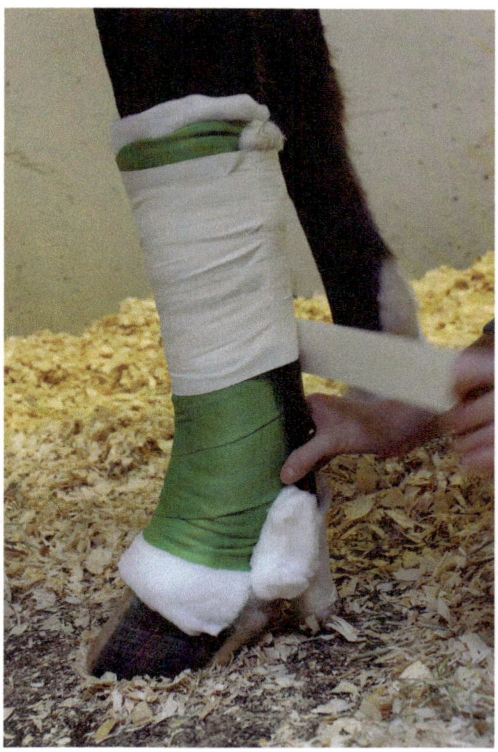

(c)

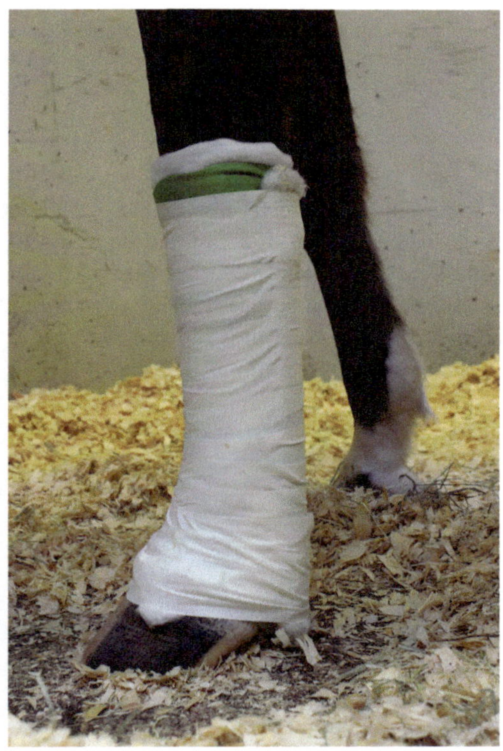

(d)

Figure 7.16 **(a)** A length of PVC pipe is placed as a palmar splint over a distal limb bandage. Splints are used to limit fetlock flexion, thereby reducing the tension sustained by wounds located on the dorsal surface of the metacarpal/tarsal area. The splint must span the distance between the floor and the proximal extremity of the cannon bone. Cotton is placed to fill the void between the splint and the palmar/plantar surface of the pastern, thereby assisting in the restriction of fetlock flexion. **(b)** Alternatively, heat may be used to enable bending of the PVC pipe so that it conforms to the angle of the pastern. **(c)** The splint is attached with white tape, overlapping each turn by 50% and running with even tension up and down in the limb. The tape should be applied only where the underlying area has been generously padded. **(d)** With the splint now in place, it is apparent that the heel bulbs remain exposed; in the long-term, this may favor the development of rub sores. Optimally, the bandage material must cover all the skin underneath the splint.

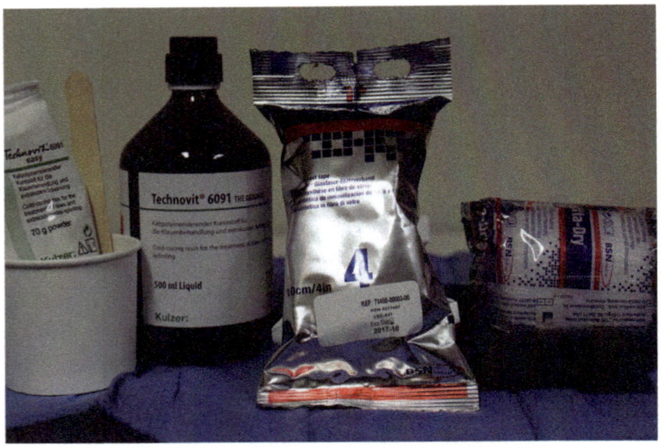

Figure 7.17 The materials required to build and apply a cast: cast padding (Delta dry), fiberglass cast material, and the components to make Technovit® (an acrylic that can be applied to the bottom of the foot to reinforce this area). Thick (black) felt is also required for placing at the top edge of the cast.

by a secondary layer of cotton, a firm tertiary layer and, finally, the cast material itself.

What to avoid

- In the case of a bandage–cast, avoid overly thick or loose bandage material because these tend to bunch or slip beneath the cast, creating areas of increased pressure and thereby predisposing to the development of sores.

Examples of common casting materials (Figure 7.17) and how they are used in the making of a cast can be found in Table 7.2. Fiberglass cast material is preferred over plaster of Paris because the time to set and cure is considerably shorter and the fiberglass material is porous, thus allowing any wound drainage to exit the cast. Box 7.1 outlines the preparation of the patient, the materials and the equipment required for the placement of a cast.

Materials

See Table 7.2.

General considerations – how to apply a cast

If a stockinette is used, it is placed over the wound dressing. A strip of felt is placed circumferentially around the limb at the level the cast is expected to reach at its most proximal extent. The cast padding is then applied, overlapping each layer by 50% and avoiding any wrinkles. The cast material is applied to cover all soft tissues and to reach the middle of the felt strip but not touch the skin proximal to it. With the newer cast paddings such as Delta-Dry cast padding, the stockinette is omitted. The cast material used in adult horses, commonly 10–12 cm wide, is submerged in water, at room temperature, for approximately

Box 7.1 Preparation of the patient, materials and equipment needed for cast application.

Preparation of the foot and limb

- **Foot**
  1. Remove shoe, trim and clean foot
  2. Treat/pack sulcus with gauze soaked in povidone–iodine (Betadine™ Solution, Purdue Frederick Co., Norwalk, CT) if thrush is a problem
- **Limb**
  1. Clip hair around wound, as required for wound management
  2. Irrigate and debride wound
  3. Suture wound if indicated
  4. Apply appropriate dressing and secure it with half roll of sterile conforming gauze

Equipment and materials needed for cast application

- Scissors to clip excessively long hair (e.g., palmar/plantar pastern region)
- Stockinette of 5–10-cm diameter, depending on the size of the limb, rolled to form a double layer
- Cast padding:
  1. Orthopedic felt: 0.5 cm thick, cut to fit the region
  2. White, non-elastic, adhesive tape (2.5 cm) to secure the felt in place
  3. Resin-impregnated cast foam
  4. Gloves
  5. Bucket of warm water
- Cast:
  1. Rubber gloves to apply the cast
  2. Fiberglass cast material needed
     a) Mature horses. In general, the number of rolls depends on the size of the horse:
        i. Phalangeal cast: one roll of 12.5-cm cast tape (bottom of the foot), two to three rolls (hoof and pastern region) of 10-cm cast tape
        ii. Lower limb cast: six to seven rolls, including material for heel wedge
        iii. Full-limb cast: seven to nine rolls of 10–12.5-cm cast tape, including the heel wedge
        iv. Sleeve cast: Four to five rolls of 10-cm or 12.5-cm cast tape
     b) Foals:
        i. Lower limb and sleeve casts: two to three rolls of 7.5–10-cm cast tape
        ii. Full-limb casts: uncommon application for wound management; four rolls of 7.5–10-cm cast tape
     c) Weanlings and yearlings:
        i. Lower limb and sleeve casts: three to four rolls of 7.5–10-cm cast tape
        ii. Full-limb: uncommon; five to six rolls of 7.5–10-cm cast tape
- Cast protection:
  1. Hoof acrylic (e.g., Technovit®)
  2. Tongue depressor
  3. Elastic, self-adhesive material:
     a) To cover the opening at the top of the cast
     b) To cover bottom of foot (Technovit®) to help prevent horse from slipping during recovery from anesthesia and while walking on slippery surface

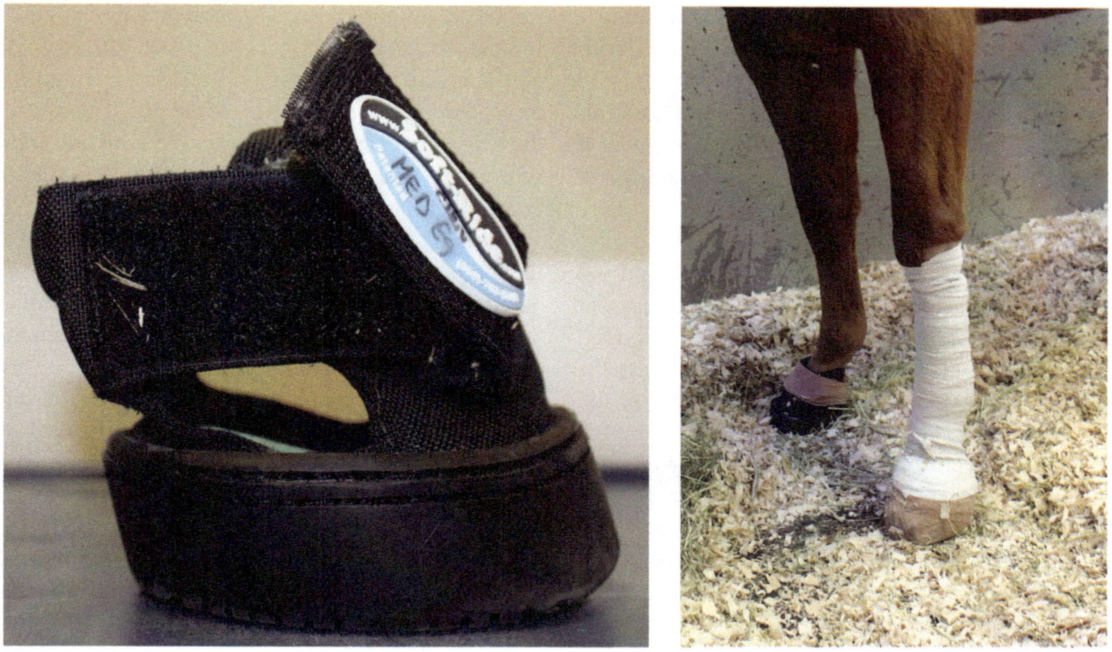

(a) (b)

Figure 7.18 **(a)** An example of a commercial boot that can be placed on the limb contralateral to that being cast, to equalize the length of the limbs. Several boot products are commercially available although a wooden block or commercial shoe can be used as an alternative. This particular commercial boot is reusable and has a soft pad on the interior. **(b)** A distal limb cast was placed on the left forelimb to assist in the treatment of a flexor tendon laceration. To equalize the length of the forelimbs and thereby avoid overloading the contralateral limb, a boot with Velcro straps (in this case reinforced with elastic tape) has been placed on the right forelimb. A soft elastic bandage has been applied around the cast to prevent abrasive trauma to the skin of the other limb if the horse lies down.

10 seconds before unwinding it around the limb. The cast material must be applied with light, even tension, as flatly as possible to avoid bunching or wrinkling, and by overlapping each turn by 50% to ensure bonding between layers as the material dries, thereby ensuring optimal strength. The top of the stockinette is folded down over the casting tape prior to applying the final layer, in order to give a soft rounded edge to the top of the cast. The cast should be handled only with flat hands to avoid leaving fingertip depressions that may cause pressure points on the soft tissues underlying the cast and subsequently lead to the development of cast sores.

Tips

- Leave the hair unclipped, as long as it does not interfere with wound healing. The hair provides extra padding and may reduce the risk of cast sores.
- Wear disposable gloves to protect your hands from the resin in the cast material.

The fiberglass cast material sets within minutes, so the casting material must be applied quickly. The distal extremity of the forelimb may be cast in either a standing horse or a recumbent (anesthetized) horse. Conversely, horses with a wound on the hindlimb that require immobilization with a cast should be anesthetized because the reciprocal apparatus makes it difficult to hold the limb off the ground for casting. When placing a cast on a recumbent (anesthetized) horse, the limb must be maintained in a position as close as possible to normal weight bearing. After the cast has set, additional protection can be provided, via the application of a product such as hoof acrylic (Technovit®), to improve the cast's resistance and reduce its permeability where it contacts the ground. Because hoof acrylic can be slippery, the bottom of the foot should be covered by elastic tape in an effort to provide better traction. A raised shoe or a commercial boot (Figure 7.18a) should be placed on the contralateral foot to equalize the length of the limbs and thereby decrease the likelihood of overloading the contralateral limb (Figure 7.18b).[12,13]

Specific casts

Foot casts

Foot casts or phalangeal casts (i.e., those that enclose the hoof and extend to just distal to the fetlock) are recommended for the treatment of heel bulb lacerations, traumatic hoof wall defects, coronary band lacerations, and distal pastern wounds. This is because expansion and contraction of the hoof wall and heel bulbs during loading and unloading of the limb cause movement sufficient to delay healing and also favor the development of EGT. The cast protects the lacerated heel bulb from movement and contamination and conveniently eliminates the requirement for frequent bandage changes. A reduced duration of treatment and a marked improvement in healing are reported for heel bulb lacerations treated with a cast as compared to those managed with bandages alone.[14,15]

A foot cast may be placed on a fresh wound immediately following primary care, or after several days of local treatment if the wound involves deeper structures. Foot casts are also useful in the management of chronic heel bulb lacerations that have failed to heal in an efficient manner after wound revision.

The shoe should be removed prior to treating the wound and applying a cast. The hoof should be trimmed, if necessary, but care should be taken to avoid further contaminating the wound or causing more trauma if the hoof wall is unstable. Prior to the application of a foot cast, the wound is cleaned, debrided, and sutured, if appropriate, and a dressing is applied. Conforming gauze or lightly applied elastic tape is used to hold the dressing in place. Following this, a stockinette may be used or this step can be replaced by covering the hoof and skin, up to the fetlock, with a thicker layer of the conforming gauze (Figure 7.19). A thick piece of felt is placed circumferentially around the limb, just distal to the fetlock, and held in place with tape. Commonly, a layer of cast foam or cast padding is then applied, followed by fiberglass casting tape.

The cast should be applied with the foot in a weight-bearing position, either in the recumbent, anesthetized horse or in the standing horse with the affected limb held off the ground.[14–16] In the anesthetized horse, the limb to be cast, whether the fore- or hindlimb, should be carefully positioned in full extension while ensuring that there is no medial or lateral deviation. In the hindlimb this is facilitated by manually locking the stifle in extension. Alternatively, two wires placed through holes made in the white line, 2 cm medial and lateral to the dorsal midline of the hoof, may be used to pull the phalanges into extension while the cast material is being applied. These wires are then cut flush with the cast.

In the standing horse, a weight-bearing position can be achieved in the forelimb by lifting at the radius and letting the distal aspect of the limb hang from the carpus while pulling the toe dorsally into extension, or by flexing the limb at the carpus and supporting it with a hand under the cannon bone. Alternatively, the limb can be flexed at the carpus to enable the placement of material around the bottom the hoof, after which the limb is replaced on the ground in a normal standing position (on a bag or towel), and the rest of the cast material is applied proximally. This is also the optimal way to place a foot cast on the hindlimb in the standing horse (i.e., raising the limb to allow placement of the cast material over the bottom of the foot, which is subsequently replaced on the ground). The easiest way to cast the bottom of the foot in a standing horse is to begin by unrolling one roll of casting tape and repeatedly folding it back and forth on itself, accordion-style, to create a multi-layered rectangular pad of a size sufficient to cover the bottom of the hoof (Figure 7.14). After immersing this rectangular pad of cast tape in warm water, it is applied to the bottom of the hoof, the foot is replaced on the ground and, with the horse bearing weight, the edges of the rectangle are wrapped around the dorsal and palmar/plantar surfaces of the hoof. The rest of the casting tape is applied around the walls of the hoof and the pastern, incorporating the curled edges of the pad. This method ensures that the cast covers the bottom of the hoof and the toe and is sufficiently thick to prevent the cast from eroding through to hoof at these sites.

Another approach to applying a phalangeal cast to the hindlimb of a standing horse is to have the horse stand with both hind feet on a block of wood (5 × 15 × 20 cm); the toe of the affected limb rests on the board. It is important that the sole of the affected limb remain parallel to the ground and that the toe does not become elevated.[16] Positioning the foot in this manner allows the majority of the cast to be applied with the limb fully bearing weight. Once this cast material has dried, more cast material is applied to the toe region while the limb is extended craniad. Technovit® is applied to the bottom of the hoof for protection.[16] Whenever a phalangeal cast is applied while the horse is standing, the patient must not walk until the cast has cured (20–30 minutes).

Tips

- Narrower cast material (such as 7 cm rather than 10 or 12 cm width) conforms more readily to the irregular shape of the hoof and the heel bulbs, thereby reducing the risk of creating wrinkles that predispose to the development of pressure sores.
- Use a wide strip of felt under the top of the cast to protect the skin around the fetlock when the horse bears weight. The cast material should extend no further than the middle of the felt ring, and the proximal edge of the cast must be smooth (Figure 7.19d).
- If the cast is applied to a standing horse, the limb should be placed on the ground and the horse encouraged to bear weight to ensure the cast hardens in a correct position on the weight-bearing limb. A towel or bag should be placed under the cast to prevent it from bonding to the floor!

What to do

- Thin areas around the toe of the cast are prone to breakage. Pleating the cast material to create a pad that covers the sole and toe helps ensure sufficient coverage with cast material.

Elastic, adhesive tape should be placed, without tension, at the proximal limit of the cast to prevent foreign material from entering under the cast. Hoof acrylic can be applied to the bottom of the foot for reinforcement and for waterproofing (Figure 7.19e); alternatively, duct tape followed by elastic, adhesive tape, can be applied to the bottom of the cast.

Foot casts used to support the healing of heel bulb lacerations are generally left in place for 2–4 weeks. Most heel bulb lacerations heal within 2–3 weeks but if, upon cast removal, it is found that healing is incomplete, then a second cast can be applied. The cast usually must be left in place longer (3–4 weeks) if the injury involves the coronary band or if a portion of the hoof wall has been lost.

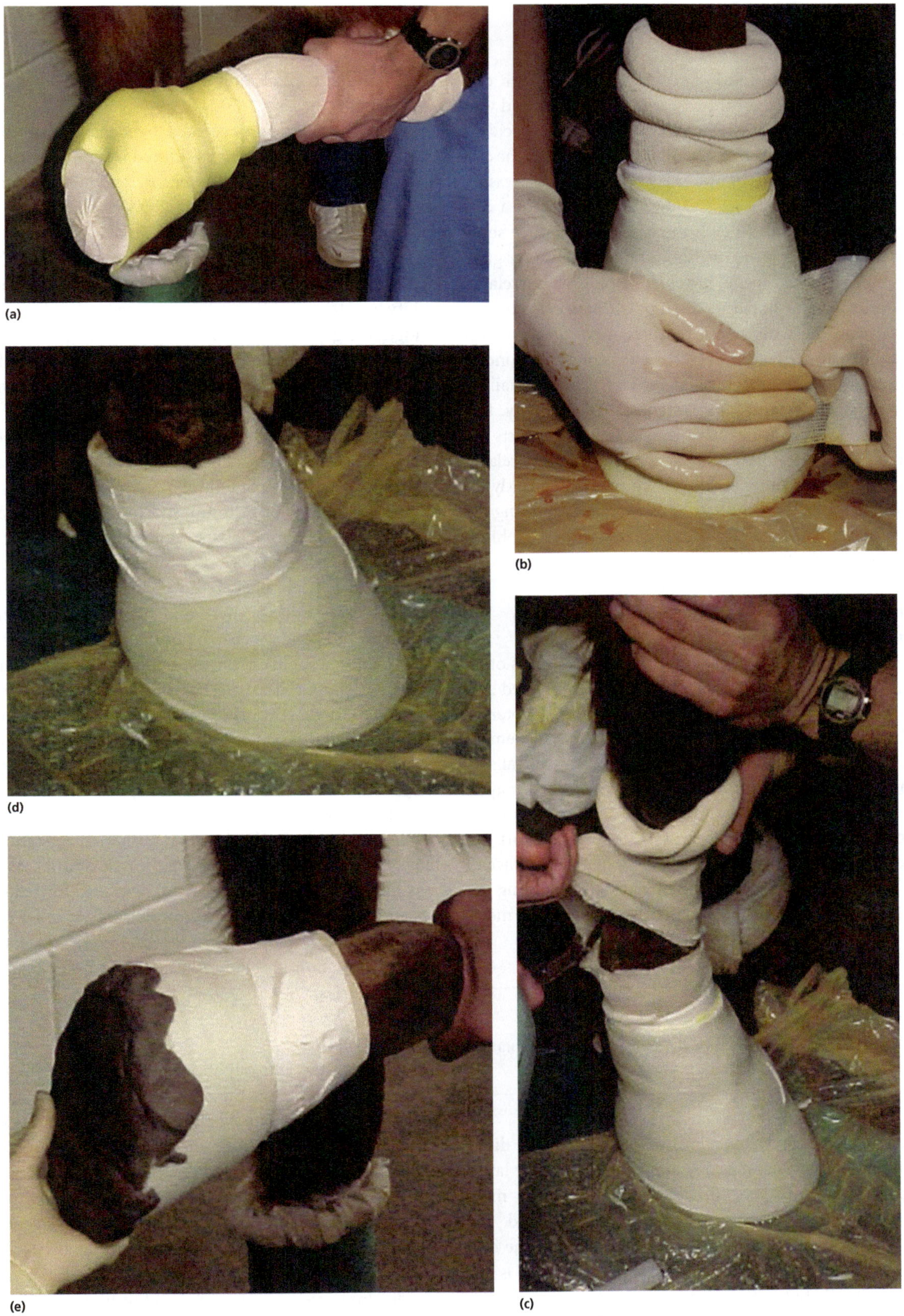

Figure 7.19 **(a)** Application of a phalangeal cast in the standing horse. The limb is held off the ground to apply a single layer of cast padding (yellow) to the pastern and hoof regions and a fiberglass cast tape to the bottom of the foot (not shown). A ring of orthopedic felt, underlying the foam, is placed at the proximal pastern. **(b)** A roll of 12.5-cm fiberglass cast tape was applied to the bottom of the foot. The remainder of the cast is being applied to the pastern up to the middle of the ring of orthopedic felt. **(c)** Excess stockinette is removed in preparation for rolling the remaining portion distally over the cast. **(d)** The rolled stockinette is secured to the cast with 5-cm white, non-elastic adhesive tape. **(e)** Technovit® has been applied to the bottom of the cast.

The horse should be comfortable immediately after cast application. When this is not the case, the clinician should wait 24–48 hours (for any tissue swelling to subside) before deciding whether or not to replace the cast. If discomfort persists, the cast should be replaced since discomfort may be caused by a pressure point that would no doubt lead to the development of a cast sore. Because the wound beneath the cast may produce some exudate, seepage through the cast should not be cause for great alarm. The degree of seepage, however, should be correlated to the comfort of the horse to distinguish between seepage emanating from the wound and that emanating from a cast sore. Seepage in an area of the cast that does not correspond to the location of the wound is a cause for concern, especially if the seepage is accompanied by lameness. Reassuringly, two separate retrospective studies have shown that when casts are used in the treatment of heel bulb lacerations, few cast-related complications are encountered and the wounds heal quickly.[15,16] The prognosis for healing and return to function following the use of foot casts to manage very contaminated wounds in high-motion areas was 80–90%.[14,15]

Distal limb casts (distal to the carpus/tarsus and including the foot)

Because degloving wounds in the metacarpus/metatarsus often involve the tendons, support more rigid than that provided by a bandage may be required (the reader is referred to Chapter 17 for more information about tendon healing and the management of tendon injuries). When degloving wounds on the dorsal surface of the canon bone are sutured, some immobilization may be desirable to prevent dehiscence from increased tension on the suture line that results from flexion of the fetlock. Support can be provided either by a splint on the palmar/plantar surface of the limb or a cast placed over the bandage, and spanning the distance from the ground to the proximal extremity of the metacarpus/metatarsus.

> **What to avoid**
>
> - Avoid ending the cast mid-metacarpus/mid-metatarsus, because this may create a fulcrum over which the bone could fracture.

The bandage is applied as previously described for the distal limb, avoiding bulkiness and firmly applying the tertiary layer. When applying a bandage–cast, the bandage material must cover all the skin down to and including the coronary band. The felt band, stockinette, and cast foam are omitted, and the cast material is applied directly to the bandage. The bandage is left exposed proximally but the cast extends past the bandage distally, on to and around the hoof, to include the foot. Hoof acrylic can be applied to the cast where it covers the bottom of the foot, to improve traction. Elastic adhesive tape is applied loosely to the top of the bandage to secure it to the skin to prevent the entry of foreign material under the bandage–cast. A shoe is placed on the contralateral foot to ensure the limbs remain of equal length (Figure 7.18b).

When the only purpose of a bandage–cast is to prevent movement during healing of a sutured wound or one healing by second intention, without extensor tendon involvement, the cast can usually be removed after 2–3 weeks.

When a cast (or a splint) is used to manage wounds involving injury to and loss of function of the extensor tendons, the length of time support is required is variable. Although the horse's ability to extend the digit is fully restored only when scar tissue bridges the gap between the severed ends of the tendon, some horses learn to extend ("flip") their limb with just a bandage, whereas other horses require more rigid support, with a splint or cast, for the first 1–3 weeks following injury.

When the function of one or both digital flexor tendons has been lost, a homemade splint from PVC pipe, a bandage–cast, or a Kimzey Leg Saver Splint (Kimzey, Woodland, CA) must be applied to the limb prior to transporting the horse to a referral hospital. The splint or bandage–cast is often the preferred mode of support during the period of intensive wound management since it can be more easily removed than a traditional cast (the bandage–cast can be bivalved and either replaced after wound treatment and bandage changes or the caudal half may be used, on its own, as a splint). Once the wound no longer requires daily treatment, support is usually continued, via casting, for a longer period (6–8 weeks). In these instances the limb is commonly cast with a support under the heel to hold the fetlock in a slightly flexed position and relieve strain on the flexor tendons. The support under the heel can be supplied by many different methods. An intact roll of cast material can be incorporated into the cast under the heel or some veterinarians prefer a wooden block incorporated into the foot of the cast. Several cast changes may be required during this period to amend for reduced soft-tissue swelling or to treat any pressure sores or other complications that may develop (the reader is referred to Chapter 17 for more information on tendon healing and the management of tendon injuries).

Full-limb casts

Immobilizing the entire limb may greatly aid healing of large transverse wounds over the dorsal surface of the carpus or the plantar surface of the hock. Nevertheless, the risk of complications relating to full-limb immobilization is high, particularly during recovery from general anesthesia. Thus, if possible and appropriate, the full-limb cast should be applied to the standing horse in an effort to avoid the risks associated with general anesthesia. Alternatively, the use of techniques of assisted recovery from general anesthesia, such as sling recovery, are recommended for horses having received a full-limb cast. The benefits of immobilization, therefore, must be carefully weighed against the potential risks incurred.[5,6,13] The risks of casting are explained more fully in the section on cast complications but, briefly, the full-limb cast may cause a fracture of the tibia or radius as it can be difficult to extend the cast sufficiently proximad to avoid the creation of a fulcrum somewhere along the long bone. Moreover, because the horse will experience more difficulty moving its cast limb and standing up or lying down, any struggling to rise, or stumbling, increases the risk of fracture. Therefore, full-limb casting can be justified only when the healing of the wound would be severely impeded by its absence. In the majority of cases, a full-limb Robert Jones bandage is an appropriate alternative.

Depending on the extent of the injury, the cast may encompass the entire limb, including the hoof, or it may end distally just proximal to the fetlock as a "tube cast." If the aim of casting is to prevent movement by flexion of the hock/carpus, then a tube cast would suffice. Conversely, if healing of a large wound involving the dorsal surface of the carpus or hock would also be impeded by flexion of the fetlock, then a full-limb cast is preferred. A tube cast, compared to a full-limb cast, facilitates advancement of the limb and its use circumvents immobilization of the fetlock and more distal regions, which may help limit the development of "cast disease." Nevertheless, tube casts can slip distad to rub on the fetlock.

A full-limb cast may be applied without the underlying three-layered bandage, however this is likely appropriate only for wounds associated with significant orthopedic injury.[13] The technique is similar to that described for the casting of wounds of the distal aspect of the limb. The wound is dressed with a light dressing held in place by conforming gauze, carefully applied to avoid wrinkling or folding. A stockinette is then placed to span the entire limb. A thick piece of felt is positioned circumferentially at the proximal extremity of the radius/tibia and held in place with white tape. A layer of cast padding is applied, overlapping each turn by 50%, beginning at the coronary band and reaching to the middle of the band of felt. A donut of felt may be placed at the level of the accessory carpal bone. Cast material (width of 10–12 cm for adult horses) is then applied using light tension and overlapping each turn by 50% to ensure good bonding between layers. The cast should incorporate the hoof and extend proximally to halfway up the felt band. If, on the other hand, a tube cast is to be used, a second thick piece of felt is positioned proximal to the fetlock at the level of the distal metacarpus/metatarsus; the distal edge of the cast material extends to the middle of this second band of felt.

What to avoid

- Avoid applying a tube cast over a thick bandage because this increases the risk of distal slippage and rubbing on the fetlock.

A full-limb cast is most easily applied with the horse under general anesthesia. When applying a full-limb cast with the horse standing, the cast material should first be applied over the foot, which is then placed on the floor (either on a towel or a plastic sheet); the rest of the cast is applied with the limb in a weight-bearing position. Because the cast material must dry before any movement is allowed, the horse should be sedated to keep it still for approximately 30 minutes after the cast has been applied.

What to do

- The full-limb cast must extend as proximad as possible (on the radius or the tibia) to reduce the risk of fracture, which is greatest when the horse is recovering from general anesthesia or rising from recumbency.
- If a full-limb cast is applied with the horse under general anesthesia, the cast limb must be uppermost while the horse recovers from anesthesia. Recovery should be assisted, if possible.

Although most horses usually adjust quickly to a full-limb cast, some may initially require assistance to advance the limb, which can be accomplished by placing a rope around the pastern region and gently pulling the limb forward. Horses with full-limb casts require intensive monitoring for signs of complications and to provide assistance in rising should they lie down with the cast limb beneath them. If the condition and behavior of the horse allow, cross-tying the horse or maintaining it in a sling to prevent it from lying down may be wise (Figure 7.20). When a

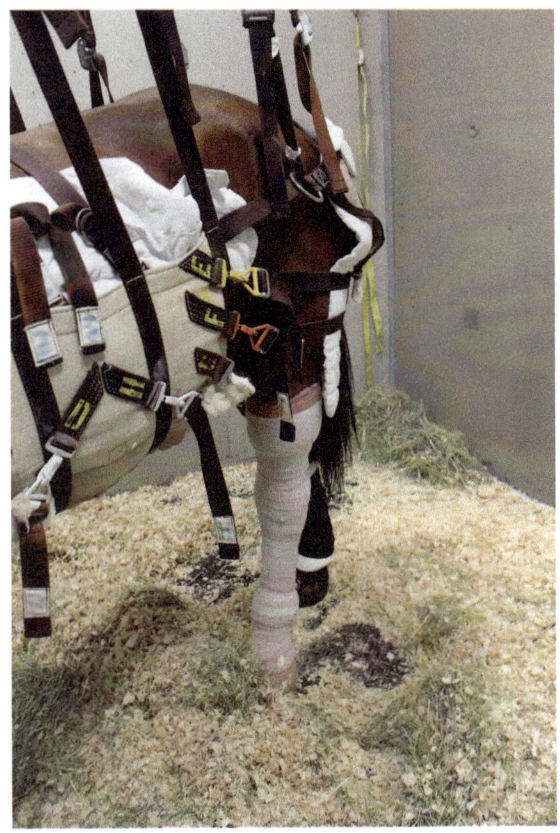

Figure 7.20 When a full-limb cast is applied to aid in the healing of a wound, a sling may be used to keep the horse standing and thereby avoid placing significant force on the bones of the immobilized limb upon lying down and rising. Potentially severe complications such as long bone fractures and rupture of the *peroneus tertius* can be minimized using this precaution. An alternative is to keep the horse cross-tied.

full-limb cast is used to aid in the healing of a wound, the cast can usually be removed, in the standing horse, after 2–3 weeks.

Cast removal

A cast is usually removed with the horse standing (see Box 7.2 for a list of the materials required for cast removal). However, if the cast must be replaced, this is done with the horse anesthetized or standing, depending on the type of cast to be applied, the horse's anticipated behavior, the available facilities, and the treatment required by the underlying wound. To remove any type of cast with the horse standing, the horse is sedated and adhesive tape, duct tape, and/or foot acrylic are removed. A cast saw is then used to cut the cast medially and laterally, from proximad to distad, into two longitudinal halves.

What to do

- Apply light inwards pressure on the saw until a loss of resistance is felt. Remove the saw, advance it distally and push inwards again. Repeat this procedure until the saw cut spans the length of the cast.

What to avoid

- Avoid running the saw proximally and distally while exerting pressure, because this tactic may lacerate the skin, especially if little cast padding is present underneath. This is particularly important when removing a cast with the horse anesthetized because the horse will not react to a skin cut.

Tip

- When removing the cast from a standing horse, activate the cast saw from a distance to allow the horse a few seconds to acclimatize to the noise.

When cutting over a bandage or cast padding and stockinette, the slight loss of resistance upon traversing the fiberglass and reaching this underlying layer helps determine the appropriate depth to cut. When a cast extends over the hoof, this indicator is lost since the hoof wall will provide the same sensation as the cast material. Care should therefore be taken when cutting a cast over the hoof; the depth of cut achieved proximally can serve as a guide, and/or making several passes over the same area until a slight opening of the cast is seen, can serve as an alternative.

When the saw cut has spanned the full thickness of the cast, the two edges separate slightly and must then be levered apart. If the cast was placed over a bandage, cutting the tertiary layer of bandage material (Vetrap™ and/or Elastikon®) with scissors may be necessary because this layer may have bonded to the cast material and will not be cut with the cast saw. After the cast and underlying bandage (where used) have been removed, the limb is cleaned thoroughly and appropriate wound care is administered. The horse may demonstrate a slight lameness for the first few days following cast removal, until the limb adjusts to an increased load. When a cast was used to assist in the healing of a flexor tendon injury, it is common to replace it by a splint, upon cast removal, and then by a special shoe, to gradually increase the load on the tendons (the reader is referred to Chapter 17 for more information about tendon healing and the management of tendon injuries).

Tip

- Use Vetrap™ for the tertiary layer of the bandage to minimize bonding between the bandage and a fiberglass cast.

Box 7.2 Material required for cast removal.

Cast saw and electric extension cord
Scissors
Screw driver to chip off foot acrylic
Cast spreader (to lever the cut edges of the cast apart)
Sedatives

Also include supplies to clean the limb and the wound: warm water and towels, isotonic saline solution, gauze, chlorhexidine soap, clean bandage material, and splint, if indicated.

Complications relating to the use of casts

Horses with casts or splints require close monitoring. Horses should be comfortable in a cast after the initial pain relating to the wound has decreased; this should occur within the first few days of trauma. Persistent discomfort (not thought to be associated with the wound) or an increase in discomfort (apparent by reduced weight bearing), drainage (not anticipated from the wound), swelling proximal to the cast, or breakage of the cast indicate that the cast should be changed as soon as possible. If a horse begins to mutilate its cast, the cast should be changed to ensure there is not an underlying problem; behavioral signs of discomfort should be taken seriously.

Tips

- A cast applied to a swollen limb may quickly loosen as the swelling dissipates; in such a situation, an early cast change must be anticipated.
- When explaining to owners why a cast may cause discomfort and require changing, it helps to compare casts to shoes – some fit and are very comfortable whereas others may pinch a little in one spot and so need to be changed.

A recent study of risk factors associated with casts suggests that bandage–casts have a lower risk of complications compared to traditional casts.[11] When bandage–casts were used, the rate of complications was 34% compared to a 52% rate for casts placed over only stockinette and cast padding or cast foam. Complications were predominantly cast sores: 26% of horses with a bandage–cast and 57% of horses with a conventional cast developed sores, respectively.

Cast sores are most common over the palmar/plantar surface of the sesamoid bones, the dorsoproximal surface of the metacarpus/metatarsus, the accessory carpal bone, and the heel bulbs.

Careful monitoring for discharge in these areas or signs of a decrease in comfort (i.e. increased lameness) is an important component of case management.[11,13] Although drainage may be a sign of underlying cast sores, interpreting its significance can be difficult when the cast was used to immobilize a limb with a wound, because some drainage from an open wound, especially a heavily contaminated one, is to be expected. In such a case, the area of the cast discolored by drainage should be outlined with a pen so that it can be monitored for enlargement. It is expected that drainage from the original wound will decrease over the treatment time; consequently, an increase may be attributed to a cast sore, especially if this coincides with discomfort. Cast sores are best managed by removal of the cast and transition to a bandage that relieves the pressure caused by the cast. A cast sore will often continue to enlarge following the replacement of the cast by a bandage, due to the pressure necrosis having caused more damage than is initially visible. If another cast must be applied, a donut may be formed from stockinette or gauze material and placed around the cast sore to protect the area from further pressure. Alternatively, a traditional cast can be replaced by a bandage–cast.

Comfort is assessed by daily observation of the horse and palpation of the limbs. The horse should not exhibit any obvious signs of lameness and should move around the stall readily. The horse can be walked for several steps outside the stall each day to assess any subtle decrease in weight bearing. The amount of time spent in sternal or lateral recumbency should not increase from normal. The digital pulse on the contralateral limb should be palpated to monitor for an increase that might signal impending laminitis. A recent study on the incidence of support limb laminitis found that 20% of the horses with a full-limb cast, used in the management of a laceration, developed clinical signs of laminitis while in the horses with only a distal limb cast, no signs of laminitis developed.[13]

The limb should be evaluated for signs of swelling above the cast and the elastic tape protecting the top of the cast should be changed every 1–2 days. Horses having received a cast for the management of a wound are not commonly given anti-inflammatory drugs for a long period and this facilitates the interpretation of observed decreases in comfort. Discomfort accompanied by drainage is always an indication to change the cast as this is usually associated with the development of a cast sore. Conversely, enlarging areas of discoloration, in the absence of obvious discomfort, more likely indicate an accumulation of exudate within the cast, possibly in relation to the original wound. In such a case, though not urgent, the cast should be changed earlier than planned since the wound and surrounding skin may become macerated.

> **Tip**
>
> - The gathering of flies at a focal area on a cast may be an early indicator of a cast sore at that site. In such a case, close monitoring of the horse and the cast are warranted so that the cast is changed before the sore enlarges and deepens.

Even with only a small amount of drainage or bleeding after wound debridement, casts usually develop a rather foul odor. If the horse is comfortable and any areas of discoloration are stable, the presence of a bad odor, on its own, is not an indication to change the cast.

In addition to the risk of a radial or tibial fracture after a full-limb cast has been applied, rupture of the *peroneus tertius* may occur in response to repeated and prolonged strain associated with flexion of the stifle while the hock is in a fixed position within the cast. This rupture will commonly go on to heal after cast removal but will require additional rest.[13]

Another complication of prolonged immobilization is the development of "cast disease." This term refers to the harmful effects of immobilization on joint health. When the limb is immobilized there is a damaging effect on bone and cartilage metabolism: bone can become osteopenic and cartilage may thin.[5,6] These effects may be compounded by increased stiffness of the joint capsule and surrounding soft tissues. A certain amount of recovery can be expected after removal of the cast but some effects may resolve incompletely.[5,6]

The use of casts in foals also merits special considerations. Because the risk of foals developing cast sores largely exceeds that of adults, the use of external coaptation in the form of splints and casts should, when possible, be avoided in very young foals. Splints should be applied over padded bandages and changed at least once daily. A cast applied to very young foals should be changed every 10–14 days because if left longer than this it may interfere with growth of the limb. In spite of this precaution, the hoof, when enclosed within a cast, frequently becomes contracted.

Conclusion

Bandaging, with or without the addition of a splint or a cast, is an important component of wound management in horses. The dressing that constitutes the primary layer must be selected judiciously to support healing of the wound. The secondary and tertiary layers must be applied with care to avoid common complications. Bandaging, splinting, and casting may be associated with various complications, and the veterinarian must always evaluate the wound, the care-giver, and the environment of the horse to determine whether the use of an external support can help or hinder recovery after wounding.

References

1. Dart AJ, Perkins NR, Dart CM, *et al.* Effect of bandaging on second intention healing of wounds of the distal limb in horses. *Aust Vet J* 2009; **87**: 215.
2. Theoret CL, Barber SM, Moyana TN, *et al.* Expression of transforming growth factor β_1, β_3, and basic fibroblast factor in full-thickness skin wounds of equine limbs and thorax. *Vet Surg* 2001; **30**: 269.

3. Céleste CJ, Deschene K, Riley CB, *et al.* Regional differences in wound oxygenation during normal healing in an equine model of cutaneous fibroproliferative disorder. *Wound Repair Regen* 2011; **19**: 89.
4. Berry DB, Sullins KE. Effects of topical application of antimicrobials and bandaging on healing and granulation tissue formation in wounds of the distal aspect of the limbs in horses. *Am J Vet Res* 2003; **64**: 88.
5. Richardson DW, Clark CC. Effects of short-term cast immobilization on equine articular cartilage. *Am J Vet Res* 1993; **54**: 449.
6. Van Harreveld PD, Lillich JD, Kawcak CE, *et al.* Effects of immobilization followed by remobilization on mineral density, histomorphometric features, and formation of the bones of the metacarpophalangeal joint in horses. *Am J Vet Res* 2002; **63**: 276.
7. Gomez JH, Hanson RR. Use of dressings and bandages in equine wound management. *Vet Clin North Am Equine Pract* 2005; **21**: 91.
8. Theoret CL, Bolwell CF, Riley CB. A cross-sectional survey on wounds in horses in New Zealand. *N Z Vet J* 2016; **64**: 90
9. Sole A, Bolwell C, Dart A, *et al.* Wound in horses: a cross-sectional survey of Australian veterinarians. *Aust Eq Vet* 2015; **34**: 68.
10. Tnibar A, Grubb Lin K, Thuroe Neilson K, *et al.* Effect of a stent bandage on the likelihood of incisional infection following exploratory coeliotomy for colic in horses: a comparative retrospective study. *Equine Vet J* 2013; **45**: 564.
11. Janicek JC, McClure SR, Lescun TB, *et al.* Risk factors associated with cast complications in horses: 398 cases (1997–2006). *J Am Vet Med Assoc* 2013; **242**: 93.
12. Stokes M, Hendrickson DA, Wittern C. Use of an elevated boot to reduce contralateral support limb complications secondary to cast application in the horse. *Equine Pract* 1998; **20**: 14.
13. Virgin JE, Goodrich LR, Baxter GM, *et al.* Incidence of support limb laminitis in horses treated with half limb, full limb or transfixation pin casts: a retrospective study of 113 horses (2000–2009). *Equine Vet* J Suppl 2011; 7.
14. Ketzner KM, Stewart AA, Byron CR, *et al.* Wounds of the pastern and foot region managed by phalangeal casts 50 cases in 49 horses (1995–2006). *Aust Vet J* 2009; **87**: 363.
15. Janicek JC, Dabareiner RM, Honnas CM, *et al.* Heel bulb lacerations in horses: 101 cases (1988–1994). *J Am Vet Med Assoc* 2005; **226**: 418.
16. Fitzgerald BW, Honnas CM, Plummer AE, *et al.* How to apply a hindlimb phalangeal cast in the standing patient and minimize complications. *Proc Am Assoc Equine Pract* 2006; **52**: 631.

CHAPTER 8
Approaches to Wound Closure

Updated by Yvonne A. Elce, DVM, Diplomate ACVS

Chapter Contents

Summary

Selection of the optimal way to manage a wound should not be based on rigid rules relating to time or conditions, but rather, it should rely on careful examination of the wound and consideration of factors relating to the patient. Each wound is unique and requires individualized care. Wounds may be closed immediately after cleansing and debridement (referred to as primary closure) or closure may be deferred for a few days to allow continued debridement and treatment (referred to as delayed primary closure). Alternatively, wounds may be revised and closed after granulation tissue has formed (referred to as delayed secondary closure) or left to heal without suturing (referred to as second-intention healing). Primary closure should be considered in all cases, and particularly when tissues underlying the skin, such as bone or tendon, are exposed, because this approach is most likely to provide the best cosmetic and functional outcome.

Introduction

When a horse incurs a wound, the goals of treatment are to reduce pain and restore a normal appearance and function to the wounded area, as rapidly as possible. The manner in which this goal is achieved varies because many options exist. Careful examination of the horse in general, and of the wound specifically, should always be performed before any therapeutic decisions are made. A complete medical history must be obtained and should include the status of tetanus vaccination, as well as details pertaining to when and how the wound occurred. The owner's goals and limitations (financial, time, technical, or facility-related) must be discussed. After a thorough history has been obtained and the horse physically examined to rule out any noteworthy systemic problems, a detailed examination of the wound may begin.

Administering some form of sedation that simultaneously provides analgesia and diminishes the anxiety of the patient, thereby facilitating a careful examination and protecting the veterinarian, is helpful. While examining the wound, special attention should be paid to the following: the involvement of underlying structures, such as joints, body cavities, bone, and tendon; the amount of gross contamination; an estimation of the manner in which the wound was incurred and the time elapsed since wounding, if not clear from the medical history (e.g., crushing or sharp trauma; fresh or chronic appearing); the location, shape, and depth of the wound; and the integrity of the local vascular supply. Because these factors contribute to the overall status of the wounded tissues, rigid guidelines based on the age or degree of contamination of a wound should not be used to dictate whether or not the wound can be sutured or must be left to heal

Equine Wound Management, Third Edition. Edited by Christine Theoret and Jim Schumacher.

Companion website: www.wiley.com/go/theoret/wound

by second intention. The options for wound management are primary closure, delayed closure (either primary or secondary), and leaving the wound unsutured to heal by second intention, with or without some form of skin grafting.

Whenever possible, wounds should be managed by primary closure because this leads to a superior cosmetic and functional outcome. Many veterinarians were taught that a wound is suitable for primary closure, without risk of infection and subsequent dehiscence, if it is less than 6–8 hours old. This "golden period" relates to the time that it takes multiplying bacteria in a surgical wound, created experimentally in laboratory animals, to reach an infective concentration, considered to be more than 10^5 organisms per gram of tissue or milliliter of exudate.[1] In fact, we now know that this time may be longer than 6–8 hours in very clean, minimally contaminated wounds, and it may be shorter in heavily contaminated, contused tissues.[2] Consequently, the concept of a "golden period" is inaccurate,[3] and the outcome of primary closure is now considered to depend predominantly on the adequacy of the host's immune response, the virulence of contaminating bacteria, and local environmental factors that might potentiate the virulence of bacteria.[4] For more information on the bacterial impact on wound healing, the reader is referred to Chapter 3. In the horse, primary closure is considered ideal for fresh, minimally contaminated wounds of the extremities, wounds of the head, and flap wounds with a good blood supply, such as those found, for example, on the neck, the flank, the thorax, or the proximal aspect of the limb. Wounds caused by contact with sharp objects often heal successfully after primary closure because this type of injury inflicts minimal trauma to the tissues and their blood supply (Figure 8.1).

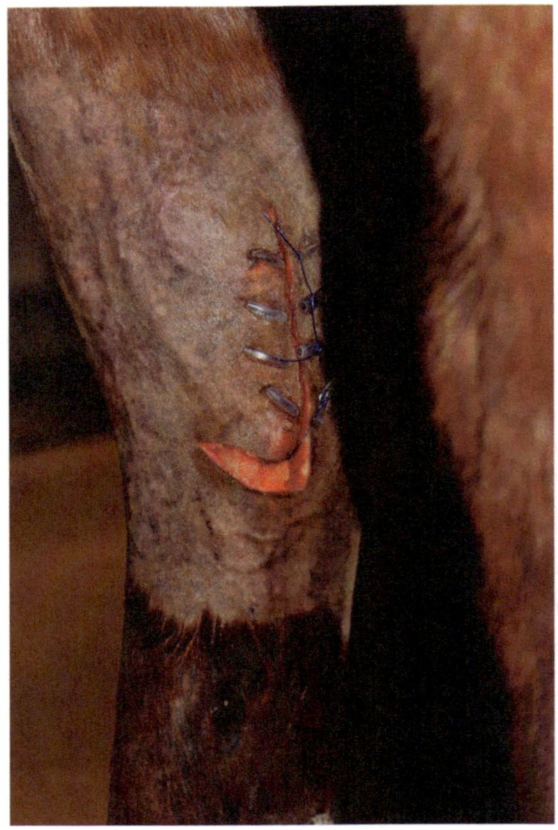

Figure 8.1 Example of a fresh skin wound on the medial surface of the right hock, with sharp edges, caused by a metal gate. The wound was partially closed primarily, leaving its ventral extent unsutured to allow drainage. A vertical mattress suture pattern, with tubing used as stents, was selected to counter the tension that results from flexion of the hock. The sutured wound was then supported by a full limb bandage. Placing a bandage over stents can result in pressure necrosis, so the wound should be monitored closely for signs of this complication. Pressure on the bandage overlying the wound should be reduced to decrease the likelihood of pressure necrosis from developing beneath the stents. If damage to skin beneath the stents appears, the limb should be left unbandaged, or the stents should be removed in a staged approach.

Delayed primary closure is defined as that carried out days after injury, but before granulation tissue begins to appear, usually 4–5 days after injury. Delayed secondary closure (secondary closure) typically refers to wound apposition, with suture, after granulation tissue is grossly apparent, usually more than 5 days after injury. Although others have suggested that delayed primary and delayed secondary closure be referred to simply as delayed closure,[5] these forms of wound management are considered, in this chapter, as distinct because the presence or absence of granulation tissue exerts an influence on the method of closure.[5] Delayed primary closure is often selected as an approach to manage fresh wounds that are moderately contaminated, contused, and swollen. Closure is achieved in a fashion similar to primary closure but after a short duration (1–3 days) of treatment aimed at diminishing swelling and/or contamination. Recent meta-analyses of the human medical literature suggest that delaying primary skin closure may reduce the incidence of infection of contaminated and dirty abdominal incisions (mostly relating to complicated appendicitis), but this trend cannot be confirmed due to a paucity of well-designed, large-numbered, randomized clinical trials.[6,7] No comparable studies have been conducted on horses to determine whether delayed primary closure leads to an outcome superior to that associated with primary closure of contaminated, accidental wounds. Nevertheless, experience in the human medical field suggests that the low incidence of infection of dirty wounds managed by delayed primary closure is attributable to repeated irrigation and debridement of the wound prior to suturing, rendered possible by delaying closure.[7,8]

Delayed secondary closure is usually appropriate for wounds that are contaminated or have a compromised blood supply. The wound is closed after it develops a healthy bed of granulation tissue. The granulating wound often must be revised to enable firm apposition of the skin edges. Granulation tissue is debulked, if necessary, the skin surrounding the wound often must be undermined, and a thin margin of skin is removed from the periphery of the wound to create fresh edges that are more likely to heal once apposed and sutured. Examples of wounds that are usually amenable to delayed secondary closure are heel bulb

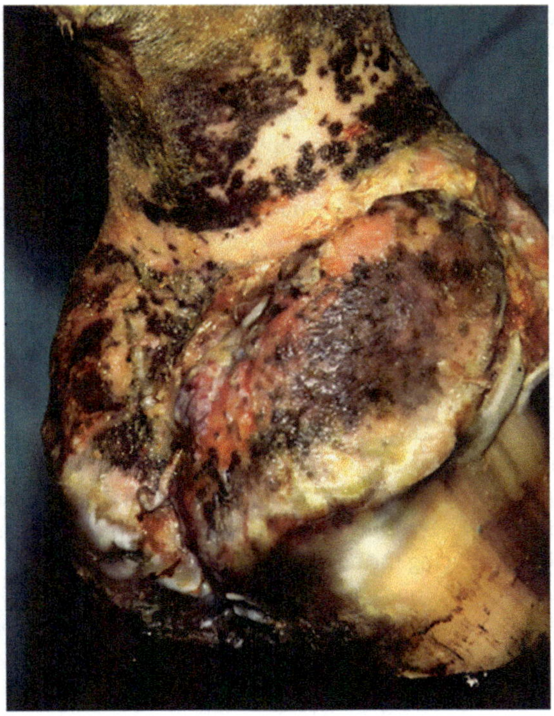

Figure 8.2 Heel bulb laceration of several days duration that was managed by delayed secondary closure. The cause was barbed wire. The horse was severely lame on the affected limb, and the wound was exudative and swollen, indicating infection.

lacerations and wounds of the body that can be revised (Figure 8.2). "Degloving" injuries, which usually involve the metacarpal/metatarsal area, are often very contaminated and have a compromised blood supply, and so, theoretically, these wounds would be good candidates for delayed secondary closure. The metacarpal/metatarsal area, however, has very little redundant skin, and consequently, revising these wounds in view of performing a delayed secondary closure is often difficult or impossible. Based on personal experience, the author recommends that degloving wounds of the metacarpus/metatarsus be sutured as early as possible, either via primary or delayed primary closure, to avoid the extended duration associated with second-intention healing and to maintain a humid healing environment to prevent desiccation of structures exposed by wounding, such as bone and tendon.[9] Because degloving injuries that are sutured are at risk of suffering partial or complete dehiscence as a result of wound infection,[10] owners must understand the reasons for electing this approach and should be made aware of the possibility of failure of the primary closure. More information on the management of degloving injuries can be found in Chapter 14.

Second-intention healing (i.e., by formation of granulation tissue, contraction, and epithelialization) is often the favored approach for the management of large wounds located over highly mobile regions (e.g., pectoral, axillary, groin, gluteal, etc.) (Figure 8.3) or for wounds that cannot be closed because of damage to surrounding soft tissues or because of loss of skin.

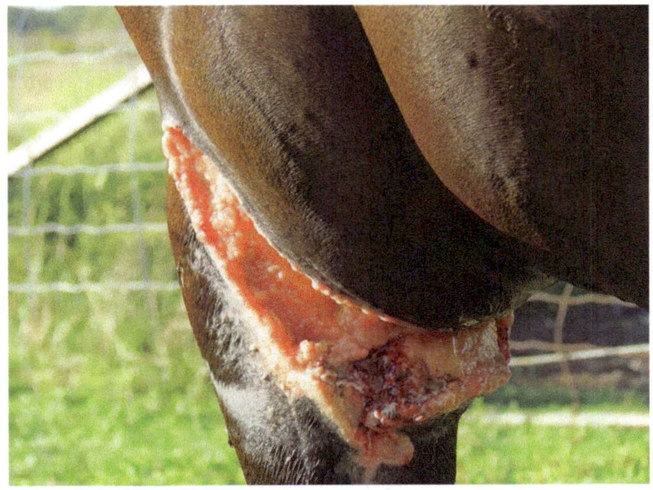

Figure 8.3 Example of a large wound in the axillary area that was managed by second-intention healing. At the time the horse was presented, granulation tissue had already filled the wound bed, and subcutaneous emphysema, which commonly accompanies wounds in the axillary region, was not observed.

These conditions are, unfortunately, common in horses. Skin grafting is useful in cases in which the tissue deficit exceeds the capability of wound contraction and epithelialization. For more information regarding skin grafting, see Chapter 18. Reconstructive surgery and revision of scar tissue may be used to achieve a superior cosmetic and functional outcome in a wound that has already healed. For more information regarding reconstructive surgery, see Chapter 10.

Evaluation and preparation of the wound

Examination and preparation of the wound are the first steps required to identify the most appropriate method of closure (See Box 8.1). The horse should be sedated to facilitate the examination, and analgesic medication may also be administered systemically, if required, to improve the patient's comfort. More information on the effects of anti-inflammatory drugs on wound healing is available in Chapter 4.

Antimicrobial drugs are commonly included in the management regimen when treating wounds at risk of becoming infected, such as contaminated wounds, penetrating wounds, wounds with devitalized tissue, or open fractures. Acute or superficial wound infections in horses are usually the result of one dominating microorganism. Conversely, chronic or deep wound infections in horses are often polymicrobial.[10,11] Antibiotics selected for use should reflect this microbial epidemiology,[10,11] bearing in mind the emergence of antimicrobial resistance and the importance of using a narrow-spectrum antibiotic, the selection of which is based on antibiotic sensitivity testing. Table 19.1 in Chapter 19 lists the common bacteria isolated from various types of wounds in horses, and Table 19.3 in Chapter 19 lists likely antibiotic sensitivities for each pathogen, as a basis for empiric antimicrobial therapy most probable to be useful. For a full discussion regarding the use of antimicrobial drugs for the management of wounds, the reader is referred to Chapter 4.

Local anesthesia and analgesia

Whether local administration of an anesthetic agent to desensitize the wound precedes or follows clipping of hair at the wound's periphery and cleansing of the wound depends on the horse's demeanor, the condition of the wound, and of the skin surrounding the wound. Ideally, the local anesthetic agent is administered after clipping and cleansing, but for horses that do not tolerate clipping and cleansing, the area may be desensitized after removing only gross debris.

The wound may be desensitized by local, regional, or intralesional anesthesia. A wound on a limb can be desensitized by placing a line or ring block proximal to the wound or by administering regional (i.e., perineural) anesthesia proximal to the wound. For wounds of the body, the local anesthetic agent can be placed in a curved line cranial to the wound; the line is extended slightly caudally around the edges of the wound to ensure complete desensitization. Wounds of the head may be desensitized by administering the local anesthetic agent subcutaneously, caudal to the wound or with more targeted perineural anesthesia.[12] Alternatively, a wound may be desensitized by direct intralesional placement of local anesthetic solution, although this should be done only after clipping and cleansing to minimize seeding of contaminants into deeper tissues.

Two percent lidocaine or mepivacaine hydrochloride is commonly used as a local anesthetic agent and provides desensitization for a sufficient time for examining, debriding, and closing the wound. Mepivacaine, rather than lidocaine, should be used if the wound is extensive and apt to require a long intervention because desensitization resulting from mepivacaine lasts longer than that from lidocaine. The duration of anesthesia, however, depends on the location and the vascularity of the wounded area; consequently, the horse must be monitored closely for signs of discomfort during manipulations.

Commercially available topical anesthetic creams or gels [e.g., Emla Cream™, containing lidocaine (2.5%) and prilocaine (2.5%), Oak Pharmaceuticals] may provide sufficient desensitization of the wound because they have been shown to be as effective as infiltration with lidocaine in providing desensitization when performing episioplasty in mares.[13] The slower onset of blockade provided by creams and gels (around 45 minutes), however, may limit their usefulness.

General anesthesia is rarely required for initial examination and cleansing of the wound, but it may be useful for foals or for horses with a large and heavily contaminated wound, or for horses with a wound that involves a critical structure underlying the skin, such as a joint or tendon. General anesthesia, administered intravenously, may be used for all stages of examination, cleansing, and treatment if the horse is not accustomed to being handled, to ensure the safety of both the horse and the veterinarian.

Cleansing and debridement

Surgeon and patient preparation

The skin adjacent to an open wound should be prepared as for aseptic surgery; this is usually done immediately prior to cleansing and debriding the wound. Involved personnel should don sterile gloves, after surgical hand antisepsis, to avoid further contaminating the wound. Three types of solutions are available for surgical hand antisepsis: aqueous scrubs; alcohol rubs; and alcohol rubs containing additional active ingredients. Although aqueous scrubs containing chlorhexidine and povidone–iodine (PI) have withstood the test of time, newer alcohol-based rubs offer the advantage of rapid and immediate action, as well as reduced skin damage after repeated use. The clinical use of an alcohol-based hand rub (Avagard, 3M Healthcare) was tested in the environment of an equine hospital and found to be as effective for presurgical hand antisepsis as the traditional water-based chlorhexidine hand scrubs in reducing the number of colony-forming units on the hands of surgeons prior to elective equine surgeries.[14] Verwilghen *et al.* recently found that a commercial alcohol-based hand rub (Sterillium, Bode-Chemie) was as effective as 4% chlorhexidine digluconate (Hibiscrub, Regent Medical) and superior to 7.5% PI (Vetclean, Ecuphar) in reducing the number of colony-forming bacterial units on the hands of equine and small animal surgeons and showed a superior sustained effect.[15] There are important differences between the various commercial alcohol-based hand rubs (concentration of alcohol, method of application, etc.); consequently, the manufacturers' guidelines for time and method of application should be followed. Using an alcohol rub may be more practical than using an aqueous scrub for achieving hand antisepsis in the field situation.

Sterile lubricating gel should be placed within the wound prior to clipping the hair on the surrounding skin. This prevents tiny hairs from accumulating within the wound, and the gel can be easily rinsed away after clipping. Placing gauzes impregnated with isotonic saline solution within the wound prior to clipping is an acceptable alternative to using a gel. The skin surrounding the wound should be scrubbed using an antiseptic detergent, such as chlorhexidine or PI, and then rinsed with sterile isotonic saline solution. Because surgical scrubs contain a cytotoxic detergent, they should not be allowed to contact the wound's surface. For more information regarding skin preparation (for both the surgeon and the patient), the reader is referred to Chapter 4.

Wound cleansing/irrigation

Wound cleansing involves the use of fluid, applied in a steady flow across the surface of the wound, to remove loosely attached cellular debris, contaminants contained in exudate, and residue from topically applied wound-care products.[16] The technique is also referred to as "irrigation" and this term is used interchangeably with wound cleansing within this textbook. Irrigating the wound is more effective than scrubbing its surface with gauze or sponges;

the negative effects of the latter technique, which damages the fragile new tissues in the wound bed, no doubt outweigh the benefits of decreasing contamination of the wound.[17,18] Pressurized wound irrigation is likely to be beneficial in reducing the bacterial count, as well as in eliminating dirt and tissue debris in heavily contaminated wounds,[19] such as those often seen in equine practice. In the author's experience, pressures ranging from 8–15 psi are beneficial in achieving the objectives of irrigation when managing wounds in horses; moreover, wound-care experts in the field of human healthcare claim that this range of pressure is strong enough to overcome adhesive forces of bacteria.[20] Pressures of 8–15 psi are unachievable with gravity flow but can be attained by using a 35- or 60-mL syringe and an 18- or 19-gauge needle.[21] Commercial irrigation devices are capable of delivering fluid under pressure and may be interesting alternatives. The volume of fluid should reflect the size and the degree of contamination of the wound. Irrigation should continue until the wound is rid of gross contaminants but stopped before the tissues take on a gray, waterlogged, edematous appearance.

The wound should initially be cleansed using sterile, isotonic, non-toxic fluids, delivered at body temperature. Unadulterated polyionic fluids, such as 0.9% saline solution or lactated Ringer's solution, are readily available and certainly appropriate but can be expensive when large volumes are required. A systematic review, conducted in human medicine, concluded that tap water offers a low-cost yet equally effective irrigation solution for acute and chronic wounds and does not seem to increase the risk of infection or delay healing beyond that which occurs when using isotonic saline solution.[22] The authors of that review, however, caution that the tap water must be of good quality (i.e., potable).[22] If large volumes of tap water are used, the wound must be monitored carefully for the development of edema. Some veterinarians perform an initial cleansing with tap water to remove the gross contamination of dirt and debris and then use polyionic fluids for a final irrigation, commonly performed in conjunction with some debridement. Some veterinarians may opt to add an antimicrobial drug to the irrigation fluids when cleansing chronic or severely contaminated/infected wounds. Antiseptics have a broad range of activity and are less likely to induce bacterial resistance than are antibiotics. Nevertheless, concentrations of PI or chlorhexidine must be kept very low to avoid the toxic effect of the antiseptic on cells and deleterious effects on healing, though what constitutes an ideal concentration remains controversial.[23–25] The concentration of PI should not exceed 0.2% (20 mL per litre of fluid), and that of chlorhexidine should be 0.05% (25 mL of the 2% concentrate diluted with 975 mL of fluid).[20,25,26] The addition of an antibiotic to irrigation fluids goes against current antibiotic stewardship, except possibly when cleansing wounds suffering from ischemia or in which the presence of a biofilm is suspected.[10,11,27]

The earlier a wound is cleansed the better, because in chronic wounds, bacteria may have formed a biofilm resistant to mechanical disruption. After a biofilm has formed, debridement is more effective than irrigation in ridding the wound of bacteria.[10]

The reader is referred to Chapters 4 and 5 for more information regarding techniques of wound cleansing and solutions used for irrigation.

Wound debridement

Debridement, ideally performed simultaneously with irrigation, consists of trimming jagged skin edges and removing necrotic debris and heavily contaminated tissue to reduce the bacterial load of the wound, thereby enhancing healing.

Although autolytic debridement occurs naturally, wounds of horses are often so heavily contaminated that this particular mode of debridement is rapidly overwhelmed, making a complementary means of debridement necessary. Sharp surgical debridement, using a scalpel, a curette, or a hydrosurgical device,[28,29] is an excellent method for rapidly cleaning wounds containing a large amount of devitalized tissue and/or bioburden and is less traumatic than is scraping the tissues with a scalpel blade or rubbing them with gauze. A narrow margin of skin at the wound's edge should be trimmed; this is followed by removal of devitalized tissues, often using a "layered" approach that begins at the wound's surface and progresses to its depths. The criteria governing removal of tissue are the tissue's color and attachment; the aim of debridement is to remove discolored and poorly attached tissue, leaving only healthy, bleeding tissue. Nevertheless, skin of questionable viability should be spared because the horse does not have an abundant supply of it and because skin contributes the most to healing. Dressing-enhanced autolytic debridement, enzymatic debridement, and biosurgical debridement (i.e., maggot debridement therapy) can be useful in wounds that are not closed primarily. More information regarding the various methods of debridement is available in Chapter 4.

After the wound is clean, it is explored to determine the extent of damage to structures deep to the skin, including bone, tendon, ligament, synovial cavity, sinus, or body cavity (thoracic, abdominal), and to rule out the presence of a foreign body. A common method of exploration is to palpate the wound with a sterile probe or a gloved finger. Particular attention should be paid to the presence of fluid within a wound located near a synovial structure. Plain or contrast radiographic examination of the region surrounding a deep wound or a wound suspected of involving bone, can be helpful; ultrasound may be used to identify an accumulation of gas or fluid or the presence of a radiolucent foreign body. More information regarding the techniques of exploration can be found in Chapter 4. Involvement of deeper structures influences the approach to closing the wound. For example, primary closure may be preferred when the injury involves the thoracic or abdominal cavity, bone, tendon, paranasal sinuses, or synovial cavity, whereas delayed primary closure may be more appropriate if one or more of these structures are involved but heavily contaminated.

Box 8.1 Initial wound management.

- Perform a complete physical examination.
- Cover the wound with a clean bandage before systemic problems are addressed.
- Provide sedation and analgesia, if indicated.
- Cover the wound with gauze soaked in isotonic saline solution or a water-soluble gel, and clip the surrounding hair.
- Clean the surrounding skin and administer local anesthesia to facilitate irrigation, debridement, exploration, and closure.
- Irrigate and surgically debride the wound.
- Explore the wound to determine involvement of deep structures.
- Select the appropriate approach to closure (primary closure, delayed primary or secondary closure) or manage by second-intention healing.

Primary closure

Primary closure is the preferred method of treatment for all wounds because suturing the wound protects it from further contamination, curtails the time required for complete healing, reduces scarring, thereby improving cosmetic and functional outcomes, and limits the cost incurred and aftercare required by the owner. For these reasons, even wounds that suffer a substantial loss of tissue can benefit from partial primary closure. When tissue has been lost, as much as possible of the wound should be closed, while avoiding excessive skin tension that might compromise the viability of tissue (Figure 8.4). This approach achieves a more cosmetic result than does leaving the entire wound open to heal by second intention.

Nevertheless, some heavily contaminated wounds and wounds containing crushed tissue are not amenable to primary closure. When closed primarily, these wounds often dehisce when contamination leads to infection, necessitating costly interventions.

The decision to perform primary closure is based on the location and conformation of the wound, the amount of residual contamination after cleansing and debridement, and the integrity of the blood supply to the wounded tissues. Closure may be performed with the horse sedated, using local anesthesia, or with the horse anesthetized. If the practitioner prefers to refer the horse for primary closure, the wound should be cleansed, and a protective bandage applied to the wound before the horse is transported. Potable tap water may be used to remove gross debris. If the horse is difficult to handle and the practitioner is unable to safely cleanse the wound with the horse standing prior to referral, a bandage should nevertheless be applied, after

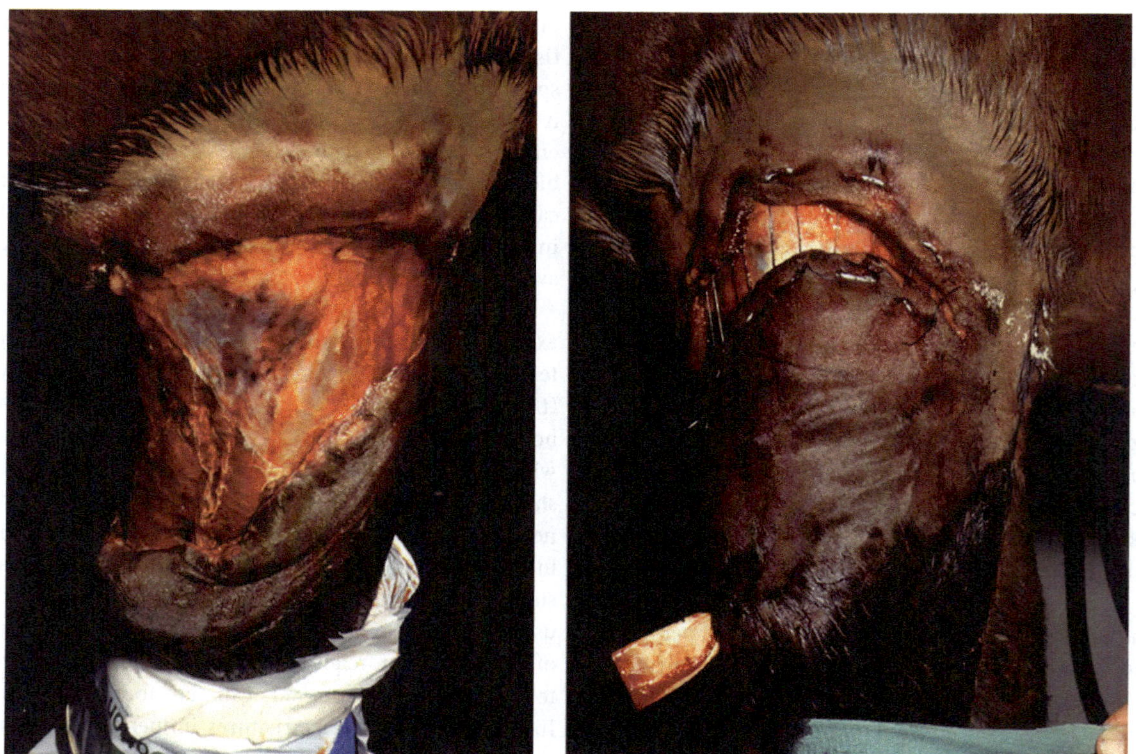

(a) (b)

Figure 8.4 Example of a wound that can be partially closed and in which a drain should be used. **(a)** Acute wound of <4 hours duration involving the proximal region of the antebrachium. Note the skin flap at the distal aspect of the wound is displaced distad. Suturing the skin flap into its normal position would create a sizeable dead space underneath the skin flap. **(b)** The wound could not be completely closed because of tension. Note the Penrose drain exiting the undermined skin flap at the distal limit of the flap. The drain was anchored by sutures attaching it to the skin, proximad and distad. The drain's exit site was covered with a sterile bandage.

sedating the horse. The bandage protects the wound from further contamination and trauma during transport and also reduces the development of edema.

Contamination

The degree of bacterial contamination of a wound is often difficult to quantify in the field or even in a referral hospital. An infective concentration of bacteria is considered to be more than 10^5 organisms per gram of tissue or milliliter of exudate.[1] The time to reach this concentration, however, may vary considerably according to the wound's characteristics; minimally contaminated, minimally damaged tissue likely takes longer to reach this concentration than does heavily contaminated, extensively damaged tissue. Even if the time elapsed since the injury is known (which is uncommon in equine patients), using time to decide whether or not to close a wound primarily is likely inappropriate.

Various methods may be used to identify the type or quantify the number of bacteria within a wound after cleansing and debridement. For instance, Gram-stained smears of the wound may be examined to identify the type of bacteria present at the surface of the wound, although examination fails to inform on the bacterial status of the deeper tissues and cannot be used to confirm infection. Alternatively, a sample of the wounded tissue may be used to provide, via serial dilution cultures of a homogenate, quantitative information on the wound's bacterial burden.[10,11] These methods of bacterial identification and quantification, however, are not practical in field situations. Moreover, bacterial virulence and the immune status of the horse exert a considerable influence on the outcome of contamination so that the actual concentration of bacteria is only one factor in determining if a wound is infected.

Therefore, in a clinical context, the veterinarian must rely on visual assessment of the wound. The amount of gross contamination within the wound should be considered. Clinical signs of infection, such as inflammation (redness, heat, pain on palpation, edema/swelling, or cellulitis around the wound) and purulent discharge, indicate that the wound is less likely to heal successfully after primary closure than is an acute, uninfected wound. The extent and nature of the inciting trauma can also guide decision making. The decision to primarily close a relatively fresh and clean wound with sharp edges is easy; these are wounds such as those caused by sharp metal objects (metal siding, hoof knives) (Figure 8.1). Conversely, crushing or repeated abrasive action usually causes more damage than is initially apparent. Because the health of tissues damaged in this manner may degrade, wounds caused in this fashion are usually not amenable to primary closure. Likewise, wounds contaminated by fecal matter or soil and/or that are edematous are unlikely to heal successfully by primary closure.

Blood supply

Sufficient blood supply to the tissues damaged by wounding is a prerequisite to successful healing. Blood flow is crucial to resistance to infection because it ensures circulation of the host's defenses, including functional neutrophils and macrophages, as well as systemically administered antibiotics. Moreover, oxygen, carried by the red blood cells' hemoglobin, is required for neutrophils to function and to nourish the healing tissues. Because infection of a sutured wound invariably leads to dehiscence, the integrity of the blood supply is an important factor to consider when deciding whether to perform primary closure or to defer closure until later.

The integrity of the blood flow may be estimated by various non-invasive methods, such as infrared thermography, which measures skin temperature as a reflection of cutaneous blood flow, or Doppler ultrasound, but equipment necessary to use these methods is not readily available in most clinical situations. Furthermore, data obtained from a fresh wound may be difficult to interpret because reflex vasoconstriction followed by vasodilation occurs in response to wounding.[30,31] Consequently, the integrity of the blood supply to wounded tissues is largely determined by clinical observation and is based on a sound knowledge of the vascular supply to the injured area.

The anatomic location and configuration of the wound should be considered, particularly if trauma has created a flap of skin. The length, thickness, and orientation of the flap have a significant influence on the flap's vascular supply. Because the blood vessels of the skin run subdermally in the subcutaneous tissues or are closely associated with the *panniculus carnosus* muscle with branching vessels reaching the surface of the upper portion of the dermis, preservation of subcutaneous tissues, fascia, or muscle within the skin flap increases the probability of conserving adequate blood supply and is especially important when the flap is long and narrow.[32] A skin flap on a limb, that has its base located proximally is ideal with regards to preservation of its blood supply, although flaps oriented in this manner are seldom seen. Conversely, a thin skin flap that has its base located distally frequently accompanies degloving injuries to the distal aspect of the limb and is predisposed to avascular necrosis. Wounds to the head, on the other hand, are often amenable to primary closure, regardless of the direction of the flap, due to the good blood supply of the area. Primary closure of wounds of the head is often necessary to protect underlying structures, such as bones or the paranasal sinuses.

General principles of primary closure

After primary closure is determined to be the best method of treatment, the wound is prepared, as described previously and discussed in detail in Chapter 4. Non-viable tissue, including the frayed ends of damaged tendons or necrotic bone, should be debrided. After the wound has been debrided, gloves and instruments should be changed, and the wounded area re-draped prior to suturing.

Although the method of closure must be adapted to the characteristics of the wound and the patient, several general principles apply to primary closure. Sutures are foreign material, and so, the smallest number of sutures required to effectively appose the tissues should be used (the reader is referred to Chapter 9 for more information regarding the selection of suture materials for wound closure). Tissues deep to the skin, such as underlying

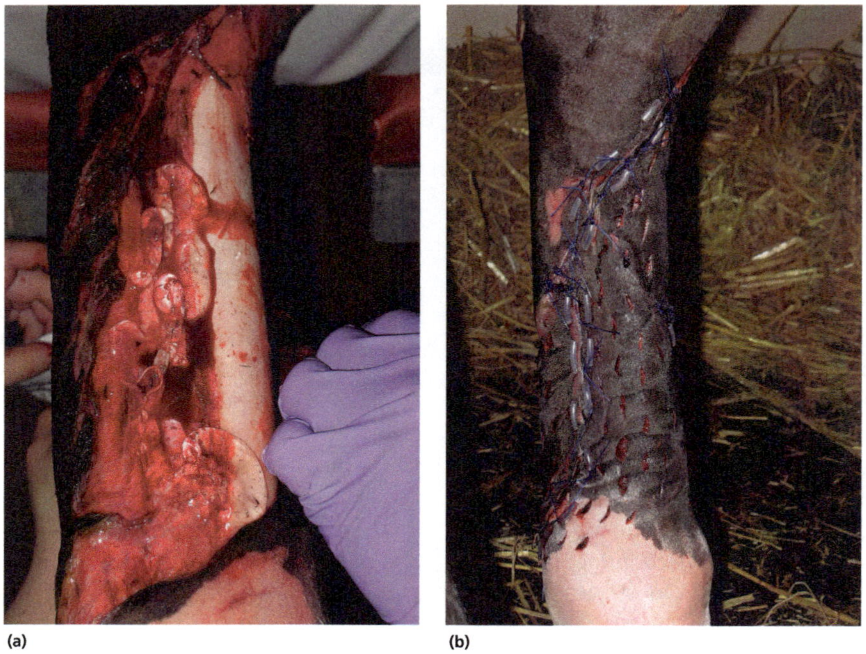

Figure 8.5 In this extensive degloving injury to the distal aspect of the limb, the extensor tendons are lacerated and the metacarpal bone stripped of its periosteum. Despite gross contamination and the likelihood that a portion of the skin flap would suffer avascular necrosis, primary closure was attempted to protect the deep tissues from desiccation until granulation tissue covered the bony surface. Healing even a small portion of a wound by primary closure reduces the amount of second-intention healing required, thereby minimizing scarring and improving functional and cosmetic outcomes. **(a)** Sterile gel has been placed in the wound during cleansing and preparation of the skin flap, prior to irrigating the wound. **(b)** Releasing incisions have been made to reduce tension on the primary closure and to allow drainage; these are best made in the skin surrounding the wound rather than in the skin flap, the blood supply to which is already compromised. Stents made of plastic tubing are used in combination with a horizontal mattress suture pattern, interspersed with sutures placed in a simple interrupted pattern. This repair was protected by a bandage–cast for 2 weeks. This wound healed well, with only a small portion of the skin flap (2 cm) at the proximal extent of the wound lost to necrosis 1 week after primary closure. Placing a bandage over stents can result in pressure necrosis so the wound should be monitored closely for signs of this complication. Pressure on the bandage overlying the wound should be reduced to decrease the likelihood of pressure necrosis from developing beneath the stents. If damage to skin beneath the stents appears, the limb should be left unbandaged, or the stents should be removed in a staged approach.

muscle, fascia, or subcutaneous tissue, should be closed to add strength to the skin closure and to reduce dead space, thereby preventing the formation of a serum pocket. Synthetic, monofilament sutures that are absorbed rapidly are preferred to appose tissues deep to the skin.

Sutures may be used to close large rents in a synovial capsule (the reader is referred to Chapter 16 for more information regarding the management of wounds involving synovial structures) or to appose the ends of a lacerated flexor tendon; suturing lacerated extensor tendons is usually not necessary (the reader is referred to Chapter 17 for more information regarding the management of lacerations of tendons and the paratenon).

If a skin flap is situated over muscle and fascia, "walking sutures" may be placed between the underside of the flap and the wound's bed to incrementally pull the flap towards the center of the wound or towards the opposite margin of the wound, while distributing tension and obliterating subcutaneous dead space. Care must be taken to align the wound's edges and to avoid pulling the flap in the wrong direction.

Tension should be relieved, if necessary, prior to completing the primary closure. Techniques used to relieve tension include: (1) undermining the skin at the edges of the wound to mobilize the skin, and (2) creating "relaxing" or "releasing incisions" in the skin parallel and adjacent to the wound's edges to allow the intervening, meshed skin to contribute to the closure of the primary defect (Figure 8.5). Creating a wound to close a wound is justified when the releasing incisions allow primary closure of a wound that exposes underlying structures (e.g., tendons, nerves, vessels, bone) in exchange for a new defect in a less obtrusive location.[32] Tension-relieving sutures may be used to lessen tension on the primary suture line although they should not replace efforts to relieve the tension on the skin using the aforementioned methods. Types of tension-relieving suture patterns include horizontal and vertical mattress tension suture patterns, with or without supports/stents placed between the suture and the underlying skin in an effort to delay the suture from cutting through the skin in places of tension. Supports can be made by cutting rubber tubing into short sections and threading these on to the suture between suture bites through the tissue. Tension sutures with supports should not be used beneath casts or pressure bandages because the supports may create pressure points on the skin, causing necrosis. As few tension sutures as possible should be used because the mattress tension sutures increase the amount of suture material placed in the wound. A simple approximating or everting suture pattern should be used in addition to the mattress tension sutures. The tension sutures should be removed within a maximum of 14 days and ideally in a staggered manner, over several days, beginning the first week after their placement. Timing of removal of tension sutures depends on the number of tension-relieving sutures used. The reader is referred to Chapters 9 and 10 for more information regarding methods to reduce skin tension during closure.

Because primary closure used to manage accidental wounds is commonly performed on tissues with some degree of contamination, the opportunity for drainage should be provided to avoid trapping within a closed space, any bacteria, tissue debris, or components of blood that provide a medium for bacterial proliferation. Moreover, drainage is required to channel unwanted fluid or gas from the wound to relieve pressure that might restrict tissue perfusion, thereby compromising healing. Drainage can be provided by leaving an opening at the most ventral portion of the wound or by temporarily implanting a drain (Figure 8.4). To avert descending bacterial contamination, the proximal or dorsal extremity of a passive drain (e.g., a Penrose drain) should not exit the skin but, rather, should be buried at the most proximal, most dorsal, or deepest extent of the wound. It should be secured at this site using a single suture, tied on the surface of the skin adjacent to the wound. Passive drains should exit the wound or the dead space distad or ventrad to the most distad or ventrad extent of the wound, through a single stab incision created in a dependent position near the wound (Figure 8.4b). This extremity of the drain should be secured to the skin, with one or more sutures to prevent it from retreating into the wound, and be covered with a sterile, absorptive dressing, which must be changed regularly.[33] The frequency with which the bandage should be changed is governed by the amount of discharge from the exit portal of the drain. The drain should be removed after 2–3 days, unless there is a strong indication (copious discharge, infection) to prolong its use, because it is irritating to the tissues. The reader is referred to Chapter 9 for more information regarding the classification of drains and the principles of using drains in wound management.

Tips

- Use a different color of suture material, and leave the suture ends extra long when securing the drain. This facilitates distinguishing the suture used to secure the drain from that used for the primary closure of the wound when the drain is removed.
- If exudate discharging via a passive drain is not absorbed by a bandage, petroleum jelly should be smeared on the skin adjacent to the exit portal of the drain to prevent skin scalding.

What to avoid

- Do not expect drainage to fully resolve as long as the drain remains within the wound; the drain is irritating to the tissues, because it is a foreign body, and elicits continued production of fluid.

What to do

- Remove the drain as soon as the drainage decreases substantially in volume and changes from purulent or serosanguineous to serous, non-odoriferous, and non-turbid.

Wounds on the distal aspect of the limb – a special situation

In most cases, degloving wounds to the distal extremities should be managed by primary closure, even in the face of considerable contamination. This is done to provide a humid environment to exposed surfaces of bone and tendon, thereby encouraging the formation of protective granulation tissue (Figure 8.5).

A large retrospective study of primary intention healing of accidental wounds in equids, more than two thirds of which were located on the distal aspect of the limb, showed that an attempt at primary closure was successful (defined as complete healing by primary intention without any degree of dehiscence) in only 26% of horses and 41% of ponies.[9] Although a portion or even all of the wound can be expected to dehisce, an attempt at primary closure must nevertheless be made with the aim to avoid prolonged healing and the development of exuberant granulation tissue (EGT) associated with second-intention healing of a wound on the limb. Indeed, another study of 129 horses suffering a wound on the distal aspect of the limb that included laceration of a digital extensor tendon, found that wounds managed by primary closure (most often supported by some form of external coaptation) had a superior cosmetic outcome (i.e., less scarring). Moreover, complete suture of the wound was significantly correlated with a positive athletic outcome, with horses treated in this manner being 2.6 times more likely to return to soundness than those in which the wound was left unsutured or was only partially sutured. No other variables, including the location of the wound, presence of a functional tendon, or involvement of a synovial structure, were significantly associated with outcome.[34]

Tip

- Owner education is critical before attempting primary closure of a degloving injury to the distal aspect of the limb because dehiscence, followed by loss of the skin flap, is common (usually occurring within 5–10 days). The skin flap should be considered a form of temporary "biologic bandage" that, even if eventually lost, encourages the formation of healthy, protective granulation tissue over the surface of exposed bone or tendon.

For more information regarding the management and complications associated with wounds of the distal aspect of the limb, the reader is referred to Chapters 13, 14, and 15.

Delayed closure

Delayed closure combines healing by primary intention with healing by secondary intention and is sometimes selected as an approach to wound management when suturing an acute wound puts that wound at high risk of infection and subsequent dehiscence. To perform delayed closure, the wound is cleansed and observed for a few days, and after determining that it displays no signs of infection, the wound is sutured. Delayed closure may be performed after several days of open wound management, before granulation tissue has formed (referred to as "delayed primary closure"), or it can be performed after granulation tissue has formed (referred to as "delayed secondary closure"). Studies in rats have shown that healing and gain in tensile strength are not significantly postponed by closure after a moderate delay (3–5 days),[35] and meta-analyses of the human medical literature suggest that delayed primary closure may reduce the likelihood of infection at the surgical site of sutured contaminated and dirty incisions, though no such data concerning horses are available.[6,7]

Delayed primary closure

Delayed primary closure is considered a suitable approach to manage a wound that is heavily contaminated or where the injured tissues are excessively swollen due to the extent or nature of trauma suffered at the time of wounding. A common example in the horse is a wound caused by crushing (e.g., trapping of a limb between boards or railings). Wounds with a contaminated synovial cavity are often best managed by delayed primary closure to provide the time required to re-sterilize the synovial cavity (e.g., via joint lavage and the administration of appropriate antimicrobial drugs, either systemically, regionally, and/or intrasynovially) prior to closing the wound.

The main disadvantage of postponing primary closure is that delay results in the temporary expansion of the wound's surface area. This expansion, which usually lasts 7–14 days in horses, may impede suturing of the wound, thereby necessitating healing by second intention.

After the wound is cleansed and debrided, it is dressed and bandaged appropriately until it is deemed ready for suturing. Because primary closure is deferred due to the probability of infection and consequent wound dehiscence, dressing and bandage materials are selected according to their ability to manage contamination and control infection (the reader is referred to Chapter 6 for more information regarding wound dressings). Bandages should be changed daily or on alternate days so that the wound can be periodically debrided, if necessary, and so that the wound's readiness for closure may be closely monitored.

To counter retraction of the wound's edges during this "waiting period," skin sutures may be placed to span the wound (from one edge to the other), thereby holding the edges loosely in place. In spite of this effort, many wounds are not entirely amenable to primary closure after a delay of several days.

If delayed primary closure is selected as the approach to manage a degloving injury in the metacarpal/metatarsal area, loosely tied sutures should be placed through the skin adjacent to the wound. These sutures draw skin over the wound to serve as a temporary biologic bandage, which reduces desiccation of underlying structures (e.g., bone and/or tendon) that would otherwise be exposed, and limit retraction of the wound's edges. Rather than placing temporary sutures to manage the wound by delayed primary closure, the veterinarian should consider closing the wound primarily if contamination can be eliminated through debridement and the establishment of ventral drainage.

> **Tip**
>
> - In the case of an injury that has caused substantial blood loss, and perhaps shock (e.g., a heel bulb laceration that has severed a digital artery or a large wound to the body (Figure 8.6), managing the wound by delayed primary closure allows the patient's systemic status to improve and stabilize prior to closing the wound. The basic principles of cleansing and bandaging apply, and the wound is closed when the systemic status of the horse has improved and stabilized.

The wound is prepared for closure after the wounded tissues are no longer edematous and the risk of infection has diminished in response to appropriate management of contamination. Clinical judgement is the most practical way to determine the point at which the wound can be closed, although quantitative methods, if available, may be used to measure the wound's bacterial load. The wound should appear healthy, swelling should be minimal, and discharge should be clear, serous, and non-odoriferous. The wound is closed in much the same way as for primary closure. The horse is anesthetized, or the wounded region is desensitized by using local or regional anesthesia administered after the horse is sedated. The hair is clipped from the skin surrounding the wound, and the skin is scrubbed with an antiseptic soap. The wound may require a new round of debridement and the wound's edges often must be undermined slightly to mobilize skin. Sutures are used to appose the tissues, as with primary closure (Figure 8.6c). Often, when the wound is managed by delayed closure, the wound can be only partially closed as a result of the skin retraction that occurs during the first few days after wounding. Nevertheless, partial (delayed) primary closure is preferable to forcing the entire wound to heal by second intention, for the reasons enumerated previously.

Delayed secondary closure

Delayed secondary closure is carried out on a wound healing by second intention after a healthy bed of granulation tissue has formed. At this point, the wound is revised, and granulation tissue is trimmed or debulked, if required, to allow apposition of the wound's edges, often with the use of a tension-relieving suture pattern (Figure 8.7). If partial resection of the granulation tissue creates a dead space, a drain should be placed to prevent

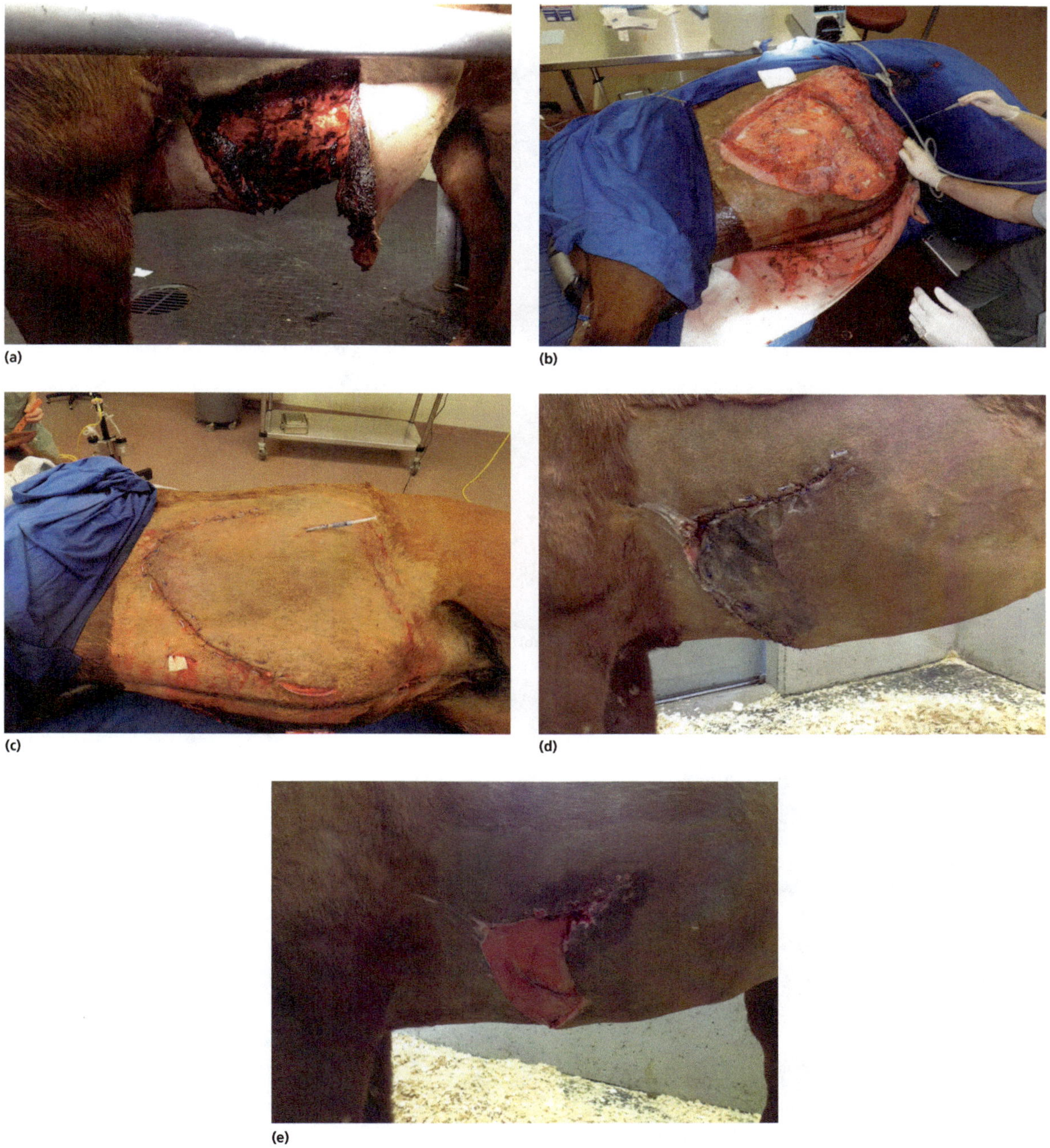

Figure 8.6 **(a)** Example of a wound in which primary closure was deferred due to the patient's compromised systemic status (i.e., shock requiring administration of fluids and a blood transfusion) and contamination of the wound with hair and soil. The wound was irrigated daily, dressed with honey, and bandaged. **(b)** Delayed primary closure was undertaken 2 days after injury, after the horse's systemic status had improved and stabilized. The flap has been debrided and is being irrigated with polyionic fluids. **(c)** A horizontal mattress suture pattern, in combination with stents made of plastic tubing, has been used to close the wound. In an effort to ensure adequate drainage of fluid produced by the wound, a passive drain (Penrose tubing) and an active drain (homemade with a syringe) have been placed, and the most ventral portion of the wound has been left unsutured. A simple approximating or everting suture pattern is commonly used, in addition to the mattress tension sutures, to maintain integrity of the sutured incision if the mattress tension sutures must be removed to avoid pressure necrosis caused by the accompanying stents. **(d)** Approximately 8 days after injury and 6 days after delayed primary closure, the cranial portion of the skin flap became necrotic (note the leathery appearance) due to insufficient blood supply. **(e)** The necrotic portion of the skin flap was excised, and the underlying wound bed, which was filled with healthy granulation tissue, was gently cleansed. The remaining wound healed by contraction and epithelialization, without complication, within 4 weeks.

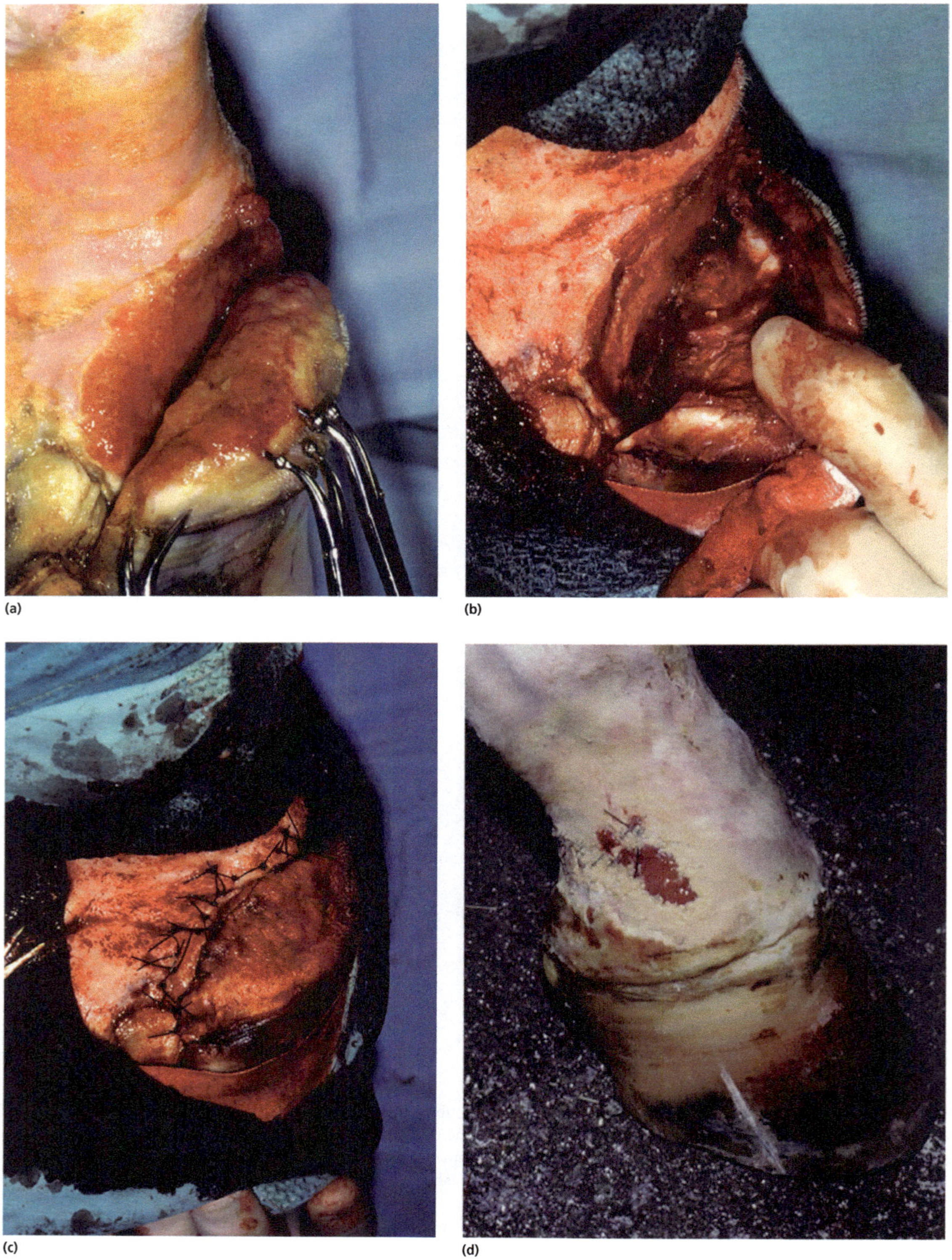

Figure 8.7 Same wound as in Figure 8.2. **(a)** The wound, 5 days later, after cleansing, debridement, and administration of antimicrobial therapy. Note the healthy bed of granulation tissue. This wound is ready for delayed secondary closure. **(b)** The wound, after excising granulation tissue. A portion of the lateral ungual cartilage was damaged and, therefore, excised (white tissue proximal to the gloved digit). **(c)** The partially sutured wound. The coronary band has been apposed at the heel bulb, but the skin at the dorsal limits of the wound (just to the right of the last suture) could not be apposed due to a tissue deficit (missing skin). A phalangeal cast was applied after surgery and left in place for 2 weeks. **(d)** The wound 2 weeks after cast removal. The sutured portion of the wound healed primarily, and the area of tissue deficit (granulating wound) healed by second intention beneath a bandage. The coronary band healed primarily, obviating the development of a defect in the hoof wall.

accumulation of fluid within the wound and subsequent separation of the tissue layers. A thick bandage or a cast is usually required to protect the repair when a wound closed by delayed secondary intention is located on the limb.

This approach to wound closure is relegated to wounds that are first seen by the veterinarian more than 1 week after injury or that are heavily contaminated or infected when first examined. The former situation arises quite frequently because many horse owners attempt to manage their horse's wound prior to consulting a veterinarian.[36–38] In the latter situation, the initial management consists of cleansing and debriding the wound and then dressing and bandaging it appropriately until healthy granulation tissue fills the wound. Various types of dressings or negative pressure therapy may be used to encourage fibroplasia (the reader is referred to Chapter 6 for more information regarding wound dressings and to Chapter 22 for more information regarding negative-pressure therapy).[39]

Delaying closure until after the appearance of healthy granulation tissue works well for contaminated or infected heel bulb lacerations; as is the case with primary closure of wounds in this area, the repair should be protected by a foot cast. The reader is referred to Chapter 7 for more information regarding techniques of bandaging and casting. Delayed secondary closure may be more challenging if the wound is located over a cannon bone, because mobilizing the surrounding skin sufficiently to suture the wound is difficult, even after the granulation tissue has been resected. Thus, primary closure, delayed primary closure, and second-intention healing are the only practical approaches to managing wounds in the metacarpal/metatarsal area. Free skin grafting of acute wounds or those that have developed a healthy bed of granulation tissue is also a useful technique to manage wounds in the metacarpal/metatarsal area and should be considered to avoid the long healing times associated with second-intention healing of degloving wounds in this area (see Chapter 18 for more information regarding skin grafting).

Second-intention healing

Healing of wounds is nearly always faster and more cosmetic when the wound is primarily closed. Moreover, experimentally created cutaneous wounds of horses healed by second intention have been shown to withstand a maximum breaking load equivalent to only 60% of the breaking force of normal, intact skin.[40] Additionally, skin appendages are usually absent in epithelial scars, resulting in the absence of pigmentation and hair as well as deficient functions, such as the production of sweat or sebum.

Unfortunately, many accidental wounds in horses are not amenable to primary closure because of massive loss of tissue or contamination. Moreover, wounds that are sutured often partially or completely dehisce. Indeed, a retrospective study of more than 500 horses with accidental skin wounds showed that primary closure was successful in only 26% of the horses and 41% of the ponies in which it was attempted.[9] Additionally, some owners are unwilling or unable to cover the immediate costs associated with primary closure of their horse's wound. Consequently, many wounds managed by equine practitioners must heal by second intention.

Second-intention healing relies on the body's ability to decrease the wound's surface area by contraction and to cover the remaining area with newly formed epithelium. Second-intention healing is selected to manage wounds characterized by extensive trauma to and/or loss of tissue and those that are heavily contaminated. Wounds caused by pressure or entrapment (e.g., a limb that has been trapped by a rope) are frequently treated by second-intention healing or by delayed secondary closure because the health of the traumatized tissue often continues to deteriorate after the injury was incurred, thereby threatening the integrity of any sutured closure. Burn injuries are another example of wounds best managed by second-intention healing and are discussed in Chapter 20.

Tip

- Allowing a wound to heal by second intention, while less expensive at the onset, usually incurs an expense similar to that incurred by primary closure because of the costs associated with labor (veterinarian's honorarium for farm visits to monitor healing or trim EGT) and with bandaging materials.

When second-intention healing is selected, the wound must still be cleansed and debrided to remove necrotic debris and reduce the bacterial burden. Good ventral drainage must be ensured to avoid accumulation of exudate and proliferation of bacteria within deep pockets underlying the skin. The wound is then dressed and bandaged, as required. The reader is referred to Chapters 5 and 6 for more information regarding dressings and the techniques of bandaging. The frequency of bandage change is dictated by the nature of the underlying wound and the selected dressing; additional cleansing and debridement may be required at bandage changes. If the wound is not bandaged, the skin ventral/distal to the wound should be kept clean, and petrolatum jelly applied to the skin to prevent scalding from serum and/or exudate draining from the wound. After healthy granulation tissue has filled the wound, the frequency and intensity of general wound care can be decreased, and at this stage of healing, many clinicians opt to leave the wound uncovered, particularly if it is located on a limb, to reduce the likelihood of having to trim EGT.

Wounds on the body left to heal by second intention often have acceptable cosmetic and functional outcomes, unless the wound was very large at the onset, necessitating healing, in large part, by epithelialization (Figure 8.8). Epithelial scars are thin and easily traumatized. Skin grafting may be useful to decrease epithelial scarring and should be considered in a wound healing by second intention as soon as the wound is covered by healthy granulation tissue (Figure 8.9); for more

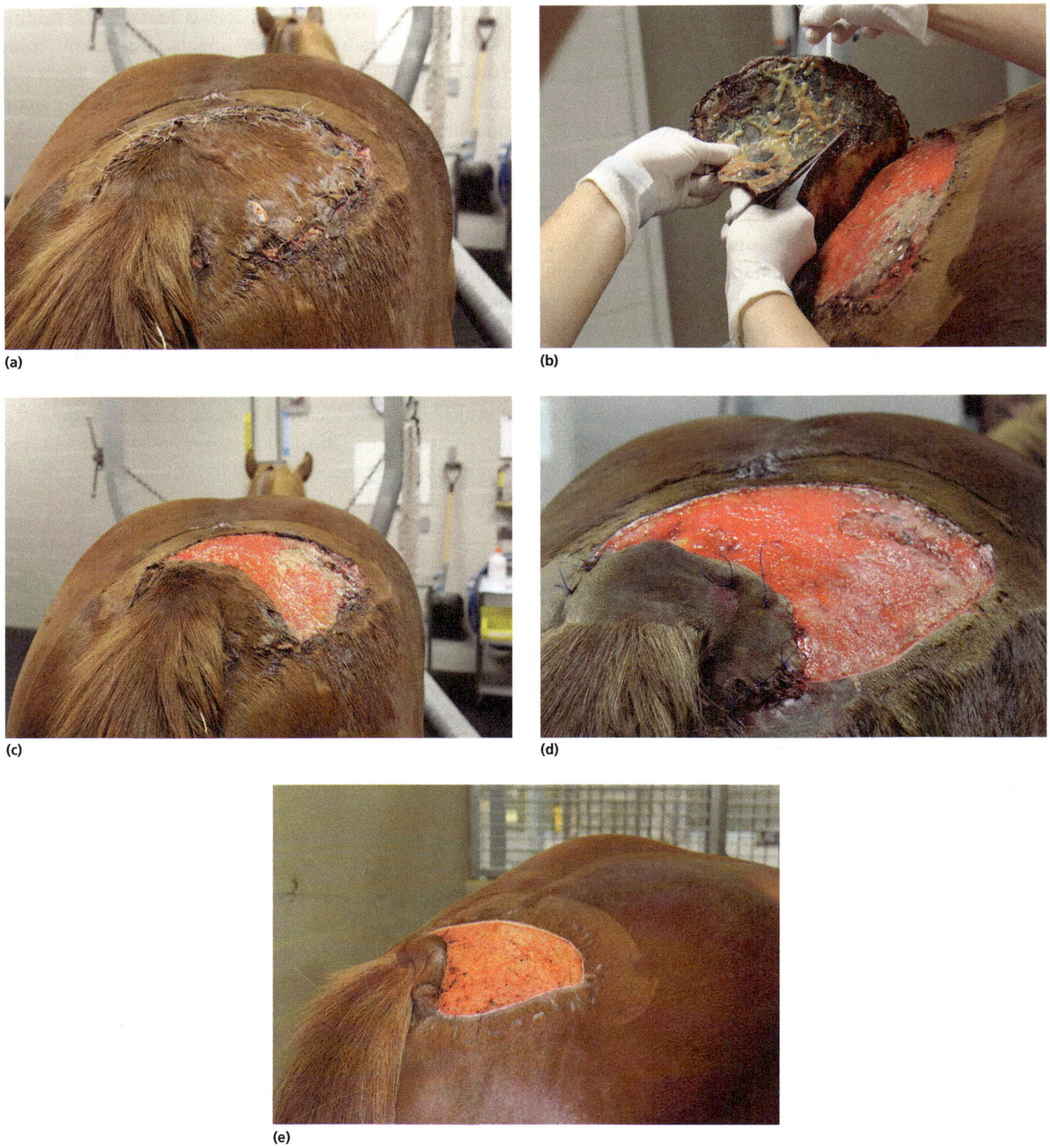

Figure 8.8 Injury at the tail head. **(a)** The large skin flap did not include any underlying muscle. The wound was closed primarily, in the field, by the referring veterinarian. Clipping of the hair initially proved difficult due to the attitude of the very young horse at the time of wounding. **(b)** The thinness and the orientation of the skin flap (the base was located caudally and the dominant blood supply arrived from the cranial extremity/apex of the flap), combined with inadequate ventral drainage, thereby trapping exudate, led to necrosis of the flap and the development of infection beneath it. Although it was ultimately lost, the flap served temporarily as a "biologic bandage." The necrotic tissue was excised. **(c)** The area beneath the necrotic skin flap is covered by healthy granulation tissue. **(d)** The wound bed, after cleansing and debridement. A few sutures were placed to anchor the skin of the tail head to prevent it from retracting further. **(e)** The wound, left to heal by second intention, has contracted and has a pink epithelial rim approximately 1 week after cleansing and debridement.

information regarding free skin grafting, the reader is referred to Chapter 18. Wounds in the axilla or groin often heal well by second intention, due to good ventral drainage and a generous blood supply to the region, whereas primary closure of wounds in these areas often fails due to excessive motion that, in the horse, is quasi-impossible to limit.

When possible, some form of immobilization (i.e., a thick bandage, splint, or cast) should be provided to support second-intention healing of a wound located in an area of high motion, such as the carpus or the tarsus. Immobilization limits the damage suffered by the early repair tissue during extension and flexion of the limb. Wounds on the distal aspect of the limb

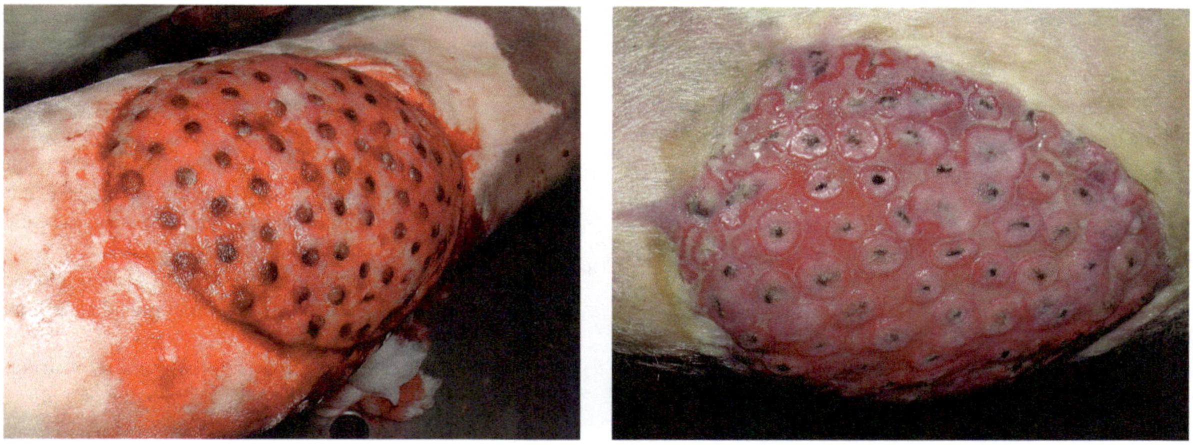

(a) (b)

Figure 8.9 This wound, located on the dorsal surface of the metatarsus in a draft horse, was initially left to heal by second intention until healthy granulation tissue filled the wound. **(a)** After this had occurred, skin grafting was considered because contraction and epithelialization appeared unlikely to result in rapid and complete healing of the wound. The wound was implanted with island grafts, rather than being covered with a sheet graft, because of the owner's financial constraints. **(b)** 10 days after island grafting. Tufts of hair surrounded by raised new epithelium are observed. In some areas, there is evidence of coalescence between the new epithelial islands. Approximately 80% of the punch grafts ultimately survived, which is the expected percent of graft "take" for island grafting. Courtesy of Dr. Christophe Celeste.

heal poorly by second intention; healing is prolonged, and EGT frequently forms.[9,41]

Conclusion

Selecting the most suitable approach to wound closure should be based on clinical assessment and experience, as well as a sound knowledge of the physiologic processes of wound repair. The aim is to provide pain relief and comfort and to return the horse, as quickly as possible, to its previous function, while achieving the best possible cosmetic outcome by minimizing scarring.

Assuming that primary closure is always the best method to achieve this goal is tempting. In some instances, however, primary closure invites wound dehiscence through infection. Tissues may be sutured when they are in a state amenable to healing, that is to say, with scant bioburden, good blood supply, and minimal edema/cellulitis in the surrounding skin. The choice of "if" and "when" to close the wound must be adapted to each wound and circumstance.

References

1. Robson MC, Heggers JP. Bacterial quantification of open wounds. *Mil Med* 1969; **134**: 19.
2. Miller M. Wound infection unravelled. *J Community Nursing* 2001; **15**: 31.
3. Zehtabchi S, Tan A, Yadav K, *et al.* The impact of wound age on the infection rate of simple lacerations repaired in the emergency department. *Injury* 2012; **43**: 1793.
4. Bowler PG. The 10(5) bacterial growth guideline: reassessing its clinical relevance in wound healing. *Ostomy Wound Manage* 2003; **49**: 44.
5. Caron JP. Management of superficial wounds. In: Auer J (ed). *Equine Surgery*, 1st edn. WB Saunders: Philadelphia, 1992: 232.
6. Bhangu A, Singh P, Lundy J, *et al.* Systemic review and meta-analysis of randomized clinical trials comparing primary vs delayed primary skin closure in contaminated and dirty abdominal incisions. *JAMA Surg* 2013; **148**: 779.
7. Siribumrungwong B, Noorit P, Wilasrusmee C, *et al.* A systematic review and meta-analysis of randomised controlled trials of delayed primary wound closure in contaminated abdominal wounds. *World J Emerg Surg* 2014; **9**: 49.
8. Rui-feng C, Li-song H, Ji-bo Z, *et al.* Emergency treatment on facial lacerations of dog bite wounds with immediate primary closure: a prospective randomized trial study. *BMC Emerg Med* 2013; **13** Suppl 1: S2.
9. Wilmink JM, van Herten J, van Weeren PR, *et al.* Retrospective study of primary intention healing and sequestrum formation in horses compared to ponies under clinical circumstances. *Equine Vet J* 2002; **34**: 270.
10. Freeman K, Woods E, Welsby S, *et al.* Bioflim evidence and the microbial diversity of horse wounds. *Can J Microbiol* 2009; **55**: 197.
11. Westgate SJ, Percival SL, Knottenbelt DC, *et al.* Microbiology of equine wounds and evidence of bacterial biofilms. *Vet Microbiol* 2011; **150**: 152.
12. Tremaine WH. Local analgesic techniques for the equine head. *Equine Vet Educ* 2007; **19**: 495.
13. Erkert RS, Macallister CG, Campbell G, *et al.* Comparison of topical lidocaine/prilocaine anesthetic cream and local infiltration of 2% lidocaine for episioplasty in mare. *J Vet Pharmacol Ther* 2005; **28**: 299.
14. Almeida da Silveira E, Bubeck KA, Rodriguez Batista E, *et al.* Comparison of an alcohol-based hand rub and water-based chlorhexidine gluconate scrub technique for hand antisepsis prior to elective surgery in horses. *Can Vet J.* 2016; **57**: 164.
15. Verwilghen DR, Mainil J, Mastrocicco E, *et al.* Surgical hand antisepsis in veterinary practice: evaluation of soap scrubs and alcohol based rub techniques. *Vet J* 2011; **190**: 372.

16. Rodeheaver GT. Wound cleansing, wound irrigation, wound disinfection. In: Krasner D, Rodeheaver G, Sibbold G (eds). *Chronic Wound Care*, 3rd edn. HMP Communications: Wayne PA, 2001: 389.
17. Mak SS, Lee MY, Cheung JS, *et al.* Pressurised irrigation versus swabbing method in cleansing wounds healed by secondary intention: a randomised controlled trial with cost-effectiveness analysis. *Int J Nurs Stud* 2015; **52**: 88.
18. Atiyeh BS, Dibo SA, Hayek SN. Wound cleansing, topical antiseptics and wound healing. *Int Wound J* 2009; **6**: 420.
19. Granick MS, Tenenhaus M, Knox KR, *et al.* Comparison of wound irrigation and tangential hydrodissection in bacterial clearance of contaminated wounds: results of a randomized, controlled clinical study. *Ostomy Wound Manage* 2007; **53**: 64.
20. Barnes S, Spencer M, Graham D, Boehm Johnson H. Surgical wound irrigation: a call for evidence-based standardization of practice. *Am J Infect Control* 2014; **42**: 525.
21. Singer AJ, Hollander JE, Subramanian S, *et al.* Pressure dynamics of various irrigation techniques commonly used in the emergency department. *Ann Emerg Med* 1994; **24**: 36.
22. Fernandez R, Griffiths R. Water for wound cleansing. *Cochrane Database Syst Rev.* 2012; **15**: 2 CD003861. doi: 10.1002/14651858.CD003861.pub3.
23. Sanchez IR, Swaim SF, Nusbaum KE, *et al.* Effects of chlorhexidine diacetate and povidine iodine on wound healing in dogs. *Vet Surg* 1988; **17**: 291.
24. Amber EI, Henderson RA, Swaim RF, *et al.* A comparison of antimicrobial efficacy and tissue reaction of four antiseptics on canine wounds. *Vet Surg* 1983; **12**: 63.
25. Berkelman RL, Holland BW, Anderson RL. Increased bactericidal activity of dilute preparations of povidine–iodine solution. *J Clin Microbiol* 1982; **15**: 635.
26. Wilson JR, Mills JG, Prather ID, *et al.* A toxicity index of skin and wound cleansers used on *in vitro* fibroblasts and keratinocytes. *Adv Skin Wound Care* 2005; **18**: 373.
27. Bowler PG. Wound pathophysiology, infection and therapeutic options. *Ann Med* 2002; **34**: 419.
28. Skarlina EM, Wilmink JM, Fall N, Gorvy DA. Effectiveness of conventional and hydrosurgical debridement methods in reducing *Staphyococcus aureus* inoculation of equine muscle *in vitro*. *Equine Vet J* 2015; **47**: 218.
29. Liu J, Ko JH, Secretov E, *et al.* Comparing the hydrosurgery system to conventional debridement technique for the treatment of delayed healing wounds: a prospective, randomized clinical trial to investigate clinical efficacy and cost-effectiveness. *Int Wound J* 2015; **12**: 456.
30. Celeste CJ, Deschesne K, Riley CB, Theoret CL. Skin temperature during cutaneous wound healing in an equine model of cutaneous fibroproliferative disorder: kinetics and anatomic-site differences. *Vet Surg* 2013; **42**: 147.
31. Di Scantolo S, Sagnelli M, Mancini M, *et al.* High resolution color-Doppler ultrasound for the study of skin growths. *Arch Dermatol Res* 2015; **307**: 559.
32. Provost PJ, Bailey JC. Principles of plastic and reconstructive surgery. In: Auer J, Stick J (eds). *Equine Surgery*, 4th edn. Elsevier Saunders: St Louis Missouri, 2012: 271.
33. Stashak TS. Selection of approaches to wound closure. In: Stashak TS, Theoret CL (eds). *Equine Wound Repair*, 2nd edn. Wiley Blackwell: Oxford, 2008: 183.
34. Mespoulhes-Riviere C, Martens A, Bogaert L, *et al.* Factors affecting outcome of extensor tendon lacerations in the distal limb of horses: a retrospective study of 156 horses (1994–2003). *Vet Comp Orthop Traumatol* 2008; **21**: 358.
35. Fogdestam I. Biomechanical study of healing rat skin incisions after delayed primary closure. *Surg Gynecol Obstet* 1981; **153**: 191.
36. Theoret CL, Bolwell CF, Riley CR. A cross-sectional survey on wounds in horses in New Zealand. *N Z Vet J* 2016; **64**: 90.
37. Sole A, Bolwell CR, Dart A, *et al.* Descriptive survey of wounds in horses presented to Australian veterinarians. *Aust Equine Vet* 2015; **34**: 68.
38. Owen KR, Singer ER, Clegg PD, *et al.* Identification of risk factors for traumatic injury in the general horse population of north-west England, Midlands and north Wales. *Equine Vet J* 2012; **44**: 143.
39. Howe LM. Current concepts in negative pressure wound therapy. *Vet Clin North Am Small Anim Pract* 2015; **45**: 565.
40. Monteiro SO, Lepage OM, Theoret CL. Effects of platelet-rich plasma on the repair of wounds on the distal aspect of the forelimb in horses. *Am J Vet Res* 2009; **70**: 277.
41. Wilmink JM, Veenman JN, van den Boom R, *et al.* Differences in polymorphonucleocyte function and local inflammatory response between horses and ponies. *Equine Vet J* 2003; **35**: 561.

CHAPTER 9

Selection of Suture Materials, Suture Patterns, and Drains for Wound Closure

Christophe Celeste, DrVet, PhD, Diplomate ECVS, Diplomate ACVS

Chapter Contents

Summary

Sutures play an important role in wound repair by supporting healing tissues. Understanding the various characteristics of suture materials enables appropriate selection. However, no single suture material is ideal, and compromises must be made. Proper suture placement, using specific patterns, generally ensures a predictable progression of wound healing and of scar formation. Drains, when properly applied, may help to prevent or at least lessen complications during healing. Sutures and drains are not substitutes for proper wound management because they cannot compensate for poor cleansing, debridement, and wound irrigation. Moreover, inappropriate use of sutures and drains may delay healing and may lead to scarring.

Introduction

Sutures serve important functions in wound repair, namely holding tissues in apposition and counteracting physiologic forces until healing progresses to the point that the tissue can take over this function. Sutures also provide hemostasis and obliterate dead space, thereby minimizing the risk of infection and promoting repair.

A broad range of suture materials is available. A sound knowledge of the properties of various suture materials, an accurate assessment of the wound's condition, an appreciation of the wound's location, as well as a good understanding of the healing process of the particular tissues involved in the wound, ensure selection of the most appropriate suture material by the surgeon, and thereby enhance the healing process.

Equine Wound Management, Third Edition. Edited by Christine Theoret and Jim Schumacher.

Companion website: www.wiley.com/go/theoret/wound

Although selection of the appropriate suture material is important, so is the surgical technique used to close the wound. Good surgical technique is mandatory because it significantly affects outcome. Proper placement of sutures allows precise approximation of the wound's edges, which helps minimize and distribute tensional forces on skin. Proper application of a drain facilitates elimination of dead space by evacuating accumulations of fluid and gas, thereby minimizing the risk of infection. Satisfactory results are best achieved when the surgeon uses the appropriate suture material and optimal suture pattern for wound closure, as well as the most suitable system of drainage.

The aim of this chapter is to review the various suture materials and patterns used to close wounds and to discuss the proper use of drains in wound management.

Suture material and selection

Optimal material

The optimal suture material should:

- be easy to handle and comfortable for the surgeon to use;
- have first-throw holding strength and good knot security;
- stimulate minimal tissue reaction to avoid creating an environment favorable to bacterial growth;
- retain adequate tensile strength until its purpose is achieved and then be absorbed without inducing complications;
- resist infection and have good elasticity to accommodate for swelling of the wound;
- be non-electrolytic, non-capillary, non-allergenic, non-carcinogenic, non-ferromagnetic, non-corrosive, and non-toxic;
- be inexpensive, readily available, and easily sterilized without altering its properties.

Although some of the newly available suture materials have many of these characteristics, none possess all of them; consequently, compromises must be made.[1–3]

Suture material characteristics

Suture materials are described and compared on the basis of their composition, morphology, and biologic and biomechanic properties. A sound understanding of the main characteristics of all suture materials is mandatory so that the appropriate suture is selected.

Composition

Sutures are made from naturally occurring substances, synthetic polymers, or metallic fibers. Natural materials, such as cotton and silk, tend to elicit a substantial inflammatory reaction and have mostly been replaced by synthetic materials.

Morphology

Sutures can be broadly classified as monofilament or multifilament. Sutures constructed of one filament (i.e. single-stranded) are referred to as monofilament, whereas those constructed of multiple filaments (i.e. multi-stranded) that are either braided or twisted together are referred to as multifilament. Multifilament sutures have greater strength and pliability than monofilament sutures of the same material and thus are easier to handle and manipulate for tying knots and are less susceptible to catastrophic damage from crushing or nicking. Moreover, less tension is required to ensure good apposition of tissues when using multifilament sutures, because they have a higher coefficient of friction than monofilament sutures; this characteristic also improves knot security. Multifilament sutures, however, have greater tissue drag and thereby injure tissue further when inserted and removed. Multifilament sutures have interstices between fibers, making them more capillary than monofilament sutures, which in turn, makes them more likely to absorb and retain fluid and bacteria.[1,2,4,5] Recent studies reported that biofilms show a preference for growing in the braid grooves formed between filaments; thus, multifilament sutures might be a predisposing factor for the formation of biofilms.[6,7]

> **What to avoid**
>
> - Avoid the use of multifilament sutures in contaminated or infected wounds.

Suture materials, especially multifilament sutures, can be coated with a variety of compounds, broadly characterized as water soluble or insoluble, including antibiotics, to increase pliability, reduce capillarity, decrease tissue drag, improve tying characteristics, facilitate knot formation, and lessen the likelihood of surgical site infection (SSI). Nevertheless, coatings, especially water-insoluble ones, tend to reduce knot security compared with similar uncoated suture.

Antibiotic coatings are now available on a number of sutures. The most common antibiotic coating contains triclosan (Coated Vicryl Plus Antibacterial; Monocryl Plus Antibacterial; Polydioxanone Plus Antibacterial – Ethicon, Johnson & Johnson Company, Inc.), a bacteriostatic drug that has been shown to inhibit the *in vitro* growth of both wild-type and methicillin-resistant *Staphylococcus aureus* and *Staphylococcus epidermidis*[8] and to reduce the incidence of SSI after clean, clean–contaminated, and contaminated surgery[9] without affecting tissue reaction, healing response, or the absorption profile of coated sutures.[10] The use of triclosan in many consumer products including soaps, toothpastes, shower gels, deodorants, etc., over the years has, however, led to the emergence of strains of bacteria that are triclosan resistant. A new synthetic antimicrobial suture coating, poly[(aminoethyl methacrylate)-co-(butyl methacrylate)] (PAMBM), inspired by natural antimicrobial peptides (AMPs), has been shown to provide bactericidal activity against both wild-type and methicillin-resistant *S. aureus* compared with the bacteriostatic property of triclosan *in vitro*. Because of their simple physical mechanism of action, AMPs display broad-spectrum activity against Gram-positive and Gram-negative bacteria, and it appears difficult for bacteria to develop resistance against them.[11] Such products have not yet been tested *in vivo* and are, therefore, not available commercially.

A variant in the morphology of suture material is the presence of surface barbs, created by placing linear nicks along the suture material. Self-anchoring, barbed monofilament sutures have been developed (V-Loc™ 90, 180 or PBT Wound Closure Device, Covidien, Medtronic; Quill™ PDO Knotless Tissue-Closure Device, Angiotech, Surgical Specialties Corporation, Inc.) in an attempt to eliminate knots, thus providing increased tensile strength and a stronger repair, and shortening surgical times. Knots are known to be the weakest portion of a suture line. Indeed, implanting, tying, and especially knotting of suture decrease its strength by up to 40%.[4] Knot-tying techniques are described later in this chapter, and the influence of various suture materials on security of the knot and suture line is summarized in Table 9.3. Contrary to expectations, studies report that knotless absorbable barbed suture devices yielded wound strength and tissue reaction scores that were comparable to traditional non-barbed sutures secured with knots.[12,13] According to Rosen,[14] barbed sutures have, however, revolutionized the approach of plastic surgeons not only by shortening surgical times but also by enhancing their ability to quilt and powerfully lift tissue and to eliminate surgical drains. Although little is yet known about the use of barbed sutures in the management of wounds of horses, the security and utility provided by this suture look promising.

Degradation behavior

Absorbable sutures degrade and lose tensile strength, usually within 60–90 days after implantation, either by hydrolysis, enzymatic digestion, or phagocytosis.[4] Their rate of absorption varies depending on their composition, coating, size, biologic environment, and species into which they were implanted. The environment surrounding the suture material is a major determinant of the rate at which the material is absorbed. Thus, although general times for absorption are offered as guidelines for clinical use, considerable variations in the rate of absorption and residual strength are noted. As an example, exposure to bodily fluids, such as urine, especially infected urine,[15] or gastric secretions, substantially accelerates the rates of degradation and absorption.

Non-absorbable sutures retain tensile strength for longer than 90 days, and, consequently, they are mainly used when extended support of the wound is required. Non-absorbable sutures are not degraded substantially after implantation and are usually encapsulated or walled off by fibrous tissue.

It is widely accepted that synthetic absorbable and non-absorbable suture materials are superior to the natural suture materials because the latter elicit more reaction, including inflammation; thus, the use of synthetic suture materials should be favored. The most important characteristics of commonly used absorbable and non-absorbable, natural and synthetic, monofilament and multifilament suture materials are summarized in Table 9.1 and Figure 9.1.

Suture size

Suture size is standardized to U.S. Pharmacopeia (USP) standards. The USP size (expressed with zeroes, with 12-0 being the smallest and 7 the largest) indicates a specific diameter necessary to produce a predetermined tensile strength, which varies among the different categories of suture material. The tensile strength of a suture material is the maximal stress that the suture can withstand before breaking. Tensile strength varies among suture materials and is correlated to suture diameter. The smaller the suture size, the less tensile strength the suture has. Sutures should be as strong as the tissue through which they are placed.[2] The tensile strength of the selected suture material, however, need not exceed that of the tissue it secures, and the rate at which the suture material loses tensile strength and that at which the wound gains strength should concord as much as possible to avoid dehiscence.[2] Consequently, the smallest-diameter suture that adequately apposes and holds the wound's edges during healing should always be preferred.[1,19]

Using an unsuitably large suture introduces more foreign material into the wound than is necessary, interferes with the blood supply, and may cause excessive inflammation, all of which alter the tissue's architecture and ability to resist infection.[1] Excessive tension on sutures leads to tissue necrosis, which favors wound dehiscence by interfering with local blood supply and increasing edema of the wound and surrounding tissues.[20–23] Most suture materials are recognized by the body as foreign and, therefore, can potentiate the risk of wound infection when used in excess (i.e., too much suture, too large a diameter, or too many knots).[1,24]

> **What to avoid**
>
> - Avoid selecting inappropriately large suture material and exerting undue tension on it.

If suturing alone cannot reduce the tissue tension to an optimal level, other tension-relieving techniques to mobilize the wound's edges should be used before closing the wound.[1,19,25] The reader is referred to Chapter 10 for more information about mobilizing skin to reduce tension upon closure.

Suture selection

The goal of suturing a wound is to provide secure partial or complete closure while minimizing morbidity. A sound knowledge of the suture material's properties, an accurate assessment of a wound's location and condition, and a good understanding of the process of repair of the particular tissues involved in the wound ensure selection of the most appropriate suture material by the surgeon, thereby optimizing healing. The following biomechanical principles should be considered in order to select the most suitable suture material and size:

- synthetic sutures elicit a weaker tissue reaction than do natural ones;
- suture material should be as strong as the intact tissue through which it is placed;
- temporal loss of tensile strength of the suture material and gain in strength of the wound tissues should concord;

Table 9.1 Characteristics of the most commonly used non-absorbable and absorbable suture materials.

Generic name	Trade name	Suture characteristics	Reduction in tensile strength*	Complete absorption (days)	Relative knot security	Handling	Tissue reaction	Comments
Polypropylene	PROLENE[a] SURGIPRO[b] SURGILENE[b] FLUOROFIL[c]	Non-absorbable Multifilament	Biologically inert No reduction after implantation		+++	– (slippage)	–	Higher knot security than all monofilament non-metallic synthetic suture materials Stable in contaminated wound environment Best suture available for skin
Polybutester	NOVAFIL[b]	Non-absorbable Multifilament	Biologically inert No reduction after implantation		++	++	–	Non-reactive in tissues Provides prolonged support for slow-healing tissues
Silk	SILK[a,d,e] SOFTSILK[b] PERMA-HAND[a]	Non-absorbable Multifilament Uncoated or coated	30% at 14 days 50% at 1 year		+++	+++	+++	Rapid loss of tensile strength Incites tissue reaction May potentiate infection Capillarity
Surgical stainless steel	FLEXON[b] STEEL[a] SYNETURE[h]	Non-absorbable Monofilament or multifilament	Biologically inert No reduction after implantation		+++	–	–	Greatest tensile strength of all sutures Inflexible ends can cause inflammation and tissue necrosis, leading to localized skin infection Tends to cut tissue
Polymerized caprolactam	SUPRAMID[f] BRAUNAMID[g]	Non-absorbable Multifilament Coated	Retains no tensile strength after 6 months		++	–	++ (if coating breaks)	Superior tensile strength compared to nylon Should not be buried since it absorbs up to 10% of its weight in fluid Elicits moderate to severe tissue reaction, swelling, and sinus tract formation
Nylon	ETHILON[a] NUROLON[a] DERMALON[b] SURGILON[b]	Non-absorbable Monofilament or multifilament	30% at 2 years (monofilament) 75% at 180 days (multifilament)		+	+	–	Incidence of infection very low, even in contaminated wounds (similar to stainless steel) Degradation products have antibacterial properties
Polyester/ polybutester	MERSILENE[a] DACRON[b] NOVAFIL[b] ETHIBOND[a] TICRON[b]	Non-absorbable Monofilament or Multifilament Uncoated or coated	Biologically inert No reduction after implantation		++	+	++ (when there is no coating or if coating breaks)	One of the strongest non-metallic suture materials available Provides prolonged support for slow-healing tissues Non-coated form has a high coefficient of friction Coating reduces friction and knot security Causes the most tissue reaction of the synthetic non-absorbable suture materials Should not be used in contaminated wounds
Surgical gut	CATGUT	Absorbable Multifilament	33% at 7 days 100% at 2–3 weeks	Unpredictable 70 days	– wet	+	+++	Rarely used Induces inflammatory reaction Rapid loss of tensile strength
Polyglactin 910	VICRYL[a]	Absorbable Multifilament Coated	25% at 14 days 50% at 21 days 100% at 35 days	Predictable 56–70 days	++	+++	+	Minimal tissue reaction, excellent handling properties, stable in contaminated wounds
	VICRYL Rapide[a]		50% at 5 days 100% at 21 days	42 days				

Polyglycolic acid	DEXON[b]	Absorbable Multifilament Can be coated	35% at 14 days 65% at 21 days	Predictable 60–90 days	++	++	+	Degradation products have some antibacterial effects Prematurely absorbed in the oral cavity and urine Tends to drag through tissues
Lactomer	POLYSORB[b]	Absorbable Multifilament Coated	20% at 14 days 70% at 21 days	Predictable 56–70 days	++	+++	–	Biomechanically superior to Polyglactin 910 High initial tensile strength
Polydioxanone	PDS II[a]	Absorbable Monofilament	25% at 14 days 30% at 28 days 50% at 42 days	Predictable 180 days	++	++	+	Maintains tensile strength over a prolonged period of time
Polyglyconate	MAXON[b]	Absorbable Monofilament	25% at 14 days 50% at 28 days 75% at 42 days	Predictable 180 days	+++	++	+	Best effective postimplantation strength and best knot security of all absorbable suture materials
Poliglicaprone 25	MONOCRYL[a]	Absorbable Monofilament	40–50% at 7 days 70–80% at 14 days	Predictable 90–120 days	++	+++	+	Very low tissue drag, minimal tissue reaction
Glycomer 631	BIOSYN[b]	Absorbable Monofilament	25% at 14 days 60% at 21 days	Predictable 90–110 days	++	+++	+	Minimal memory and excellent handling properties
Polyglytone 6211	CAPROSYN[b]	Absorbable Monofilament	40–50% at 7 days 70–80% at 14 days	Predictable 56 days	+++	+++	+	Provides short-term tensile strength combined with very rapid absorption

Source: Adapted from Celeste,[1] Kümmerle,[3] Schmiedt,[4] McPhail,[5] Toombs,[16] Blackford.[17,18]
*Values are approximate. Actual loss of tensile strength may vary
[a] Ethicon, Johnson & Johnson company, Inc.
[b] Covidien, Medtronic
[c] Mallinckrodt Veterinary, Schering Plough, Merck & Co
[d] Merck & Co
[e] C.P. Medical
[f] S. Jackson, Inc.
[g] Jorgensen Laboratories
[h] United States Surgical

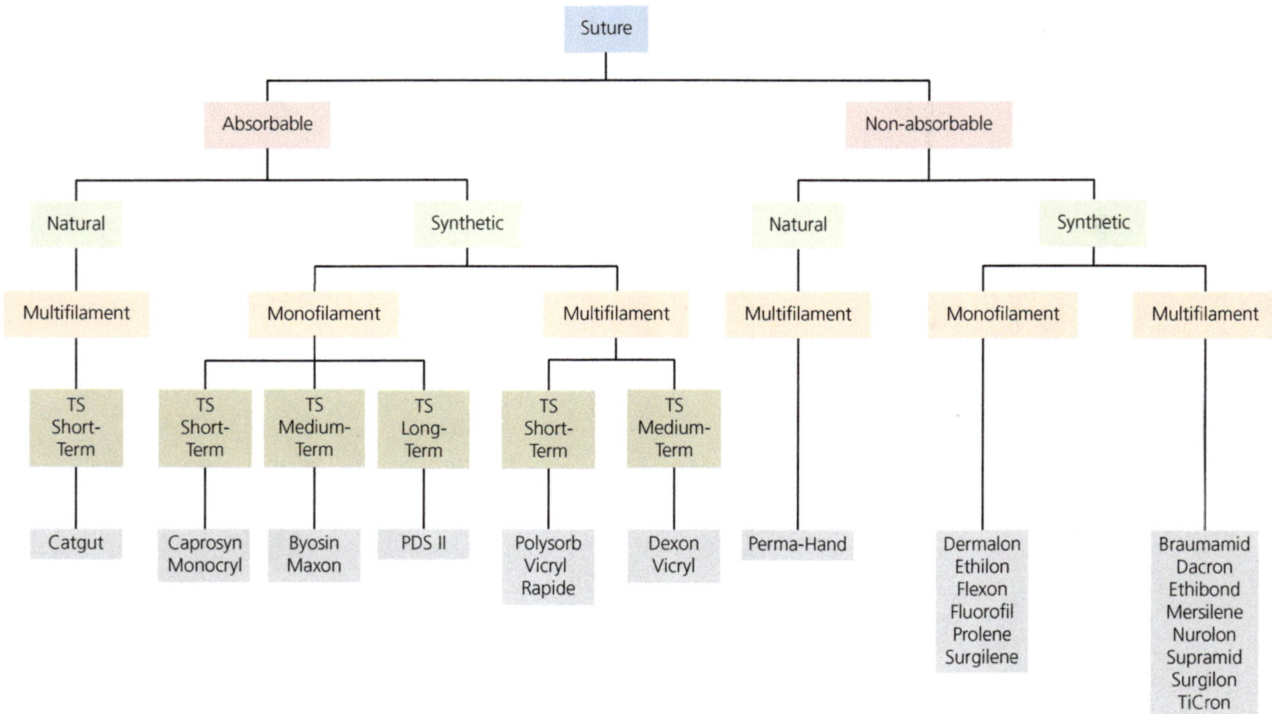

Figure 9.1 Characteristics of sutures most commonly used in veterinary medicine. TS, tensile strength. Source: Adapted from McPhail 2013.[5] Reproduced with permission of Elsevier.

- selecting inappropriately large suture material and exerting undue tension result in excessive tissue reaction;
- increasing the number of sutures apposing the wound edges and/or using tension-relieving techniques is preferable to increasing the size of suture material in wounds sutured under tension;
- the strength of a wound is more dependent on the injured tissue's ability to retain suture materials and the trauma created at the time of surgical repair than on the strength of the suture material itself;
- environmental variables, such as tissue pH, temperature, infection, or exposure to bodily fluids (digestive secretions, blood, milk, urine, etc.), can dramatically alter the performance of suture materials and should be considered when choosing the optimal suture for a given application.[1,15,16,25]

> **Tips**
>
> - Exposure of absorbable sutures to urine, and especially to urine infected with *Escherichia coli* or *Proteus* bacteria, results in a dramatic increase in degradation and absorption rates.
> - Exposure of absorbable sutures to either sterile or infected milk results in decreased suture strength.
> - Sutures with a glycolide component degrade more rapidly in an alkaline environment, whereas sutures with a dioxanone component lose tensile strength more rapidly in an acid environment.[4]

Guidelines for selecting the type and size of suture material for use in large-animal surgery have not been officially established. Table 9.2 reflects the author's preferences for suturing wounds of horses.

Surgical needles

Suture needles are manufactured from surgical steel and are usually described by the geometric shape of the body and point, the taper ratios associated with the point section, and the method by which the suture is attached to the needle.

Surgical needle characteristics

Surgical needles can be straight, half-curved, or curved into a 1/4-, 3/8-, 1/2-, or 5/8-circle configuration (Figure 9.2). The type of tissue and the wound's depth, size, and accessibility for suturing are factors that guide the selection of a needle's shape.[1,4] Straight and half-curved needles are most often used for suturing close to the surface of the body and are used almost exclusively to suture skin, whereas 5/8-curved needles are preferred for suturing in confined, deep locations. In most situations, the 3/8- or 1/2-circle needle is used because it is easier to handle within tissues than are the straight, half-curved, and 5/8-circle needles. The needle should be long enough to penetrate both edges of the wound in one bite. Its diameter should be the smallest that allows it to penetrate tissue without buckling or bending; the length-to-diameter ratio should be less than 8:1 to limit tissue trauma.[31]

The shape of the needle's point and body determines the needle's ability to penetrate tissue (Figure 9.3). Non-cutting (i.e., taper-point) needles have a sharp point and cylindrical body; they should be used whenever possible to minimize tissue trauma and inadvertent damage to vessels and nerves. Cutting needles are designed to penetrate dense connective tissues. The following types of cutting needles are available: (1) the

Table 9.2 Guidelines for suture material selection in equine wound management.

Tissue type	Suture size (USP)	Suture type
Skin – appositional suture	2–0 to 0	Non-absorbable monofilament (polypropylene, nylon, polybutester)
Skin – tension suture	0 to 2	Non-absorbable monofilament (polypropylene, nylon)
Subcutis	3–0 to 2–0	Absorbable monofilament (poliglecaprone 25, glycomer 631) or multifilament (polyglactin 910, polyglycolic acid)
Fascia	0 to 3	Slow absorbable monofilament (polyglyconate, polydioxanone) or multifilament (polyglactin 910)
Muscle	2–0 to 2	Absorbable monofilament (polyglyconate, polydioxanone) or multifilament (polyglactin 910)
Tendon	2	Slow absorbable monofilament (polydioxanone, polyglyconate)
Vessel (ligatures)	3–0 to 0	Absorbable monofilament (poliglecaprone 25) or multifilament (polyglycolic acid, polyglactin 910)
Vessel (sutures)	6–0 to 5–0	Non-absorbable monofilament (polypropylene, nylon)
Nerve	10–0 to 7–0	Non-absorbable monofilament (polypropylene, nylon) or multifilament (silk)
Eye – eyelid	6–0 to 4–0	Non-absorbable monofilament (nylon) or multifilament (silk)
Eye – sclera	8–0 to 6–0	Non-absorbable monofilament (nylon)
Eye – conjunctiva and cornea	9–0 to 7–0	Absorbable monofilament (polydioxanone) or multifilament (polyglactin 910, polyglycolic acid)

Source: Adapted from Boothe,[2] Blackford,[17,18] MacKay,[26] Miller,[27] Millichamp,[28,29] Nasisse.[30]

conventional curved cutting needle, the cutting edge of which lies on the needle's concave surface; (2) the reverse curved cutting needle, the cutting edge of which lies on the needle's convex surface so that the suture lies within the hole created by the needle and is less likely to cut through tissue; (3) the tapered cutting needle, which combines a round shaft with a reverse cutting point to make the needle useful for suturing delicate yet dense tissue (e.g., fascia, periosteum, tendons).[31,32]

Tips

- Non-cutting needles are designed to suture muscle, subcutaneous tissue, fat, and viscera.
- Cutting needles are designed to suture fascia, periosteum, tendon, ligament, and skin.

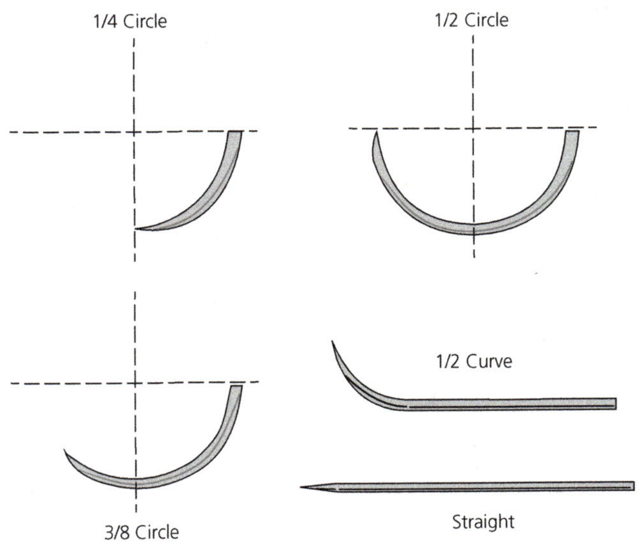

Figure 9.2 Various shapes of surgical suture needles.

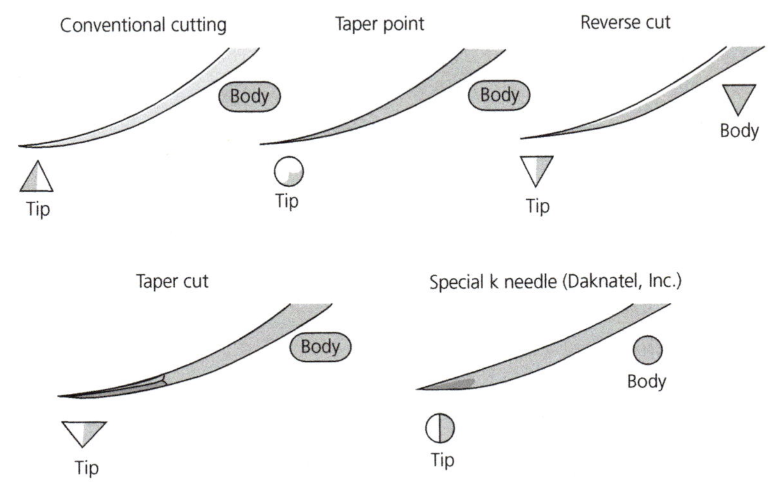

Figure 9.3 Various point and body designs of surgical suture needles.

Suture needles can be classified as non-swaged (i.e., eyed) and swaged (i.e., eyeless). Non-swaged needles have a closed eye or a ridged slit to hold suture as the needle is passed through tissue, whereas a swaged needle is attached to the suture by a crimp so that the needle and suture form a single, continuous unit. Non-swaged needles, which are reusable, are more traumatic to tissues than are swaged needles, because when using a non-swaged needle, a double strand of suture is pulled through tissues, whereas when using a swaged needle only one strand is pulled through tissue. In addition, non-swaged needles become dull with reuse and repeated cleaning and sterilization. Swaged needles are used more commonly because they are less traumatic to tissue, easier to handle, for single use only (and thus always sharp), and make surgery quicker, since threading the suture on to the needle is obviated.

Selecting the surgical needle

Selecting an appropriate suture needle is important for optimal healing of sutured wounds. Factors to be considered when selecting a surgical needle include: (1) characteristics of the tissue to be sutured; (2) configuration of the wound; and (3) size of the suture material.[1]

The needle should meet the following specific requirements: (1) the hole made by the needle should be just large enough to permit the passage of the suture material; (2) the design and diameter of the needle should minimize tissue damage (i.e. the sutured tissue should not be weakened by passage of the needle); and (3) the needle should have the appropriate design to permit rapid, accurate, and precise suturing.[32]

Suturing techniques

Because the blood supply at the margin of the wound is inversely proportional to the tension on the closed wound, sutures must be placed accurately and without tension to maximize blood flow to the edges of the wound, which in turn optimizes healing and minimizes the likelihood of scarring.

Suture placement

The choice of where the suture is placed in relation to the wound is often influenced by the configuration and biomechanical properties of the wound. A common recommendation is to place sutures at a distance from the wound's edge equal to the thickness of the wound's edge. Factors, such as tension on the edges of the wound and the thickness and stiffness of the lacerated tissues, however, must also be considered. Inflammation and lysis of collagen by collagenases occur during the early phases of wound healing and remain high within 0.5 cm of a skin incision. These processes weaken the suture-holding power of a wound, so sutures should be placed at least 0.5 cm from the wound's edge for improved security.[33] Because new epithelium lacks holding power, sutures should be placed well back from the wound's edge to ensure optimal holding strength when repair is to be achieved by delayed secondary closure.

For both human and veterinary patients, placing interrupted sutures 0.5 cm apart generally ensures good apposition of tissue, minimal tension on individual sutures, and maximum holding strength.[1,3,33,34] Placing interrupted sutures closer together than this may result, in some instances, in delayed healing, because of excessive reaction by the tissue to the suture and interference to the blood supply of the wound's edges.[1] Spacing between sutures can be increased in thick-skinned regions and regions where incisions or lacerations are parallel to the skin's lines of tension. The opposite is true in thin-skinned regions and regions where incisions or lacerations are perpendicular to the lines of tension.[1]

> **Tip**
>
> - Place sutures in sufficient number to provide good apposition of edges of the wound (Figure 9.4).

Suture knots

Sutures are most commonly tied in a square knot because this knot is among the most secure. When the first throw of a square knot does not accurately appose the wound's edges, the knot can be modified into a surgeon's knot (Figure 9.5a). The surgeon's knot, however, places more suture material within the wound, thus potentiating the likelihood of infection. Moreover, use of a surgeon's knot with some suture materials (e.g., chromic catgut) may decrease the structural stiffness of the knot; therefore, the surgeon's knot should be used only when needed to achieve accurate apposition of the wound's edges. The influence of knot-tying techniques and the characteristics of suture materials on the security of the knot and suture line are summarized in Table 9.3. The three techniques of knot-tying, the one-handed tie, the two-handed tie, and the instrument tie, are discussed

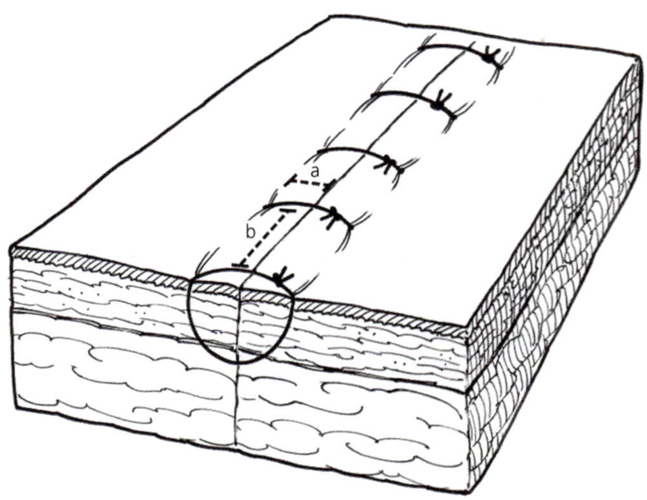

Figure 9.4 Simple interrupted suture pattern. Knots should be offset so they do not rest upon the apposed skin margins. Sutures should be placed close enough to prevent gaping. a = distance from the wound edge the suture should be placed to ensure optimal holding strength (>0.5 cm). b = minimal distance between two consecutive suture bites (±0.5 cm).

in depth elsewhere (ETHICON Knot-Tying Manual – freely available online) and, therefore, are not discussed here.

Knots, when placed in subcutaneous or intradermal tissue, must be buried (Figure 9.5b and Figure 9.6) to reduce irritation caused by rubbing of the knot against superficial tissue and to prevent extrusion of the suture. To decrease the likelihood of extrusion of buried suture, the volume of suture material should be kept to a minimum, useless throws should be avoided (Table 9.3), the knots should be as flat as possible and positioned perpendicular to the suture line, and the suture end length should not exceed 3 mm, which is the minimum recommended length to optimize knot integrity.[1,3,36] The use of inappropriately large suture material increases the size of knots buried immediately beneath or within the skin. These knots can cause excessive pressure on overlying skin leading to local skin necrosis, extrusion of the suture, infection of the wound, and a poor cosmetic outcome.

Table 9.3 Minimal number of throws required (including the first) for a secure square knot in interrupted suture patterns and continuous suture patterns. abs, absorbable; non-abs, non-absorbable; mono, monofilament; multi, multifilament.

Suture type	Interrupted suture pattern	Beginning continuous suture pattern	Ending continuous suture pattern
Polydioxanone abs, mono	4	4	7
Catgut abs, multi	3	4	5–6
Polyglycolic acid abs, multi	3	3	5–6
Polyglactin 910 abs, multi	3	3	5–6
Polypropylene non-abs, mono	3	3	5–6
Nylon non-abs, multi/mono	4	4	6–7

Source: Adapted from Rosin 1998.[35]

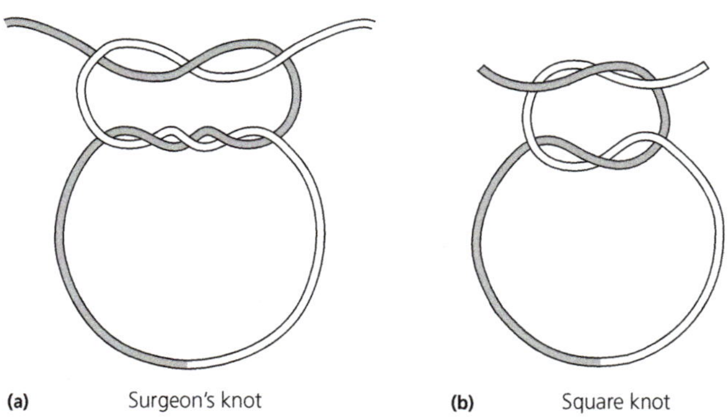

Figure 9.5 Surgical knots. (a) Surgeon's. (b) Square.

Suture patterns

A wide variety of suture patterns has been described for use in animals and people. The patterns are classified as interrupted or continuous by the way in which they appose tissue, or as appositional, everting, inverting, or tension-relieving by the way they overcome tension that may disrupt accurate approximation. Inverting sutures are rarely used in wound management and, therefore, are not discussed in this chapter. Sutures can further be classified according to the tissues they appose (e.g., muscular or subcutaneous).

In wounds characterized by no loss of tissue, such as most surgical wounds, an appositional suture pattern provides superior approximation of the edges of the wound, leading to secure closure and good cosmetic results. Wounds with large defects or loss of tissue, such as most accidental wounds in horses, are much more difficult to close without creating tension on the suture line. Tension sutures redistribute tension across the edges of the wound, minimizing interruption of blood flow and necrosis. Everting sutures are sometimes useful to close skin because skin edges apposed with appositional sutures tend to invert during healing.[1]

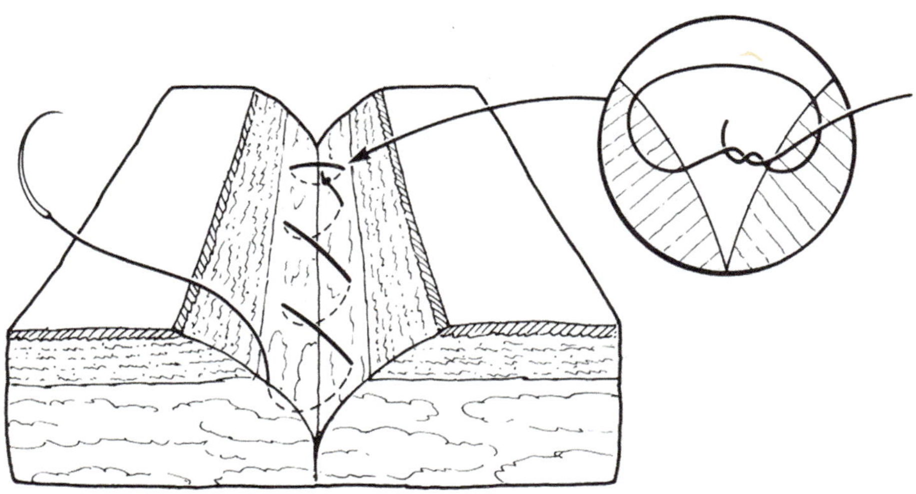

Figure 9.6 Suture placement for a subcutaneous continuous or running suture pattern. The initial knot is buried in the subcutaneous tissues.

The reader is referred to Table 9.4 and Table 9.5 for the general features and the common uses of appositional (Figures 9.7, 9.8, 9.9, 9.10, 9.11, 9.12, 9.13, 9.14, 9.15, and 9.16), everting (Figures 9.10a and 9.12a), and tension sutures (Figures 9.17, 9.18, 9.19, 9.20, 9.21, 9.22, and 9.23).

Interrupted versus continuous suture patterns

The choice of an interrupted over a continuous suture pattern is somewhat contentious because both types of patterns have advantages and disadvantages. The major advantages of using an interrupted suture pattern are the ability of interrupted

Table 9.4 Appositional suture patterns for wound management.

Suture type	Advantages	Disadvantages	Common uses
Simple interrupted (SI) (Figure 9.7)	Easily and quickly applied Precise suture tension possible Minimally alters the skin architecture Provides secure, anatomic closure Concurrent closure of skin, subcutis, and underlying fascia may reduce dead space Minimal alteration in blood supply	Requires increased time for placement Excessive tension causes inversion of skin margins	Skin, subcutis, fascia, blood vessels, nerves
Interrupted intradermal (II) or subcuticular (Figure 9.8)	Similar to SI (upsidedown SI suture placed in dermis and subcutis)	Requires increased time for placement compared to SI and continuous suture patterns	Intradermal skin closure Rarely used
Interrupted cruciate or cross mattress (Figure 9.9)	Easiest of all mattress sutures to apply, more rapidly applied than SI No alteration of blood supply even when placed under tension Provides stronger closure than SI Resists tension Prevents eversion of wound edges at fascia level	Excessive tension causes inversion of skin margins Skin margins tend to gap between sutures	Fascia (occasionally skin)
Interrupted vertical mattress (IVM) (Figure 9.10)	Provides precise wound edge-to-edge apposition with slight eversion when tied Minimal alteration in skin blood supply A single layer can be used for concurrent closure of skin and subcutis to eliminate dead space	Takes longer to apply and creates slightly more inflammation because suture passes through tissue four times	Skin, subcutis, fascia Can be alternated with SI sutures to prevent inversion and gaping
Allgöwer corium vertical mattress (Figure 9.11)	Minimal trauma (through dermis only) Perfect alignment of skin margins without inversion and with minimal or no eversion Cosmetically superior closure	–	Skin
Interrupted horizontal mattress (IHM) (Figures 9.12)	Appositional to everting suture, depending on suture tension and whether suture penetrates tissue full or split thickness Requires less suture material than IVM	Tends to reduce skin blood supply Potential for tissue strangulation (can be reduced with stents) Excessive scar formation when used alone because of skin eversion and gaping	Skin, subcutis, fascia, muscle, tendon
Simple continuous (SC) (Figure 9.13)	Saves time Promotes suture economy Provides good apposition of wound edges or skin margins Provides airtight or watertight seal	Good only for layers under low tension Provides less strength than SI Gain in wound tensile strength delayed compared to SI Excessive tension causes puckering and strangulation of skin	Skin, subcutis, fascia, blood vessels
Continuous intradermal or subcuticular (Figure 9.14)	Similar to II Saves time Promotes suture economy	Provides less strength than skin closure	Intradermal skin closure
Continuous mattress; horizontal (Figure 9.15a) and vertical (Figure 9.15b)	Horizontal: appositional to everting suture, depending on suture tension; facilitates rapid closure Vertical: minimal alteration in blood supply; precise edge-to-edge contact	Horizontal: can cause skin eversion/gaping Vertical: difficult to apply; rarely used	Skin, subcutis, fascia
Continuous lock or Ford interlocking (Figure 9.16)	Similar to SC Provides greater security than SC if broken	Similar to SC Requires large amount of suture Time consuming to apply May cause pressure necrosis and become buried when placed under tension	Skin

Source: Adapted from Celeste,[1] Toombs,[16] Blackford,[17] Provost.[19]

Table 9.5 Tension suture patterns for wound management.

Suture type	Advantages	Disadvantages	Common Uses
Interrupted vertical mattress (IVM) (Figure 9.17)	Minimal alteration to cutaneous blood supply Adding more, widely placed rows of IVM suture reduces tension on appositional primary suture line Stronger than IHM in tissues under tension	Occasionally suture will cut out when placed under excessive tension	Undermined skin under tension Used with supports (bandage, buttons, stents)
Interrupted horizontal mattress (IHM) (Figure 9.18)	Placed widely, IHM suture reduces tension on appositional primary suture line Less suture material than IVM	Tends to compromise skin blood supply Does not reduce tension as effectively as IVM Potential for tissue strangulation (can be reduced with stents)	Skin, subcutis, fascia, muscle, tendon Supports are added to reduce cutting out of sutures in regions that cannot be bandaged
Quilled or stented (Figure 9.19)	Similar to IVM (variation of IVM that loops over a stent on either side of incision) Very effective in reducing tension on appositional primary suture line Everting mainly Can also be a variation of the IHM	Skin necrosis underneath the quilled/stented sutures can occur if too much suture tension Should not be used under a cast	Combined with appositional suture for skin in areas of extreme tension where bandage cannot be applied
Near and far (or far and near) (Figure 9.20)	Combines tension suture (far portion) and appositional suture (near portion) Higher tensile strength than either SI or mattress pattern Provides necessary tension for wound edge approximation without applying tension to wound edge itself	Excessive tightening can cause inversion Leaves large amount of suture material in wound	Skin, subcutis, fascia
Looking loop (LL) (Figure 9.21)	Provides good apposition compared with other tendon sutures, with equal holding strength	May compromise intrathecal blood supply	Tendons
Three loop pulley (Figure 9.22)	Has slightly higher tension strength compared to LL Minimal alteration to blood supply	More suture is exposed compared to LL	Tendons
Intraneural (Figure 9.23)	Centrally placed neurorrhaphy suture anchored externally with silicone buttons	N/A	Nerve

Source: Adapted from Celeste,[1] Toombs,[16] Blackford,[17] Provost.[19]

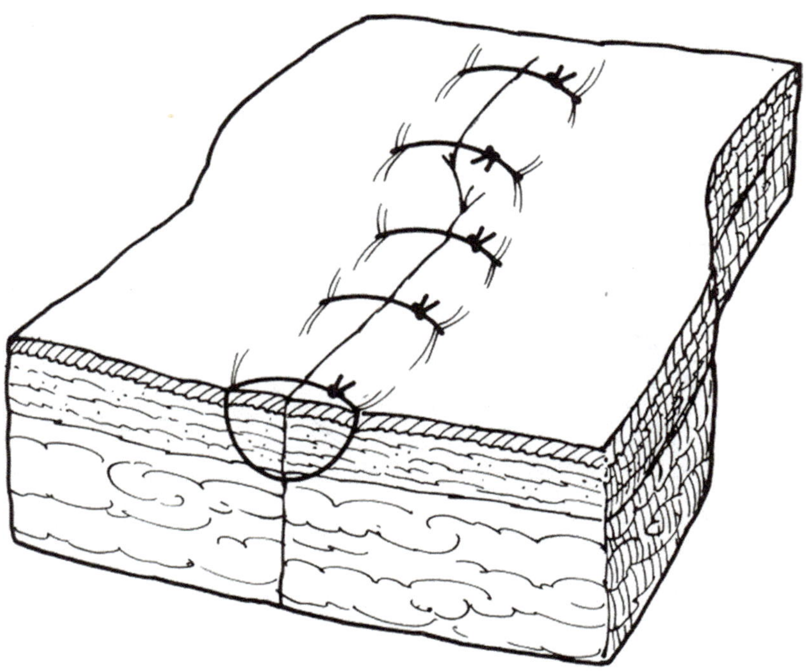

Figure 9.7 Simple interrupted suture pattern. The independent nature of each suture allows for mobility and use in irregularly shaped areas.

sutures to precisely control tension at each point along the wound, the possibility of making adjustments to improve alignment of the edges of an irregularly shaped laceration, and the minimal interference of the suture pattern with the skin's blood supply.[1,19] Disadvantages of using an interrupted suture pattern include increased surgical time (to tie multiple knots and cut the suture ends), increased volume of foreign material within the wound when the sutures are buried, increased risk of wound dehiscence,[37] and poor economic use of suture material.[16]

In contrast, a continuous suture pattern is quickly placed, thus reducing surgical time; distributes tension evenly along the entire length of the wound; uses less suture material, thus reducing cost; and minimizes the number of knots, thus reducing the amount of foreign material within the wound (Figure 9.13).[16] A continuous pattern also forms a better seal against fluid and air.[38] On the downside, the tension on a continuous suture line cannot be varied to the same degree as can tension on an interrupted suture pattern, and failure of the knot or suture material can have a disastrous effect on the closure. Suture used in a continuous pattern, therefore, must be handled carefully. Instrument-induced trauma to the suture should be avoided (e.g., grasping the suture with needle holders or thumb forceps), throws of the knots should be applied correctly, and the knots should be secure. Because of their design, continuous suture patterns tend to compromise the microvascular supply to the edges of the wound.[39] If the compromise is marked, it may lead to the formation of edema that, in turn, can prolong the inflammatory phase of wound healing and delay the wound's gain in tensile strength. The Ford interlocking suture pattern represents a compromise between interrupted and continuous suture patterns (Figure 9.16).

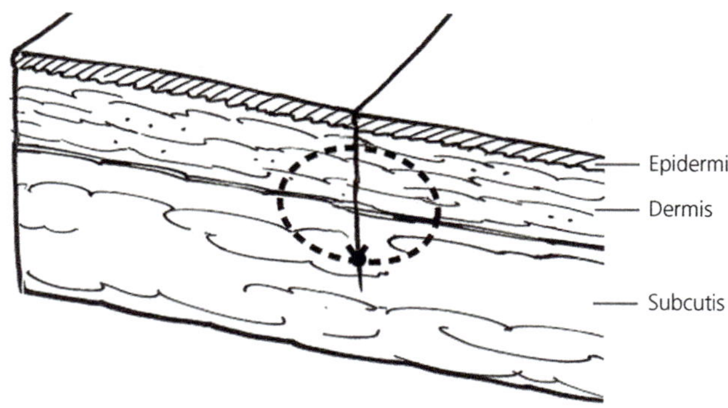

Figure 9.8 Interrupted intradermal suture.

Inverting versus everting suture patterns

Disrupted tissue may be apposed using a suture pattern that inverts or everts tissues, depending on the wound's location. Inversion is usually desirable only to close hollow viscera to prevent leakage, but excessive inversion reduces luminal diameter. Slight eversion to counter the tendency of edges of a cutaneous wound to invert during healing is desirable because slight eversion leads to the most cosmetic outcome after sutures are removed.[1]

Tension sutures

Wounds suffering from a substantial loss of tissue are difficult to close without creating tension on the suture line. Some suture patterns offer mechanical advantages over others, by requiring less force to close the wound.[40] Although clinical experience suggests that a moderate amount of tension is acceptable in sutured wounds of horses,[19] when the forces exerted by individual sutures increase to the point where sutures cut through tissue and restrict blood flow, tension sutures should be used. Tension sutures draw the wound edges together while minimizing the risk of vascular damage, which leads to necrosis and dehiscence.

Tension sutures, which are usually everting sutures (Figures 9.10a, 9.12a), placed well away from the wound edges to avoid strangulation of tissue, can be used either alone

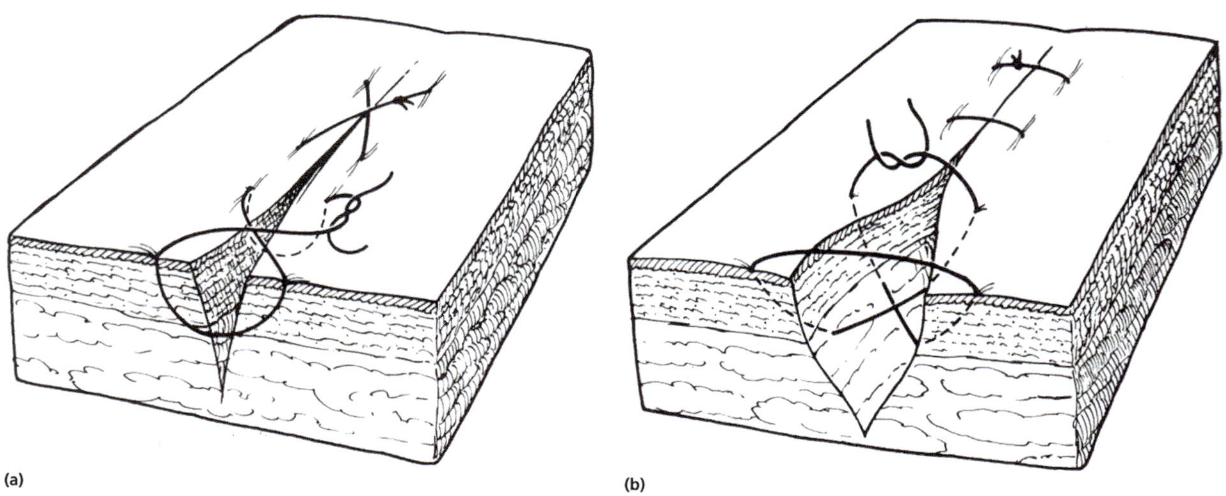

Figure 9.9 (a) Cruciate mattress suture pattern. (b) Inverted cruciate mattress suture pattern.

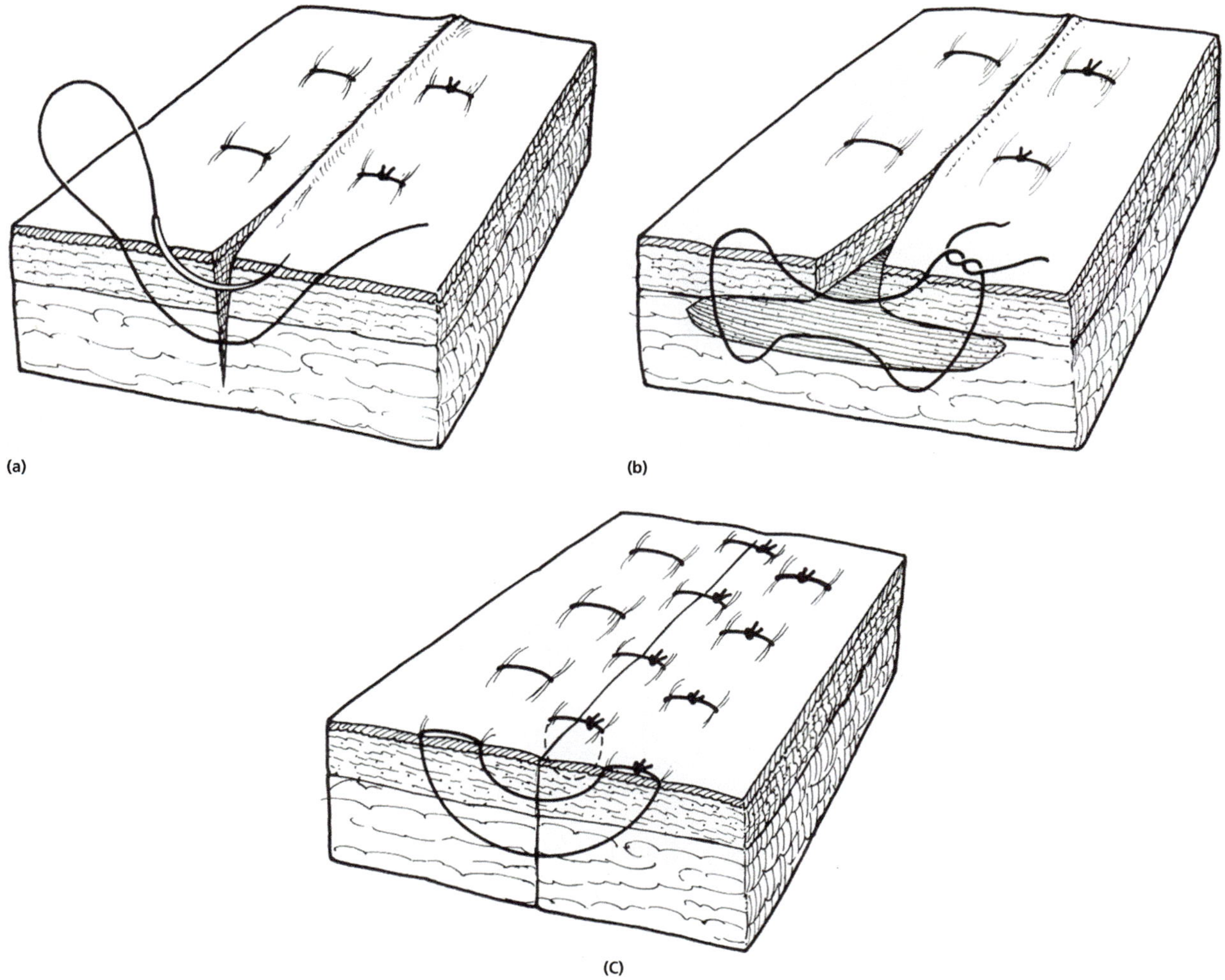

Figure 9.10 (**a**) Interrupted vertical mattress suture pattern. These sutures provide precise edge-to-edge skin apposition with slight eversion after they are tied. They also minimally compromise skin vasculature. (**b**) Interrupted vertical mattress suture pattern used to decrease dead space. (**c**) Alternating vertical mattress and simple interrupted suture patterns to prevent skin inversion. Note: There is no biomechanical advantage over a simple interrupted suture pattern when placed as described. The alternating vertical mattress suture pattern can however be placed widely to reduce tension on the primary suture line or associated with rubber "stents" or buttons.

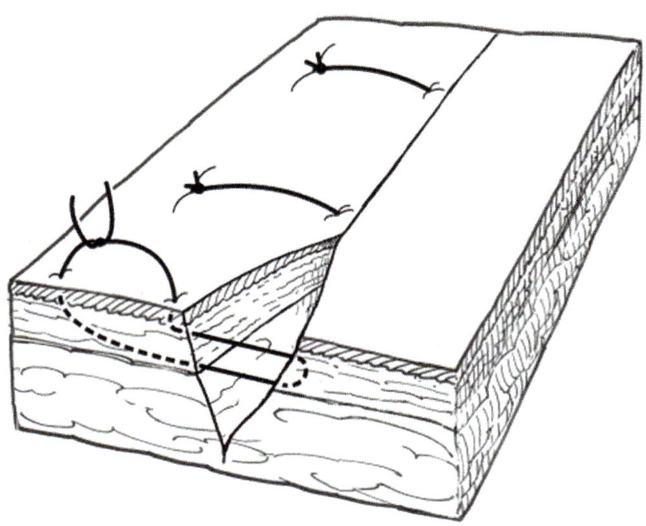

Figure 9.11 The Allgöwer corium vertical mattress suture pattern. This minimally traumatic suture pattern provides good apposition of skin margins with minimal or no eversion of the skin edges.

(Figure 9.20) or in combination with an appositional suture pattern (Figures 9.17, 9.18, 9.19). Tension sutures are usually preplaced. Skin edges are brought into apposition with the aid of towel clamps, and the preplaced tension sutures are tied. The edges of the laceration or incision are apposed using an appositional suture pattern (Figures 9.17b,c, 9.18, 9.19).[1]

Walking sutures (Figure 9.24) are buried tension sutures that: (1) move skin progressively toward the center of the wound or the opposite margin of the wound; (2) distribute tension; and (3) obliterate subcutaneous dead space, thereby preventing the formation of a serum pocket.[3]

Tips

- Walking sutures do not penetrate the skin surface.
- Walking sutures are placed no closer than 1–2 cm apart in a staggered fashion.
- The number of walking sutures should be minimized to prevent compromising circulation.

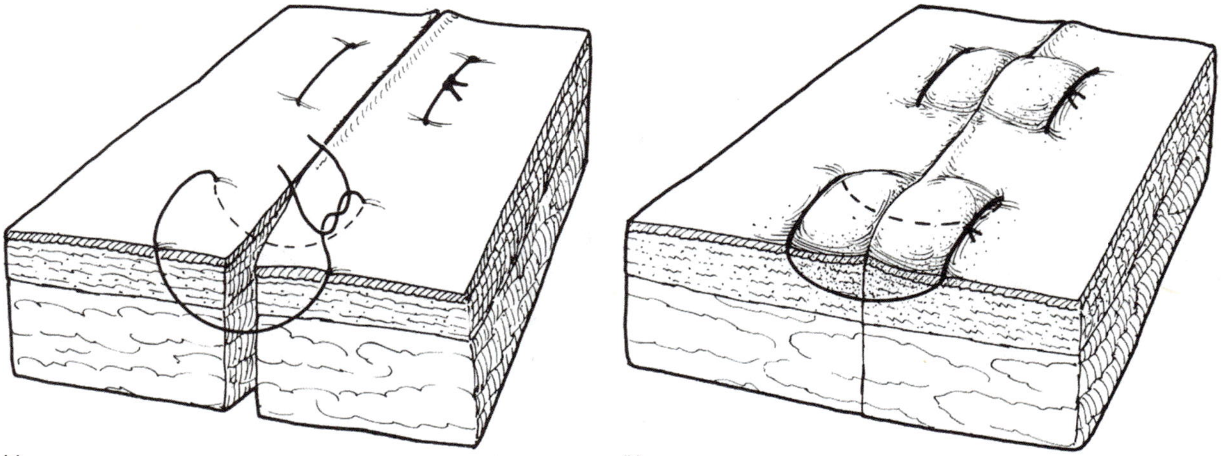

(a) (b)

Figure 9.12 (**a**) Horizontal mattress suture pattern. Slight eversion and some gaping of the wound edges occur after they are tied. (**b**) If the sutures are tied too tightly or if tissues swell excessively after placement, reduction of the skin blood supply occurs (elevated tissue and dashed lines within the suture pattern) and can impair wound healing.

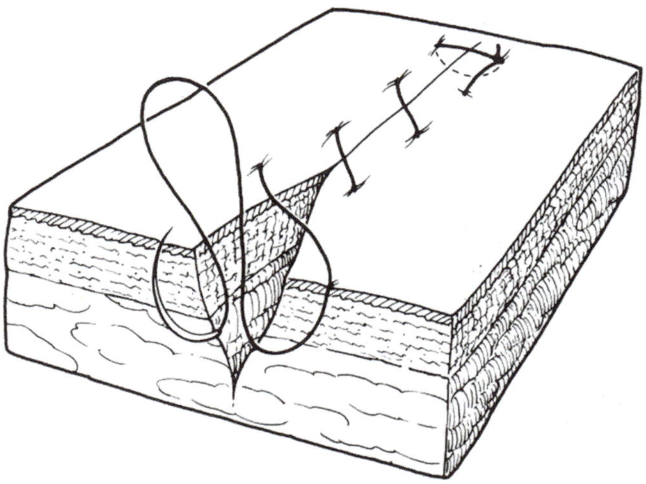

Figure 9.13 Suture placement through all skin layers in a simple continuous suture pattern.

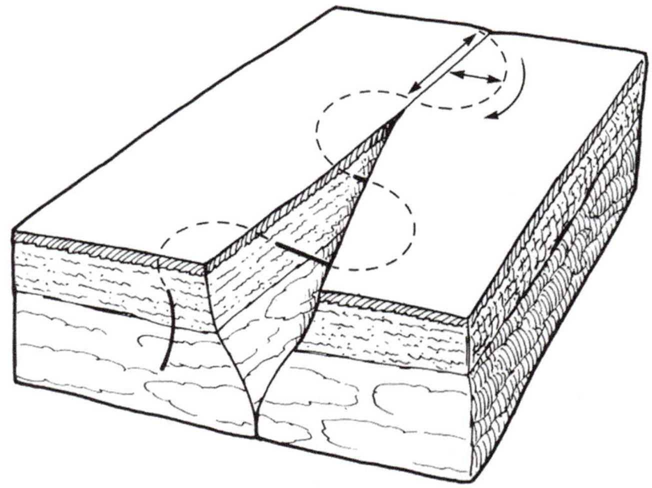

Figure 9.14 Continuous intradermal suture pattern. The suture should pass through the dermis perpendicular to the long axis of the wound. Suture bites in the dermis should be of equivalent depth. Spacing between bites should also be regular.

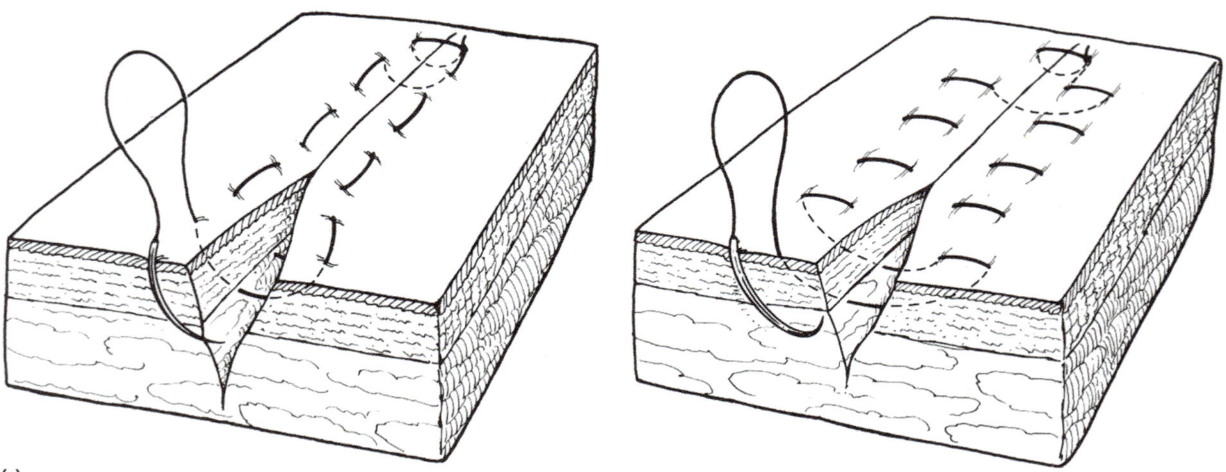

(a) (b)

Figure 9.15 Continuous mattress suture pattern. (**a**) Horizontal mattress. (**b**) Vertical mattress.

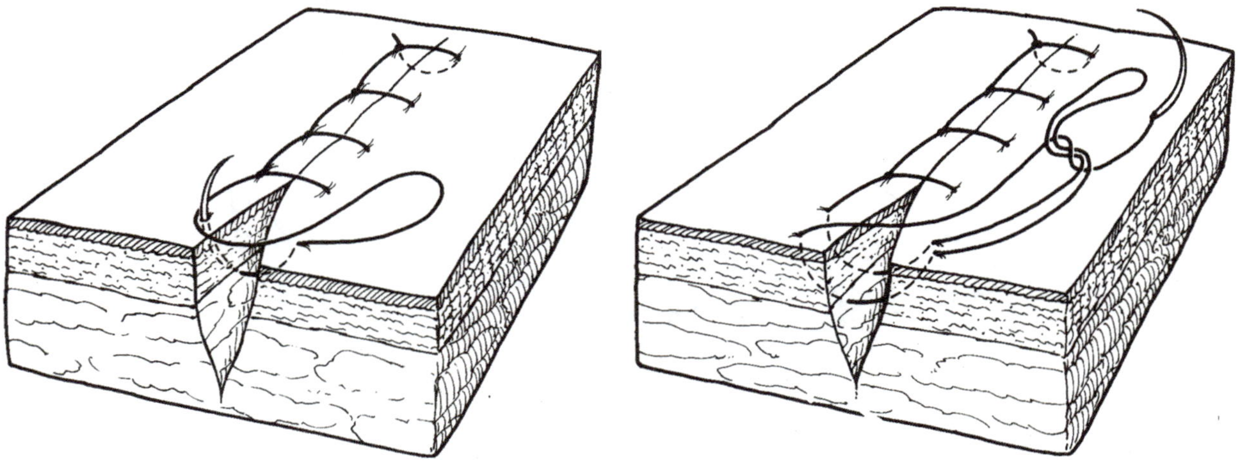

(a) (b)

Figure 9.16 Continuous locking or Ford interlocking suture pattern. (**a**) Passage of the suture. (**b**) Tying the suture after completion.

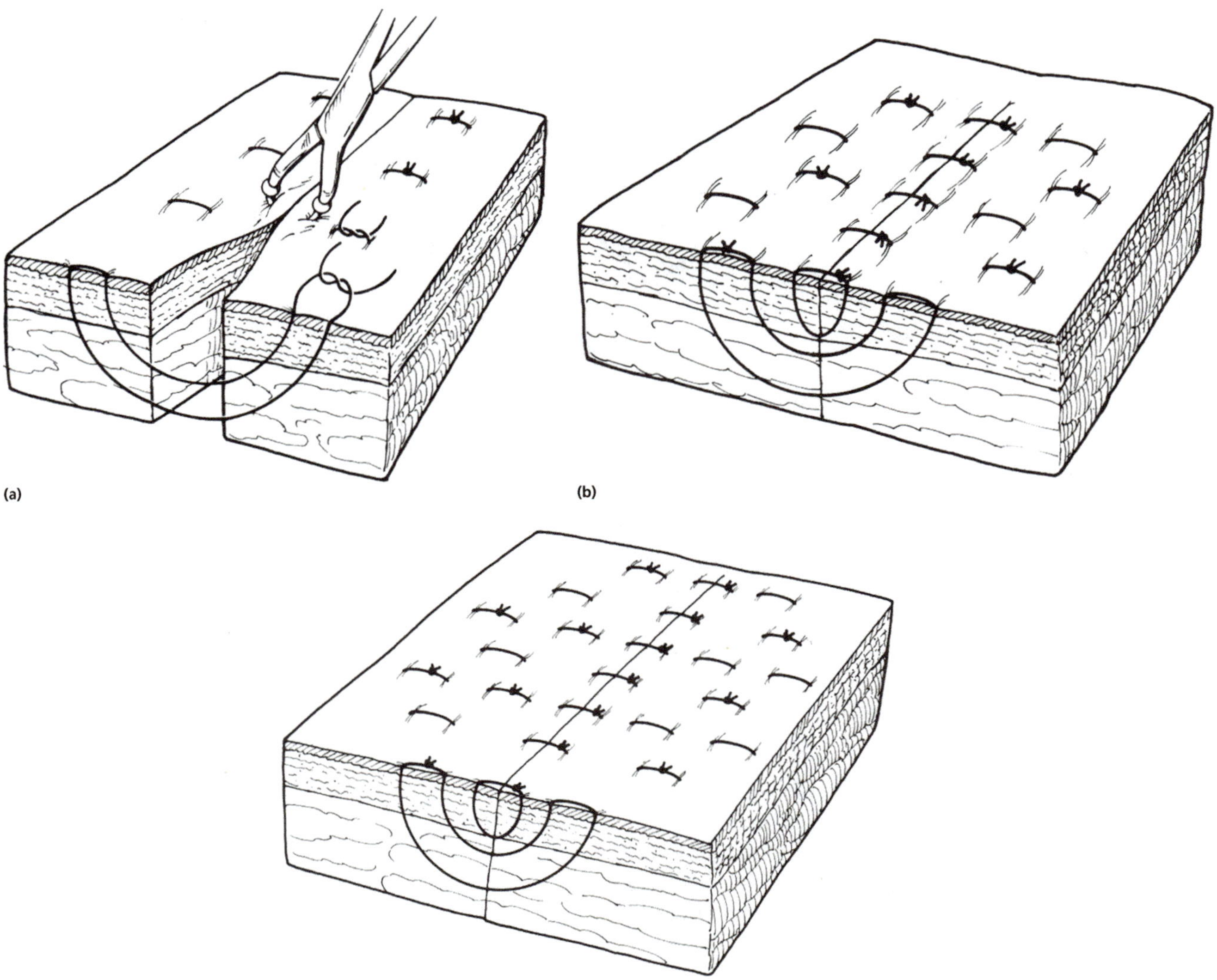

(a) (b) (c)

Figure 9.17 (**a**) Vertical mattress sutures are preplaced and the skin edges apposed with towel clamps. (**b**) Two rows of vertical mattress sutures are used to reduce the tension at the site of primary closure. (**c**) Three rows of vertical mattress suture are used to reduce the tension at the site of primary closure. In both **b** and **c**, placement of interrupted vertical mattress sutures is in an "echelon" pattern.

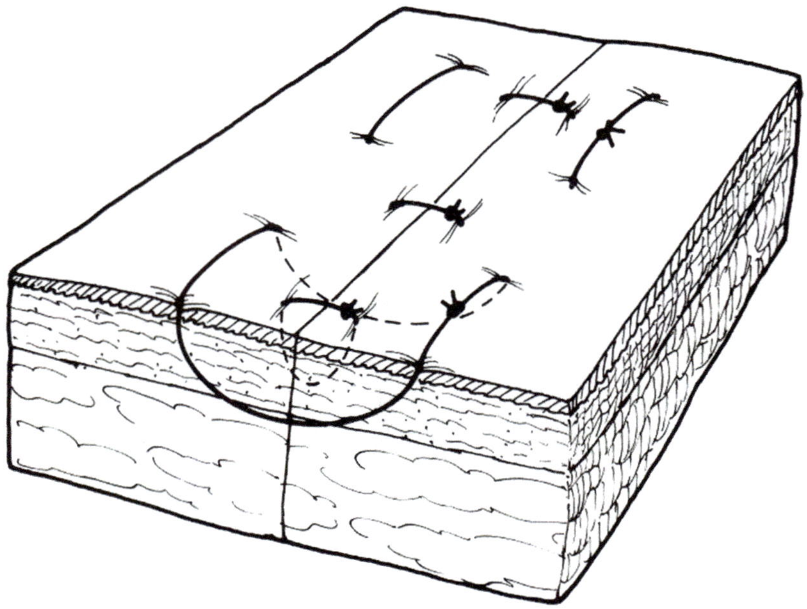

Figure 9.18 Widely placed interrupted horizontal mattress and simple interrupted sutures reduce tension on the primary repair site and prevent eversion of the skin edges.

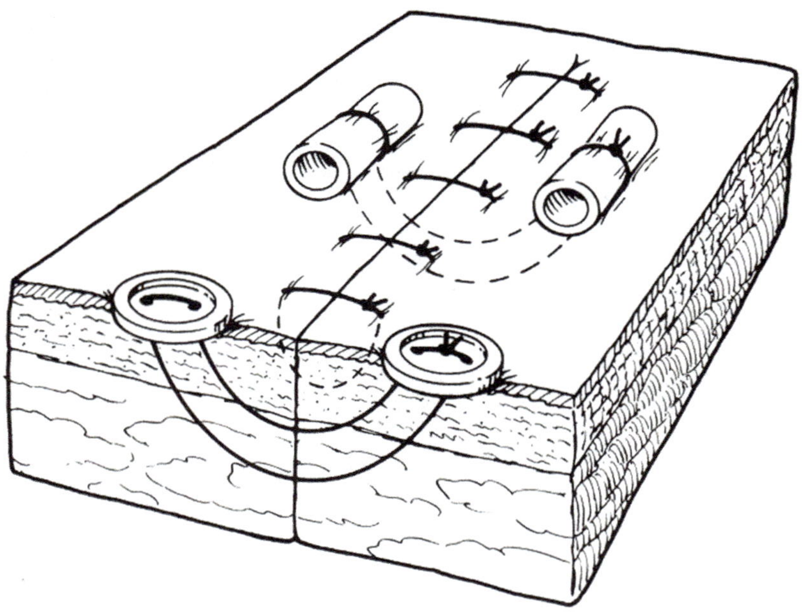

Figure 9.19 Quilled or stented tension sutures augmented by supports (rubber stents or buttons).

Additional support, in the form of buttons, rubber tubing, and/or gauze placed beneath the loops of the tension sutures or incorporated into them before the sutures are tied, reduces the risk of the sutures cutting through skin (Figure 9.19 and Videos 9.1 and 9.2 on companion website: www.wiley.com/go/theoret/wound). Sutures supported in this manner are referred to as a quilled or stented sutures. Quilled/stented sutures are best used in wounds that suffer from excessive tension (such as on limbs, near joints) or where bandages are difficult to apply, such as the neck and trunk.

Tip

- Place several rows of tension sutures, rather than using buttons, rubber tubing, or gauze as suture supports, when applying a cast over the sutured wound in order to prevent areas of skin necrosis beneath the supports.

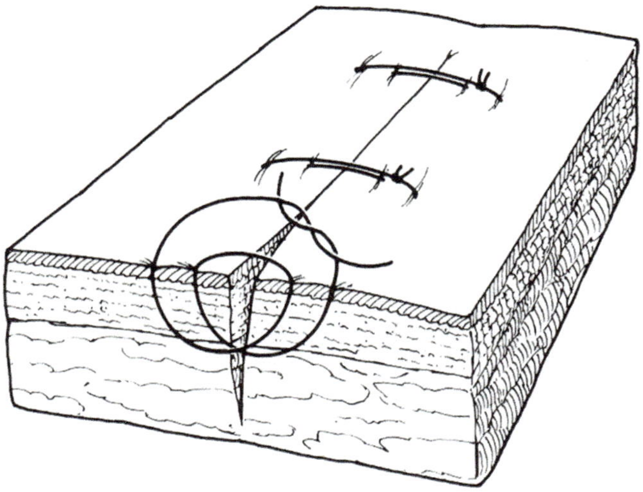

Figure 9.20 A far–near near–far suture pattern. The far component reduces tension while the near component holds the tissue edges in apposition.

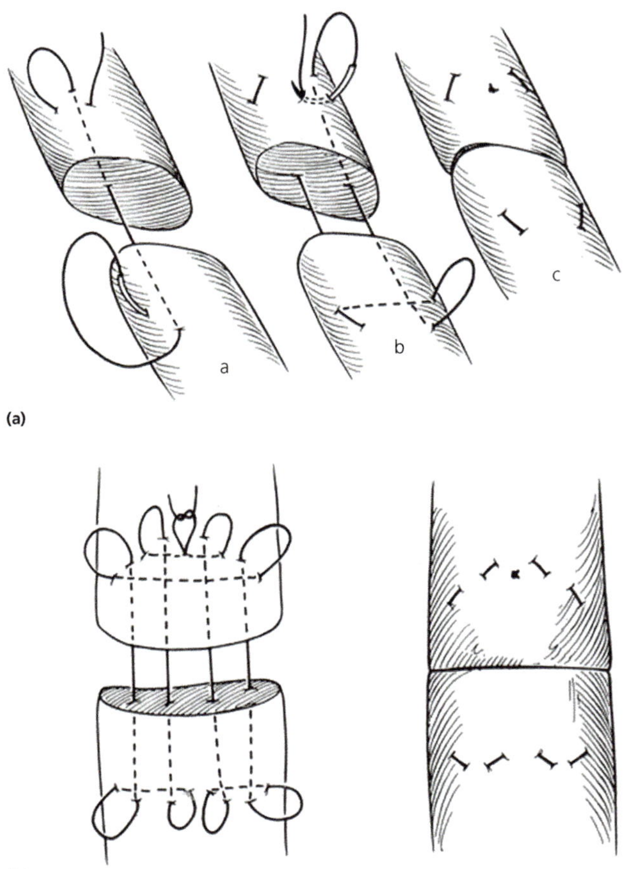

Figure 9.21 (a) Single modified locking loop suture pattern. (b) Double modified locking loop suture pattern.

Suture removal

Skin sutures should be removed after healing is sufficient to prevent dehiscence. In the case of a surgical wound healing by primary intention, skin sutures are usually removed

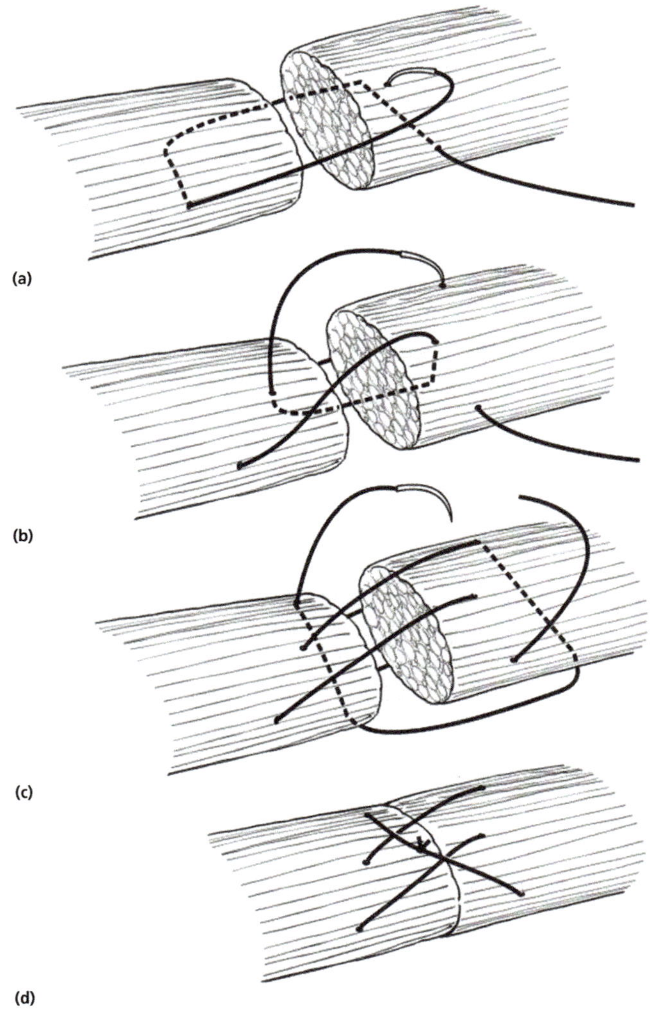

Figure 9.22 The three-loop pulley suture pattern. Each loop is oriented 120 degrees relative to the others. The first loop is in a near-far suture pattern (a), the second loop is equidistant from the transected ends of the tendon (b), and the third loop is placed in a far–near pattern (c, d).

within 12–14 days of application. In the case of an accidental wound with extensive tissue damage and loss requiring sustained support, the sutures may need to be left in place for a longer period of time. Several criteria will dictate suture removal in such a case: (1) filling of the wound defect with healthy granulation tissue; (2) firm adhesion between skin and underlying tissues; and (3) tension sutures starting to cut through skin.

Staples

In equine practice, non-absorbable skin staples made of 316L stainless steel are the most commonly used. They allow for rapid closure of clean cutaneous wounds that are not subjected to substantial tensile forces, with excellent cosmetic and functional results. Clinical advantages of skin stapling

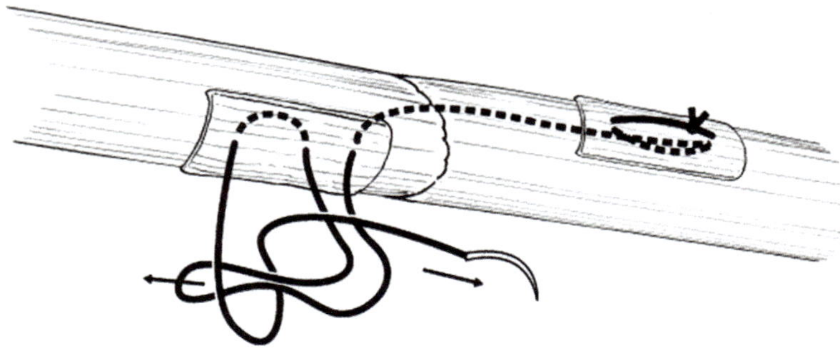

Figure 9.23 Intraneural suture pattern.

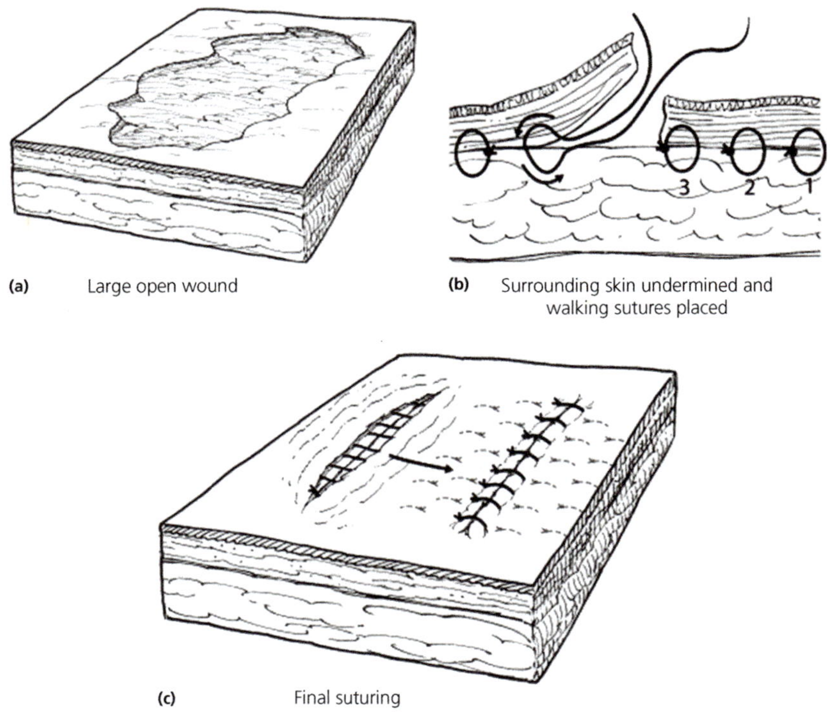

Figure 9.24 Walking sutures. Skin around the initial wound is undermined. Using absorbable suture material, the first bite is taken deep within the dermis (without penetrating the epidermis). The second bite is taken in the underlying fascia toward the center of the wound or the opposite wound margin. Tying the suture advances the skin flap in the chosen direction. Walking sutures are placed on both sides of the wound until the skin margins are close enough to allow closure with an appositional suture pattern placed without tension.

include excellent wound edge eversion without strangulation of tissue, more favorable blood flow and oxygenation at the wound site, minimal tissue reaction, less pain, and reductions in surgical time and cost.[3,4,41–43] A clinical disadvantage of staples is difficulty during removal, especially when staples twist within the wound and staples' legs exit the skin, which usually results in increased wound trauma and patient discomfort.

Several studies conducted in humans[44] and other mammals, including horses,[45,46] provided confounding and conflicting data about the use of non-absorbable staples to close cutaneous wounds. A meta-analysis[47] recently concluded that, on the one hand, there is clear evidence that wound closure with staples reduces the mean operating time but, on the other hand, there is no clear evidence of superiority for either non-absorbable staples or sutures with respect to SSI, post-surgical complications, or duration of hospital stay.

Absorbable skin staples (e.g., co-polymer of polyglycolic and polylactic acids) have recently been developed. These staples are not apposed against the skin surface but are rather inserted into the subcutaneous tissue to securely approximate wound edges. Absorbable skin staples produce less of an inflammatory response in the early stages of skin healing than do other methods of wound closure, they provide a rapid and cosmetic skin closure, and they eliminate the need for staple removal.[5,42,43]

Tip

- Although their application is rapid, absorbable or non-absorbable surgical staples are not as strong as sutures; therefore, they should not be used when skin is under tension, unless they are supported by tension sutures.

Tissue adhesives

Currently, the use of topical tissue adhesives in the equine patient is scarce because of limited indications and possible unawareness of their potential applications.

Skin incisions or lacerations that benefit from closure using tissue adhesives alone are: (1) small (<5 cm in length) superficial skin incisions or lacerations; (2) located in non-mobile areas; (3) in which clean and sharp edges are separated less than 5 mm; and (4) that would normally require sutures of size 4-0 or smaller in diameter for repair.[5] Such wounds are rare in horses and are often left to heal by second intention. The use of tissue adhesives is contraindicated in the management of wounds in mucous membranes, contaminated wounds, large or deep wounds, and wounds under tension,[3] which are the most frequently encountered wounds in equine practice.

Tissue adhesives can be used in combination with other materials, including suture materials, to improve closure of wounds or incisions. Examples of combination procedures used or that could be used in the horse include stabilizing cutaneous edges after subcutaneous suturing in wounds managed under casts, attaching split-thickness grafts to graft sites, stabilizing grafts to repair acute and chronic hoof injuries, and also carrying healing cells to injured tissues.[3,48]

Cyanoacrylate glues

Cyanoacrylate glues (2-cyanoacrylate, Vetbond, 3M; N–butyl-2-cyanoacrylate, Indermil, United States Surgical; 2-octylcyano-acrylate, Dermabond, Ethicon) are commonly used for tissue adhesion in small-animal and human surgery. They are quick and easy to apply, requiring only one tenth to one fourth of the time required for skin suture placement. Cyanoacrylate glues rapidly polymerize in an exothermic reaction on contact with skin moisture to form a three-dimensional, strong, flexible, waterproof bond to skin cells. Bonding generally takes less than 1 minute if there is no hemorrhage. Cyanoacrylate glues slough with epidermis; thus, there is no need for removal.

Correct application of cyanoacrylate glue is critical to success. Before application, the skin must be defatted, the skin edges must be perfectly apposed, without any tension, and held in precise apposition. The glue is applied over the top of the entire wound, extending 5–10 mm beyond the wound edge in order to form an occlusive seal all over the wound. Octylcyanoacrylate is applied in a thin layer. Once the first layer has dried (10–30 seconds), a second layer is applied. Three to four layers are usually necessary. N-butyl-2-cyanoacrylate requires only a single application by droplet that sets in 30 seconds and requires no direct contact with the wound. Entry or persistence of cyano-acrylate glue inside the wound usually causes a chronic local inflammation secondary to foreign body reaction and elution of toxic by-products, leading to either granuloma formation or dehiscence.[4,5]

In addition to their indication for use as tissue adhesives, cyanoacrylate glues are approved by the US Food and Drug Administration for use as barriers against common bacterial microbes, including certain staphylococci, *Pseudomonas*, and *Escherichia coli*. Thus, they may be used either to close a full-thickness wound after buried sutures have been placed in the subcutaneous layer, or to reinforce incisions fully closed with suture or staples to protect them against bacterial colonization. The main disadvantages, but by no means the least, are (1) the cost per unit of cyanoacrylate, which is higher than that of any comparable suture, and (2) that sutures are significantly better than tissue adhesives for minimizing dehiscence.[49]

Fibrin-based glues

Fibrin-based glues (e.g., Tisseel, Baxter) are mainly composed of separate solutions of concentrated fibrinogen, thrombin, and calcium chloride, that, when combined, replicate the end stage of the coagulation cascade. Fibrin-based glues can be either autologous (e.g., Vivostat, Cavaleo) or heterologous (e.g., Tisseel, Baxter), with or without a platelet component.[50] The final composition of fibrin-based glues may vary considerably depending on their anticipated use. Higher fibrinogen concentrations boost the clot strength, whereas higher thrombin concentrations enhance the speed of clotting and addition of factor XIII increases the tensile strength and stability of the clot, thus improving hemostatic properties.[48]

The main advantages of fibrin-based glues are tissue compatibility, biodegradability, and efficacy when applied to wet surfaces.

Fibrin-based glues are used for a variety of surgical procedures, including minimally invasive surgery, in both humans and small animals (e.g., as an hemostatic agent or as a sealant for gastrointestinal, vascular, and nerve anastomoses). Few studies have specifically evaluated the application of fibrin-based glues in equine surgery. Use of fibrin glue as a carrier matrix for mesenchymal stem cells for the treatment of soft tissue[51,52] and cartilage[50] injuries represents, at the moment, a promising application in horses.

New directions

The bonding of wounds using laser energy, known as laser welding, has been developed as an alternative to traditional wound closure. Compared with suturing, laser welding decreased surgical time, provided an immediate watertight tissue closure, and eliminated foreign-body reactions to suture materials. Collateral thermal injury has, however, prevented its regular clinical use.

To minimize this side-effect, laser soldering was introduced. This process consists in the application of a biologic "solder" (e.g., bovine serum albumin, chromophores) prior to temperature-controlled laser welding. Preliminary results look promising, but additional studies are necessary to determine the practical use of laser soldering in wound management.[53,54]

Support for sutured wounds

The support provided to the sutured wound can determine success or failure of a repair. Bandages (regular, pressure, or stent) and casts may be used to support a sutured wound by immobilizing surrounding skin and adjacent joints, minimizing accumulation of edema, and obliterating dead space.[34] A balance should be sought between providing adequate support to the sutured wound and interfering with the regional cutaneous blood supply.[19] The reader is referred to Chapter 6 for more information about bandage materials and to Chapter 7 for more information about the techniques for bandaging, splinting, and casting.

Drains

Drains are temporary implants designed to channel unwanted tissue debris, fluid, or gas from a body cavity or wound; they can be used prophylactically or therapeutically. Drains serve a number of important functions, but they are not benign, however, and, when used inappropriately they may delay healing and cause other complications, including retrograde bacterial migration, inflammation, and hemorrhage. An improperly anchored drain can be lost prematurely or become trapped within the wound.

Optimal material

The ideal drain should:

- efficiently channel unwanted fluid or gas from a body cavity or a wound;
- be sterile, non-reactive, non-allergenic, non-carcinogenic, non-corrosive, non-toxic, and pyrogen-free to avoid creating an environment favorable to bacterial contamination and growth;
- be soft and compliant;
- be inexpensive, readily available in different sizes, and easily sterilized without altering its properties;
- be easy to handle and comfortable to the patient;
- be radiopaque so that it can be identified radiographically if it accidently disappears within a wound or a body cavity.[1]

The ideal drain material does not exist, but materials commonly used to make drains possess many of these properties.

Principles of drain usage

Benefits of drains include the following:

- removal of accumulations of components of blood that provide a medium for bacterial proliferation, not readily attained by the immune system or antimicrobial drugs;
- relief of pressure that can restrict tissue perfusion and may cause pain;
- evacuation of inflammatory mediators, bacteria, tissue debris, and foreign bodies that perpetuate infection.[4]

Drains are not a substitute for proper wound management. They do not preclude the need to:

- follow Halsted's principles of surgery;
- properly cleanse, debride, and irrigate contaminated wounded tissues;
- use delayed primary or secondary closure, rather than primary closure, when indicated.[4]

Drains are foreign bodies that increase the wound's susceptibility to infection and can cause mechanical injury to tissue. Consequently, they should not be placed in the immediate vicinity of delicate tissues (e.g., blood vessels and nerves), and nor should they lie directly beneath or exit a sutured incision.[1,55–57] The most frequent complication associated with the use of drains is retrograde infection of the wound by environmental multi-resistant bacteria. The risk of drain-associated infection can be minimized by the following steps: (1) using aseptic technique when placing, handling, and removing the drain; (2) using the smallest number and size of drains possible; (3) choosing a flexible and soft drain; (4) using an active drain; (5) covering the wound and the exit site of the drain with a sterile absorptive dressing and changing the dressing frequently; and (6) removing the drain as soon as it no longer benefits the patient.[1,4]

The amount of drainage and its consistency dictate the frequency with which protective and absorptive bandages must be changed (passive drains) or vacuum containers emptied (active drains). The sterile absorptive dressing is held in place using standard bandaging techniques for the extremities; a stent or tie-over bandage can be used in areas that are not easily covered with a standard bandage.

Classification of drains

The mechanism of drainage can be passive, relying on gravity, body movement, pressure differentials, capillary action, and overflow, or active, relying on continuous or intermittent suction. Passive drains are typically open (exudate flows down the outer surface of the drain to collect in a bandage), whereas active drains are most commonly closed (exudate flows through the lumen of the drain and is collected in a reservoir.[4]

Passive drains

Passive drains are composed of soft collapsible radiopaque latex (e.g., a Penrose drain) or a more rigid tube composed of rubber, polypropylene, or silicone. Although a Penrose drain is tubular, drainage occurs along the outside of the drain; therefore, Penrose drains should not be fenestrated because fenestration decreases the surface area available for drainage. To avert descending bacterial infection, the proximal or dorsal extremity of the passive drain should not exit the skin, but rather should be buried at the most proximal, most dorsal, or deepest extent of the wound. It should be secured at this site by a single penetrating suture tied on the surface of the skin adjacent to the wound. Passive drains should exit the wound or dead space distad or ventrad to the most distal or ventral extent of the wound through a single stab incision in a dependent position near the wound (Figure 9.25 and Videos 9.3, 9.4, 9.5, and 9.6 on companion website: www.wiley.com/go/theoret/wound). This extremity of the drain should be secured with sutures to prevent it from retreating into the wound.

Tips

- Ensure sutures securing the drain can be easily distinguished from sutures used to close the wound to avoid inadvertently removing sutures apposing the wound's edges.
- The external component of a passive drain should emerge far enough from the wound to ensure that the drain does not disappear completely into the wound when the horse moves (Figure 9.26).
- It is advisable to protect the skin adjacent to the exit portal of the passive drain with a thin layer of petroleum jelly to prevent exudate from excoriating the skin around the drain's exit portal.
- Because round wounds heal more slowly than triangular or square/rectangular wounds, it is recommended to create a round drainage opening to ensure a patent exit portal for a long period of time.[56]

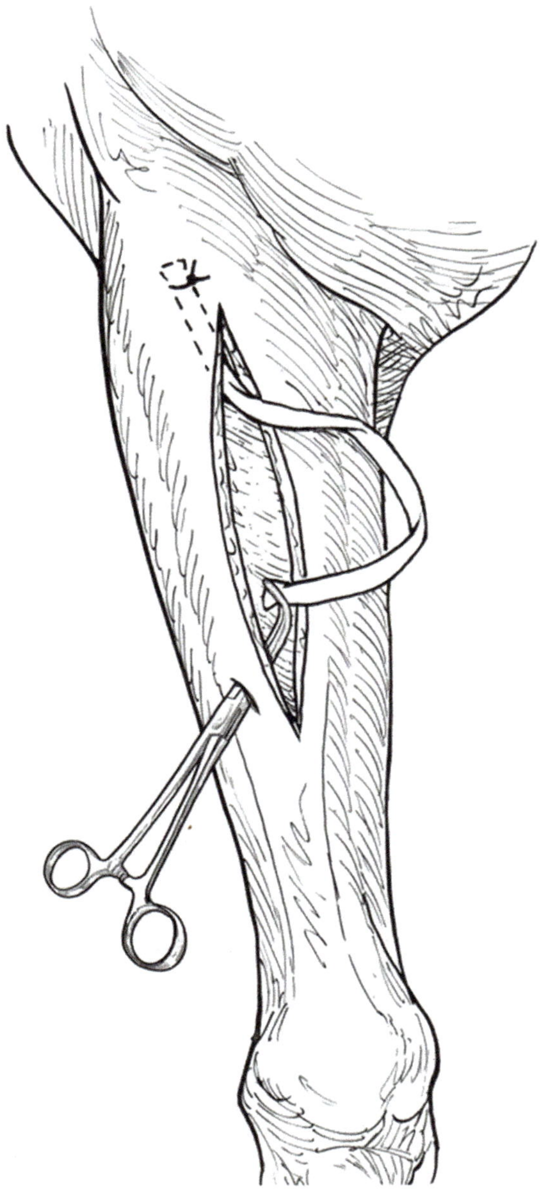

Figure 9.25 Proper placement of a Penrose drain to facilitate passive drainage. The proximal end of the drain is buried within the proximal aspect of the wound and is secured with a single penetrating suture tied on the outside of intact skin adjacent to the wound. The distal end exits the wound below its most distal aspect through a single stab incision in a dependent position near the wound. The wound is subsequently closed.

An exception to exiting only one extremity of the drain should be made when placing a drain in a wound in the axillary or inguinal region. For these wounds, exiting the proximal or dorsal extremity of the drain through a proximal or dorsal skin incision prevents entrapment of subcutaneous air, thereby averting the development of emphysema as the horse moves. Having cranial and caudal exit sites for a drain placed in a

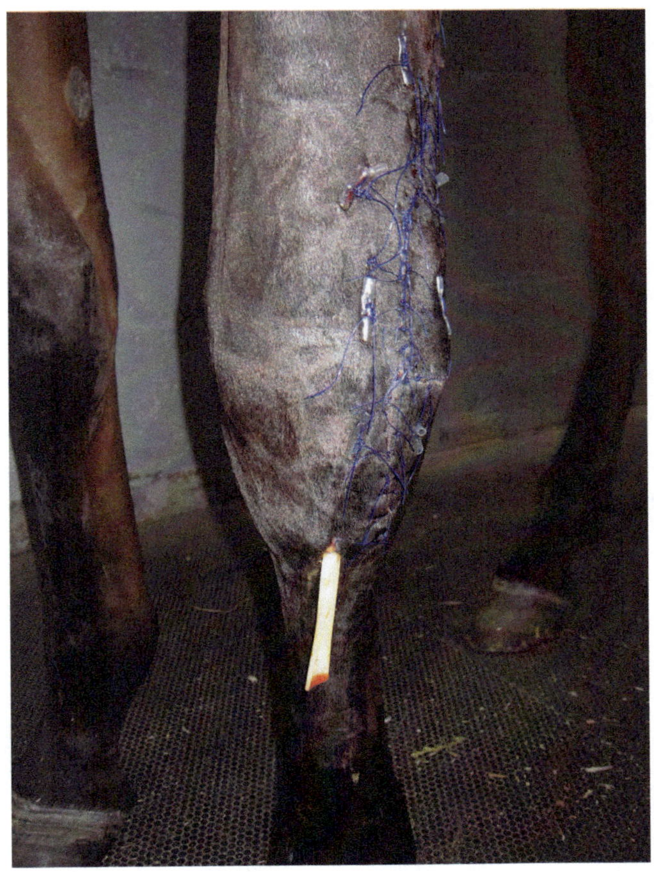

Figure 9.26 Wound over the carpus managed with multiple tension sutures and a Penrose drain exiting the wound distally through a stab incision in a dependent position near the wound. The drain was removed within 5 days and the wound healed by primary intention under a full limb Robert Jones bandage.

wound in the throatlatch region facilitates drainage no matter the position of the head and neck (i.e., extension, flexion, or neutral).

A sterile absorbent dressing should be placed over the external component of the passive drain. The bandage collects the exudate, allowing an assessment of the quality/quantity of drainage, provides a barrier to environmental contamination, and prevents exudate from excoriating the skin around the drain's exit site.[4] The sterile absorptive dressing is held in place using standard bandaging techniques for the extremities; a stent or tie-over bandage may be used in areas that are not easily covered with a standard bandage. Table 9.6 provides more details about passive drains commonly used in equine wound management.

Active drains

Active drains create an artificial gradient for evacuating fluid and gas by applying negative pressure to the wound, sometimes against gravity. Refer to Table 9.7 for details about active drains commonly used to manage equine wounds.

Closed suction is useful for evacuating fluid and collapsing dead space within large cavities. Closed suction drains are frequently used in the management of infected synovial cavities, large and deep wounds, and to evacuate the pleural space.[56] They usually consist of a multi-fenestrated drain with a non-fenestrated extension (drain tube) that is connected to a suction device and a drain reservoir (Figures 9.27, 9.28, 9.29). Most multi-fenestrated drains are composed of polyvinylchloride (Redon-type drain) or silicone or silastic elastomer (Black

Table 9.6 Characteristics of the most commonly used passive drains.

Type	Raw material	Mechanism of action	Advantages and uses	Disadvantages
Gauze drains[c]	Fine mesh gauze	Drainage occurs by gravity and capillary action	Economical May be soaked with antibiotics or antiseptics or made from commercially available antimicrobial dressing material (Kerlix® Antimicrobial Dressing[b]) May be applied as packing in profusely bleeding cavities or in abscesses Adherence of surrounding tissues and fibrin clots to gauze exerts a debriding action	Strong foreign body reaction increasing inflammation and potential for infection Prolonged use can result in fibrous tract Wicking effect facilitates ascending infection Should not be used in abdominal or thoracic cavities
Penrose drains[d]	Soft and pliable latex	Drainage occurs mostly extraluminally by gravity and capillary action (hollow tube) **WARNING**: Fenestration weakens drain and reduces surface area of drainage thereby decreasing efficacy	Economical Easily sterilized Readily available in various sizes Weak foreign body reaction Radiopaque Many applications: in contaminated wounds not completely debrided, in fluid-filled dead spaces, underneath skin grafts, in second-intention healing, in synovial cavities left open for lavage	Kink easily Cannot be used in abdominal or thoracic cavities Cannot be used with suction May facilitate ascending infection Some contain zinc diethyldithiocarbamate, a vulcanizing accelerator, shown to be toxic
Silicone Penrose drains[a]	Soft and pliable non-reactive silicone	As regular Penrose drain	As regular Penrose drain Less irritating Latex-free for sensitive patients Contains radiodense markers	As regular Penrose drain
Sheet drains	Waved sheet of red rubber Smooth surface	Drainage occurs by gravity and capillary action	Relative stiffness: gap between the two layers of drain, when folded, resists obstruction Can be cut to size	Increased foreign body reaction Impurities can support bacterial growth
Stiff tubular drains	Red rubber Smooth surface	Drainage occurs by gravity and capillary action	Relative stiffness: rarely compressed or occluded Suction can be applied	Increased foreign body reaction Impurities can support bacterial growth Easily obstructed by debris
Soft tubular drains (Flexi-Drain[a], J-VAC Drain[c])	Soft and pliable non-reactive silicone	Drainage occurs by gravity and capillary action Drainage is increased when tubes are joined together	Contains radiodense markers Can be split longitudinally to size Suction can be applied	Easily obstructed by debris

Source: Adapted from Celeste,[1] Blackford,[17] Auer[56].
[a]Benson Medical Industries, Inc.
[b]Tyco Healthcare Kendall
[c]Ethicon, Johnson & Johnson company, Inc.
[d]Sherwood Medical

Table 9.7 Characteristics of the most commonly used drains in active drainage.

Type	Material	Material description	Mechanism of action	Advantages and uses	Disadvantages
Redon drain[a]	Polyvinylchloride (PVC)	Round multi-fenestrated tube at its distal end with non-fenestrated extension Length of multifenestrated part: 14 cm Total length of drain: 50–80 cm Diameter: 3–6 mm	Active or passive drainage intraluminally	Can be used as closed or open drainage system Excellent for evacuation of fluids from body cavities Available in different diameters	Attaching suction device may be difficult depending on wound location Fibrin may plug/clog the drain. This can be prevented by flushing tube with full-strength sterile heparin prior to implantation
Jackson–Pratt drain[b]	Silastic, Teflon	Flat multi-fenestrated drain at its distal end with non-fenestrated plastic extension	Active or passive drainage intraluminally	Can be used as closed or open drainage system Excellent for evacuation of fluids from body cavities Less reactive (may be left in place for longer period of time)	Attaching suction device may be difficult depending on wound location
Black drain[c]	Silicone	Flat or round drains with four channels along sides with solid core center connected to extension tubing. Available either ¾ fluted or full fluted, with or without trocar	Active or passive drainage intraluminally	Available in wide variety of sizes Greater tissue contact area than regular perforated drains Offers multiple drainage routes to resist clogging Minimal tissue irritation so greater patient comfort Removal may be less traumatic to surrounding tissues	Relatively voluminous, making it hard to fix to horse's body and limbs Suction possible only when skin suture is tight Single use only

Source: Adapted from Celeste,[1] Auer[56].
[a]Zimmer, Inc.
[b]Cardinal Health
[c]Ethicon, Johnson & Johnson company, Inc.

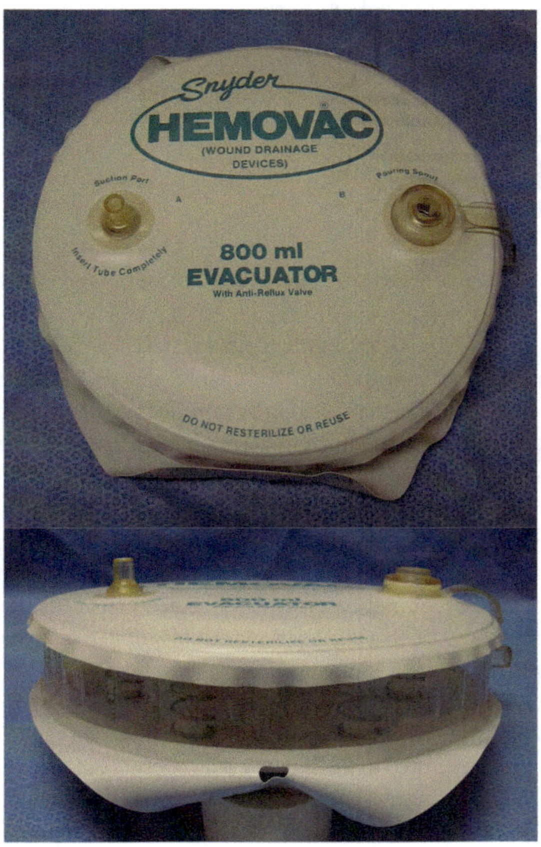

Figure 9.27 Snyder Hemovac wound drainage device – 800 mL. Bellows-type drain reservoir, used as active drainage system.

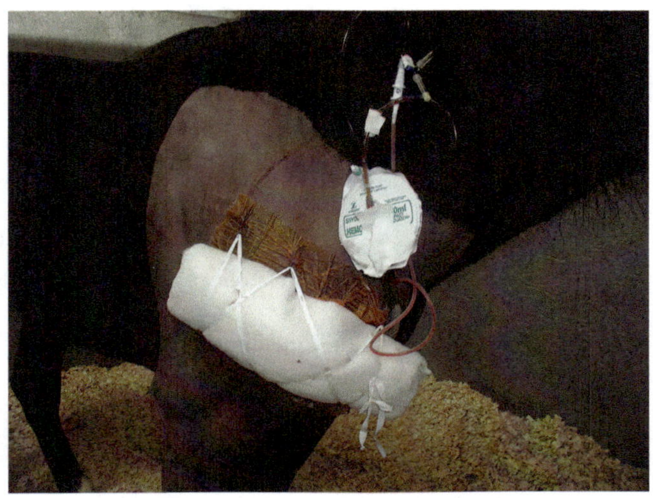

Figure 9.28 Active drainage system (Jackson–Pratt drain connected to a bellows type Snyder Hemovac reservoir) being used in the management of septic arthritis (shoulder joint). Photo courtesy of Dr. Florent David.

drain, Ethicon; Jackson–Pratt drain, Cardinal Health). Closed-suction systems eliminate saturation of bandages with fluid from the wound, significantly decrease the likelihood of ascending infection, a common problem with passive drains, and avoid excoriation of skin by fluid draining from the wound.

Suction can be either continuous or intermittent. Continuous suction is usually more efficient because it prevents the drain

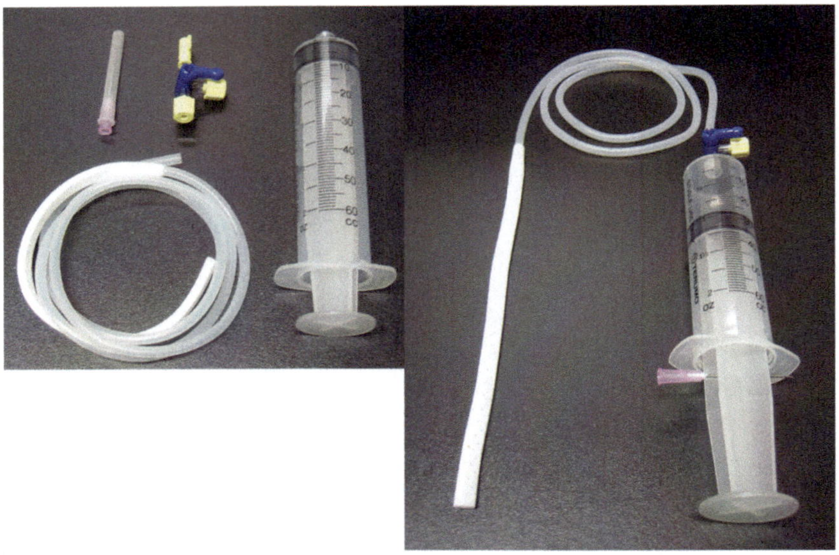

Figure 9.29 Homemade active drain constructed by connecting one end of a tube to a Jackson–Pratt drain and the other end to a three-way stopcock. The stopcock is attached to a 60-mL syringe that acts as a drain reservoir. The plunger of the syringe is withdrawn to achieve the desired negative pressure and held in that position by introducing a large needle through the syringe plunger.

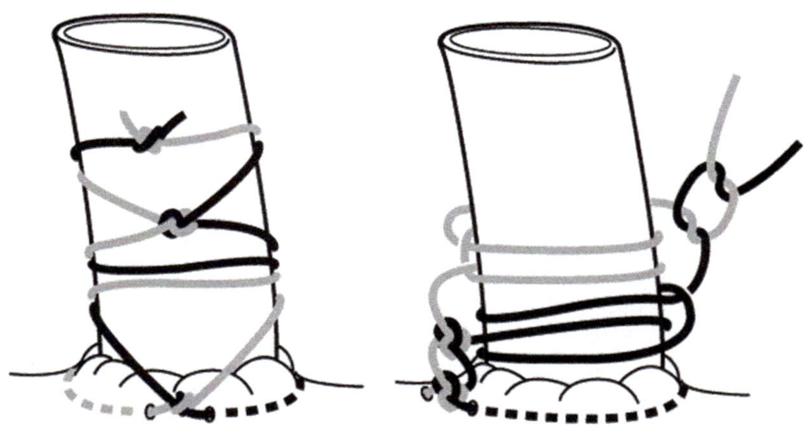

(a) (a)

Figure 9.30 Suture patterns commonly used to secure a suction drain to the body or limb. **(a)** "Chinese finger trap" suture pattern. **(b)** "Double clove hitch" pattern.

from occluding and reduces the amount of time that the drain must remain in place. Several portable continuous-suction devices are available commercially and consist of a bellows-type drain reservoir (Figures 9.27, 9.28). The reservoir is compressed to evacuate air, attached to the drain tube while compressed, and then compression is released to create a vacuum within the reservoir. The negative pressure generated by these units varies according to their size and filling; suction slowly decreases as the reservoir fills up. The bigger the reservoir, the smaller the negative pressure, peak suction, and suction capacity (100 mL drainage system = peak suction of −117.6 mmHg; 400 mL drainage system = peak suction of −71.4 mmHg).[58] An average negative pressure of 70–80 mmHg is usually sufficient to evacuate fluid and collapse dead space without damaging tissues.[59] Homemade active drains (Figures 9.29) can be constructed by connecting the external end of a drain tube, through a three-way stopcock, to a large syringe (e.g., 60 mL), which acts as a reservoir. The plunger of the syringe is withdrawn to achieve the desired negative pressure and held in that position by introducing a large needle or a small pin across the plunger at the top of barrel of the syringe through a predrilled hole. The pin keeps the plunger withdrawn from the barrel thereby maintaining negative pressure in the syringe. The syringe, when filled with exudate, can be emptied through the three-way stopcock.[55,56] It is extremely important that the drain reservoir not become disconnected inadvertently from the drain, because this results in sudden loss of negative pressure and introduces environmental bacteria into the tubing.

Multi-fenestrated drains are positioned into the wound or body cavity and secured to the skin at the level of the drain tube. Drain tubes may be sutured to the skin using a variety of suture patterns. The "Chinese finger trap" suture pattern and the "double clove hitch" are the patterns most frequently used (Figure 9.30).

Reservoirs are usually secured to the skin at a remote site and protected with bandages. Reservoirs should be monitored frequently to ensure that sufficient negative pressure is maintained, particularly during the first 24 hours after insertion when production of fluid is maximal. The desired initial suction, the anticipated volume of drainage, the frequency of reservoir emptying, and the fragility of surrounding tissues dictate the size of the reservoir (from 60-mL syringe to 400-mL drainage reservoir).

Tips

- Smaller reservoirs are more successful in generating a high initial suction than larger reservoirs, especially when the volume of fluid in the drain is relatively low.
- Larger reservoirs do tolerate higher volumes of fluid collection and allow for longer times to elapse before emptying.[58]

A special closed suction system has been used successfully to promote production of granulation tissue in wounds of people and horses with exposed bone (i.e., vacuum-assisted closure). The reader is referred to Chapter 22 for more detail.

What to avoid

- Passive drains should never be back-flushed.
- Active drains should not be back-flushed unless obstructed, because of (1) the risk of transporting microorganisms into the wound and (2) mechanical disturbance of the wound-healing process.

Drain removal

The decision to remove a drain is usually based on the quantity and quality of collected fluid and whether or not the drain is functioning properly. Because the risk of bacterial colonization increases with the length of time a drain is maintained in the wound, drains should be removed, in an aseptic manner, as early as possible. A good indication that the drain can be removed is a substantial decrease in the volume of drainage and a change from purulent or serosanguinous fluid to a serous, non-odoriferous, non-turbid fluid. Because drains, passive or active, are foreign, they may elicit production of fluid; consequently, drainage rarely ceases completely.

The time for which a drain should remain within a wound varies according to the situation. As a rule, the average time for maintaining a drain within a wound is 2–4 days (i.e., during the inflammatory phase of wound repair). But the following situations are exceptions to this rule: (1) when drains are placed in small cavities to evacuate capillary bleeding, they can usually be removed within 24 hours; (2) when drains are placed to treat bacterial infection, they are usually maintained for 48–72 hours; and (3) when drains are placed into large body cavities to promote the union of local tissues, their presence may be necessary for a week or more.[55] Drains can be cultured upon removal to assess resolution of infection. The drain, after it is removed, should be carefully examined to verify its integrity. When a portion of the drain has been accidentally left in the wound, drainage persists until that portion has been removed.

Conclusion

Sutures and drains serve important functions in wound repair; proper use usually speeds healing and allows for a better cosmetic and functional outcome. A broad range of suture and drain materials is available. Knowledge of the advantages and disadvantages of each material, assessment of a wound's location and condition, as well as familiarity with the rate of healing of the tissues involved in the wound to be managed dictate the appropriate selection for optimal outcome. Although this choice is important, more vital is the fundamental approach in managing the wound. Indeed, sutures and drains are not a substitute for proper wound management. They cannot compensate for proper cleansing, debridement, and irrigation; inappropriate use of sutures and drains may delay healing and occasionally may even increase morbidity or lead to mortality.

References

1. Celeste C, Stashak TS. Selection of suture materials, suture patterns and drains for wound closure. In: Stashak TS, Theoret CL (eds). *Equine Wound Management*, 2nd edn. Wiley Blackwell: Ames, 2008: 193.
2. Boothe HW. Suture materials, tissue adhesives, staplers, and ligating clips. In: Slatter D (ed). *Textbook of Small Animal Surgery*, 7th edn. WB Saunders: Philadelphia, 2003: 235.
3. Kümmerle JM. Suture materials and patterns. In: Auer J, Stick J (eds). *Equine Surgery*, 4th edn. Elsevier Saunders: St Louis, 2012: 181.
4. Schmiedt CW. Suture material, tissue staplers, ligation devices, and closure methods. In: Tobias KM, Johnston SA (eds). *Veterinary Small Animal Surgery*, 1st edn. Elsevier Saunders: St Louis, 2012: 187.
5. McPhail CM. Biomaterials, suturing, and hemostasis. In: Welch Fossum T (ed). *Small Animal Surgery*, 4th edn. Elsevier Saunders: St Louis, 2013: 64.
6. König L, Klopfleisch R, Kershaw O, *et al.* Prevalence of biofilms on surgical suture segments in wounds of dogs, cats, and horses. *Vet Pathol* 2015; **52**: 295.
7. Limbert G, Bryan R, Cotton R, *et al.* On the mechanics of bacterial biofilms on non-dissolvable surgical sutures: a laser scanning confocal microscopy-based finite element. *Acta Biomater* 2013; **9**: 6641.
8. Rothenburger S, Spangler D, Bhende S, *et al. In vitro* antimicrobial evaluation of Coated Vicryl Plus Antibacterial Suture (coated polyglactin 910 with triclosan) using zone of inhibition assays. *Surg Infect (Larchmt)* 2002; **3**: S79.
9. Daoud FC, Edmiston CE Jr, Leaper D. Meta-analysis of prevention of surgical site infections following incision closure with triclosan-coated sutures: robustness to new evidence. *Surg Infect (Larchmt)* 2014; **15**: 165.

10. Barbolt TA. Chemistry and safety of triclosan, and its use as an antimicrobial coating on Coated Vicryl Plus Antibacterial Suture (coated polyglactin 910 with triclosan). *Surg Infect (Larchmt)* 2002; **3**: S45.
11. Li Y, Kumar KN, Dabkowski JM, *et al.* New bactericidal surgical suture coating. *Langmuir* 2012; **28**: 12134.
12. Oni G, Brown SA, Kenkel JM. A comparison between barbed and nonbarbed absorbable suture for fascial closure in a porcine model. *Plast Reconstr Surg* 2012; **130**: 535.
13. Zaruby J, Gingras K, Taylor J, *et al.* An *in vivo* comparison of barbed suture devices and conventional monofilament sutures for cosmetic skin closure: biomechanical wound strength and histology. *Aesthet Surg J* 2011; **31**: 232.
14. Rosen AD. New and emerging uses of barbed suture technology in plastic surgery. *Aesthet Surg J* 2013; **33**: 90SS.
15. el-Mahrouky A, McElhaney J, Bartone FF, *et al. In vitro* comparison of the properties of polydioxanone, polyglycolic acid and catgut sutures in sterile and infected urine. *J Urol* 1987; **138**: 913.
16. Toombs JP, Clarke KM. Basic operative techniques. In: Slatter D (ed). *Textbook of Small Animal Surgery*, 7th edn. WB Saunders: Philadelphia, 2003: 199.
17. Blackford LW, Blackford JT. Suture materials and patterns. In: Auer J and Stick J (eds). *Equine Surgery*, 3rd edn. Saunders Elsevier: Philadelphia, 2006: 187.
18. Blackford JT, Blackford LW, Disegi J, *et al.* Biomaterials, surgical implants and instruments. In: Jorg Auer and John Stick (eds). *Equine Surgery* 3rd ed. Saunders Elsevier: Philadelphia, 2006: 96.
19. Provost JP, Bailey JV. Principles of plastic and reconstructive surgery. In: Auer J, Stick J (eds). *Equine Surgery*, 4th edn. Elsevier Saunders: St Louis, 2012: 271.
20. Stashak TS. Suture patterns used for wound closure in veterinary surgery. *Proc Am Assoc of Equine Pract* 1978; **24**: 383.
21. Moy LS. Management of acute wounds. *Dermatol Clinics* 1993; **11**: 759.
22. Trostle SS, Wilson DG, Stone WC, *et al.* A study of the biomechanical properties of the adult equine *linea alba*: relationship of tissue bite size and suture material to breaking strength. *Vet Surg* 1994; **23**: 435.
23. Hendrickson D, Virgin J. Factors that affect equine wound repair. *Vet Clin North Am Equine Pract, Wound Management* 2005; **21**: 33.
24. Hendrickson DA. Management of superficial wounds. In: Auer J, Stick J (eds). *Equine Surgery*, 4th edn. Elsevier Saunders: St Louis, 2012: 306.
25. Hendrickson D, Virgin J. Factors that affect equine wound repair. *Vet Clin North Am Equine Pract, Wound Management* 2005; **21**: 33.
26. MacKay RJ. Peripheral nerve injury. In: Auer J, Stick J (eds). *Equine Surgery*, 3rd edn. Saunders Elsevier: Philadelphia, 2006: 684.
27. Miller TR. Eyelids. In: Auer J, Stick J (eds). *Equine Surgery*, 3rd edn. Saunders Elsevier: Philadelphia, 2006: 702.
28. Millichamp NJ. Conjunctiva. In: Auer J, Stick J (eds). *Equine Surgery*, 3rd edn. Saunders Elsevier: Philadelphia, 2006: 716.
29. Millichamp NJ. Principles of ophthalmic surgery. In: Auer J, Stick J (eds). *Equine Surgery*, 3rd edn. Saunders Elsevier: Philadelphia, 2006: 693.
30. Nasisse MP, Jamieson VE, Brooks DE. Cornea and sclera. In: Auer J, Stick J (eds). *Equine Surgery*, 3rd edn. Saunders Elsevier: Philadelphia, 2006: 731.
31. Heath MM. Needle selection in veterinary surgery. *Anim Health Tech* 1983; **4**: 45.
32. Trier WC. Considerations in the choice of surgical needles. *Surg Gynecol Obstet* 1979; **149**: 84.
33. Forrester JC. Suture materials and their uses. *Nurses Mirror* 1975; **140**: 48.
34. Swaim SF. Management and reconstruction in the dog and cat. In: Swaim S (ed). *Surgery of Traumatized Skin*, 1st edn. WB Saunders: Philadelphia, 1980: 165.
35. Rosin E, Robinson GM. Knot security of suture materials. *Vet Surg* 1998; **18**: 269.
36. Drake DB, Rodeheaver PF, Edlich RF, *et al.* Experimental studies in swine for measurement of suture extrusion. *J Long Term Eff Med Implants* 2004; **14**: 251.
37. Gurusamy KS, Toon CD, Allen VB, *et al.* Continuous versus interrupted skin sutures for non-obstetric surgery. *Cochrane Database Syst Rev* 2014; **2**: CD010365.
38. Knecht CD. Fundamental techniques in veterinary surgery. In: Knecht C, Allen A, Williams D, Johnson J (eds). *Fundamental Techniques in Veterinary Surgery*, 3rd edn. WB Saunders: Philadelphia, 1987: 205.
39. Speer DP. The influence of suture technique on early wound healing. *J Surg Res* 1979; **27**: 385.
40. Austin BR, Henderson RA. Buried tension sutures: force-tension comparisons of pulley, double butterfly, mattress, and simple interrupted suture patterns. *Vet Surg* 2006; **35**: 43.
41. Graham DA, Jeffery JA, Bain D, *et al.* Staple vs. subcuticular Vicryl skin closure in knee replacement surgery: a spectrophotographic assessment of wound characteristics. *Knee* 2000; **7**: 239.
42. Pineros-Fernandez A, Salopek LS, Rodeheaver PF, *et al.* A revolutionary advance in skin closure compared to current methods. *J Long Term Eff Med Implants* 2006; **16**: 19.
43. Fick JL, Novo RE, Kirchhof N. Comparison of gross and histologic tissue responses of skin incisions closed by use of absorbable subcuticular staples, cutaneous metal staples, and polyglactin 910 suture in pigs. *Am J Vet Res* 2005; **66**: 1975.
44. Smith TO, Sexton D, Mann C, *et al.* Sutures versus staples for skin closure in orthopaedic surgery: meta-analysis. *BMJ* 2010; **340**: c1199.
45. Torfs S, Levet T, Delesalle C, *et al.* Risk factors for incisional complications after exploratory celiotomy in horses: do skin staples increase risk? *Vet Surg* 2010; **39**: 616.
46. Colbath AC, Patipa L, Berghaus RD, *et al.* The influence of suture pattern on the incidence of incisional following exploratory laparotomy. *Equine Vet J* 2014; **46**: 156.
47. Hemming K, Pinkney T, Futaba K, *et al.* A systematic review of systematic reviews and panoramic meta-analysis: staples versus sutures for surgical procedures. *PLoS One* 2013; **8**: e75132.
48. Wilson DA. New and innovative approaches to wound closure. In: Stashak TS, Theoret CL (eds). *Equine Wound Management*, 2nd edn. Wiley Blackwell: Ames, 2008: 225.
49. Dumville JC, Coulthard P, Worthington HV, *et al.* Tissue adhesives for closure of surgical incisions. *Cochrane Database Syst Rev* 2014; **11**: CD004287.
50. Grissom MJ, Temple-Wong MM, Adams MS, *et al.* Synovial fluid lubricant properties are transiently deficient after arthroscopic articular cartilage defect repair with platelet-enriched fibrin alone and with mesenchymal stem cells. *Orthop J Sports Med* 2014; **2**: doi:10.1177/2325967114542580.

51. Ferris D, Frisbie D, Kisiday J, *et al.* *In vivo* healing of meniscal lacerations using bone marrow-derived mesenchymal stem cells and fibrin glue. *Stem Cells Int*; **2012**: 691605.
52. Lacitignola L, Crovace A, Rossi G, *et al.* Cell therapy for tendinitis, experimental and clinical report. *Vet Res Comm* 2008; **32**: S33–S38.
53. Hu L, Lu Z, Wang B, *et al.* Closure of skin incisions by laser-welding with a combination of two near-infrared diode lasers: preliminary study for determination of optimal parameters. *J Biomed Opt* 2011; **16**: 038001.
54. Gabay I, Barequet I, Varssano D, *et al.* Bonding surgical incisions using a temperature controlled laser system based on a single infrared fiber. *J Biomed Opt* 2013; **18**: 111416.
55. Miller CW. Bandages and drains. In: Slatter D (ed). *Textbook of Small Animal Surgery*, 7th edn. WB Saunders: Philadelphia, 2003: 244.
56. Auer JA. Drains, bandages, and external coaptation. In: Auer J, Stick J (eds). *Equine Surgery*, 4th edn. Elsevier Saunders: St Louis, 2012: 203.
57. Baines SJ. Surgical drains. In: Fowler D, Williams JM (eds). *Manual of Canine and Feline Wound Management and Reconstruction*, 1st edn. Br Small Anim Vet Assoc: London, 1999: 44.
58. Carruthers KH, Eisemann BS, Lamp S, *et al.* Optimizing the closed suction surgical drainage system. *Plast Surg Nursing* 2013; **33**: 38.
59. Hampel NL, Johnson RG. Principles of surgical drains and drainage. *J Am Animal Hosp Assoc* 1985; **21**: 21.

CHAPTER 10

Principles and Techniques for Reconstructive Surgery

Ted S. Stashak, DVM, MS, Diplomate ACVS and **Jim Schumacher**, DVM, MS, Diplomate ACVS, MRCVS

Chapter Contents

Summary

The aim of reconstructive surgery is to primarily close a wound created by accident or by excision of a lesion. Reconstructive surgical techniques allow tension-free closure of many wounds that may seem impossible to suture. The advantages of these techniques over managing an open wound by second-intention healing are a reduced healing time, an increased percentage of the wound's surface being covered by full-thickness skin, a more cosmetic outcome, and an earlier return to function. When indicated, mobilizing adjacent tissue to cover a skin defect is preferable to skin grafting of an open wound because it provides more reliable healing and better cosmetic and functional results.

Introduction

When a full-thickness skin wound, caused by trauma or excision of a lesion, cannot be closed by suturing alone, mobilization of adjacent skin should be considered, particularly if the objective is to achieve the best functional and cosmetic outcome.[1–3] The ability of a surgeon to successfully close a wound is dictated by the extent of skin loss and the amount of loose skin surrounding a wound.[4]

That said, reconstructive surgical techniques (e.g., presuturing, adjustable sutures, and tension suturing techniques) allow tension-free closure of many wounds heretofore deemed impossible to close. Techniques to expand skin (e.g., intraoperative tissue expansion and implanted elastomers) allow the surgeon

Equine Wound Management, Third Edition. Edited by Christine Theoret and Jim Schumacher.

Companion website: www.wiley.com/go/theoret/wound

to stretch the skin adjacent to a lesion to be excised, thus reducing the tension created by primary closure. Additional relief of tension may be obtained by simply undermining the skin surrounding the wound, making one or more longitudinal relaxing incisions, using a skin mesh expansion technique, or using a V–Y or Z plasty. Combining tissue debulking (i.e., excision of granulation tissue or scar tissue) with techniques for mobilizing skin and relieving tension may be necessary to cosmetically reconstruct a large, open wound, such as one created in an accident or one created by removing a large cutaneous lesion (e.g., scar or tumor).

The shape of the wound is also an important consideration. Whereas fusiform (i.e., spindle-shaped – wide in the middle with tapered ends) skin wounds often can be closed after only undermining surrounding skin to relieve tension, closure of large rectangular, square, triangular, or circular skin wounds typically requires a combination of strategically placed incisions with local undermining to create a skin flap capable of covering the wound. In some cases, a rotation flap or a transposition flap may be needed to cover a circular wound in a tight-skinned region.

A skin flap differs from a skin graft in that a flap retains its blood supply through its attachment to a pedicle of skin and subcutaneous tissue. Randomly based pedicle flaps, also referred to as random-pattern skin flaps, derive their blood supply from many small, direct arteries (described later under Cutaneous blood supply), whereas axial-pattern flaps rely on a single neurovascular trunk (i.e., a named vascular pedicle) for blood supply to the raised and transferred tissue. Randomly based pedicle flaps are used more commonly in equine surgery.[5] Types of randomly based pedicle flaps include rotation flaps and transposition flaps, which are flaps that are rotated in an arc about a pivot point into an adjacent wound, and advancement flaps, which are flaps that are moved directly into a defect without rotation.[6] The rotation flap is semicircular, whereas the transposition flap is rectangular or square. Randomly based pedicle flaps are classified according to their design (Table 10.1). Often, the defect created by advancing or rotating a cutaneous flap into a wound cannot be approximated with sutures and, consequently, is allowed to heal by second intention or is healed by applying a free skin graft. For information regarding the methods used for skin grafting, see Chapter 18.

Because a significant direct relationship between width and viable length of a randomly based flap has been demonstrated in an experiment using ponies, the skin flap should be designed so its base is as broad as possible.[7] The viability of a randomly based pedicle flap is adversely affected by extrinsic factors, such as infection, but the blood supply to the flap is probably the most important factor in the flap's survival.[7] A flap raised in two stages is more likely to survive than is a flap lifted and transplanted at the first operation.[8] This increase in likelihood of survival is termed the *delay phenomenon*. Delay either conditions the flap to ischemia, allowing it to survive on less blood flow than is normally needed, or more likely, delay improves vascularity of the flap, perhaps by causing an increase in expression of cytokines that stimulate growth of vascular endothelium.[9] To increase the likelihood of survival of a skin flap when the flap's survival may be precarious, the flap is created but only partially undermined, and at a later date (e.g., 7–14 days later), the flap is completely elevated and inserted into the wound to be covered.

Table 10.1 Classification of local skin flaps according to their design.

Flap design	Definition	Best use
Rotation flap		
Unilateral	A semicircular or three-fourths circular flap of skin and subcutaneous tissue that rotates about a pivot point into a defect to be closed	Triangular defects with skin available on one side. Of limited use in the horse, in the authors' experience. May be most useful to cover defects of skin over the maxilla and nasal bones
Bilateral	Rotation flaps designed on both sides of the wound	Triangular defects with skin available on two sides. Of limited use in the horse, in the authors' experience. May be most useful to cover defects of skin over the maxilla and nasal bones
Pedicle advancement flap	Flap of skin that is mobilized by undermining and advancing it into a defect without altering the plane of the pedicle	Rectangular or square defect
Single (French flap)	Skin that is available for closure on one side of the defect (e.g., eyelid)	Half H-plasty (Figure 10.33)
Modified single	Skin that is available for closure on one side of the defect	To cover irregular or unequal angular defects (Figures 10.36, 10.37) To cover triangular-shaped defects (Figures 10.39, 10.40, 10.41) More practical than rotation flaps, in the authors' experience
Two opposing	Skin that is available for closure on two sides of the defect	H-plasty (Figure 10.32). Use primarily for large defects
Transposition flap	Usually a rectangular piece of skin and subcutaneous tissue that is rotated on a pivot point to cover an adjacent defect	To cover defects in tight-skinned regions, such as the face To be most effective, the flap is developed close to the defect so minimal rotation is required (Figure 10.43)

Free-transfer skin flaps, or axial-pattern skin flaps, when compared to randomly based pedicle flaps, have been shown to have superior vascular perfusion and a greater ability to maintain a larger percentage of baseline perfusion when subject to tension.[10] Relatively few axial-pattern flaps have been identified in horses compared to the number identified in dogs, cats, and humans. A type of axial-pattern flap referred to as the Estlander flap was used to repair a large, chronic lip laceration in a foal.[11] Free-transfer skin flaps are discussed later under that heading.

Reconstructive techniques may be used in conjunction with primary closure (the exception is skin expansion using a silicone elastomer) and delayed closure, and for closure after excision of a tumor or revision of scar tissue. The advantages of these techniques over open wound management are an overall reduction in healing time, an increased percentage of the wound's surface being covered by full-thickness skin, and a more cosmetic outcome with an earlier return to function. When indicated, mobilizing adjacent tissue to cover a skin defect is preferable to skin grafting of an open wound because it provides more reliable healing and better cosmetic and functional results.[12]

Before undertaking a reconstructive procedure, the surgeon should be aware of the owner's expectations, and the owner should be informed of the potential complications, the expected outcome, and the financial costs associated with the procedure. Such a discussion is especially important when performing an elective cosmetic procedure where failure to accomplish an esthetic outcome can lead to considerable client dissatisfaction. This said, a successful outcome can be very rewarding professionally and especially pleasing to the client. This chapter reviews cutaneous reconstructive surgical techniques and describes their clinical applications.

Cutaneous blood supply

An understanding of the cutaneous blood supply is crucial to successful reconstructive surgery. Whereas detailed descriptions of the vascular supply to the skin of humans[13,14] and dogs[15,16] have been the basis for substantial advancement of cutaneous reconstructive surgery, little information detailing the vascular supply to the skin of horses is available. Two types of cutaneous blood supply have been identified in mammals: perforating musculocutaneous vessels and direct cutaneous vessels. Perforating musculocutaneous arteries pass though the body of a muscle to supply the overlying skin. These arteries are larger and sparser in areas where the skin is loose, and smaller and more densely packed in regions where the skin is less mobile.[14] Microangiograms[7] and latex vascular injections[17] have demonstrated that, similar to dogs and cats, horses and ponies do not have perforating musculocutaneous arteries.

Direct cutaneous arteries pass through fascial septa between muscles and supply a larger area of skin than do the perforating musculocutaneous vessels found in some mammals. Direct cutaneous arteries are found in loose-skinned regions, running parallel to the skin surface in close association with the *panniculus carnosus* muscle, where present, whereas in the distal extremities of most animals, they run beneath and parallel to the dermis. Smaller vessels branch off these direct cutaneous arteries and in the dog, and perhaps in the horse, arborize in the dermis, forming three interconnected plexuses: the subcutaneous (deep) plexus, the cutaneous (middle or intermediate) plexus, and the superficial (subepidermal or subpapillary) plexus, which together supply the dermis and the adnexa directly and the epidermis by passive diffusion.[18] All three of these vascular plexuses are important to consider when manipulating and/or undermining skin.

Physical and biomechanical properties of skin

Interaction between the skin's structural components, collagen and elastic fibers, as well as ground substance, provides skin with its natural tension and its viscoelastic properties. Knowledge of these properties allows the surgeon to select the appropriate direction in which to excise a mass or reconstruct a wound to create the least amount of tension upon closure and to enable stretching of the skin to overcome the forces of tension. Tissues can be stretched to overcome tension because of the following physical, biomechanical, and viscoelastic properties: (1) inherent extensibility; (2) mechanical and biologic creep; and (3) stress relaxation. The surgeon must have an understanding of these properties and of the lines of skin tension to be able to stretch skin to reconstruct a wound.

Lines of skin tension

The normal tension that exists in skin is a result of elastic fibers in the dermis. These fibers cause the edges of the wound to retract when the skin is incised, converting a linear wound into an elliptical wound. Lines of skin tension (i.e., Langer's lines) have been referred to as lines of maximal skin tension. However, because skin is anisotropic (i.e., lacking similar properties in all directions) and because these lines of tension can be influenced by movement of an anatomic part, Langer's lines are more accurately referred to as static or relaxed lines of skin tension.[19] Different from static forces but also important are the dynamic forces on skin, which are created by the contraction of underlying muscles. Wounds that are at right or oblique angles to these static and dynamic forces gape more widely and heal with a wider scar than do wounds created parallel to these lines. Incisions or lacerations made at oblique angles to the static or dynamic lines of tension take on a curvilinear shape. Incisions made perpendicular to these lines tend to gape widely, are subject to greater tension, and require more sutures to approximate their edges, and consequently tend to develop a wider epithelial scar. A surgeon can determine the direction in which to close a wound or to create a fusiform incision to remove a lesion by assessing the direction of maximal extensibility of the skin. Both static and dynamic lines of tension should be determined. Thus, the ideal incision is made parallel to these lines of tension, and wounds should be closed in a direction that averts or minimizes skin tension.[20] Lines of tension of humans[21] and dogs[22] have been well described, but those of horses have been investigated only to a small extent.[23]

Inherent extensibility

Inherent extensibility refers to the skin's normal capacity to stretch while an anatomic part is at rest.[24,25] This property allows the surgeon to excise a small fusiform-shaped piece of skin and perform primary closure of the resultant wound. A skin biopsy punch wound model showed that lines of maximal skin extensibility of the equine carpus, upon flexion and extension, run in the same direction as Langer's lines, which are parallel to the limb's long axis.[26] The best direction for an incision, therefore, is straight and parallel to the lines of maximum extensibility. The edges of the wound have the least tension when they are approximated parallel to the direction of maximal extensibility.

Pinching the skin to elevate it over the proposed site of excision of a tumor or scar or over a site of proposed reconstruction of a wound provides a rough estimate of the skin's inherent extensibility.[4,25,27] Maximal skin extensibility should be assessed with the anatomic part in its normal position, at rest, followed by movement of the part (e.g., flexion and extension of the joints of the limb), which can greatly influence extensibility.[28]

Mechanical creep and stress relaxation

Mechanical creep and stress relaxation represent two different kinds of biomechanical events that occur, within minutes to hours, in viscoelastic tissue placed under a constant load or strain.[29] Mechanical creep is the biomechanical property that allows skin, when placed under a constant load, to stretch, over time, beyond its normal limits of extensibility.[25] Creep is calculated by applying a constant amount of tension or load on the tissue and measuring the amount of tissue deformation that occurs over time. Creep is, therefore, described as tissue deformation per given length of time at a constant load. Creep occurs because randomly oriented collagen fibers in the dermis straighten longitudinally and become aligned parallel to the stretching force, allowing the skin to stretch.[30]

Stress placed on skin, when skin is loaded rapidly to a finite strain while its length is held constant, decreases with time.[29] This viscoelastic property of skin is referred to as stress relaxation. To measure stress relaxation, a fixed amount of tension that results in a certain degree of deformation or elongation is applied to the skin. The tension is held constant for a period of time, after which the tension within the tissue is measured. The decrease in tissue tension during this time period represents the stress relaxation of the tissue.[29] Stress relaxation can be achieved during surgery by placing the skin under constant or cyclic strain. Over time, the amount of strain required to maintain elongation decreases, and the skin becomes less taut. This biomechanical property of skin explains why the tension on a suture line decreases within hours after surgery.[4,25] The amount of tension required to successfully achieve stress relaxation in the clinical situation is unknown, but excess tension on a suture line may compromise blood flow to the skin edges, resulting in ischemia and dehiscence. Sound clinical judgment is required, therefore, to make use of this important property of skin.

The time-dependent reorientation of collagen fibers that occurs within a viscous matrix was assumed to account for all of the viscoelastic behavior of extensible connective tissue.[30] A recent study, however, found no obvious reorientation of collagen fibers, when *low loads* of tension were applied to skin during the time course of the stress-relaxation and creep experiments. These results suggest that viscoelastic properties of skin reside not only within the collagen fibers but also at the fiber–extracellular matrix interface.[31] The skin's time-dependent deformation is significantly influenced by the dermal viscoelasticity primarily, up to a critical load beyond which it is controlled by the outermost aspect of the epidermis, particularly the *stratum corneum*.[32]

Biologic creep

Biologic creep is different from mechanical creep in that the skin is expanded rather than stretched and thinned.[25] Biologic creep is the slow expansion of tissue, over weeks to months, that accompanies pregnancy or obesity. It also occurs when a subcutaneous mass, such as a tumor, enlarges slowly. The skin is not thinned, as with mechanical creep, but gradually responds by increasing epidermal mitotic activity and in-growth of blood vessels and cells into the dermis in proportion to the growth of the mass; both of these processes allow more skin to develop and an increase in the blood supply to the expanded skin.[25,33]

General principles of reconstructive surgery

Developing a surgical plan

Mobilizing adjacent tissue to cover a full-thickness skin defect requires careful planning. Skin extensibility should be determined while the affected anatomic part is in a normal relaxed position (inherent extensibility), as well as during movement (maximal extensibility) by puckering the skin either over or adjacent to the wound or lesion to be removed (Figure 10.1). In some cases, extensibility can be evaluated sufficiently by elevating a lesion to be excised with the thumb and forefingers. Evaluating skin extensibility in a systematic manner delineates the regions of skin available for relief of tension and mobilization and for forming a skin flap.

The lines of skin tension and maximum skin extensibility on the limbs are parallel to the long axis.[12,26] Wounds that are parallel to the limb's long axis, therefore, are not subjected to the same amount of tension during flexion or extension as are wounds that are oblique or at a right angle to the limb's long axis.[3] Wounds located on the dorsal or palmar/plantar surface that are perpendicular or oblique to the limb's axis typically separate widely when the limb is flexed or extended (Figure 10.2), and consequently, postoperative immobilization of such wounds is usually required. When removing a lesion from a limb, the

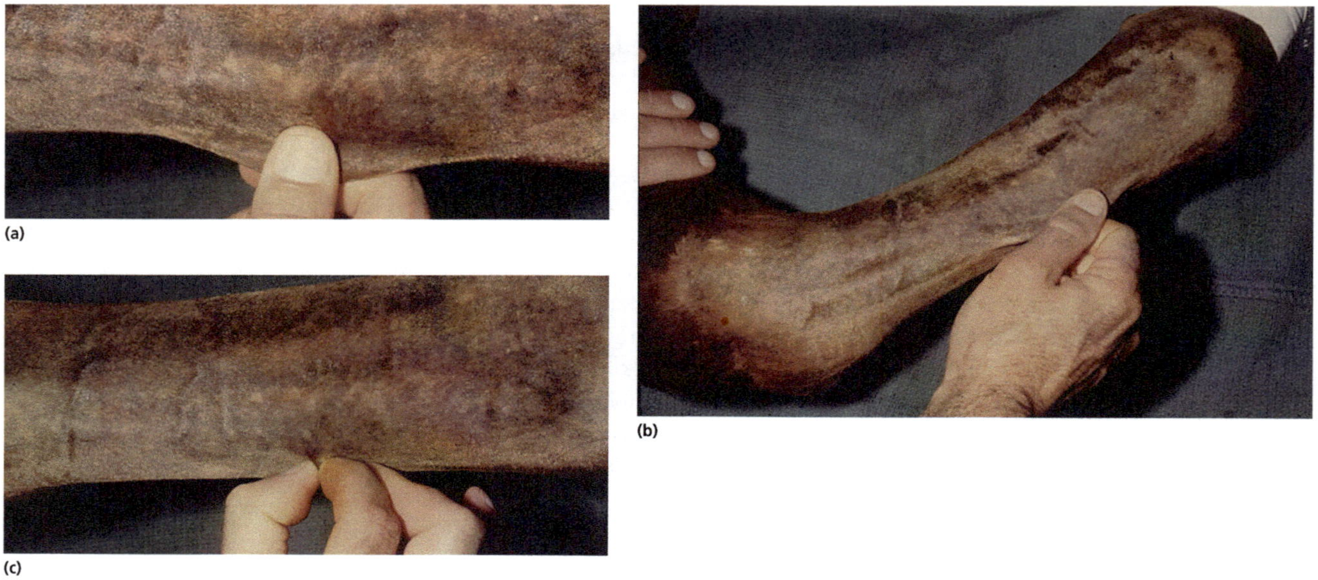

Figure 10.1 Tension lines and maximal extensibility of the skin of the forelimb are parallel to the limb's long axis. **(a)** Forelimb in its normal position at rest. Skin extensibility is evaluated by pinching the skin, parallel and perpendicular to the limb's long axis, over the dorsal mid-metacarpal region. **(b)** Carpus and fetlock flexed. Skin extensibility and tension remains the same. **(c)** Carpus and fetlock flexed. Skin extensibility is assessed perpendicular to the limb's long axis over the dorsal mid-metacarpal region. Compared to skin tension with the limb in its normal position, skin tension has increased markedly, and the extensibility has decreased.

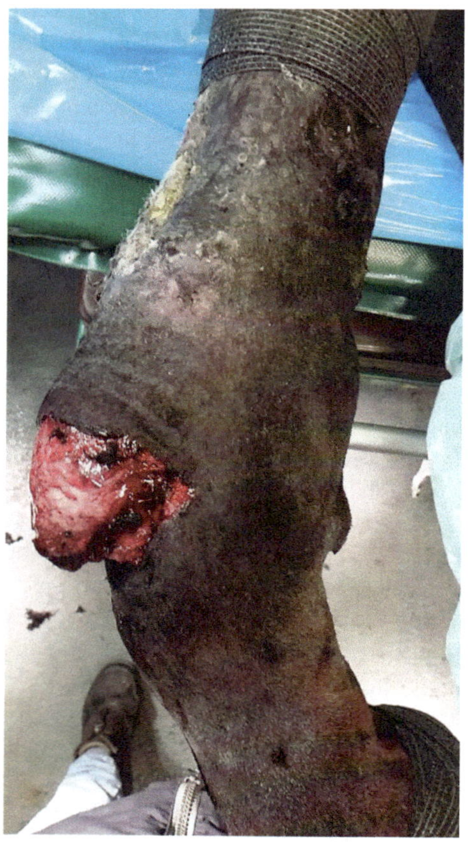

Figure 10.2 Transverse laceration involving the dorsal surface of the fetlock joint. The wound gapes widely while the joint is flexed, whereas the wound's edges were in contact when the fetlock was extended. The severed end of the common digital extensor tendon protrudes from the wound. Courtesy of Dr. Tom O'Brien.

longitudinal axis of excision should be parallel to the long axis of the limb whenever possible. Skin is then mobilized in a transverse plane (lateral to medial) rather than from proximal to distal, which would subject the wound to greater stress.

To determine in what direction to suture a wound or excise a lesion from the proximal portion of a limb, the trunk, or the neck, the affected structure should be manipulated through its full range of motion prior to making a final decision regarding skin extensibility (Figure 10.3a). During surgery, the affected structure should be maintained in a position that creates the greatest tension so that the appropriate surgical approach is selected to close the wound and reduce the risk of postoperative dehiscence (Figure 10.3b). The choice of direction of excision is dictated by available skin and the configuration of the defect. A sterile ruler, sterile marking pen, or sterile methylene blue applied with a sterilized instrument can be used to draw this pattern on the skin (Figure 10.4). After incision, the skin is mobilized, or flaps are created by separating tissues in their natural cleavage planes deep within the subcutaneous tissue.

What to do

- Surgical incisions should be made parallel to the direction of maximal extensibility, which, on the limbs, is parallel to the long axis of the limb.
- The maximum extensibility of skin should be determined with the anatomic part in its normal position and also in maximum flexion and extension.
- At surgery, the affected structure should be maintained in a position that creates the greatest tension so that the appropriate surgical approach is selected to close the wound.

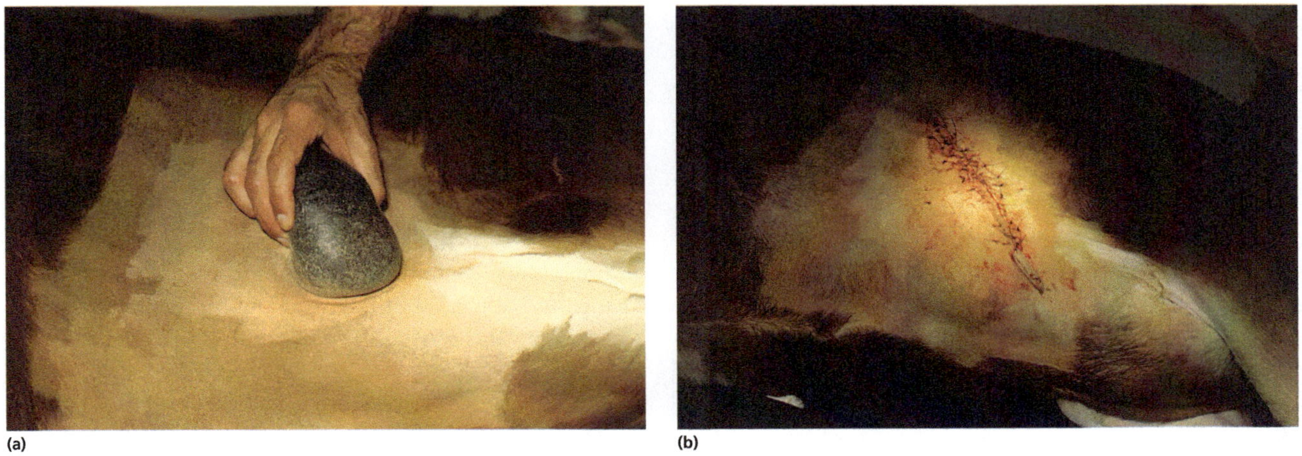

Figure 10.3 This large solitary melanoma on the right ventrolateral thoracic region in a cow is used to illustrate the value of movement of a part to determine the correct axis for excision and to predict the extent of excision required to remove this lesion. The melanoma was freely movable, somewhat pedunculated, and appeared to be attached by a stalk of skin approximately 10 cm in diameter while the cow was standing. **(a)** With the cow anesthetized and in left lateral recumbency, the right limb was extended forward as would occur during walking or when resting in sternal recumbency. The lesion became sessile when the limb was extended. **(b)** The extent of excision required to remove the melanoma was greater than would have been predicted while the animal was standing. The limb was maintained in extension during surgery to ensure that the appropriate surgical approach, skin mobilization, and suturing techniques to close the wound were selected.

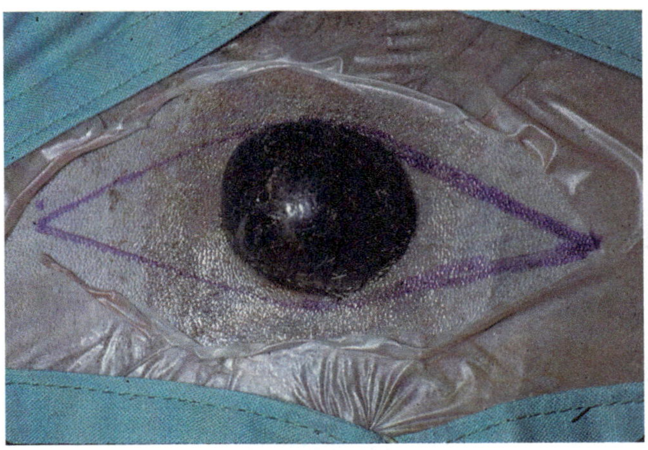

Figure 10.4 Solitary melanoma on the caudal thigh of a horse. A sterile marking pen was used to draw this fusiform pattern on the skin in preparation for excision.

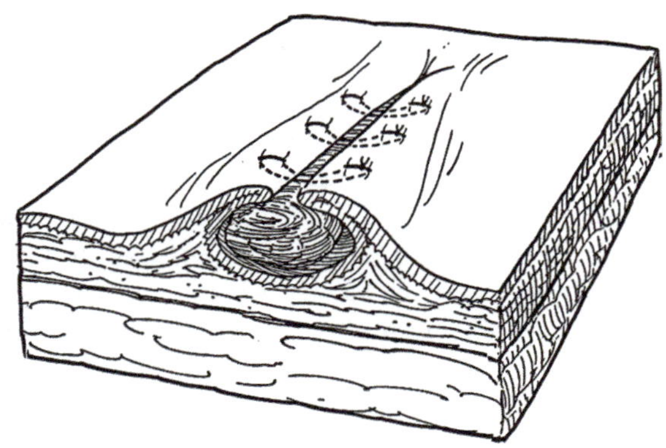

Figure 10.5 Illustration of the presuturing technique. Adapted from Liang 1988.[36]

Tension-reducing suturing techniques

Suturing techniques that allow tension-free closure of a defect rely on two biomechanical properties of skin: mechanical creep and stress relaxation.

Presuturing

Presuturing is a technique whereby sutures are placed preoperatively to plicate skin over a proposed site of excision or to relieve tension on the wound's margin.[34,35] The technique is performed by spanning the wound with heavy sutures, placed in an interrupted or mattress Lembert suture pattern, hours before a lesion is to be excised or a wound is to be debrided and sutured. It is most applicable to lesions or wounds of the body and proximal region of the limbs but sometimes may be useful for closing wounds of the distal portion of the limb.

Using heavy, non-absorbable suture material, such as size 1 or 2 polypropylene or nylon, suture bites are placed in the skin perpendicular and 2 cm to 6 cm from each side of the lesion or the edges of the wound.[34,35] Tension applied to the sutures elevates and folds skin over the lesion or wound (Figure 10.5). The procedure is performed between 2 and 8 hours before surgery, with the horse sedated, after desensitizing the surgical site by using local or regional anesthesia. Placing these sutures 24 hours or more in advance of surgery may cause tissue surrounding the wound to become edematous, complicating closure.[25,26,30,33–35,37] Presuturing relies on creep, which permits skin to be stretched beyond its inherent ability to stretch.[38] When skin is stretched to a certain length, the force required to maintain that length gradually diminishes via stress relaxation. Presuturing experimentally created wounds on pigs showed that closing a presutured wound required 40% less force than that required to close a non-presutured wound.[25] When compared with simply undermining the surrounding skin, presuturing resulted in some tissue gain and an initial decrease in closing tension.[37]

Although the original description of this technique suggests that presuturing avoids the potential complications of undermining,[25] the combination of presuturing and undermining (discussed later in this chapter) may provide advantages beyond presuturing alone. Because presuturing reduces skin tension, less undermining of adjacent skin is required to close a defect.[4]

Tips

- Imbricating skin over a lesion to be excised (i.e., presuturing), between 2 and 8 hours before surgery stretches the skin, thereby decreasing the force required to close the wound created when the lesion is excised.
- Presuturing can usually be performed with the horse sedated after desensitizing the site of surgery using regional or local analgesia.
- Combining presuturing with undermining provides greater relief of tension.

Mesh overlay

Just as mesh can be used to bolster repair of an abdominal incisional hernia, so too can it be used to bolster repair of a wound sutured under excessive tension (Figure 10.6) or of a wound located in an area subjected to constant movement, such as a nostril or lip. Using this technique, a mesh [e.g., woven polypropylene (Bard, Davol), or knitted polyester (Mersilene, Ethicon)] is placed over the sutured wound. One edge of the mesh is sutured to the skin using 2-0 non-absorbable suture material placed in a simple interrupted pattern (Figure 10.6b). The open side of the mesh is sutured to the skin on the opposite side of the sutured wound using pre-placed sutures of the same material, placed in a Mayo mattress pattern (Figure 10.6c). The pre-placed sutures are tightened in unison and tied to transfer tension from the sutured wound to the mesh. To distribute tension over a wider area, two or more staggered rows of simple interrupted sutures anchoring the mesh to skin can be placed axial to each sutured edge of the mesh (Figure 10.6d). To minimize interruption of blood supply to the sutured wound, sutures anchoring the mesh should be placed perpendicular to the sutured wound, unless the mesh is placed in a highly vascular area, such as a lip or nostril.

Adjustable suture technique

Problems associated with delayed closure of a wound – particularly a wound on the distal aspect of a limb of a horse, such as retraction and reduced pliability of the wound margins and ineffective wound contraction – can be obviated to a large degree by placing constant tension on the wound's margin with an adjustable suture, a technique referred to as augmented wound contraction.[38] To perform this technique, the wound and surrounding tissue are desensitized using local infiltration of anesthetic solution or regional anesthesia, after which a heavy suture is placed intradermally to span the wound's margins using a continuous horizontal mattress pattern. Each suture bite is advanced slightly, so that the suture passes at an angle across the wound, allowing the suture to slide easily through the dermis. Each end of the suture exits the skin, and by applying tension to these suture ends, the skin on one side of the wound is drawn toward that of the opposite side. Each end of the suture is threaded through a button, and after tension has been applied to the margin of the wound by tightening the suture, the ends are anchored to the button using an umbilical clamp or split-shot.

The margins of the wound are pulled closer together by tightening the suture daily. The most rapid decrease in the size of the wound occurs during the first 3 days.[38] Subsequently, the skin edges are apposed, if possible, or the wound is left to heal by second intention. The technique can be used not only to augment contraction but also to prevent a fresh wound from expanding. A commercially available wound closure system (Dynamic Tissue Systems™, Southmedic Inc) uses multiple anchors that are inserted in the skin on opposite sides of the wound. Tension on the wound's edges is created when elastomer bands are affixed to the anchors.

What to do

- A wound that cannot be completely closed at the time of surgery can sometimes be closed gradually, over the course of 3 or 4 days, by using an adjustable suture, a technique referred to as "augmented wound contraction."

Tips

- An adjustable suture is a heavy suture placed intradermally, from one edge of the wound to the other, using a continuous horizontal mattress pattern. Each end exits the skin and is threaded through a button. After tension has been applied to the margin of the wound by pulling on the ends of the suture, the ends are anchored to the button with an umbilical clamp or split-shot.
- An adjustable suture applied to a fresh wound too large to close keeps the wound from expanding.

Tension suturing techniques

Tension suturing techniques are most often used in conjunction with other skin mobilization techniques (e.g., undermining, which is discussed later).

Tension on skin sutures may be relieved by inserting deep dermal sutures with buried knots before inserting superficial skin sutures. These dermal sutures also align the skin edges, easing insertion of the superficial skin sutures. The surgeon should place only as many sutures as are necessary to reduce tension on the wound, especially when the wound is contaminated, because these deep dermal sutures act as foreign bodies and can become a nidus for infection.

Sutures placed in a horizontal or vertical mattress pattern, well away from the skin margins, can also be used to decrease

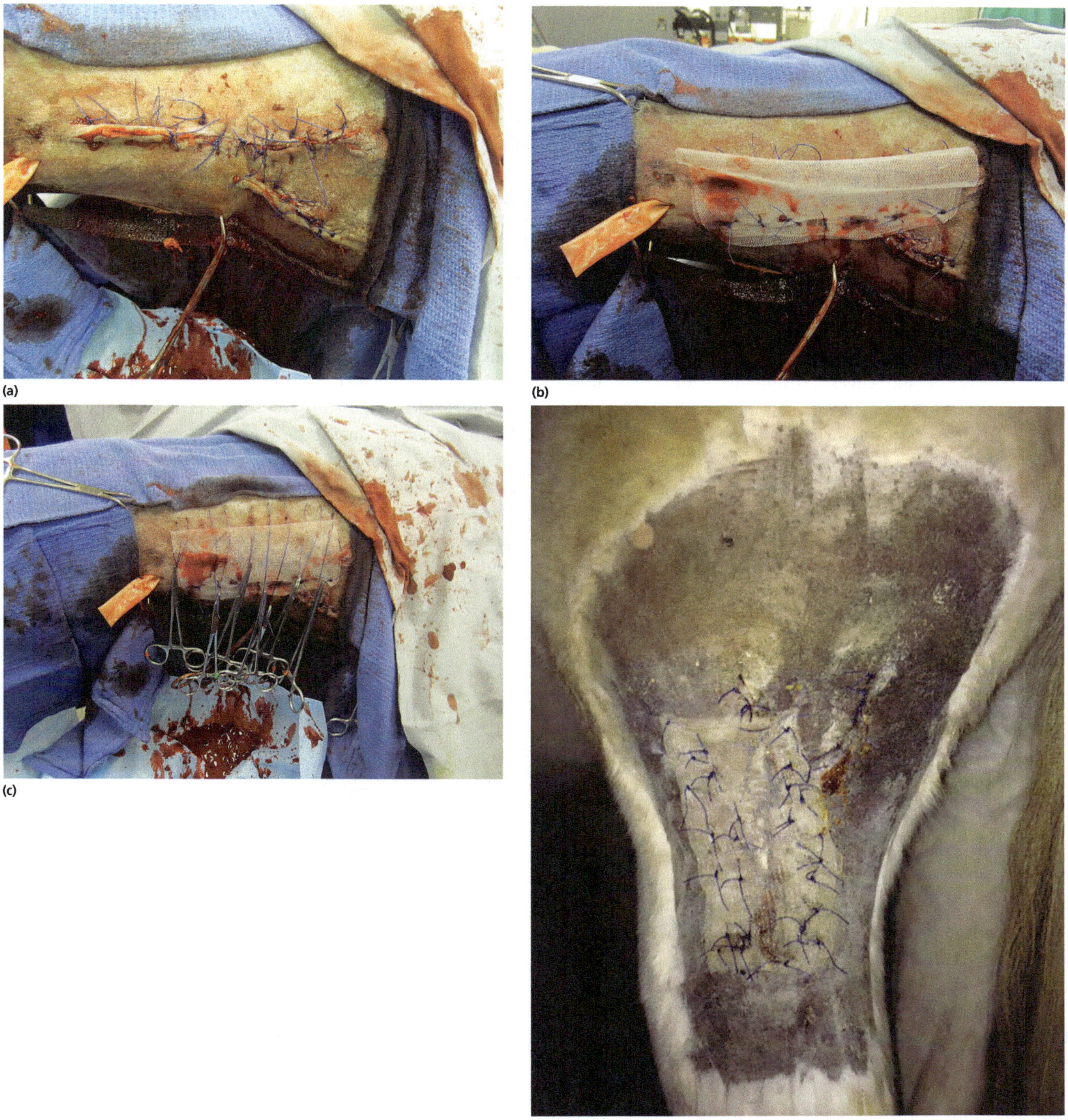

(a) (b) (c) (d)

Figure 10.6 Technique of mesh overlay used to decrease tension on a sutured wound on the thigh of horse. **(a)** This wound was sutured under great tension. **(b)** Using the technique of mesh overlay, a polypropylene mesh was placed over the sutured wound, and one edge of the mesh was sutured to the skin on one side of the wound. **(c)** The other side of the mesh was sutured to the skin on the opposite side of the wound using pre-placed Mayo sutures. When the sutures were tightened and tied, tension on the sutured incision was transferred to the mesh. Tension was distributed over a wider area by placing two or more staggered rows of simple interrupted sutures anchoring the mesh to the skin. **(d)** The mesh overlay 10 days after surgery.

tension at the wound margins. The wound margins are then approximated, without tension, with sutures placed closer to the margin, using a simple interrupted or a vertical mattress pattern. The vertical mattress pattern is less likely to interfere with blood supply than is the horizontal mattress pattern. Sections of rubber tubing (supports) placed under the loops of the tension sutures distribute pressure and may prevent interruption of blood flow to skin underlying these sutures (see Figure 9.19).

The use of rubber tubing to distribute pressure, however, should be reserved for regions that cannot be supported by bandaging (e.g., the neck, trunk, and proximal portion of the limb) because placing a pressure bandage over the sections of rubber tubing may cause pressure necrosis in the skin underlying these supports. The tension sutures are removed in 5–7 days, by which time tension on the approximating sutures should have greatly dissipated.

The far–near–near–far pattern serves as both a tension suture, by providing a pulley-like effect, and an approximating suture.[39] The far component relieves tension on the near component, which approximates the margins of the wound. The loop in the suture greatly increases the strength of the suture and of the tissue in which it is placed. Excessive tightening of the suture tends to invert the skin edges. Tension on a sutured wound may also be relieved by closing it with a walking suture pattern. For a complete discussion of suturing patterns and techniques, see Chapter 9.

Tips

- More than one row of sutures placed in a mattress pattern may be required to adequately reduce tension on the margins of a wound.
- Far-and-near suture patterns approximate tissue and, by providing a pulley-like effect, relieve tension on the margins of the wound.

What to avoid

- Sections of tubing should not be placed beneath the loops of sutures if the sutured wound is to be covered with a bandage because pressure placed on the tubing from the bandage may cause the skin underlying the tubing to become necrotic.

Skin stretching and expansion techniques

As with tension-reducing suturing techniques, skin stretching and expansion techniques rely on the skin's biomechanical properties of mechanical creep and stress relaxation to achieve the desired outcome of tension-free closure of a defect.

External stretching devices for primary or delayed primary closure

Externally applied devices designed to pull, thus stretch, the skin surrounding a wound or excisional site are commercially available (e.g., Sure-Closure™, SyntheMed, Inc.; Wisebands Skin Closure Device™, 4 Med Ltd; TopClosure®, IVT Medical Ltd).[40–42] These skin-stretching devices apply controlled traction to skin surrounding a large tissue deficit thereby allowing the deficit to eventually be sutured.

The use of a skin-stretching apparatus composed of Velcro (Velcro USA Inc) has been described in dogs. This apparatus uses pads of Velcro, attached to the skin using cyanoacrylate glue and connecting cables of Velcro.[42] Placement of the adherent pads in relation to the skin edge can be adjusted according to the amount of skin needed to cover the wound; thus, large areas of skin may be mobilized adjacent and more distant to the wound. Tension on the cables is adjusted every 6–8 hours, and in most cases, enough skin is recruited to allow closure within 48–72 hours. The system can also be left in place for 2–4 days after wound closure to offset excessive tension at the suture site. Separation of the pad from the skin during the process of stretching is the most common complication associated with the use of this system. This apparatus may be applicable to horses, although to the authors' knowledge, its use to stretch the skin surrounding wounds of horses has not been reported.

Another system (Sure-Closure™) attaches the skin to the undersurface of the device using hooks that face the wound and abut against an 8-cm long intradermal needle inserted on each side and parallel to the wound. A 7.5-cm long screw-driven tension rod is used to increase the tension (Figure 10.7).[41] A tension-gauge on the device is not engaged until tension applied to skin exceeds 1 kg, and when the tension exceeds 2.5 kg, a safety clutch disengages the device, thus neutralizing tension. The advantages to this system are that: (1) the device can be applied, using sterile technique, by local infiltration of anesthetic solution or regional anesthesia; (2) undermining of the skin edges is not required; (3) the stretching force on the skin margin is spread over a wide area (i.e., over 8-cm long intradermal

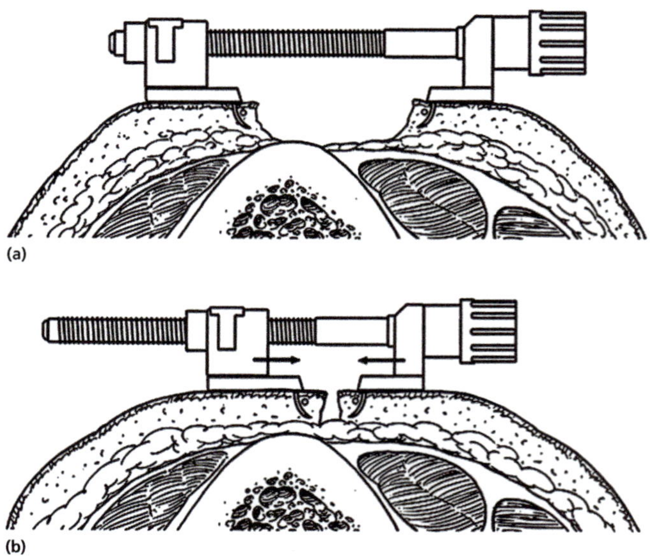

Figure 10.7 Schematic drawing of a skin stretching system (Secure Closure™) being used to stretch skin and the underlying subcutaneous tissue over exposed bone without undermining the skin. **(a)** Application of the system involves placement of two straight 8-cm long needles in the dermis opposite each other and 0.5 cm from the wound edges (small circles axial to the hooks in the skin contact plate). The skin contact U-shaped arms are secured to the skin by two inward-facing intradermal hooks (two hooks on each U-shaped plate) that, after insertion through the skin, abut against previously placed intradermal pins. **(b)** The threaded screw is tightened to increase tension, which is monitored by a tension gauge located on the device, and the wound is brought into apposition, ready for suturing. Source: Adapted from Hirshowitz *et al.* 1993.[44]

needles); (4) traction can be applied incrementally with periods of tension relaxation; and (5) the skin can be sutured while the device is in place. The disadvantage is that applying tension to a wound wider than 7.5 cm is difficult.

The Wisebands Skin Closure Device™ is composed of a stretching device and a 50-cm long polypropylene band that encircles the skin and underlying tissues (subcutaneous fat, fascia, and muscle), allowing closure of complex wounds.[40] A gauge permits application of 1 kg/cm^2 of tension to tissues surrounding the wound; if tension on the tissue exceeds 1 kg/cm^2, the tension placed by the device relaxes to a lesser tension. Tissue is stretched intraoperatively by tightening the band, pausing until the tissue relaxes, thereby releasing tension on the device. The band is then retightened until the wound edges can be approximated with sutures. The device may be left in place for several days if the sutured wound is at risk of dehiscence because of moderate tension. If the edges of the wound cannot be approximated completely during the operation, the open wound is dressed appropriately, and the wound is stretched daily until the wound can be sutured. The advantage to this system is that it may be applied to assist the closure of complex wounds, no matter their shape or depth, and it can be applied to most regions of the body. The disadvantages are that the horse must be anesthetized for the device to be applied, and, because the gauge allows only 1 kg/cm^2 of tension to be applied, which is considerably less than the 3 kg/cm^2 of tension that can be safely applied to stretched skin (at least in humans),[41] a longer period is required to close the defect than when using the Sure-Closure™ device. The Wisebands device™ is supplied for single use only.

The TopClosure® system is comprised of two attachment plates, which are placed on either side of the wound and opposite each other, and a connecting approximation strap, which spans the wound. The attachment plates are secured to the skin, 1.5–2 cm from the wound edge, using the adhesive on the underside of the attachment plate, and can be further secured, if skin tension is great, by using skin staples inserted through holes in the application plate. After the application plates are secure, the approximation strap is inserted through the lock/release mechanism (LRM) on one attachment plate and crossed over the wound to lock in the opposite attachment plate's LRM. The number of TopClosure® sets needed, the incremental stretch intervals, and the period of application, depend on the elasticity of the skin, the size of the wound, and the location of the defect. The TopClosure® system incorporates a safety mechanism to limit tension to ~3 kg, which prevents over-stretching of the skin and collapse of LRM on the system. Heavy nylon sutures (size 0 to 2) may be indicated for high-tension closure.[43]

Tension sutures, using non-absorbable 0 to 2 nylon or polypropylene, can be applied to this system to further reduce tension for high-tension skin closure. Tension sutures are placed by penetrating the skin through one of the designated holes in the attachment plate, passing the suture through the deep subcutaneous tissue on both sides of the wound, and exiting the suture through the skin and the hole in the attachment plate on the opposite side of the wound. Advantages to this system are that: (1) it can be applied using local anesthesia; (2) undermining of the skin edges is not required; (3) traction can be applied incrementally with periods of tension relaxation; (4) the skin can be sutured while the device is in place; and (5) the device can be left in place for days to weeks to reduce the tension on the sutures used to close the wound primarily.

A simple mechanically assisted method of closure that uses hypodermic or spinal needles or Kirschner wires (K-wires) combined with sutures has been described for use in dogs (Figure 10.8).[45] Using this technique, the Kirschner wire or long needle is inserted along each side of the wound, approximately 0.5 cm from the wound's edge. The wire or needle is inserted parallel to wound's margin in such a manner that the wire or needle is exposed at regular intervals. The wound is covered with an appropriate dressing, a gauze pad, and a cylinder, such as the barrel of a syringe or a syringe case, into which holes have been drilled. Heavy, simple interrupted non-absorbable sutures are passed around the exposed portions of the needles or wires on each side of the wound and passed through the holes in the cylinder and tied together under tension. As with the TopClosure® system, the incremental stretch intervals and the tension applied to the needles or wire depend on the elasticity of the skin, the size of the wound, and the location of the defect.

These mechanically assisted systems of closure rely on mechanical creep and stress-relaxation properties of skin. In general, the greatest gain in skin stretching is achieved within 48–72 hours after applying any one of these systems.[42] When skin and subcutaneous tissue of acute clean wounds are normal, however, the skin can be stretched rapidly (~20–30 minutes).[41] In a clinical study, using the TopClosure® system, acute stress relaxation was achieved during surgery by repeated load cycles of 2–3 minutes of high tension, which inflicted either blanching or shininess at the wound edges, followed by 5 minutes of relaxation. Mechanical creep was achieved by daily pulling the wound edges toward each other in increments of a few millimetres over a period of a few days.[43] The time required for

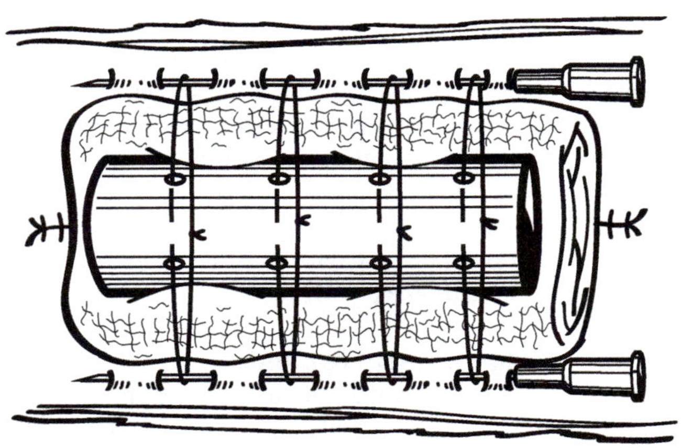

Figure 10.8 A simple, mechanically assisted method of closure that uses hypodermic or spinal needles or Kirschner wires (K-wires) combined with sutures. Source: Adapted from Tsioli *et al.* 2015.[45]

stretching skin surrounding chronic wounds is often prolonged as a result of edema and fibrosis along the wound's margin. Applying tension in cycles, with periods of relaxation between loadings, allows for far greater elongation of tissues, beyond their intrinsic capabilities to extend.[41,46,47] The use of these devices, to the authors' knowledge, has not been reported in the horse. Regardless, the authors believe these systems may hold some promise for difficult-to-close wounds of the body, proximal portion of the limbs, and possibly some wounds of the head.

Intraoperative tissue expansion

Intraoperative tissue expansion has been advocated as a means of decreasing tension on a wide wound while the wound is sutured. The technique involves rapid expansion of skin surrounding a wound by applying tension with towel forceps attached to the skin edges or by advancing the skin edges by inserting sutures in a near-and-far pattern temporarily until the edges of the wound have been approximated. Skin on either side of a wound can also be expanded intraoperatively by inserting a monofilament suture in a simple continuous pattern across the wound.[48] Both ends of the suture are left free. One free end is grasped at the surface of the skin with a hemostat, and tension is placed on the suture by pulling on the other end with a second hemostat. A third hemostat is placed proximal to the second hemostat, just above the skin, and is left in place long enough to produce stretching by stress relaxation. The second and third hemostats are then used in an alternating pulling-and-holding fashion until the skin can be approximated with interrupted sutures placed within the simple continuous suture. These techniques of intraoperative tissue expansion cause creep and stress relaxation but to a lesser extent than does preoperative tissue expansion.

Another intraoperative technique of wound expansion involves inserting an inflatable balloon (e.g., a Foley catheter) subcutaneously for several minutes before beginning suturing.[49] The original theory, postulating that this technique causes mechanical creep, has been challenged because the histologic changes normally attributed to mechanical creep are lacking.[50] The undermining of the skin required to place an inflatable balloon probably accounts for the decrease in closing tension on sutures.[51,52] An experiment designed to compare the amount of force required to close a wound before and after undermining its edges and after intraoperative expansion using an inflatable balloon, found that undermining resulted in a significant decrease in the force required to close the wounds, whereas intraoperative expansion did not significantly decrease the closing tension on sutures.[52]

Silicone elastomer (bag) expander

A technique that expands the normal tissue adjacent to the defect by stretching it 2- to 3-fold has been described.[53–55] This is accomplished by inserting a silicone bag (Tissue Expander™, Cox UpHoff) into the subcutaneous tissues adjacent to a cosmetic defect that is to be reconstructed (Figure 10.9a). As a rule of thumb, the area of the elastomer expander's base should be 2.5 times that of the defect to be closed.[56,57] Attached to the expander by a tube is a self-sealing injection dome, which is implanted conveniently nearby, yet remote to the silicone expander (Figure 10.9b). After the incision created to insert the implant has healed (~15 days), tissue is expanded by injecting sterile saline solution into the injection dome to inflate the expander until the skin becomes taut (Figure 10.9c). The skin over the injection portal is cleansed with alcohol prior to administering the injection. Similar injections are carried out at 4–7-day intervals until the skin has expanded sufficiently to permit closure of the wound (Figure 10.9d). The volume injected is dependent on the size of the expander and on signs of discomfort displayed by the horse. To account for skin retraction, which occurs after the removal of the expander, the area of expanded tissue should be at least 20% greater than that estimated to be required to cover the defect.[58] After expansion is sufficient, the expander and injection dome are removed, and the expanded skin is mobilized to cover the defect. Microscopic changes seen in the skin are consistent with biologic creep.[50]

Generally, the skin can be expanded to three times its original surface area, but this must be done slowly to prevent ischemic necrosis. The epidermis responds to tissue expansion by increasing its mitotic activity, resulting in a net increase in epidermal tissue. The dermis thins in response to expansion, and the thinning is compensated for by formation of a thick fibrous capsule surrounding the expander.[59] The thickness of expanded skin plus the fibrous capsule, which forms in a matter of days, is the same thickness as normal unexpanded skin.[50] The fact that normal skin with the same hair color and texture directly adjacent to the wound can be used to cover the defect makes this technique somewhat attractive, although more experience is required before its full benefit and limitations for use in horses become known.

Skin mobilization procedures to reduce tension

Excess tension on a suture line may result in considerable discomfort to the horse, ischemia of the cutaneous margins of the wound, and suture pull-through resulting in partial or complete dehiscence of the wound and excessive scarring. These consequences can be ameliorated, to a large extent, by undermining the skin surrounding a lesion, by using tension sutures (previously discussed under Tension-reducing suturing techniques), or by using techniques to mobilize skin. These techniques can be used alone or in combination to reduce tension on the suture line.

Undermining surrounding skin

Undermining the skin can be used alone or in combination with other tension-relieving techniques (e.g., mesh expansion, skin flaps, etc.) and is a time-honored approach for reducing tension

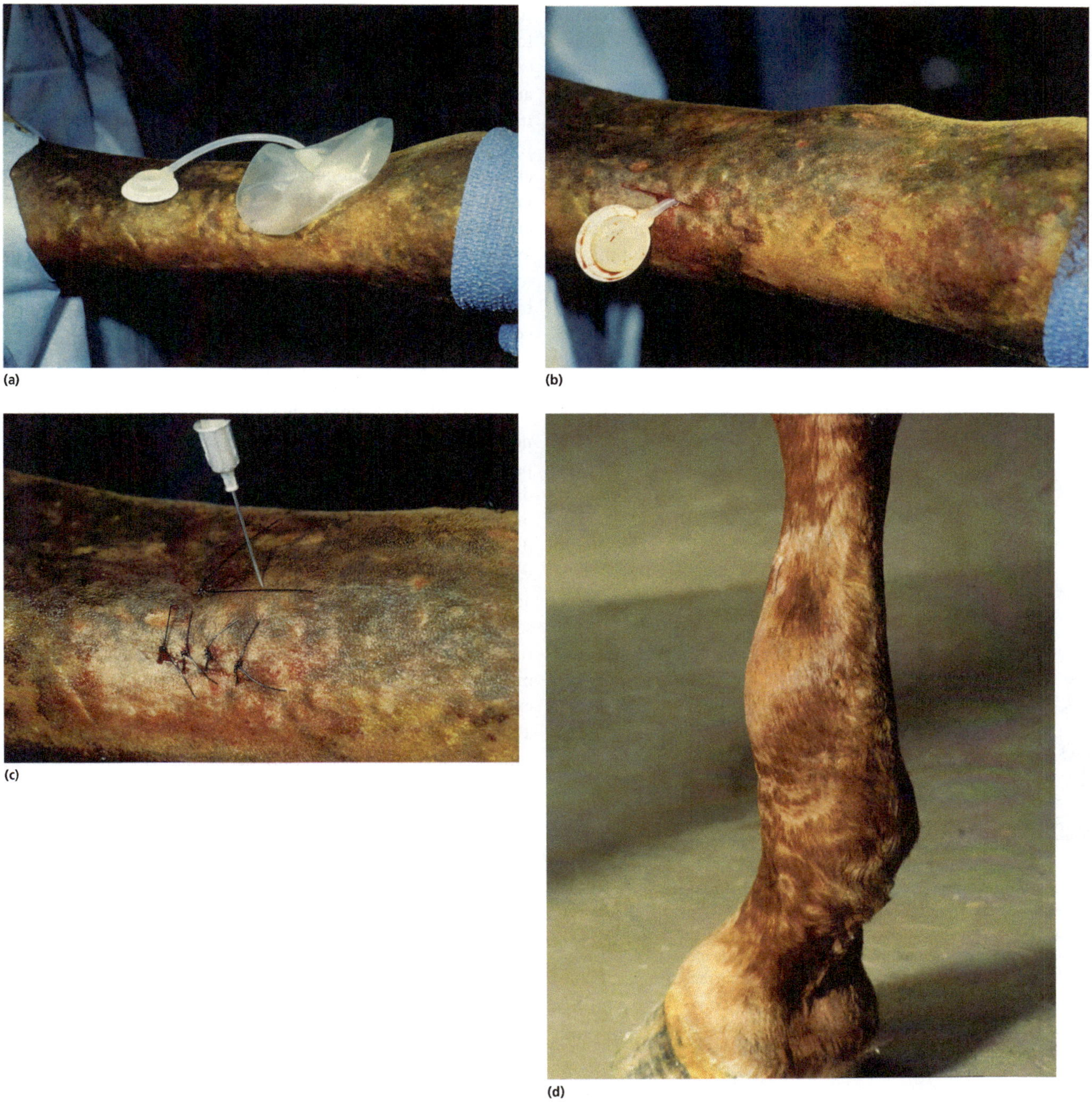

Figure 10.9 **(a)** A silicone elastomer tissue expander is positioned on the limb at the proposed site of implantation. The clear expander is to the right and the injection dome is to the left. **(b)** The tissue expander has been inserted in the subcutaneous tissue, and the injection portal will be implanted nearby. **(c)** Sterile isotonic saline solution is being injected into the injection dome to inflate the expander until the skin becomes taut. **(d)** Note the tissue expansion (swelling) on the lateral surface of the metacarpus. Courtesy of Dr. L. Booth.

on a sutured wound. Undermining releases the dermis from its attachments, permitting the edges of the wound to be approximated with less force. It is commonly used in conjunction with suturing techniques that reduce tension on the primary suture line (i.e., the sutures that approximate the skin edges).

The skin surrounding a wound on an extremity is undermined by separating the skin and subcutaneous tissue from their underlying attachments to fascia; occasionally, the cutaneous muscle is also undermined where it exists in the neck and trunk. As with any surgery, the tissue should be handled gently, and every effort made to protect its blood supply. The wound should be debrided and cleaned before its edges are undermined so that undermining does not spread debris and bacteria deeper into tissues.

Skin can be undermined using blunt or sharp dissection. Blunt dissection is accomplished by opening the blades of a scissor after the scissor has been inserted, with its blades closed, into the desired tissue plane. The procedure is repeated along the margin of the wound until the tissue has been adequately undermined. Tissue can also be separated bluntly by inserting the handle of a scalpel and moving the handle in a back-and-forth motion. Blunt dissection has the advantage of minimizing the damage to the cutaneous blood supply, but it tears tissue, creating more trauma, and is of little use when attempting to undermine the margin of chronic fibrotic wounds. The authors find this approach most useful when undermining skin surrounding a wound in a relatively loose-skinned region (e.g., the neck and some parts of the trunk).

Even though sharp dissection using a scalpel (Figure 10.10) or scissor (Figure 10.11) has the disadvantage of potentially transecting blood vessels, disruption of blood supply is unlikely to be consequential when undermining skin surrounding a wound on an extremity of a horse, making this technique the authors' preferred method of undermining skin of the extremities. When using a scalpel, one deep, cleanly made incision, following the contour of the anatomic part, to separate the attachment of the subcutaneous tissue from the underlying fascia, is preferred to multiple small, shallow incisions, which create more trauma and a greater likelihood of hemorrhage. When using a scissor, rather than making multiple small snips to separate the tissue, the authors prefer to insert the sharp blades in a partially open position, which, with pressure, converts it into a cutting instrument (Figure 10.11). In the authors' opinion, multiple snips with a scissor creates more tissue trauma and, therefore, should be avoided.

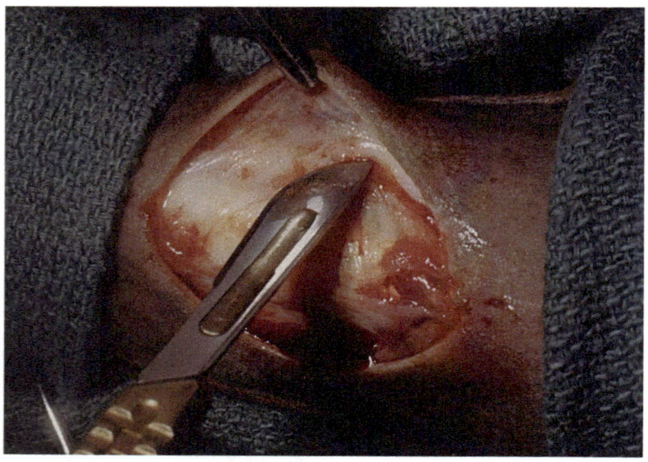

Figure 10.10 Undermining the skin using a scalpel. The scalpel blade is oriented flat against the fascia; it is then used to make a clean incision, following the contour of the anatomic part, which separates the attachment of the subcutaneous tissue from the underlying fascia. One cleanly made incision is preferred to multiple small shallowly made incisions, which create more tissue trauma and a greater risk of hemorrhage.

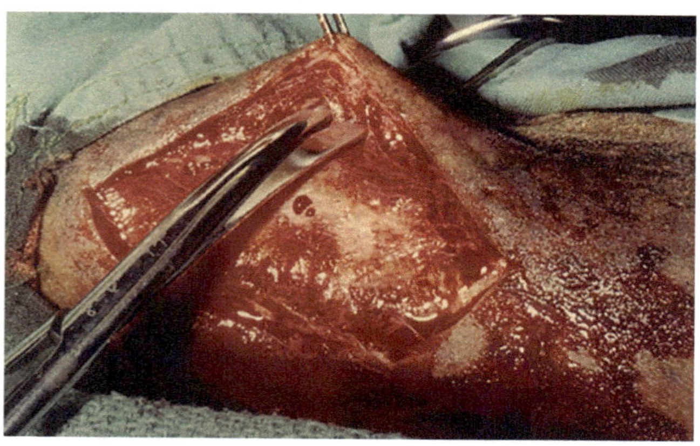

Figure 10.11 A scissor is being inserted with the blades in a half-closed position. This position allows the scissor to be used as a cutting instrument to separate the subcutaneous tissue from its attachments to the underlying fascia.

The depth at which the skin is undermined depends on the neurovascular anatomy of the region, so this should be reviewed prior to surgery to avoid injury to neurovascular structures. The dissection should be as deep as possible between the subcutaneous tissue and deep fascia when undermining skin of the distal portion of the limbs.[12,20,27] Skin of the trunk should be elevated beneath the cutaneous muscle when that muscle is adhered to the dermis; if subcutaneous tissue is present, it is dissected in the manner described for dissection of subcutaneous tissue surrounding a wound in the distal portion of the limb. In most cases, these planes of tissue are easily identified; an exception is an old, scarred wound in which readily identifying a tissue plane is difficult until dissection has been continued for some distance. In this situation, beginning with an incision in normal skin adjacent to the wound, or extending the dissection until normal skin is encountered, is appropriate. This enables the surgeon to identify the proper tissue plane.[27]

The amount of skin that must be undermined can be roughly determined by pulling the skin edges together with towel forceps. As a general rule, for fresh wounds, a distance equal to the width of the defect itself should be undermined on each side of the wound.[20] For instance, if the defect is 5 cm from edge to edge, each edge can be undermined 5 cm. The skin edges are then drawn together using towel forceps, and the tension is assessed. If the tension appears too great, undermining can be extended half as much again (i.e., 2.5 cm on each side of the wound).[4,20] Given the potential for disrupting the cutaneous blood supply when undermining skin, careful judgment is needed. If continued undermining is likely to compromise the blood supply to the skin, combining undermining with another skin mobilizing procedure (e.g., relaxing incisions, Z or V-Y plasty) should be considered.

The extent to which the skin of horses can be undermined without damaging the blood supply and causing necrosis has not been established. The skin of companion animals may be undermined quite extensively without causing necrosis as long as the blood supply remains intact, and clinical experience suggests the same is true for horses.[27,39,60] Used in conjunction with a mesh expansion technique on the limbs of dogs, 360-degree undermining of the skin was not associated with any major complication.[61]

If hemorrhage appears to be a problem after undermining skin, the surgeon should consider using a drain and a properly applied pressure bandage to prevent the deleterious effects of a hematoma, such as increased tension/pressure on the suture line and the presence of a medium for bacterial growth. For more information regarding the use and application of drains, see Chapter 9. For information regarding pressure bandaging, see Chapter 7.

Severing subcutaneous tissue attachments to the underlying fascia allows the wound's edges to be pulled toward one another and makes use of the elastic properties of skin. The closing tension for a defect varies greatly among anatomic regions and is correlated to the amount of loose skin in the area.[52] The amount of tension relief derived from undermining diminishes as the extent of undermining increases. Frequently checking the amount of tension relief achieved is important to avoid unnecessary undermining or to prompt the decision to use other methods of relieving tension prior to the onset of deleterious effects of undermining (e.g., interruption of the cutaneous blood supply and formation of a hematoma). Much of the elasticity of skin surrounding a chronic, scarred wound has been lost, making extensive undermining necessary to achieve the desired result.

What to do

- When undermining normal skin, undermine as deeply as possible between the subcutaneous tissue and deep fascia of the distal portion of the limbs. Skin of the trunk should be undermined beneath the cutaneous muscle when that muscle is adhered to the dermis.

Tips

- To identify a proper tissue plane when undermining an old scar, begin with an incision in normal skin adjacent to the wound or extend the dissection until normal skin is encountered.
- The amount of skin that must be undermined on each side of a fresh wound that cannot be closed is a distance equal to the width of the defect itself. The skin edges are then drawn together using towel forceps, and the tension is assessed. If the tension appears too great, undermining can be extended half as much again.

Tissue debulking

Although not classically considered a tension-relieving procedure, removing exuberant granulation tissue or fibrous tissue (debulking) and undermining of the adjacent skin provide considerable relief of tension and allow cosmetic reconstruction of many wounds of the distal portion of the limb (Figure 10.12). Skin incisions should extend beyond the margins of the wound into normal tissue so the thickness of the skin can be identified. Using the normal skin

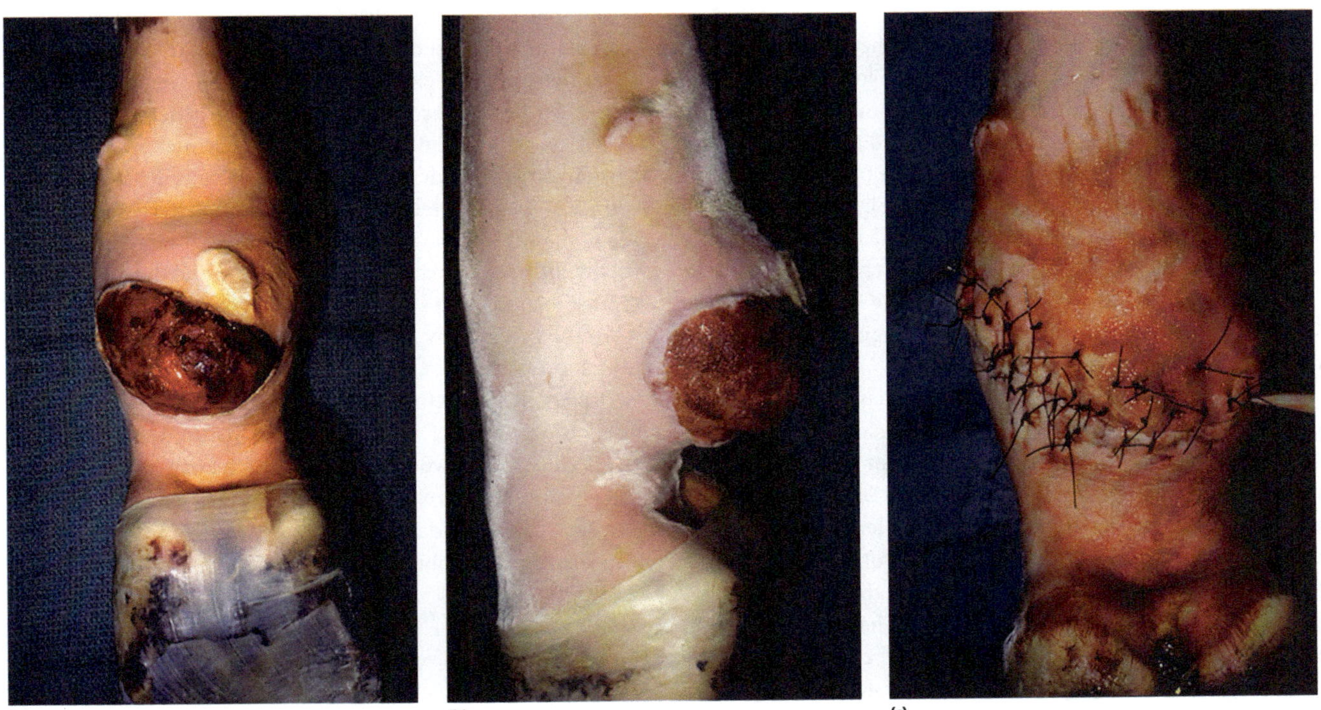

(a) (b) (c)

Figure 10.12 Example of how removal of exuberant granulation tissue (debulking) allows wound closure. **(a)** Plantar view of a non-healing wound of ~6 months' duration. The chronic exuberant granulation was acting as a barrier, which prevented healing by second intention (epithelialization and/or contraction) of the wound. **(b)** Side view of the same. Note how the skin has attempted to heal over the chronic granulating mass. At this point, it is likely that skin has undergone biologic creep that will allow closure of the wound with little tension on the suture line, following excision of the granulation tissue. **(c)** Following removal of the exuberant tissue, the skin edges were easily apposed with sutures. Because there was considerable dead space in which blood could accumulate, a drain was used. A distal limb cast was applied and left in place for 2 weeks. The cast was removed by the referring veterinarian, and the distal portion of the limb was maintained in a bandage for 1 week after cast removal. Primary healing was ultimately achieved.

thickness as a guide, the skin overlying the granulation or scar tissue (Figure 10.12b) is dissected free until a normal subcutaneous tissue plane is encountered. After the surrounding skin is freed, excessive tissue (granulation or scar) within the wound is excised to conform the wound bed to the normal underlying tissues. Care must be taken to maintain the blood supply to the undermined skin and to avoid transecting a vital support structure (e.g., a tendon, joint capsule) or entering a synovial cavity.

Skin tension is tested after undermining; if more undermining is needed, it should be performed at this time. A Penrose drain placed beneath the resultant skin flap is used to drain the undermined region. The drain is exited through a stab incision distal to the surgical site and secured with sutures at each end of the undermined tissue. The incision for the distal/ventral exit site for the drain should be separate from the wound's edges, and the hole through which the drain exits should be large enough to allow free drainage. Orienting the drain perpendicular to the exit incision allows the drain to lie flat, which in turn, maximizes drainage (see Figure 9.25). The drain should not reside directly beneath the sutured incision because this might hinder the subcutaneous tissue's contribution to healing. If required, tension sutures are used to reduce the tension on the primary incision line, after which the skin is closed with non-absorbable suture material placed in an interrupted pattern (Figure 10.12c). See Chapter 9 for more information on drains and suturing patterns and techniques.

The method of physically restraining the wounded region (e.g., bandage versus bandage splinting versus cast) is dictated by the location of the wound and the amount of tension on the primary suture line. Stent bandages and tie-over bandages are useful in regions that are not amenable to routine application of a bandage or cast (see Figure 7.11). They protect the wound from external contamination, and if secured tightly with sutures, they reduce the tension on the primary suture line and provide uniform pressure to the surgical site. See Chapter 7 for more information on bandaging, splinting, and casting techniques.

Generally, a drain is removed after 1–2 days unless drainage persists, in which case it may be left in place longer. A compressive bandage is maintained for 4–5 weeks for the best cosmetic result. A cast is usually removed after 14 to 21 days, depending on the amount of skin mobilization and tension required to close the wound and the horse's tolerance of the cast. A compression bandage should be maintained on the limb for several weeks after the cast has been removed. The greater the skin mobilization and suture tension required to close a wound, the longer the cast is left in place, if well tolerated by the patient. Tension sutures and drains are removed when the cast is removed, whereas tension sutures used under bandages are usually removed after 7–10 days, depending on the amount of tension required to close the wound and the amount of movement in the region. The more the tension and the greater the movement of the region (e.g., a sutured wound on the dorsum of the carpus), the longer the sutures are left in place.

What to do

- Scars and granulation tissue commonly adhere to vital structures deep within a wound. To identify the vital structures located deep to the scar or granulation tissue, make an incision in normal skin, proximal/dorsal or distal/ventral to the lesion to be removed, then dissect until the vital structure is identified.

What to avoid

- Do not exit a drain through a sutured wound and do not place the drain directly beneath the suture line.

Tips

- Maintain a compressive bandage for 4–5 weeks for the best cosmetic result.
- Stent bandages and tie-over bandages are useful in regions that are not amenable to routine application of a bandage. If a large dead space in a sutured wound cannot be compressed with a routine bandage, it should be compressed with a tie-over bandage.

Longitudinal relaxing incisions

Longitudinal relaxing incisions made adjacent to the wound's margin can aid in advancing skin to cover the wound.[24] A single incision created parallel to the long axis of the wound is termed a simple relaxing incision. The skin between the relaxing incision and the wound is undermined and advanced toward the wound. The width of the skin between the simple relaxing incision and the wound should be equal to the width of the wound.[38] When the wound is closed by creating only one relaxing incision, the defect created by that incision is generally about the same size as the original wound, whereas making a relaxing incision on both sides of the wound results in two smaller wounds. When two relaxing incisions are created, one on each side of the wound, the sum of the distance between the original wound and each relaxing incision should equal the width of the original wound.

Wounds created by relaxing incisions heal by second intention, and one large relaxing incision heals more slowly than do two smaller relaxing incisions. Creating one or two relaxing incisions to close a wound may be justified if the incision allows closure of a wound that exposes a ligament or tendon. When planning for relaxing incisions, efforts should be made to create the secondary defect over healthy tissue, thereby minimizing the problems associated with second-intention healing.

Mesh expansion

A mesh expansion method, which allows greater mobilization of adjacent skin than can be achieved by undermining alone, has been described.[60] With this method, the skin is undermined to free the attachment of the subcutaneous tissue to the underlying fascia, after which rows of staggered, 10–15 mm long, tension-relieving incisions are made parallel to the wound in the undermined skin adjacent to the wound's edges (Figure 10.13). As the skin is drawn over the wound, the tension-relieving

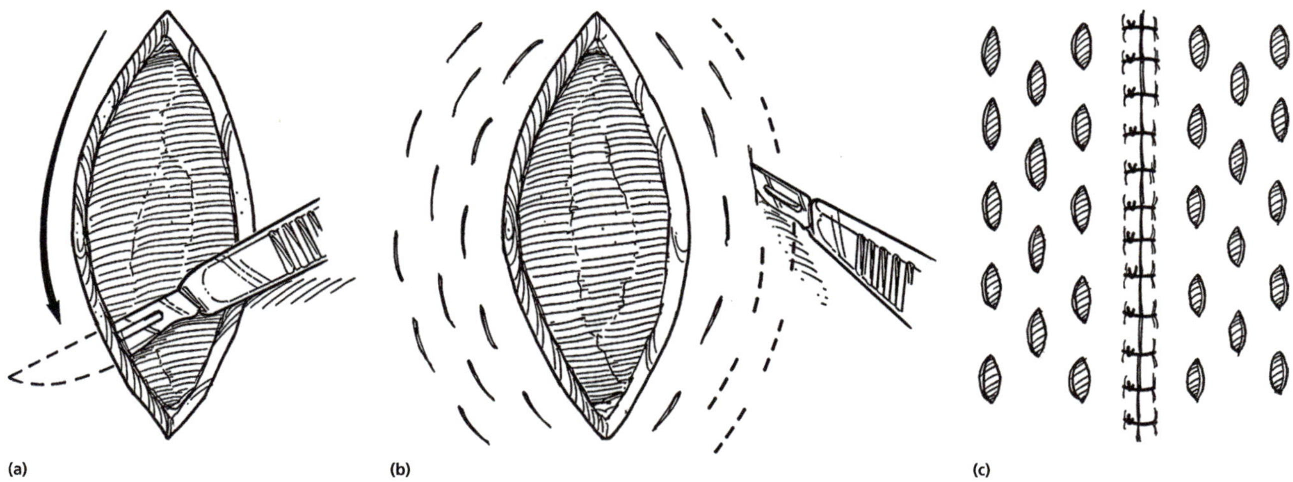

Figure 10.13 Illustration of the mesh expansion method. **(a)** The skin adjacent to the fusiform defect is being undermined to separate the subcutaneous tissue attachments to the underlying fascia. **(b)** Strategically placed stab incisions, 10–15 mm long, are made through the full thickness of the undermined skin. **(c)** Following apposition of the skin edges with simple interrupted sutures, the stab incisions open in a mesh fashion to reduce tension on the primary suture line. Source: Adapted from Bailey and Jacobs 1983.[60]

incisions widen, as would occur with a meshed skin graft, and the tension required for closure is reduced. The incisions should be 15 mm long when the skin is thickened and fibrotic and shorter when it is not. Although these small wounds heal much faster and impart a better cosmetic appearance than do one or two long relaxing incisions,[38] they do not provide as much skin relaxation as do long relaxing incisions.

> **Tip**
>
> - Mesh expansion is not as effective in mobilizing skin as is making one or two long relaxing incisions, but the small wounds created by meshing the skin heal much more rapidly and cosmetically.

V–Y plasty

V–Y plasty provides tension relief when the apex of the V-shaped incision is directed away from the undermined skin defect to be closed. After the original defect has been closed, closure of the V incision is completed by converting it to a Y, thereby gaining length and relieving tension. In the authors' experience, this technique provides very little tension relief for a large defect in the distal portion of the limb of horses. The authors find the technique most useful for closing chevron-shaped (upsidedown "V") lacerations where the tip of the V has been lost (Figure 10.14) and to offset contracture of scar tissue associated with the palpebrum (Figure 10.15). A Y–V closure can be used to increase skin tension, if needed.

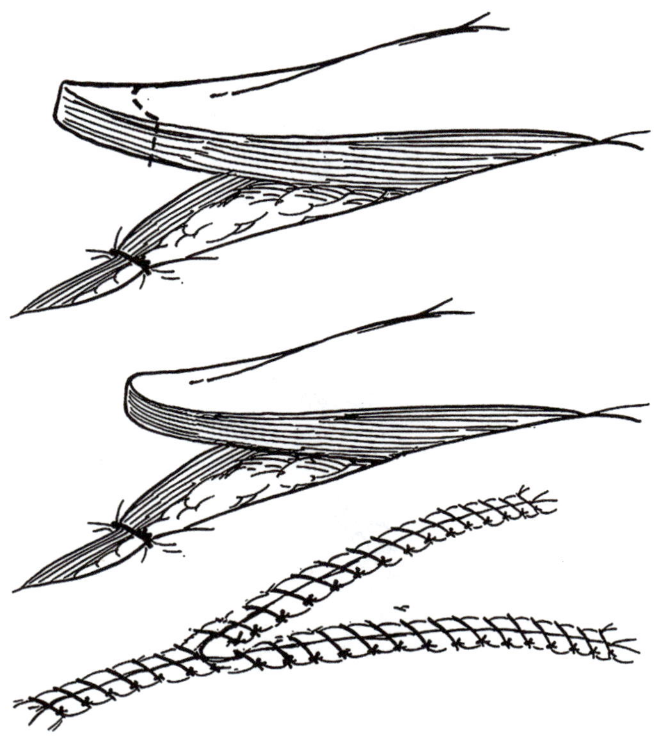

Figure 10.14 Closure of a chevron-shaped skin laceration where the tip of the chevron has been lost.

Z plasty

A Z plasty is composed of a central limb, two arms, and two angles formed where the two arms join the central limb (Figure 10.16a). Each of the two arms should be the same length as the central limb. Although the angles can range from 30° to 90°, in the authors' experience, angles of 60° work best in the horse, and angles greater than 60° are difficult to transpose. The Z plasty is developed by making a Z-shaped skin incision, the central limb of which is usually the scar itself, and undermining and then transposing the two triangular skin flaps created by the incision. This results in a change in the orientation of the central limb of the Z and a gain in length in the direction of the central limb (Figure 10.16b).[62] The gain in length achieved by the procedure is in the direction of the original central limb prior to

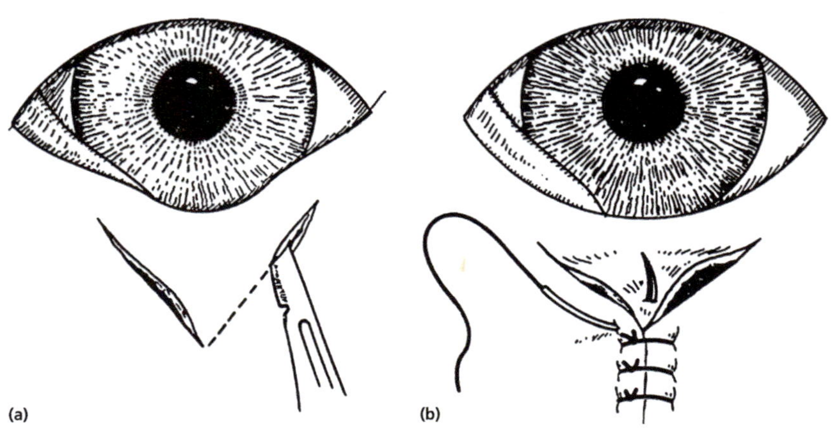

Figure 10.15 V–Y plasty being used to reduce skin tension at the ventral palpebrum. (**a**) The apex of the V-shaped incision is directed away from the palpebrum and the V is undermined. (**b**) The apex of the V is advanced toward the palpebrum, and the Y-shaped incision is apposed with sutures placed in a simple interrupted pattern.

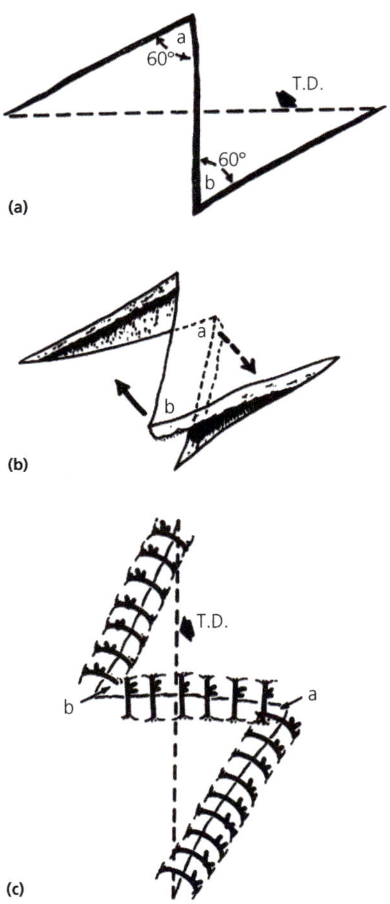

Figure 10.16 Z plasty. (**a**) Line a–b is the central limb. Two arms attach to the central limb at angles of 60°. Transverse diagonal (TD; dotted line) is an imaginary line drawn to connect the ends of the arms. TD is 75% longer than the central limb. The TD will be reoriented vertically after the flaps are undermined and transposed. (**b**) Undermined skin flaps are being transposed. (**c**) A simple interrupted pattern of sutures is used to appose skin. Note the TD (dotted line) is oriented vertically, and the central limb is now oriented horizontally.

transposition. This may be more easily understood if an imaginary line connecting the ends of the limbs, referred to as the transverse diagonal (TD) measurement, is visualized or drawn (Figure 10.16a). If the angles where the arms join the central limb are 60°, the TD will be 75% longer than the central limb. When the flaps are transposed, the TD reorients itself to replace the central limb, while the central limb is reoriented to replace the TD.[20] Although gain in length in the direction of the original central limb is dictated somewhat by the angles of the Z plasty (larger angles give more relaxation), in the authors' experience, a gain of only 50% in length can be expected in most instances due to the relatively inelastic properties of equine skin.

Z plasty can be used to lengthen or excise a contracted (bowstring) scar (Figure 10.17), dilate a scarred stenotic orifice (e.g., stenotic nares; Figure 10.18),[63] and relieve tension associated with closing a fusiform excision (discussed later under cosmetic closure of elongated defects; Figure 10.19).[20,27] In all instances, the gain in length or relaxation is in the direction of the central limb of the Z after the flaps of the Z have been transposed.

When Z plasty is used to lengthen a bowstring scar, the central limb is oriented in the direction of the scar (Figure 10.17). In this case, the scar is most often excised at the site of the central limb, after which the arms are incised and the flaps are undermined and transposed. In the case of a scarred stenotic orifice, more than one Z plasty may be required to achieve the desired dilation (relaxation) (Figure 10.18).

To relax a wound involving the trunk, the skin surrounding the wound should be elevated to determine whether there is sufficient skin in one plane to allow the required relaxation. Because the skin of the distal portion of the limb has minimal inherent extensibility, the Z plasty is simply oriented with the central limb in the direction in which relaxation is needed (Figure 10.19). When Z plasty is used to relieve tension associated with fusiform excision of a wound, the undermining should extend from the defect to include the Z plasty.

In all cases, after undermining is complete, the flaps of the Z are transposed, and the apices are secured with non-absorbable

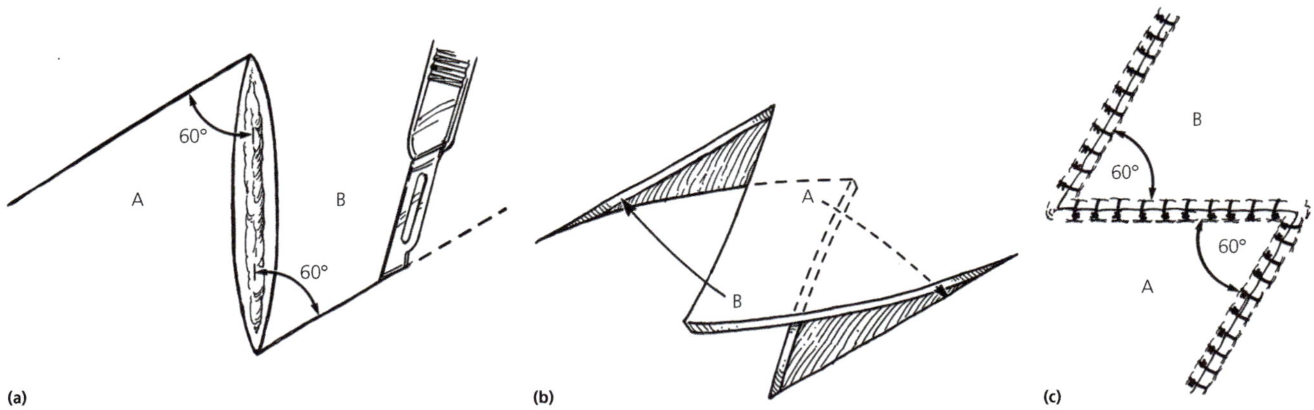

Figure 10.17 Drawings (**a**)–(**c**) illustrate how Z plasty can be used to remove a contracted (bowstring) scar and release tension from the site at which the scar resided.

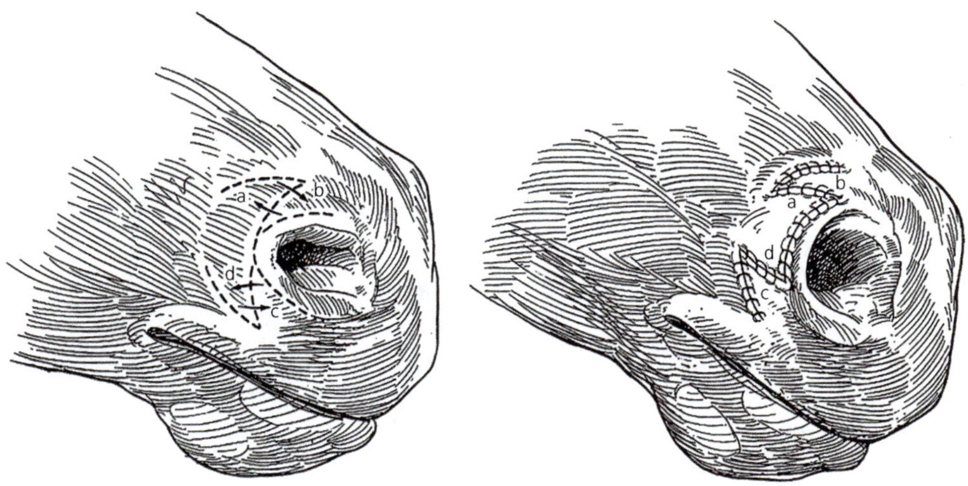

Figure 10.18 Left, a constricted right nostril due to scar formation following injury. Dotted lines indicate the site where two connected Z-plasty incisions will be made. Right, Z plasties complete. The diameter of the nostril is enlarged.

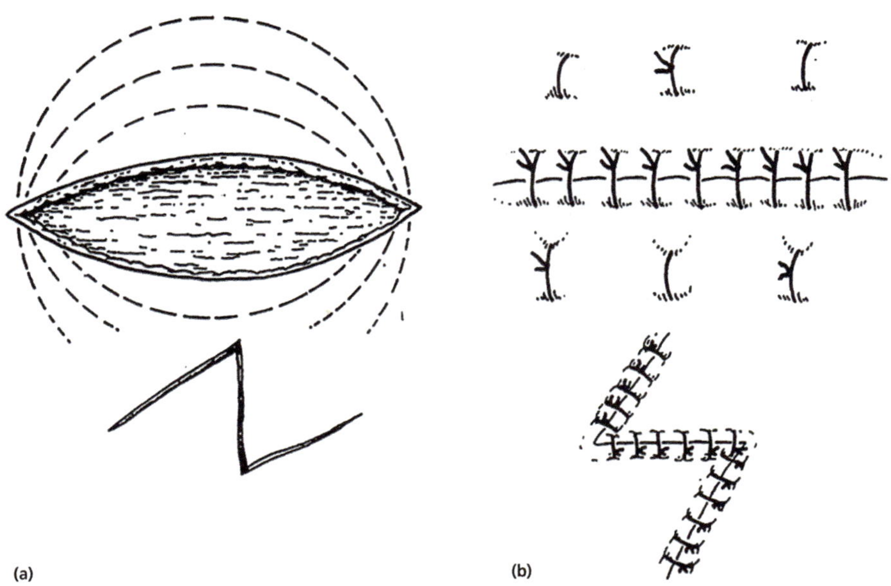

Figure 10.19 Z plasty being used to relieve the skin tension associated with a fusiform defect. (**a**) The central limb of the Z plasty is centered over the region of greatest tension, which is perpendicular to the long axis of the defect. Dashed lines indicate undermining. (**b**) Tension sutures placed in a vertical mattress pattern are used as support for the closure of the fusiform defect itself, accomplished with sutures placed in a simple interrupted pattern. Flaps of the Z plasty were transposed and sutured.

sutures placed in a vertical mattress pattern. If Z plasty was used to excise a bowstring scar, the rest of the Z plasty is apposed with non-absorbable sutures in a simple interrupted pattern. On the other hand, if Z plasty was used to reduce suture tension for closure of a fusiform defect, the defect is sutured before the Z plasty is sutured. In the latter case, a drain is often used because considerable dead space is created after the defect and Z plasty are undermined. For more information regarding the indications and use of drains, refer to Chapter 9.

A drawback to using the Z plasty to relieve tension associated with closure of a fusiform excision is that suturing the Z plasty prolongs surgery time considerably, and therefore, the Z plasty is used by the authors only as a last resort. Although it has been reported that the most common complication of Z plasty in the horse is necrosis of the tips of the triangular skin flaps as a result of ischemia,[4] this is not a problem, in the authors' experience, as long as the angles of the Z plasty are equal to or greater than 60°.

What to avoid

- To avoid dog ears when performing a Z plasty, the length of the arms of the Z plasty must be equal to the length of the central arm.

Tip

- When performing a Z plasty on a horse, the most appropriate angle between each arm and the central limb of the Z is 60°.

Cosmetic closure of defects of various shapes

Elongated defects

Elongated wounds can be converted to a fusiform shape (Figure 10.20), and circular or elongated lesions can be removed by a fusiform excision, as described later under triangular, circular, and V-shaped defects (Figure 10.21). The term fusiform is preferred over the term ellipse because the ends of the incision are tapered, whereas a true ellipse is oval. The shape of the fusiform excision lends itself to a cosmetic closure superior to closure of an ellipse because the fusiform shape adapts readily to a straight line when closed (Figure 10.22).

The correct axis for removal is determined by the shape of the lesion, its position, tension lines, and extensibility of the surrounding skin. Pre-marking reference points or drawing the fusiform pattern at the site of excision, prior to incising, reduces the likelihood of removing excess tissue and improves mirror imagery; as a result, a superior cosmetic closure can be anticipated (Figure 10.4, Figure 10.23a–c). In most instances, closure requires support from tension sutures and sometimes an additional tension-relieving procedure (Figure 10.22, Figure 10.23d–f).

One of the most rewarding applications of fusiform excision, in the authors' experience, is for cosmetic revision of scars on the distal portion of limbs of horses (Figure 10.24).

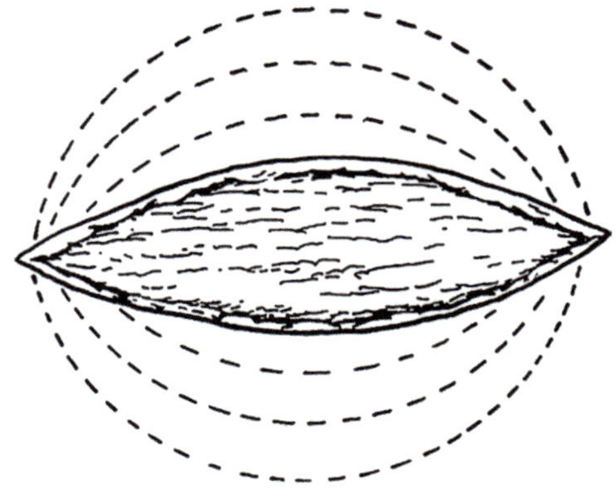

Figure 10.20 Fusiform-shaped defect. The dotted lines represent the required extent of undermining of the skin to allow tension-free closure.

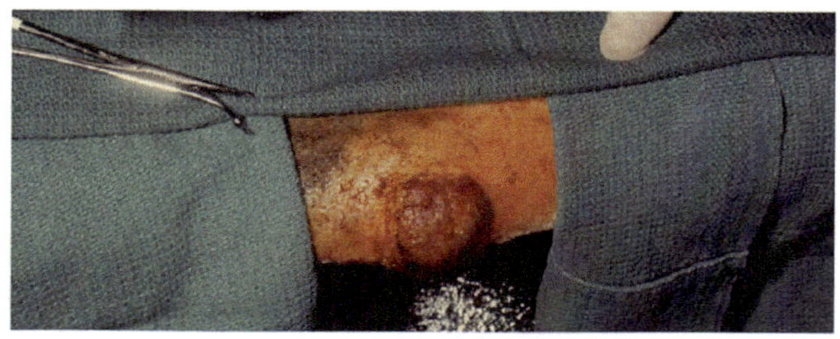

(a)

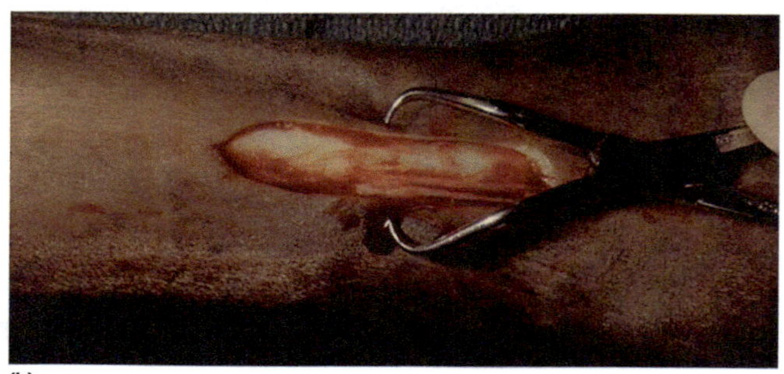

(b)

Figure 10.21 **(a)** Circular mass of exuberant granulation tissue on the dorsal surface of the metacarpus. The owners requested reconstructive surgery to improve cosmesis. **(b)** A fusiform excision was used to remove the mass and facilitate tension-free closure. Towel forceps were used to estimate skin tension and the amount of undermining required to reduce tension for closure.

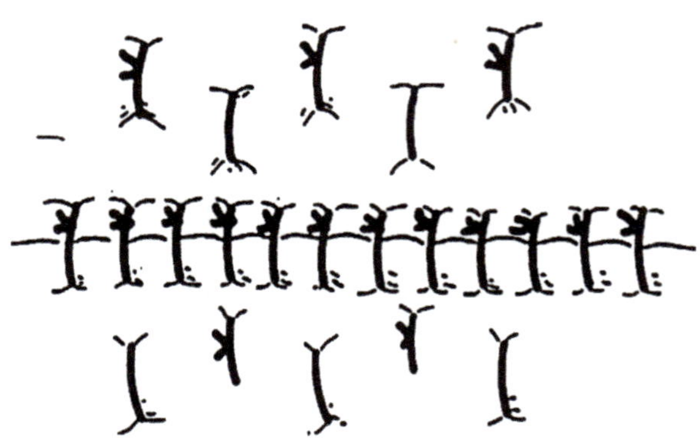

Figure 10.22 Following undermining of the skin, as illustrated in Figure 10.20, the fusiform excision is apposed with sutures placed in a vertical mattress pattern to reduce the tension on the sutures placed in a simple interrupted pattern to appose the skin edges.

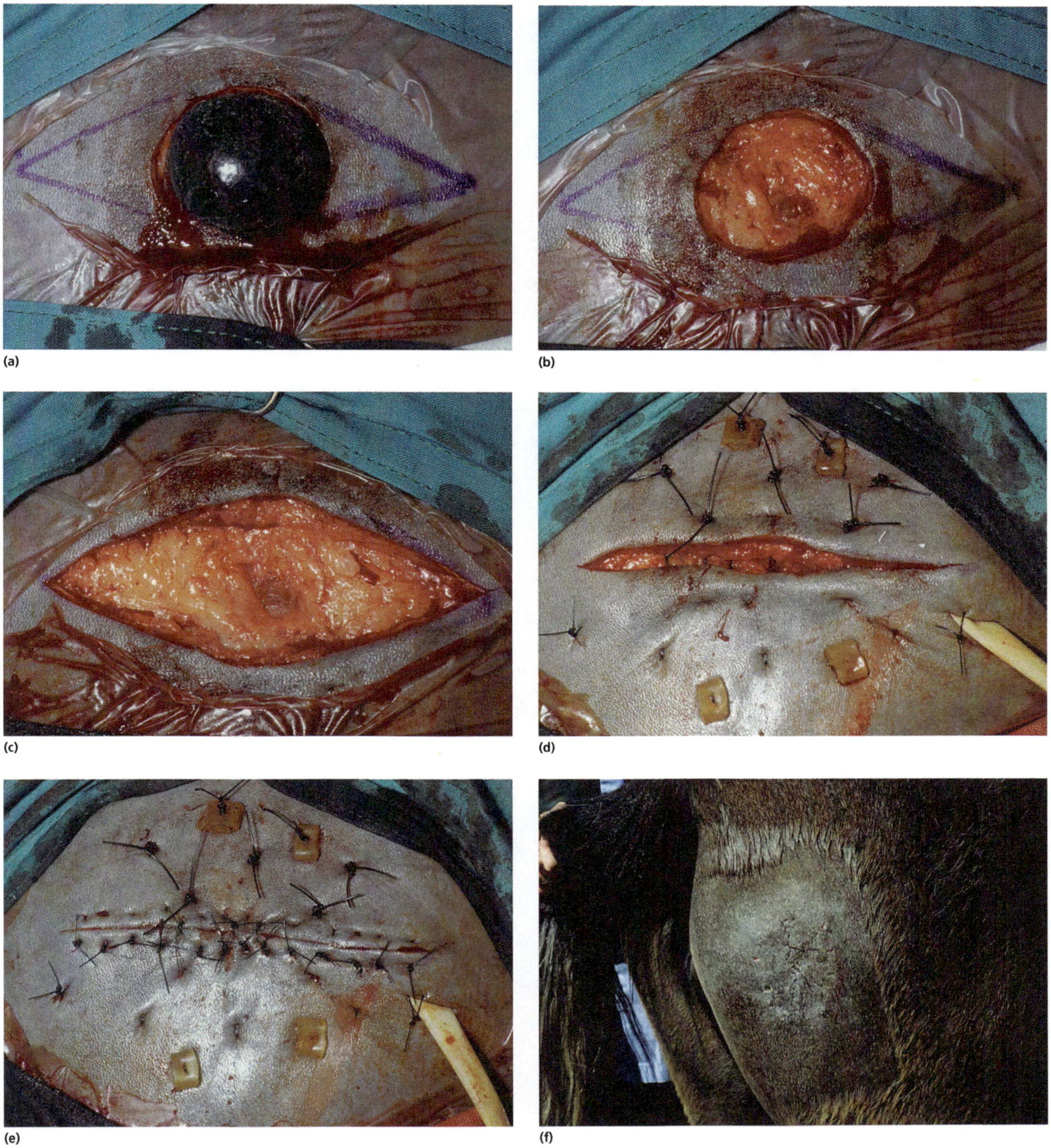

(a) (b) (c) (d) (e) (f)

Figure 10.23 Same case as in Figure 10.4. The horse was anesthetized and in left lateral recumbency. **(a)** A circular incision was made around the border of the melanoma. **(b)** The melanoma was completely removed. **(c)** A fusiform excision was completed, and the skin was undermined. **(d)** Widely placed sutures in a vertical mattress pattern were used to reduce tension on the primary suture line. The mattress sutures subjected to the greatest tension were supported with soft rubber tubing. A Penrose drain was placed in the wound. **(e)** The skin was apposed using an interrupted vertical mattress suture pattern. **(f)** The surgical site, in the standing horse, following suture removal 2 weeks postoperatively.

For large scars, the outline for the proposed fusiform excision should be drawn with a sterile marker before the incisions are made (Figure 10.25a). The incision along the pre-marked site is begun proximal or distal to the scar so that the thickness of normal skin can be determined, and any important anatomic structures (e.g., tendons, joint capsules, etc.) underlying the scar are identified before the scar tissue is removed and undermining begins (Figure 10.25b). Knowing the thickness of normal skin provides the surgeon with a guideline as to how deep to undermine the skin that is adhered to the scar,

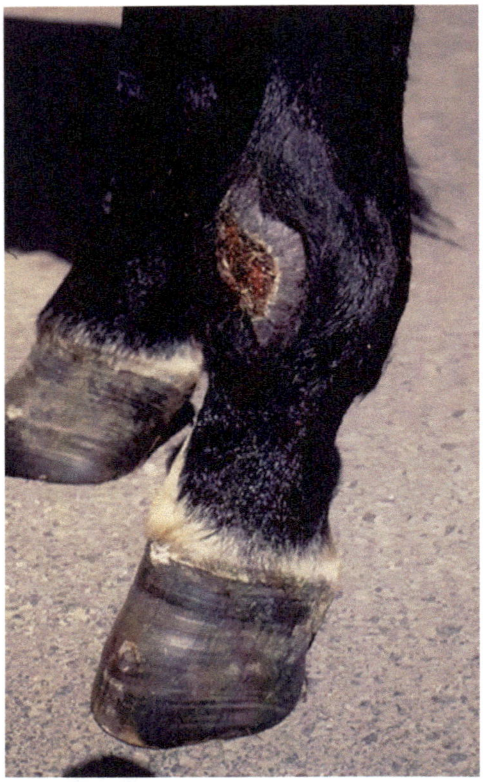

(a)

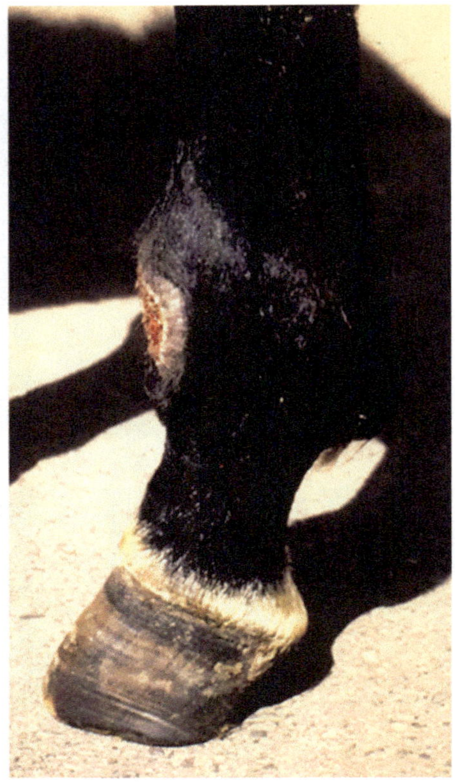

(b)

Figure 10.24 (**a**) Wound of 1 year's duration over the dorsal aspect of the fetlock. The wound cracked and bled periodically, particularly after forced exercise. (**b**) Lateral view of the same. Note the swelling deep to the wound and haired skin overlying the fetlock. Biologic creep of the skin presumably occurred because of slow enlargement of the scar tissue associated with this swelling. Tension-free closure after excision of the underlying scar would be expected.

whereas identifying important structures in advance of removing the scar from the wound bed minimizes the risk of severing a support structure or entering a synovial cavity (Figure 10.25c).

After the scar tissue has been completely excised, the decision is made as to whether the skin should be undermined further to allow its approximation or whether more skin should be excised to achieve proper tension on the approximated skin (Figure 10.25d–f). Closure involves placement of a drain, in most cases, the use of tension sutures to approximate the skin, and sometimes application of a cast (Figure 10.25 g, Figure 10.26). This approach has also been rewarding for the removal of extensive scar tissue deep to the skin (Figures 10.27).

Most horses require immobilization of the distal portion of the affected limb with a cast or a bandage splint to achieve the most cosmetic result. For information regarding the techniques for applying a cast or bandage splint see Chapter 7. A good cosmetic result is usually achieved without complications.

Correction of "dog ears"

Although "dog ears" (i.e., bunching [redundancy] of the skin at the end of the incision) may accompany skin closure of any geometrically shaped wound or a skin flap that is rotated into position, in the authors' experience, dog ears most commonly accompany skin closure after fusiform excision and repair of a curved wound.

Figure 10.25 Same case as in Figure 10.24. The horse was anesthetized and placed in lateral recumbency. Proximal is to the left. (**a**) The outline for the proposed fusiform excision was drawn with a sterile marker. Note the unhaired epithelium and centrally located, non-healed wound. A major surgical objective was to remove the non-healed wound. (**b**) The incision along the pre-marked site was completed. The thickness of normal skin and the extensor tendon in this region were identified prior to removal of the scar in the wound. (**c**) Scar tissue overlying the extensor tendon was removed. (**d**) The skin was undermined until normal subcutaneous tissue was encountered. (**e**) Pushing the undermined skin edges toward each other, using finger pressure, identified tension-free skin. Note the non-haired epithelium axial to the thumb; this was removed prior to suturing. (**f**) Hairless epithelium was excised, and the wound bed irrigated in preparation for suturing. (**g**) Following closure. Note that the drain exit site was separate from the sutured incision. The drain was sutured at its proximal and distal limits and was placed in the dead space adjacent to the sutured incision. Betadine ointment was applied to the drain exit site after which sterile dressing and conforming gauze were applied in preparation for application of a distal limb cast.

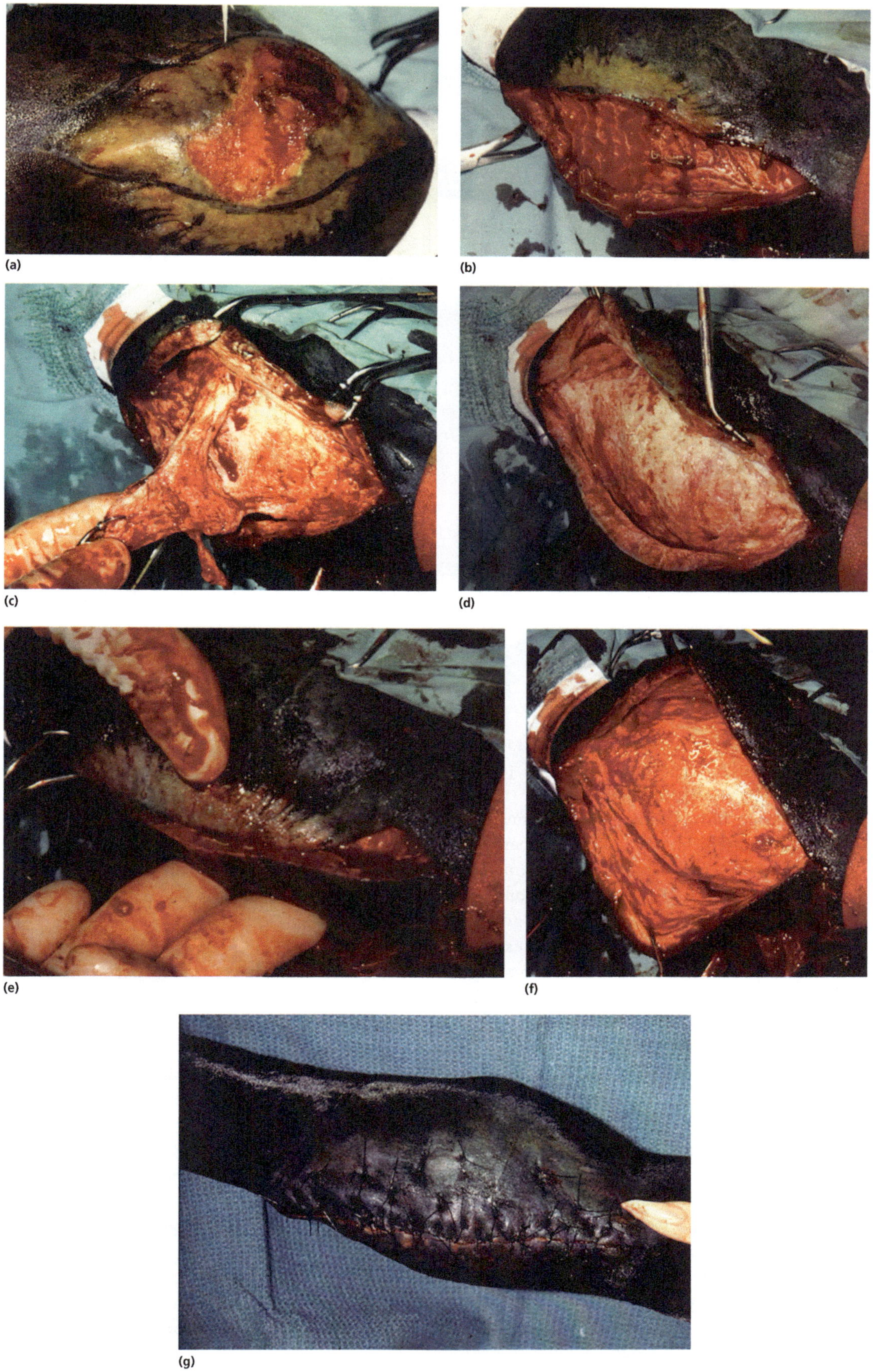
(a)
(b)
(c)
(d)
(e)
(f)
(g)

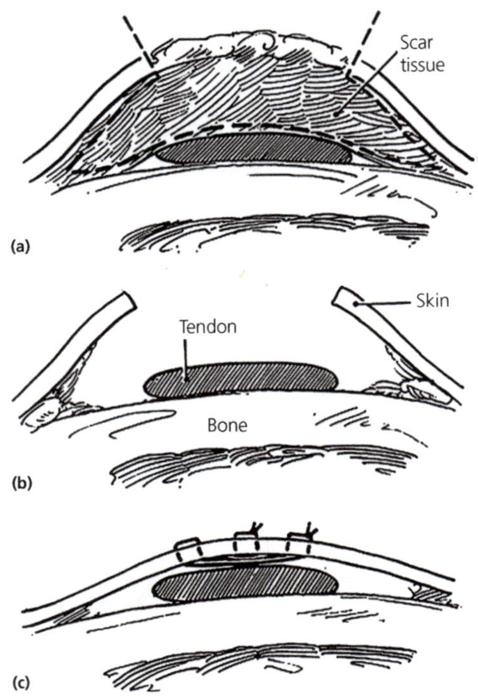

Figure 10.26 Technique used in Figure 10.25 illustrated in cross-section. **(a)** Dotted line illustrates excision of the scar tissue overlying the extensor tendon. **(b)** Following removal of scar tissue and undermining of the skin, sufficient skin is available for tension-free closure. **(c)** Skin closure complete.

In the design of a fusiform excision, the length-to-width ratio should approach 4:1, whenever possible, to prevent formation of dog ears.[20] Smaller ratios, however, have resulted in cosmetic closure after fusiform excision of scar tissue in the distal portion of the limbs of horses (authors' experience) (Figure 10.27). When dog ears occur after symmetrical closure of a wide fusiform wound, the bulging tissue on either side, at the end of the incision, can be removed by grasping the centermost prominent (elevated) part of the dog ear, with thumb tissue forceps which, after lifting the tissue, creates a triangular fold of skin (Figure 10.28). An incision is made at the base of the triangle first on one side, then on the other side, to remove the dog ear (Figure 10.28). Alternatively the redundant tissue may be removed by simply extending the incision through the center of the elevated dog ear, thus creating two triangular pieces of skin, which are excised at their bases (Figure 10.29). In both situations, the remaining linear defect is approximated with sutures.

Closing a curved wound evenly is difficult, and uneven closure leads to a redundancy of skin (dog ear), on one side, at one or both ends of the wound. A curved wound can be sutured evenly, thus avoiding dog ears, by placing the first suture in the center of the wound and then placing subsequent sutures at bisecting intervals between the central suture and the ends of the wound, until the margins of the wound are approximated (Figure 10.30). When dog ears occur as a result of one side of the excision being longer than the other, they can be removed by incising the skin at the end of the dog ear at a 45° angle to the axis of the sutured wound (Figure 10.31). The excess skin that overlaps the wound is excised along an imaginary line parallel to the 45° incision, and the margins of the extended wound are approximated.

Tip

- To avoid "dog ears" when suturing a curved wound, place the first suture in the center of the wound and subsequent sutures at bisecting intervals until the margins of the wound are approximated.

Square and rectangular defects

Sliding H plasty can be used to repair/reconstruct square and rectangular defects (Figure 10.32). Normally, two flaps are created. If skin is available on only three sides of a defect, however, one-half of the H plasty is used (Figure 10.33).[20,27,65] Using this technique, a rectangular or square piece of skin and subcutaneous tissue adjacent to the defect is mobilized and advanced into the defect. Advancement is aided by creating a Bürow's triangle on each side of the flap at the flap's base. These triangular excisions are created to equalize the length between the sides of the flap and adjacent margins of the wound. Creating Bürow's triangles is usually unnecessary when performing an H plasty to cover a cutaneous defect of the skin of a cat or a dog because the skin of cats and dogs is much looser than that of a horse. If two sliding flaps are used, the base of each Bürow's triangle should equal at least half the width of the defect (Figure 10.32a), whereas if a single flap is used, the base of each triangle should equal the width of the defect (Figure 10.33a). Advancement can also be enhanced by increasing the width of the base of the flap and back-cutting each side at the base so that each cut opens into a V when the flap is advanced (Figure 10.34).[6]

The skin flap(s) are undermined to separate their subcutaneous tissue attachments to the underlying fascia. For old wounds, scar tissue usually must be removed (i.e., debulked) to mobilize skin (Figure 10.35a,b). Tension sutures are required in most cases. Sutures are placed in a vertical mattress pattern in the mobilized skin flaps, the edges of the wound are approximated by applying towel clamps, then the sutures are tied (Figure 10.32b,c, Figure 10.35c,d). Next, the bases of the triangles are sutured (Figure 10.32c). A drain is often used beneath these flaps (Figure 10.35c). Primary suture approximation of the rest of the plasty then follows. A modification of the one-half H plasty can be used to cover unequal or irregularly shaped defects where limited skin is available for creating a sliding flap (Figure 10.36, Figure 10.37). An advantage to this technique is that, for a narrow defect, the base of a sliding flap can be made wider to ensure that the blood supply to the reconstructed site is adequate.

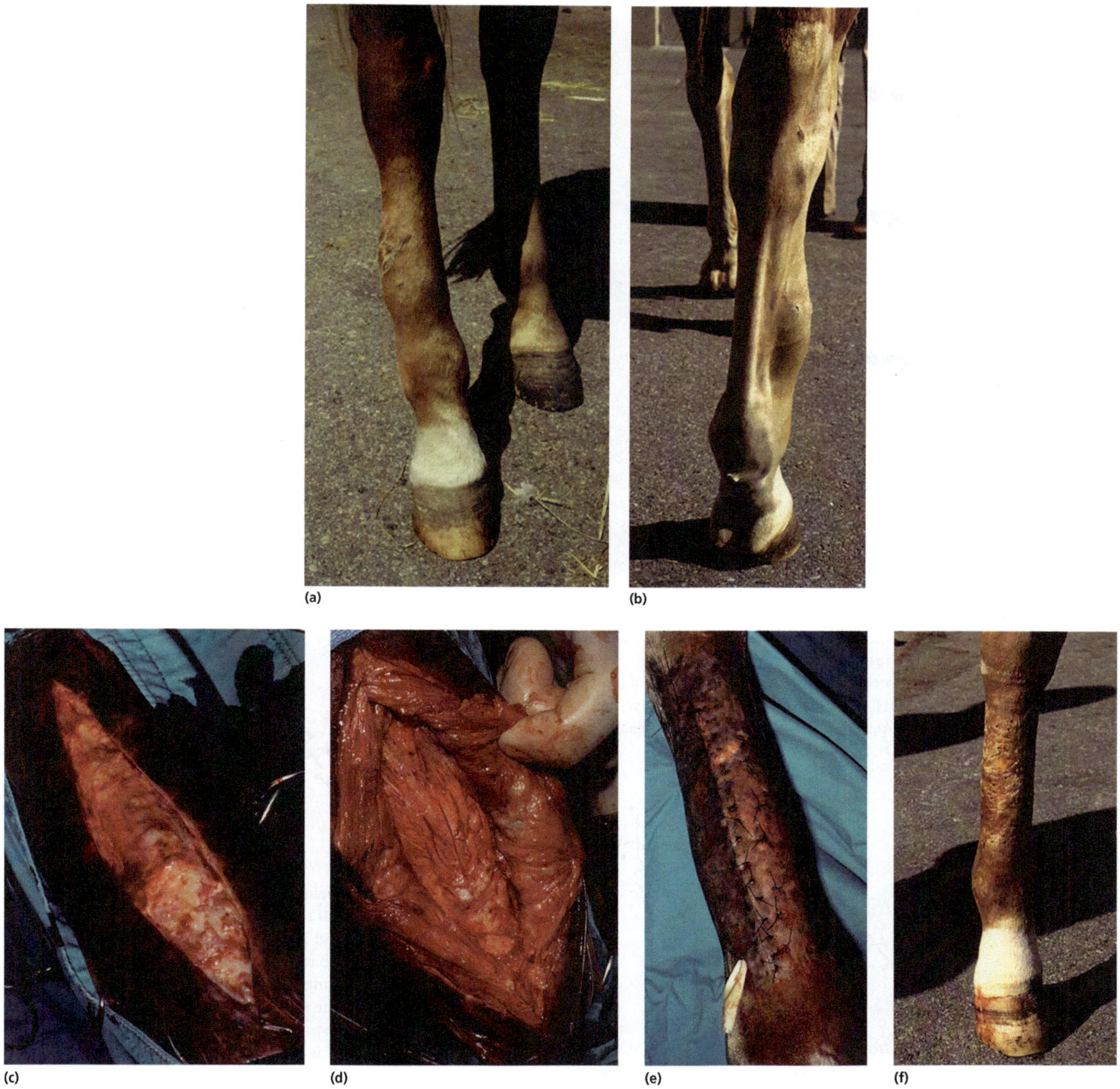

Figure 10.27 This horse sustained multiple kicks to the right metatarsus during transport in a trailer with another horse ~6 months earlier. The owner was interested in cosmetic reconstruction. **(a)** Dorsal view of the site of injury. Note that the skin is intact but significant swelling is present deep to the skin. The horse was not lame at exercise. Radiographs revealed slight bony proliferation from the cortex of the third metatarsal bone. **(b)** Plantar view of the same. **(c)** At surgery, a long fusiform skin excision was used to expose the underlying scar tissue. **(d)** Scar tissue was bisected down to the underlying tendon after which the skin was undermined and the scar removed. **(e)** Closure complete including a drain, which was removed after 2 days, prior to applying a cast. A distal limb cast was applied for 2 weeks, immediately after drain removal, 2 days after the wound was sutured. **(f)** Appearance of the reconstructed site at the time of dismissal 2.5 weeks after surgery.

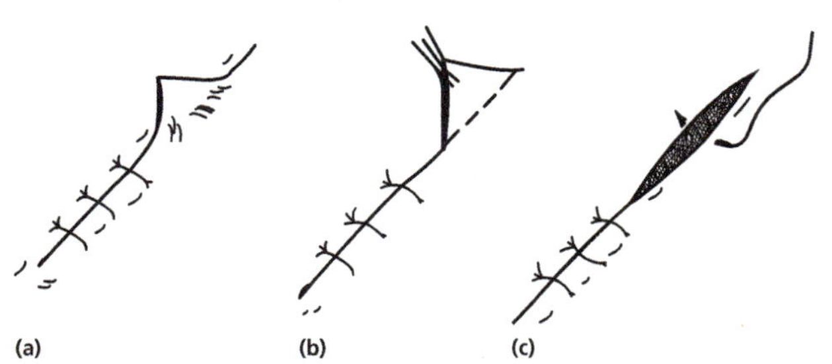

Figure 10.28 Removal of a "dog ear" by making an incision on either side of its base. **(a)** The scalpel is used to incise one side of the base of the dog ear. **(b)** An incision is made in the base on the opposite side of the dog ear. **(c)** Closure after removal of the dog ear. Original drawings by Dr. Faith Riley.

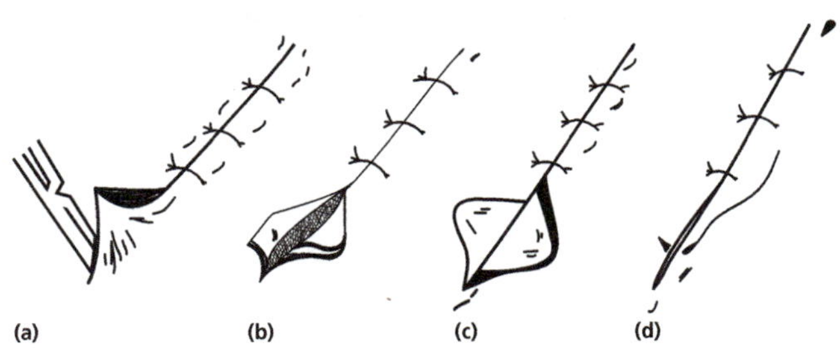

Figure 10.29 Removal of a dog ear by extending the incision through the bunched tissue. **(a)** Extending the incision through the dog ear. **(b)** The incised dog ear. **(c)** Excision of the two skin triangles. **(d)** Closure after dog ear removal. Drawings by Dr. Faith Riley, adapted from Swaim and Henderson 1990.[20]

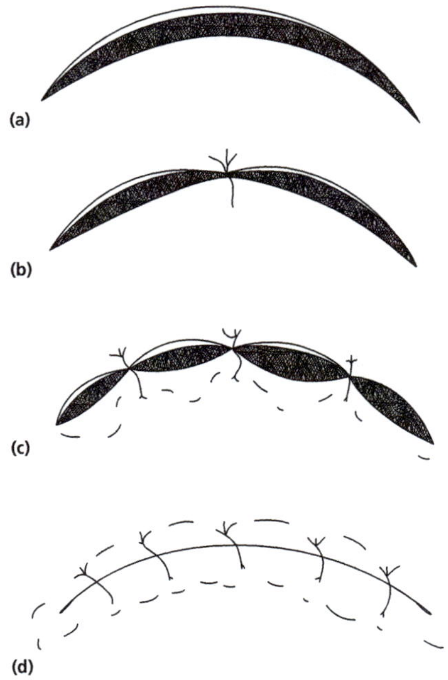

Figure 10.30 To suture a curved wound evenly, thus avoiding dog ears, the first suture should be placed in the center of the wound and then subsequent sutures placed at bisecting intervals until the margins of the wound are approximated. **(a)** First bisecting suture. **(b)** Second bisecting sutures. **(c)** Third bisecting sutures. **(d)** The wound has been completely sutured. Original drawings by Dr. Faith Riley.

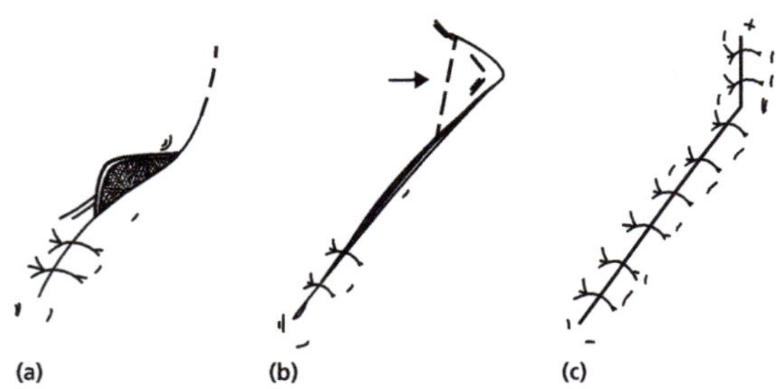

Figure 10.31 Dog ear resulting from one side of the wound being longer than the other. **(a)** One-sided dog ear. **(b)** Short, right-angle incision made at the base of the dog ear; the dotted line defines the skin to be excised. **(c)** Closure after dog ear removal. Drawings by Dr. Faith Riley, adapted from Trott 2005.[64]

Tips

- When performing a sliding H plasty, the base of each Bürow's triangle should equal at least half the width of the defect.
- Tension sutures are usually required when suturing an H plasty.

Triangular defects

A triangular defect may be sutured as a simple single suture line by converting the triangle into a fusiform incision (Figure 10.38). To close the incision without excessive tension, the length of the incision should exceed its width by a ratio of at least 3:1.[64] Tissue adjacent to a triangular defect can also be

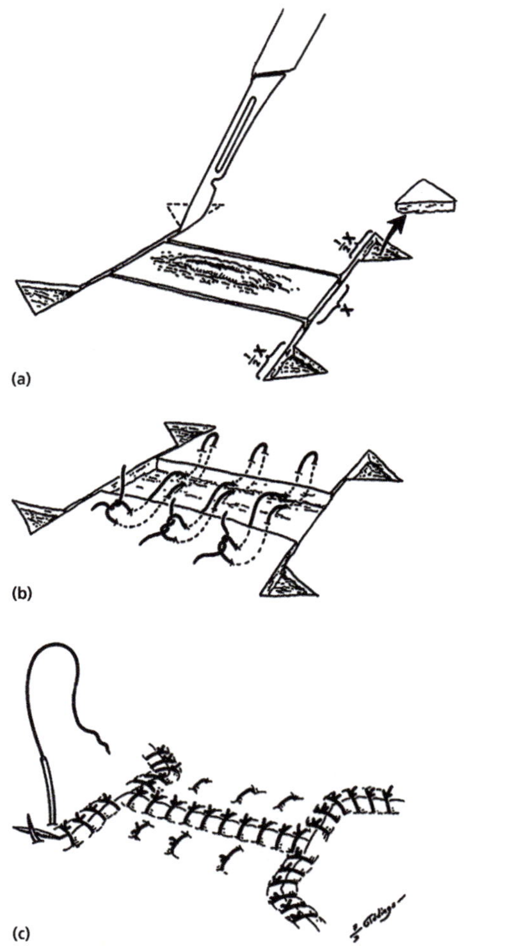

Figure 10.32 Sliding H flaps being used to reconstruct a rectangular defect. **(a)** Rectangular defect is excised (center, width = X) and the two arms of the H incision extend at least 1–1.5 base widths away from the excision site. Triangles whose base equals 0.5X are created at the end of each arm to prevent puckering after the skin edges are sutured. **(b)** Following undermining, the skin flaps are drawn together using a vertical mattress tension pattern. **c)** A simple interrupted suture pattern completes the closure. A drain is often placed under the skin flaps.

used to cover the defect (Figure 10.39). If excessive tension is encountered while closing the defect, one (Figure 10.40) or two inverted triangles (Figure 10.41) can be made two to three triangle base widths away from the lesion; skin flaps are then undermined, pulled into position, and sutured. The decision to create one or two flaps is dictated by tension and the amount of available loose skin. In most cases, creating two inverted triangles, each with a base of one-half the width of the original defect, relieves more tension than does creating one large inverted triangle.

Tip

- A triangular defect can be closed most easily by converting the triangle into a fusiform incision.

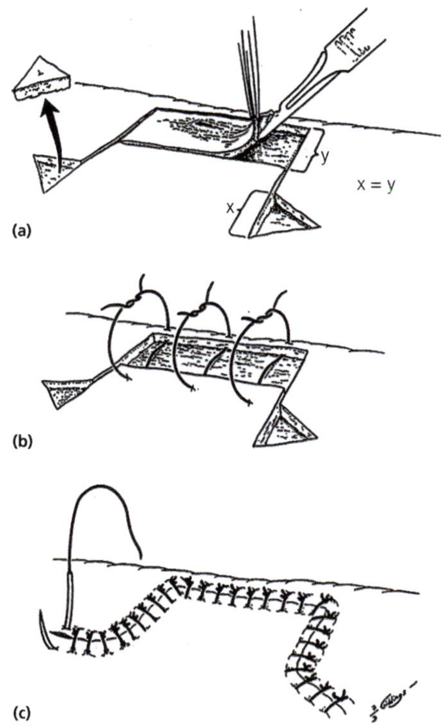

Figure 10.33 Example of a half H plasty being used when skin is available on only three sides of the defect. **(a)** Y = the width of the defect created by excision. Note the base of the triangle. X = the width of the excised defect, Y. **(b)** Following undermining, a simple interrupted suture pattern is used to hold the top of the flap in place. The bases of the triangles are then apposed. **(c)** Suturing is complete.

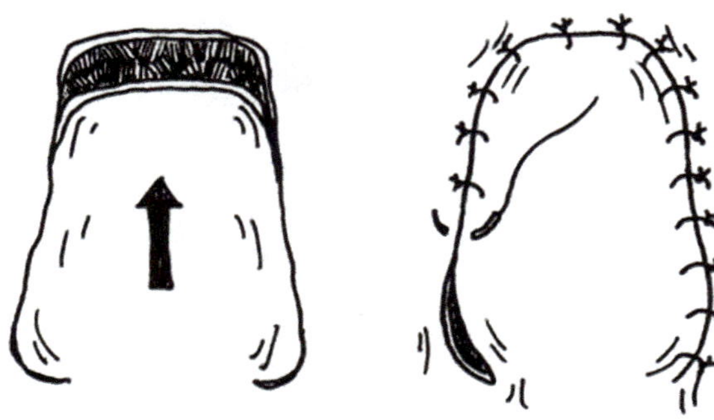

Figure 10.34 Advancement of an H flap may also be enhanced by increasing the length of the base of the flap and by back-cutting each side at the base. Drawing by Dr. Faith Riley, adapted from Grabb 1975.[6]

V-shaped defects

V-shaped wounds are fairly common, and often the tip of the V-flap is lost or is devitalized, requiring its removal prior to closure. After it is debrided, the chevron-shaped wound can be closed in a Y pattern similar to that of the V–Y plasty (Figure 10.14). An alternative method for closing a long, narrow, V-shaped wound with ample loose skin surrounding it is to convert it into a fusiform excision (Figure 10.20), as described previously for suturing a triangular defect, after which the fusiform wound is closed as a linear defect (Figure 10.22).

> **What to do**
>
> - A V-shaped wound can be sutured in a V–Y configuration.
> - If the V-flap is very narrow, it can be excised and the wound converted into a fusiform incision for easy closure.

Circular defects

The simplest method of closing a circular defect (or excising a circular lesion) is to convert it into a fusiform incision (Figures 10.20 and 10.21). If the defect is too large to convert into a fusiform incision, the circular defect may be closed by using a double V–Y closure technique (Figure 10.42).

A local pedicle flap, such as a rotation flap or transposition flap (Table 10.1), can also be used to close or cover circular wounds (Figure 10.43). Although these techniques are best used in regions where the skin is more freely moveable, such as the neck and trunk, the rotation flap or transposition flap is occasionally used in tight-skinned regions, such as on the head, to cover a defect (e.g., nasocutaneous or sinocutaneous fistula) (see Figure 11.46). The length and width of a transposition flap should be slightly longer and wider than the defect itself. In the case of pedicle skin flaps, the work of Hinchcliff *et al.* showed a positive correlation between the flap's width and viable length.[7] Because the transposition flap's length decreases as the arc of rotation increases, and because the horse's skin lacks the extensibility of skin of cats and dogs, the flap should be created as close to the lesion as possible (Figure 10.43). Often, in tight-skinned regions, a small defect may remain that must heal by second intention or by application of a free skin graft. For more information regarding the use of a transposition flap for the repair of a facial fistula, see Chapter 11.

> **What to do**
>
> - The simplest method of closing a circular defect is to convert it into a fusiform incision.
> - A large, circular defect can be closed by using a double V–Y plasty.

Vascularized free-tissue transfers (axial-pattern skin flaps)

Large wounds, particularly those involving the distal portion of the limb, are difficult to close in spite of reconstructive surgical techniques. Vascularized free-tissue transfers, based on axial-pattern flaps and using microvascular anastomosis, are commonly used in small animals.[15,66–68] Attempts have been made to adapt this approach for use in the horse.[69] In equids, a large, free axial-pattern skin flap and microvascular anastomosis using the deep circumflex iliac artery and vein[70,71] and a smaller skin flap using the saphenous artery and medial saphenous vein[72] have been described. In these experimental studies, none of the transferred skin flaps survived longer than 6 days. Failure was believed to result from ischemia reperfusion

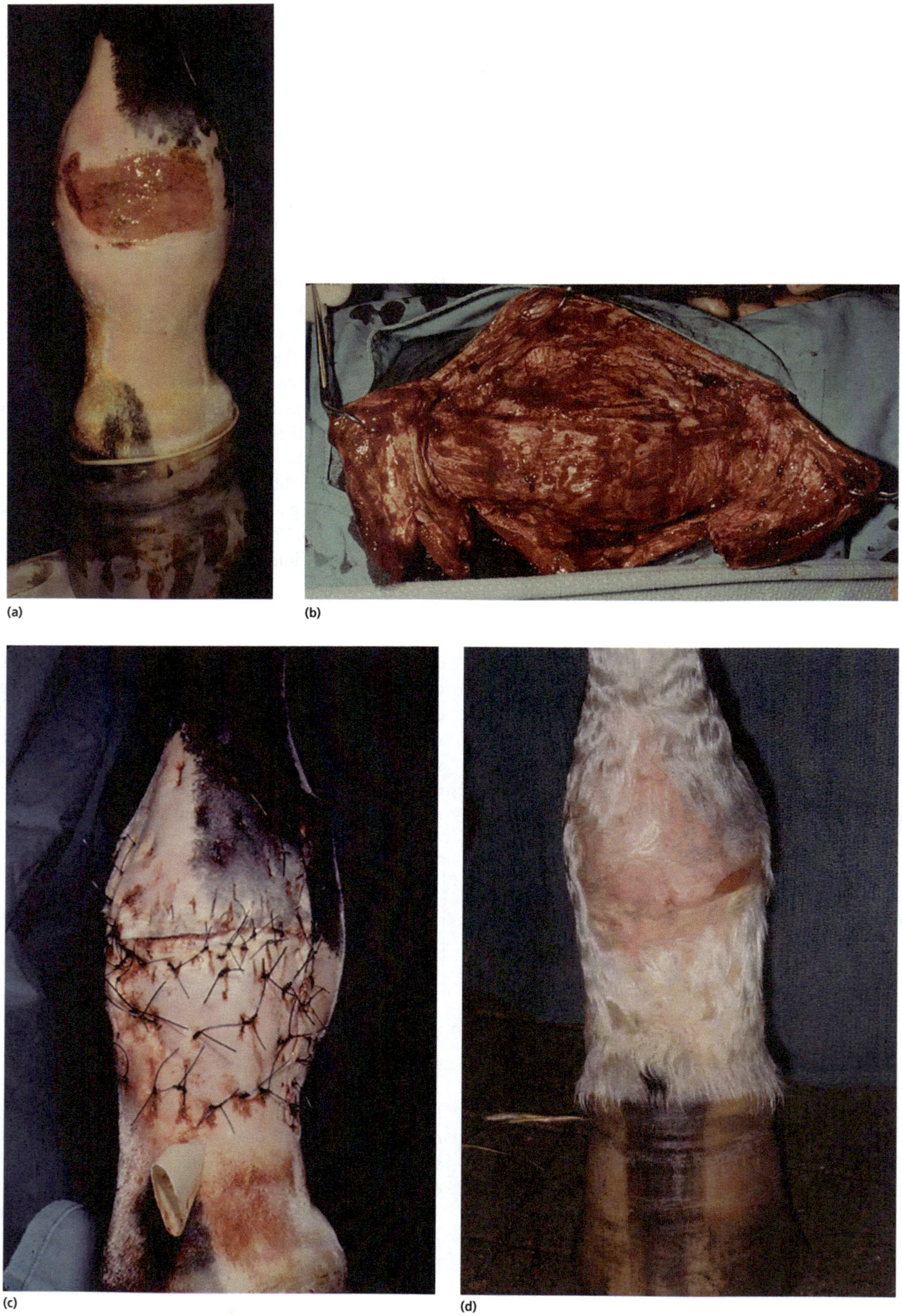

Figure 10.35 **(a)** Non-healing wound on the dorsal aspect of the fetlock of ~6 months' duration. **(b)** At surgery, the central lesion was excised, the skin flaps were undermined, and the scar tissue in the wound was removed in preparation for closure of the H plasty. **(c)** After placement of a drain and skin closure. Three rows of sutures placed in a vertical mattress pattern were required to substantially reduce the tension on the primary suture line. A distal limb cast was applied for 3 weeks. **(d)** Healed wound ~8 weeks after surgery. A small portion of the skin flap on the right side dehisced, resulting in a wound that had to heal by second intention. Note that the pigmentation is markedly diminished just proximal to the surgical site on the right side. Note the alopecia. The loss of pigmentation and alopecia may have been due to a reduced blood supply to the area, either from the extensive undermining of the skin or as a result of the tension required to close the skin.

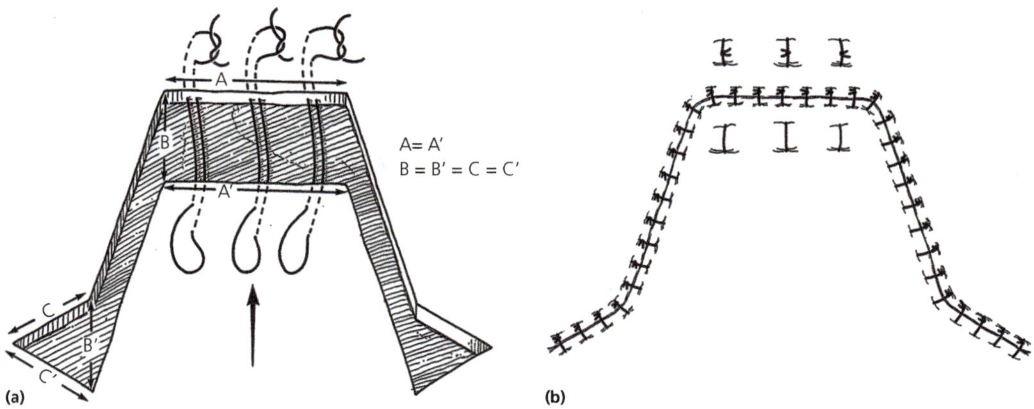

Figure 10.36 Modified half H plasty, which can be used to cover an irregular (unequal) angular defect. (**a**) After removing an angular defect, incisions in normal skin are extended at the same angle from the defect. Triangles, whose base B′ = that of B, are excised. The skin flap has been undermined, and sutures are preplaced in a vertical mattress pattern. The arrow indicates the direction in which the skin flap will be pulled. (**b**) The preplaced sutures are tied, and a simple interrupted suture pattern is used for skin closure.

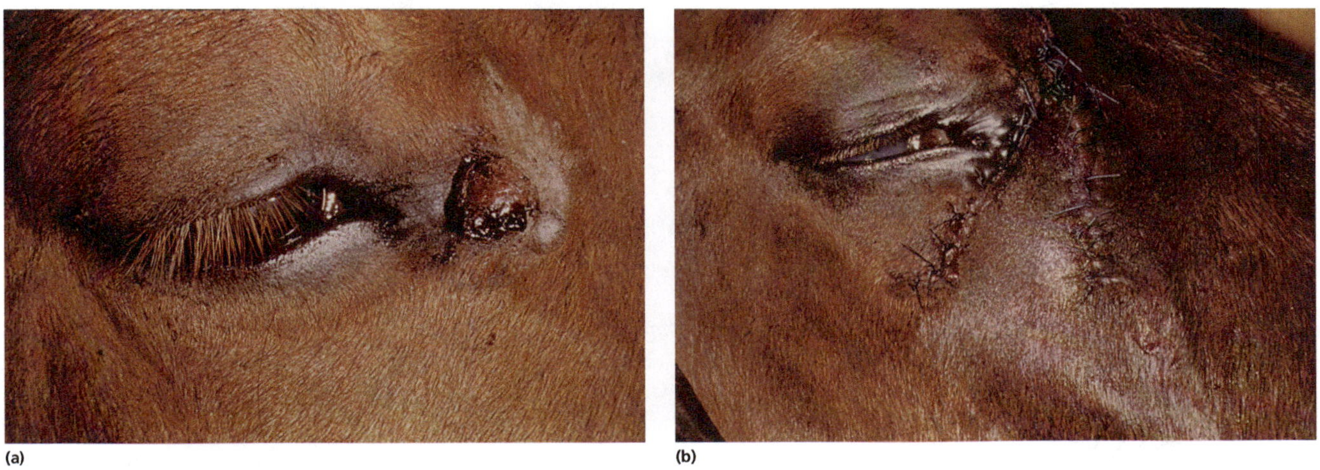

Figure 10.37 (**a**) A lesion adjacent to the medial canthus of the eye that would be amenable to removal and coverage with full thickness skin using a modified half H plasty. (**b**) After excising the lesion, the skin rostral to the medial canthus was mobilized to allow coverage of the defect.

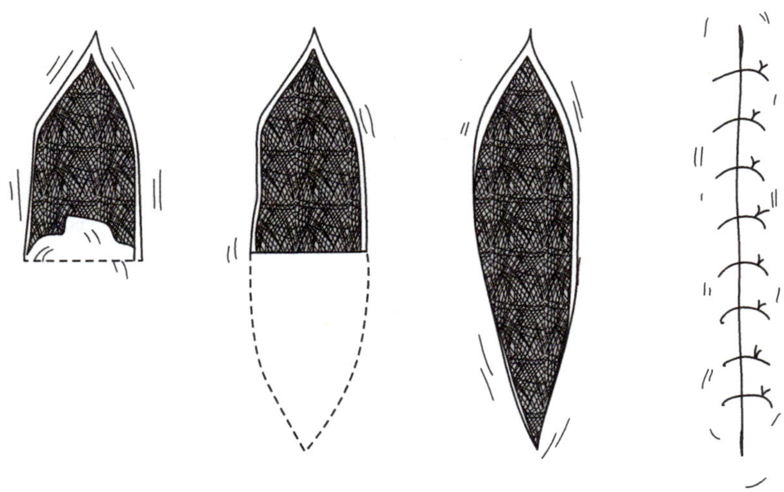

Figure 10.38 A triangular defect can be sutured as a single suture line by converting the triangle into a fusiform incision. Original drawings by Dr. Faith Riley.

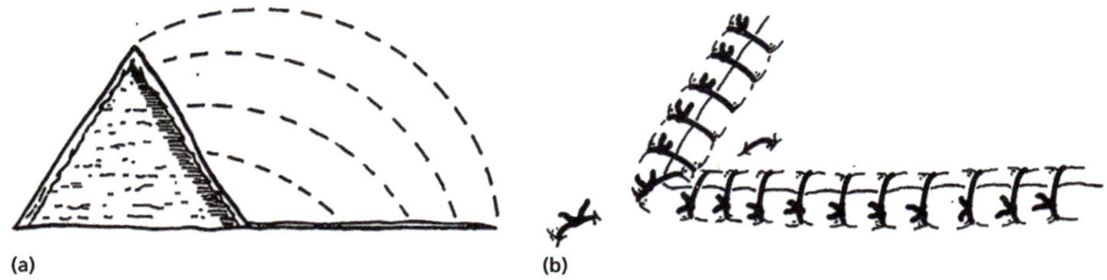

Figure 10.39 Triangular defect with adjacent loose skin. (a) Adjacent skin is undermined (dotted lines). (b) Sutures placed in a vertical mattress pattern secure the apex of the flap, and a simple-interrupted suture pattern is used for closure.

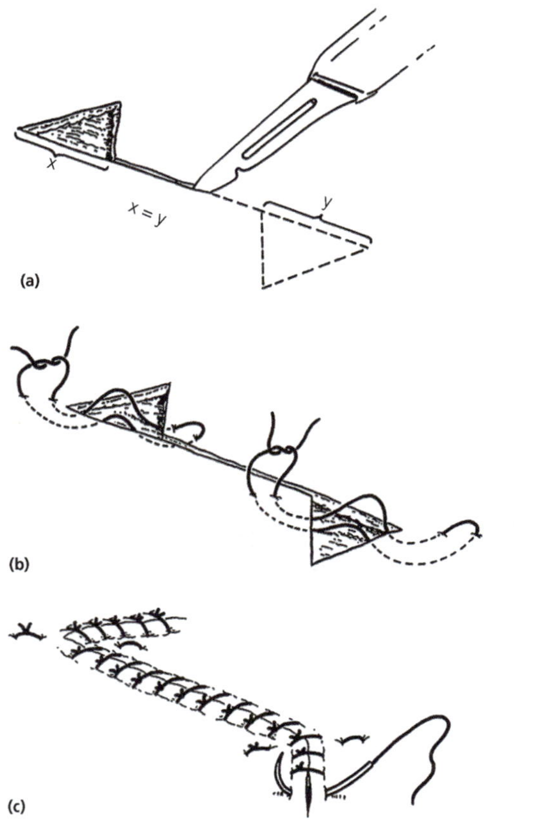

Figure 10.40 Triangular defect with loose skin available ventral to the defect. (a) One inverted triangle is created several base-widths away from the original triangular defect. (b) Following undermining of the skin, sutures are placed in a vertical mattress pattern at the base of the triangles to pull them into apposition. (c) A simple interrupted suture pattern is used to appose the skin.

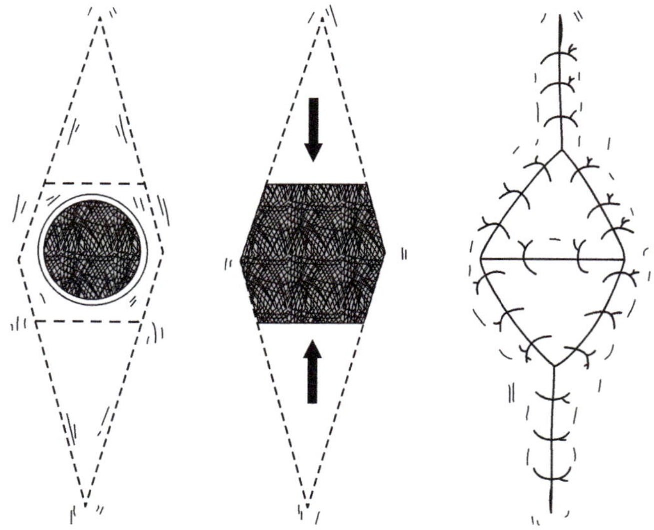

Figure 10.42 A circular defect too large to convert into a fusiform incision may be closed using a double V–Y technique. Original drawings by Dr. Faith Riley, adapted from Trott 2005.[64]

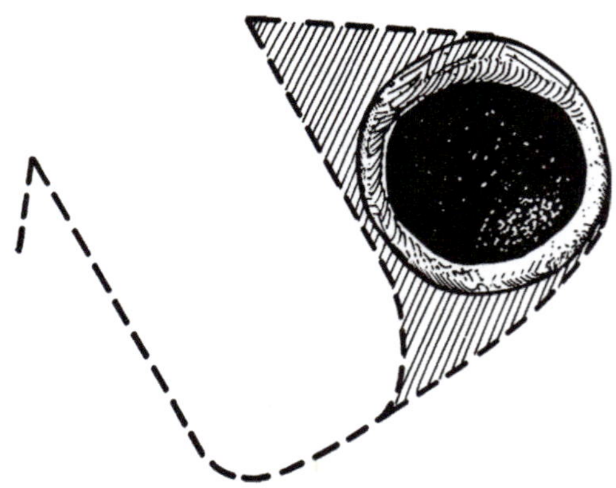

Figure 10.43 A transposition flap is created to cover a full-thickness circular defect (solid black). Dotted lines indicate incisions. The solid line indicates the circular defect. Oblique lines surrounding the circular defect represent further skin removal required to accommodate transposition of the skin flap from left to right.

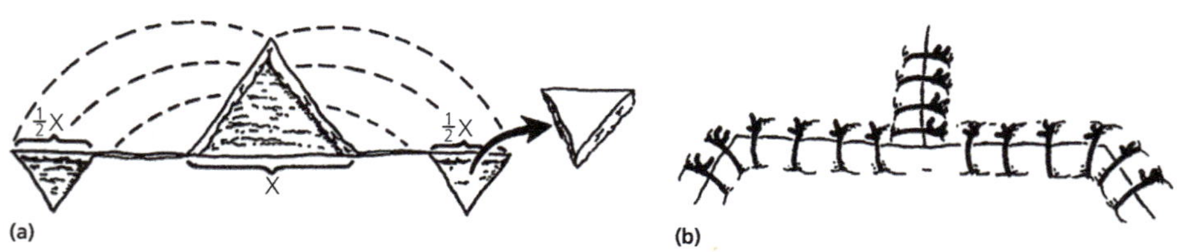

Figure 10.41 Triangular defect with loose skin available on either side. (a) Two inverted triangles, equaling 1/2 X, are created several base-widths away from the defect. The skin is undermined (dotted lines) in preparation for mobilization and closure. (b) A simple interrupted suture pattern is used for skin apposition.

injury, vascular thrombosis, and poor perfusion as a result of vasospasm, known as "no-reflow" phenomenon, within the skin flap. An experimental study showed no difference in the accumulation of neutrophils, a significant source of oxygen free radicals, between the control myocutaneous flap and those subjected to ischemia and reperfusion.[73] More work is needed to define the potential benefits of vascularized free-tissue transfers in horses.

Conclusion

The aim of reconstructive surgery is to shorten healing time, to improve cosmesis of the wounded site over that which would be achieved by second-intention healing, and to return the horse to performance as soon as possible. Reconstructive techniques range from the use of simple tension-relieving measures to complex vascularized free-tissue transplants. Although most skin wounds should be closed using the simplest approach, considering the scarceness of loose skin in the equine patient, the various methods described in this chapter to mobilize surrounding skin to cover a defect are often overlooked in practice. By successfully applying these techniques, the potentially deleterious effects associated with second intention healing (e.g., slow contraction, excessive and unsightly scarring, and reduced function) can be avoided. This chapter has provided the practical information required to successfully apply the various techniques of reconstructive surgery with the aim to stimulate interest and encourage the use of reconstructive techniques in practice.

References

1. Kirk MD. Selective scar revision and elective incision techniques applicable to the legs of horses; part 1. *Vet Med Small Anim Clin* 1976; **71**: 661.
2. Kirk MD. Selective scar revision and elective incision techniques applicable to the legs of horses. part 2. *Vet Med Small Anim Clin* 1976; **71**: 801.
3. McGuire MF. Studies of the excisional wound: I. Biomechanical effects of undermining and wound orientation on closing tension and work. *Plast Reconst Surg* 1980; **66**: 419.
4. Bailey JV. Principles of reconstructive surgery. In: Auer J, Stick J (eds). *Equine Surgery*, 3rd edn. Elsevier Saunders: St. Louis, 2006: 254.
5. Peyton LC, Campbell ML, Wolf GA, *et al.* The use of random skin flaps in equine reconstructive surgery. *Equine Vet Sci* 1983; **3**: 80.
6. Grabb WC. Introduction to the clinical aspects of skin flaps. In: Grabb WC, Myers MB (eds). *Skin Flaps*. Little, Brown and Company: Boston, 1975: 135.
7. Hinchcliff KW, MacDonald DR, Lindsay WA. Pedicle skin flaps in ponies: viable length is related to flap width. *Equine Vet J* 1992; **24**: 26.
8. Myers MB. Attempts to augment survival in skin flaps – mechanism of delay phenomenon. In: Grabb WC, Myers MB (eds). *Skin Flaps*. Little, Brown and Company: Boston, 1975: 145.
9. Lineaweaver WC, Lei MP, Mustain W, *et al.* Vascular endothelium growth factor, surgical delay, and skin flap survival. *Ann Surg* 2004; **239**: 866.
10. Bristol DG. The effect of tension on perfusion of axial and random pattern flaps in foals. *Vet Surg* 1992; **21**: 223.
11. Smyth GB, Brown RG, Juzwiak JS, *et al.* Delayed repair of an extensive lip laceration in a colt using an Estlander flap. *Vet Surg* 1988; **17**: 350.
12. Stashak TS. Mobilization of adjacent skin to cover full surface defects for the practice of large animal surgery. In: Jennings P (ed). *Large Animal Surgery*, 1st edn. WB Saunders: Philadelphia, 1984: 305.
13. Taylor GI, Palmer JH. The vascular territories (angiosomes) of the body: experimental study and clinical applications. *Br J Plast Surg* 1987; **40**: 113.
14. Taylor GI, Minabe T. The angiosomes of the mammals and other vertebrates. *Plast Reconstr Surg* 1992; **89**: 181.
15. Pavletic MM. Canine axial pattern flaps using the omocervical thoracodorsal and deep circumflex iliac direct cutaneous arteries. *Am J Vet Res* 1981; **42**: 391.
16. Pavletic MM. Vascular supply to the skin of the dog. *A review. Vet Surg* 1980; **9**: 77.
17. Lindsay WA. Wound treatment in horses: healing by third intention. *Vet Med* 1988; **83**: 506.
18. Hughes HV, Dransfield JW. The blood supply to the skin of the dog. *Br Vet J* 1959; **115**: 199.
19. Borges AF. *Elective Incisions and Scar Revision*, 1st edn. Little, Brown and Company: Boston, 1973: **316**.
20. Swaim SF, Henderson RA. Management of skin tension. In: Swaim S, Henderson R (eds). *Small Animal Wound Management*, 1st edn. Lea and Febiger: Philadelphia, 1990: 87.
21. Kraissl CJ. The selection of appropriate lines of elective surgical incisions. *Plast Reconstr Surg* 1951; **8**: 1.
22. Irwin DHG. Tension lines in the skin of the dog. *J Small Anim Pract* 1966; **7**: 593.
23. Wakuri H, Sakuma Y, Mutoh K, *et al.* Cleavage line patterns of the skin in the horse. *Okajimas Folia Anat Jpn* 1990; **67**: 351.
24. Gibson T, Kenedi RM. Biomechanical properties of skin. *Surg Clin North Am* 1967; **47**: 279.
25. Liang MD, Briggs P, Heckler FR, *et al.* Presuturing – a new technique for closing large skin defects: clinical and experimental studies. *Plast Reconstr Surg* 1988; **81**: 694.
26. Cartee RE, Cowles WR. Surgical implications of extensibility of the skin of the equine carpus. *Am J Vet Res* 1978; **39**: 387.
27. Stashak TS. Reconstructive surgery in the horse. *J Am Vet Med Assoc* 1977; **170**: 143.
28. Stashak TS. Full thickness sliding skin flaps for reconstructive surgery in the horse. *Proc Am Assoc Equine Pract* 1978; **24**: 395.
29. Turgut G, Ozcan A, Sümer O, *et al.* Reconstruction of complicated scalp defects via skin traction. *J Craniofac Surg* 2009; **20**: 263.
30. Gibson T, Kenedi RM, Carik JE. The mobile microarchitecture of dermal collagen: a bioengineering study. *Br J Surg* 1965; **52**: 764.
31. Purslow PP, Wess TJ, Hukin DWL. Collagen orientation and molecular spacing during creep and stress-relaxation in soft connective tissues. *J Exp Biol* 1998; **201**: 135.
32. Jee T, Komvopoulos K. Skin viscoelasticity studied in vitro by microprobe-based techniques. *J Biomechanics* 2014; **47**: 553.
33. Madison JB. Tissue expansion. *Vet Clin N Am Equine Pract* 1989; **5**: 633.

34. Bigbie RB, Shealy P, Moll D. Presuturing as an aid in the closure of skin defects created by surgical excision. *Proc Am Assoc Equine Pract* 1990; **36**: 613.
35. Harrison IW. Presuturing as a means of reducing skin tension in excisional biopsy wounds in four horses. *Cornell Vet* 1991; **81**: 351.
36. Liang MD, Briggs P, Heckler FR, *et al.* Presuturing – a new technique for closing large skin defects: clinical and experimental studies. *Plast Reconstr Surg* 1988; **81**: 694.
37. Neves RI, Saggers GC, Mackay DR, *et al.* Assessing the role of presuturing on wound closure. *Plast Reconstr Surg* 1998; **97**: 807.
38. Scardino M, Swaim SF, Henderson RA. Enhancing wound closure on the limbs. *Compend Contin Educ Pract Vet* 1996; **18**: 919.
39. Swaim SF. Management of skin tension in dermal surgery. *Compend Contin Edu Pract Vet* 1980; **2**: 758.
40. Barnea Y, Gur E, Amir A, *et al.* Our experience with wisebands: a new skin and soft-tissue stretch device. *Plast Reconstr Surg* 2004; **113**: 862.
41. Hirshowitz B, Lindenbaum E, Har-Shai Y. A skin-stretching device for the harnessing of the viscoelastic properties of skin. *Plast Reconstr Surg* 1993; **92**: 260.
42. Pavletic MM. Use of an external skin-stretching device of wound closure in dogs and cats. *J Am Vet Assoc* 2000; **217**: 350.
43. Topaz M, Carmel NN, Topaz G, *et al.* A Substitute for skin grafts, flaps or internal tissue expanders in scalp defects following tumor ablative surgery. *J Drugs Dermatol* 2014; **13**: 48.
44. Hirshowitz B, Lindenbaum E, Har-Shai Y. A skin-stretching device for the harnessing of the viscoelastic properties of skin. *Plast Reconstr Surg* 1993; **92**: 260.
45. Tsioli V, Papazoglou LG, Papaioannou N, *et al.* Comparison of three skin-stretching devices for closing skin defects on the limbs of dogs. *J Vet Sci* 2015; **16**: 99.
46. Melis P, Noorlander ML, Bos KE, *et al.* Tension decrease during skin stretching in undermined versus not undermined skin: an experimental study in piglets. *Plast Reconstr Surg* 2001; **107**: 1201.
47. Wihelmi BJ, Blackwell SJ, Mancoll JS, *et al.* Creep vs. stretch: a review of the viscoelastic properties of skin. *Ann Plast Surg* 1998; **41**: 215.
48. Casparian JM, Rodewald EJ, Monheit GD. The "modified" winch stitch. *Dermatol Surg* 2001; **27**: 891.
49. Johnson TM, Brown MD, Sullivan MJ, *et al.* Immediate intraoperative tissue expansion. *J Am Acad Dermatol* 1990; **22**: 283.
50. Johnson TM, Lowe L, Brown MD, *et al.* Histology and physiology of tissue expansion. *J Dermatol Surg* 1993; **19**: 1074.
51. Hochman M, Branham G, Thomas RJ. Relative effects of intraoperative tissue expansion and undermining on wound closing tensions. *Arch Otolaryngol Head Neck Surg* 1992; **118**: 1185.
52. McKay DR, Saggers JC, Kotwal N, *et al.* Stretching skin: undermining is more important than intraoperative expansion. *Plast Reconstr Surg* 1990; **86**: 722.
53. Austad ED, Pasyk KA, McClatchey KD, *et al.* Histomorphologic evaluation of guinea pig skin and soft tissue after controlled tissue expansion. *Plast Reconstr Surg* 1982; **70**: 704.
54. Booth L. Tissue expanders for mobilizing skin. *Proc Ann Surg Forum* 1987; **15**: 55.
55. Madison JB, Donawick WJ, Johnston DE, *et al.* The use of skin expansion to repair cosmetic defects in animals. *Vet Surg* 1989; **18**: 15.
56. Morgan RF, Edgerton MT. Tissue expansion in reconstructive hand surgery: case report. *J Hand Surg* 1985; **10**: 754.
57. van Rappard JH, Molenaar J, van Doorn K, *et al.* Surface-area increase in tissue expansion. *Plast Reconstr Surg* 1988; **82**: 833.
58. Pamplona DC, Weber HI, Leta FR. Optimization of the use of skin expanders. *Skin Res Technol* 2014; **20**: 463.
59. Austad ED, Rose GL. A self-inflating tissue expander. *Plast Reconstr Surg* 1982; **70**: 588.
60. Bailey JV, Jacobs KA. The mesh expansion method of suturing wounds on the legs of horses. *Vet Surg* 1983; **12**: 78.
61. Vig MM. Management of integumentary wounds of extremities in dogs: an experimental study. *J Am Anim Hosp Assoc* 1985; **21**: 87.
62. Furnas DW, Fischer GW. The Z plasty: biomechanics and mathematics. *Br J Plast Surg* 1971; **24**: 144.
63. Bowman KF. Double apposing Z plasty for correction of stenotic nares in a horse. *J Am Vet Med Assoc* 1982; **180**: 772.
64. Trott AT. *Wounds and Lacerations*, 3rd edn. Elsevier Mosby: Philadelphia, 2005: **135**.
65. Peyton LC. Reconstructive surgical techniques in the horse. *J Am Vet Med Assoc* 1981; **179**: 460.
66. Fowler JD, Miller CW, Bowen V, *et al.* Transfer of the vascular cutaneous flaps by microvascular anastomosis: results in six dogs. *Vet Surg* 1987; **16**: 446.
67. Miller CW, Bowen V, Change P. Microvascular distant transfer of a cervical axial pattern flap in a dog. *J Am Vet Med Assoc* 1987; **190**: 203.
68. Remedios AM, Bauer MS, Bowen CV. Thoracodorsal and caudal superficial epigastric axial pattern skin flaps in cats. *Vet Surg* 1989; **18**: 380.
69. Bristol DG, Hudson LC, Spaulding KA. The use of a barium gelatin mixture to study equine vasculature with potential application to free flap transfer. *Vet Radiol* 1991; **31**: 19.
70. Lees MJ, Bowen CV, Fretz PB, *et al.* Transfer of deep circumflex iliac flaps to the tarsus by microvascular anastomosis in the horse. *Vet Surg* 1989; **18**: 292.
71. Lees MJ, Bowen CV, Fretz PB, *et al.* Identification of a free skin flap from the region vascularized by the deep circumflex iliac artery of horse. *Am J Vet Res* 1990; **51**: 796.
72. Miller CW, Hurtig M. Identification and transfer of free cutaneous flaps by microvascular anastomosis in the pony. *Vet Comp Orthop Traumatol* 1989; **1**: 21.
73. Scott MW, Fowler D, Matte G, *et al.* Effect of ischemia and reperfusion on neutrophil accumulation in the equine microvascular tissue flaps. *Vet Surg* 1999; **28**: 180.

CHAPTER 11

Management of Wounds of the Head

Spencer Barber, DVM, Diplomate ACVS and Ted S. Stashak, DVM, MS, Diplomate ACVS

Chapter Contents

Summary

Injuries to the head are common and can result in a significant loss of function if a vital structure is involved. The head is highly prominent, so cosmetic repair of a wound to the head is often important esthetically and may help retain the horse's resale value. Injuries to the head generally heal well, but the repair of such injuries requires skilled treatment to obtain optimal results. Meticulous attention to repair is necessary when repairing a laceration of a lip, eyelid, or nostril because proper function of these highly mobile structures is important. Although injuries to ears are not common, restoring the cosmetic appearance and function of an injured ear is challenging. Facial and orbital fractures are usually depressed, creating a conspicuous deformity, but they generally can be reconstructed successfully. Nasocutaneous and sinocutaneous fistulas have significant functional and cosmetic implications and can be very challenging to repair, especially if large.

Introduction

The head is commonly wounded, and most often when the horse attempts to flee from a frightening situation while being restrained with a halter and lead rope. This chapter describes commonly encountered injuries to the head, and factors important to their successful management.

Lacerations

Lacerations, the most frequently encountered head injury, often are treated by primary or delayed closure, for the following reasons:

Equine Wound Management, Third Edition. Edited by Christine Theoret and Jim Schumacher.

Companion website: www.wiley.com/go/theoret/wound

1. Wounds of the face that are left to heal by second intention (i.e., by contraction and epithelialization) develop a larger epithelial scar than do wounds in other anatomic regions because the mobility of facial skin for healing by contraction is poor.
2. Epithelial scars, which can be large, lack hair, sebaceous and sweat glands, and pigmentation.[1,2] Because the head is highly visible, a wound that heals largely by epithelialization is esthetically unacceptable and decreases the horse's value.
3. Several body systems (e.g., respiratory, digestive, auditory, and ocular) can be injured so severely that the performance and even the life of the horse are in jeopardy.[3–6] Consequently, surgical repair is preferred so that proper function of the traumatized body system can be maintained.

A wound of the head is usually minimally contaminated, at least when compared to a similar wound on the distal portion of the limb, because horses with a head wound often are presented promptly, and because wounds in this location are a remote distance from debris and feces found on the ground. A good understanding of principles of plastic and reconstructive surgery is beneficial when treating a horse for a severe or chronic injury to the head.[7,8] Clinical experience suggests a wound to the head can be closed more successfully than can a similar wound on the limb or the body, possibly because the blood supply to the head is more abundant.[3–6]

Lip

A laceration to the lip is usually caused by a sharp, protruding object (e.g., a nail) (Figure 11.1). Partial-thickness wounds to the lip can be treated by primary or delayed primary closure, or the wound can be left unsutured to heal by second intention, although the outcome may not be cosmetically appealing.[3–5] Restoring good cosmesis and function to a lip with a full-thickness wound is challenging,[3–5,9] but leaving a full-thickness wound unsutured to heal by second intention can result in drooling of feed and/or saliva. Dehiscence is common if the technique of repair is poor, because the intimate attachment of the muscles of the lip to the dermis and the oral submucosa subjects the lips to forceful movement (Figure 11.2). Sharply undermining the skin and mucous membrane from the muscle, along with the use of tension sutures to bolster repair, can largely prevent dehiscence.[3–5] Because lips have a copious blood supply, lip lacerations rarely become infected following injury, unless blunt trauma has compromised blood supply to the wound.

Treatment

Preoperative preparation usually includes verification that the horse has been vaccinated against tetanus, initiation of antimicrobial therapy, administration of a non-steroidal anti-inflammatory drug (NSAID), lavage of the oral cavity with a dilute antiseptic solution (e.g., 0.1–0.2% povidone-iodine), and routine surgical preparation of the lip.

The skin and oral mucosa are undermined 1–1.5 cm from the margin of the wound, using a #10 scalpel blade to separate them from underlying musculature (Figure 11.3a,b). Non-absorbable, monofilament, size 0 or 1 suture material is preplaced in a vertical mattress pattern, with stents, through the isolated musculature centrally so the knots and supports, when later tied, remain on the outside of the lip (Figure 11.3c,d).

The mucosa is apposed with a simple interrupted or continuous suture pattern using size 2-0 or 3-0 synthetic absorbable suture material (Figure 11.3e), except at the mucocutaneous junction where one or more vertical mattress sutures are placed

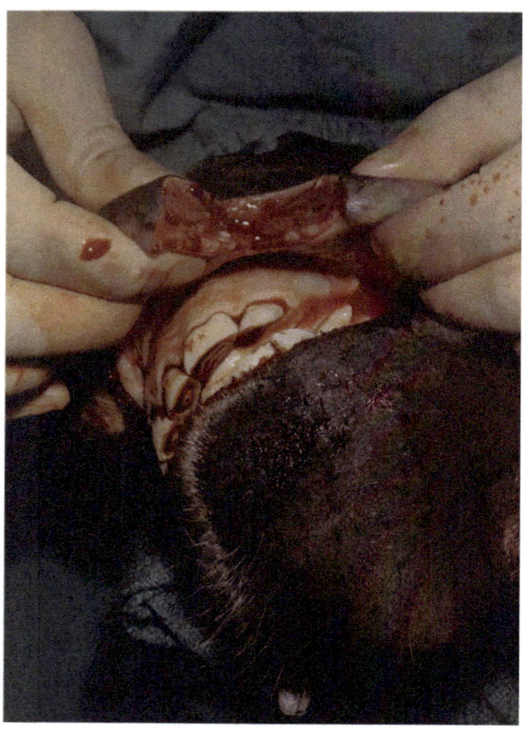

Figure 11.1 Acute, sharp laceration of the rostral aspect of the upper lip.

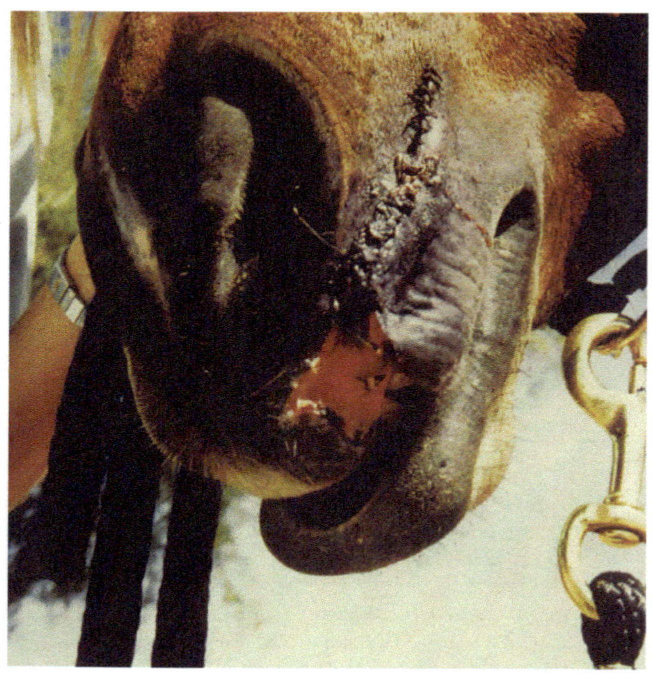

Figure 11.2 Sutured lip laceration that dehisced 6 days after reconstruction.

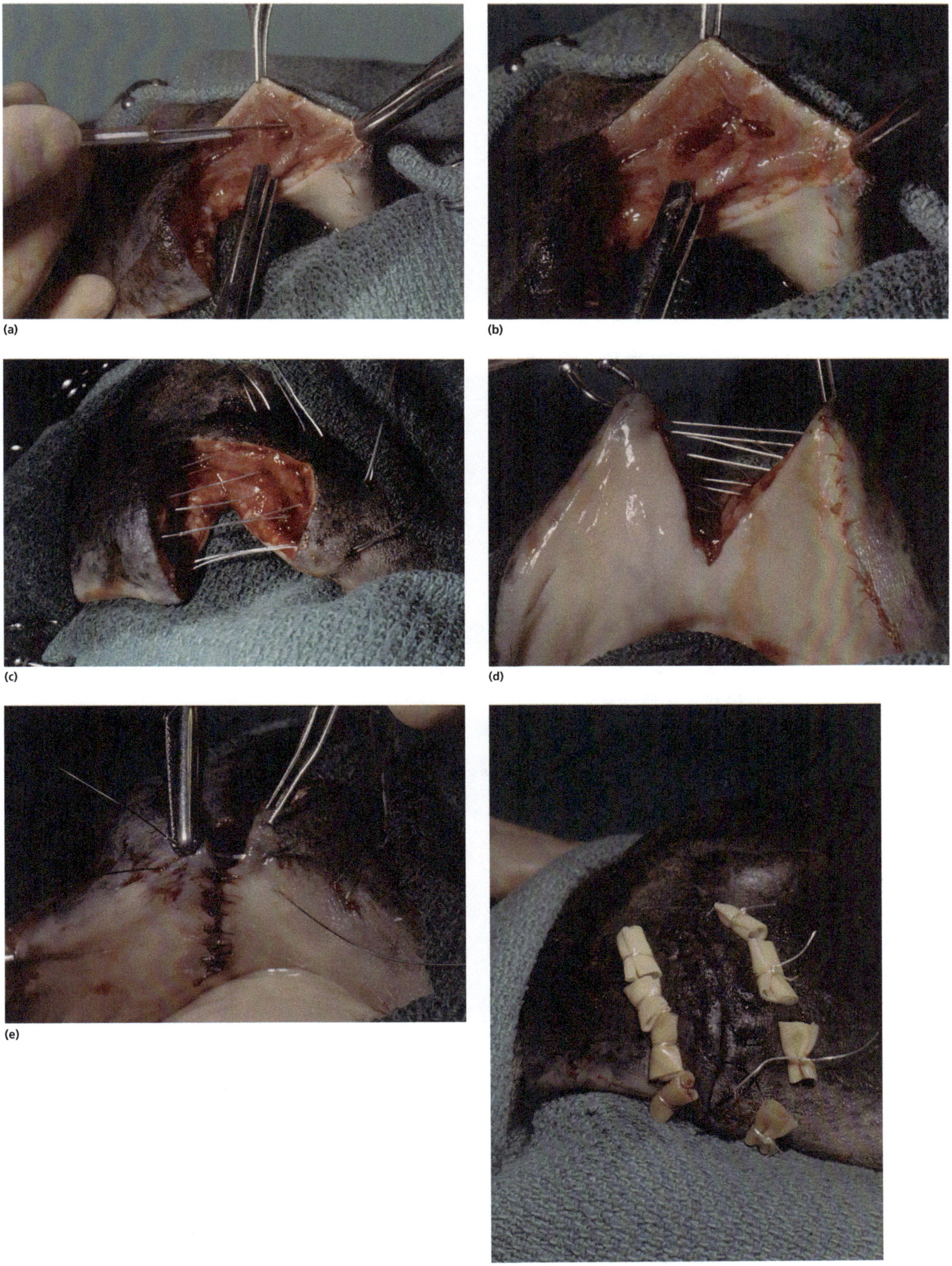

Figure 11.3 Same horse as in Figure 11.1. **(a)** Sharp dissection of the muscle from the skin and oral mucosa. **(b)** Dissection is complete except for the muscle at the mucocutaneous junction. **(c)** External view of the placement of vertical mattress tension (quill) sutures. Both suture passages should include the muscle. **(d)** Oral view of the placement of the vertical mattress tension (quill) sutures. **(e)** The oral mucosa is apposed with sutures in a simple interrupted pattern, and the mucocutaneous junction is sutured using a vertical mattress pattern. **(f)** Vertical mattress sutures appose the skin and vertical mattress quill sutures are tied over soft rubber tubing.

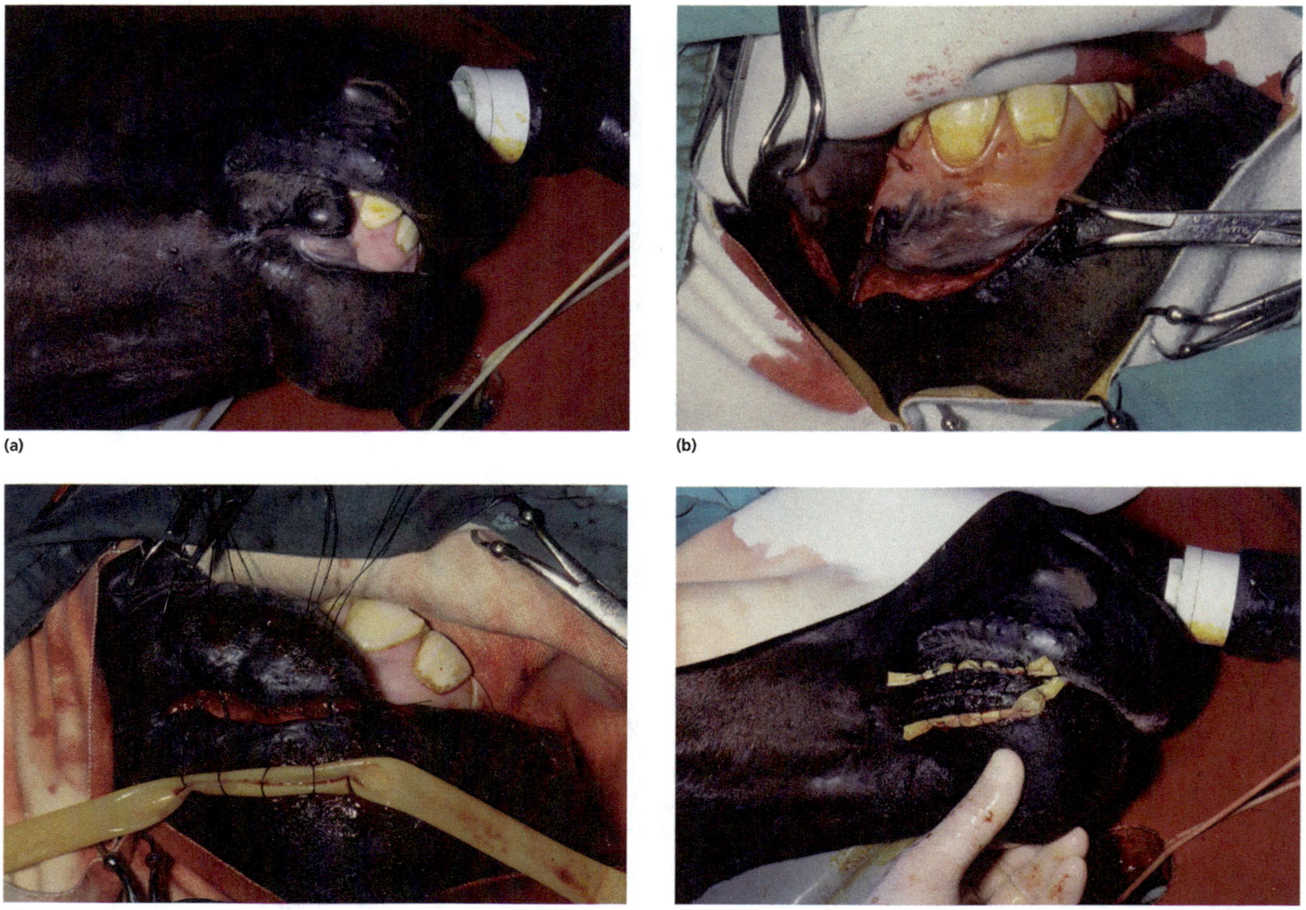

(a) (b) (c) (d)

Figure 11.4 **(a)** Chronic lower lip laceration that was sutured on two separate occasions and dehisced after repair. **(b)** Incision at the mucocutaneous junction. The skin and oral mucosa must be dissected from the scarred muscle. **(c)** Placement of the vertical mattress (quill) tension sutures at least 2 cm from the repair site. The oral mucosa and scarred muscle have been apposed with sutures. **(d)** Repair complete.

to minimize the likelihood of dehiscence. The preplaced sutures are then tied, over soft rubber tubing, and the skin apposed with an interrupted vertical mattress pattern of 2-0 monofilament, non-absorbable suture. Using a vertical mattress pattern to close the skin, rather than a simple interrupted pattern, prevents inversion of the skin edges.

A similar approach is used to revise a laceration that has healed by second intention, except that dissection of the skin and mucosa begins at the scarred mucocutaneous junction (Figure 11.4a,b) and is continued until the skin and mucosa have been undermined approximately 1.5–2 cm from the margin of the wound. The preplaced vertical mattress sutures should exit the skin at least 2 cm from the skin edges (Figure 11.4c). The rest of the closure is the same as for an acute laceration (Figure 11.4d).

Tension on a sutured laceration at the commissure of the lips increases tremendously when the mouth is opened (Figure 11.5a,b). To counter this tension, at least two additional vertical mattress sutures, with stents, of size 1 or 2 monofilament non-absorbable suture material should be placed rostral to the repair, through the uninjured lips (Figure 11.5c,d).

The horse should receive antimicrobial therapy and a NSAID postoperatively for 3–4 days, and can be fed its normal ration.

What to do

- Place draping material in the mouth to isolate the wound from the oral cavity.
- Use soft rubber tubing (e.g., a Penrose drain) to support the tension sutures (Figure 11.3f and 11.4d).
- Separate the skin and mucosa from the underlying musculature to protect against dehiscence.
- Sutures should be preplaced, in a vertical mattress pattern, through the musculature of the lip to achieve first-intention healing.

Tip

- A full-thickness axial pattern skin flap (i.e., Estlander flap), should be used to repair an extensive laceration to the lateral region of the lip when a portion of the lip has been lost.[9]

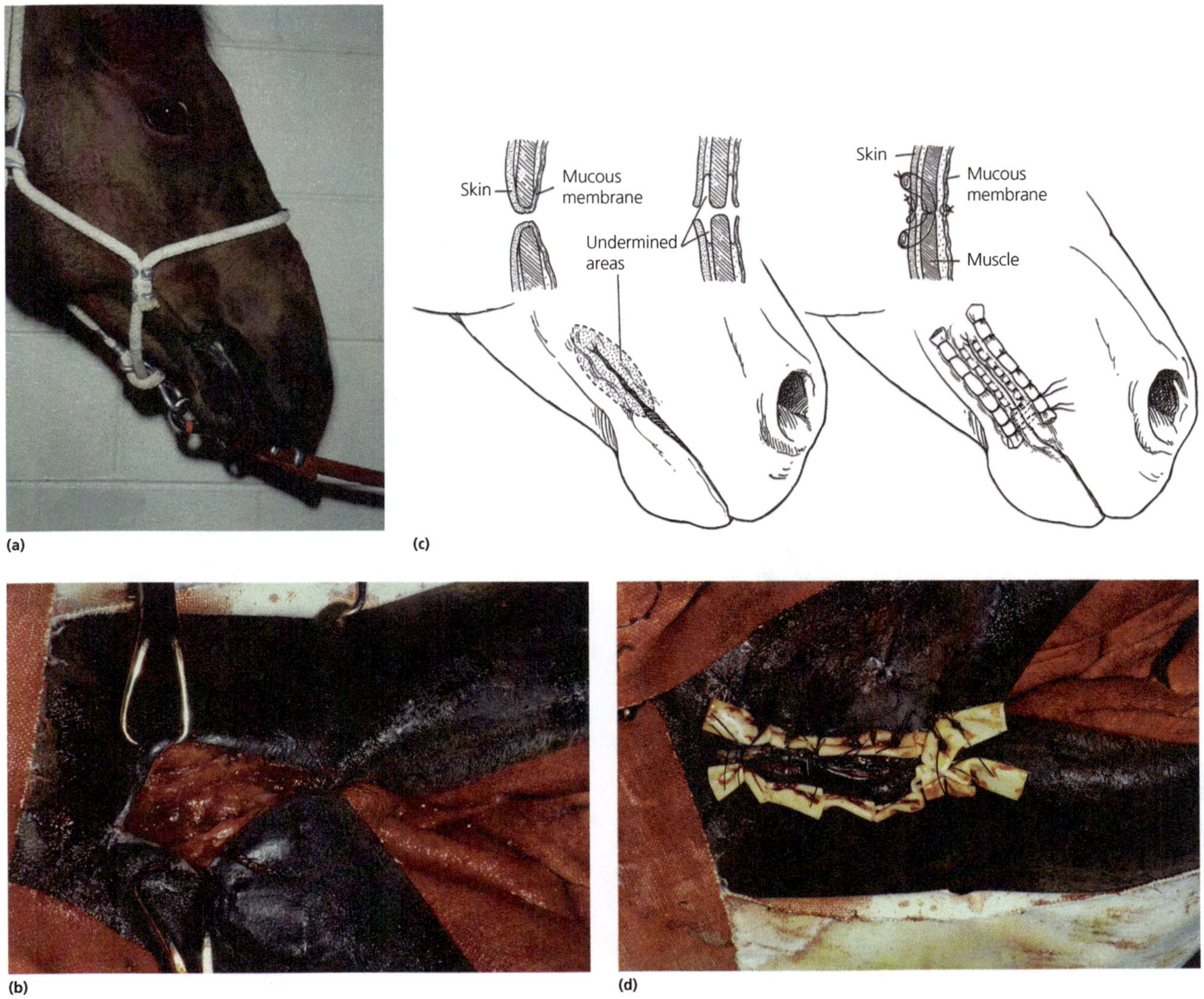

Figure 11.5 (a) Chronic laceration involving the right commissure of the lip and cheek. (b) Dissection of skin from the muscles of the cheek. (c) Left bottom: dotted line and dotted area illustrate the extent of undermining of the lip and cheek; left top: two cross-sections illustrating the undermining procedures; right bottom: the laceration is sutured, and two vertical mattress quill tension sutures are placed rostral to the repaired commissure to further stabilize the region; right top: cross-section illustrating suture apposition of the various layers. (d) Closure complete.

The patient can be cross-tied, and even sedated or tranquilized, if it attempts to rub the repaired lip. The additional tension sutures with stents, placed rostral to the repair, can be removed in 7–10 days, and skin sutures are removed in 14 days. Dehiscence, if it occurs, usually starts at the mucocutaneous junction. When a lip laceration is sutured using proper surgical technique, healing is by primary intention, and cosmesis and function are good.

Parotid salivary gland and duct

The parotid salivary gland and its duct, being located superficially, are more prone to injury than the better protected sublingual and mandibular glands and ducts. Laceration, direct blunt trauma, and iatrogenic surgical injury are the most common causes of injury to a salivary duct or gland.[10–12] The parotid duct is vulnerable to injury at the caudal border of the mandible (Figure 11.6) and is especially vulnerable at the ventral border of the mandible (i.e., at the vascular notch) where the duct and facial vessels course from medial to lateral. The duct then follows the rostral border of the masseter muscle for about 5 cm, turns rostrad beneath the facial artery and vein, and perforates the cheek obliquely to empty at a papilla located in the buccal vestibule opposite the third or fourth maxillary premolar,[11,12] but its location is variable. Laceration of the gland or duct should be suspected if a large volume of serous fluid discharges from the wound, especially when the horse is fed (Figure 11.7). The salivary glands of a 500-kg horse produce ~38 L of saliva in 24 hours, and because the parotid gland is the major producer, discharge of saliva is readily apparent when its duct is lacerated.[13]

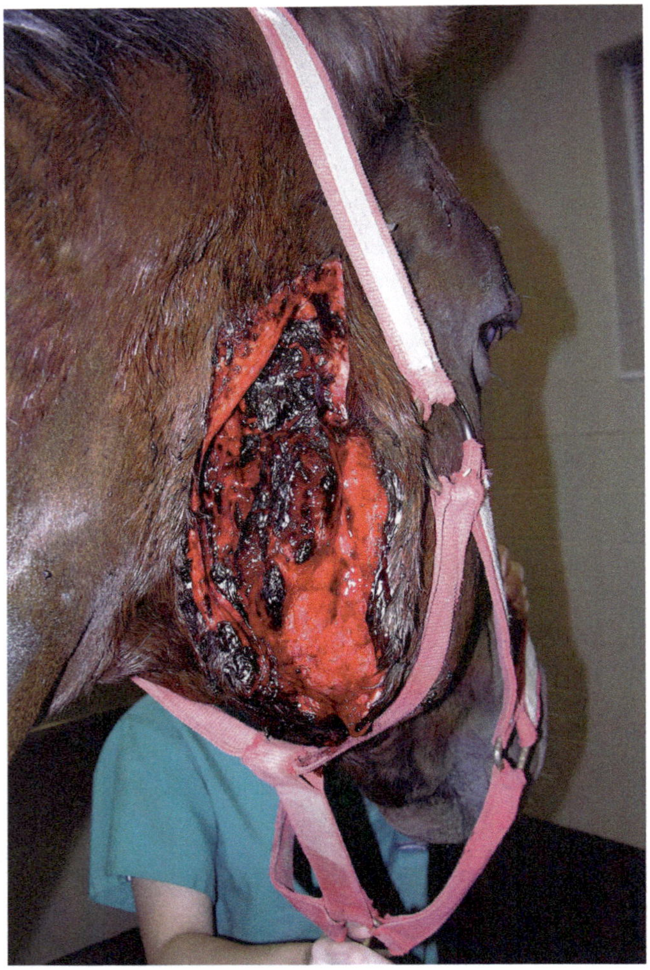

Figure 11.6 The parotid salivary duct is vulnerable to injury where it travels over the tendon of the *sternomandibularis* muscle and proceeds ventrally and rostrally at the caudal border of the mandible. An extensive wound at the caudal border of the mandible, such as the one suffered by this horse, is very likely to involve the parotid salivary duct. Courtesy of Dr. Reid Hanson.

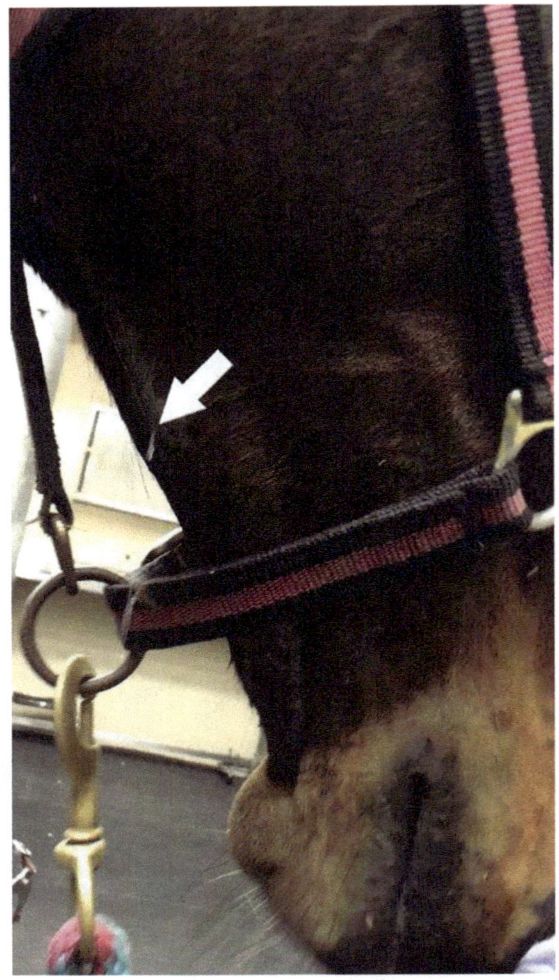

Figure 11.7 This horse suffered a laceration to the parotid salivary duct at the ventral aspect of the mandible where the duct and facial vessels course from medial to lateral (i.e., at the vascular notch). Saliva is flowing from a fistula into the duct. Leakage of saliva from a lacerated duct was especially copious when the horse ate. Courtesy of Dr. Reid Hanson.

The site of disruption of a parotid duct within a large wound (Figure 11.6) can be determined by passing a catheter retrograde, with the horse anesthetized, from the oral papilla and watching it exit the wound. Locating the papilla for catheterization occasionally requires a buccotomy slightly rostral to the maxillary premolar adjacent to where it lies.[11] To place the catheter, a small cutaneous incision can be created a few centimeters rostral to the buccotomy, through which the catheter is tunneled subcutaneously to the buccotomy. The catheter is inserted in the exposed papilla and advanced into the duct. Contrast radiography can also be used to establish patency of the parotid duct and its radicles that enter the gland (Figure 11.8).

Treatment

Surgical management of an injured salivary gland or duct is aimed at repairing the injured structure or eliminating the secretion of saliva. Many acute salivary fistulas heal by second intention within 1–3 weeks, and thus, deferring treatment can be a worthwhile option.[12] A fresh wound involving glandular tissue can be repaired by primary closure following standard preparation, irrigation, and debridement of the wound. The wound is reconstructed using a multilayer closure starting with the capsule of the gland. Care is taken not to penetrate the glandular tissue with suture because the suture could act as a nidus for formation of a calculus.[14] The wound should be allowed to heal by second intention if it is heavily contaminated or chronic, or if the owner imposes a financial constraint. If discharge from a wound over the parotid gland persists, laceration of one of the several large radicles that form the parotid duct should be suspected.[12]

A lacerated duct may be treated by primary closure, delayed primary closure, or second-intention healing. Horses with a lacerated duct are often presented for treatment after the epithelium of the duct has healed to cutaneous epithelium, causing

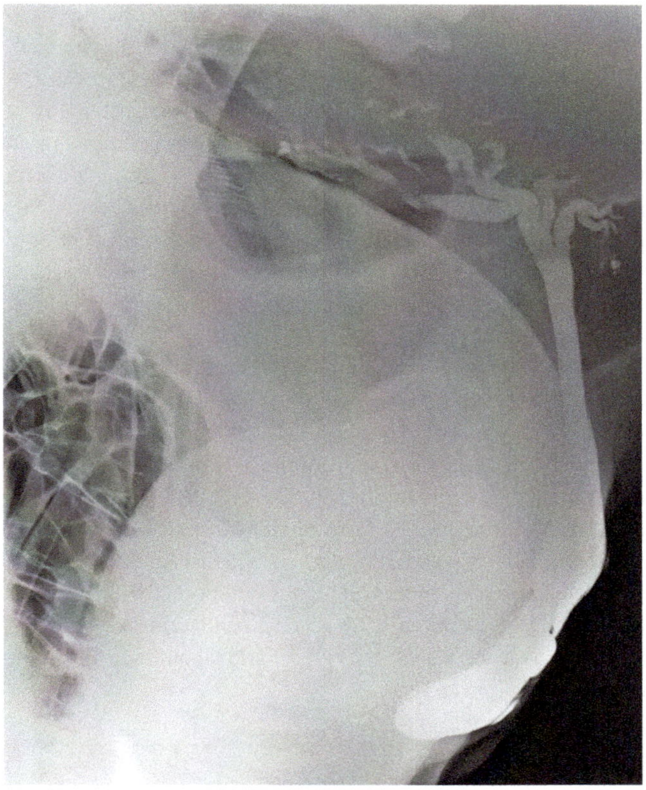

Figure 11.8 Contrast radiograph of parotid salivary duct and its radicles. Courtesy of Dr. Reid Hanson.

a salivary fistula. Primary closure of a freshly lacerated duct or a non-healing salivary fistula can be facilitated by suturing the defect over an intraluminal catheter placed in the duct (authors' recommendation). Cannulating the duct's papilla can sometimes be difficult or impractical. In this situation, a size 2 nylon suture can be threaded normograde, through the laceration or fistula, into the distal portion of the duct and exited through the papilla into the mouth. A catheter is then passed through a 14-gauge needle, used as a cannula, inserted through the cheek to enter the oral cavity just rostral to the papilla. The catheter is then guided over the nylon suture into the duct. When the tip of the catheter emerges from the laceration or fistula, it is directed retrograde into the proximal aspect of the duct to the level of the ventral aspect of the parotid gland. The lacerated duct is reconstructed using 5-0 or 6-0 absorbable suture material placed in a simple interrupted pattern.[10,11]

Alternatively, the duct can be reconstructed by placing three interrupted sutures of 5-0 or 6-0 monofilament absorbable suture material that appose the cut ends of the duct. The three sutures are placed an equal distance apart to form a triangle, and 5-0 or 6-0 sutures are placed between the apices of the triangle.[11,14] The external end of the catheter is sutured to the side of the face to provide visible evidence of continued flow of saliva and to allow for easy removal of the catheter when the duct has healed. The catheter is left in place for 4–5 weeks. [10,11] Leaving the catheter in place this long helps prevent stricture of the duct, ensures continued flow of saliva, and the catheter acts as a support for healing. If the cut ends of the duct cannot be anastomosed because too much tissue has been lost, an interposing polytetrafluoroethylene tube graft (Gore.com/medical) may be sutured to each cut end to bridge the gap.[15] The latter technique is recommended for salivary duct defects greater than 2.5 cm in length. Alternatively, a soft, smooth polyvinylchloride catheter (liberatormedical.com/catheters/8-Fr.), acting as a temporary intraluminal stent to bridge the tissue gap for shorter defects (less than 2.5 cm in length), can be used to allow healing of the defect over the stent, restoring ductal continuity.[10] Other options for maintaining salivary secretion are to create a fistula from the duct proximal to the injury into the oral cavity or to translocate the parotid duct to another site. Because of inconsistent results, these procedures are not recommended by the authors.[12]

The horse should receive antimicrobial therapy and a NSAID postoperatively for 4–5 days and can be fed its normal ration. The horse can be made to reduce production of saliva to enhance healing, especially if the ends of the duct cannot be completely apposed with sutures. To do this, the horse should be isolated, in a box stall, from other horses being fed, and fed small amounts of soaked hay pellets several times daily. The head is often bandaged to prevent the horse from dislodging an externally sutured catheter (see Chapter 7 for more information about bandaging techniques). The bandage is maintained until the catheter is removed.

The alternative method of resolving a fistula of the parotid duct is to eliminate the source of saliva. Horses readily tolerate the loss of one parotid gland.[12] The source of saliva can be eliminated by ligating the parotid duct or by chemically ablating the gland. Excising the gland is difficult to impossible because of the intimately associated large vessels and nerves located adjacent to and embedded within the glandular tissue.[12] Chemical ablation and ductal ligation are easier procedures to perform and more economical than reconstructing the duct.

To bring about physiologic destruction of the parotid gland, the duct is ligated between the gland and the fistula. A catheter is advanced into the proximal portion of the duct through the fistula, and an incision is made over the catheter, which can be palpated beneath the skin. Several sutures are placed around the catheterized duct and tied after the catheter is withdrawn. The duct should be ligated with heavy suture material (i.e., 0 or 1) because, if fine suture material is used for ligation, the suture may cut through the duct causing its lumen to be re-established. If the wound is fresh, hampering locating the severed end of the duct, the duct can be located and ligated where it crosses the tendon of insertion of the *sternomandibularis* muscle. To locate and ligate the duct where it crosses the tendon, an incision is made caudal to the vertical ramus of the mandible over the longitudinal axis of the tendon. The duct can be located by palpation through this incision. Because one or two radicles often exit the gland distal to the duct at this location, the duct should also be ligated further distally. To locate the duct further distally, the lumen of the duct is catheterized through a small incision in the duct, a second incision is made over the catheter 3–4 cm distal to the first incision, and several sutures are placed around the portion of the catheterized duct exposed in the second incision and tied after the catheter is withdrawn. The cutaneous incisions are sutured.

The parotid gland may be chemically ablated by infusing the gland, via a catheter placed into the duct, using 10% formalin, 2% chlorhexidine, or 2 or 3% silver nitrate.[12,14,16] Of these chemicals, 10% formalin produces the least amount of inflammation and necrosis and is, therefore, the solution of choice.[16] Water-soluble, iodinated contrast solution is also capable of eliminating glandular tissue.[12,16] This should be taken into consideration when performing retrograde contrast radiography. To avoid destroying the gland when examining the duct and gland using contrast radiography, the contrast material should be allowed to drain from the gland and duct, and the duct and gland should then be irrigated with sterile isotonic saline solution. When using 10% formalin to destroy the gland, 35–40 mL are infused into the gland by inserting a catheter into the proximal extent of the duct at the fistula. The solution is maintained within the gland for about 90 seconds before it is allowed to drain. Secretion of saliva is eliminated usually within 3 weeks.[16]

Tips

- Laceration of the gland or duct should be suspected if a large volume of serous fluid discharges from the wound, especially when the horse is fed.
- Many acute salivary fistulas heal by second intention within 1–3 weeks, so deferring treatment can be a worthwhile option.
- Use a 14-gauge needle as a cannula, instead of a buccotomy, to place the catheter into the oral cavity just rostral to the papilla.
- Chemical ablation and ductal ligation are easier to perform and more economical than surgical reconstruction of the duct.

Facial nerve

Lacerations that transect the facial nerve cause permanent sagging of the lower lip and a wry upper lip (Figure 11.9a,b), collapse of the ipsilateral nostril during exercise and result in unsightly drooling and slobbering of feed and water due to the loss of a buccal seal.

Treatment

Although motor function to the lips cannot be restored, a wedge resection of the lower lip aligns the lips sufficiently to restore a buccal seal, which prevents slobbering and drooling and often improves the cosmetic appearance of the lip.[3–5] The amount of lower lip to excise is estimated by comparing the lower lip to the upper lip when the two are pressed together so that they become aligned in a normal position. Because both the upper and lower lips droop when the horse is anesthetized, the preferred technique is to push them both back from their sagged position by applying pressure on the muzzle, thus causing the lower lip to bulge laterally, allowing an estimate of the amount of tissue to be removed.

A full-thickness, triangular wedge of lip, the apex of which is directed ventrad, is excised to the reflection of the mucosa on to the gum, (Figure 11.9c). The mucosa and skin are sharply separated from the underlying atrophied muscle for 1–1.5 cm from the right and left aspects of the margins of the wound. Sutures are preplaced in the musculature using a vertical mattress pattern, with stents, as described earlier. The mucosa is sutured from within the oral cavity, using 2-0 synthetic absorbable suture material placed in a simple interrupted or simple continuous pattern, so that the knots are located orally. The skin is apposed with 2-0, non-absorbable monofilament suture material placed in a vertical mattress pattern, and the preplaced tension sutures are tied (Figure 11.9d).

Antimicrobial therapy and a NSAID are administered before surgery, and administration is continued for a few days postoperatively. The horse should be observed closely for signs of rubbing at the surgical site; if observed, administering a tranquilizer and continuing the administration of the NSAID usually prevent rubbing. If they do not, the horse should be cross-tied for a week to prevent rubbing of the surgical site. Dehiscence, if it occurs, usually begins at the mucocutaneous junction. Tension sutures can usually be removed at 7–10 days, and skin and mucosal sutures at 14 days. A cosmetic and functional outcome is usually achieved (Figures 11.9e,f).

What to do

- The skin and mucosa should be separated from the underlying musculature to protect against dehiscence.
- Sutures should be preplaced in a vertical mattress pattern through the musculature of the lip to achieve first-intention healing.

What to avoid

- Tension on a sutured laceration at the commissure of the lips can be avoided by inserting two or more sutures, through undamaged lip, rostral to the commissure.

Tip

- When estimating the amount of tissue to remove from a paralyzed lower lip, the lower lip should be pressed against the upper lip so that the lips become aligned in a normal position.

Tongue

The tongue can be lacerated by the teeth during recovery from anesthesia, by the bit when a horse pulls back when tied fast by the reins, or when a sharp object enters the mouth.[3–5] The laceration commonly extends transversely across the dorsal surface of the tongue into the musculature. Healing by second intention produces a defect on the dorsum of the tongue, the extent of which depends on the depth and width of the laceration.

This defect can cause three problems: (1) the bit may periodically lodge in the defect, causing problems with control of the horse's head and, hence, performance; (2) the tongue may be re-injured at the defect causing bleeding; and (3) if the defect is deep, the tongue may not remain between the dental arcades (i.e., a flail tongue) causing it to be injured by the teeth. The

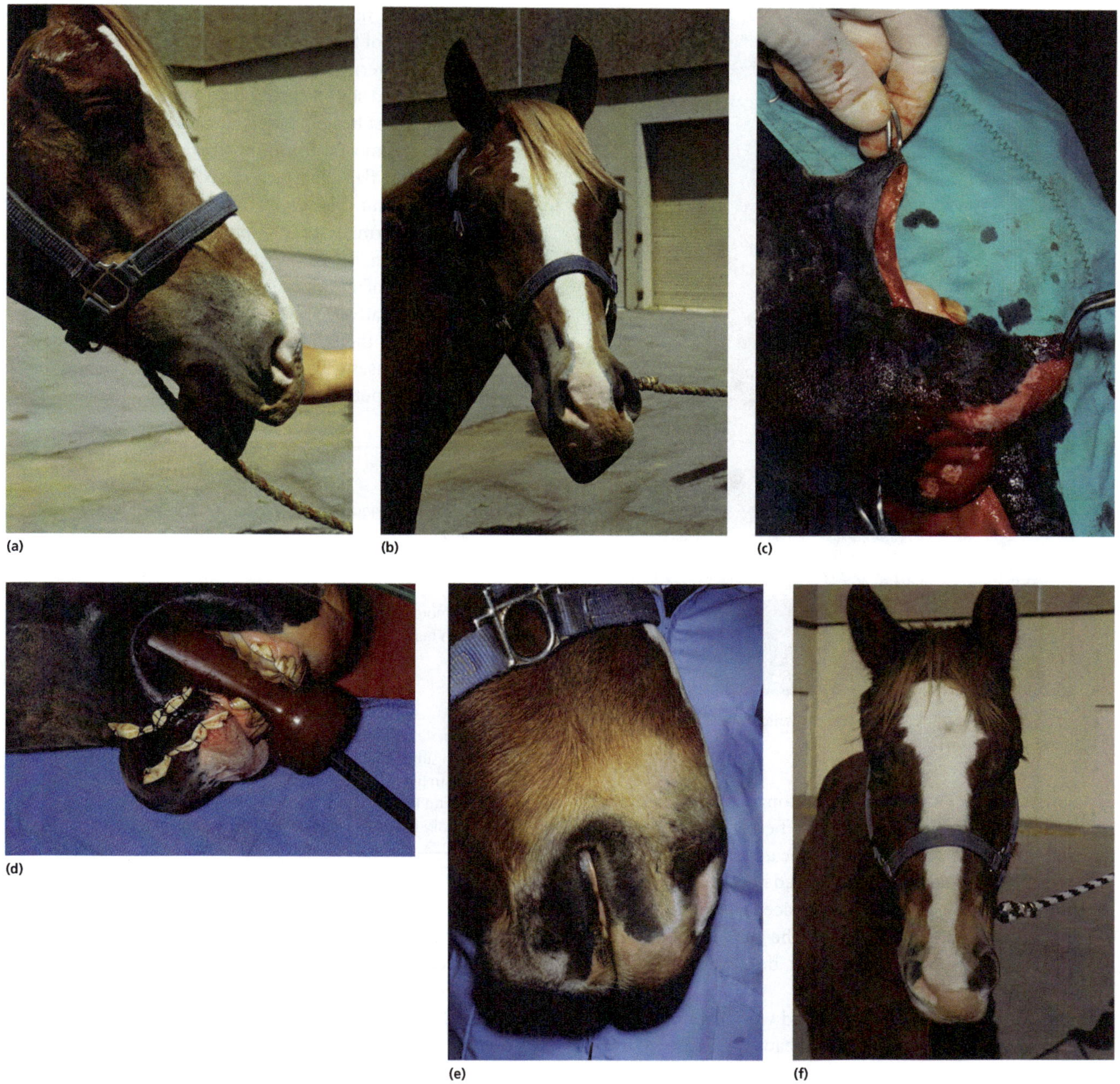

Figure 11.9 (a) Lateral view of a horse with transection of the facial nerve. The lips on the right side droop, and the tongue protrudes slightly. (b) Frontal view of the same horse. Note the wry appearance to the right lips and nostril. (c) Wedge resection of the lower lip completed. (d) Sutured lip. (e) Lateral view 1 year later. Note the good apposition of the lips. (f) Frontal view 1 year later.

depth and location of the wound and the intended use of the horse are considered to determine if the wound should be sutured. Lacerations involving less than 30% of the tongue's thickness can be left to heal by second intention, but deeper lacerations should be sutured (Figure 11.10).[4]

Because the tongue's vascular and nervous supply is located in the ventral half of the tongue, even deep lacerations can be sutured successfully because the blood vessels and nerves are rarely damaged by the injury. Assessment of the vascular supply is usually based on color, temperature, and bleeding from the edges of the wound during debridement, or less commonly by fluorescence after fluorescein dye (1.2 mg/kg) is administered intravenously. If avascular, that portion of the tongue rostral to the laceration must be amputated.

Treatment

Preoperative preparation includes administration of an antimicrobial drug and a NSAID. The oral cavity is lavaged to remove feed, and the tongue and wound are gently scrubbed with a mild antiseptic solution using a gauze swab.

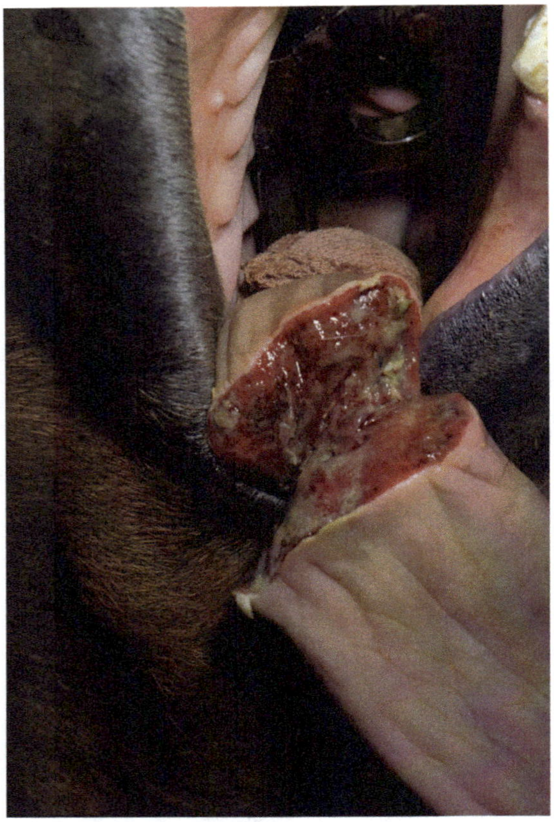

Figure 11.10 Deep laceration of the tongue, which would likely result in a flail tongue if not sutured.

Small lacerations at the tip of the tongue can sometimes be repaired with the horse standing, but the horse should be anesthetized if the injury is extensive or located more caudally than at the tip. The tongue of the anesthetized horse is exteriorized by exerting traction on a towel clamp placed through the tongue, or on a gauze loop, placed around the tongue, caudal to the laceration. The exposed wound can be isolated by draping (Figure 11.11a).

The margin of the wound is excised with a scalpel. Excising anything more than a narrow margin causes the sutured tongue to deviate dorsally or laterally. Accurate closure of dead space and approximation of tissue edges are imperative to prevent dehiscence, because constant movement of the tongue and the presence of saliva, bacteria, and feed hinder healing. The lacerated sides of the tongue must be apposed accurately.

The mucosa of the dorsal surface of the tongue is thick and dense and has great strength and, therefore, holds tension sutures well. The tongue should be sutured using absorbable suture material to eliminate the necessity for removing sutures. A vertical mattress tension pattern using 0 or 1 monofilament, absorbable suture should penetrate the laceration into the musculature centrally so the knots, when later tied, reside on the dorsal aspect of the tongue (Figure 11.11b). This layer provides great strength to the repair. Before tying the vertical mattress sutures, synthetic absorbable monofilament sutures (0 or 2-0), are used to appose the lacerated muscles and eliminate dead space. The mucosa of the tongue is also apposed with a vertical mattress suture pattern (Figures 11.11c,d) or a combination of vertical mattress and simple interrupted suture patterns.

If the tongue must be amputated, a transverse wedge-shaped piece of tissue is removed from the remaining stump, creating dorsal and ventral flaps that are closed with a horizontal or vertical mattress suture pattern.[3–5] Horses can be expected to eat and handle a bit normally after amputation of the tongue to the level of the frenulum.[17]

Administration of antimicrobial therapy and a NSAID is continued postoperatively for 3–5 days. Feeding a soft food may ease the comfort of the horse. A good functional result can be expected in most cases (Figure 11.11e), even if a portion of the tongue requires amputation.

What to do

- The sides of the tongue must be accurately apposed if the laceration is sutured.

What to avoid

- Excising more than a narrow margin of tissue at the edge of the laceration may cause the tongue to deviate dorsally or laterally when sutured.

Tips

- Most superficial lacerations of the tongue do not require suturing.
- A tension suture pattern on the dorsum of the tongue provides great holding strength.
- Amputating the tongue to the level of the frenulum does not substantially impair function of the tongue or use of the horse.

Nostril

Lacerations of the nostril, more common in head-shy horses, are usually caused by a protruding object, such as an angled bolt protruding from a gate or a horse trailer.[3–5] The soft tissues collapse during inspiration and flutter during expiration if the laceration is extensive and full-thickness, because the horse is unable to properly dilate the nostril and because negative inspiratory pressure collapses the nostril. A good blood supply to the region usually facilitates healing, even if the laceration is chronic.

Laceration to the lateral margin (i.e., base) of the nostril can be problematic because of tension/shearing forces resulting from muscle contractions associated with movement of the upper lip when the horse eats and movement of the ipsilateral alar cartilage when the nostril dilates. Repair of a full-thickness laceration to the arch of the nostril is fairly straightforward and rarely problematic. The horse can be discouraged from rubbing the repaired nostril by administering a NSAID, by cross-tying it, or by applying a half-muzzle.

Occasionally, a horse develops a stenotic nostril when the laceration is left to heal by second intention (Figure 11.12a) or when the normal arch to the nostril is not restored with

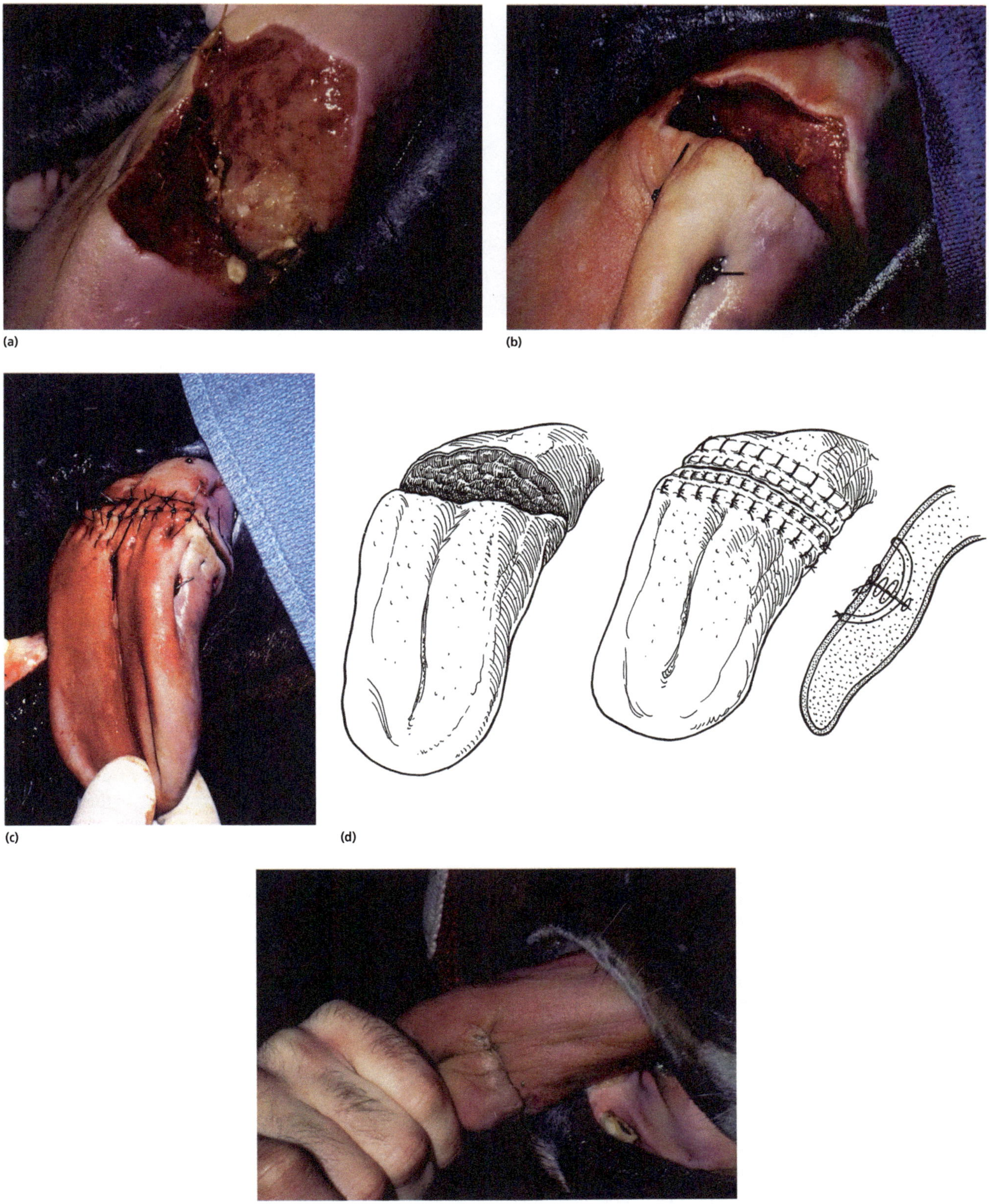

(a) (b) (c) (d) (e)

Figure 11.11 **(a)** Laceration involving two-thirds of the tongue. **(b)** Vertical mattress sutures are placed, and the muscles are apposed with a simple interrupted suture pattern. **(c)** Repair complete. **(d)** Combination of vertical mattress and simple interrupted suture patterns. **(e)** Top view of healed tongue laceration. (a) Courtesy of Dr. G.W. Trotter.

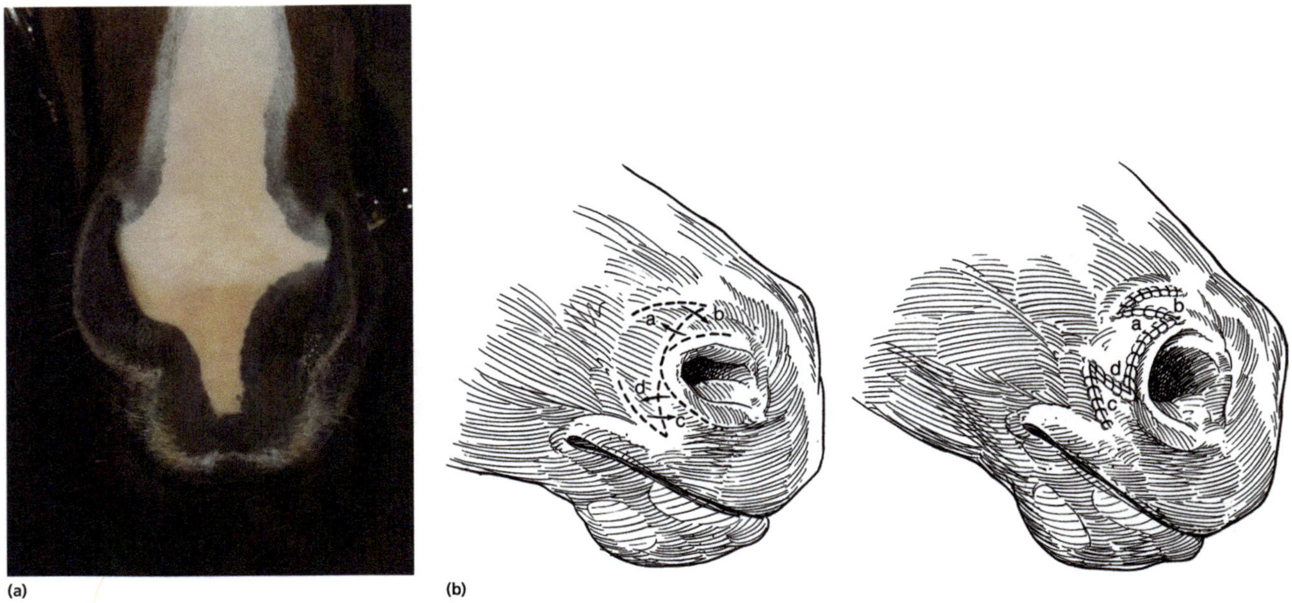

Figure 11.12 **(a)** Reduced opening of the left nostril after suture repair 3 months earlier. This racehorse was presented because of inadequate and noisy airflow through the left nostril. **(b)** Left: constricted nostril due to scarring (dotted lines illustrate incisions for Z plasties); right: Z plasties complete and sutured. The diameter of the nostril is enlarged.

suturing. If only the most rostral aspect (external orifice) of the nostril is stenotic, two Z plasties can be used to increase the diameter of the opening (Figure 11.12b).[18] If, however, the stenosis extends caudally to involve the false nostril, the stenotic nostril must be incised along the healed scar and re-apposed so that the normal arch of the nostril is restored.[4]

Treatment

Acute lacerations of the dorsal arch of the nostril (Figure 11.13a) should be sutured with 2-0 monofilament nylon in an interrupted, modified figure-of-eight pattern to appose the skin on the outside of the nostril and skin within the false nostril (Figure 11.13b-d).[3–5] The advantages of this approach to suturing are speed of application, good apposition of all tissue layers, and the ability to remove the sutures by cutting a single loop. Alternatively, simple interrupted sutures can be used, but gaping of the wound between the sutures is common.

Acute lacerations of the base of the nostril are usually best handled by primary closure (Figure 11.14a).[3–5] After the site is prepared for surgery, the nostril is packed with sterile gauze, and drapes applied to the area (Figure 11.14b). The wound should be debrided, but care must be taken to not further compromise the blood supply to the flap (Figure 11.14c). Because this area is subjected to high motion from movement of the upper lip and alar cartilage, a three-layer suture closure is recommended (Figure 11.14d) to provide security and good approximation of tissue. The skin inside the false nostril is sutured from within using a continuous-horizontal mattress suture pattern of 2-0 synthetic absorbable suture material (Figure 11.14d). The deep tissue is apposed in a simple interrupted fashion, and the skin is sutured with 2-0 monofilament non-absorbable suture using an interrupted vertical mattress pattern (Figure 11.14d,e).

A chronic laceration of the base of the nostril presents a special problem because the flap of tissue may be smaller than its original size due to contraction (Figure 11.15a,b).[3–5] The flap must be incised to create fresh edges that are then undermined to reform the inner and outer epithelial layers at the base of the nostril. When creating these fresh edges, only a minimal amount of tissue should be excised (Figure 11.15c).

The first step is to make an incision in the base of the nostril that extends rostrally along the line of injury from the base of the flap to the site where the most rostral tip of the flap should reside, without reducing the luminal diameter of the nostril. The skin on the dorsum and on the ventrum of the base of the wound is undermined to produce two edges of tissue for internal and external closure (Figure 11.15c). Inner and outer edges are created in the tissue flap in a similar manner (Figure 11.15c). The fresh edges produced by these incisions

What to do

- Tissue flaps should be debrided sparingly to conserve tissue and protect vascularity.

What to avoid

- Failure to restore the normal arch to the nostril results in a nostril that functions improperly.

Tips

- The modified figure-of-eight interrupted suture pattern nicely apposes both epithelial surfaces of the arch of the nostril.
- The horse should be closely monitored postoperatively to prevent rubbing that may lead to wound dehiscence.

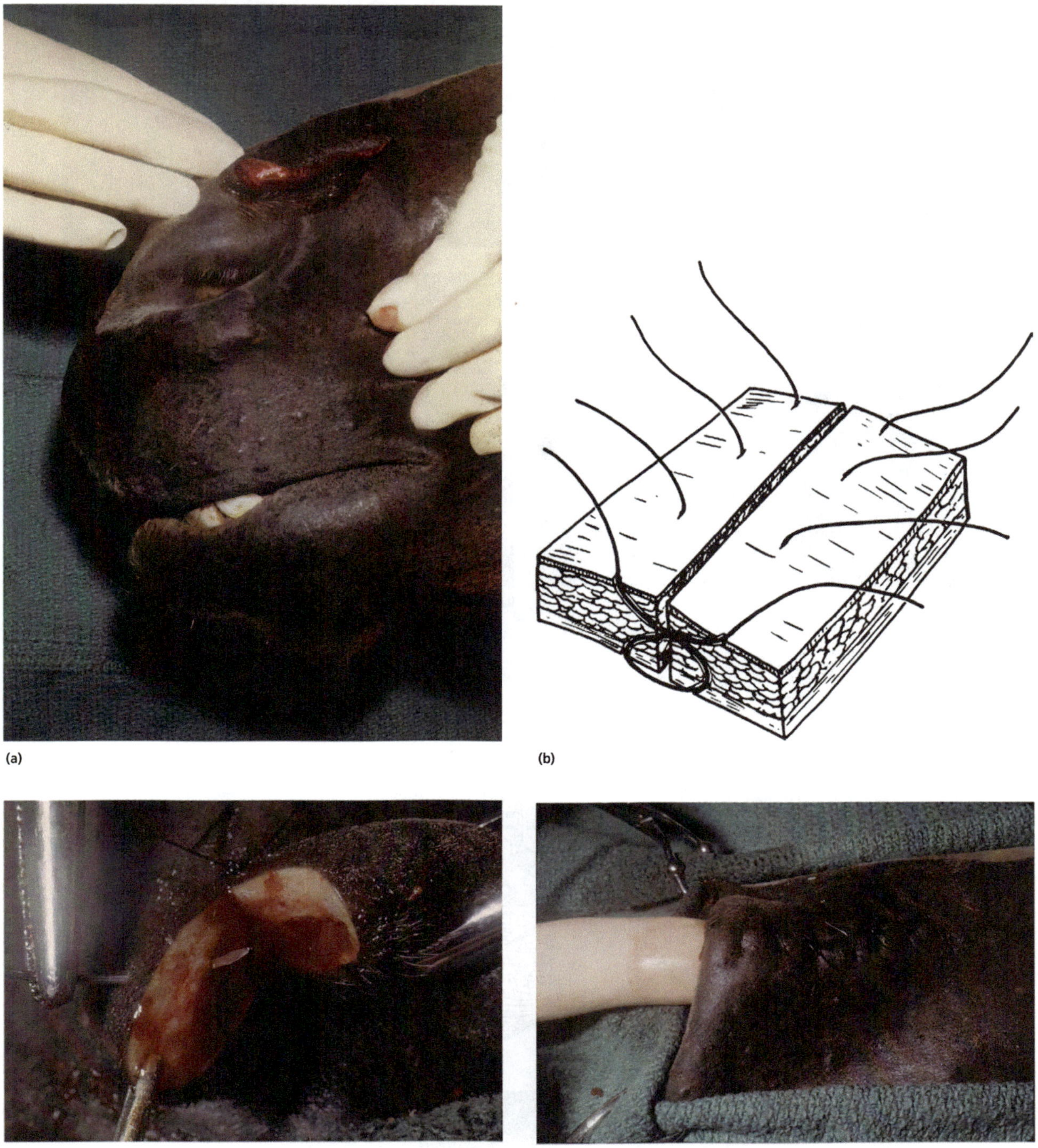

(a) (b) (c) (d)

Figure 11.13 (**a**) Sharp laceration of the dorsal arch of the left nostril. (**b**) Placement of the modified figure-of-eight interrupted suture pattern that apposes both epithelial surfaces. (**c**) Passage of the suture through half the thickness of tissue. The suture then enters the tissue on the opposite side and exits through the skin within the false nostril. (**d**) Suturing is complete.

are sutured as described previously for acute lacerations. The freshened edges are apposed by suturing from the base of the flap toward the tip of the flap (Figure 11.15d,e). Alternatively, closure can be started by suturing the tip of the flap to the appropriate site on the base of the nostril. Pulling the flap too rostrad may result in stenosis of the nostril and increases tension on the sutured wound.

Postoperative care is similar to that for repair of other lacerations of the nostril. A muzzle that covers the nostril, while allowing the horse to eat and drink, can be applied to prevent the horse from rubbing the surgical site (Figure 11.15f). Lacerations of the nostril generally heal well, and a good functional and cosmetic result can be obtained if the principles in this section are followed; otherwise, results can be very disappointing.

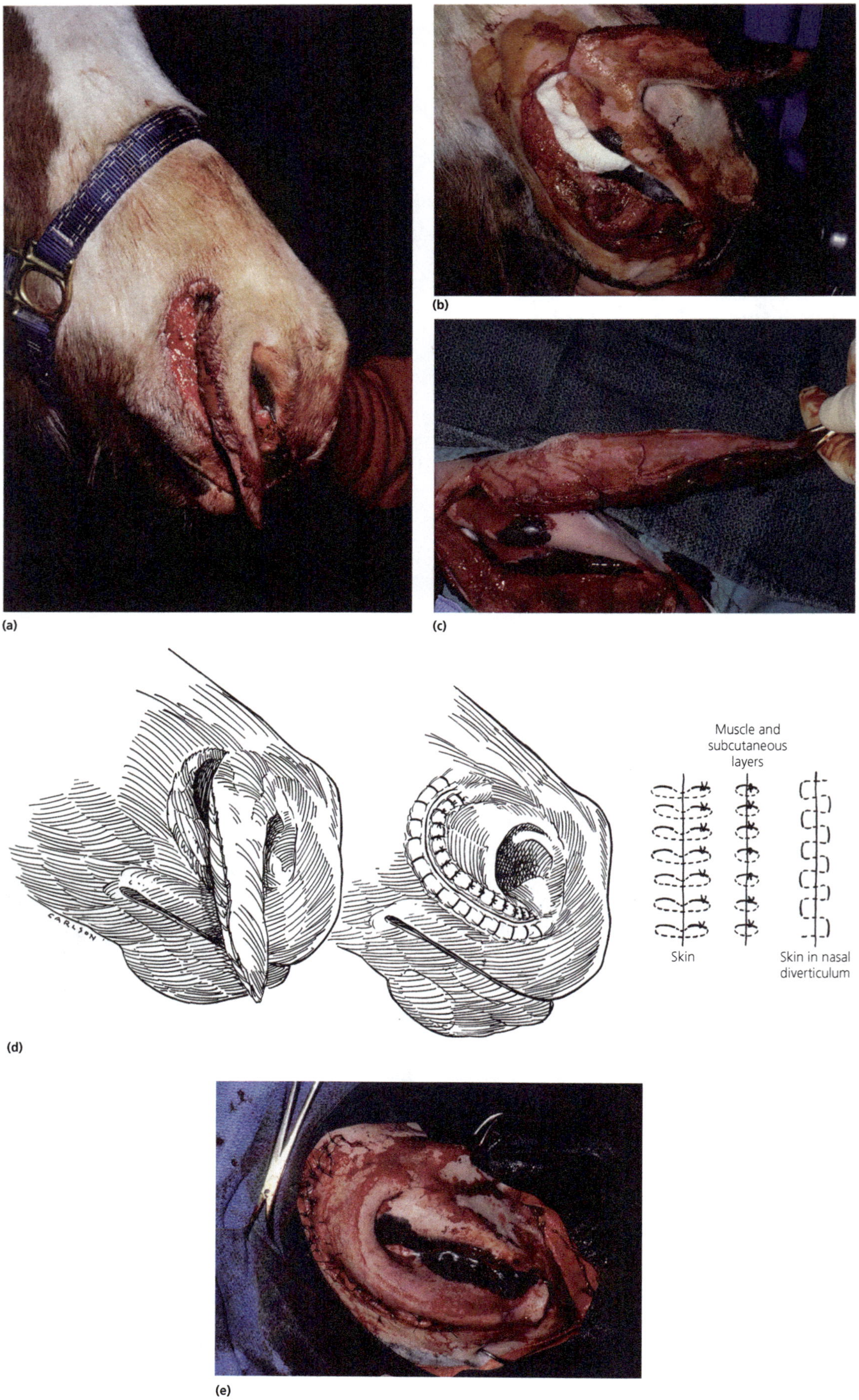

Figure 11.14 (**a**) Laceration at the base of the nostril. (**b**) The nostril is packed with sterile gauze after clipping hair, scrubbing with surgical soap, and irrigating with an isotonic saline solution. (**c**) Debridement is complete. Note the limited attachment of the caudal extent of the skin flap. (**d**) Left: laceration; middle: sutures placed in the nostril; right: suture patterns used for the three-layer closure. (**e**) Suturing complete.

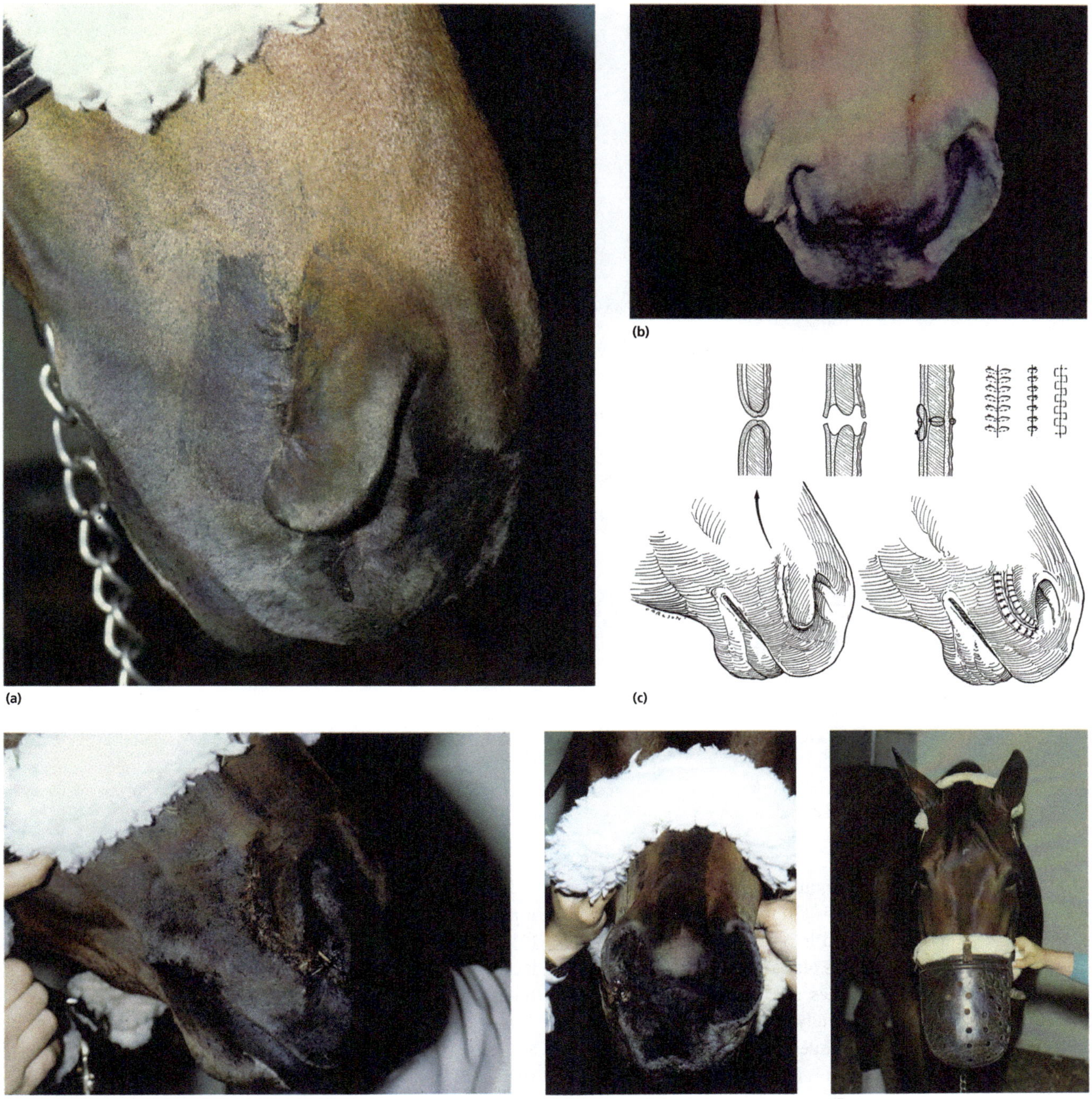

(a) (b) (c) (d) (e) (f)

Figure 11.15 **(a)** Side view of a chronic laceration at the base of the right nostril. **(b)** Cranial view of this chronic laceration. Note the reduction in diameter of the external naris. **(c)** Top: dissection planes and layers of closure; bottom left: laceration at the base of the nostril; bottom right: nostril reconstruction is complete. **(d)** Lateral view of the reconstructed nostril. **(e)** Cranial view of the reconstructed nostril. Note that the nostril's diameter is almost equivalent to that of the opposite, normal side. **(f)** A half-muzzle covering the nares to protect the repair site from trauma; it was attached to the halter, and because it covered only the nostrils, the horse could still eat and drink.

Eyelid

Lacerations of the upper and lower eyelids are relatively common and usually occur when the eyelid contacts a sharp object.[3–5] If the wound is caused by a blunt object, however, the eye should be examined, and the bony orbit evaluated (see Management of fractures of the medial aspect of the orbital rim and zygomatic [supraorbital] process, later in this chapter). Because eyelids have a generous blood supply that is conducive to healing, repair is always attempted (Figure 11.16) to preserve the mucocutaneous junction of the margin of the eyelid, an appropriate palpebral fissure, and a functional blink response.[19,20] Even flaps with a very small base often survive.

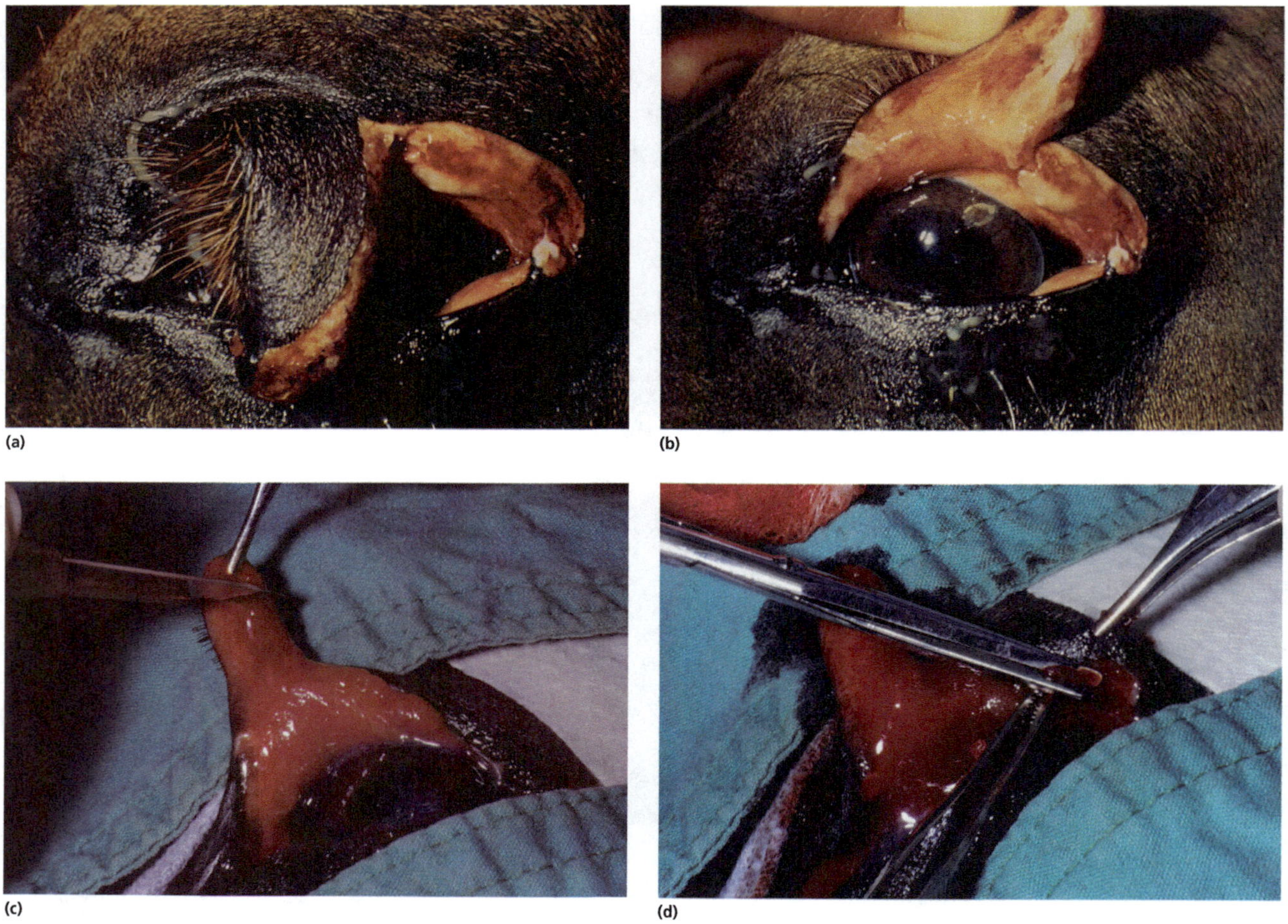

Figure 11.16 **(a)** Acute, full-thickness, oblique laceration of the upper eyelid. **(b)** Lacerated margin is elevated to expose the laceration of the conjunctiva. **(c)** A #11 Bard Parker blade is used to debride the laceration. **(d)** Scissors are used to complete the debridement. Courtesy of Dr. G. Severin.

Eyelid lacerations less than 3 hours old can usually be sutured immediately, as can lacerations 3–12 hours old, provided edema is not excessive and the wound is not severely contaminated. Lacerations more than 12 hours old are treated by delayed primary closure the next day, as described under Treatment. The eye should be examined carefully. A tractable horse with a minor injury may be treated while standing, but anesthetizing the horse is best if the laceration is full thickness or involves the margin of the lid.

Treatment

The hair is clipped, but not shaved, because shaving might create enough irritation to cause swelling. The eyelashes are trimmed with scissors. The skin is prepared using a mild antiseptic solution (0.1–0.2% povidone–iodine is recommended), and the eye is rinsed with a sterile eye wash for surgery.[19,21] The edges of the wound are debrided minimally, removing only tags of obviously dead tissue. Although ophthalmologic instruments are ideal, the eyelid can be repaired with straight and curved mosquito hemostats, Brown Adson thumb tissue forceps, and a #10, #11, or #15 Bard Parker scalpel blade.

Basic principles for surgery of the eyelid include the following:[3–5,19,20] (1) remove as little tissue as possible (Figure 11.16c,d); (2) accurately align and carefully appose the tissues; (3) suture lacerated conjunctiva so that the knots are buried within the tissue and do not rub on the cornea (Figure 11.17a,b).

A support skin suture must sometimes be placed first to align the tissues and reduce tension. To assure correct apposition and restoration of eyelid function, the first skin suture is placed along the sharp edge of the lid through the Meibomian gland and tied so that the knot does not contact the cornea (we recommend 4-0 to 6-0 non-absorbable suture material) (Figure 11.17c,d, Figure 11.18a). The next suture should be placed deeply, 2 mm from the edge of the eyelid, to penetrate the tarsal plate (Figure 11.17g); this suture absorbs most of the tension. Alternatively, tissues at the margin of the eyelid may be apposed using suture inserted in a figure-of-eight pattern (Figure 11.17i). The rest of the closure is routine, using either an interrupted or continuous suture pattern (Figure 11.17j, 11.18b).

To perform delayed primary closure, the laceration and skin are cleaned with dilute povidone–iodine solution (0.1–0.2% is

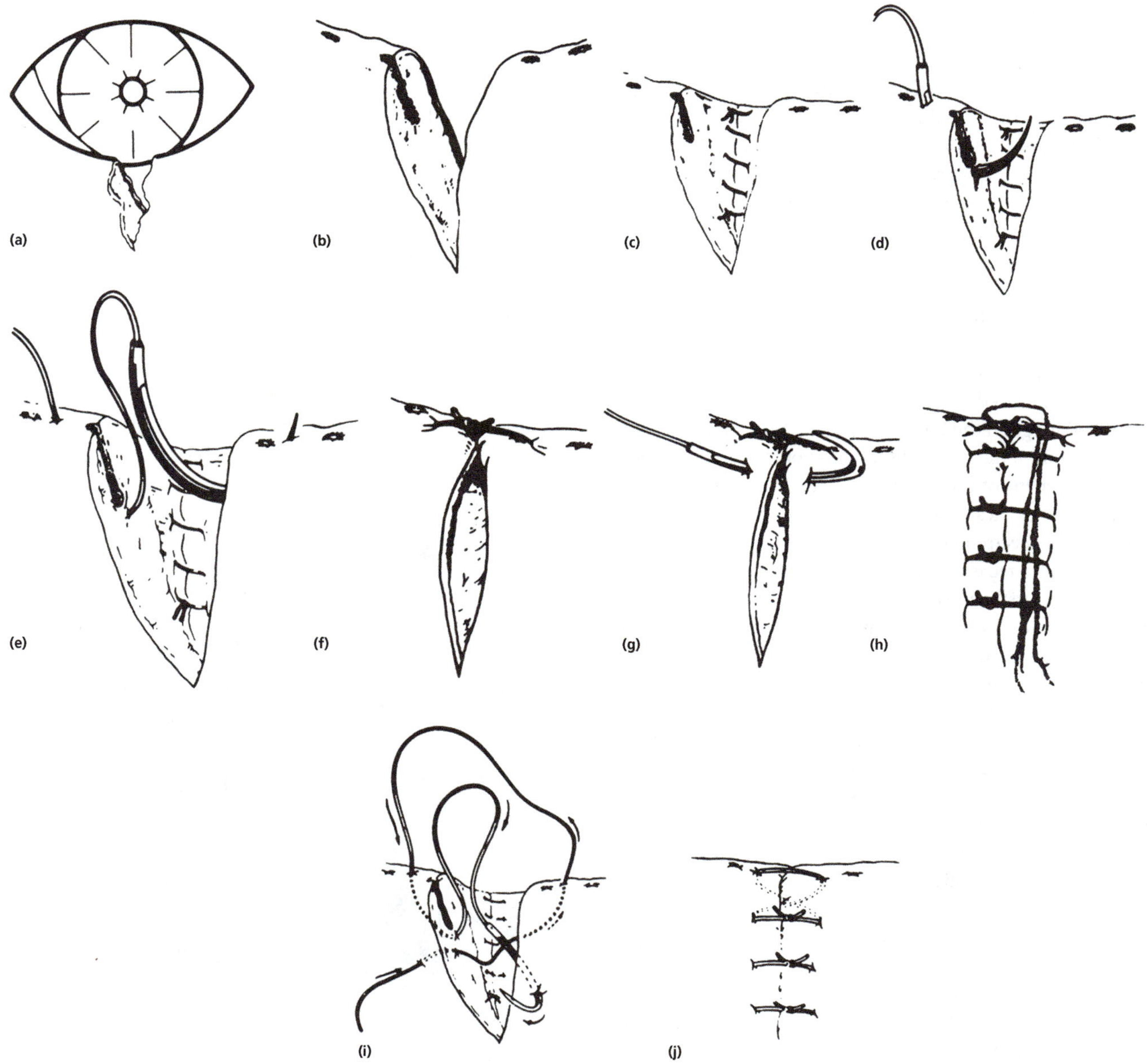

Figure 11.17 Repair of an eyelid laceration. **(a)** Full-thickness lower eyelid laceration. **(b)** Close-up of **(a)**. Dark lines at the eyelid margin illustrate the tarsal plate. **(c)** Continuous sutures are used to appose the conjunctiva. Note that the knots are placed so they are buried in tissue, preventing them from rubbing on the cornea. **(d,e,f)** Suture is placed along the lid margin through the Meibomian glands and tied so the knot does not contact the cornea. **(g)** The second skin suture is placed through the tarsal plate and tied to take up the tension. **(h)** Simple interrupted sutures appose the skin. **(i)** Illustrates a figure-of-eight suture pattern to appose the lid margin and the tarsal plate. **(j)** Simple interrupted suture closure. Courtesy of Dr. G. Severin.

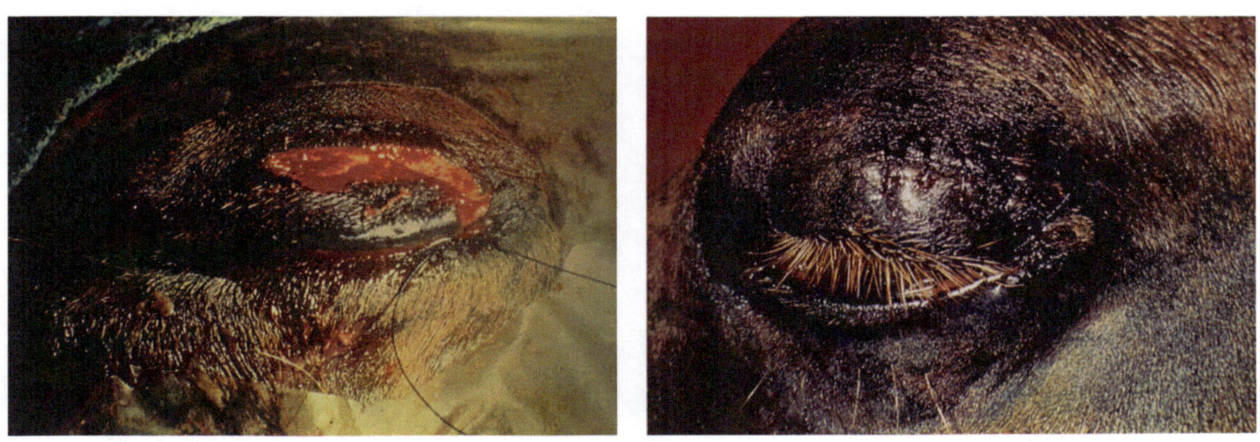

Figure 11.18 Same horse as in Figure 11.16. **(a)** The apex of the laceration was sutured into its normal position to assure good alignment. **(b)** The eyelid 14 days postoperatively. Courtesy of Dr. G. Severin.

recommended). Silver sulfadiazine cream 1% is applied to the laceration liberally, and the laceration and eye are covered by a bandage that encircles the head.[21] Antimicrobial therapy and a NSAID are administered systemically to the horse. This treatment is very effective in reducing edema, and in most cases, the wound can be sutured after 24 hours of treatment, as previously described.

The horse should receive antimicrobial and analgesic therapy, systemically, for 24 hours postoperatively if the wound was fresh when sutured. Antimicrobial therapy should be continued for 5–7 days if the wound was contaminated or infected. A NSAID can be administered for 3–5 days, and administration should be continued longer if the horse displays signs of uveitis. Excessive manipulation of the eyelid should be avoided to reduce the risk of malalignment of the mucocutaneous junction, which could contribute to corneal disease.

Entropion or ectropion may result from a failed or inappropriate repair of a lacerated eyelid. Either condition can result in irritation of the ocular surface and corneal ulceration, and, in an aged horse, chronic irritation can lead to formation of a squamous cell carcinoma or a cataract.[22,23] In one report, entropion and ectropion developed in the same horse. Entropion developed after a repaired lower eyelid laceration dehisced, and an attempt to correct the entropion by removing tissue from the lower eyelid resulted in a cicatrix that, in turn, resulted in ectropion. Because the ectropion was too severe to repair by using a lateral eyelid wedge excision or the V-Y plasty, a modified Kuhnt-Szymanowski procedure was used to correct the ectropion and repair the margin of the eyelid.[22,24]

Applying an antibiotic solution or ointment to the eye is not necessary unless the cornea was injured and/or the wound was infected. If the upper eyelid was sutured, the antibiotic can be instilled beneath the lower eyelid by displacing the lower lid rostrad, or a subpalpebral lavage system can be installed beneath the lower eyelid. If the lower eyelid was sutured, topical medication can be administered by using a subpalpebral lavage system placed beneath the upper eyelid. Bandaging, a fly mask, protective goggles, or cup ("Eye Saver", http://www.naghorseranch.com), and cross-tying may be necessary to protect the wound from trauma produced by rubbing.[4,5,19,20] Skin sutures are removed 14 days after closure. Eyelid lacerations heal well, and success is good if surgical closure is meticulous.

What to do

- Fluorescein stain should always be applied to the cornea to assess its integrity following an eye injury.
- When closing a torn eyelid, first close the subconjunctiva.
- Place the first suture along the lid edges to align the margins of the eyelid to avoid creating a deficit.
- Ensure sutures at the margin of the eyelid do not contact the cornea.

What to avoid

- Avoid excessive manipulation of the eyelid after surgery.

Tip

- Use a subpalpebral lavage system for local delivery of an antibiotic after surgery, if needed.

Ears

Injury to an ear results from freezing, bites, and lacerations.[3–5] Injury caused by freezing or a bite is usually confined to the tip of the ear (Figure 11.19, Figure 11.20), but occasionally, a larger portion of the ear is affected (Figure 11.21a). A lacerated ear, if untreated, may curl or flop over causing it to become unsightly and, in some cases, useless (Figure 11.21a, Figure 11.22).[25,26]

Treatment

General principles in treating an ear laceration include: (1) minimally debriding the soft tissues (Figure 11.23a,b); (2) removing

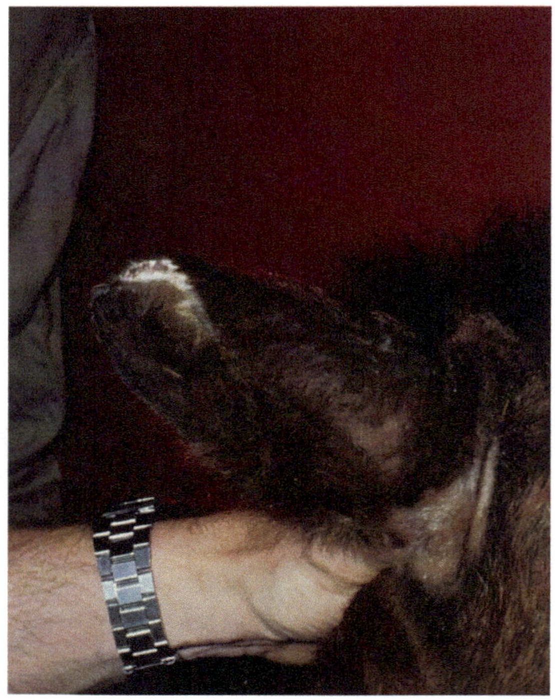

Figure 11.19 The tip of an ear was lost due to frostbite.

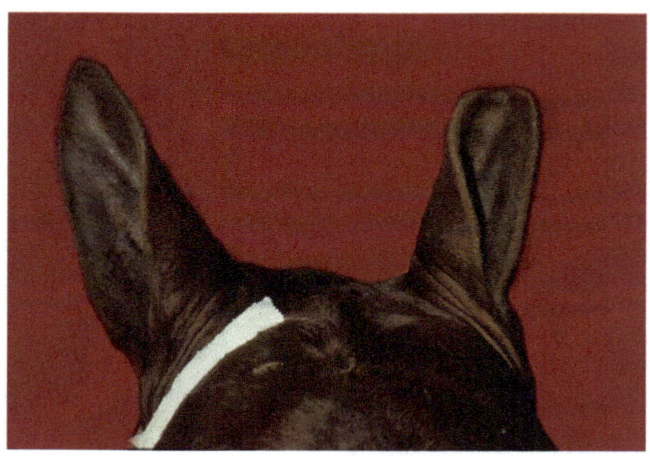

Figure 11.20 The tip of the left ear was bitten off by the dam.

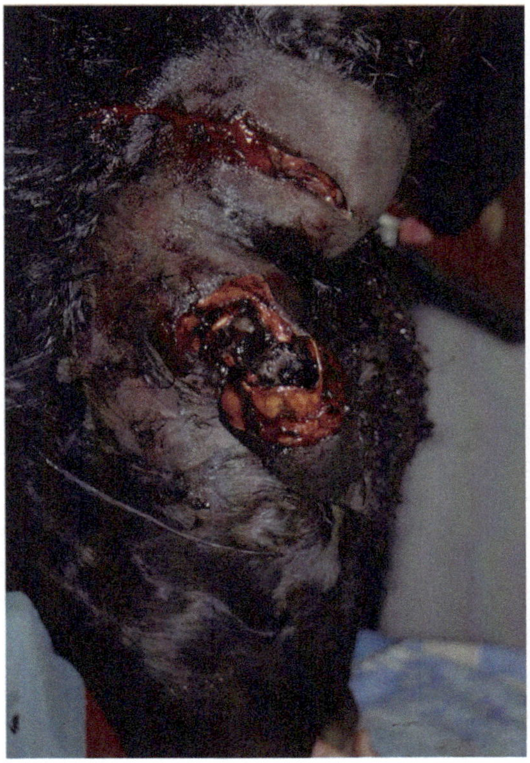

(a)

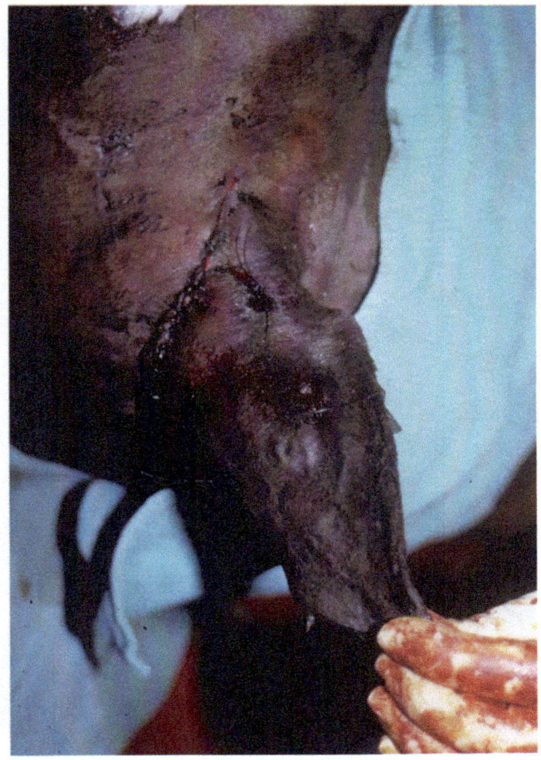

(b)

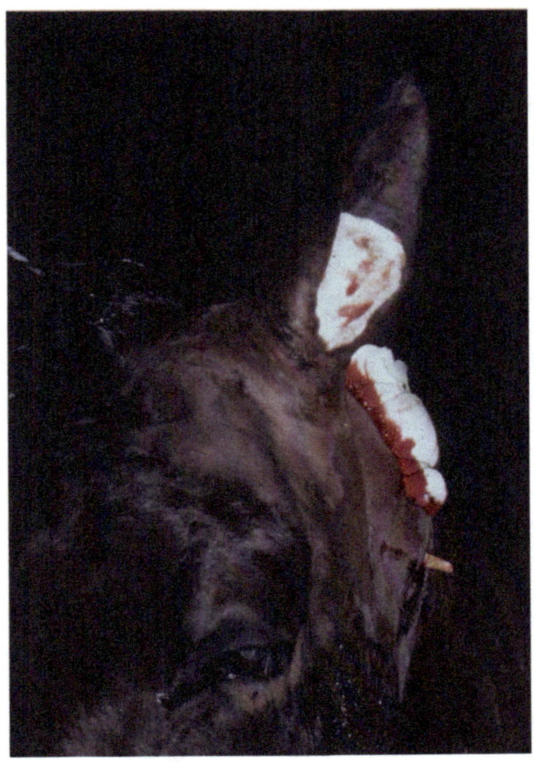

(c)

Figure 11.21 **(a)** The base of the ear was lacerated slightly >50% of its circumference. Bottom center: the ear was flopped forward, and the tip resided above the lateral canthus of the eye. Muscles transected included *parietoauricularis*, *scutuloauricularis superficialis*, and *scutuloauricularis supeficialis accessories*. Another laceration was present caudal (upper center) to the lacerated ear. **(b)** After suturing the muscles, skin at the base of the ear was sutured. **(c)** Rolled gauze was packed into the ear canal and sutured to support the ear in an upright position until healing was complete. A head bandage was applied to encircle the affected ear. The drain was removed within 2 days. The gauze stent was removed from within the ear 4 weeks postoperatively.

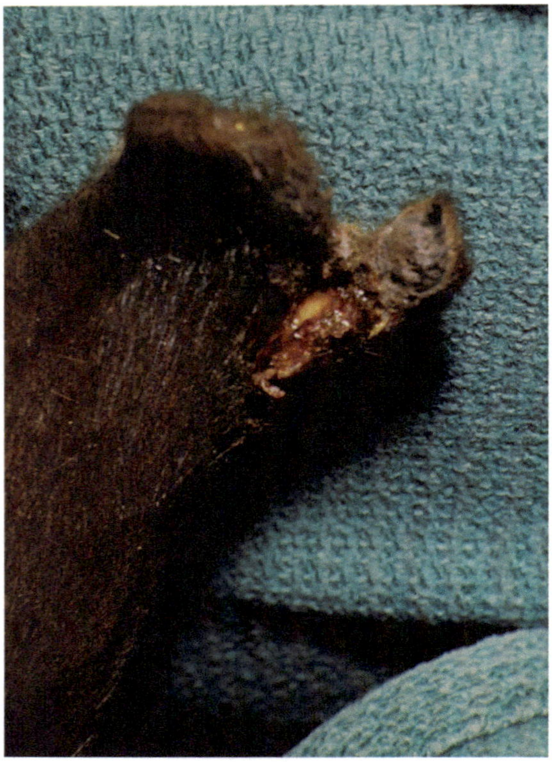

Figure 11.22 A chronic ear laceration. If left untreated, the ear would thicken and curl and have a forked tip. Courtesy of Dr. G.W. Trotter.

a narrow edge of the cartilage on either side of the laceration; (3) suturing only the soft tissues. Cartilage should not be penetrated by suture material (Figure 11.23c,d), except when a stent bandage is applied to the sutured wound. When suturing a stent bandage to the ear, the sutures penetrating the cartilage should be placed far from the wound (Figure 11.23e). If the ear bends, curls, or flops (Figure 11.21a), a support stent made of X-ray film, rolled gauze, or thermoplastic material can be applied to the inside of the ear after the wound is repaired (Figure 11.21c, Figure 11.23e).[26,27] The stent can be left in place for up to 4 weeks, if necessary, to provide time for the cartilage to heal sufficiently to hold the ear in an upright position.[3–5,24]

Owners occasionally request cosmetic reconstruction of the tip of the ear after injury caused by a bite or freezing. The ear should be completely healed before attempting reconstruction so that inflammation and infection do not interfere with healing of the surgical repair (Figure 11.19, Figure 11.20).[3–5] If only one ear is involved, the other ear serves as a template for reconstruction of the damaged ear. The normal ear is laid flat, and its contour is traced on to sterile paper or sterile X-ray film. The silhouette of the normal ear is reversed and applied to the damaged ear.

Because the affected ear is shorter than normal, the length of the template must be adjusted appropriately. To do this, the length of the affected ear is measured from its base to its tip. The template is then cut to that length by trimming the base portion of the template, and the shortened silhouette of the normal ear is drawn on to the damaged ear, using a sterile marker or sterile methylene blue, with the silhouette reversed (Figure 11.24a). The same shortened silhouette is drawn on to the normal ear, but the silhouette is not reversed. If the symmetry appears satisfactory, the ears are trimmed following the marking (Figure 11.24b).

The thumb and forefinger are used to tighten the skin by pulling it toward the side of the ear opposite that being cut. This not only facilitates cutting because the ear is held rigid, but it also ensures that enough skin is available to cover the exposed cartilage. Sharp Mayo scissors are used to trim skin and cartilage. Trimming all layers at once with the scissors reduces hemorrhage and prevents the skin edge from retracting from the cartilage. When trimming the other side of the ear, the skin is pulled in the opposite direction. The two skin surfaces are then apposed, in close approximation, with a continuous suture pattern using 3-0 synthetic monofilament non-absorbable suture (Figure 11.24c,d).

Postoperative management is as described previously for lacerations of the ear and includes administration of antimicrobial therapy and a NSAID. The horse may require tranquilization or cross-tying to prevent rubbing. Sutured injuries of the ear heal well, and generally, the cosmetic result is good. Nevertheless, it is a challenge to make an ear, deformed by freezing, look normal.

What to avoid

- Avoid removing too much tissue during debridement to avoid creating a noticeable defect.
- Avoid gapping between sutures.
- Avoid inserting sutures through the cartilage, if possible, except when applying a support stent to prevent the ear from curling.

Scalping and degloving injuries of the head

Forehead

V-shaped "scalping" injuries are one of the most common types of laceration seen on the head. They are often on the forehead overlying the neurocranium (Figure 11.25a, Figure 11.26a) and most often occur when the horse throws its head while being handled, causing contact with an overhead roof, archway, or gate.[3–5] The flap, typically restricted to the skin and subcutaneous tissue, usually has a broad base. The apex of the V-shaped flap may point caudad or rostrad. The periosteum of the frontal or nasal bones may also be exposed or lacerated and attached to the flap (Figure 11.25, Figure 11.26). Movement of the head causes repeated displacement of the flap, and the tip may curl under, exposing the surface of the wound. The skin is usually minimally retracted, allowing the skin edges to be easily apposed.

Treatment

Acute scalping wounds are generally minimally contaminated and can usually be sutured with the horse sedated. The wound is prepared for surgery in a routine fashion following the principles outlined in Chapter 4.

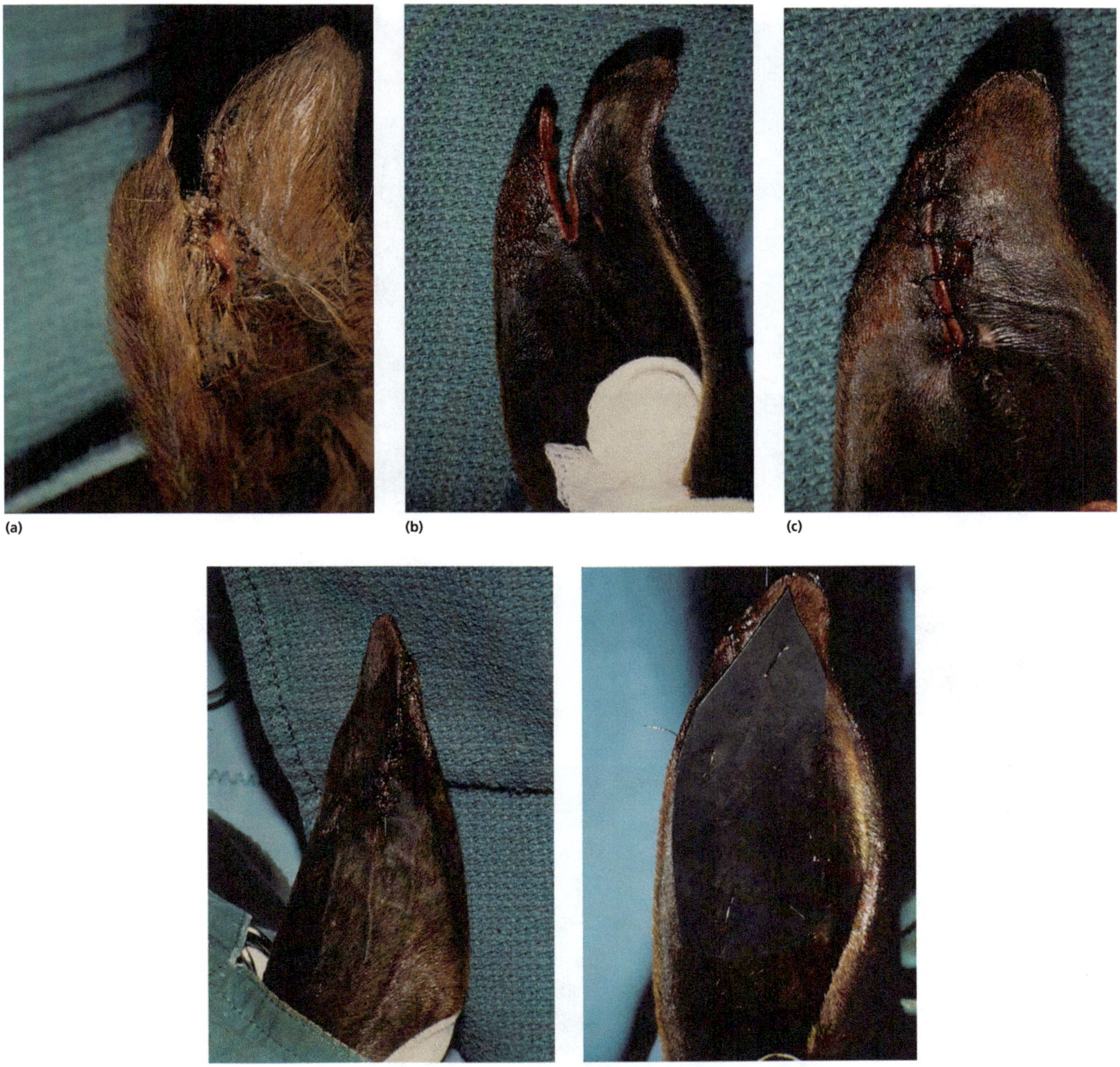

Figure 11.23 Same case as Figure 11.22. **(a)** Laceration of the ear, cranial view. **(b)** After clipping and antiseptic preparation, the laceration (skin and cartilage) was debrided. The ear canal was packed with sterile gauze. **(c)** The skin on the concave surface of the ear was apposed with 3-0 nylon placed in a simple interrupted suture pattern. Cartilage was not included in the suture. **(d)** The skin on the convex surface of the ear was apposed with 3-0 nylon in a simple interrupted suture pattern. Cartilage was not included in the suture. **(e)** Widely placed, through-and-through 2-0 nylon sutures were used to hold a piece of X-ray film on the concave surface of the ear to hold it in an upright position. Courtesy of Dr. G.W. Trotter.

Lifting (or elevation) of periosteum from the underlying bone creates conditions conducive to the formation of a bone sequestrum. This is because periosteum supplies blood to and forms a protective barrier over cortical bone. Its elevation may, therefore, cause ischemia within the underlying external cortex and may allow entry of bacteria into the cortex via the Volkmann canals.[3–5,28,29]

The authors believe curettage to be ineffective at removing bacteria from the irregular bone surface and recommend irrigation (at 15 psi) or "partial decortication" — the removal of the outer ischemic and contaminated cortex with a pneumatic-driven burr or a hip arthroplasty rasp. If the wound is acute, irrigation is likely adequate, but partial decortication is preferred when the bone is grossly contaminated or when it is discolored or has a chalky appearance (Figure 11.27a). Only a fine layer can be removed because these flat bones are very thin (Figure 11.27b). The decorticated cortical surface is irrigated with isotonic saline solution applied at 10–15 psi and covered with viable tissue (e.g., muscle, subcutaneous tissue, or skin) to prevent the formation of a sequestrum (Figure 11.27c).

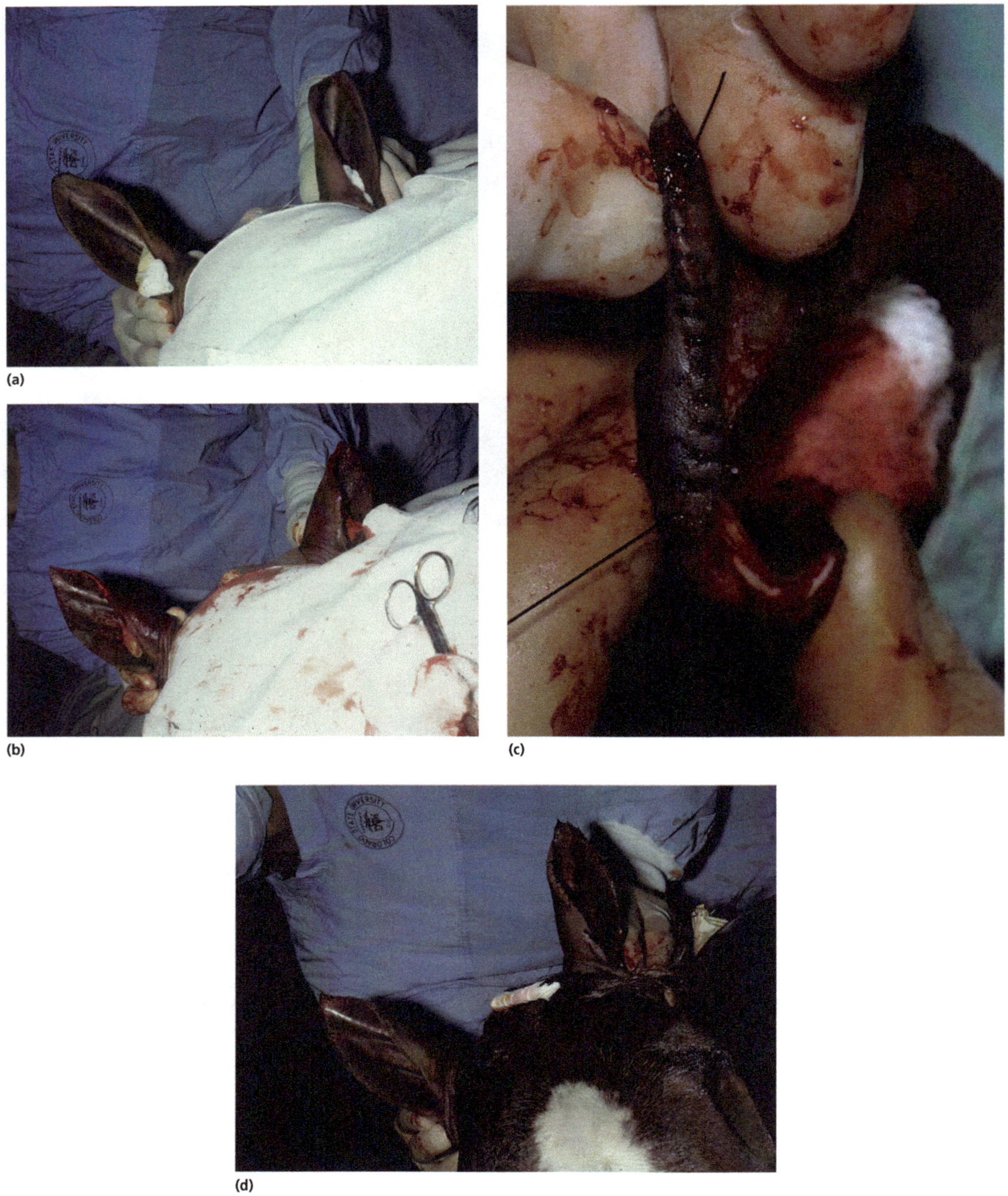

Figure 11.24 Same horse as in Figure 11.20. **(a)** Sterile methylene blue was used to draw the contour on the concave surface of the ear to adjust the height of the affected ear. **(b)** Both ears were trimmed and rechecked for symmetry. **(c)** The ear was sutured so that the skin completely covered the cartilage. The suture bites were placed close enough together so that the subcutaneous tissue was completely covered. **(d)** Suturing complete.

In some cases there is insufficient subcutaneous tissue to be closed as a separate layer. With acute flaps, the skin edges can usually be easily apposed with synthetic non-absorbable suture material (e.g., 2-0 nylon, polypropylene, or polybutester) placed in a simple interrupted pattern. If tension arising from closure is excessive, the skin edges are undermined using scissors, and the skin is apposed using a near–far suture pattern. Cosmetic repair is best achieved by placing the first suture in the tip of the flap after it is pulled into the point of the V. Sutures are then placed in the arms of the V, which often are different in length. Dead space is minimal, and a drain is rarely necessary.

A horse with a chronic scalping wound often must be anesthetized for treatment because chronic wounds are inevitably desiccated and contaminated, and the flaps are often folded and fibrotic. Extensive debridement, partial decortication, and irrigation are often required before the wound can be sutured. Closing the skin may be challenging because both the flap and surrounding skin

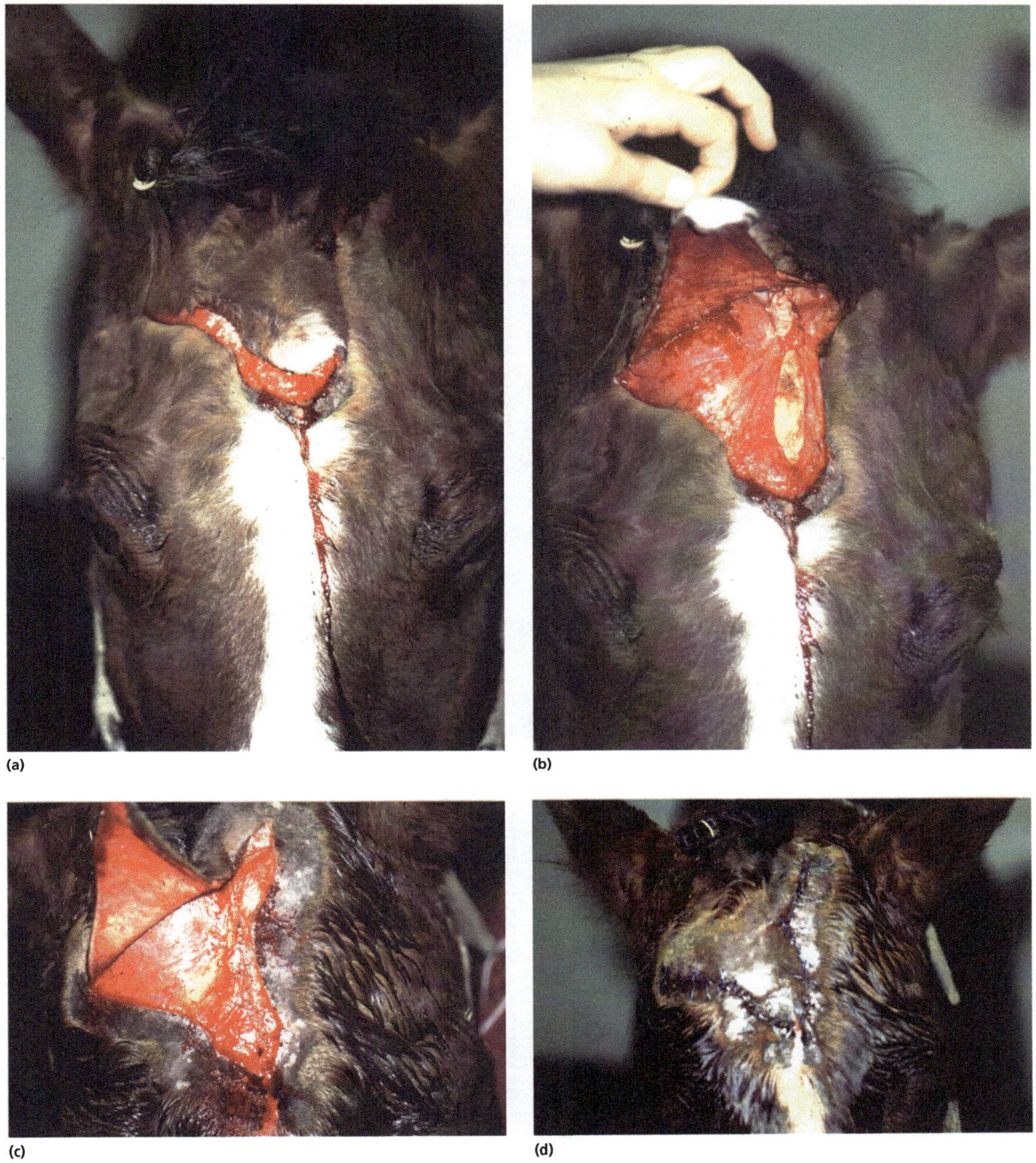

Figure 11.25 **(a)** Acute scalping injury from a trailer loading accident. Note that the skin flap was only slightly retracted from its normal position. **(b)** The wound was fresh (<3 hours) and minimally contaminated, but the periosteum was lacerated, and a portion of the frontal bone was exposed. **(c)** After irrigation of the bone surface, the periosteum was closed over the bone. (d) The wound was closed by suturing the flap with an interrupted suture pattern placed without excessive tension. A drain was not needed.

become less extensible with time. A 2–3-mm strip of skin should be removed from the wound's edges to expose viable tissue prior to closure. Subcutaneous tissue can be extensively dissected to relieve tension while ensuring that it is elevated along with the skin and that major vital structures are avoided. Tension, if excessive, can be relieved by mesh expansion of the surrounding skin edges (preferred) or by the development of a skin flap.[3–5,7,8] If a portion of the skin flap has been lost, the defect may be closed by using a transposition flap or a single or bi-pedicle advancement flap.[1,3–5,8] The latter type of flap exposes subcutaneous tissue adjacent to the wound, but this

What to do

- Exposed bone should be covered with viable tissue, if possible.

Tips

- Proper debridement of exposed cortical bone is as important as that of the soft tissues.
- Partial decortication of the bone is especially indicated if exposed bone appears chalky or discolored.
- The first suture should be placed through the tip of the flap after it is pulled into the apex of the V.

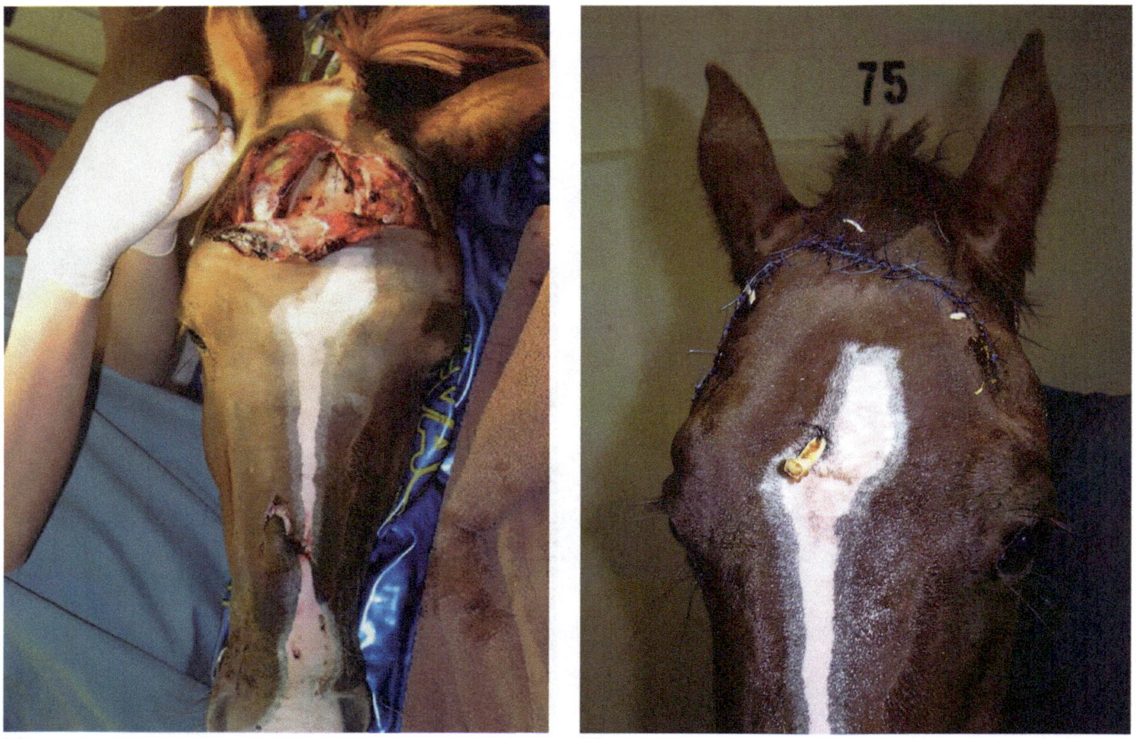

(a) (b)

Figure 11.26 (**a**) Large scalping injury in a foal. The periosteum was elevated with the skin flap, but the temporal muscles were intact. After irrigation and partial decortication of the bone surface, a Penrose drain was placed deep within the wound to drain the dead space underlying the base of the flap. (**b**) Because there was some tension after closure, a few sutures, placed in a near-and-far pattern, were used along with the simple interrupted suture pattern.

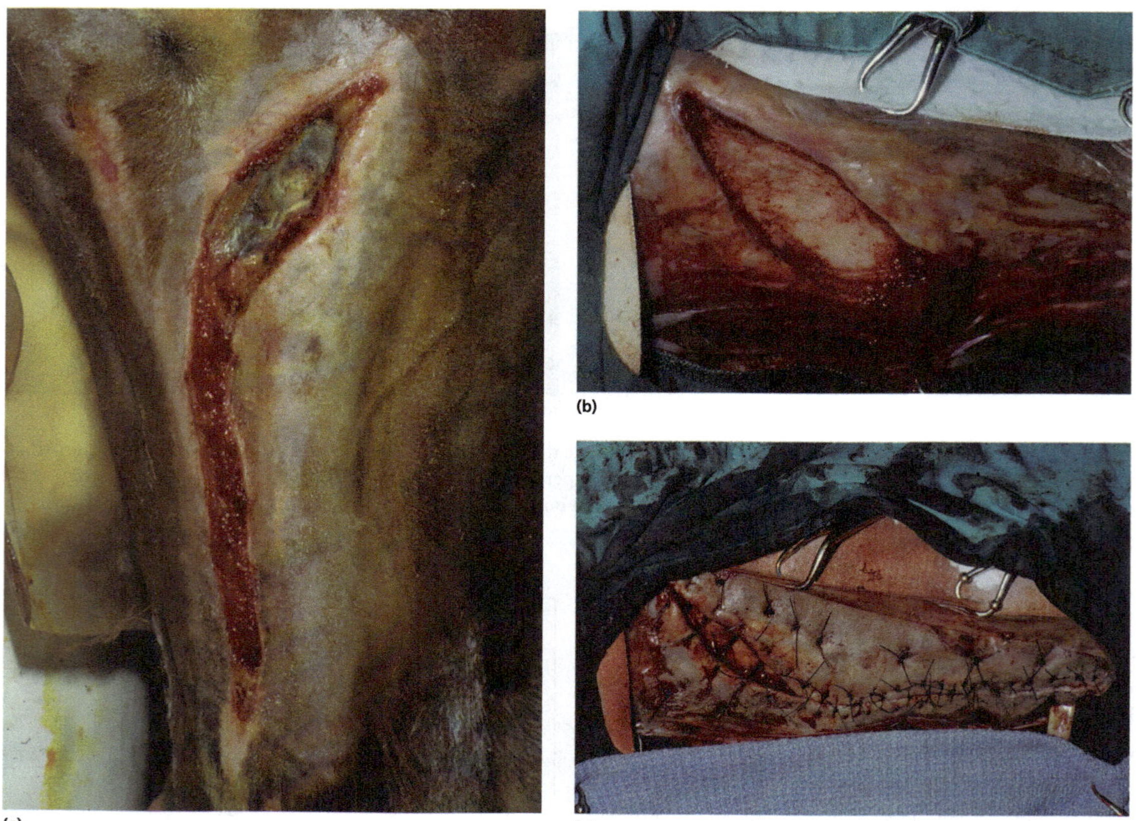

(a) (b) (c)

Figure 11.27 (**a**) Four-day-old scalping injury to the face with exposed, discolored bone. (**b**) Forehead to the left. The wound, after debridement of the soft tissues and partial decortication of the discolored bone using a hip arthroplasty rasp. After debridement, the wound edges were undermined and mobilized to reduce skin tension for wound closure. (**c**) The skin was apposed using a combination of vertical mattress and simple interrupted suture patterns. Alternatively, a near-and-far suture pattern could have been used. Only a narrow strip of the facial bone remained exposed. The region of exposed bone healed uneventfully by second intention.

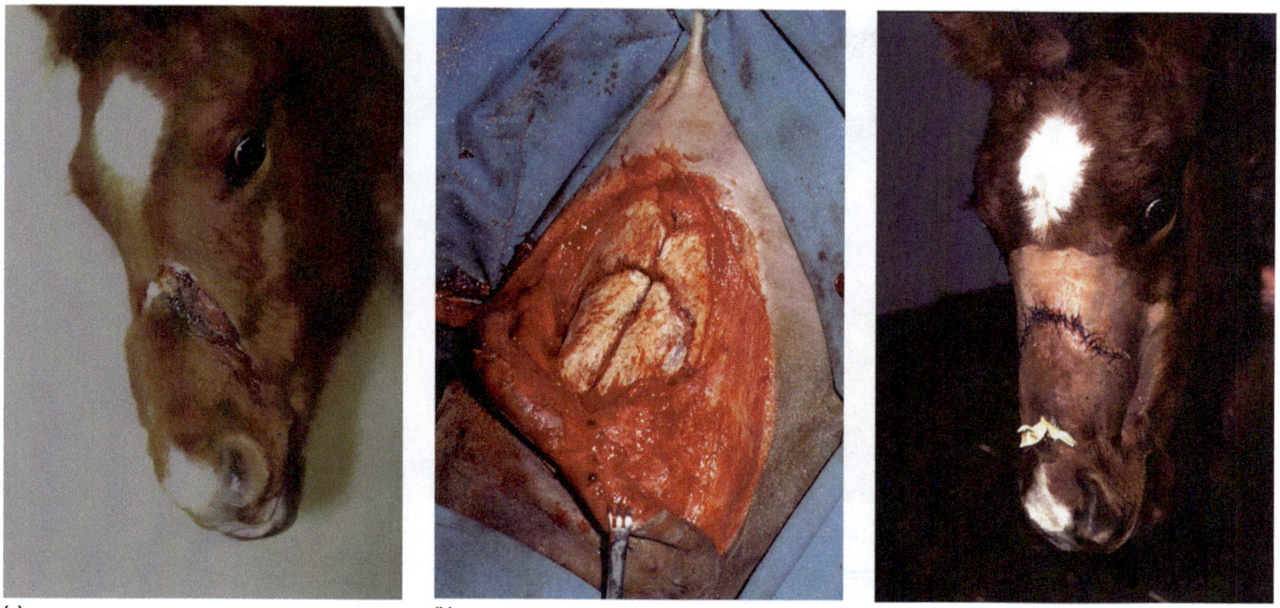

(a) (b) (c)

Figure 11.28 Typical degloving laceration of the face. **(a)** The laceration was fairly large and had a rostral base, and the flap was retracted to expose the nasal bones. The wound was less than 12 hours old. **(b)** Wound after debridement. Periosteum was lost from the nasal bones, which nonetheless looked healthy after partial decortication. There was a non-displaced fracture of both nasal bones, which was stabilized with suture material placed through holes drilled in the nasal and adjacent frontal bones. **(c)** Soft tissue was closed over the exposed fracture site in two layers. Penrose drains were inserted to provide ventral drainage.

is preferable to leaving cortical bone uncovered.[3–5] See Chapter 10 for more information regarding techniques to relieve tension.

Nasal region

Degloving injuries that expose bone, are very similar to "scalping" injuries and occur on the dorsal rostral portion of the face or caudal to the lower lip (Figure 11.28, Figure 11.29). When the dorsal surface of the face is involved, the apex of the V-shaped laceration usually points caudad, and the skin and subcutaneous tissue are reflected. This exposes the nasal bones, which may be stripped of their periosteum or even fractured.

Treatment

The comments regarding debridement and closure of scalping injuries apply to degloving injuries of the nasal region. If the nasal bones are fractured and displaced, however, the fracture must be reduced to achieve a cosmetic repair and to prevent impairment of airflow through the nasal cavity. The fragments should be levered or elevated into position using a bone hook, and the nasal septum examined and repositioned, if necessary. Fractured nasal bones commonly separate from the nasal septum without damaging it. When the fragments of nasal bone are unstable they can be secured with stainless steel wire or other suture material placed through holes drilled in the bone. Dry, dirty, or discolored bone should be decorticated, irrigated, and, if possible, covered with soft tissue. If a small fragment is lost, the soft tissue can usually be closed over the osseous defect without loss of function. Penrose drains are often placed deep in the wound to allow drainage of the dead space present beneath the rostral extent of the skin flap. Even dirty wounds with unstable fragments heal well after liberal debridement, stabilization of fragments, and closure of the wound.

What to do

- Cover exposed bone with viable soft tissue.
- Stabilize unstable fracture fragments.

Lower lip

Degloving injury to the lower lip with displacement of the tissue from the rostral extent of the mandible can occur from forceful contact of the lower lip and chin with the ground. The injury results in a "flail" lower lip, difficultly eating, and an unsightly blemish (Figure 11.29).[3–5]

Treatment

Reconstruction usually involves drilling holes in the rostral extent of the mandible, while avoiding the roots of the incisors, for placement of a single row of through-and-through, modified tension sutures of size 2 monofilament non-absorbable suture material (Figure 11.29b). One arm of the suture extends from the skin, through the predrilled hole in bone, into the oral cavity, and from the oral cavity, through another predrilled hole in bone and exits the skin to create a mattress suture (Figure 11.29b). A Penrose drain, exiting ventrally, should be placed to drain the large dead space beneath the avulsed flap (Figure 11.29b). The tension sutures (quill sutures) are preplaced in a rostral-to-caudal direction to assure accurate approximation of the edges of the mucosa. After all the sutures are placed, they are tied over segments of Penrose drain to stabilize the lip flap. A single row of the modified sutures is usually all that is needed, but if the lip appears unstable, more rows of tension sutures can be added. The mucosa is apposed with 2-0

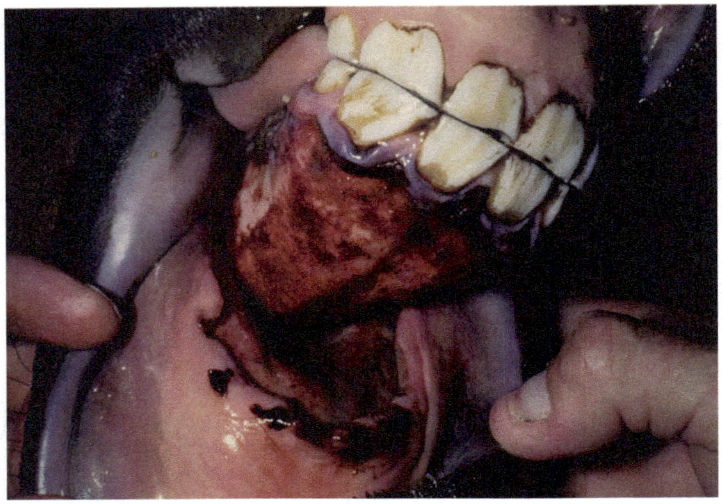

(a)

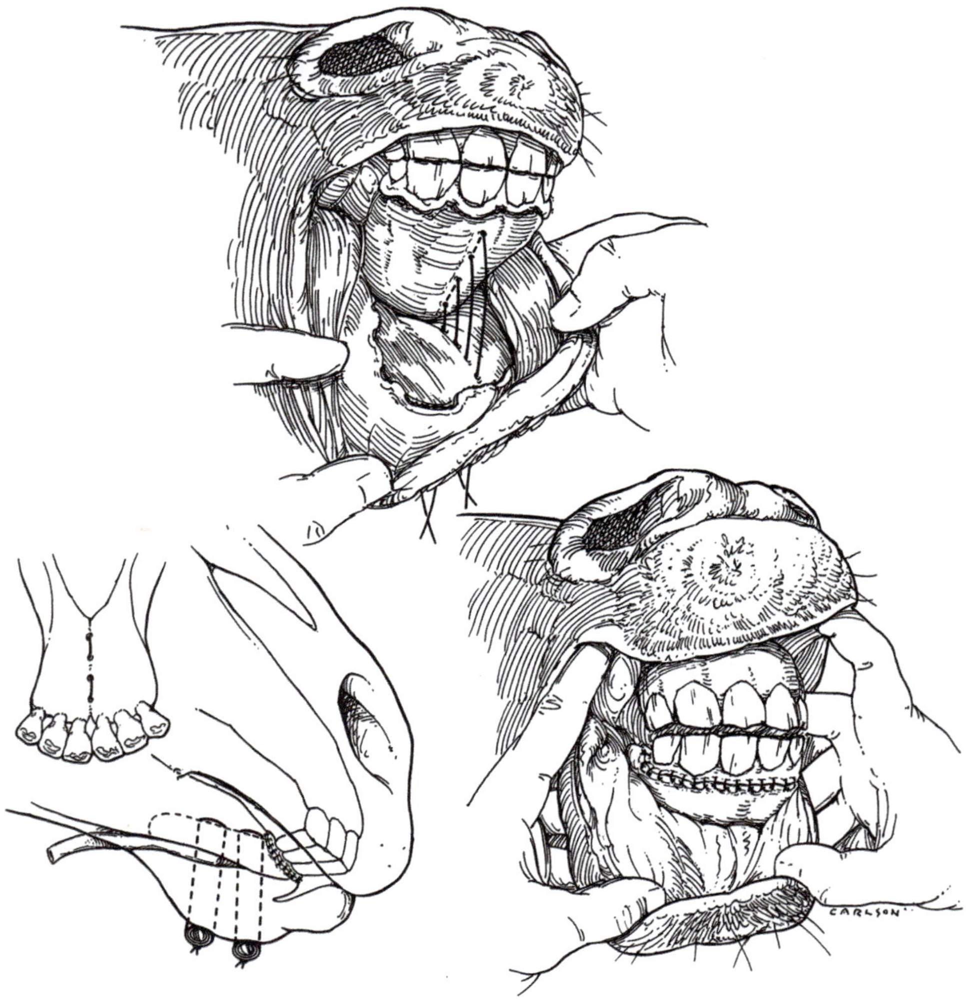

(b)

Figure 11.29 (a) Degloving injury of the lower lip exposing the rostral extent of the mandible. (b) Top: illustration of the degloving injury; holes have been drilled through the rostral extent of the mandible, and nylon sutures have been inserted through the holes; bottom left: placement of the mattress sutures as quills (i.e. over stents) and insertion of the Penrose drain; the oral mucosa has been sutured; bottom right: frontal view illustrating sutures in the oral mucosa.

synthetic absorbable suture material placed a simple interrupted pattern (Figure 11.29b). Sometimes the mucosa of the flap must be undermined to free it sufficiently for suturing. Although the mucosa may partially dehisce, healing usually occurs without major complications.

Postoperatively, the horse is fed a moist gruel, the mouth is lavaged between feedings, and a muzzle is applied. The Penrose drain is removed when discharge is minimal, usually within 2 days. Antibiotic therapy is continued for 5–7 days, and a NSAID is administered, as needed. The modified quill sutures are removed in 7–10 days, and complete healing occurs in 15–21 days. Proper positioning and securing of the flap and prevention of rubbing in the postoperative period are imperative, and, if achieved, the result is good.

Tips

- Ensure accurate placement of the tension (quill) sutures through the avulsed lip so that, when tightened, the mucosal edges are in close enough approximation that they can be sutured.
- Place additional tension sutures to obliterate the dead space beneath the flap.
- Lavaging the oral cavity between feedings and the application of a muzzle are important.

Ear

Degloving injuries to the ear are uncommon but usually involve the convex surface and expose auricular cartilage (Figure 11.30a). This type of injury is seen most commonly in young horses and is usually the result of a bite. If left to heal by second intention, the ear curls as the healing wound contracts.

Treatment

In the authors' opinion, skin grafting is the best option for treatment. If cartilage is exposed, the ear is bandaged until a layer of healthy granulation tissue covers it (Figure 11.30a), but the ear can be grafted immediately if subcutaneous tissue covers the cartilage. A full-thickness graft, meshed or unmeshed, is preferred (see Chapter 18 for more information about skin grafts) because it is better at preventing secondary graft contraction and is less susceptible to tissue mismatch than a split-thickness graft.[30] A template of the auricular skin defect can be obtained at surgery by using sterile X-ray film or paper (Figure 11.30b). This template is used to harvest a section of skin that approximates the dimensions of the wound. The pectoral region is a common site used to harvest a full-thickness graft. The graft is held in place with the least number of sutures possible (Figure 11.30c).

Bandaging of the grafted ear is important. The graft is covered with a non-adherent dressing, and the ear splinted to prevent curling. A non-adherent, semi-occlusive dressing, or one that has its contact layer lightly coated with an ointment, suffices as the primary dressing. The ear is bandaged and splinted with conforming gauze after applying rolled gauze to the concave surface of the ear and into the ear canal. The conforming gauze and dressing are secured with elastic self-adhesive tape applied around the ear with minimal circumferential pressure to prevent ischemia of the graft. The throat latch region is incorporated

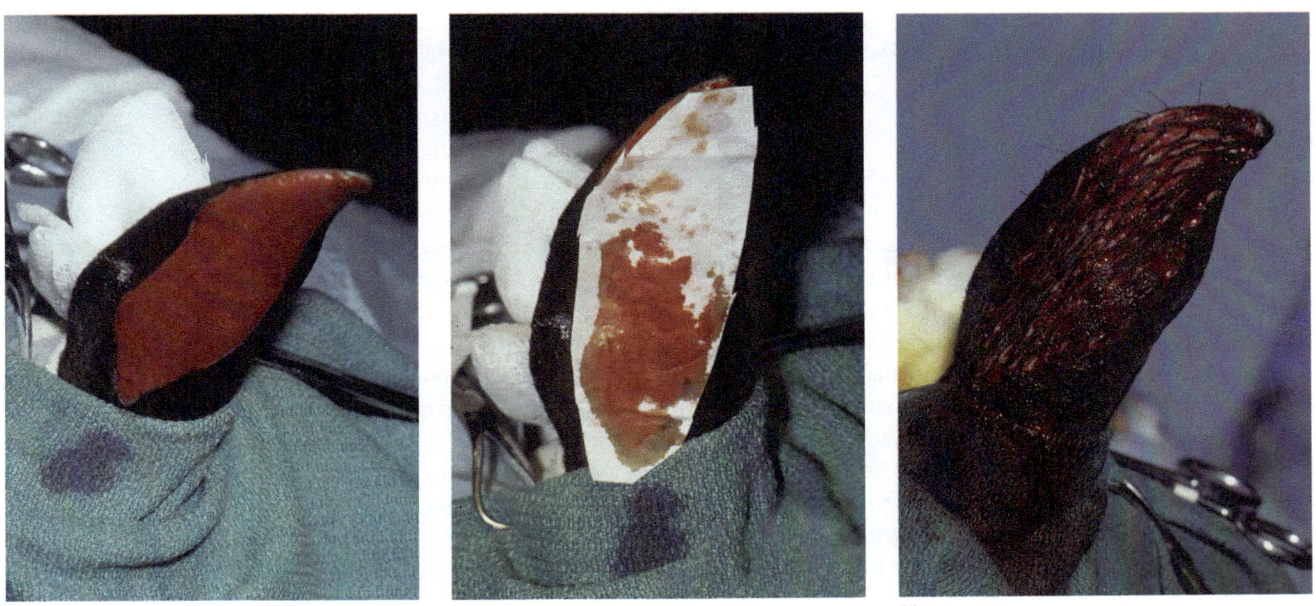

(a) (b) (c)

Figure 11.30 Avulsion injury to the ear of a foal caused by a bite from the dam 4 days earlier. The ear had been bandaged after the injury. **(a)** At surgery; note the healthy bed of granulation tissue which will facilitate graft acceptance. **(b)** A template using surgical glove paper is made to document the dimensions of the degloving defect so a piece of skin of appropriate size may be harvested from the pectoral region for grafting. **(c)** The full-thickness meshed skin graft is held in place with as few sutures as possible. The referring veterinarian reported that the graft was completely accepted and that the ear healed without a tendency to curl.

into the bandage to prevent the elastic adhesive tape from slipping. This bandage is usually left in place for 5–7 days.

Antimicrobial therapy is continued for 24 hours, and a NSAID is administered for 5–7 days. Tranquilization and cross-tying (provided the horse is adult) help prevent the horse from rubbing its grafted ear. Sutures are removed at 10–12 days, bandaging is continued for at least 3 weeks, and the graft protected from direct sunlight for at least 2 months.

A good cosmetic outcome is expected if the wound is grafted before the ear curls and scarring occurs, and, of course, if the skin graft is accepted. Some blemish should nevertheless be expected.

What to avoid

- Bandaging a skin-grafted ear too tightly causes ischemia of the graft.
- The horse must not be allowed to rub its grafted ear.

What to do

- Incorporate the throat latch region into the bandage to prevent the elastic self-adhesive wrap around the ear from slipping.

Tip

- Intimate contact of the graft with the granulation bed is imperative.

Fractures of the facial bones

The facial bones are commonly fractured by external trauma – occasionally from the horse impacting a solid stationary object but usually from a blow, such as a kick. Because of the complex anatomy of the head, clinical signs vary, and treatment is challenging.[3–5,28,29]

Anatomic considerations

The bones most commonly fractured are the nasal, maxillary, lacrimal, frontal, and zygomatic (malar) (Figure 11.31).[3–5] These flat, relatively thin bones form the external limits of the nasal cavities and paranasal sinuses, and because they are sparsely covered with muscle, they are vulnerable to trauma.

The nasal bones cover the nasal cavities, whereas the frontal bones overlie the frontal sinus. The bones that form the external wall of the maxillary sinuses are the maxillary, lacrimal, and zygomatic bones. The limits of the maxillary sinus are important clinically (Figure 11.31); they are the orbital rim caudally, the facial crest laterally, an imaginary line from the infraorbital foramen to the facial crest rostrally, and an imaginary line from the infraorbital foramen to the medial canthus of the eye dorsally. The location of the maxillary septum, which divides the rostral and caudal maxillary sinuses, varies and the septum is often incomplete. The maxillary sinuses drain into the middle meatus of the nasal cavity through a slit-like opening, the nasomaxillary aperture. The frontal sinus does not drain directly into the nasal cavity; rather it drains via the frontomaxillary aperture into the caudal maxillary sinus.[28] The lacrimal and zygomatic bones form a large portion of the medial surface of the orbital rim. The lacrimal bone contains the fossa for the lacrimal sac, and the nasolacrimal duct traverses the maxillary and lacrimal bones in a direction parallel to the facial crest and slightly dorsal to the infraorbital foramen.[28]

Flat bones

A blow to the face may produce a complete fracture, with complete separation of a fragment from the parent bone, or an incomplete fracture, that leaves the fragment attached, along one of its sides, to the parent bone. An incomplete fracture is depressed into the nasal cavity or paranasal sinuses and is stable, whereas a complete fracture produces depressed, unstable fragments. Often a combination of complete and incomplete fracture fragments is present.[3–5] The flat bones of the skull are formed by intramembranous ossification, and, therefore, have a greater blood supply than other bones of the skeleton.[28] This may explain the clinical impression that the flat bones of the skull heal more rapidly than do other bones.

The clinical signs displayed by a horse with a facial fracture depend on the location, severity, and cause of the injury. Injuries caused by sharp objects lacerate the skin and expose bone (Figure 11.32). The presence of a fracture (or fractures) and involvement of the nasal cavity or the paranasal sinuses in the injury can usually be determined by digital and visual examination, but this approach seldom defines the full extent of damage.

Most commonly, the injury is caused by a blunt object, and the skin is intact (Figure 11.33).[3–5] Facial asymmetry is obvious if the injury is chronic, especially if the fragments are depressed into the nasal cavity or sinuses, but if the injury is acute, soft tissue swelling may obscure this sign.[3–5,29] Crepitus can sometimes be detected if the fracture is acute, comminuted, and unstable. Tenderness, unfortunately, makes a thorough digital examination difficult, even when the horse is sedated.[3–5]

Epistaxis is common and indicates that the mucosa of the nasal cavity or paranasal sinuses has been damaged.[3–5] Bilateral epistaxis indicates bleeding has occurred into both nasal cavities or both paranasal sinuses or that the nasal septum has been damaged. Dyspnea is uncommon but indicates bilateral nasal obstruction from fracture of the nasal bones or nasal septum. Subcutaneous emphysema is uncommon but may occur when a bony fragment penetrates the airway.

An orbital rim fracture, especially one involving the maxillary, zygomatic, or lacrimal bone, causes abnormal shape and function of the orbital structures.[3–5] Depressed fragments can impinge on the globe or its muscles and prevent the eye from moving normally within its orbit when the head is moved (i.e., an "entrapped eye"). The fracture may cause the eye to protrude, and swelling of the eyelids may prevent their closure (Figure 11.34).[3–5,31] Transection of the nasolacrimal duct may not be readily apparent because lacrimal secretions are discharged into the open wound. The transected duct may become stenotic causing chronic epiphora as the injury heals.[3–5,32]

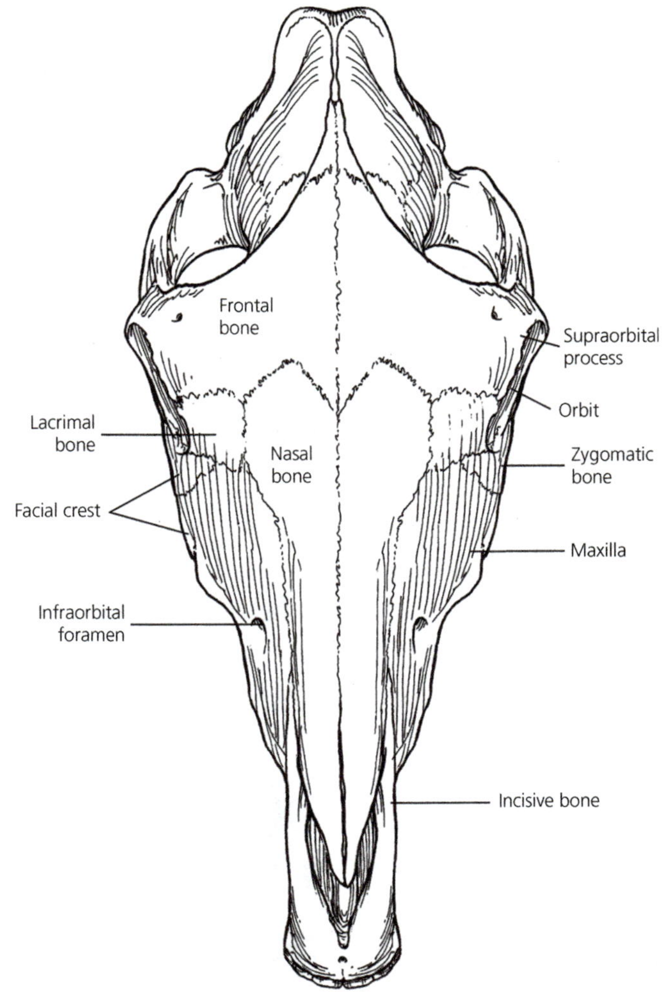

(a)

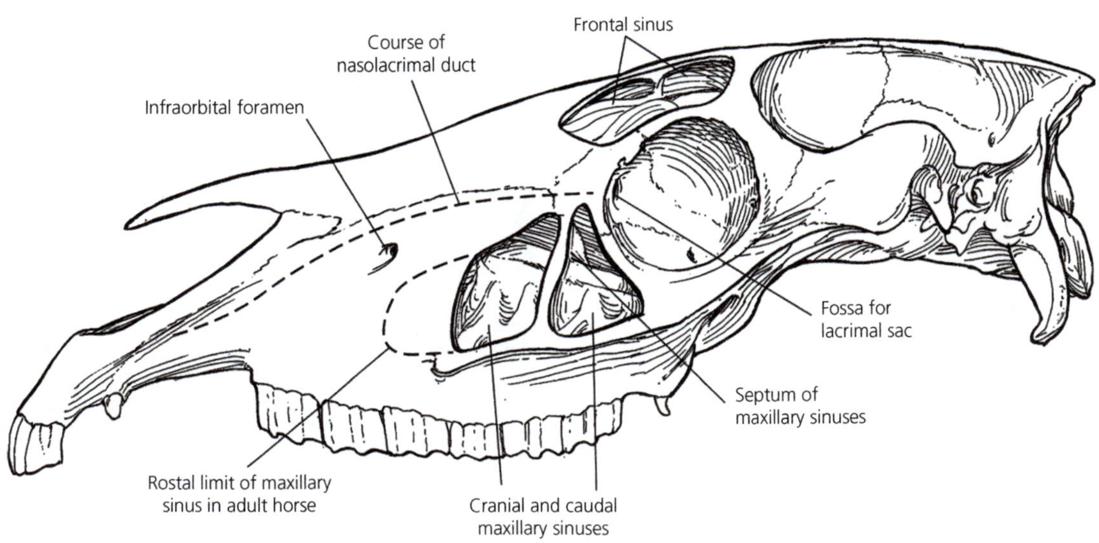

(b)

Figure 11.31 (**a**) Dorsal view of a horse skull showing the bones of the face that commonly are fractured by facial trauma. (**b**) Lateral view of the skull with portions of the facial bones removed to demonstrate the location of the sinuses. Note the location of the rostral limit of the maxillary sinuses and the location of the nasolacrimal duct.

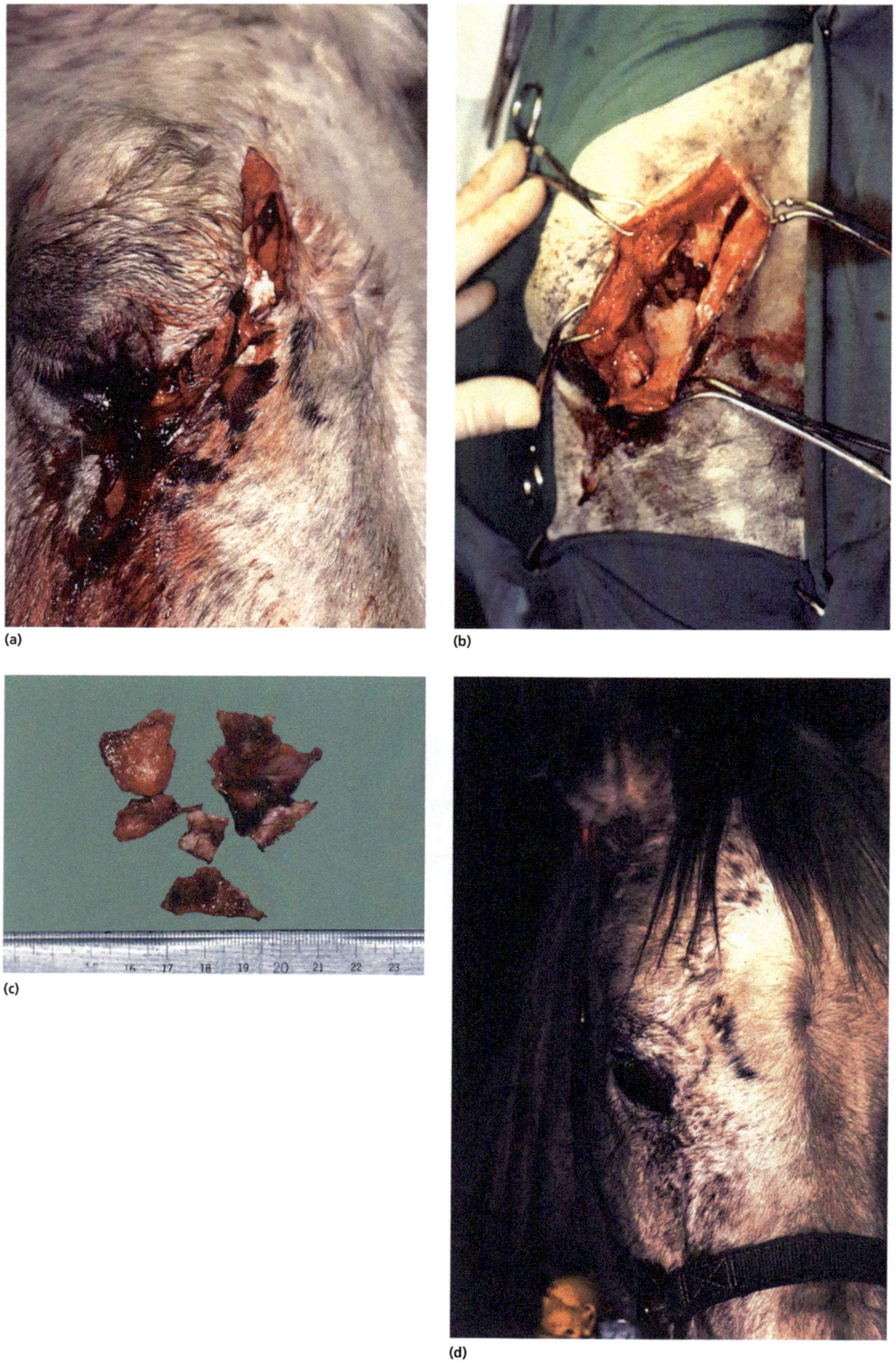

Figure 11.32 (**a**) This horse impaled its head on a metal bolt, lacerating the skin and fracturing the frontal and lacrimal bones over the frontal sinus. (**b**) The laceration, when slightly enlarged, gave excellent exposure for surgical manipulations. The supraorbital process required stabilization with wire sutures. (**c**) Several small fragments of loose bone were removed, and the defect was covered with soft tissue. (**d**) Excellent appearance 13 weeks postoperatively.

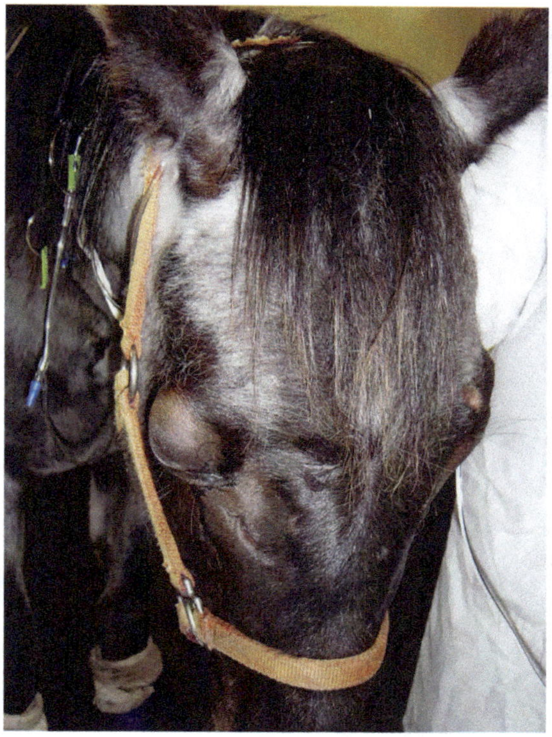

Figure 11.33 This yearling was kicked in the face by an older horse. Note the intact skin and depression in the facial bones rostral to the right eye. The eye was entrapped and partially proptosed.

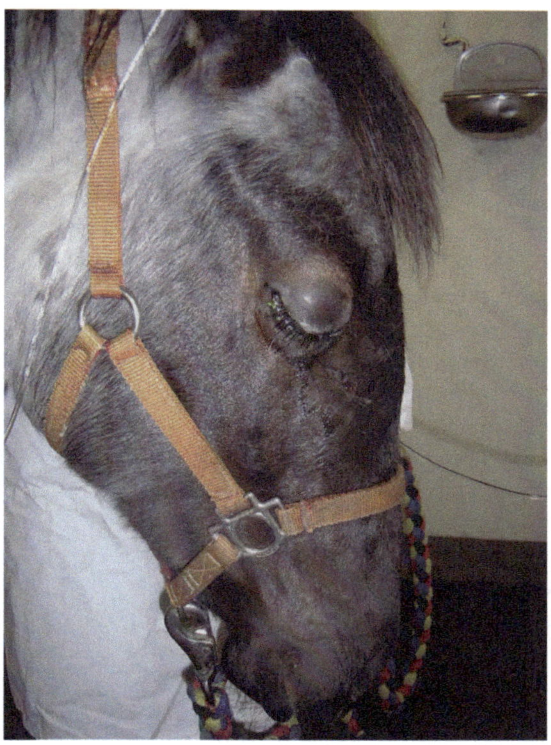

Figure 11.34 Same horse as in Figure 11.33. Note the swelling in the orbital area. The swollen eyelids could no longer completely cover the cornea, which developed exposure keratitis. After reconstruction of the facial bones, the eye was no longer entrapped or proptosed, and the corneal defect healed after topical medication was administered via a subpalpebral lavage system.

Passing a nasogastric tube helps to evaluate patency of the nasal cavities. Endoscopic examination is useful for observing the nasal septum and the nasal bones and if drainage or hemorrhage stems from the paranasal sinuses. Digital examination of the rim of the orbit, performed with the horse sedated, is indicated to determine if the orbit has been fractured. The contralateral eye, as well as the eye associated with an orbital fracture, should be examined because retinal detachment of both eyes is possible.[32] The patency of the nasolacrimal duct can be determined by passing a catheter normograde or retrograde through the duct, by lavage, or by instilling fluorescein dye onto the globe and watching it exit the nasolacrimal aperture in the nasal vestibule.[3–5,32]

Radiographic examination of the head is always indicated (Figure 11.35). The presence of a fluid-line within the paranasal sinuses, which are normally filled only with air, indicates hemorrhage into the sinuses.[3–5] A dorsoventral radiographic projection is needed to examine the nasal septum, and several radiographic views of varying obliquities are required to identify facial fractures. The full extent of injury often cannot be determined by radiographic examination, however, because of the complexity of fractures and of the anatomy of the head.[3–5] The nasal bones and lateral surface of the orbital rims are the easiest regions to profile radiographically, but these bones are less commonly fractured than are the maxillary, lacrimal, and zygomatic bones. Radiographs are best used to determine if the paranasal sinuses contain fluid and to confirm the existence of a fracture, rather than to determine the number of fragments and the relationship of the fragments to one another. Additional fractures are usually identified at surgery.[3–5] Computed tomography (i.e., a CT scan) is an excellent means of identifying and characterizing fractures and should be considered, especially when the injury involves the orbital rim, but its use is not required for treatment to be successful.

Indications for surgery

Horses with an open sinus or nasal cavity, an entrapped or damaged eye, or a displaced nasal bone or nasal septum, and horses in which the cosmetic appearance must be restored, require surgery.[3–5] Although many facial injuries heal without surgery, surgery minimizes the following complications: (1) unacceptable cosmetic appearance after swelling recedes; (2) bone sequestration from comminution and contamination; and (3) sinus infection from blood clots occluding normal drainage of the sinuses.

Treatment

Antimicrobial therapy and a NSAID are administered for several days. A lavage system should be placed into the paranasal sinuses if the fracture is open and extends into the sinuses or when the sinuses contain blood. The sinuses should be lavaged twice daily with isotonic saline solution or a dilute antiseptic solution, and the horse should be fed off the ground to enhance gravity-assisted drainage.[3–5]

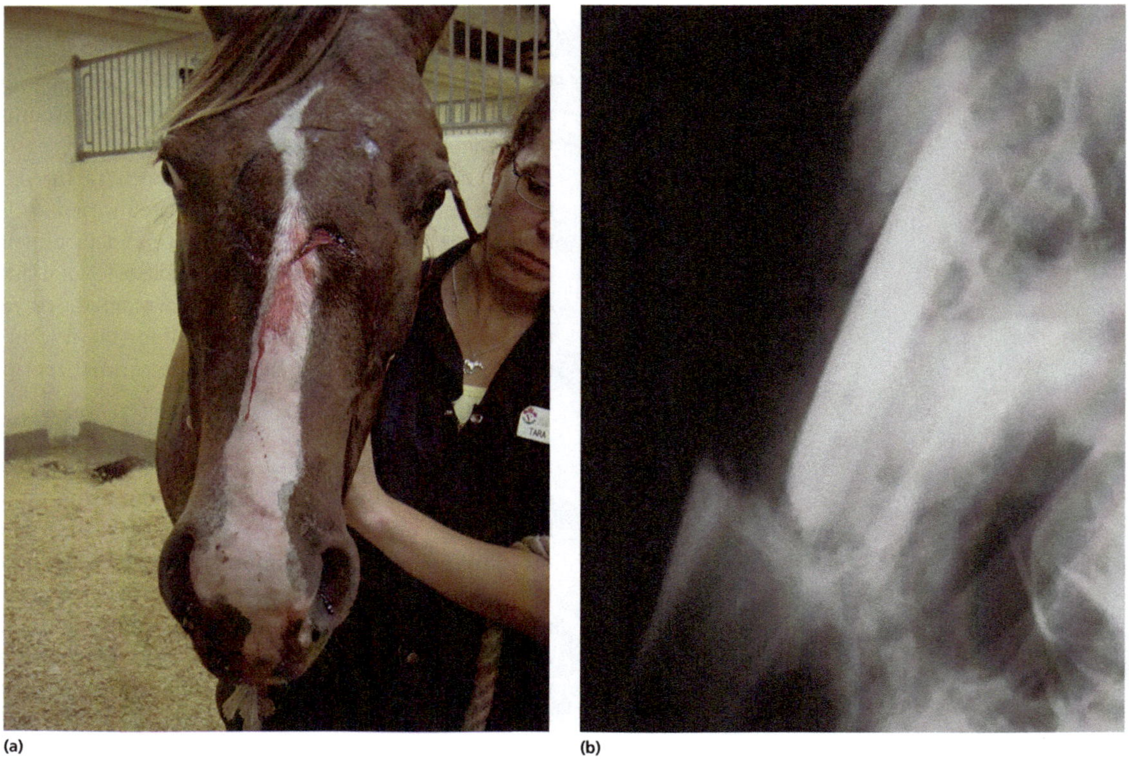

Figure 11.35 **(a)** This horse ran into a heavy metal gate head first. The only abnormality seen clinically was a small cut and some exposed nasal bone. **(b)** Radiographic examination shows a large fragment of bone greatly displaced into the frontal sinus. No cavitation of the face was seen clinically, likely because of swelling.

A lavage system can be easily installed through a small stab incision in the skin where the catheter is to be inserted. An intramedullary pin just slightly larger than the catheter to be inserted is placed through the bone using a hand chuck.[3-5] The catheter may be inserted directly into a maxillary sinus through a hole in the maxillary bone or into the frontal or caudal maxillary sinus (via the frontomaxillary aperture) through a hole in the frontal bone or the caudal extent of the nasal bone. A silastic catheter is fed several inches into the sinus, secured by suturing butterfly tape to the skin, and an extension set is attached to the catheter and extended to the withers or neck region for remote instillation of fluid. After lavaging the sinuses for approximately 5 days, the catheter is removed, and the incision in the skin is closed with a suture or skin staple or left to heal by second intention.

Surgical approaches

The surgical approach to reduce and stabilize a facial fracture depends on the type of injury and the surgeon's preference.[8] A highly invasive approach may be necessary to reduce and stabilize a complex, unstable, comminuted fracture (Figure 11.35), whereas a simple incomplete depressed fracture can often be reduced and stabilized through one or more small stab incisions.[3-5,33] Retraction of the wound's edges may adequately expose the fracture if the wound is large, whereas a small skin wound may need to be enlarged to expose the fracture (Figure 11.32b). These approaches provide excellent exposure of the fracture, but closing the wound directly over the repaired fracture increases the risk of dehiscence. To reduce and stabilize a closed fracture or an open fracture accompanied by a small skin opening, the authors prefer to make a curved skin incision adjacent to the area of trauma (Figure 11.36, Figure 11.37).[3-5] Small holes in the skin associated with the original injury should first be debrided and closed (Figure 11.36a). A curved skin incision is created adjacent to the area of trauma, and skin and subcutaneous tissue are undermined and reflected to gain access to the fracture. Periosteum should be left attached to the bone fragments, but if the periosteum was stripped from the depressed bone fragments, as is often the case, it should also be reflected (Figure 11.36).

Reduction

1. Blood clots at the fracture site and within the sinus should be removed by irrigation and suction before the fracture is reduced (Figure 11.36). If the fracture is subacute, fibrin must be removed to obtain an accurate anatomic reduction, and, if the fracture site is healed or nearly healed, cutting or breaking bones may be necessary to accurately reposition fragments.
2. Completely separated fragments are highly mobile and, therefore, are usually easily reduced, but they may need to be retrieved from the sinuses or nasal cavity, and their edges

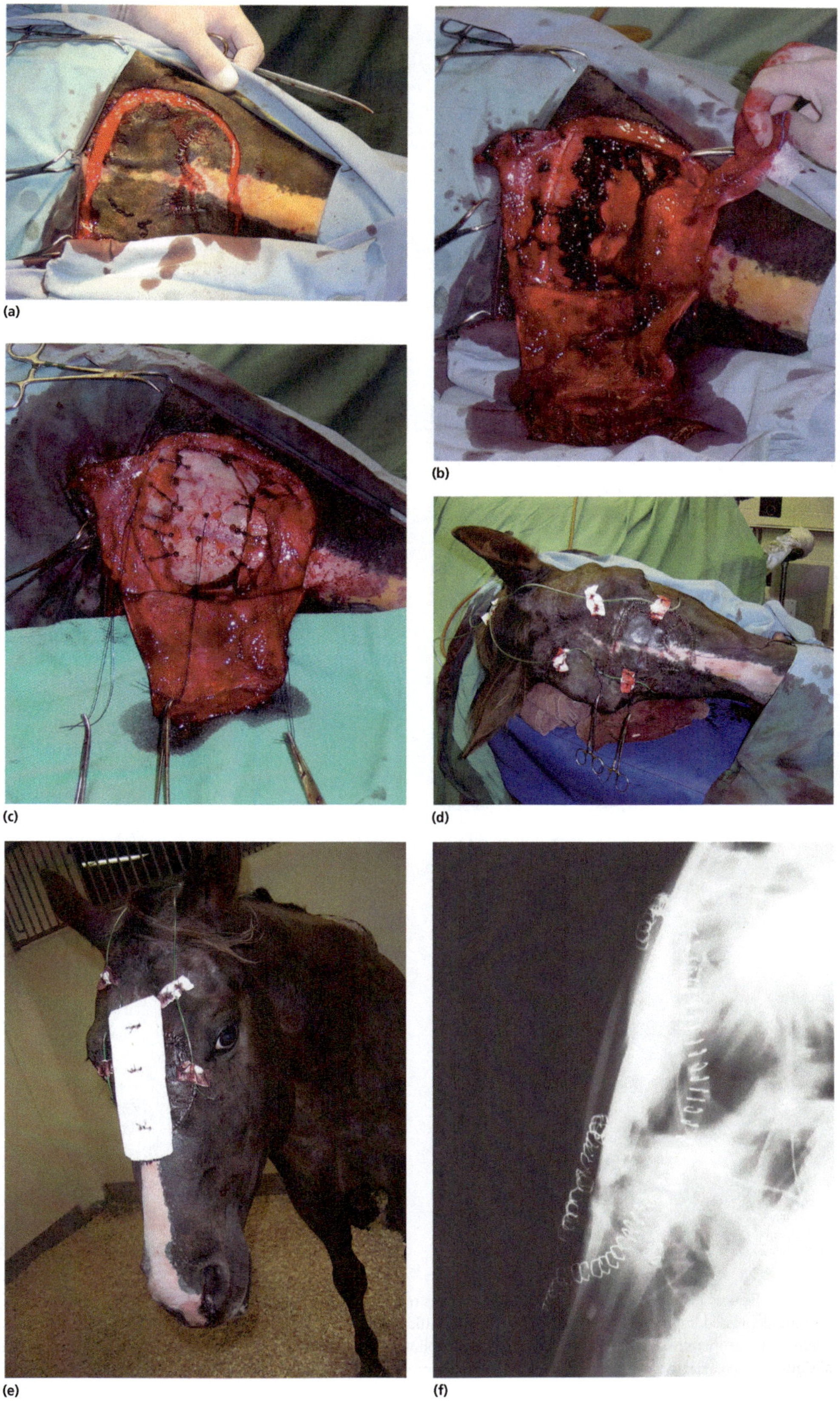

Figure 11.36 Same horse as in Figure 11.35. **(a)** A large curved incision was made to obtain the surgical access required to reduce the large fracture seen on the radiograph in Figure 11.35b. Note: the small wounds over the nose were debrided and closed with staples. **(b)** Although the periosteum was torn during injury, the creation of a large periosteal flap was still necessary to expose the fracture. Notice the large piece of nasal bone imbedded in the frontal sinus and the blood clots. **(c)** The large fragment was reduced and stabilized with suture material placed through predrilled holes. Note the bony defects left from discarding small bony fragments. Three horizontal mattress sutures were preplaced in the fragment and surrounding stable bone to secure an external splint after closing the skin. **(d)** The skin flap was closed, and lavage systems were placed in both sinuses with extensions along the neck. **(e)** The horse on the first postoperative day. Note the external plastic splint that was secured with the horizontal mattress sutures that were preplaced through the bone and skin at the time of surgery. **(f)** Radiographic appearance of the head postoperatively. The fragment was stabilized with absorbable suture material. Note the metal skin staples.

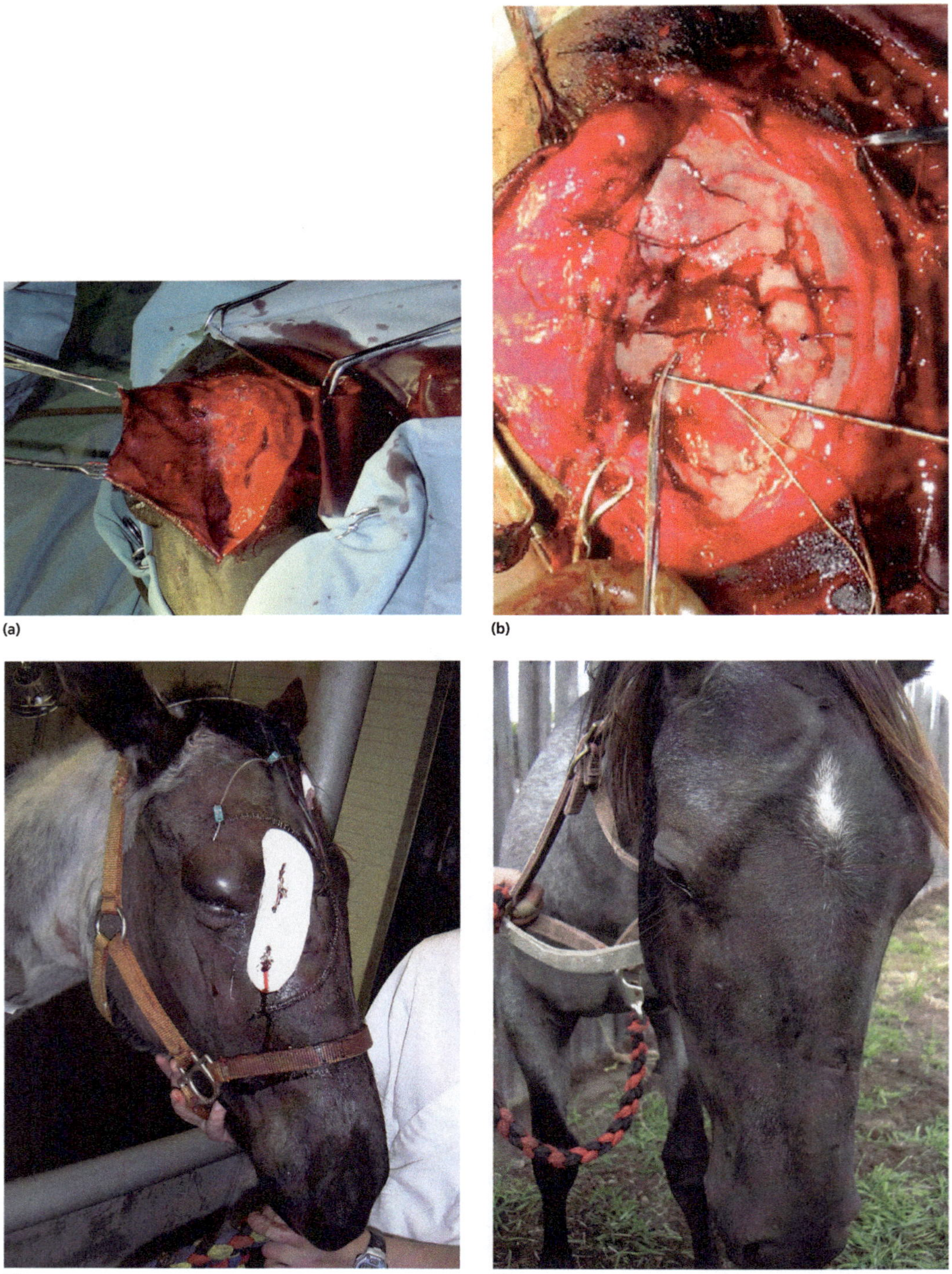

(a) (b) (c) (d)

Figure 11.37 Same horse as in Figures 11.33 and 11.34. **(a)** A large skin flap was required to gain sufficient access to observe and reduce the fracture. **(b)** Several comminuted and depressed fragments were seen. Reduction was difficult, and the fracture fragments remained somewhat unstable, even after wiring. **(c)** Appearance of the horse on postoperative day 1. Note the external plastic splint that was used to prevent collapse of the fracture fragments, the lavage system into the conchofrontal sinus (located axial to the plastic splint), and the catheter in the medial canthus of the eye that passed through the lacrimal duct into the maxillary sinus. **(d)** Appearance 4 months after surgery. The face looks symmetrical, there is minimal blemish from the surgical repair, and epiphora is absent.

cleaned prior to stabilization. Incomplete depressed fractures are usually stable and, after being elevated into position, may not require additional stabilization.[3–5,33] Most facial fractures are a combination of complete unstable fragments and incomplete depressed stable fragments.

3. Numerous instruments can be used to lever, or pry, displaced fragments into position, including periosteal elevators, retractors, bone hooks, and even scissor blades (Figure 11.38c).[3–5,33] Usually, the instrument is inserted into the fracture or through a space created by a displaced or discarded small fragment.

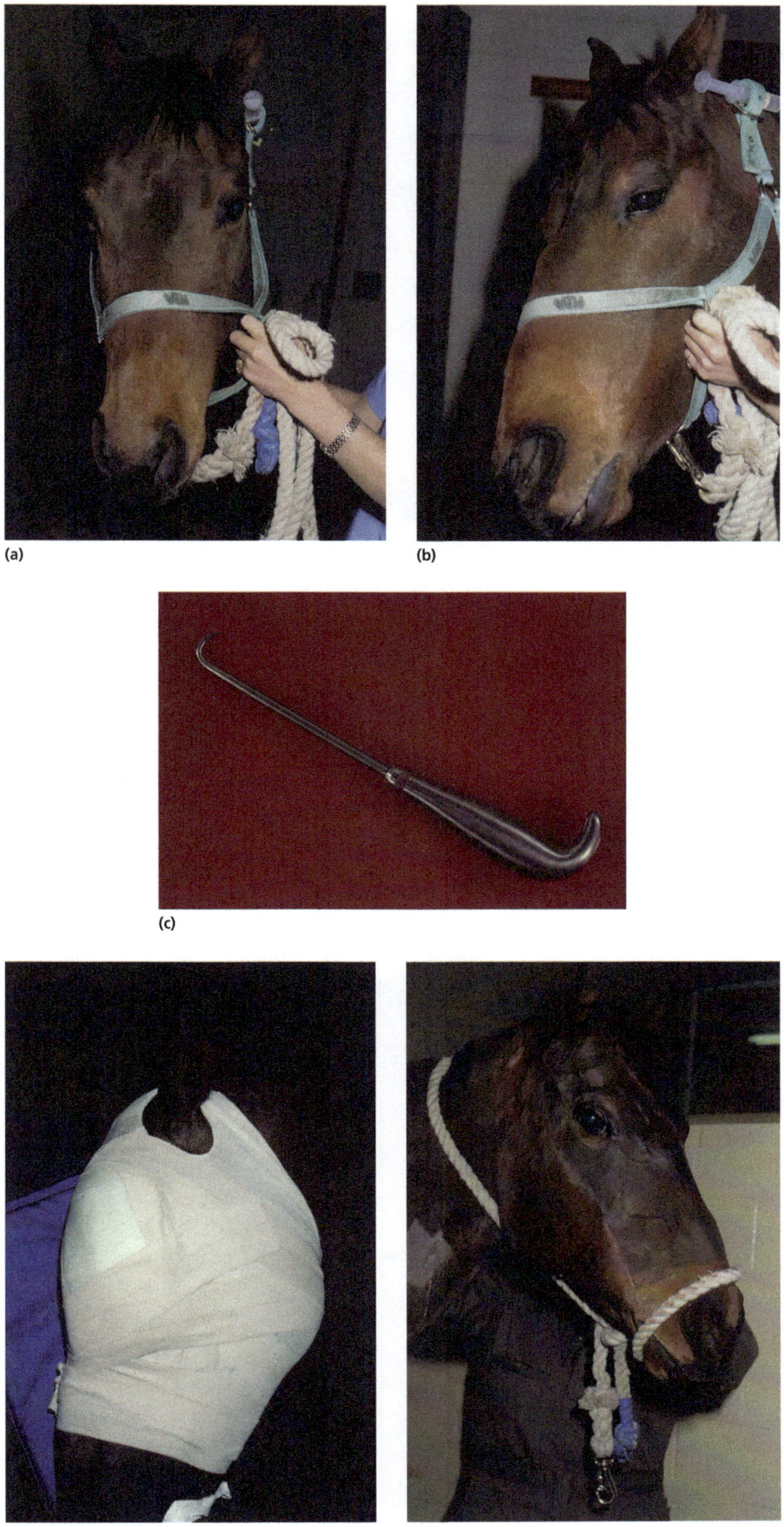

(a) (b) (c) (d) (e)

Figure 11.38 **(a)** Example of a simple depressed incomplete fracture of the facial bones that can be reduced without using wire or bone plates for stabilization. **(b)** Side view of the same fracture. **(c)** The bone hook that was used to elevate the depressed incomplete fracture. Several small stab incisions were used to gain access to the fragment, and a bone rongeur was used to create an opening in the parent bone to allow introduction of the bone hook. **(d)** A cast helmet was used to recover the horse from general anesthesia. **(e)** Lateral view taken the day after surgery. Note the good cosmetic outcome.

Prying on the edge of the fragment should be avoided because this can cause the fragment to fracture. If there is no space to insert an instrument for prying, one can be created at the fracture line with a rongeur, or a hole may be drilled into the fragment. Traction on a bone hook or a bent intramedullary pin inserted through the space or hole elevates the fragment.[3–5,33] Another method of elevating a fragment is to lift on the head of a screw inserted into the fragment.

4. Incomplete depressed fragments usually have sufficient interdigitations to remain stable after they are reduced (Figure 11.38).[3–5,33] Some fractures occur obliquely through the bone, and small pieces of the bone's edge may need to be removed with rongeurs before the fragment can be reduced.[3–5] If some instability persists, particularly at the site of a bony prominence, a cast helmet can be applied to protect the fractured region while the horse recovers from anesthesia (Figure 11.38d).

Stabilization

Unstable fragments should be secured with monofilament suture material (size 0–1) or orthopedic wire (20 gauge) placed through drill holes made along the edge of the fragment and the adjacent edge of parent bone (Figure 11.36c, Figure 11.37b). Suture material is preferred because it is easier to manipulate, absorbable, less irritating to the overlying soft tissue, less likely to cut through the bone, and is easier to preplace. After the fragments have been reduced, not many sutures are required to hold them in position. The holes are best made before the fracture is reduced completely.

Some comminuted fractures remain unstable after suturing and tend to collapse into the underlying sinus or nasal cavity. To enhance stability, a bone plate(s) may be used; complications, such as drainage, screw loosening, and the need for implant removal, however, have been reported.[34,35] To avoid complications associated with implants, the authors prefer to apply an external splint if enhanced stability is required (Figure 11.36e, Figure 11.37c).[3–5] To place a splint, holes are drilled in the fragments and adjacent stable bone prior to reducing the fracture. Heavy suture material (size 1–2) or orthopedic wire is preplaced in a mattress pattern, through the periosteum, subcutaneous tissue, and skin. After reducing and stabilizing the fragments and suturing the skin, the suture/wire for the external splint is placed through holes made in the splint. Moldable plastic works well for splinting and can be shaped and trimmed to fit the face.[3–5] Little force is usually needed to maintain reduction, and the splint should not be applied too tightly against the skin. The splint is easily removed in 2–4 weeks.

Small fragments that are completely free can be discarded, and healing occurs as long as sufficient viable soft tissue is available to close the defect (Figure 11.32c, Figure 11.36c).[3–5] Application of an external splint is required to enhance stability if there are large spaces between fragments (Figure 11.37c). If the defect created by removing a loose fragment is located in a dependent portion of the sinuses, the sinuses should not be lavaged postoperatively or the volume of lavage should be minimal to prevent the lavage solution from draining into the subcutaneous tissue, predisposing the wound to infection and/or dehiscence. Large pieces of bone completely devoid of periosteum are reduced, stabilized, and covered with soft tissue. Although they lack a blood supply, they are needed for structural support of the soft tissues to prevent deformity. Formation of bone sequestra is uncommon if the horse receives antimicrobial therapy, if the surgical site and underlying sinuses are lavaged vigorously, if fragments have been stabilized, and if the bone has been covered with viable soft tissue.

Closure

All available portions of the periosteum should be closed over the fracture site because the periosteum protects and supports the repair, may enhance blood supply to the underlying bone, and has osteoprogenitor cells in its cambial layer that may facilitate healing. If a large bony defect is present, a flap of periosteum from adjacent intact bone can be reflected over the opening,[36] or the opening bridged with absorbable, synthetic mesh.[37]

The repaired fracture site should be covered with viable soft tissue, but often an insufficient amount of skin is available for easy closure. In that case, subcutaneous undermining of skin adjacent to the incision can allow the skin to be closed without excessive tension. If skin has been lost, tension-relieving incisions, transposition skin flaps, single pedicle or bi-pedicle advancement flaps, or sliding H flaps may be used (see Chapter 10).[3–5,7,8] Leaving a cutaneous defect a few centimeters adjacent to the fracture site is better than having a cutaneous defect directly over the fracture site. These skin defects usually heal well by second intention. Rubbing of the surgical site is uncommon but may cause reduced bone fragments to become displaced. With a good knowledge of the anatomy of the head, thorough preoperative evaluation, and application of the principles discussed in this chapter, the horse's prognosis for return to full function and a good cosmetic outcome is excellent.

What to do

- Always evaluate the eye for entrapment or internal injury. The retina of the contralateral eye should also be evaluated.
- Lavaging the paranasal sinuses, through a lavage system, for a few days after surgery ensures that the sinuses are cleared of blood clots.

Tip

- Stabilizing fragments with sutures is much easier than stabilizing them with wire.
- An external splint is easy to apply and worth the effort if stability of the reduced bone fragments is questionable.
- Preventing rubbing postoperatively is crucial to ensure that reduced bone fragments do not become displaced.

Medial surface of the orbital rim

Fractures of the facial bones often occur rostral to the medial canthus of the eye. If, however, the zygomatic bone or, more commonly, the lacrimal bone, is depressed into the sinuses, a portion of the bone that forms the orbital rim or comprises a portion of the orbit may be displaced, causing proptosis, entrapment, or damage to the globe (Figure 11.33).[3–5,33,38] Pieces of bone that form the orbit should be reduced and stabilized, but an impinging fragment that cannot be reduced and stabilized should be exposed by subconjunctival dissection and removed. Each globe should be examined thoroughly because injury to the contralateral eye is possible.[32]

Fracture of the lacrimal or maxillary bones can result in damage to the lacrimal sac or nasolacrimal duct. The lacrimal sac is contained within the lacrimal fossa of the lacrimal bone, and the nasolacrimal duct passes from the lacrimal sac through the lacrimal and maxillary bones.[28] No associated clinical signs are seen when the injury is acute because the lacrimal fluid drains into the wound or into a sinus. Epiphora develops after the transected duct becomes occluded by fibrosis or a bony callus.[3–5,33] In the authors' experience, minimal displacement of these bones does not usually result in loss of integrity of the nasolacrimal duct. The patency of the duct, nevertheless, should always be checked by catheterizing it or by flushing it with fluorescein dye. If the duct has been transected, silicone tubing can be placed through it to act as a stent while it heals, provided both ends of the duct can be identified within the fracture site.[31,37]

Another technique to resolve epiphora when the nasolacrimal duct has been severed is to create a permanent communication between the nasolacrimal duct and the maxillary sinus by placing a segment of silastic tubing (i.e., catheter) through the orbital puncta and into the caudal maxillary sinus, either through a bony defect created by the fracture or through a hole created surgically (Figure 11.37c).[3–5,31] A bony defect created by the surgeon is less likely to become occluded by fibrosis or bony callus. The catheter is left in place for 2–3 weeks, and the horse should be cross-tied to prevent it from dislodging the catheter by rubbing.

The prognosis for proper movement of the eye and unimpeded drainage of lacrimal secretions is good following the removal of impinging fragments and creation of lacrimal drainage into a sinus.

Zygomatic (supraorbital) process

The zygomatic (supraorbital) process is that portion of the frontal bone that forms the dorsocaudal part of the orbital rim.[28] Because of its prominence, it is frequently the only portion of the orbit that is injured, and, typically, the skin over it is intact. Usually, a single fragment is displaced medially and ventrally,[3–5,33] resulting in asymmetry of the orbital region and swelling and tenderness over the zygomatic process.[3–5] The depressed bone fragment may damage or entrap the eye. If entrapped, the eye remains in a fixed position when the head is moved. The eye may be swollen, and the globe may be proptosed. The fracture can usually be identified on a skyline radiograph of the orbit.[3–5,31]

Fractures that do not interfere with the globe can be left to heal without being reduced, but healing of a non-reduced fracture may not always lead to a cosmetic appearance. The authors recommend surgical treatment to reduce the

> **What to do**
>
> - If a fracture of the orbit cannot be reduced, simply break off and remove that portion of bony fragment impinging on the globe.
> - Always check the nasolacrimal duct's integrity.
> - A horse with a catheter in the nasolacrimal duct should be cross-tied to prevent it from dislodging the catheter by rubbing.
>
> **Tip**
>
> - Establishing a communication between the nasolacrimal duct and the sinuses is much easier than placing a stent in the nasolacrimal duct.

likelihood of ocular damage that may occur if the fragment becomes more displaced before it heals.

Simple fractures can be reduced non-invasively by using a bone hook (Figure 11.38c).[3–5,39] With the horse anesthetized, the interior of the orbit is digitally palpated, and, using a finger as a guide, the surgeon places the end of the bone hook on the ventral extent of the bony fragment. The fracture is reduced by pulling the fragment dorsally with the bone hook. Traction can be applied to the fragment at various sites by repositioning the hook (Figure 11.40).

The accuracy of the reduction is determined by visual inspection and digital palpation. No other treatment is necessary if the reduced fragment is stable, but if the fragment is unstable, an incision is made over the fracture, and the fragment is stabilized with wire or absorbable suture material passed through holes drilled in the fragment and the adjacent parent bone, as described earlier in this chapter (Figure 11.39, Figure 11.41).[3–5,33] An unstable fracture may also be stabilized with a reconstruction plate and screws.[39] The horse's head should be protected with a cast helmet (authors' preference) or a padded hood during recovery, or the horse can be hand recovered (Figure 11.38d).

The horse is cross-tied and given antimicrobial therapy and a NSAID for several days. A stable repair is usually easily obtained by using an open approach, and an excellent prognosis for cosmesis and function should be expected. If the fracture cannot be stabilized, depression of the facial bones may be evident (Figure 11.39c).

> **What to do**
>
> - Perform an ophthalmic examination in all cases.
> - Opt for an open approach if quality of reduction or stability is in doubt.
>
> **Tip**
>
> - Equine skin is thin, so synthetic absorbable or non-absorbable suture material is preferred over wire to stabilize fragments.

Imbedded foreign bodies

Occasionally a horse is presented with a foreign body imbedded in the skull (Figure 11.42a). Establishing which anatomical structures have been injured is important, and, by examining

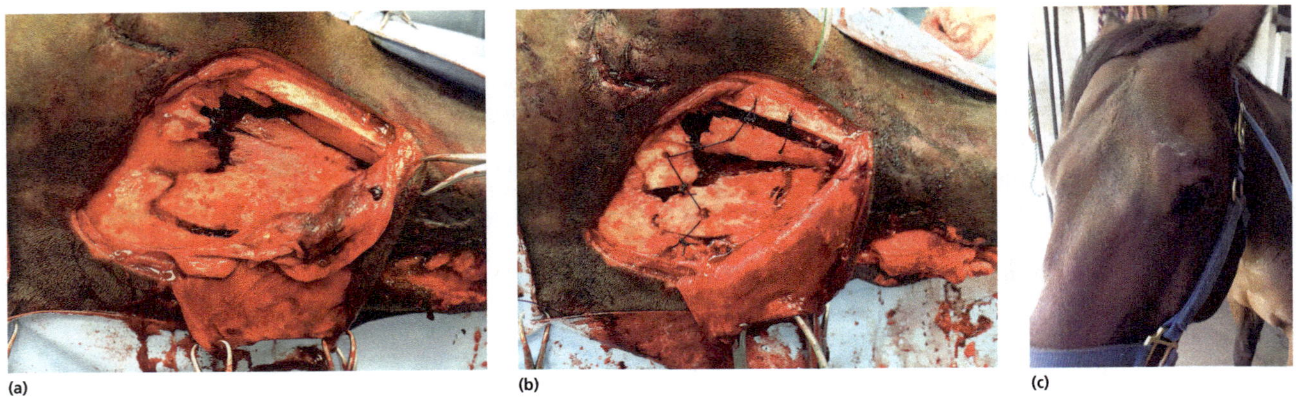

Figure 11.39 (**a**) An intraoperative view of a large depressed facial fracture. Removal of the bone from the sinus was difficult and resulted in splintering of the fragments. (**b**) These fragments were retained and secured with suture placed through holes drilled in the bones. The periosteum and skin were closed over the defect, and the face had a normal appearance after recovery from general anesthesia. (**c**) There was a substantial depression 6 months after surgery caused by the horse continually rubbing its head on objects after discharge. This deformity could possibly have been prevented by using an external splint and/or cross-tying the horse.

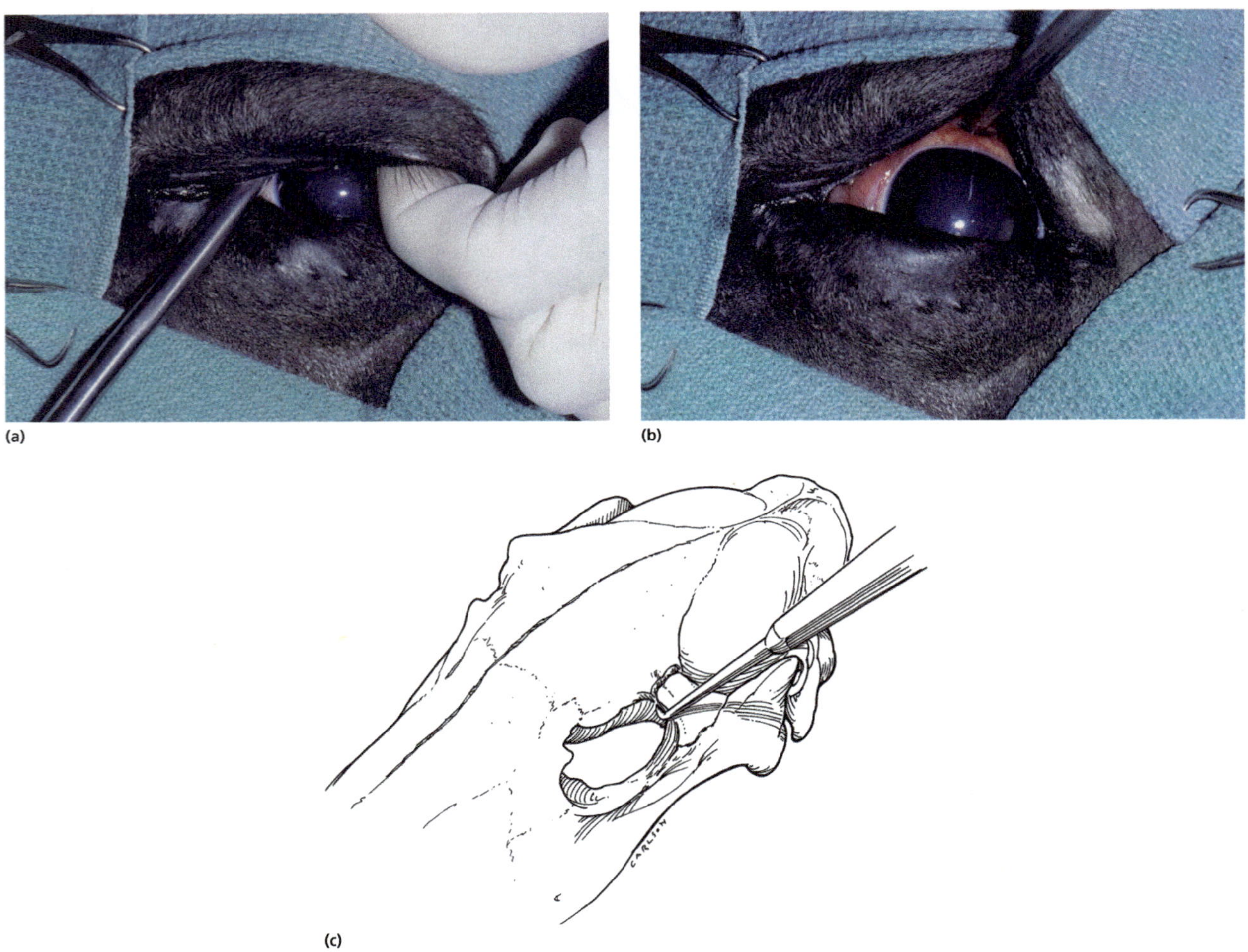

Figure 11.40 This horse has a displaced orbital process. (**a**) A gloved finger is used to palpate the fornix of the conjunctiva prior to placing the bone hook. (**b**) The bone hook is positioned beneath the fracture fragment for elevation. (**c**) Drawing showing the positioning of the bone hook for elevating the fracture fragment.

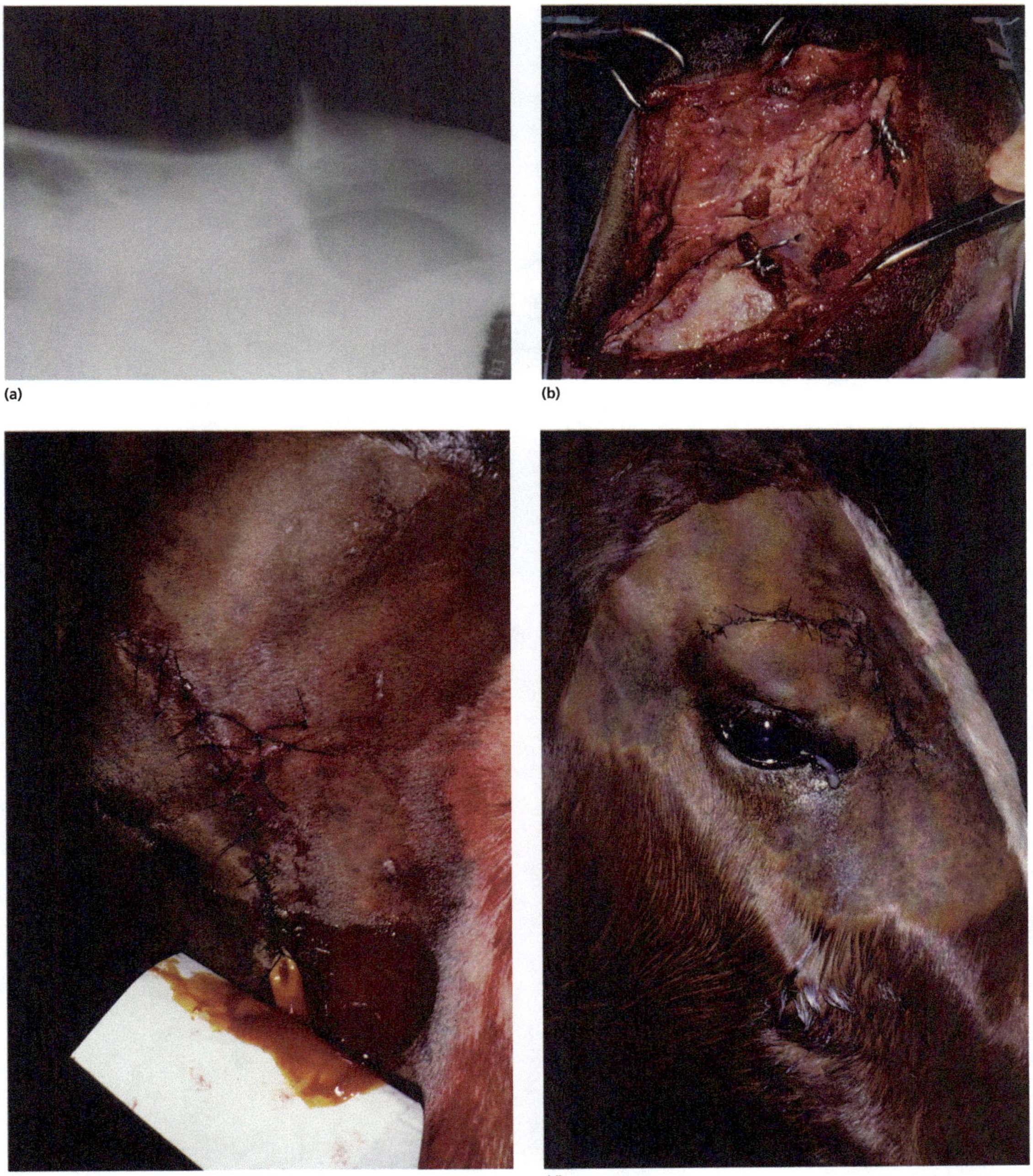

(a) (b) (c) (d)

Figure 11.41 This horse had a displaced supraorbital process that was not stable after being reduced. (**a**) Oblique radiograph of the skull showing a displaced fracture of the supraorbital process. (**b**) The fragment was elevated into position and stabilized with orthopedic wires placed at each end. (**c**) Immediately after surgery. Note the size and location of the incision required for surgical exposure and the placement of the Penrose drain. (**d**) Two days postoperatively. A stent bandage, originally placed over the incision, and the Penrose drain have been removed. Good cosmetic and functional outcomes were achieved.

lateral, skyline, and dorsoventral radiographic projections, the depth and location of the foreign body can be determined, and hemorrhage or exudate within the paranasal sinuses can be identified (Figure 11.42b). A foreign body lodged in the nasal cavity can be identified during endoscopic examination of the nasal cavities (Figure 11.42c). Endoscopic examination may also help identify blood or exudate draining from the paranasal sinuses into the middle nasal meatus or from a guttural pouch into the nasopharynx at the nasopharyngeal opening of the pouch. The paranasal sinuses can be examined directly through a trephine hole created in the frontal or maxillary bone. Computed tomographic examination of the head is ideal for determining the extent of injury, if this modality is available and the owners can afford it. The horse should also receive a neurologic examination.

Preoperative preparation includes administration of antimicrobial therapy and a NSAID. Many foreign bodies can be extracted with the horse sedated, using a large bone-holding forceps or channel-lock pliers (Figure 11.42d). Packing material should be

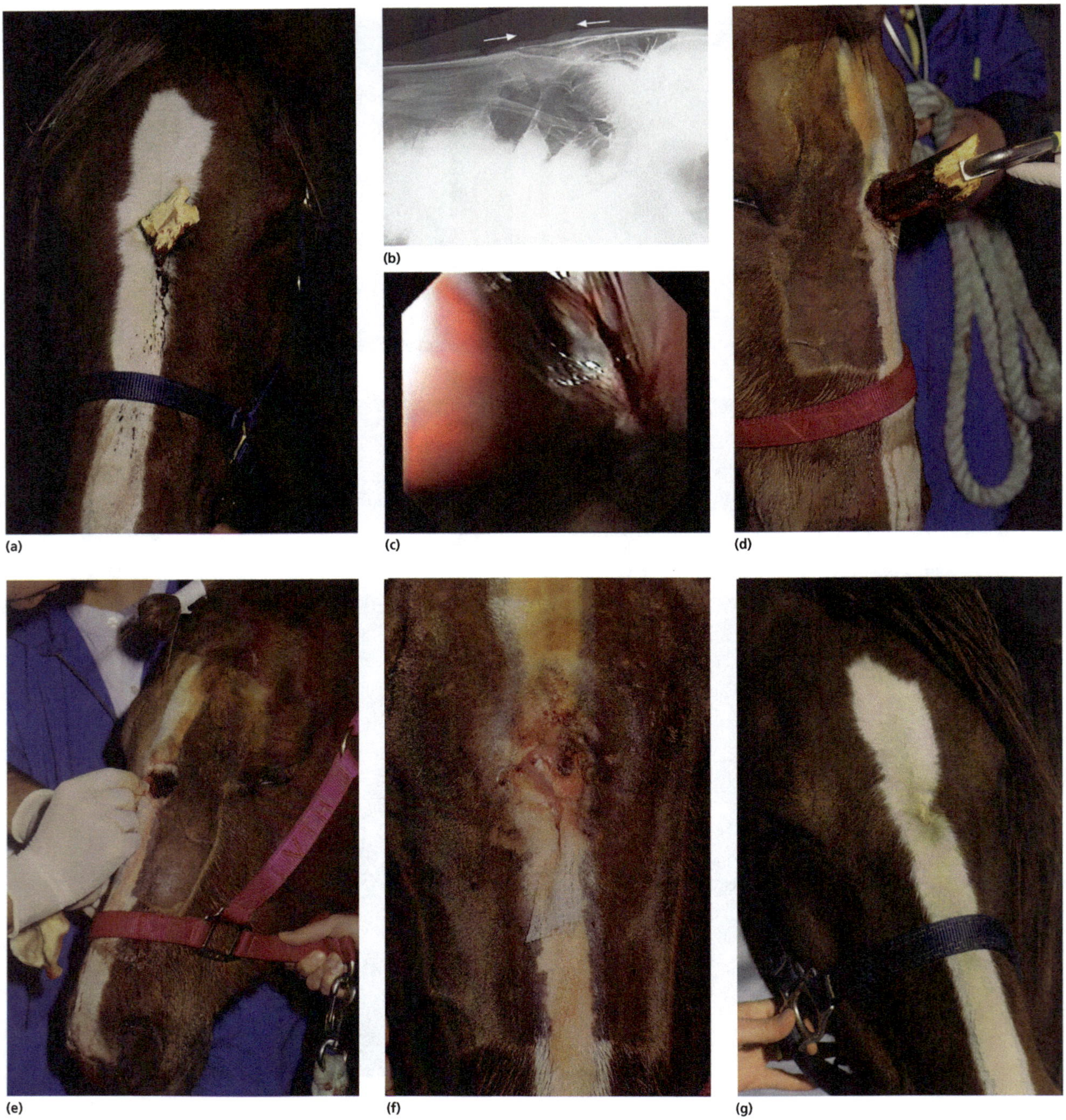

Figure 11.42 (**a**) Example of an imbedded piece of wood in the skull of a horse. The injury occurred less than 12 hours previously. Blood dripped from the horse's left nostril. (**b**) Radiographic examination identified fluid within the left dorsal conchal and rostral maxillary sinuses. The outline of the piece of wood was seen (arrows) with what appeared to be an incomplete depressed fracture of the nasal bone. (**c**) An endoscopic view of the nasal cavity showed blood entering the nasal cavity after exiting the nasomaxillary aperture. (**d**) Removing the piece of wood using channel-lock pliers. (**e**) Wound after removal of the imbedded wood fragment. The tract was debrided, irrigated, and packed with Kerlix AMD gauze. The packing was changed daily for 2 days, after which time the incomplete fracture was elevated into position using a bone hook. (**f**) Appearance of the bone after reduction. Although suturing the soft tissues would have been ideal, the owner did not wish to incur the additional expense. (**g**) Follow-up, 1 year. Note the dimple-like scar. This probably could have been prevented by suturing the wound after reducing the bone flap.

made available for the unlikely event that hemorrhage is substantial. If used, packing should be left in place for 2–4 hours, by which time hemorrhage is unlikely to occur when the packing is removed.

The wound is examined to determine the extent of soft-tissue and osseous injury after the foreign body has been removed. Usually, dirt, hair, and other debris have been driven into the depths of the wound, making it inadvisable to reduce the fracture and suture the wound immediately. The wound is irrigated, debrided, and packed with an anti-microbial dressing in preparation for a delayed closure.

Changing the packing daily rids the wound of hair, necrotic tissue, and/or debris within 2–3 days. The wound is ready for repair after a healthy bed of granulation tissue appears. Often, a depression fracture of a facial bone is identified (Figure 11.42b). The depressed fragment can often be elevated with the horse sedated by placing traction on a bone hook or a bent Kirshner wire inserted through a fracture gap created with rongeurs or a hole created with a drill bit. The reduced fragment is usually stable (Figure 11.42f). The wound is covered by suturing available periosteum and skin, or the wound is left to heal by second intention (Figure 11.42f). Full recovery is common, and the blemish is usually acceptable to the owner.

Tips

- If there is potential for severe hemorrhage when the foreign body is removed, a suitable blood donor for the horse should be available, and the foreign body should be removed with the horse anesthetized.
- The wound should be examined thoroughly to ensure all foreign material has been removed.

Nasocutaneous and sinocutaneous fistulas

A fistula, an abnormal passage from one epithelialized surface to another, can result from a facial fracture, especially if the injury is complicated by infection, sequestration of bone, or substantial loss of skin or bone over the paranasal sinuses or nasal cavity (Figure 11.43, Figure 11.44).[3–5,32,33]

Most facial wounds into the paranasal sinuses or nasal cavity should be closed, using primary or delayed primary closure, but wounds less than 3 cm wide or long can be left unsutured to heal by second intention. A fistula forms when epithelium advancing from the edge of the mucosa of the sinuses or nasal cavity fuses with epithelium advancing from the edge of the skin wound.[1,2] To prevent this from happening, the edge of the wound should be curetted frequently, or a strongly angiogenic extracellular matrix scaffold can be applied to the wound (see Chapter 6 for more information about biologic dressings).[40] Conservative management may be successful but is more time consuming and labor intensive, and usually results in a larger scar than does surgical repair.

Numerous techniques can be used to close an acute wound or fistula.[3–5,31,37,41–44] An important principle of repair is to provide a tissue barrier between the contaminated cavity and the skin to prevent dehiscence. If the wound is fresh, subcutaneous tissue, fascia, or muscle can be used to close the defect. A fistula may be closed with one or two mucosal flaps (Figure 11.45), inverted or reversed skin flaps (Figure 11.46b,c), periosteum (Figure 11.47, Figure 11.48c,d), and/or muscle flaps (Figure 11.49). After the barrier has been created, the skin must be mobilized to cover the barrier.

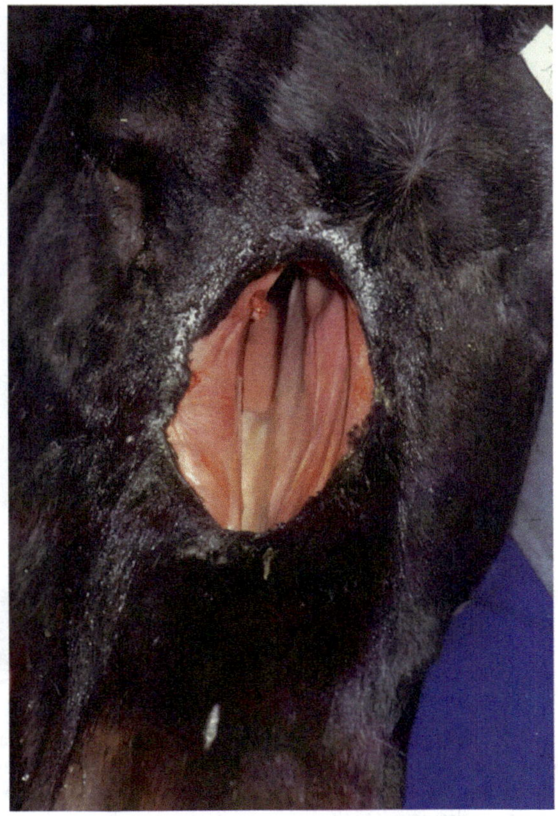

Figure 11.43 Example of a large nasocutaneous fistula.

Management of the acute injury

Antimicrobial therapy and a NSAID are administered to the horse, and the wound is debrided and irrigated. For primary closure, a barrier should be created at the site of the bony defect, using any or all of the tissues previously mentioned. Because tissue surrounding the wound is sparse, debridement must be conservative. After a barrier to the contaminated cavity has been established, skin surrounding the wound must be mobilized to cover the barrier (see section on Selected techniques for mobilizing skin, later in this chapter and in Chapter 10). When the fistula involves a sinus, a lavage system is placed into the sinuses (Figure 11.44b).

If the wound is highly contaminated, closure of the defect can be delayed for several days, during which time the wound is irrigated and debrided, as needed. Packing the wound and sinus with an antiseptic dressing for a few days can sometimes be helpful to reduce contamination. After the wound begins to fill with granulation tissue, the same steps as described for primary closure are used to close the wound.

Management of chronic fistulas

Inverted periosteal flaps and rotational skin flaps have been used to close fistulas (Figure 11.46, Figure 11.47, Figure 11.48, Figure 11.49).[3–5,36,41,43] The periosteum from the wound's margin provides a viable soft-tissue barrier and a healthy surface on which to place a transposition flap or skin graft. Although

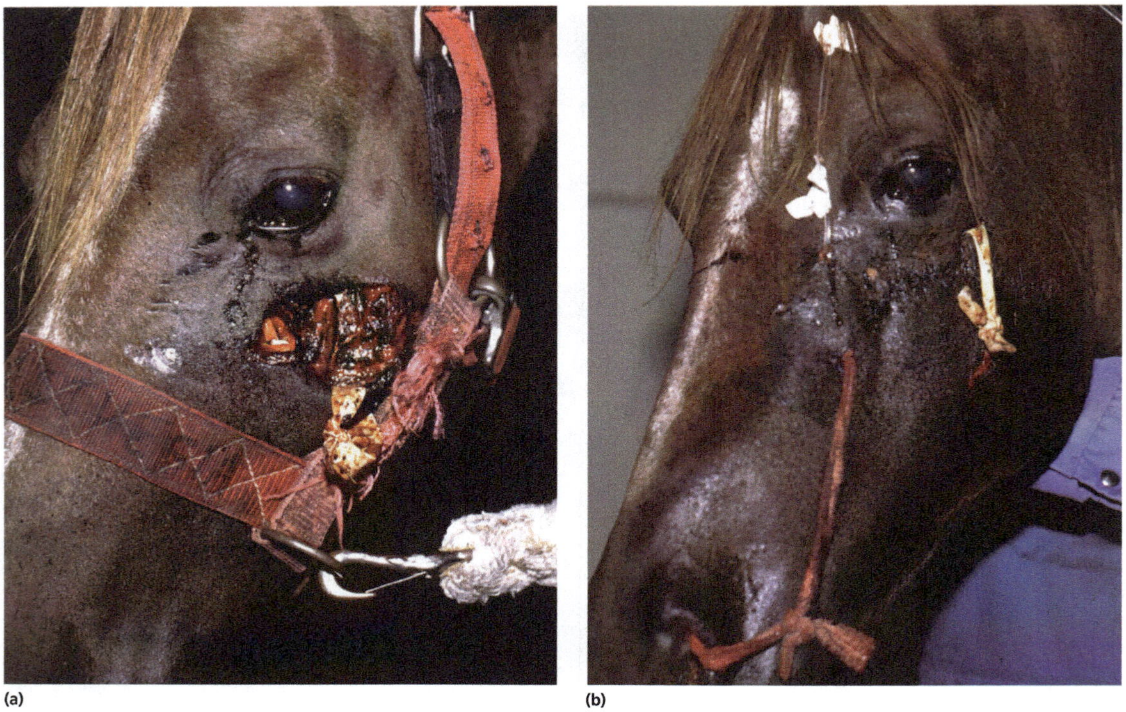

Figure 11.44 **(a)** Example of a facial injury with loss of several bone fragments and a large opening into the maxillary sinuses. Note the Penrose drain placed for drainage. **(b)** Postoperative appearance after wound debridement, sinus lavage, and wound closure. The soft tissues could be apposed over the bony defect after the subcutaneous tissue was undermined. Note the lavage system placed in the sinuses, the gauze placed through the sinus into the nasal cavity to assure drainage into the latter, and the Penrose drain in the subcutaneous tissue.

osteoprogenitor cells of the cambial layer of a periosteal flap have the potential to produce bone, a bone graft can be placed between the periosteal barrier and skin flap(s) to encourage bone formation. A myocutaneous transposition flap placed over a free, autologous mucosal graft has been used to repair a sinocutaneous fistula.[44]

To close the fistula with inverted skin flaps, a skin incision is made along the periphery and parallel to the edges of the fistula at least one half of the diameter of the fistula away from its edges (Figure 11.46). The skin, which is often scarred and unpliable, is undermined on both sides of the fistula toward its edges, and each skin flap is elevated and reflected toward the center of the defect. The inverted flaps are sutured together and covered with a transposition flap.[3–5,7,8]

The fistula can be covered in a similar manner with a single, large, inverted periosteal flap created from one side of the fistula or with a smaller inverted periosteal flap elevated from each side of the fistula and reflected toward the center of the fistula (Figure 11.48c,d).[3–5,36] The advantage of covering the defect with a single large flap of periosteum, rather than two flaps that meet in its center, is the absence of suture holes over the covered defect, through which air can move, predisposing to dehiscence. Both techniques require elevation of skin and subcutaneous tissue.

Free, autogenous periosteal grafts, taken from adjacent or remote sites, have been used by one of the authors (SB) to cover the fistula. Both reflected and free periosteum contract considerably after being elevated, so the elevated flaps should be large enough to account for some shrinkage; this is less apparent with thickened periosteum adjacent to the fistula. A cancellous bone graft[36] or a scaffold of extracellular matrix (ACell Vet® scaffold, ACell, Inc.) can be placed over the periosteum before the periosteum is covered with a skin flap.[40]

A flap composed of the *interscutularis* and *temporalis* muscles has been used to close a frontocutaneous fistula.[42] Using this technique, the caudomedial attachment of the superficial *interscutularis* muscle and fascia are elevated, rotated to cover the fistula and sutured to the periosteum. The ventral border of the *temporalis* muscle and fascia is incised (split) in a sagittal plane to create a split-thickness muscle flap, which is rotated to cover the *interscutularis* muscle (Figure 11.49). Because the flaps retain their blood supply, they can be covered with a skin graft or a skin flap, or the muscle-covered defect can be allowed to heal by second intention. One author (SB) has placed a flap of the *levator labii maxillaris* muscle directly over a defect or placed it over reflected or transplanted periosteum if the fistula was located close to the muscle. Although a muscle flap provides a thick barrier with a good blood supply, it is uncommonly used because seldom is a fistula located close to an available muscle.

Small sinocutaneous or nasocutaneous fistulas can usually be easily repaired with minimal blemish, but large defects require excellent planning and sometimes a series of surgeries; a substantial blemish should be anticipated if multiple surgeries are required.

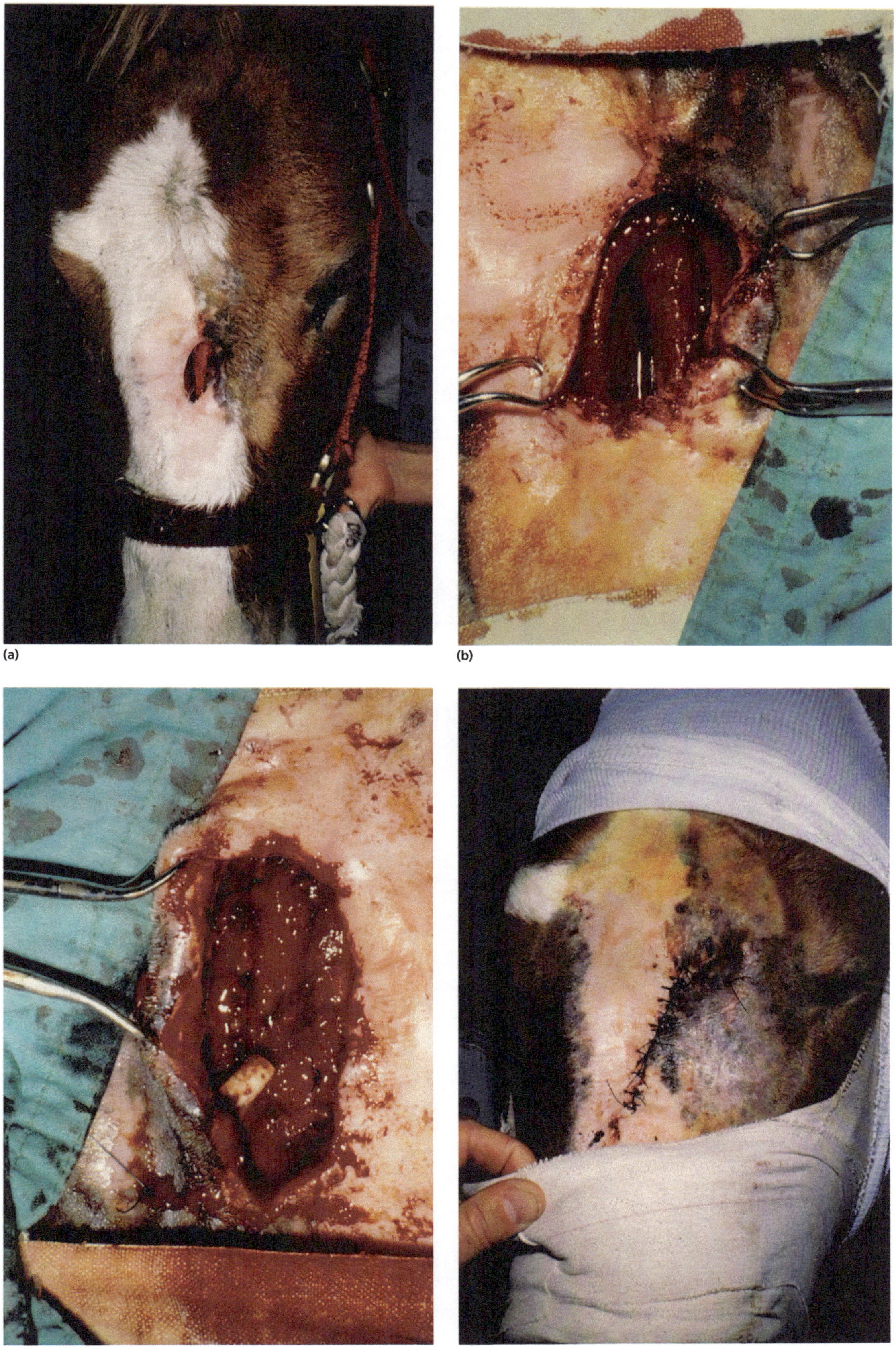

(a) (b) (c) (d)

Figure 11.45 (**a**) Example of a chronic nasocutaneous and sinocutaneous fistula. (**b**) The skin around the wound's margin has been separated from the mucosa. The mucosa will be undermined from the nasal septum (left side) and the maxillary sinus (right side). The mucosa overlying the dorsal concha (central) will be incised and undermined to create two mucosal flaps – one lateral, the other medial. (**c**) The mucosal flap from the nasal septum has been sutured to the medial mucosal flap from the dorsal nasal concha, and the mucosal flap from the maxillary sinus has been sutured to the lateral mucosal flap of the dorsal nasal concha. Note the Penrose drain. (**d**) The skin was undermined to allow closure of the defect.

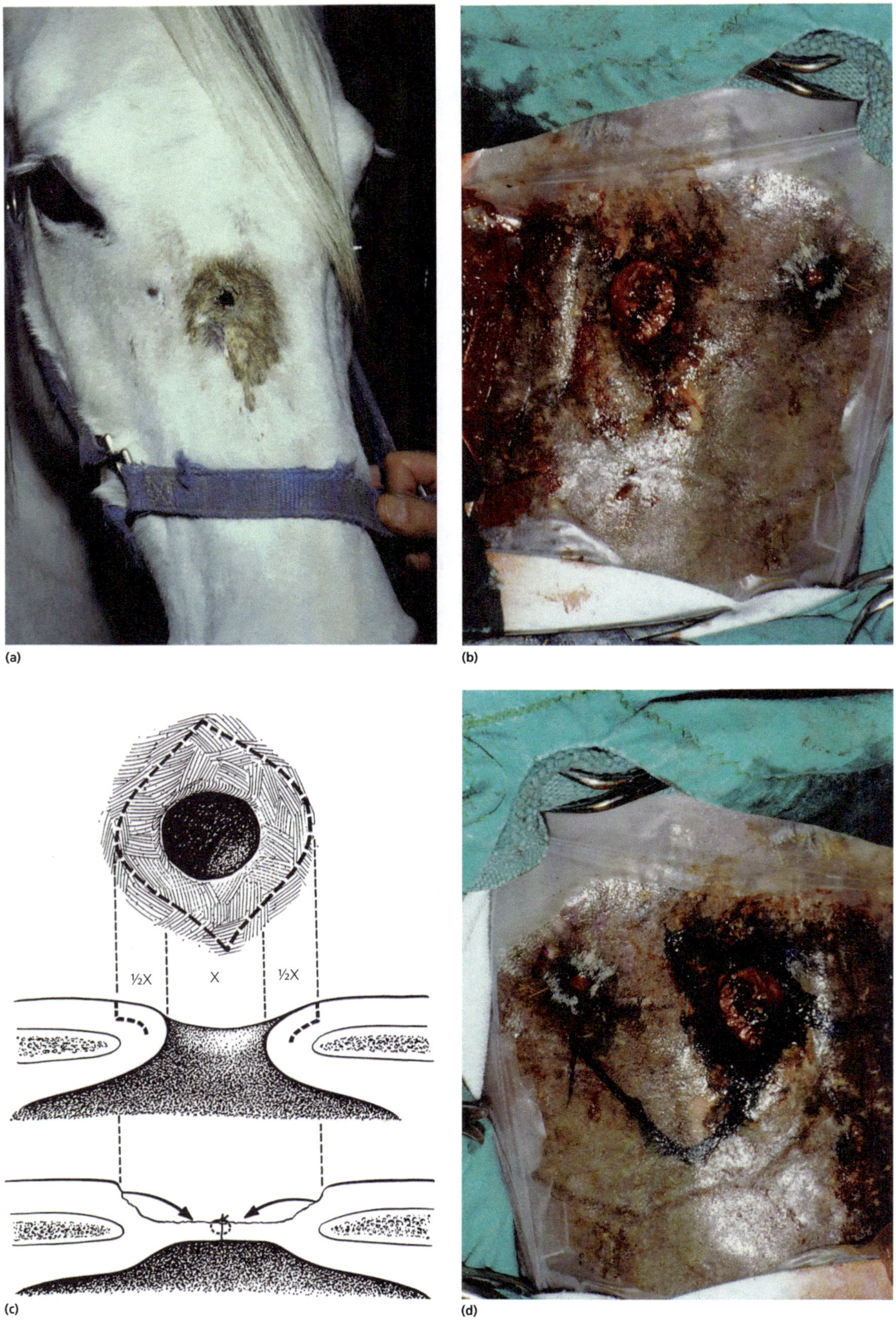

Figure 11.46 **(a)** Chronic nasocutaneous fistula. **(b)** The nasocutaneous fistula has been closed with two inverted periosteal flaps. **(c)** Illustration of inverted skin flaps. Top: the dotted lines indicate the fusiform skin incision adjacent to the fistula necessary to create two skin flaps; middle: cross-sectional view of the fistula; X = the width of the fistula; ½X = the distance the skin incisions must be located adjacent to the fistula to create flaps large enough to close the defect; the heavy dotted line indicates the depth and direction of the dissection to create the skin flaps; bottom: the flaps have been everted to close the defect, resulting in the cutaneous tissue now lining the nasal cavity. **(d)** Transposition flap developed from adjacent tissue. The outline of the flap has been drawn to the left of the fistula.

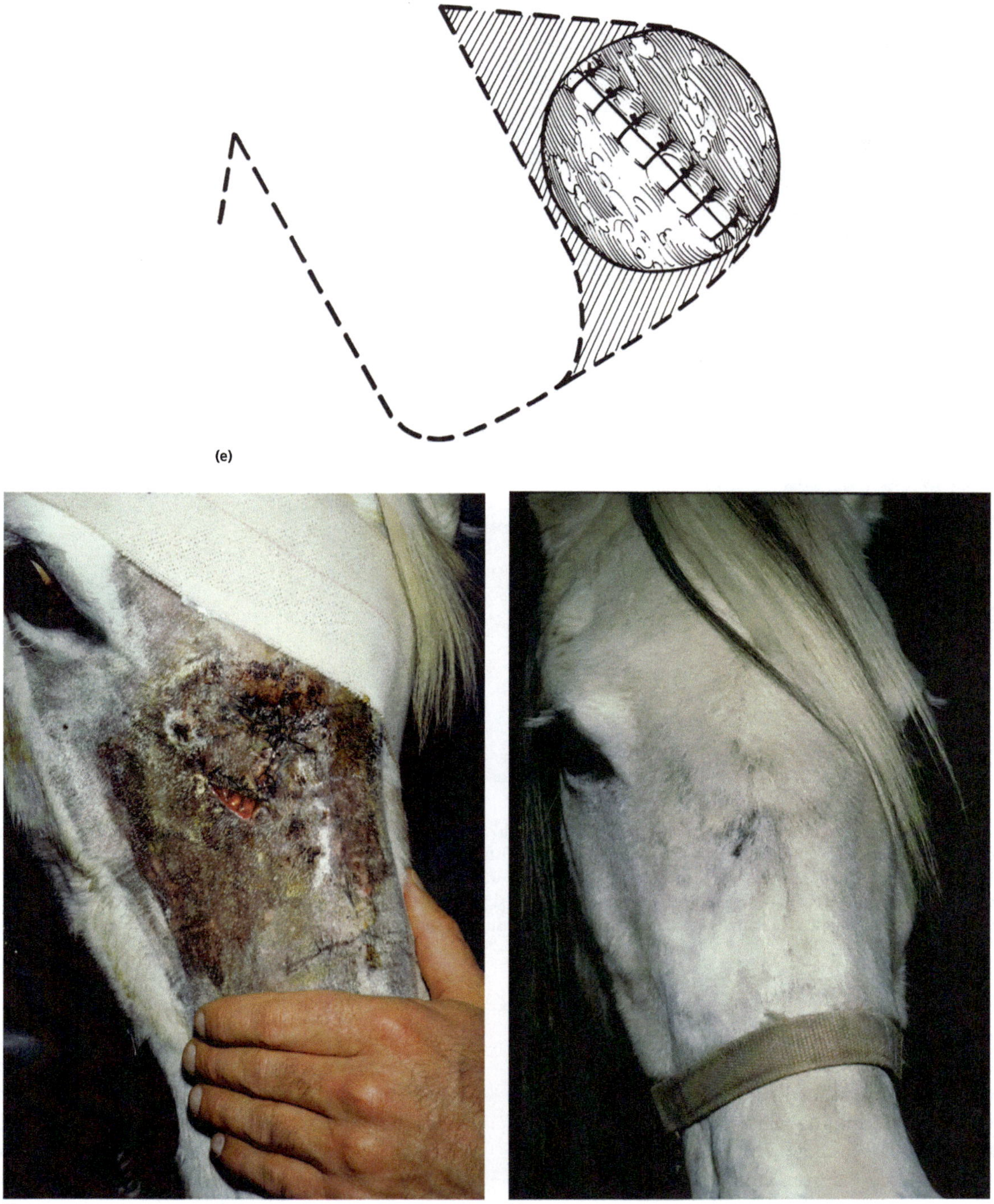

(e)

(f)

(g)

Figure 11.46 (*Continued*) (**e**) Illustration of the formation and mobilization of a transposition skin flap. The transposition flap is developed as close to the repair site as possible to minimize required rotation. Oblique lines surrounding the closed fistula represent skin that must be removed to accommodate the skin flap. (**f**) The transposition flap has been sutured in place. Vertical mattress sutures were used to reduce the size of the remaining defect lateral to the transposition flap. Four days after surgery. (**g**) Follow-up at 3 years. A reasonably good cosmetic and functional end result was achieved.

What to do

- Surgical planning to close a sinocutaneous or nasocutaneous fistula should be extensive and, if the fistula is large, should include a "dry-run" on a cadaver.
- Periosteal flaps shrink considerably, so they should be made larger than anticipated to avoid a difficult closure.

Tip

- Creating large flaps of nasal mucosa can cause extensive hemorrhage.
- Preventing air "blow through" from a defect into the nasal cavity is imperative to prevent dehiscence of the skin closure.
- A multi-layered closure (mucosa, periosteum, muscle flap, skin) is ideal.

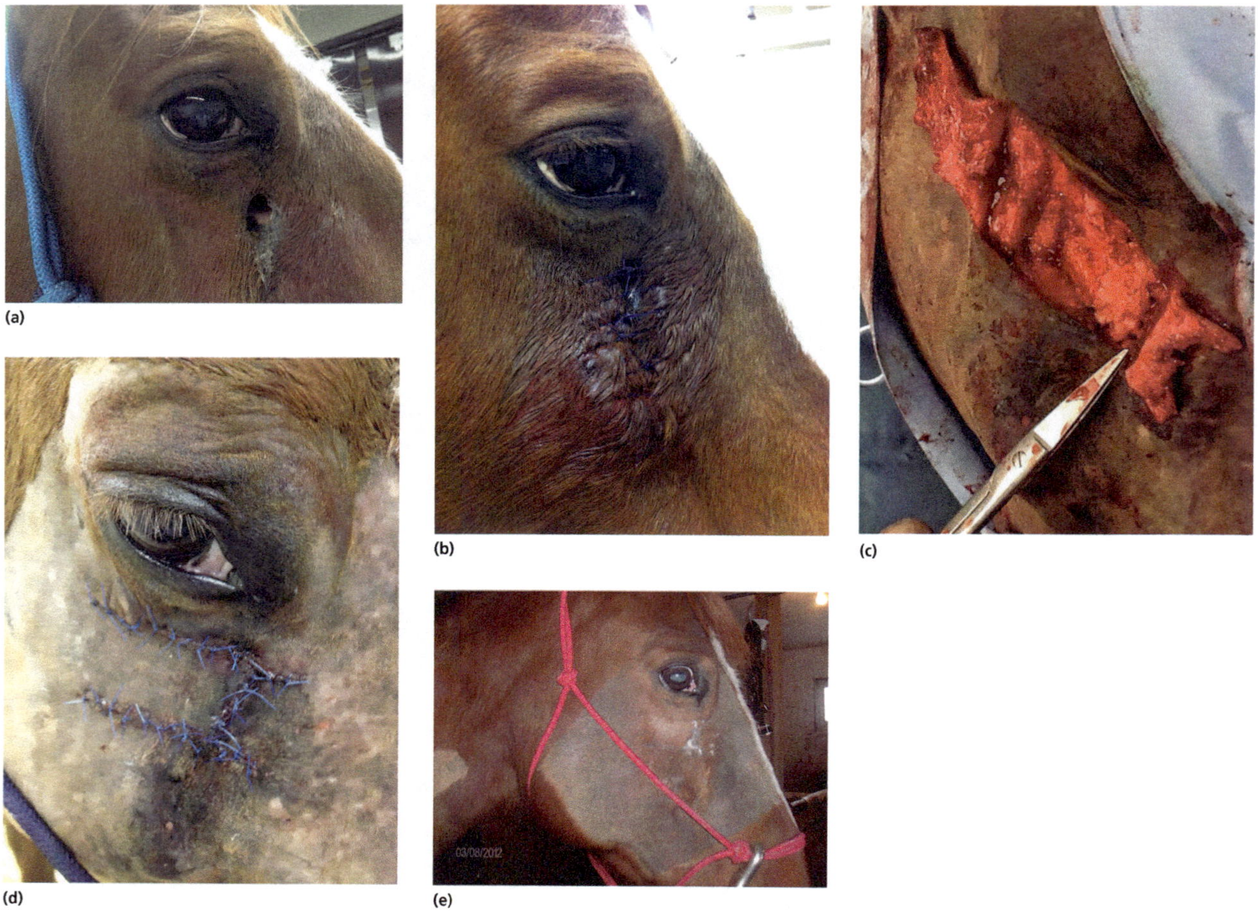

Figure 11.47 **(a)** A chronic sinocutaneous fistula of the maxillary sinuses. **(b)** Simple interrupted sutures were preplaced 24 hours prior to surgical repair. **(c)** Two sliding H flaps were made, one cranial and the other caudal to the fistula. A rectangular flap of periosteum caudal to the fistula, with its base along the fistula, was elevated and inverted over the fistula. The periosteum was thickened as a result of trauma, and provided a substantial barrier. **(d)** Appearance of the wound 1 day after surgery. With undermining of the skin, the H flaps were advanced over the periosteum without having to create Burrow's triangles at the base of the skin flaps. **(e)** Appearance 60 days after surgery shows minimal scarring.

Selected techniques for mobilizing skin

The skin can be undermined several centimeters without the risk of producing necrosis, as long as subcutaneous tissue is elevated with it. Undermining releases the skin from some of its normal attachments and allows it to be advanced towards the defect, but skin scarred from injury is difficult to mobilize. Undermining works best when the defect to be closed is small.[7,8] The subcutaneous tissue and skin are closed separately following undermining, and if the wound contains dead space, a Penrose drain should be placed into it (Figure 11.44, Figure 11.45c).

"Meshing" the skin adjacent to a wound is a good technique to enhance its mobilization, especially if the defect is not large and the skin has also been undermined (see Figure 10.13). Meshing is of limited use for repairing a large fistula, however, because the fenestrations should not lie over the soft tissue barrier that was created adjacent to the fistula to cover the opening into the nasal or sinus cavity or cavities, because doing so weakens the repair and may delay healing.[33] Pre-suturing, another technique used to decrease tension on a sutured wound, is based on the principles of mechanical creep and stress relaxation to release tension (see Chapter 10).[3–5,7,8,41] Sutures are placed in the skin on either side of the defect 2–8 hours prior to repair and tightened to force skin relaxation. This technique is probably more applicable to wounds of the body, upper limb, and neck, where the skin is more loosely attached, than to wounds of the head or the distal portion of the limb, where the skin is more tightly attached.

Skin expanders may be inserted subcutaneously, adjacent to the defect, and gradually expanded to cause biologic creep. Although they may be helpful in providing skin for closure, their use requires repeated surgeries, they are expensive, and implantation can be accompanied by numerous complications (see Chapter 10).[43]

Skin flaps

Skin flaps are indicated when undermining and/or meshing provides insufficient skin to cover a defect. A bi-pedicle advancement flap is easy to use and is created by making a

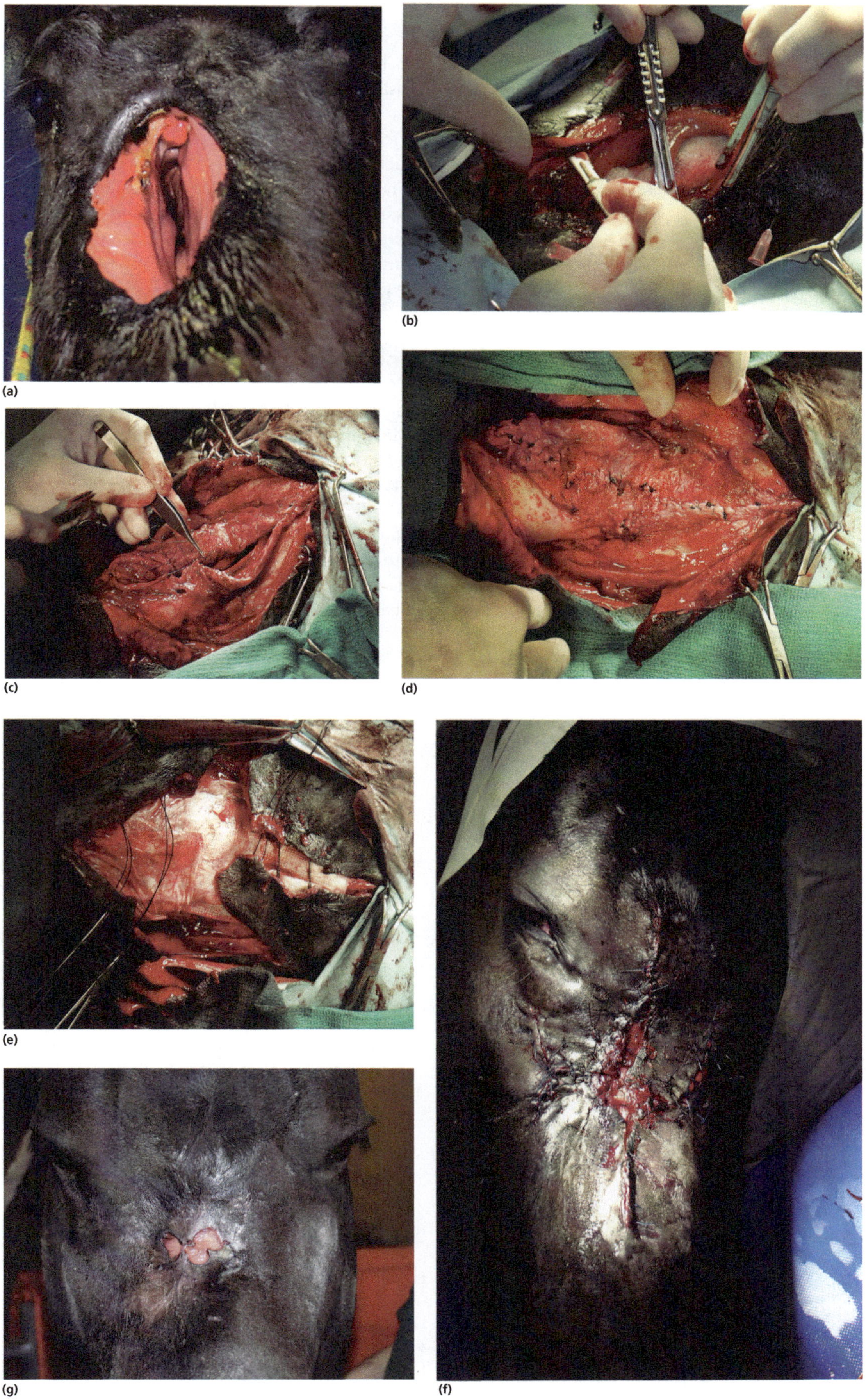

Figure 11.48 **(a)** Example of a large nasocutaneous fistula. **(b)** Undermining of the skin edges to expose the periosteum. **(c)** The formation of large inverted periosteal flaps. **(d)** The periosteal flaps are sutured. **(e)** Application of an extracellular matrix scaffold (ACell Vet® Scaffold, ACell, Inc,) over the inverted sutured periosteal flaps. **(f)** Skin flaps were created to increase skin coverage of the wound. Skin and skin flaps were closed using a vertical mattress suture pattern. **(g)** Appearance of the forehead 1 year after several surgeries.

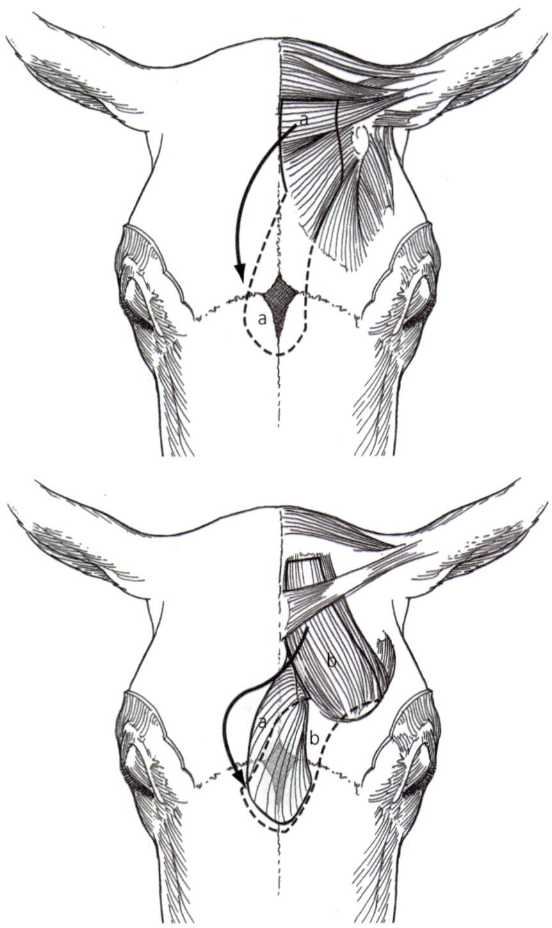

Figure 11.49 Illustration of a frontocutaneous fistula (center black lozenge). Top: the *interscutularis* muscle and fascia (a) were separated from their origin and incised laterally to form a muscle flap. The muscle flap was rotated to cover the fistula and sutured to the periosteum. Bottom: the *interscutularis* muscle (a) was sutured in place. The *temporalis* muscle (b) was incised in a sagittal plane then rotated to overlie the *interscutularis* muscle and the fistula. Source: Campbell and Peyton 1984.[42] Reproduced with permission of John Wiley & Sons.

linear incision in the skin a few centimeters adjacent to the defect.[7,8] The skin and subcutaneous tissue are elevated together, and the flap is slid over the defect. The skin defect produced by moving the flap is allowed to heal by second intention if it cannot be closed.

Sliding H flaps have been used by the authors to close a sinocutaneous fistula. Two rectangular flaps of skin are created adjacent to the defect, Burrow's triangles are removed at the base of the flaps to eliminate "dog ears," and the flaps advanced over the defect (see Chapter 10). Creating Burrow's triangles may not be necessary when the techniques of pre-suturing and undermining are used in addition to the sliding H flaps (Figure 11.47).

A rotational skin flap, which involves making a semicircular incision through the skin and subcutaneous tissue at the wound's edge, undermining the flap, and rotating it to cover the defect, is of limited use in horses because of the tautness of the skin, but it may be effective if the defect is small.[7,8] An advantage of using a rotational skin flap to cover a wound is that its use does not cause an adjacent skin defect, provided there is sufficient skin for rotation, but this is rarely the case when the wound is on the head.

Transposition skin flaps are rectangular pieces of skin and subcutaneous tissue created adjacent to the defect and rotated to cover the wound,[3–5,7,8] creating a skin defect beside the wound that must heal by second intention (Figure 11.46e,f) (see Chapter 10).

Conclusion

The horse, a flight animal, commonly sustains head injuries while in its artificial environment (i.e., stall), and while being handled or used for work or sport. The head is a complex area containing many body systems, and, consequently, injuries to the head can result in serious health problems, impair performance, or cause serious cosmetic deformities. Many horses with an injury to the head can be treated successfully, and early identification and appropriate treatment enhance the probability of a successful outcome.

References

1. Provost PJ. Wound healing. In: Auer JA, Stick JA (eds). *Equine Surgery*, 4th edn. Elsevier Saunders: St Louis, 2012: 47.
2. Stashak TS. Principles of wound healing. In: *Equine Wound Management*. Lea and Febiger: Philadelphia, 1991: 1.
3. Barber SM. Management of neck and head injuries. *Vet Clin N Am Equine Pract* 2005; **21**: 191.
4. Barber SM, Stashak TS. Management of wounds of the head. In: Stashak TS, Theoret CL (eds). *Equine Wound Management*, 2nd edn. Wiley Blackwell: Ames, 2008: 273.
5. Stashak T. *Wound management and reconstructive surgery of the head region*. Lea and Febiger: Philadelphia, 1991: 89.
6. Stashak TS. Selection of approaches to wound closure. In: Stashak TS, Theoret CL (eds). *Equine Wound Management*, 2nd edn. Wiley Blackwell: Ames, 2008: 177.
7. Provost PJ, Bailey JV. Principles of plastic and reconstructive surgery. In: Auer JA, Stick JA (eds). *Equine Surgery*, 4th edn. Elsevier Saunders: St Louis, 2012: 271.
8. Stashak TS. Principles of reconstructive surgery. In: *Equine Wound Management*. Lea and Febiger: Philadelphia, 1991: 70.
9. Smyth GB, Brown RG, Juzwiak JS, *et al.* Delayed repair of an extensive lip laceration in a colt using an Estlander flap. *Vet Surg* 1988; **17**: 350.
10. Lempe A, Brehm W, Scharner D. Stent reconstruction of an injured parotid duct in a Thoroughbred colt. *Vet Surg* 2012; **41**: 536.
11. Olivier A, Steenkamp G, Petrick SW, *et al.* Parotid duct laceration repair in two horses. *J South African Vet Assoc* 1998; **69**: 108.
12. Schumacher J, Schumacher J. Diseases of the salivary glands and ducts of the horse. *Equine Vet Educ* 1995; **7**: 315.
13. Banks W.J. *Applied Veterinary Histology*, 3rd edn. Mosby: London, 1993: **361**.

14. Dixon PM, Gerard MP. Oral cavity and salivary glands. In: Auer JA, Stick JA (eds). *Equine Surgery*, 4th edn. Elsevier Saunders: St Louis, 2012: 361.
15. Kannegieter KM, Ecke P. Reconstruction of a parotid duct in a horse using a polytetrafluoroethylene tube graft. *Austr Vet J* 1992; **69**: 62.
16. Schmotzer WD, Hultgren BD, Huber MJ, *et al.* Chemical involution of the equine parotid salivary gland. *Vet Surg* 1991; **20**: 128.
17. Lang HM, Panizzi L, Smythe TT, *et al.* Management and long-term outcome of partial glossectomy in 2 horses. *Can Vet J* 2014; **55**: 263.
18. Bowman KF. Double opposing Z-plasty for correction of stenotic nares in a horse. *J Am Vet Med Assoc* 1982; **180**: 772.
19. Barnett KC, Crispin SM, Lavach JD, *et al.* Ocular and adnexal emergencies and trauma. In: Barnett KC, Crispin SM, Lavach JD, Matthews AG (eds). *Equine Ophthalmology*, 2nd edn. Saunders: Philadelphia, 2004: 36.
20. Mowat F, Bartoe JT. Adnexal surgery. In: Auer JA, Stick JA (eds). *Equine Surgery*, 4th edn. Elsevier Saunders: St Louis, 2012: 744.
21. Personal Communication. Dr. Mary Lassaline, 2015.
22. de Linde Henriksen M, Plummer CE, Brook DE. Modified Kuhnt–Szymanowski surgical procedure for secondary cicatricial ectropion in a horse. *J Vet Ophthal* 2012; **16**: 276.
23. Giuliano EA, Equine ocular adnexal and nasolacrimal disease. In: Barnett KC, Crispin SM, Lavach JD, Matthews AG (eds). *Equine Ophthalmology*, 2nd edn. Saunders: Philadelphia, 2004: 133.
24. Van der Woerdt A. Adnexal surgery in dog and cats. *J Vet Ophthalmol* 2004; **7**: 284.
25. Howard RD, Stashak TS. Reconstructive surgery of selected injuries of the head. *Vet Clin Equine Pract* 1993; **9**: 185.
26. Massoni S, Vlaminck LE, Cokelaere SM, *et al.* Surgical correction of ear curling caused by scar tissue formation in a horse. *J Am Vet Med Assoc* 2005; **227**: 1130.
27. Hendrickson DA. Management of deep and chronic wounds. In: Auer JA, Stick JA (eds). *Equine Surgery*, 4th edn. Elsevier Saunders: St Louis, 2012: 317.
28. Hillmann DJ. Equine osteology. In: Getty R (ed). *Sisson and Grossman's, The Anatomy of the Domestic Animals*, 5th edn. WB Saunders: Philadelphia, 1975: 255.
29. Tremaine H. Management of skull fractures in the horse. *In Pract* 2004; **26**: 214.
30. Pham TV, Early SV, Park SS. Surgery of the auricle. *Facial Plast Surg* 2003; **19**: 53.
31. Caron JP, Barber SM, Bailey JV, *et al.* Periorbital skull fractures in five horses. *J Am Vet Med Assoc* 1986; **188**: 280.
32. Cruz AM, Barber SM, Grahn BH. Nasolacrimal duct injury following periorbital trauma with concurrent retinal choroidal detachment in a horse. *Equine Pract* 1997; **19**: 20.
33. Auer JA. Craniomaxillofacial disorders. In: Auer JA, Stick JA (eds). *Equine Surgery*, 4th edn. Elsevier Saunders: St Louis, 2012: 1456.
34. Burba DJ, Collier MA. T-plate repair of fractures of the nasal bones in horses. *J Am Vet Med Assoc* 1991; **199**: 909.
35. Dowling BA, Dart AJ, Trope G. Surgical repair of skull fractures in four horses using cuttable bone plates. *Austr Vet J* 2001; **79**: 324.
36. Schumacher J, Auer JA, Shamis L. Repair of facial defects with periosteal flaps in two horses. *Vet Surg* 1985; **14**: 235.
37. Martin GS, McIlwraith CW. Repair of a frontal sinus eversion in a horse. *Vet Surg* 1981; **10**: 149.
38. McIlnay TR, Miller SM, Dugan ST. Use of canaliculorhinostomy for repair of nasolacrimal duct obstruction in a horse. *J Am Vet Med Assoc* 2001; **218**: 1323.
39. Blackford JT, Hanselka DV, Heitmann JM, *et al.* Noninvasive technique for reduction of zygomatic process fractures in the horse. *Vet Surg* 1985; **14**: 21.
40. Badylak SF, Park K, Peppas N, *et al.* Marrow-derived cells populate scaffolds composed of xenogeneic extracellular matrix. *Exp Hematol* 2001; **29**: 1310.
41. Bristol DG. Skin grafts and skin flaps in the horse. *Vet Clin N Am Equine Pract* 2005; **21**: 125.
42. Campbell ML, Peyton LC. Muscle flap closure of a frontocutaneous fistula in a horse. *Vet Surg* 1984; **13**: 185.
43. Madison JB, Donawick WJ, Johnston DE, *et al.* The use of skin expansion to repair cosmetic defects in animals. *Vet Surg* 1989; **18**: 15.
44. Waldridge BM, Bradley DM, Scardino MS, *et al.* Repair of a sinocutaneous fistula in a horse using a mucosal-lined myocutaneous transposition flap. *Equine Pract* 1997; **19**: 7.

CHAPTER 12

Management of Wounds of the Neck and Body

Spencer Barber, DVM, Diplomate ACVS

Chapter Contents

Summary

Most wounds of the body and/or neck heal well; consequently, horses with a neck or body wound have an excellent prognosis for return to full function when the wound does not involve structures underlying the skin. Second-intention healing is often the most appropriate method of managing wounds of the body and/or neck, but some wounds with a large skin flap or lacerated muscle heal faster and more cosmetically after they are completely or partially sutured. If the horse has extensive muscle loss, especially from the forearm or thigh, surgical reconstruction of the remaining muscle and skin may be required to minimize the amount of function lost. Some wounds, especially those in the axilla, thorax, or abdomen, have life-threatening implications (e.g., pneumothorax and evisceration) that require immediate surgical intervention. Horses with wounds of the esophagus and trachea can be difficult to manage. The presence of foreign bodies in wounds of the body and neck can be a diagnostic challenge, and good surgical planning is required to find and remove them.

Introduction

A wide variety of wounds involving the neck and body are encountered in horses, and many of the factors contributing to the high incidence of these injuries are related to the nature and the use of the horse. As a "flight" animal, the horse often reacts to frightening circumstances by running into objects (e.g., a wooden post or fence, barbed wire). Additionally, horses housed on premises that are not properly maintained (e.g., protruding nails, broken boards, broken tin sheds) are at a greater risk of injury. Because the horse's skin is relatively thin, impact with objects commonly leads to large skin wounds. Although most wounds of the neck and body are superficial, some wounds involve structures underlying the skin. It is therefore important for the attending veterinarian to be familiar with the anatomy of deeper structures, particular in the thoracic and abdominal regions. Moreover, understanding the biology of wound repair, as well as possessing a sound knowledge of the principles of wound management and the factors that affect healing, facilitates the management of wounds involving the neck and the body.

Equine Wound Management, Third Edition. Edited by Christine Theoret and Jim Schumacher.

Companion website: www.wiley.com/go/theoret/wound

Wounds of the neck

Lacerations

Lacerations to the neck are especially common when horses are placed in pastures fenced with barbed wire. Injury occurs when the horse runs into the fence, causing a horizontal laceration that is usually located at the base of the neck. The skin edges retract as a result of the elastic fibers in skin, the normal skin tension lines,[1] and the natural movement of the neck.

Lacerations caused by wire often involve only the skin and subcutaneous tissue and are characterized by minimally retracted, relatively sharp edges, but if the laceration extends deeper, and especially deep into the *brachiocephalicus*, *sternocephalicus*, and *sternothyrohyoideus* muscles, the edges of skin and muscle retract a considerable distance. If the injury is caused by contact with a wooden object (e.g., a tree branch or fence), the wound edges are often ragged, irregular in depth, and highly contaminated.

Treatment options include primary closure, delayed closure, and second-intention healing. Many factors must be considered prior to selecting the most appropriate treatment, and these are discussed in Chapter 8 of this book. Horses with a wound of the neck are usually presented in a timely fashion, and the wound is often minimally contaminated and has sharp edges with viable tissue. Although the tension produced by closing the wound and that produced by movement of the head and neck may cause dehiscence of the suture line, primary closure is the ideal treatment in many cases, although suturing is not always required.

A narrow wound (0.5–3 cm wound gap) can usually be closed successfully, in the standing horse, without creating excessive tension on the suture line. Lacerations of the neck caused by wire do not usually involve underlying muscle, but if they do, the muscle is often lacerated only superficially and does not require closure. The subcutaneous tissue and skin are closed in one or two layers using an interrupted suture pattern. In some cases, the number of small wounds is so great that primary closure would be impractical and cost-prohibitive; such wounds usually heal uneventfully by second intention. With intermediate-sized lacerations (10–15 cm wound gap), tension suture patterns (e.g., widely placed vertical or horizontal mattress or near–far–far–near), with or without the use of stents/supports, might be needed to counteract the tension created on the skin by closure (Figure 12.1). Stents/supports can cause skin necrosis if the sutures are applied too tightly or too close to the wound's edges (more information on tension suture patterns can be found in Chapter 9 of this book). Wounds that are parallel to the long axis of the neck, especially those accompanied by a skin flap, are best managed by primary closure because skin tension is minimal and closure of the skin defect maintains the skin in position for rapid and cosmetic healing (Figure 12.2). Wounds that are several days old require more extensive debridement and often are more difficult to close because of loss of pliability of the skin edges. Because these intermediate-sized wounds usually provide a cosmetically acceptable outcome when left to heal by second intention, many clients opt for this approach, over primary closure.

Fortunately, large wounds (wound gap greater than 15 cm), or those with complete transection of the *brachiocephalicus* or *sternocephalicus* muscles, are uncommon (Figure 12.3a,b). Horses with such wounds are usually treated by primary or delayed closure of the wound, if possible, because second-intention healing is often protracted and labor intensive and because unsutured wounds can result in significant scarring and loss of

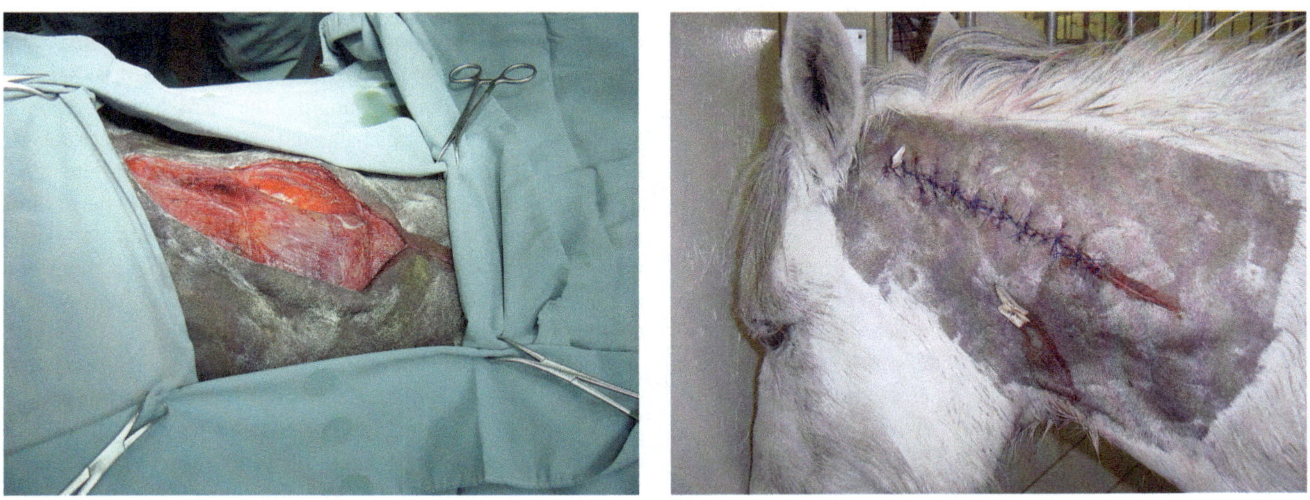

(a) (b)

Figure 12.1 This type of wound is expected to heal well by second intention but also could be treated successfully by primary closure. **(a)** This is a linear laceration parallel to the long axis of the neck. The wound was fresh, clean, and although the edges gaped moderately, they could be apposed without creating excessive tension on the skin. **(b)** After debridement and irrigation, the wound was closed in two layers: the skin closure consisted of simple interrupted sutures and near-and-far tension sutures. A Penrose drain was placed subcutaneously with one of its ends exiting ventral to the incision. The caudal portion of the incision was left open to enhance drainage.

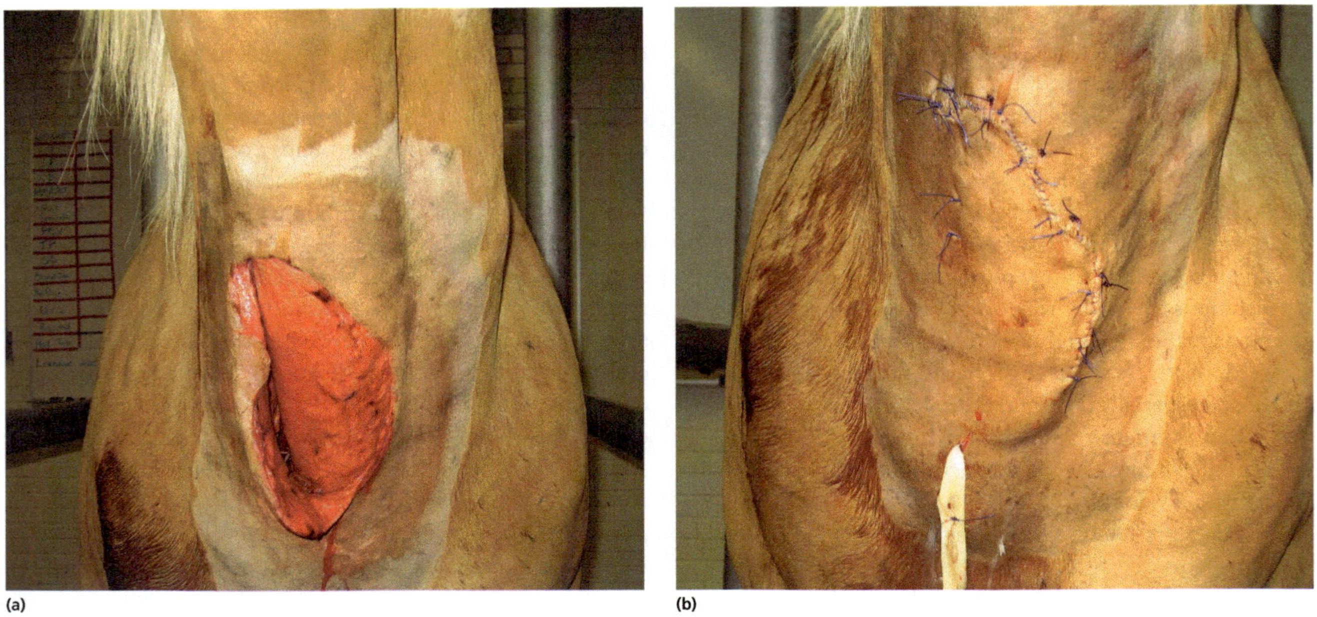

Figure 12.2 **(a)** This laceration, parallel to the long axis of the neck, resulted in a large skin flap based over the right jugular groove. The laceration was fresh and clean, and the edges could be apposed without creating excessive tension on the skin. **(b)** After debriding the wound, a Penrose drain was placed to encourage drainage of the dead space, with its exit point located ventral to the wound. The subcutaneous tissue was closed using interrupted segments of a simple continuous suture pattern. The skin was closed using several horizontal mattress tension sutures interspersed with interrupted segments of a simple continuous suture pattern.

function. If, in the standing horse, wound edges can be approximated without generating excessive tension, prognosis for primary-intention healing is good as long as the horse is cooperative; horses that accept the use of a Martingale to limit head elevation are the best candidates for primary closure. Surgical repair of large wounds should be undertaken with the horse under general anesthesia to ensure optimal debridement and primary closure. Thorough, layered (excisional) debridement of the entire wound is important and is discussed in Chapters 4 and 8.

If either the *brachiocephalicus* or *sternocephalicus* muscle is completely transected (Figure 12.3b,c), its ends should be approximated using a tension suture pattern, incorporating as much fascia as possible. The use of a drain is necessary because dead space is inevitable. Penrose drains are inexpensive, easy to place, and provide good passive drainage (Figure 12.3d). Most commonly, they are used as a single-exit drain, whereby the proximal end is sutured within the depth of the wound and the distal end exits through a skin opening ventral to the wound. With a double-exit technique, one end of the drain exits dorsal to the wound and the other, ventral to the wound. The advantage to the double-exit technique in the ventral aspect of the neck is that drainage occurs regardless of whether the neck is flexed, extended, or in a neutral position. The Penrose drains are generally removed after 2–3 days, provided drainage is minimal, but can be retained for 5–7 days if drainage persists. Importantly, the longer the drains are left in place the greater is the risk of ascending infection; thus, sterility at the exit sites of drains should be maintained. More information on the use of drains in wound management can be found in Chapter 9 of this book.

A stent bandage may be placed to protect the exit site(s) of the Penrose drain from contamination and the sutures from excessive tension (Figure 12.3d). For the stent bandage to effectively protect the skin closure sutures from tension, the lacing material (e.g., umbilical tape) must be pulled tightly enough to transfer tension on to the loops of suture securing the stent bandage to the surrounding skin; this will produce some discomfort for the conscious horse, thereby also discouraging head movement. The use of a Martingale is also advised. When the wound dressing requires changing, the stent bandage can be loosened and the dressing changed with the horse sedated. Anti-inflammatory drugs may be used during the first postoperative week, although some tenderness at the wound site helps limit head extension. Moreover, a robust acute inflammatory response is essential to wound healing; consequently, unless the horse displays serious discomfort, it is best to avoid administering a NSAID in the first week following wounding.

Wounds involving the crest of the neck are uncommon but occasionally result from impact when the neck is placed beneath a sharp object. A full-thickness cutaneous laceration results in retraction of the skin edges and the formation of a gap between the hair follicles of the mane. The skin edges should be apposed to obtain the best cosmetic outcome for the mane (Figure 12.4).

Wounds of the neck that are not sutured heal by second intention and, therefore, fill with granulation tissue, contract, and epithelialize (Figure 12.5, Figure 12.6). All wounds should be thoroughly debrided and cleansed/irrigated when initially seen

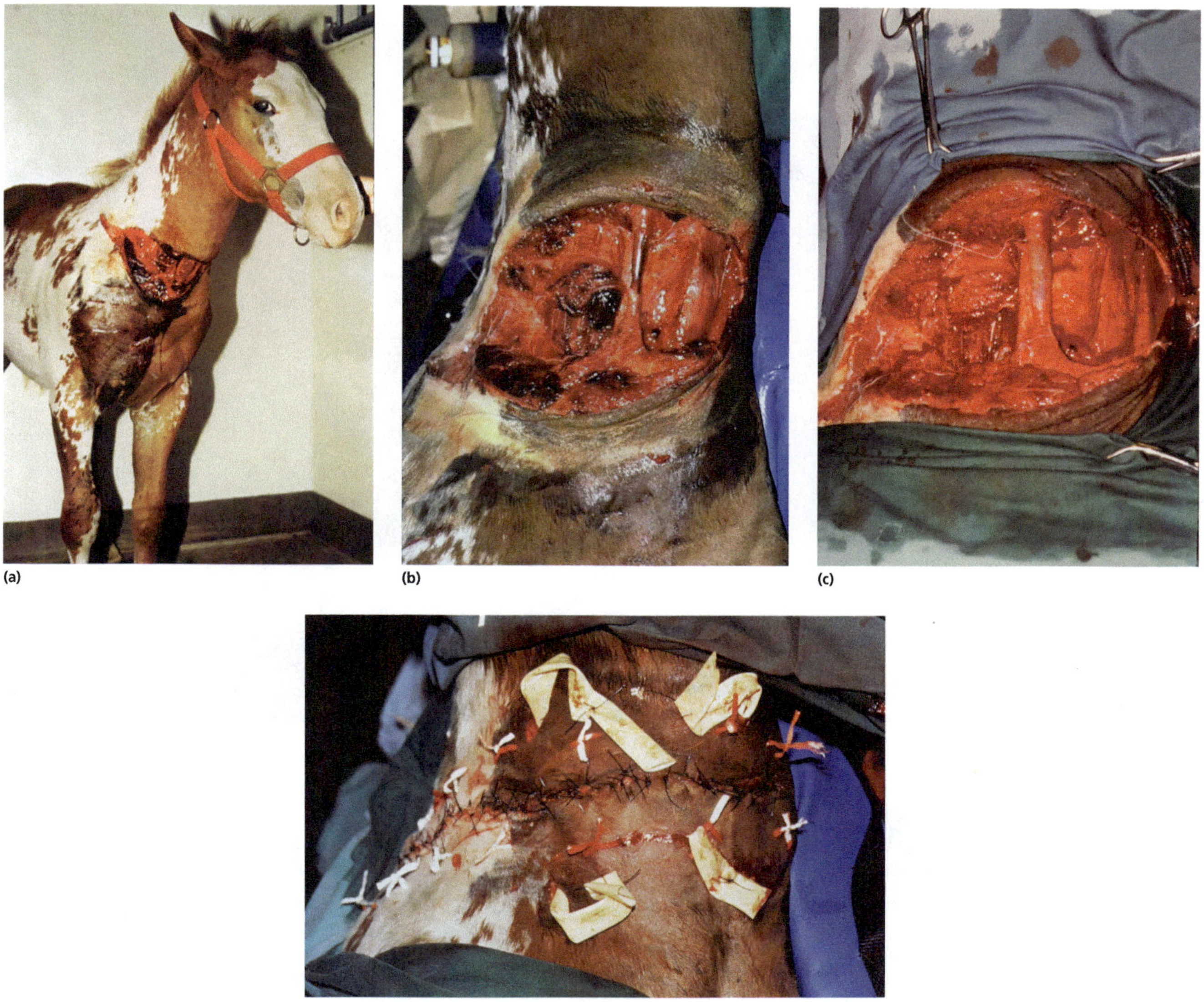

Figure 12.3 **(a)** This foal was presented a few hours after sustaining an extensive laceration caused by barbed wire. The wound appeared clean and fresh, and the skin edges, which were sharply cut, could be easily apposed. **(b)** The foal was positioned in dorsal recumbency, under general anesthesia, for wound reconstruction. The exposed jugular vein was missing much of its perivascular tissue but was judged to be viable. The proximal ends of the transected muscles were retracted beneath the skin edge and the distal ends appeared dark (bottom left of wound). **(c)** Appearance of the wound after debridement in preparation for primary closure. **(d)** Two Penrose drains were placed into the depth of the wound, and their ends exited through slits in the skin proximad and distad to the wound. Care was taken to not place the drains in close proximity to the neurovascular structures. The transected muscles were apposed with a near–far–far–near suture pattern. The jugular vein was covered with viable tissue, and subcutaneous tissue and skin were closed separately using an interrupted suture pattern. Loops of umbilical tape were placed parallel to the skin closure in preparation for a stent bandage.

by the veterinarian. With the aim to encourage filling of the defect with granulation tissue, the author often instructs the owner to spray the wound for 30 minutes with tap water from a garden hose (pressure unknown) once or twice daily. It is speculated that this "hydrotherapy" keeps the wound clean, moist and might stimulate granulation tissue formation through tissue massage or changes to tissue circulation. Although commonly prescribed, it is unclear whether this treatment is helpful or harmful. In fact, wounds in horses irrigated with isotonic saline solution or tap water administered by gentle pressure from a rubber hose showed increased collagen production, a blunted edge to the epithelium, and no enhancement of healing.[2] Because tissue injury is known to cause the release of mediators that stimulate granulation tissue formation, the author advocates hydrotherapy with strong hose pressure, or scraping the surface of the granulation tissue lightly with the fingertips of a gloved hand or with a sterile gauze sponge, once or twice daily, to produce light surface bleeding. This treatment is continued until the surface of the granulation tissue is level with the surrounding skin. Although bandages have been shown to enhance the formation

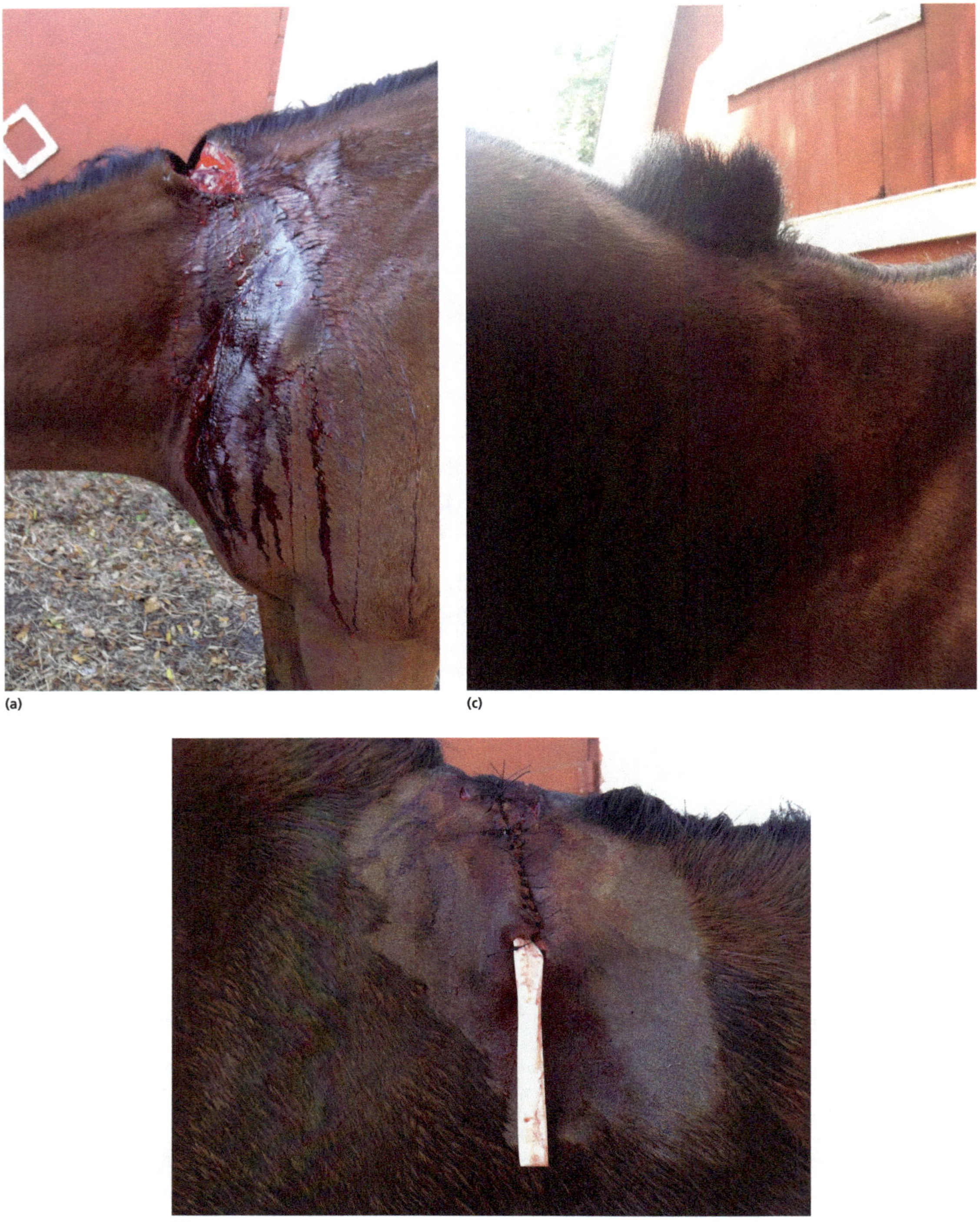

Figure 12.4 (a) This laceration resulted in complete transection of the skin on the dorsal surface of the neck and retraction of the skin edges, which contain the hair follicles for the mane. Fortunately there was no damage to the nuchal ligament. Primary closure of this wound is preferred as it would closely approximate the skin edges containing the hair follicles, whereas leaving the wound to heal by second intention would likely result in a scar devoid of hair follicles, which would produce a noticeable gap in the mane. (b) The wound, which was fresh and clean, was debrided, and a Penrose drain placed within its cavity. To relieve the tension resulting from primary closure, the soft tissues surrounding the wound were undermined, and a few tension-relieving incisions were placed in the skin near the mane. Interrupted tension (vertical mattress) and simple interrupted suture patterns were used to close the skin. (c) Several months after repair, the wound had healed well, with no gap in hair growth noticed along the mane. Courtesy of Suzanne Mund.

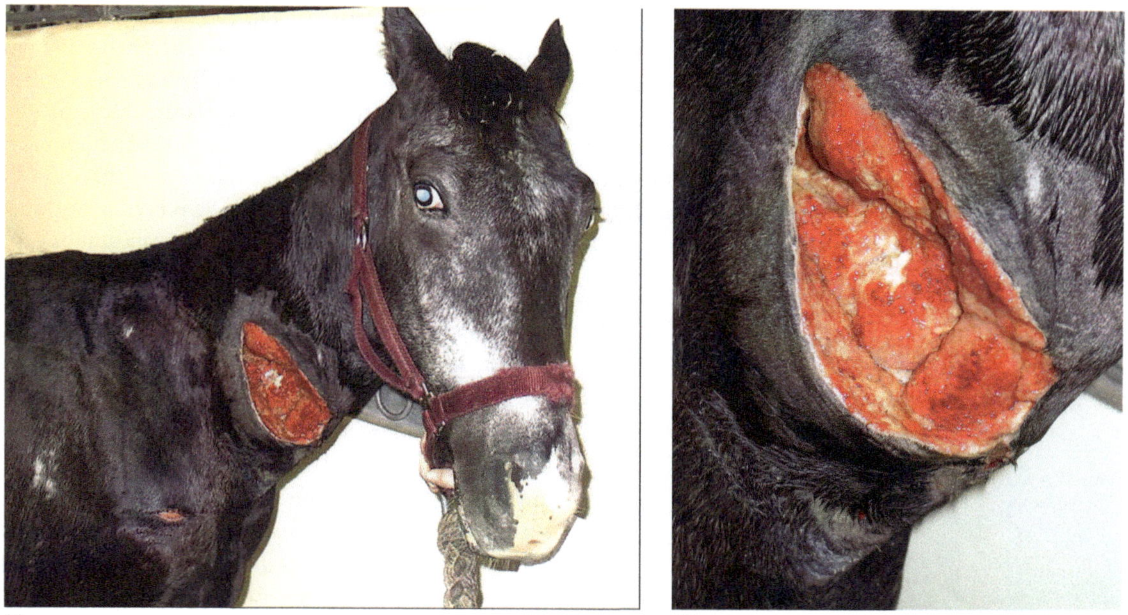

(a) (b)

Figure 12.5 **(a)** A wound of the neck, presented a week after injury, healing by second intention. **(b)** The wound cavity should be encouraged to fill with granulation tissue for wound contraction to proceed rapidly and to a maximum extent, to produce cosmetic healing.

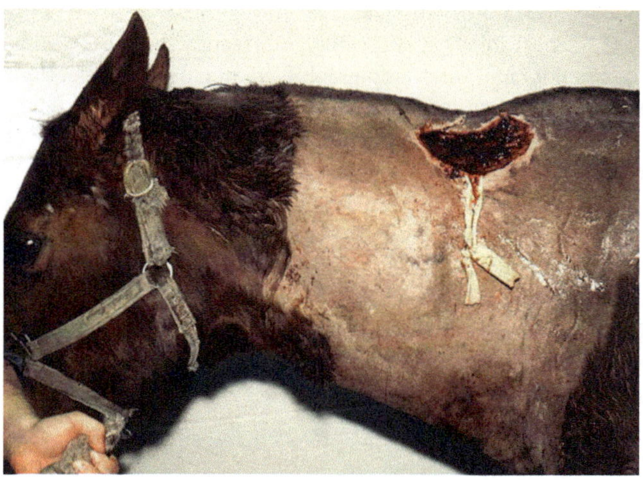

Figure 12.6 This gelding was attacked by a stallion and suffered bilateral bite wounds to the dorsolateral aspect of the neck. Because of tissue loss, the wounds could not be closed without creating undue tension. A Penrose drain was placed within the wound cavity to ensure good ventral drainage from the dorsally located wound. The blemish, after healing, was minimal.

of granulation tissue, many body wounds, including those in the neck area, are difficult to bandage.[3] A topical wound-care product may be applied in the absence of a dressing to keep the wound surface moist (the reader is referred to Chapter 5 for more information on topical wound-care products and the benefits of moist wound healing). The author stops all treatment when the surface of the granulation tissue filling the wound bed is level with the surrounding skin. Most horses with a laceration to the neck, except those with major muscle or skin loss, are expected to return to normal use with a minimal blemish.

What to do

- Large wounds and those extending through the dermis underlying the mane should be sutured, if possible.
- Only horses that tolerate a Martingale should have their wound managed by primary closure if restricted neck movement is expected to be necessary postoperatively to ensure healing by primary closure without dehiscence.

Injuries of vessels and nerves

Laceration to the cranial region of the neck has the potential to damage important neurovascular structures, including the jugular vein, common carotid artery, recurrent laryngeal nerve, and vagosympathetic trunk (Figure 12.3b,c). Of these structures, the jugular vein is the most superficial. Fortunately, it is protected within the jugular groove formed by the *sternocephalicus* and *brachiocephalicus* muscles. The jugular vein may, however, be transected along with these muscles, resulting in severe hemorrhage. More commonly, perivascular tissue is stripped away from the intact vessel, which becomes ischemic, leading to delayed rupture. Deeper wounds may affect the carotid artery, whose complete laceration results in rapid exsanguination and death. If at all possible, viable soft tissue should be used to cover an exposed vessel to protect its wall from desiccation and further trauma. Horses can survive with a single jugular vein and a single carotid artery, so, if the integrity of one or both of these vessels is of concern, the vessel should be ligated prophylactically.[4]

The recurrent laryngeal nerve and vagosympathetic trunk are most likely to be injured in wounds of the lower cervical region, where they are no longer covered by the *omohyoideus* muscle and, consequently, are more superficial. Endoscopic examination of the larynx allows evaluation of arytenoid abduction, which depends on innervation by the recurrent laryngeal nerve. Numerous clinical signs accompany damage to the vagosympathetic trunk, including abnormal intestinal motility, colic, alteration in heart rate, abnormal esophageal function, sweating, and changes in skin temperature. If the carotid artery or jugular vein must be prophylactically ligated, as mentioned previously, care must be taken to prevent injury to these nerves when performing the procedure.

What to do

- Cover exposed vessels or nerves with viable soft tissue, if possible, or with a moist dressing.

Tip

- Prophylactically ligate vessels that appear non-viable or seem to be developing an aneurism.

Injuries of the trachea

The superficial location of the trachea predisposes it to various types of injury. It is located on the midline throughout the length of the ventral surface of the neck; the common carotid arteries, recurrent laryngeal nerves, and vagosympathetic trunks lie on its dorsolateral surfaces (Figure 12.7). The esophagus lies dorsal to the trachea in the proximal portion of the neck, to its left at the mid-cervical region, and ventral to it at the base of the neck. The trachea is covered with musculature throughout the entire cervical region, and this musculature is especially thick in the caudal aspect of the neck. In the cranial cervical region, the trachea is more susceptible to injury because the left and right *sternocephalicus* muscles diverge in this region, leaving the trachea more exposed.[5] The trachea is a flexible tube composed of cartilaginous rings that are incomplete dorsally where they are bridged by the dorsal tracheal ligament. Although the trachea may be lacerated, its rigid structure makes it more susceptible to damage by crushing, such as that caused by a kick, rope pressure, or impact with a solid object, or by puncture from internal or external forces (e.g., endotracheal tube).

The tracheal mucosa, cartilaginous rings, dorsal tracheal ligament, and/or annular tracheal ligaments may be traumatized. The most common clinical signs of tracheal damage are subcutaneous emphysema and changes to the respiratory rate and sounds. External examination of the trachea through an open wound may be difficult if the wound is small, or if the site of injury is swollen or tender. A hole into the tracheal lumen allows air to escape from the trachea, possibly into the surrounding subcutaneous tissue. This may lead to extensive subcutaneous emphysema if the skin wound is small, but if the skin wound is large, emphysema may be minimal or absent. If cartilaginous rings or the dorsal tracheal ligament become invaginated into the tracheal lumen, increased inspiratory and expiratory noises are heard over the site of injury; marked obstruction causes an elevated heart rate and, occasionally, respiratory distress.

If tracheal injury is suspected, the trachea should be examined radiographically. Radiographic examination may identify a narrowed lumen, intraluminal masses, peritracheal air, pneumomediastinum, or pneumothorax. Endoscopic examination of the trachea is useful to assess luminal integrity.

Treatment depends on the structures involved and the severity of the injury. Full-thickness tears of the tracheal wall, with only minimal or no accompanying subcutaneous emphysema, may heal without treatment. In this case, second-intention healing can be assisted by confining the horse to a

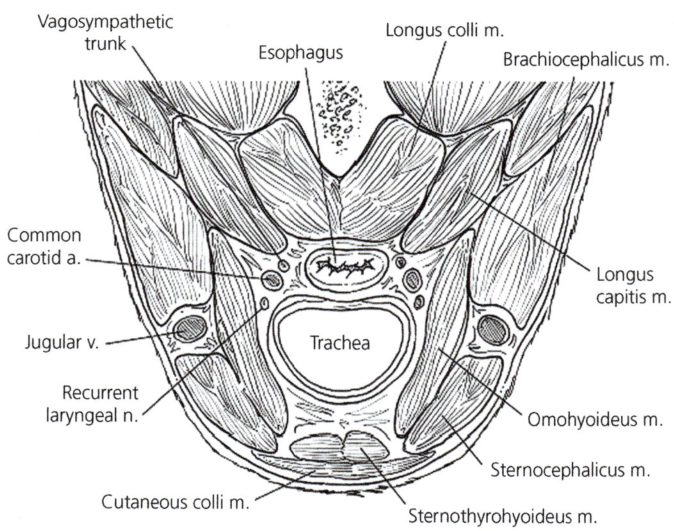

Figure 12.7 Drawing of the cross-sectional anatomy of the proximal aspect of the cervical region of the horse, showing the location of the esophagus, trachea, overlying musculature, and neurovascular structures. Lacerations to the cranial aspect of the neck could cause injury to these structures.

stall and by applying a pressure bandage over the injured area. If subcutaneous emphysema is extensive but the skin over the wounded trachea is intact, a horse with a tracheal wound may be treated in one of three ways: (1) the skin and soft tissue over the tracheal defect may be incised to release trapped air and prevent more air from becoming trapped in the subcutaneous tissue; (2) a tracheotomy may be performed adjacent to the defect; or (3) the tracheal defect may be sutured if adequate tissue is available for primary closure. With the first two approaches, all the wounds are allowed to heal by second intention. An attempt should be made to close the tracheal defect if the dorsal tracheal ligament or extraluminal connective tissue has prolapsed into the tracheal lumen.

Rarely is the trachea transected completely, and rarely is the tracheal defect large. A large defect or complete transection is an emergency because it causes severe respiratory compromise. Severed or nearly severed tracheas of horses have been repaired successfully by primary closure. Absorbable suture material (e.g., size 2 polydioxanone) rather than stainless steel suture (25–30 gauge) should be used, because steel sutures tend to cut through the cartilaginous rings and damage the soft tissues. Penetration of the tracheal mucosa with the suture material should be avoided.

Broken tracheal rings may project into the tracheal lumen thereby obstructing airflow. If the trachea is not collapsing, the portions of the ring protruding into the lumen may be excised through the original wound or through an incision over the damaged tracheal rings, and the tracheal and skin wounds allowed to heal by second intention, or, if several tracheal rings are ruptured at the ventral aspect of the trachea, a permanent tracheostomy may be performed.[6–8] Conversely, if the trachea is collapsing, each collapsing ring should be supported by suturing a polypropylene hoop to it. Horses with a severely damaged section of trachea have been treated successfully by resection of the damaged section followed by anastomosis.[9] The site of anastomosis is subject to excessive tension if more than four or five tracheal rings are removed. Applying a Martingale to the horse decreases tension at the site of anastomosis. If resection and anastomosis are not performed as an emergency procedure, conditioning the horse before surgery to tolerate the Martingale is helpful.[9] Overall, the vast majority of tracheal wounds heal uneventfully, by second-intention healing, with proper treatment.

Tips

- Tracheal injury should be suspected in any horse with cervical trauma accompanied by increased respiratory noise or subcutaneous emphysema.
- Endoscopic and radiograph examinations are indicated if tracheal injury is suspected.
- Intraluminal masses, such as torn cartilaginous rings, must be removed for healing to proceed properly.

Injuries of the esophagus

The esophagus can suffer either intraluminal damage, when feed or a foreign body becomes impacted within its lumen, or extraluminal damage, from impact with a sharp or blunt object. This section focuses on the clinical signs, diagnostic procedures, and treatment options when the esophagus suffers damage from impact with a sharp or blunt object.

Anatomic considerations

The cervical portion of the esophagus, that portion most often traumatized, is well protected from external trauma proximally because of its location dorsal to the trachea. Its location lateral to the trachea in the mid-cervical region and ventral to the trachea in the lower cervical region, however, leave it vulnerable to damage from blows or lacerations. Adjacent to the esophagus are the recurrent laryngeal nerves, vagosympathetic trunks, and common carotid arteries, which may also be injured (Figure 12.7). The esophagus is lined by abundant mucosa arranged in longitudinal folds that allow the esophagus to dilate. The mucosa and submucosa possess the greatest amount of collagen and, therefore, are the strongest layers for surgical closure. In the cervical portion of the esophagus there are two layers of striated muscle covered by a *tunica adventitia*.[10]

Clinical signs

Clinical signs displayed by a horse with a damaged esophagus depend on the nature of the injury. Rupture of the esophageal musculature from blunt trauma produces a pulsion diverticulum, which may cause a discrete swelling, the size of which is dependent on the quantity of food and water residing within it. A full-thickness rupture or laceration of the esophageal wall results in discharge of saliva, food, air, and bacteria into the peri-esophageal fascial planes. If the skin is intact, a diffuse, hot, cervical swelling accompanied by subcutaneous emphysema may develop. Crepitus can be detected when the swelling is palpated, and palpation of the swelling may elicit signs of discomfort from the horse. If the skin is open, signs of infection may be less evident, but saliva and food material can be seen exiting the wound (Figure 12.8). In either case, cellulitis is present, and infection gravitates toward the thoracic inlet. Increased respiratory rate and abnormal respiratory sounds suggest that the horse has aspiration pneumonia or that infection has extended into the mediastinum or pleural cavity.[11]

Extension of the injury into the adjacent carotid artery could result in fatal hemorrhage, whereas damage to a recurrent laryngeal nerve causes ipsilateral laryngeal hemiplegia, while injury to the vagosympathetic trunk causes Horner's syndrome. Lacerations of the esophagus lead to the loss of large volumes of saliva, and, without continued intake of food and water, hyponatremia, hypochloremia, metabolic alkalosis, and dehydration ensue.[11]

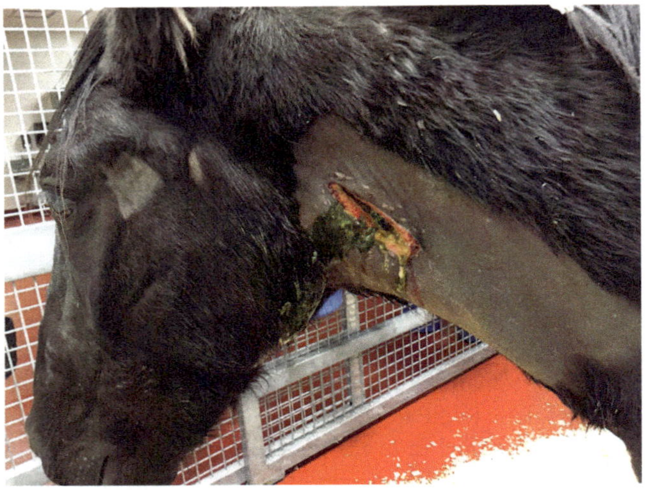

Figure 12.8 Discharge of feed from a ruptured esophagus. Courtesy of Melissa Hines.

Diagnostic considerations

A wound located at a site where the esophagus could be involved in the injury should be examined visually and digitally to determine if the esophagus has been damaged, taking care to avoid injuring adjacent neurovascular structures. A nasogastric tube may be passed to assess the patency and integrity of the esophagus. The nasogastric tube may occasionally travel normally past a pulsion diverticulum or full-thickness esophageal wound, while at other times the tip of the tube may lodge itself within the diverticulum or exit the lumen into the peri-esophageal tissue.

Endoscopic examination, using a flexible, 3-m endoscope capable of irrigation and insufflation, is helpful in identifying an esophageal injury and evaluating its severity. Normal esophageal mucosa is white to light pink, and, except at the most proximal extent of the esophagus, it has longitudinal folds that flatten when the lumen is dilated with air. Saliva or feed present within the lumen should be removed by irrigation to allow a detailed inspection of the esophagus. A pulsion diverticulum appears as an outpouching of the esophageal wall, and a defect in the mucosa is seen if the wound in the esophageal wall is full thickness.[11]

Plain radiographic examination is important even though a normal esophagus is not radiographically visible. With a pulsion diverticulum, gas, food, and saliva mixed together proximal to the obstruction produce an irregular mottled gas shadow or a gas dilation of the proximal extent of the esophagus. Metallic foreign bodies or masses external to the esophagus (e.g., abscess), although rare, may also be identified radiographically. The presence of air outside the esophageal lumen when the skin is intact suggests that the esophageal wall has been ruptured. Conversely, when the skin has been penetrated, the presence of air in the depth of the wound is normal, and contrast radiography is necessary to demonstrate a concomitant luminal defect. A negative contrast radiograph, obtained by passing a cuffed nasogastric tube into the proximal extent of the esophagus and injecting air to dilate the esophagus, helps to identify foreign bodies, a diverticulum, or a full-thickness perforation of the esophagus. A positive-contrast radiograph, obtained by administering barium sulfate paste orally, coats the normal longitudinal folds of the esophagus. Contrast material collects within the lumen of a pulsion diverticulum and is disseminated into peri-esophageal fascial planes if the esophagus is ruptured. A double-contrast study is the method of choice to evaluate mucosal lesions and can be performed by injecting barium sulfate, followed by air, through a cuffed nasogastric tube. The air dilates the esophagus and the barium coats the longitudinal folds. Swallowing while the esophagus is distended may produce peristaltic waves that resemble a stricture; this can be prevented by premedicating with xylazine (Rompun, Bayer Inc.), which attenuates the swallowing reflex.[11]

Tips

- Rupture of the esophagus should be suspected in any horse with trauma to the cranial portion of the neck.
- Endoscopic, and plain and contrast radiographic examinations are valuable diagnostic aids.

Esophageal healing

Constant tension, motion, and dilation, as well as the presence of saliva, food, and bacteria, challenge healing of esophageal wounds. Tissue strength is also limited by the absence of a serosal layer and a scant blood supply, features of a normal intact esophagus. Furthermore, the healed esophagus must be dilatable to function properly. The most common complications during healing are dehiscence and stricture formation, and the long-term rate of survival after esophageal injury is low.[12]

Injuries that cause only destruction of the mucosal epithelium heal without scar formation because of the epithelium's excellent regenerative capabilities.[13] Injury to the submucosal, muscular, or adventitial layers, however, leads to the formation of granulation tissue, which is followed by wound contraction and scar formation.[13]

Experimental studies in horses have shown that a linear esophagostomy can heal without causing a clinically significant stricture.[14] This outcome is likely because the amount of damage produced by an experimentally created incision is minor compared to that accompanying a naturally occurring injury. Because wound contraction is a concern during esophageal healing, circumferential injuries are potentially more serious than linear incisions. Indeed, when 3-cm long esophageal mucosal resections and anastomoses were performed experimentally, mucosal repairs dehisced, and all horses subsequently developed a stricture.[15] Fortunately, the severity of strictures often decreases over time. For example, maximal reduction in luminal diameter was shown in seven horses with an esophageal injury to occur at approximately 30 days after wounding.

The luminal diameter increased spontaneously to normal size in five of these horses by day 60.[16] This increase in diameter was the result of scar remodeling and luminal dilation from eating. These results show that surgical correction of a stricture, unless severe to the point of hindering feeding, should be delayed until at least 60 days post injury since the stricture may resolve spontaneously.

Sutured, experimentally created linear esophagotomies of horses healed faster than non-sutured esophagotomies, and a traction diverticulum was less likely to develop at the site of esophagotomy. Horses in which the esophagotomy was sutured, however, had a higher incidence of complications, including death, because of dehiscence, fistula formation, and/or formation of an abscess at the esophagotomy site.[17] Sutured esophagotomies are more likely to dehisce if a nasogastric tube is retained within the esophageal lumen following repair,[15] and horses fed hay are more likely to experience dehiscence of the sutured esophageal wound than are horses fed a soft diet.[17] Placement of an esophagostomy tube distal (aboral) to a sutured esophagotomy site allows better healing at the repair site, but complications, including thrombophlebitis, thoracic infection, and death, have been reported.[15,18]

Tips

- All esophageal layers, except the mucosa, heal with scar formation, limiting dilation. Therefore, surgical treatment of a horse with an esophageal injury should be avoided, if at all possible.
- Naturally occurring injuries are often circumferential, and contraction of a circumferential wound results in a stricture.
- The luminal diameter of an injured esophagus is maximally reduced by day 30 after injury but may increase spontaneously to near normal by day 60 after injury.

Management of esophageal lacerations and ruptures

Esophageal laceration or puncture is most likely when a wound is located in the lower half of the cervical region, where the esophagus lies more superficially. Ruptures, which can be caused by kicks or penetration with a foreign body, are commonly in the extent of the esophagus and result in the escape of food, saliva, and bacteria into the peri-esophageal tissue (Figure 12.8).[19]

Important considerations in determining the best approach to wound management are the type and extent of damage to the esophageal wall, the age of the injury, the degree of contamination, and the presence of infection or necrosis of the peri-esophageal tissue. Linear lacerations and acute ruptures with minimal esophageal trauma and contamination and with no signs of infection or necrosis may heal successfully following primary closure.

If the esophagus is not visible through the skin wound, it should be exposed through an incision created over the jugular groove or on the ventral midline of the neck. The esophagus is best exposed with the horse anesthetized and in dorsal recumbency. The esophagus is more easily identified if a nasogastric tube has been placed within it. Debridement of esophageal tissue should be conservative in an effort to preserve as much tissue as possible for a subsequent tension-free closure. The mucosa and submucosa are closed in a simple continuous pattern using 3-0 suture material with the knots tied in the lumen, and the muscular layers are closed with an interrupted suture pattern using 2-0 suture material.[11] Because of contamination of the peri-esophageal tissue, tissue superficial to the esophagus can be left to heal by second intention. Mucosal healing takes approximately 7 days,[11] therefore feed should be withheld for several days after suturing, after which water-soaked pellets are fed for a few days before transitioning to small amounts of softened roughage. Alternatively, an esophagostomy tube may be placed either through the esophageal rupture, if it was not sutured, or distal to the repair site. The esophagostomy tube is removed either after the sutured mucosa at the rupture or laceration site has healed or, in non-sutured cases, after a granulation tissue stoma forms at the rupture and esophagostomy sites. These stomas are then left to heal by second intention.[11]

Closure of the esophageal wound should not be attempted if the esophageal wall is extensively damaged. If the skin is intact, feed, saliva, and bacteria become trapped within the fascial planes, resulting in marked cellulitis, which can cause the overlying skin to slough. If the skin does not slough, feed and bacteria dissect ventrally into the mediastinum or pleural cavity. Ventral drainage, therefore, should be established early, and the fascial planes debrided surgically, followed by wound irrigation. An esophagostomy tube placed either through the site of rupture or through an opening created surgically distal to the rupture can be used to provide nutritional support, thereby preventing contamination of peri-esophageal tissue at the site of rupture from leakage of feed ingested orally.[11,19] Loss of food, water, and saliva from the esophageal rupture site may also be prevented by placing a temporary patch of dental acrylic over the hole.[19] Fluid therapy is used to correct hyponatremia, hypochloremia, and metabolic acidosis.[20] Broad-spectrum antibiotics (see Table 19.1), including those effective against anaerobic bacteria, must be administered and continued until the esophageal mucosa is healed or a stoma has formed, thereby preventing ingesta from draining into the subcutaneous tissue.

Esophagostomies have been associated with the development of traction diverticulum, including a mucosal web obstruction from a traction diverticulum, and death.[18,19] Despite the best efforts and care, the horse's prognosis for survival after esophageal rupture remains guarded to poor.[12] Rarely can injuries be successfully repaired. Simple injuries, with good drainage, may heal by second intention with minimal stricture formation, but horses with extensive cellulitis rarely survive.

Tips

- Most esophageal ruptures are best left to heal by second intention.
- Early identification of rupture and establishment of ventral drainage is imperative to reduce the risk of severe infection.
- Management of fluid and electrolyte abnormalities is crucial.

Esophageal strictures

Esophageal strictures are a frequent complication of naturally occurring esophageal trauma, or surgery, because lesions are usually circumferential and because, aside from the mucosal epithelium, esophageal tissue heals by fibroplasia and contraction. A stricture involving only the mucosa and submucosa is termed an esophageal ring or web; one involving only the muscular wall is termed a mural lesion; and one involving all layers of the esophagus is termed an annular stenosis.[11]

Because scar tissue is dynamic and undergoes considerable remodeling, treatment of a horse for an esophageal stricture should be delayed more than 60 days after injury.[16,21] Several techniques have been employed in an effort to resolve an esophageal stricture, including bougienage or balloon dilation, esophagomyotomy, partial resection and anastomosis of the mucosa, complete resection and anastomosis of the esophageal wall, and muscular patch grafting.[11,22] Reports of success using these procedures are few, and complications abound, leading to a low long-term rate of survival.[12]

Wounds of the body

Wounds of the body are common and, in some areas of the world, are primarily caused by contact with barbed wire. Narrow objects (e.g., wire) or sharp objects (e.g., nail, tin) usually cause linear skin lacerations followed by retraction of the wound's edges or production of a skin flap. When a wound is caused by collision with a blunt object (e.g., fence post, rail), the injured tissues suffer greater trauma, and the edges of the wound are less regular. Lacerations extending into the musculature produce multiple dissecting planes, and the cut portion of the muscle retracts. Fortunately, a muscle is rarely transected completely or damaged sufficiently to result in permanent loss of function. The most common sites of injury on the body are the forearm, pectoral region, axilla, medial aspect of the thigh, ventral aspect of the abdomen, and lateral aspect of the thorax.

Many factors must be considered when selecting the most appropriate method of treatment (the reader is referred to Chapter 8 for more information about the various approaches to wound closure). Generally, wounds to the body are less contaminated than those to the distal aspect of the limb and thus possibly more amenable to primary closure. However, complete closure of a wound on the body, while desirable, often is not possible because tissue is lost, retracted, nonviable, or adjacent to other lacerations, or because the wound is located in an area of high motion where protection of the repair from tension is difficult (Figure 12.9). Moreover, a sutured repair of a wound on the body is difficult to protect with a bandage. Fortunately, wounds of the body contract more rapidly and to a greater degree than do wounds of the distal aspect of the limb.[23] Second-intention healing of body wounds, therefore, occurs more rapidly and with fewer complications. Because a body wound can heal by second intention with acceptable cosmetic and functional results, the client often choses this approach over primary closure, which is a more costly alternative, at least initially.

All wounds should be carefully evaluated and thoroughly debrided and cleansed via irrigation, regardless of the treatment ultimately selected (the reader is referred to Chapter 4 for more information about wound evaluation and debridement). The objectives, when managing a wound by second intention healing, are to: (1) stimulate the formation of granulation tissue to fill the wound and produce a smooth surface; and (2) enhance

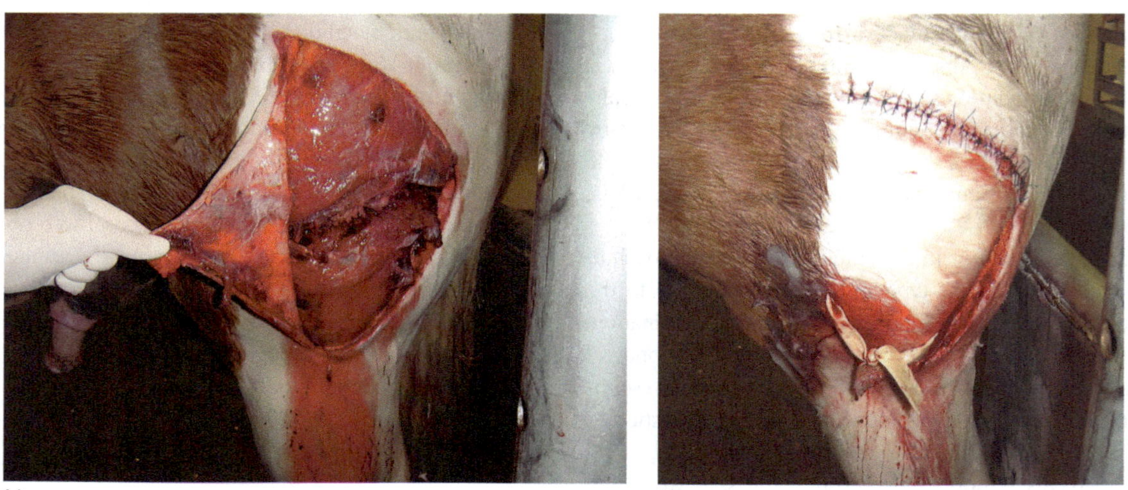

(a) (b)

Figure 12.9 **(a)** This wound was the result of the horse impaling itself on a hinge of a large metal gate. There is a sizable L-shaped skin laceration over the buttocks and a horizontal, 6-cm deep laceration of the *biceps femoris* muscle. **(b)** Partial primary closure was performed. The wound was clean, muscle tissue was minimally frayed, and all except the caudal edge of the skin flap appeared viable. After debridement, a Penrose drain was placed to facilitate drainage. The muscle was not sutured, but the subcutaneous tissue and skin were closed along the dorsal edge of the wound. The caudal edge of the skin flap died and was resected a few days later. The wound healed with minimal blemish.

wound contraction and epithelialization. Granulation tissue contains myofibroblasts required for wound contraction, and a smooth surface produces a superior final appearance once epithelialization has proceeded.

Once the surface of the wound is covered with granulation tissue, the author advocates using "hydrotherapy" or scraping the surface of the granulation tissue with the fingertips of a gloved hand or with a sterile gauze sponge, once or twice daily, to produce light surface bleeding (as described earlier in this chapter in the section on wounds of the neck). This treatment is continued until the granulation tissue has grown to a level that is even with the surrounding skin, to prevent a concavity at the wound site once epithelialization proceeds.

Epithelialization occurs more rapidly in wounds that are bandaged because contamination and desiccation are reduced, and because a bandage provides a warm, moist environment, all of which favor the migration of keratinocytes required for epithelialization. Body wounds often cannot be bandaged, so a topical wound-care product may be applied in an attempt to limit desiccation (the reader is referred to Chapter 5 for more information on topical wound-care products). The author stops all treatments once the granulation tissue is level with the surrounding skin, and allows the wound to continue to heal by second intention without topical wound-care products or bandages (Figure 12.10).

Tip

- Encouraging the formation of granulation tissue within the defect might enhance the rate of contraction and minimize the final blemish.

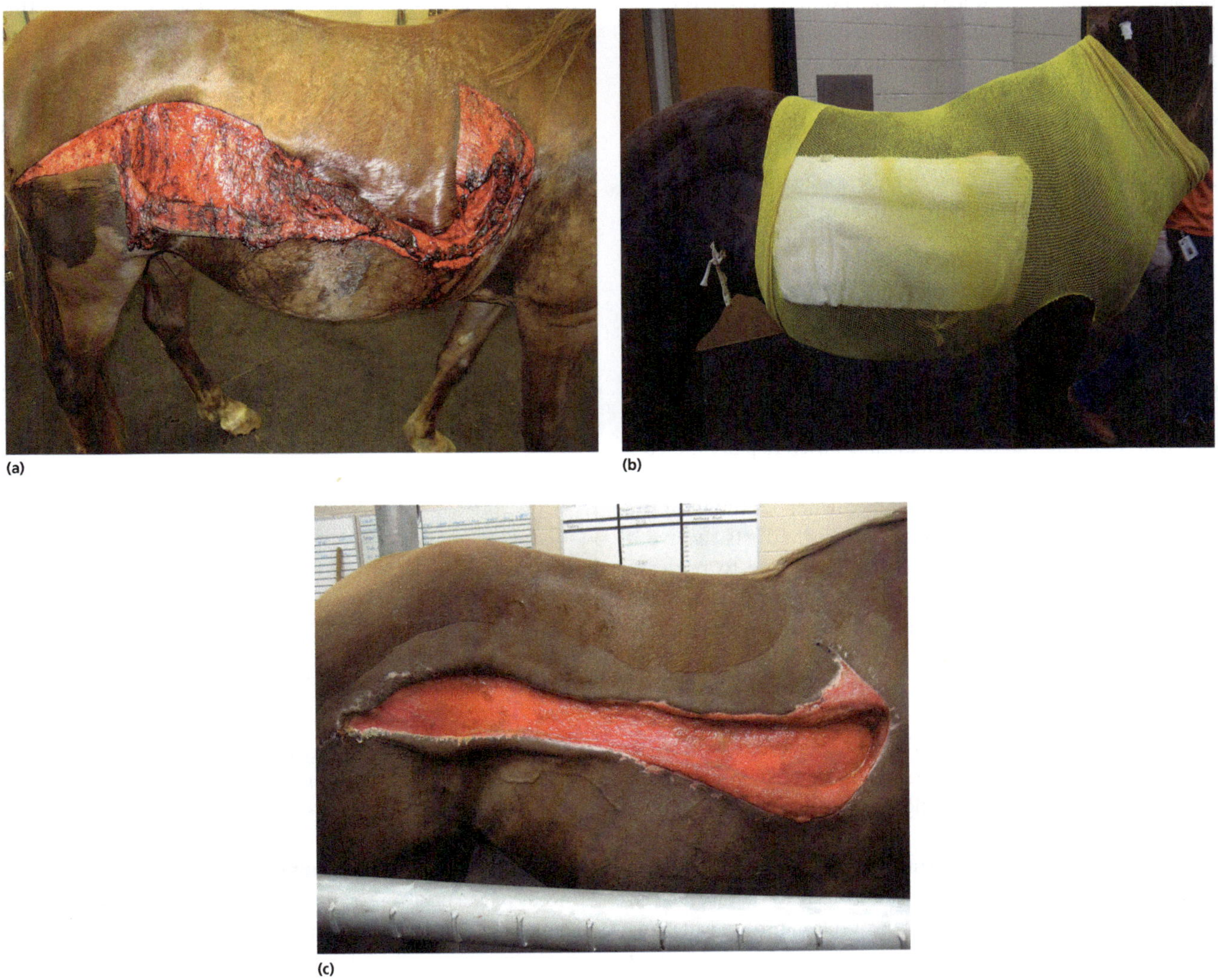

Figure 12.10 **(a)** Laceration of the right hemi-thorax and abdominal wall secondary to a high-speed collision with a metal fence post. The laceration did not enter the thoracic or abdominal cavities. The wound was sutured and bandaged but dehisced in 9 days and developed pyogranulomatous inflammation. **(b)** The wound was extensively debrided and then packed with honey, daily, for 30 days. A self-retaining mesh bandage was used to secure the dressing. **(c)** Seventy-five days after injury the wound contained healthy granulation tissue and was rapidly contracting.

Lacerations of the forearm

Lacerations of the forearm are common, and typically occur at the cranioproximal aspect of the forearm in a horizontal (transverse) plane; the skin edges may retract considerably proximad and distad. Often, only the skin and subcutaneous tissues are lacerated, but the *extensor carpi radialis* muscle and/or the common digital extensor muscle may be lacerated superficially, and a portion of the lacerated muscle may protrude over the distal skin edge (Figure 12.11a).

Horses with a large muscle flap develop considerable swelling of the carpal region and may suffer from loss of extensor function. However, it may be difficult to assess the amount of muscle damage based on stance and lameness, since even horses with a superficial wound are quite sore and advance the limb carefully due to the marked pain that occurs during motion.

Apposing the edges of a wound on a forearm is difficult because of retraction and loss of skin, but most wounds of the forearm heal well by second intention. Any muscle or skin protruding over the ventral border of the wound should be excised (Figure 12.11b). The wound is treated with hydrotherapy twice daily to encourage the formation of granulation tissue, to fill in the wound so it does not heal with a depression (Figure 12.11c). A topical wound-care product may be applied to the wound in an attempt to limit desiccation. Petroleum-based jelly is placed ventral to the wound to prevent serum scald of the skin. The portion of the limb distal to the wound may be bandaged to prevent or reduce swelling, and an analgesic may be administered to the horse for a few days, if lameness is marked.

If the wound is fresh and the tissues can be apposed without creating excessive tension, or if the wound has a large, viable, distally based flap of skin and/or muscle, primary closure may be attempted. The viability of a distally based flap is estimated clinically by its warmth, and whether the flap bleeds when poked with a needle or its edges bleed when trimmed. If the flap is cold and does not bleed when cut, efforts to save it are not worthwhile. Attempts should be made to preserve the flap, however, if it has some warmth or if it bleeds, even slightly, when cut. Although the edge of a distally based flap may eventually die, suturing the skin flap helps preserve some portions of it.

When the wound contains a large flap of extensor muscle (Figure 12.12), the muscle edges should be sutured together to preserve as much muscle as possible and thereby limit loss of extensor function. Sutures should be placed, in an interrupted pattern, within the subcutaneous tissue, when possible. Because of the high tension created by suturing wounds of the forearm, large suture material (e.g., size 1 or 2) and a tension suture pattern should be used in the skin flap. A near–far–far–near pattern is very effective at relieving tension on the sutured flap, and passing the suture material through segments of rubber tubing (stents) dissipates tension on the skin exerted by the suture material (the reader is referred to Chapter 9 for more information on suture materials and suture patterns). Some sloughing of the tip of the flap occurs commonly after closure, so the sutures should not be placed too close to the edges of the skin flap. Even if complete approximation of the skin edges is impossible, sutures retain the flap proximally, thereby minimizing the area of the wound that must heal by second intention.

When the periosteum of the radius is stripped during injury, a sequestrum may develop because nourishment of the cortical bone is compromised and because protection against bacterial contamination has been lost.[24,25] The exposed bone should be cleansed thoroughly via irrigation,[26] and the cortical surface should be debrided ("partially decorticated") with a power-driven burr or bone rasp, down to bleeding or oozing canaliculi, if, after irrigation, the cortex appears dirty or "chalky" (for more information on the management of wounds containing sequestered bone, the reader is referred to Chapter 14). The exposed bone should be covered, if possible, with viable soft tissue or a moist dressing. Penrose drains that exit the skin distal to the wound should be placed before the wound is sutured, if this is required to prevent fluid accumulation in the remaining dead space.

Restricting the horse's movement postoperatively is critical to prevent wound dehiscence. The limb is bandaged with a full-limb, modified Robert Jones bandage with a full-length, caudally positioned splint, and the horse is cross-tied to prevent walking or lying down, or tied to an overhead wire so that it may walk back and forth but not lie down. The bandage and splint are changed every 3–4 days, with the horse sedated, if necessary. The limb is maintained in a bandage and splint for a minimum of 3 weeks, and the sutures are removed at 3 weeks.

Unless there is extensive loss of muscle, the prognosis for return to full function and for a cosmetic result is excellent.

What to do

- Be conservative when debriding large skin or muscle flaps of questionable viability, in order to retain sufficient tissue for primary closure.
- Large wounds to the forearm, with skin and/or muscle flaps, should be managed by primary closure, by suturing as much as possible of the defect.

Tip

- Postoperative restriction of movement is crucial to healing of the primary closure without dehiscence.

Lacerations of the pectoral region

Wounds of the pectoral region are generally oriented in either a transverse or a sagittal plane. Laceration of the underlying musculature is usually minor if the wound is oriented transversely, but the laceration can be quite deep if oriented sagittally. The skin edges do not usually retract much if the wound is oriented transversely, and retraction is even less if the wound is oriented sagittally.

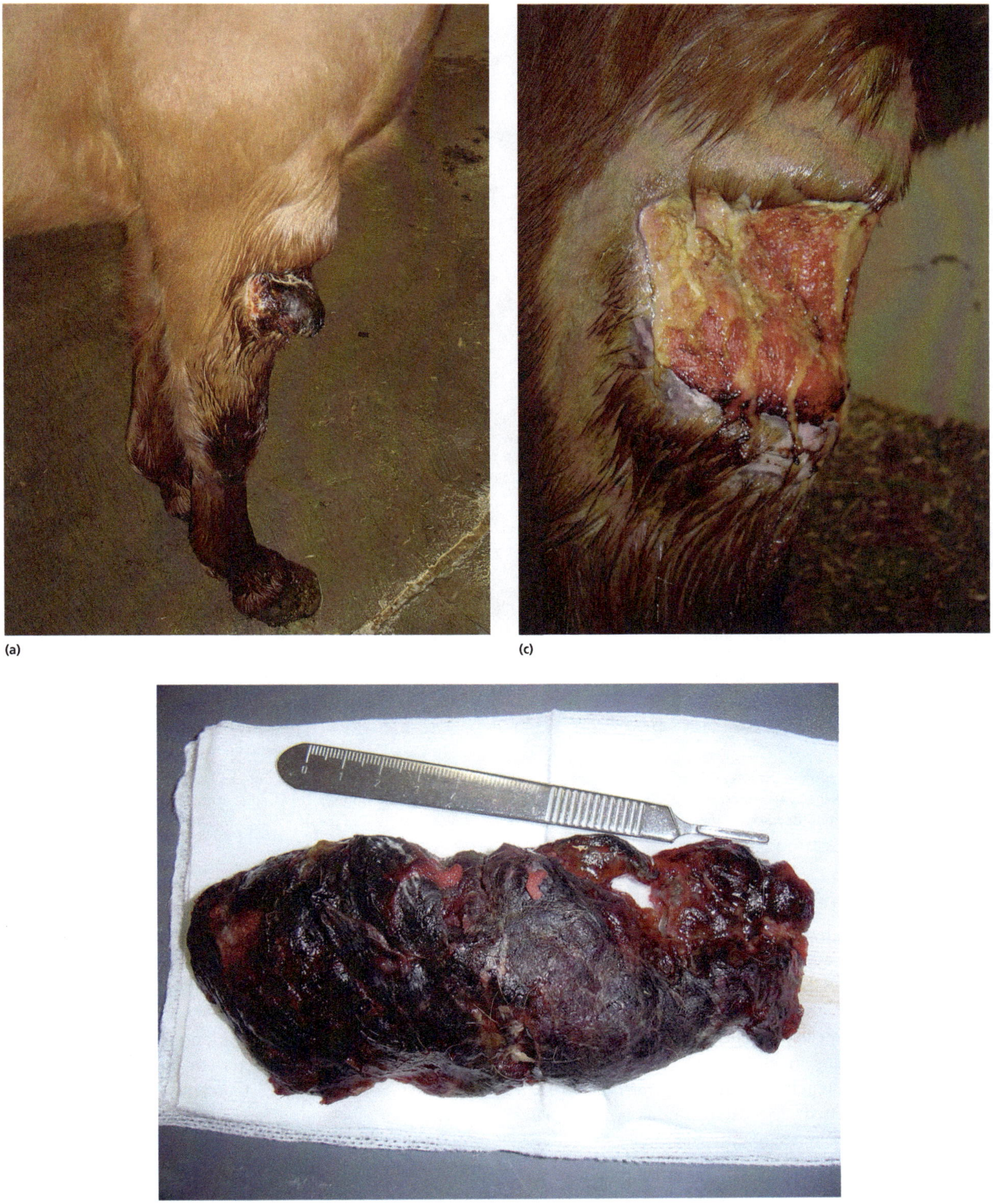

(a) (c) (b)

Figure 12.11 This horizontal laceration of the proximal aspect of the forearm occurred a few days prior to presentation. **(a)** Although the location of this laceration was not unusual, the laceration was deeper than most in this location, and a portion of the common digital extensor muscle protruded over the ventral skin edge. Closure was not possible because the suture line would have been under excessive tension due to movement of the limb. This wound healed well by second intention after the protruding portion of the muscle belly was excised. **(b)** The portion of the muscle belly excised. **(c)** Appearance of the wound 5 days after excision of the protruding lacerated muscle, at which time the wound was filling in with granulation tissue. The wound healed with almost no blemish, and the horse returned to full use.

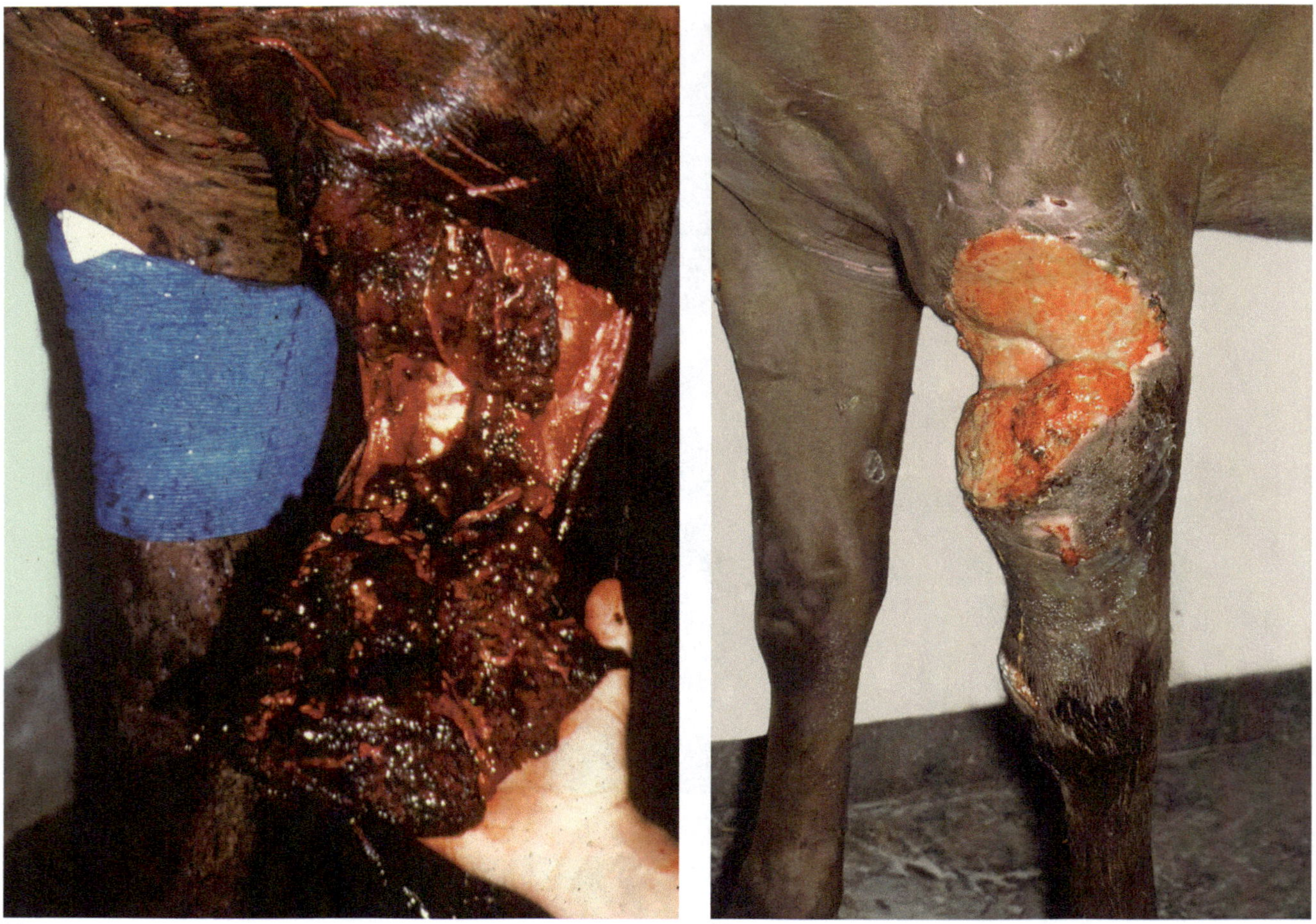

(a) (b)

Figure 12.12 (a) Fresh laceration of the forearm resulting in a large, ventrally based flap composed of skin and muscle. The extensor muscle bellies were deeply lacerated, and their viability was questionable. The radius was exposed (white area in the wound). (b) Despite primary closure and immobilization of the limb with a full-limb modified Robert Jones bandage and a caudally placed splint, a portion of the flap sloughed. The remaining wound healed by second intention, but compromised extensor function ended this horse's athletic career.

A wound to the pectoral region, if superficial and fresh, can often be sutured and heal successfully by primary closure (Figure 12.13). Because most pectoral lacerations in the sagittal plane extend deep into the muscle and are associated with extensive tissue damage, they usually are left unsutured; some, however, can be partially closed to speed healing (Figure 12.14). If a wound is left to heal by second intention, small tags of tissue (either muscular or cutaneous) protruding over the wound margins should be excised. The use of drains is not usually necessary if the wound is not sutured, and exercise need not be restricted. Pectoral wounds heal well by second intention, and loss of function from muscle damage, and production of a substantial blemish, are rare.

Lacerations of the axilla

Lacerations of the axilla are usually short (circa 5–10 cm), but can be longer, and are oriented in the sagittal plane between the pectoral muscles and the forearm. The wound edges gape minimally and the laceration involves a variable amount of muscle (Figure 12.15a). Because these wounds are typically deep, they are usually left to heal by second intention, unless subcutaneous emphysema occurs. Although lacerations of the axilla often seem relatively minor, they occasionally lead to significant complications.[27,28]

The most common complication is subcutaneous emphysema, identified by its characteristic crackling feel, known as crepitus (Figure 12.15b,c). A recently published case series reported that seven out of seven horses with axillary wounds developed subcutaneous emphysema,[28] but in the author's experience, many axillary wounds do not develop this complication. Emphysema occurs when movement of the limb causes a one-way valve effect, drawing air into the wound while it is agape, then forcing the air from the wound cavity into the surrounding tissue planes as the muscles of the limb contract. Emphysema first appears close to the wound's edges but may quickly spread over the entire body, elevating the skin by as much as 5–7 cm. The air trapped in the subcutaneous space can be absorbed within a few days after the

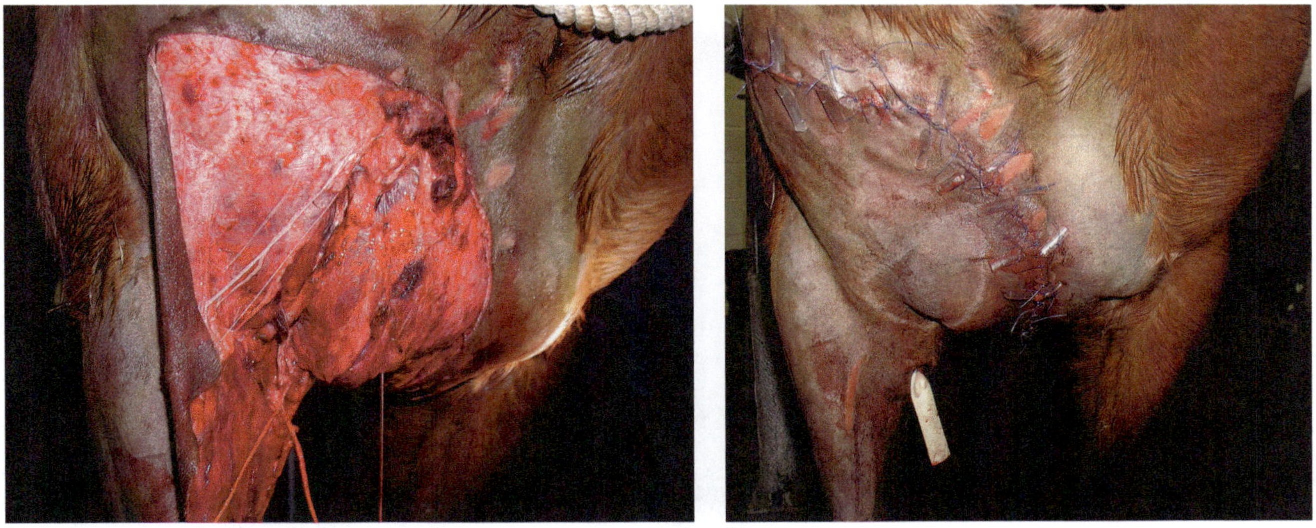

(a) (b)

Figure 12.13 (**a**) Fresh, superficial wound to the pectoral region, creating an L-shaped skin flap. (**b**) The wound edges were easily approximated because there was no tissue loss. However, a tension suture pattern (vertical mattress, with stents) was used in view of the tension that would inevitably arise postoperatively due to swelling and movement. A Penrose drain was placed into the wound and exited distad, to drain any exudate accumulating in the most ventral portion of the subcutaneous pocket caused by the wound. Courtesy of Dr. Sheila Laverty.

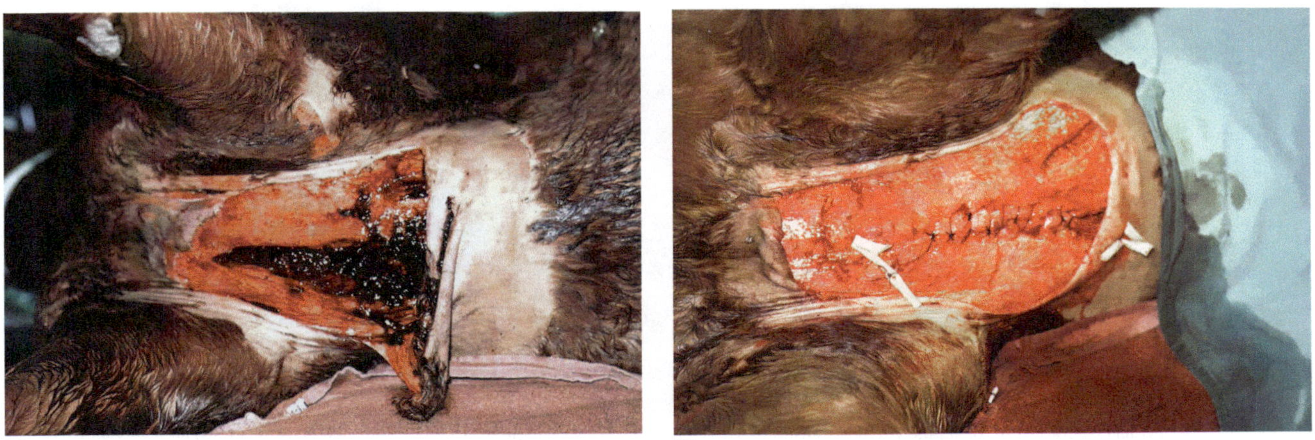

(a) (b)

Figure 12.14 (**a**) Major skin degloving injury of the ventral pectoral region (cranial to the left), including laceration of the *pectoralis* muscle in the sagittal plane. (**b**) The muscular wound was closed, after placing a Penrose drain, because the laceration was fresh, had sharp edges, and muscular trauma was minimal. The skin flap, however, was non-viable and hence was excised.

wound stops acting as a one-way valve. Neither ischemia of the skin overlying the accumulated gas, nor infection from bacteria migrating along subcutaneous fascial planes has been observed by the author. However, pneumomediastinum and pneumothorax were reported to occur commonly in a small cases series.[28] The author has observed emphysema, respiratory difficulty, and sudden death secondary to pneumothorax in association with an axillary wound in only one horse. Horses should be monitored closely for these life-threatening complications, and the thorax of horses that exhibit an elevated respiratory rate or dyspnea, should be examined radiographically for pneumomediastinum and pneumothorax.[27,28]

If the wound is not deep, or is fresh and can be sutured, subcutaneous emphysema is unlikely to develop. If the wound cannot be completely sutured, it should be partially closed then packed with sterile gauze, and the axillary region bandaged, either with a stent bandage or with tape wrapped around the horse's neck and shoulders to hold it in place. The management of a horse with an axillary wound that is left unsutured is more difficult. While packing the wound has been advocated[28] and is a good practice, in the author's experience,

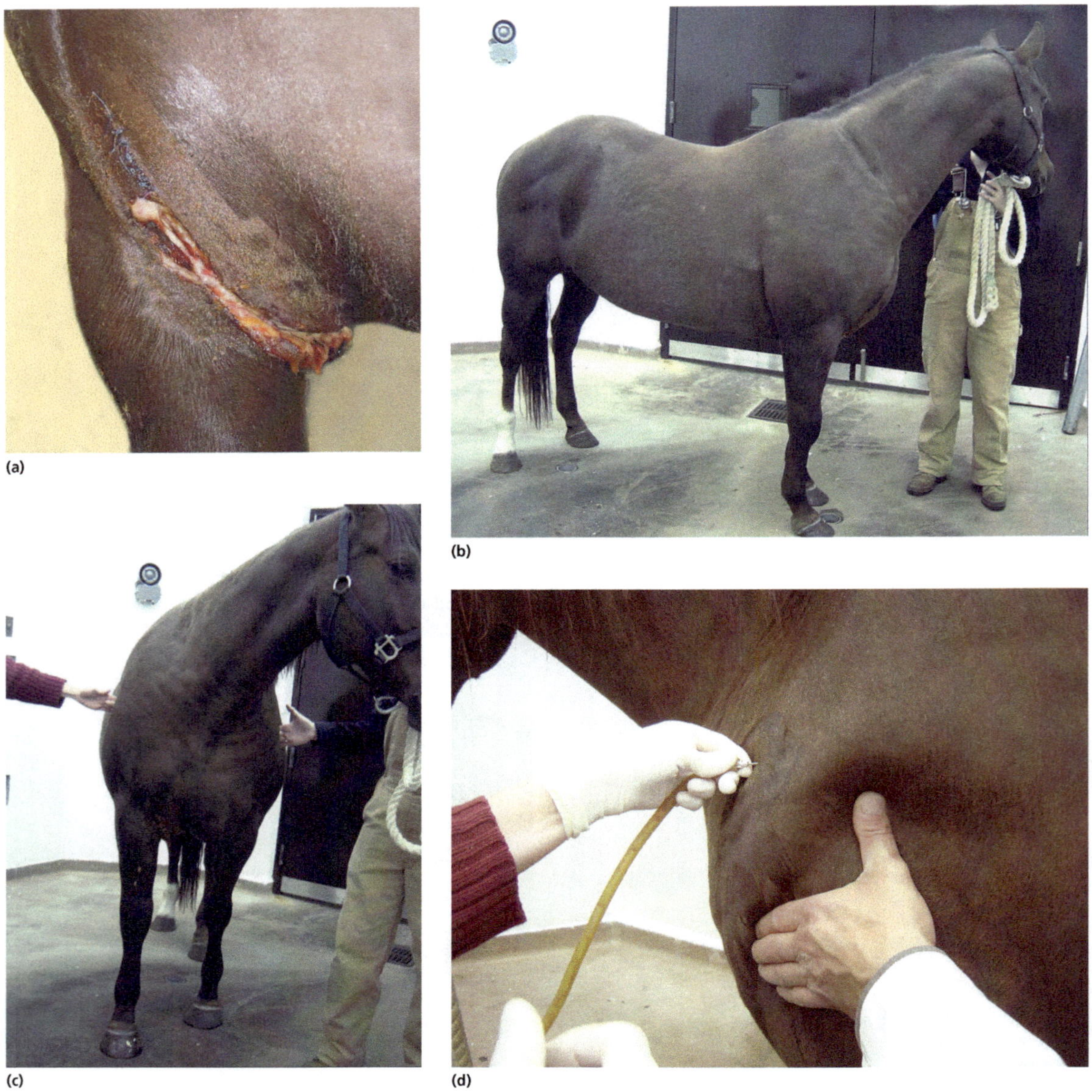

Figure 12.15 **(a)** Typical laceration of the axillary region caused by wire. The wound edges gape minimally, and the wound is not excessively deep. The proximal portion of the wound was partially closed. **(b)** Severe subcutaneous emphysema developed a few days after injury. The emphysema was progressive and extended over the entire body. The horse's vital signs, including respiratory rate and sounds, were normal. **(c)** Notice how far the examiners' fingers can push the skin inward before contacting the musculature. **(d)** Much of the air was removed by aspiration via needles placed in the subcutaneous space. The remaining subcutaneous air was resorbed over the next few days.

packing the opening with bandage material does not always limit the progression of emphysema after it has developed. Debriding the wound and enlarging its opening, on the other hand, can eliminate the valve effect and has been effective in preventing or ameliorating subcutaneous emphysema. Preventing subcutaneous emphysema is not always possible, but all horses should be cross-tied after treatment to limit the pumping action caused by walking.

If subcutaneous emphysema is extensive and progressing, the air may be removed by inserting a hypodermic needle into the subcutaneous space and attaching it to a suction unit (Figure 12.15d). Three to four sites are prepared for aseptic insertion of a needle, desensitized, and the subcutaneous air is "massaged" by the clinician's hands toward the inserted needle. This procedure may be repeated, as required, and seems to limit the progression of emphysema and hasten resolution. Pneumothorax can be resolved by removing the pleural air using a chest drain and suction.[28] Repeat treatment might be necessary if air continues to be sucked into the chest.

Horses with an axillary wound complicated by emphysema require intensive monitoring and, sometimes, additional diagnostic testing, such as thoracic radiography and ultrasonography.[27–29] The situation should be taken seriously because pneumothorax can lead to death.

What to do

- The activity of a horse suffering from an axillary wound must be restricted, and as much of the wound as possible should be closed primarily, and the remainder packed and bandaged.
- If an axillary wound is complicated by subcutaneous emphysema, the horse should be monitored closely for the development of pneumothorax.

Tip

- Subcutaneous air may be removed by suction via needle aspiration.

Lacerations of the shoulder region

Large lacerations of the cranial surface of the shoulder are less common than those of the pectoral region or forearm. Wounds in the shoulder region are often caused by several strands of barbed wire, resulting in multiple and short skin lacerations. The skin edges are usually minimally retracted. Many lacerations of the shoulder can be sutured and will heal successfully by primary closure, whereas some are so minor they heal quickly by second intention with minimal or no care. Occasionally, a large portion of skin is lost (Figure 12.16), but rarely is there substantial injury to the underlying musculature. The wound usually contracts rapidly. When a laceration is close to the point of the shoulder, an area of high motion, the horse should be confined to a box stall, and perhaps cross-tied, until a smooth bed of granulation tissue, without fissures, has filled the wound. The horse is expected to recover full function and be left with a minimal blemish.

Lacerations of the medial aspect of the thigh

These lacerations, usually caused by barbed wire, may be multiple and may go undetected for a few days because they are hidden from sight. Debriding the wound in a standing horse is difficult because of the wound's location. Consequently, general anesthesia should be considered to allow thorough debridement if required by the nature and duration of the wound (Figure 12.17). Primary closure of the wound is rarely attempted because tension from movement in this area is extensive.

In some cases, only the skin is lacerated, but a cleavage plane develops between the skin and medial muscles of the thigh. This plane often extends distally, thereby forming a pocket in which exudate accumulates. Moreover, the skin glides over underlying musculature as the limb flexes, preventing the skin from adhering to the underlying musculature. Consequently, exercise should be restricted, and a Penrose drain should be placed through a skin incision at the ventral extent of the subcutaneous pocket to encourage drainage. The drain should be left in place until the cleavage plane has disappeared and the ventral pocket

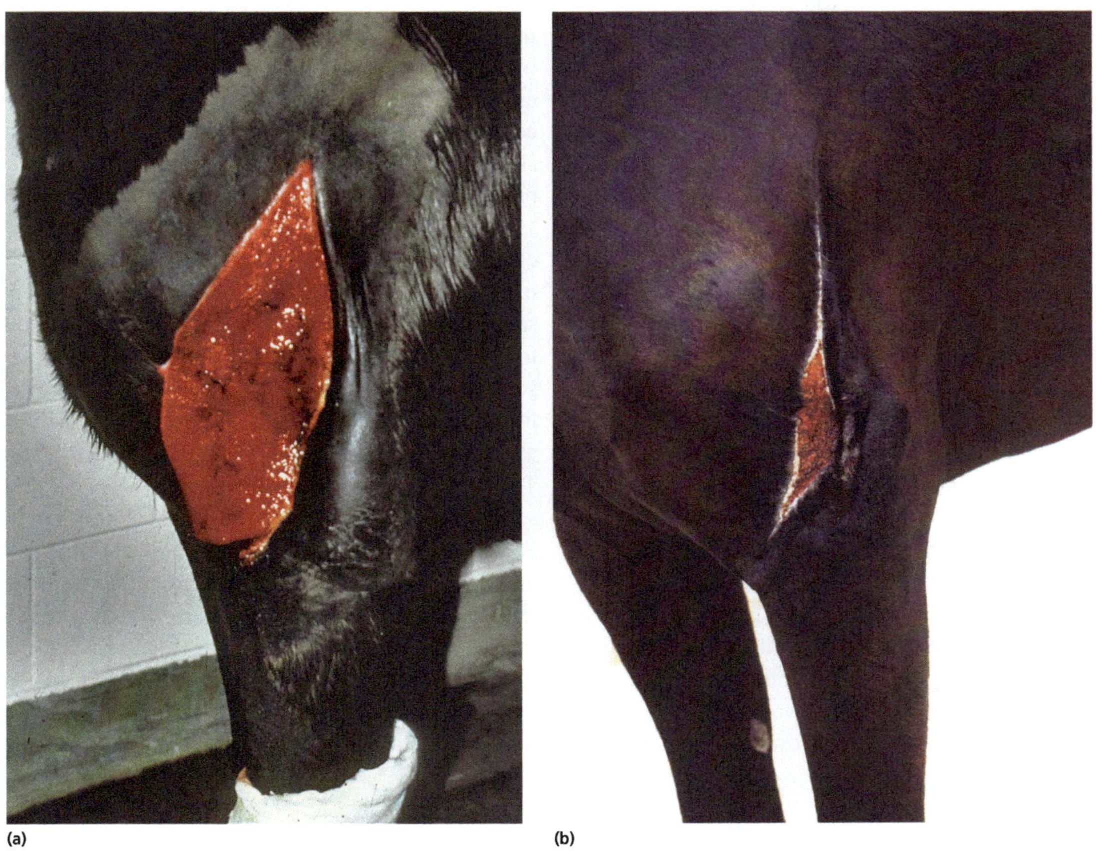

Figure 12.16 (a) Laceration of the lateral aspect of the shoulder region with substantial retraction of the skin edges. (b) The wound has almost completely healed by second intention, leaving only a minor blemish.

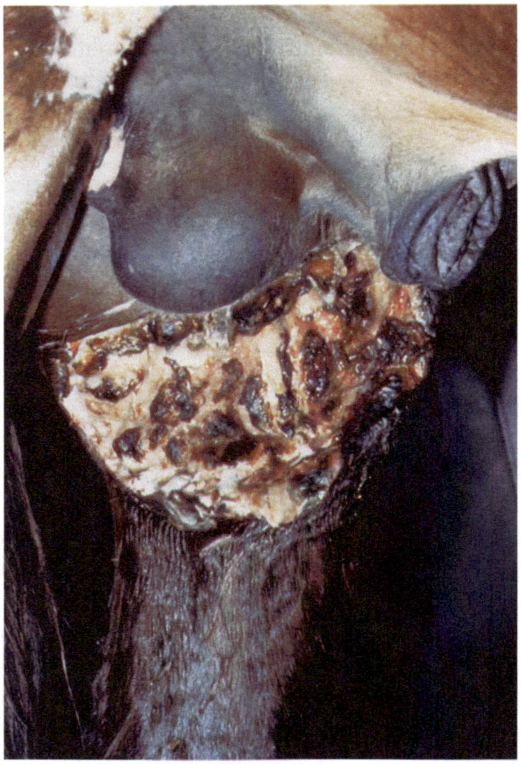

Figure 12.17 Laceration of the medial region of the thigh (cranial to the right) showing major retraction and loss of skin. Following thorough debridement of the wound, the horse was confined to a small corral to limit movement at the laceration site. The wound was cleaned daily with tap water administered from a garden hose. The wound healed uneventfully by second intention.

is filling with granulation tissue. Although primary closure is rarely possible, most wounds heal rapidly with minimal scarring once drainage is managed correctly.

Lacerations of the lateral aspect of the chest and the ventral aspect of the abdomen

Cutaneous injury to the lateral aspect of the chest and the ventral aspect of the abdomen commonly creates a viable, broad-based cutaneous/subcutaneous flap that hangs away from the body. The skin flap, if small, may be excised and the wound left to heal by second intention, since wounds in this area typically heal rapidly and cosmetically (Figure 12.18). Even wounds as large as 25 cm in diameter can heal by second intention with minimal scarring if the wound is cared for properly. Larger wounds or those with a large pendulous flap should be closed to avoid major delays in healing and to provide a more cosmetic outcome, provided that the wound is suitable for primary closure and the skin can be apposed without excessive tension (Figure 12.19).

Lacerations that penetrate the abdominal or thoracic cavity are rare, but serious complications can result from such wounds, including pneumothorax, hemothorax, septic peritonitis or pleuritis, evisceration, and herniation, among others

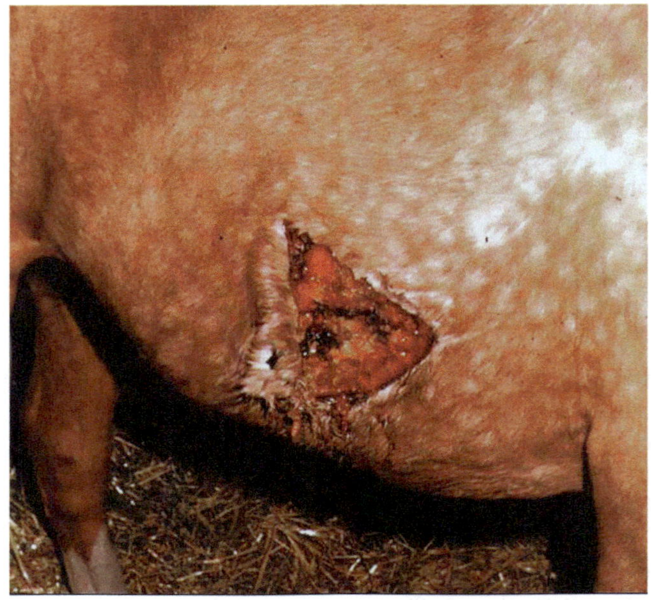

Figure 12.18 Skin flap on the thorax. This wound was partially closed by suturing the skin flap along its dorsal border and leaving the ventral area open to drain. A wound this size would easily heal by second intention, with a minimal blemish, if the skin flap was necrotic and had to be excised.

(Figure 12.20a).[27,29] The wound should be explored after aseptic preparation, using the fingers of a gloved hand or a sterile probe, to ascertain the depth and the extent of the injury. Diagnostic imaging should be considered part of a comprehensive examination if a penetration is suspected. The management of complications arising from penetration of the thoracic or abdominal cavity are described elsewhere,[29] and the remainder of this section will focus on the management of the wound itself.

The major challenges, when closing a wound into the abdominal or thoracic cavity, are to provide a secure closure and to eliminate dead space, because these wounds cannot be protected or supported easily with a bandage. Using a tension suture pattern to close the wound is crucial, and the surgeon should select suture material of sufficient size and strength to withstand the forces placed on the closure. The muscles of the thoracic or abdominal wall must be closed meticulously (Figure 12.20b). The subcutaneous tissue should be closed separately for added security, using an interrupted suture pattern. Vertical mattress and near–far–far–near patterns are ideal for apposing tissues under tension. The skin is closed using a combination of large tension sutures, sometimes placed through rubber stents, and interrupted appositional sutures (Figure 12.20c,d). Tension sutures should be placed a sufficient distance away from the skin edge so that closure is not lost if the skin edges necrose, and sutures should not be pulled so tightly that they contribute to necrosis.

If the skin edges cannot be easily apposed, undermining skin adjacent to the flap may relieve tension sufficiently to allow closure. The subcutaneous tissue should be undermined with the skin to preserve cutaneous blood supply. Because undermining

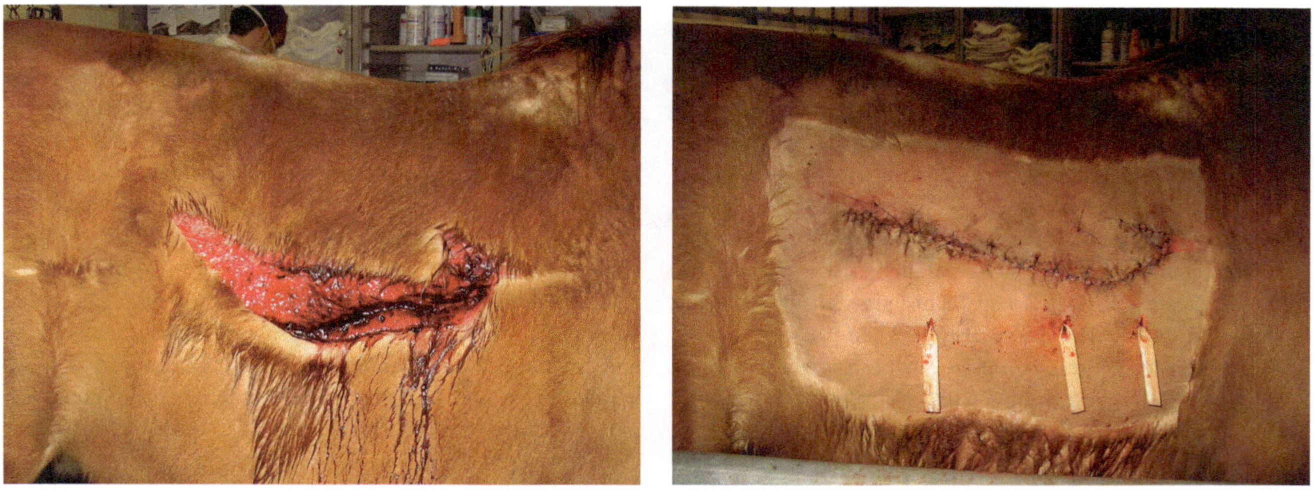

(a) (b)

Figure 12.19 **(a)** Laceration to the thoracic wall, extending into muscle, with moderate distraction of a ventrally based skin flap. The wound was fresh and clean, and the wound edges could be apposed without creating excessive tension. **(b)** The wound after primary closure. The lacerated muscle and fascia were apposed with an interrupted suture pattern, and the skin was closed using a combination of an interrupted appositional suture pattern and a few tension sutures. Penrose drains were placed in the wound cavity and exited ventrally to ensure adequate drainage of dead space.

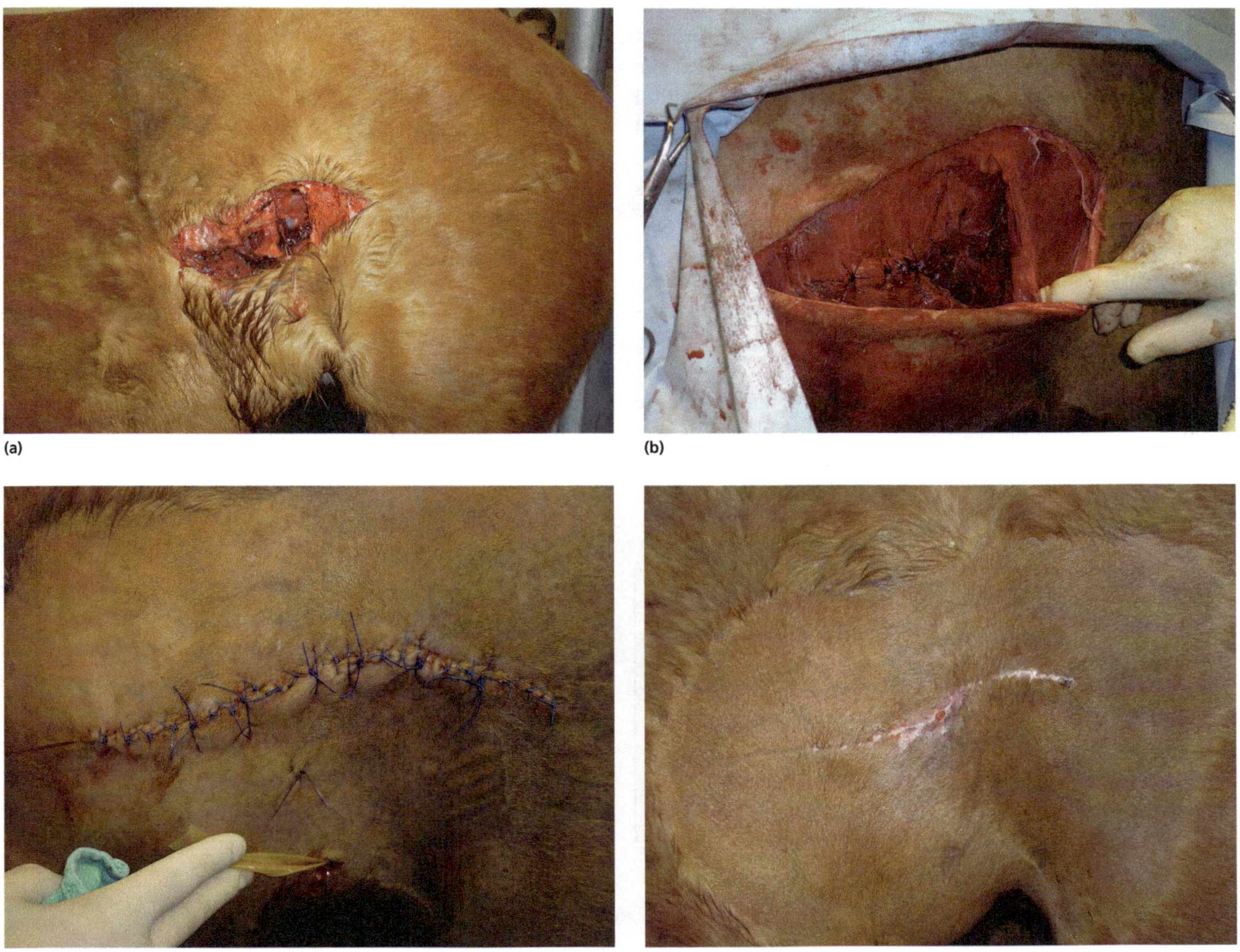

(a) (b) (c) (d)

Figure 12.20 This horse was injured by a bale spear on the bucket of a tractor. **(a)** The laceration extended deeply into the abdominal wall, and the edges of the severed muscle were retracted. The peritoneum was torn, exposing small intestine, but contamination of the abdominal cavity appeared to be minimal and no damage to the abdominal contents was identified. **(b)** The peritoneum could not be closed, but care was taken to securely close the muscle layers of the abdominal wall. Interrupted appositional and tension suture patterns were used, incorporating as much fascia as possible. **(c)** The skin wound was closed with interrupted and appositional suture patterns after closing the subcutaneous tissue with an interrupted suture pattern. Antimicrobial drugs and a NSAID were administered systemically during the perioperative period. **(d)** The wound healed well with little scarring, as seen 41 days after repair.

produces more dead space and allows the wound edges to retract further if the wound dehisces, the extent of undermining should be limited to what is required to appose the skin edges without tension. Another way to manage tension is to create many small staggered incisions, parallel to the skin edge, on both sides of the wound.[30] If greater tension relief is required, a large skin incision can be made parallel to one edge of the wound to create a bi-pedicle flap.[30] This large tension-relieving incision can double as a drainage port when it is placed ventrally. Alternatively, the skin edges can be brought as closely together as possible and secured with tension sutures, reducing the area of the wound left to heal by second intention.

Closing dead space and providing ventral drainage is important. Although walking sutures have been proposed to help reduce dead space by attaching the subcutaneous tissue of the flap to the deeper tissues of the wound, the author has not found these sutures helpful because they frequently pull out of large flaps. The author instead favors placing multiple large vertical mattress sutures, with stents, through the skin and underlying musculature. Penrose drains should be preplaced in the depth of the wound, and should exit below the sutured wound through an exit hole that is sufficiently large to allow easy drainage. The drain should be secured to the skin, at the exit portal, with a suture. Drainage may be required for several days. The exposed portion of the drain and the exit site should be cleaned daily. The wounded region should be covered with a bandage, such as a stent bandage, when possible, to compress the dead space.

Lacerations that enter the thoracic or abdominal cavity are life threatening if the horse is not treated promptly and effectively; success of treatment often depends on the veterinarian's ability to resolve ensuing complications and to create a strong wound closure. If presented early and managed correctly, most horses with a penetrating wound to the thorax or abdomen have a good prognosis for survival. Wounds with large skin flaps heal well even when the wound is only partially closed or when its edges cannot be completely approximated. Small cuts heal uneventfully, by second intention.

What to do

- Examine the wound carefully to determine if the thoracic or abdominal cavity has been penetrated. Diagnostic imaging is often useful to complement digital exploration of the wound.

Tip

- Closure of defects into the abdominal or thoracic cavity is more important than closing the rest of the wound.

Puncture wounds

Puncture wounds are caused when the horse contacts a sharp object. The puncture may be deep when the area punctured is heavily muscled, such as the chest, shoulder, or thigh. Puncture wounds are a concern because: (1) they often mistakenly appear innocuous since the skin opening is small; (2) bacteria are driven deep into the wound upon injury; (3) deep musculature may be damaged extensively; (4) they often have poor ventral drainage; and (5) the thoracic, abdominal, or a synovial cavity may have been penetrated. Consequently, puncture wounds usually are not closed primarily.

After the wound is cleaned and aseptically prepared, it should be explored with a sterile flexible probe to determine the depth and direction of penetration. This exploration helps to establish whether the wound is in proximity to a cavity, a major neurovascular structure, or a bone, for example. A flexible plastic urinary catheter is preferred to a malleable metallic probe because wound tracts are not completely linear and a plastic catheter can follow the tract to its end without causing further injury. A foreign body, if present, may sometimes be detected when it is contacted by the tip of the catheter. A small opening should be enlarged to allow more complete probing and to facilitate irrigation and drainage of the tract.

Radiographic and ultrasonographic examinations may be helpful and should be performed prior to probing or irrigating the tract to avoid imaging artifacts created by the introduction of air or fluid. Inserting a metallic probe or a plastic catheter loaded with contrast material into the tract may yield useful information about the direction, depth, and limits of the tract. A contrast fistulogram is often inconclusive if the wound is acute because the tract is not walled off, resulting in dispersal of the contrast medium throughout adjacent tissue planes. A wooden foreign body cannot be seen on a radiograph, but during ultrasonographic examination it appears as a linear, hyperechoic shadow, which is often surrounded by fluid.[31] If the presence of a foreign body close to the skin surface is confirmed by probing and medical imaging, the opening can be enlarged to allow removal of the body (Figure 12.21).

Irrigating a puncture wound is important to expel bacterial and small debris. Sterile isotonic saline solution is injected through a catheter placed into the depths of the wound, using light pressure to prevent forcing the fluid through tissue planes. Flushing should be discontinued if the irrigation fluid does not easily exit the opening. The horse should receive systemically delivered antimicrobial drugs effective against anaerobic bacteria because deep tissue trauma and contamination of the puncture wound create an environment within the wound conducive to the development of anaerobic infection. Penicillin and metronidazole provide excellent coverage against clostridial infection.[32,33] (The reader is referred to Tables 19.1 and 19.3 for more information about common bacterial isolates from wounds in horses, recommendations for interim systemic antibiotic therapy and antibiotic sensitivity patterns.) The horse's vaccination status against tetanus must be verified and updated as required. A Penrose drain should be placed though the most ventral aspect of the penetrated tissue, if possible, to promote drainage (Figure 12.22). The horse should receive a NSAID for 2–3 days to reduce swelling and relieve pain, thereby encouraging exercise, which, in turn, enhances drainage.

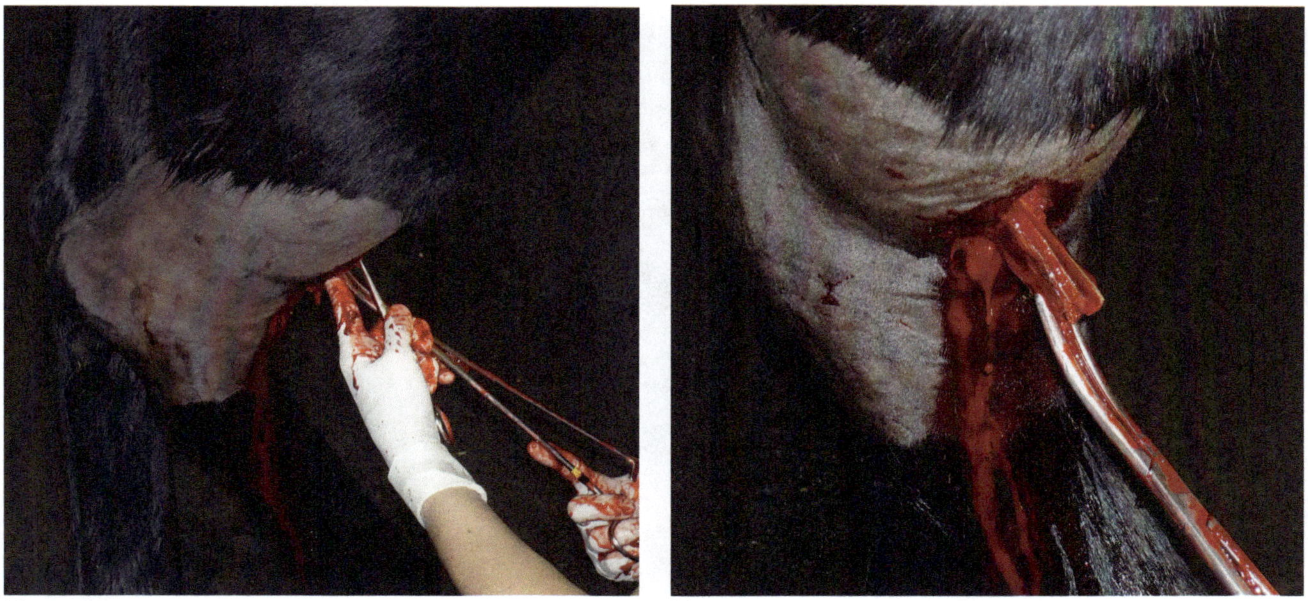

(a) (b)

Figure 12.21 Fresh puncture wound to the cranial aspect of the gaskin. The wound was approximately 6 cm deep, as determined by probing it with a flexible catheter, and a foreign body was felt with the tip of the catheter. **(a)** The foreign body was relatively shallow, easily palpated, and not encased by fibrous tissue, simplifying its extraction from the puncture site. The puncture holes in the skin and subcutaneous tissue were enlarged slightly with a scalpel and scissors to allow introduction of a forceps to grasp the foreign body. **(b)** A piece of wood was grasped with forceps and removed.

Tips

- A flexible plastic catheter is more effective than a metal catheter to determine a tract's direction and extent.
- When a puncture wound overlies a body cavity, the body cavity should be considered penetrated until proven otherwise.
- Contrast radiographic and ultrasonographic evaluations of penetrating wounds are helpful in determining the direction, depth, and limits of the tract caused by the puncture wound.

Puncture wounds into a synovial cavity

If a puncture wound is in close proximity to a joint or a tendon sheath, it is imperative to establish whether or not the synovial structure has been penetrated. This may be ascertained using careful visual or digital (using a sterile glove) examination, if the opening of the puncture wound is large. The free flow of synovial fluid from the wound, after flexing the limb, or following application of direct pressure to the synovial structure, indicates that the synovial cavity was penetrated. It may be helpful to insert a needle into the synovial cavity, at a site remote from the wound, to forcefully inject sterile fluid into the cavity to see if the fluid drains from the wound. This technique should not be used if the needle must pass through contaminated tissue. Sterile blue dye can be added to the fluid to more easily identify it leaking from the wound.

An infected synovial structure contains fluid that has a very high concentration of white blood cells (WBC) (>50 × 10^9/L), most of which are neutrophils (>90%), and a high concentration of protein (>4.0 g/dL).[34] Aggressive therapy, including arthroscopic/tenoscopic lavage and regional and systemic administration of antimicrobial drugs, is indicated to prevent septic arthritis/tenosynovitis if a synovial structure has been penetrated (the reader is referred to Chapter 16 for a complete discussion of the diagnosis and the management of wounds involving synovial structures).

What to avoid

- A needle should never be inserted into a synovial structure through inflamed/contaminated soft tissue.

Tip

- A synovial structure adjacent to a wound should be considered penetrated until proven otherwise.

Puncture wounds into the thoracic cavity

Penetration of the thorax is uncommon but dangerous because the horse may develop ipsilateral or bilateral pneumothorax and/or pleuritis. Pneumothorax may be identified radiographically and sonographically and is characterized by collapse of the lung (Figure 12.23). Unilateral pneumothorax can compromise the function of the contralateral lung by displacing the mediastinum into the contralateral pleural space.[27–29] Penetration of the thorax is often accompanied by an elevated respiratory rate or dyspnea, but the author has seen horses with an open pneumothorax that suffered neither respiratory difficulty nor an elevated respiratory rate.

The wound must be carefully examined for foreign bodies and fracture of a rib, and the chest should be auscultated for

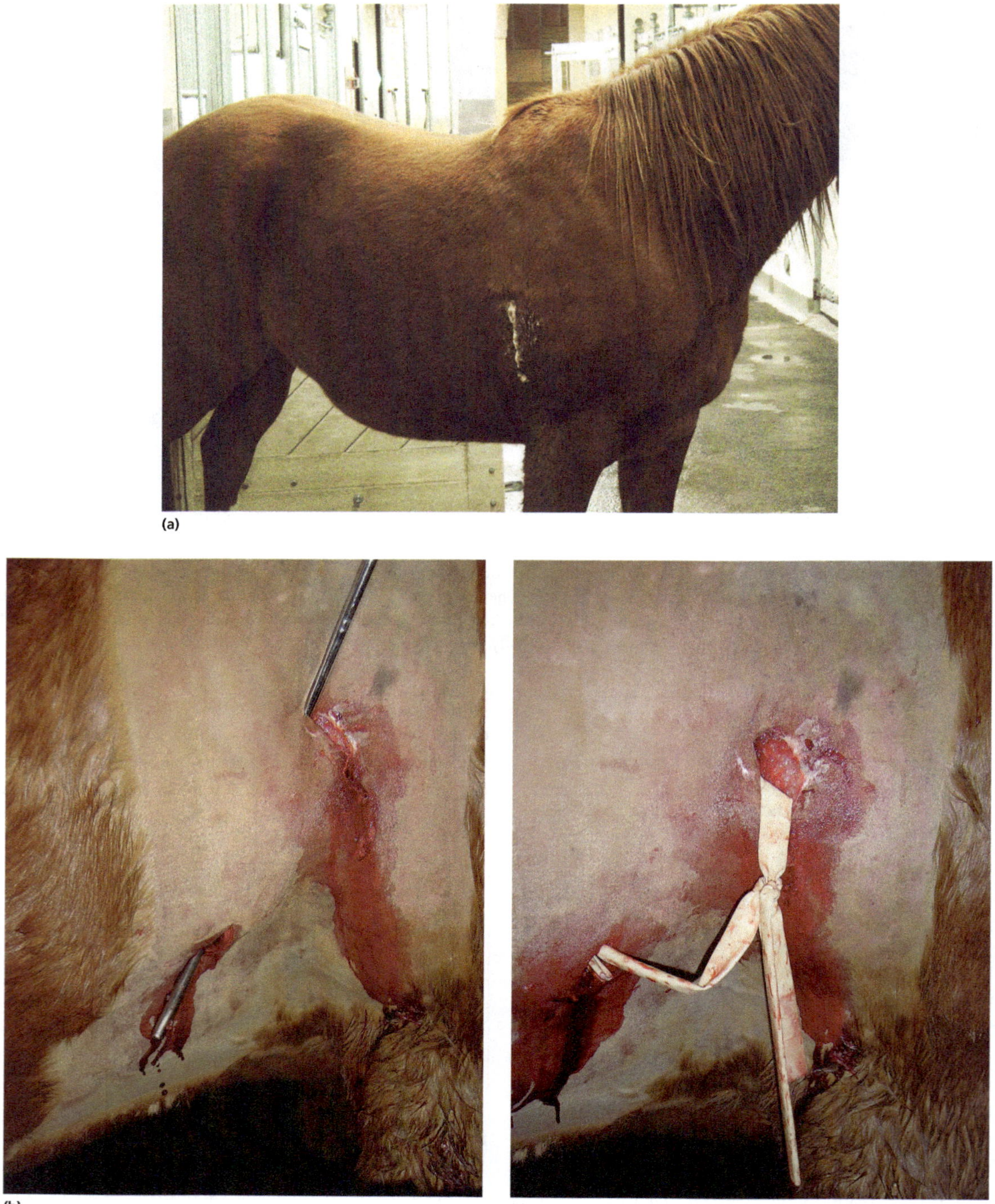

(a) (b) (c)

Figure 12.22 (a) A 1-week-old puncture wound on the thorax from which purulent material drained. While probing the puncture wound with a gloved finger, a piece of wood was identified directly beneath the skin. This piece of wood was easily removed after enlarging the hole and grasping the wood with forceps. (b) A Chamber's mare catheter was used to determine the extent of the ventral pocket, which was subsequently opened to provide drainage. (c) A Penrose drain was placed within the cavity and retained for several days to ensure adequate drainage.

evidence of pneumothorax. The wound should be thoroughly debrided, irrigated, and, if possible, the wound should be closed to prevent further contamination. Wounds that perforate the pleural cavity must be sealed to prevent collapse of the lung, and the patient should be suspected of having pneumothorax or hemothorax, and treatment to improve respiratory capacity should take precedence over examining the wound.[27,29] If the wound penetrates the pleura, the pleural cavity can be evaluated thoroughly by thoracoscopy, which should be performed at a site remote from the wound.[35] The abdomen of a horse with a

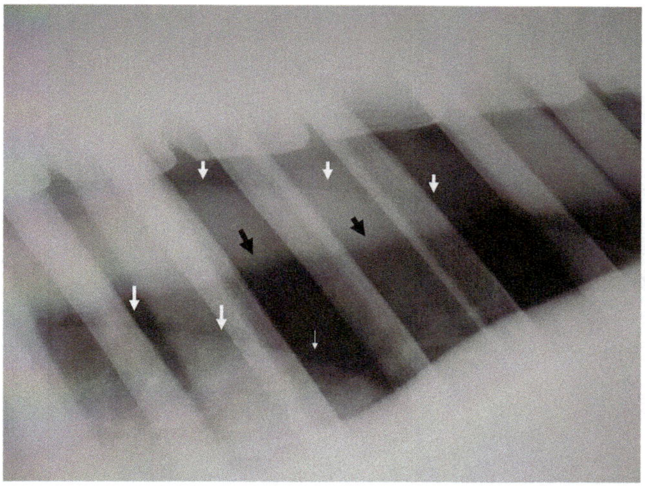

Figure 12.23 Bilateral pneumothorax, caused by a penetrating wound to the chest. White arrows indicate the retracted dorsal border of the lung lobes that no longer fill the thoracic space, and black arrows indicate the unusually clear ventral margin of the aorta.

thoracic wound, especially a wound at or caudal to the sixth rib, should also be carefully examined sonographically for free fluid or other manifestations of hemorrhage or injury to an internal abdominal organ because intra-abdominal injuries are not unusual in horses with thoracic injury.[29]

Negative pressure within the pleural space can be re-established by removing air by thoracocentesis. The pleural space can be drained or lavaged postoperatively, if necessary, via a thoracostomy tube. Reconstructive procedures may be required to close a large wound. The use of muscle pedicle flaps from the *longissimus dorsi* and external abdominal oblique muscles has been described for this purpose.[36] If the wound cannot be closed, it should be covered with a stent or thoracic bandage and allowed to heal by second intention. The horse should receive antimicrobial therapy, administered systemically, and a NSAID to lessen pleural pain and facilitate breathing. In the author's experience, the prognosis for healing and return to function is quite good if the horse does not develop septic pleuritis.

> **Tip**
>
> - Puncture of one pleural space does not necessarily cause an increased respiratory rate or dyspnea.

Puncture wounds into the peritoneal cavity

Most punctures of the abdominal wall do not penetrate the peritoneal cavity, but those that do can result in contamination of the abdominal cavity or injury to its viscera. Any wound in the abdominal region should be examined carefully for the presence of foreign material. Careful probing of the wound can usually be accomplished with the horse standing, but a safer and more thorough examination can be conducted with the horse anesthetized. Peritoneal fluid, obtained by abdominocentesis, should be examined to determine its concentrations of WBCs and protein; elevations of WBCs (>5 × 10^9/L) and protein (>2.5 g/dL) are seen with peritoneal contamination. Small wounds that do not breach the peritoneum heal best by second intention. A penetrating wound that is fresh and minimally contaminated should be debrided thoroughly and closed (Figure 12.24).

The horse should receive systemically administered antimicrobial therapy and be closely monitored postoperatively. An exploratory midline celiotomy may be indicated if injury to abdominal viscera is suspected. This allows careful examination of the viscera and thorough lavage of the abdominal cavity prior to closing the wound. Sometimes, a large defect in the abdominal wall may be impossible to close because of a lack of viable tissue, but using a mesh to close such a wound is contraindicated because of the risk of infection around the mesh. Such a wound should instead be bandaged to prevent evisceration or herniation, and allowed to heal by second intention before using a mesh to repair the resultant hernia.

Chronic draining tracts

Chronic draining tracts are usually the result of a bone sequestrum or an embedded foreign body. Sequestra associated with a wound of the body are uncommon because the bones of the body are covered by more muscle than are those of the extremities. Foreign bodies, on the other hand, are frequently the cause of a draining tract on the body. Wood is the most common foreign body encountered in wounds, but other objects found embedded in tissue include metal, plastic, or plant material.[37] Areas with a large muscle mass, especially the shoulder region, are most likely to harbor a foreign body.

The most prominent clinical sign associated with the presence of a foreign body within a wound is drainage of large amounts of purulent material from a small skin opening. There is often a history of the horse having incurred a puncture wound or laceration. The drainage may exit the original wound or it may exit from a lanced abscess or tract that developed spontaneously at a site remote from the injury (Figure 12.25a). Although most tracts caused by a sequestrum or foreign body drain constantly, the wound is sometimes characterized by transitory healing followed by repeated episodes of drainage. The horse is systemically normal and does not usually exhibit signs of discomfort when the wound is chronic and the foreign body has been "walled off."

The draining tract should be probed, and the site examined by using plain and contrast radiography and ultrasonography (Figure 12.25b,c). The author uses a long flexible plastic catheter to probe the tract, because a flexible catheter can follow the tract without puncturing its wall. While probing, one should ascertain the direction of the main tract, if the tract branches, the relationship of the tract to bones, joints, and other vital structures, and, if possible, the length of the tract. Shallow foreign bodies can be balloted with the catheter tip, whereas

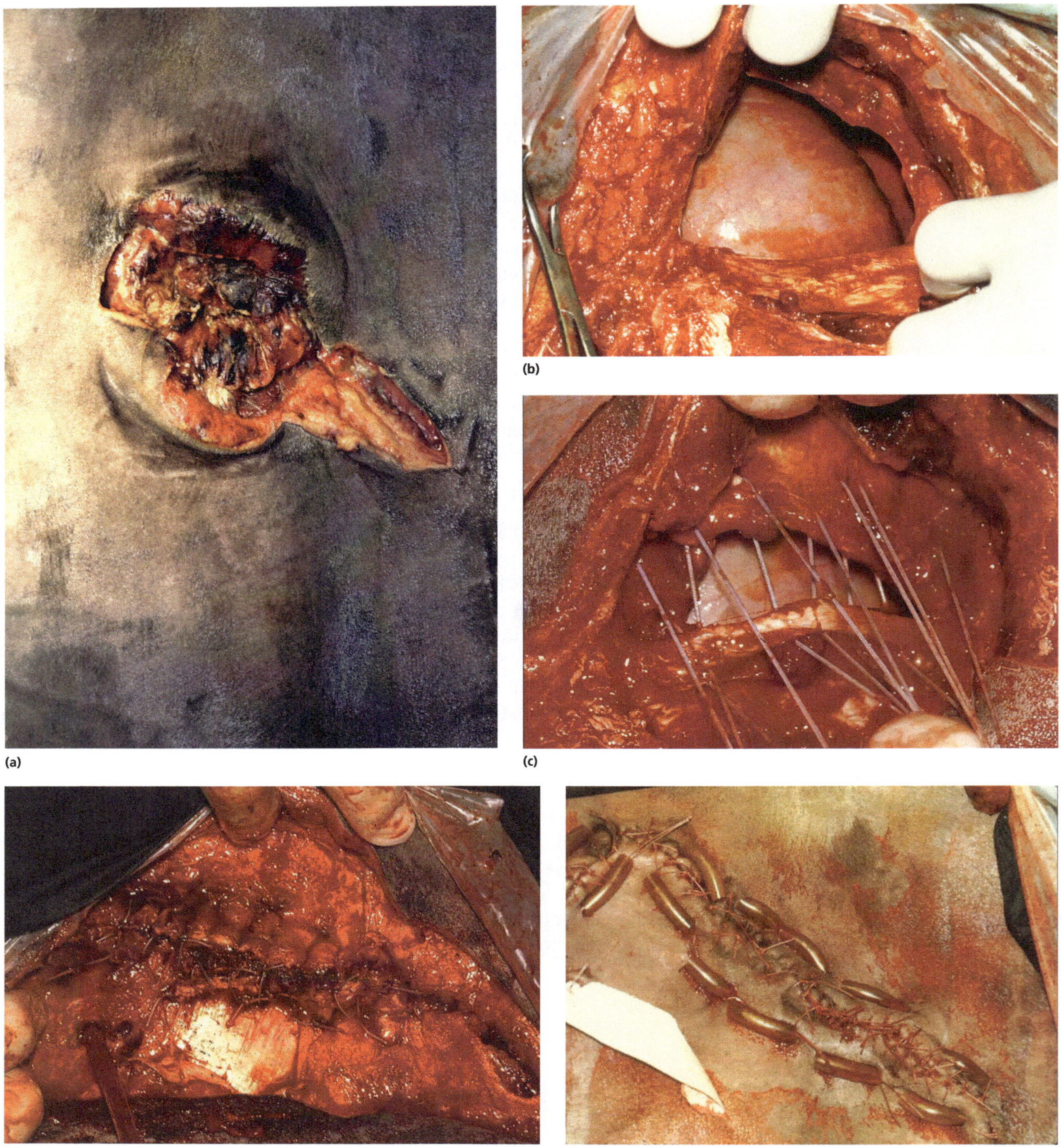

(a) (b) (c) (d) (e)

Figure 12.24 (**a**) Acute puncture of the ventral aspect of the abdomen, caused by a sharp metal post. Omentum was apparent in the depth of the wound. (**b**) The wound was debrided, and the exposed omentum amputated. A 10 × 2.5 cm annular defect was present on the ventral midline. (**c**) The abdominal musculature was closed in two layers; note the preplacement of the sutures (size 5 polyester) in the internal sheath of the *rectus abdominus* muscle. (**d**) A "relieving incision" of the *rectus abdominus* muscle and its external sheath (not shown) was required to enable closure of the abdominal defect without creating excessive tension. Note the tube placed into the abdominal cavity to facilitate postoperative drainage (bottom left).
(**e**) Horizontal mattress sutures with pieces of rubber tubing used as stents were placed in the skin for reinforcement. The intra-abdominal drainage tube was secured with sutures placed through tape positioned around the tube (bottom left).

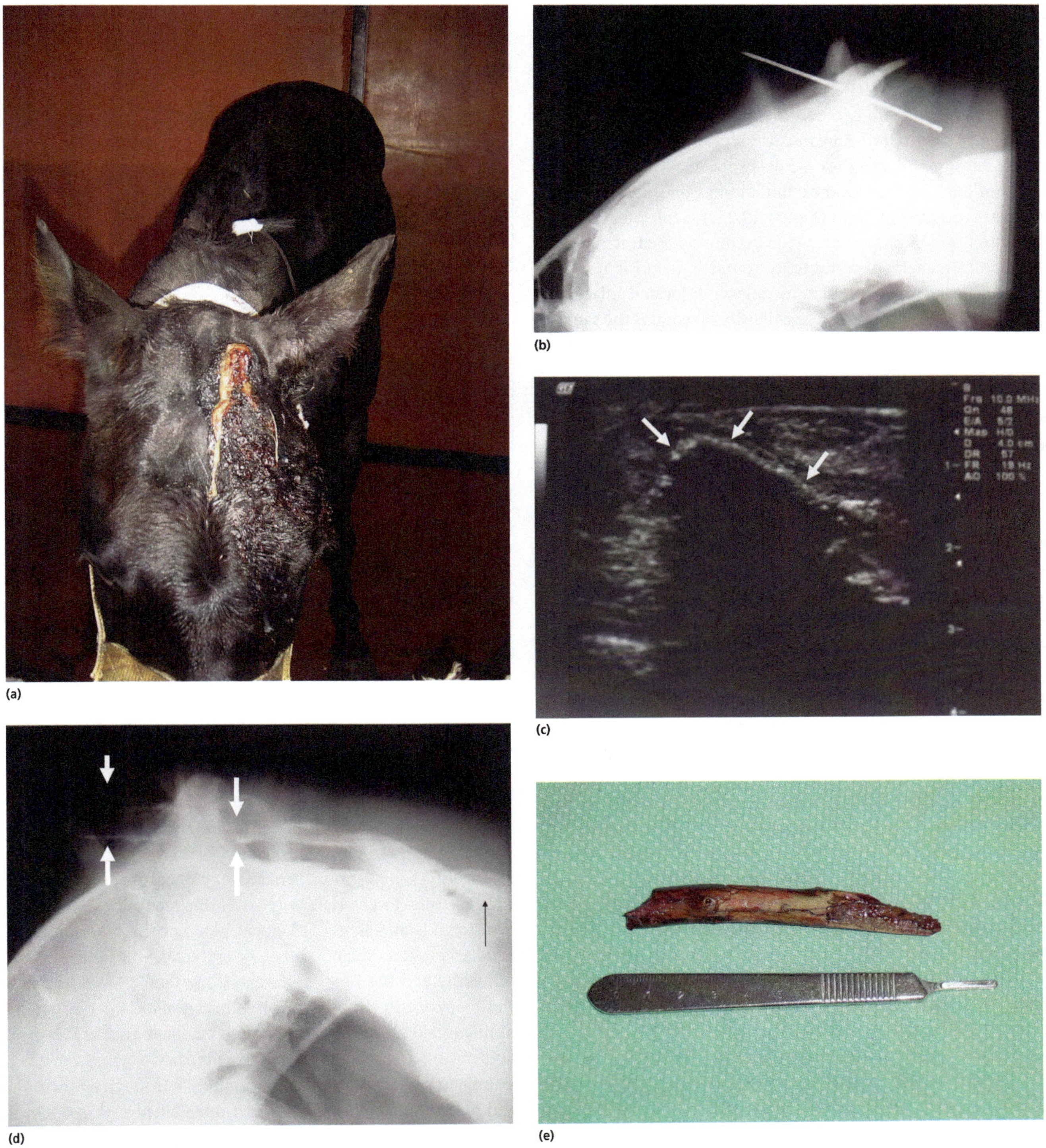

Figure 12.25 **(a)** This horse was presented with a 6-week history of purulent discharge from an opening adjacent to the left ear. Neither digital examination nor probing enabled identification of a foreign body within the tract, which extended several inches caudally towards the poll. **(b)** No foreign body was seen on plain radiographs taken with a metallic probe placed in the tract. **(c)** Ultrasonographic examination of the area immediately caudal to the opening showed a linear shadow indicative of a foreign body. **(d)** A contrast fistulogram showed a filling defect within the draining tract. **(e)** A large wooden foreign body, located within 3 cm of the opening, was removed with forceps after enlarging the skin opening.

a deep foreign body may lie beyond the reach of the catheter. A superficially located foreign body can often be found by probing the tract, but to locate a deep foreign body, additional diagnostic procedures are necessary.

The wounded region should by examined using ultrasonography and radiography before the tract is probed, to avoid artifacts created by introducing air while probing. Wooden objects are seen during ultrasound examination as linear, hyperechoic zones surrounded by fluid (Figure 12.25c).[31] Injecting isotonic saline solution into the tract, while examining the tract ultrasonographically, helps determine its course.[31] Wood is not seen during radiographic examination, unless it is located adjacent to the air-filled trachea, because the density of wood is the same as that of muscle. Air within a tract, however, may be visible during radiographic examination.

A positive-contrast fistulogram is often helpful in identifying the number of foreign bodies and their location. Contrast material should be injected under pressure, using a catheter with an inflatable cuff at the tip. If the opening of the tract is too large to occlude, or if the tract is too shallow to fully insert the cuffed catheter tip, contrast material may be injected through a flexible polyethylene catheter placed into the depths of the wound. This might allow leakage of contrast medium on to the skin, but useful information is still obtained. Foreign bodies appear as linear or rectangular radiolucent zones, or filling defects, in a tract otherwise filled with radiopaque contrast material (Figure 12.25d).

Superficial foreign bodies are often identified during probing and removed by simply incising the overlying tissue. Most foreign bodies, however, are deeply embedded, and a full work-up is required to determine the number and location of foreign bodies, as well as the least traumatic approach for removing the foreign body/bodies. A chronically embedded foreign body is encased in a fibrotic tract smaller than the diameter of the foreign body, which prevents extraction of the foreign body without first enlarging the fibrous tract.

A foreign body can be removed by dissecting along the tract (Figure 12.25e) or through an incision created at a site remote from the draining tract. When dissecting along the tract to reach the foreign body, one may inadvertently transect the tract and lose sight of the distal segment going to the foreign body. Injecting a small volume of dilute methylene blue into the tract before surgery to stain the tract renders it more easily identifiable in the event that it is accidentally transected during dissection. However, too much dye can flood the wound site and stain all the tissues, thereby obscuring the distal segment of the tract. As an alternative to the dye method, the author prefers to place a catheter within the draining tract prior to surgery, and to dissect towards the foreign body by following this guide while avoiding penetrating the lumen of the tract.

For some horses, the least traumatic approach is to incise over the foreign body at a site remote from the tract where it may be closer to the skin surface (Figure 12.26). Intraoperative ultrasonography can be helpful in locating the foreign body. Alternatively, lead markers may be placed on the skin when a fistulogram is performed prior to surgery. The location of the foreign body is determined relative to the lead markers, and the ideal location for a surgical incision is marked on the skin with skin staples or a skin suture, which is left in place during aseptic preparation of the area. Preoperative antimicrobial therapy is administered systemically to counter the risk of contamination of dissected tissue planes by the discharge exiting the chronic draining tract.

What to do

- Deeply embedded foreign bodies can often be removed less traumatically by incising directly over the foreign body, rather than by dissecting along its associated draining tract.

What to avoid

- Surgical removal of a deeply embedded foreign body should never be attempted without first accurately locating the foreign body with the use of ultrasound or contrast radiography.

Tip

- Probing a draining tract with a flexible plastic catheter can yield a wealth of information.

Abscesses, hematomas, and seromas

Hematomas usually develop subsequent to blunt trauma or to overstretching of a muscle (Figure 12.27), and their size depends on the vessel torn and the ability of surrounding tissue to restrict enlargement. Seromas result from shearing forces between skin and muscle (Figure 12.28), whereas abscesses are secondary to puncture of the skin or from hematogenous spread of bacteria to traumatized tissue (Figure 12.29).

Hematomas and seromas usually arise quickly after trauma, reach their maximum size rapidly, are soft, fluctuant, and do not feel hot. The horse usually shows no signs of pain when the seroma or hematoma is palpated. Abscesses develop more slowly, are less fluctuant, feel thicker walled, and palpation of the abscess causes the horse to show signs of pain. Ultrasonography may help distinguish a seroma from a hematoma or abscess; a seroma appears anechoic (due to low cellularity) with fine loculations, whereas a hematoma is initially echogenic but becomes anechoic and loculated when clots form. Abscesses are echogenic, due to high cellularity and inspissation, have swirling fluid on ballottement, and may contain gas. An organized hematoma cannot always be distinguished ultrasonographically from an abscess;[31] in this case, fluid obtained by centesis must be examined cytologically.

An abscess can be resolved by draining it through an incision, and patency of the incision may be maintained with a drain, if necessary. Treatment of a horse for a hematoma or seroma is less straightforward. Seromas eventually reabsorb and usually need not be drained. The author drains a confirmed seroma only if it is large and located where it may be traumatized (e.g., hip). Drainage should be established through a large incision created at the most ventral aspect of the seroma. The author believes hematomas should never be drained unless they become infected. The larger the hematoma the greater is the risk of hemorrhage when the hematoma is drained. The author has seen cases where the post-drainage hemorrhage from a deep cavity could not be located and permanently stopped in spite of repeated attempts, and the clients elected euthanasia, for financial reasons.

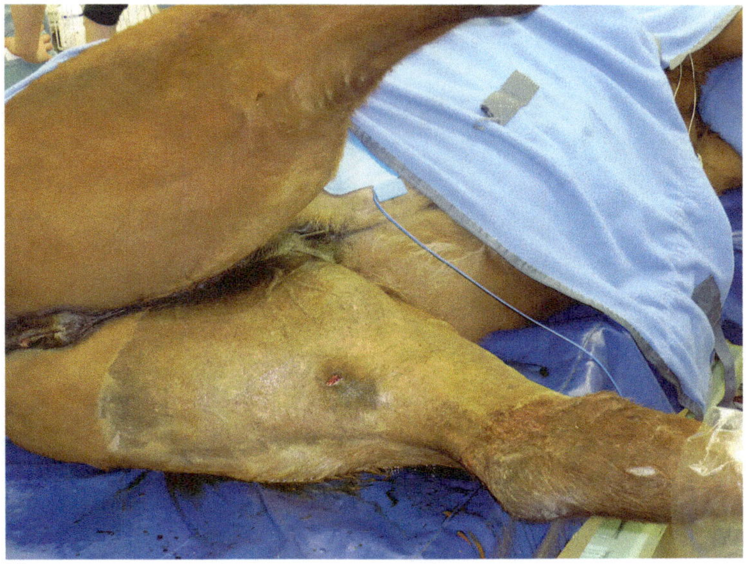

(a)

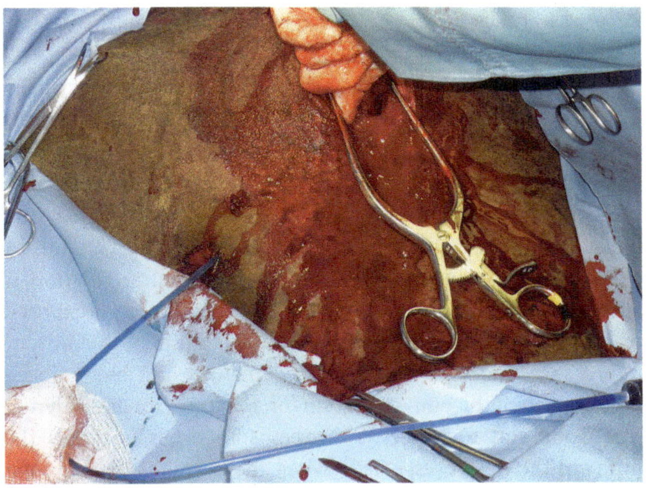

(b)

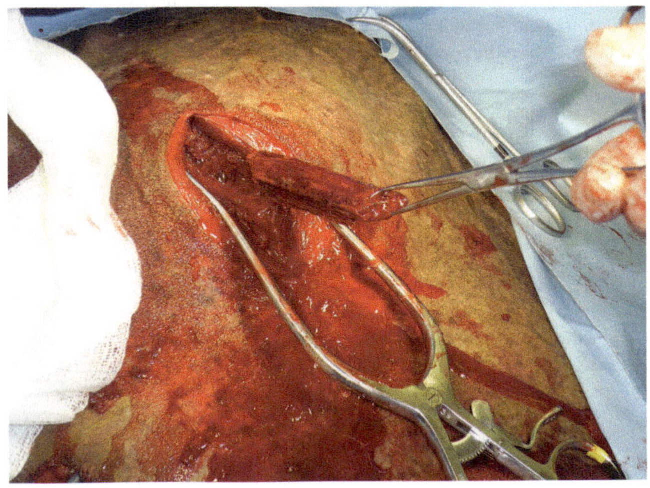

(c)

Figure 12.26 **(a)** This horse was presented with a draining tract, of several weeks duration, on the caudal aspect of the mid-gaskin area. By probing the tract with a flexible catheter, the tract was found to be approximately 25 cm long and to extend cranially into the muscles of the medial aspect of the limb. Based on sonographic and contrast-radiographic examinations, a foreign body was determined to reside within the deepest portion of the tract. The horse was positioned in lateral recumbency for diagnostic imaging and removal of the foreign body. **(b)** A catheter filled with methylene blue was placed into the draining tract to aid identification of the tract's path. An incision was made cranial to the puncture site at a location determined appropriate by the sonographic and contrast-radiographic examinations. Spinal needles were used to "probe" for the foreign body prior to incising the skin. **(c)** A piece of wood several centimeters long was removed after incising the fibrous capsule lining the tract. The wood was approximately 6 cm deep to the skin and was removed through an 8-cm long incision. This approach resulted in much less tissue damage than that which would have occurred if the wood had been extracted through the draining tract.

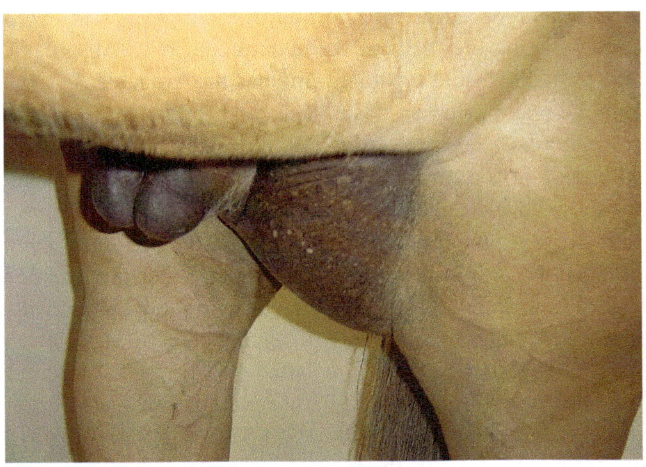

Figure 12.27 A large hematoma developed on the medial aspect of the thigh after the horse fell with the limb abducted. The mass was hard and, when palpated, caused the horse to show signs of pain. This mass persisted for several weeks.

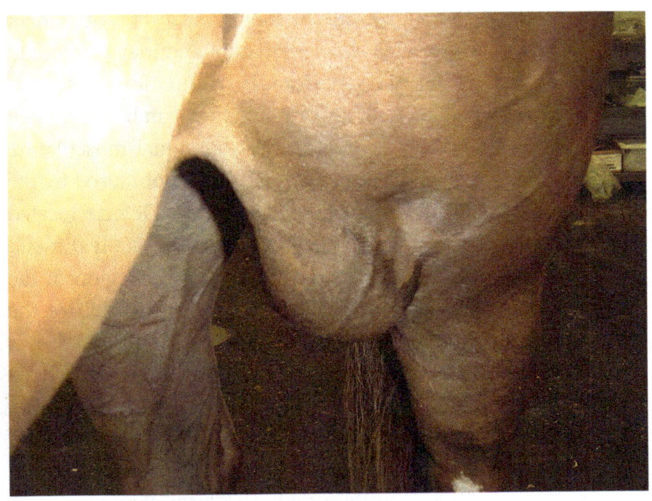

Figure 12.28 The stifle is sometimes struck when a horse jumps a fence, causing a seroma to develop. The seroma shown in this figure was soft and fluctuant but was not drained.

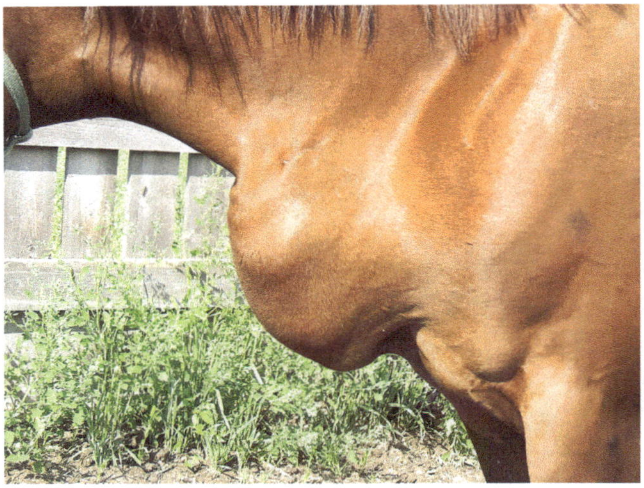

Figure 12.29 Large abscess on the ventral aspect of the neck of a breeding stallion thought to result from hematogenous inoculation of a chronic hematoma, itself the result of a kick. The abscess was lanced, and Penrose drains were placed within its cavity to ensure drainage.

Aside from rare exceptions, hematomas and seromas resolve gradually, and abscesses resolve when they are drained through an incision.

What to avoid

- Seromas and hematomas need not be drained; moreover, draining a hematoma can result in severe hemorrhage.

Traumatic abdominal hernias

Rupture of the abdominal wall, usually from a blunt object, such as a foot or fence post, usually occurs between the flank and the prepubic tendon (Figure 12.30) or on the ventral aspect of the abdomen (Figure 12.31). The skin is usually intact, but abdominal viscera escape into the subcutaneous space via a rent in the abdominal musculature.

The rupture is rarely accompanied by intestinal strangulation because the defect in the abdominal wall is typically large (~15–20 cm in diameter) because of muscle retraction. Mild transient colic may develop initially but subsides without treatment. A fluctuant swelling occurs immediately after herniation and may increase in size during the first few days after injury. Herniation, often suspected based on ballottement and auscultation, can be confirmed with ultrasonography. The defect in the abdominal musculature often cannot be palpated externally because it is obscured by the presence of viscera in the subcutaneous space. Defects located near the prepubic tendon are common and are especially difficult to palpate. The defect, when located in the caudal region of the abdomen, can sometimes be identified during palpation of the abdominal wall performed per rectum. The extent of a defect is best determined with the horse anesthetized. An abdominal hernia must be differentiated from cellulitis, a seroma, a hematoma, or an abscess. Centesis of hernial contents can result in leakage of intestinal contents into the subcutaneous tissue, thereby causing serious infection, which greatly complicates surgical repair.

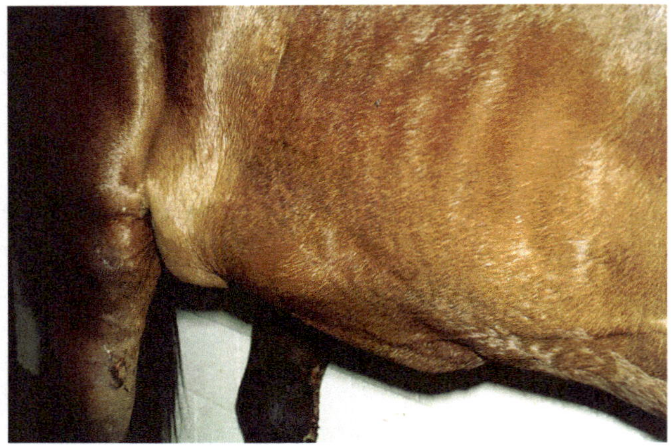

Figure 12.30 Swelling in the fold of the flank of a horse with a rupture of the ventral aspect of the body wall caused by the horse landing on a fencepost. The skin was intact, but intestine had herniated into the subcutaneous space through a rent in the body wall, located close to the pelvic brim.

If the skin over the hernia is intact, the intestines are usually uninjured and can remain in the subcutaneous space for months with little risk of strangulation or adhesion formation. The defect in the body wall should nevertheless be repaired because the herniated intestines are susceptible to further trauma, and because a horse with a hernia is of limited use. The author prefers to postpone repair unless intestinal strangulation is suspected or the skin is open and the abdominal cavity is exposed or contaminated. This is because, following injury, the musculature surrounding the defect is edematous and has reduced holding strength, and retraction of the muscles in different directions and to different degrees sometimes obscures the limits of the defect, especially when the hernia is located near the superficial inguinal ring. Although successful repair of abdominal hernias using interrupted mayo mattress or cruciate suture patterns, within 21 days of initial injury, has been reported,[38] the author has found that hernia repair is most secure when a synthetic mesh is overlaid onto the strong fibrotic hernial ring that is present several months after injury.[39–41]

Because a foreign body (synthetic mesh) is to be implanted, broad-spectrum antibiotics should be administered systemically to the horse, preoperatively and for several days postoperatively. Strict adherence to aseptic technique is important to avoid contaminating the mesh or the abdominal cavity. Absorbable and non-absorbable prosthetic meshes are available, but the author prefers using an absorbable mesh because the risk of chronic infection surrounding the implant is greatly reduced. Although various techniques regarding the site for placing the mesh have been described,[39] most surgeons place the mesh retroperitoneally to reduce the risk of adhesions developing between the mesh and abdominal viscera.[40,41] The mesh can be placed in a single or double layer, with a double layer resulting in a stronger repair with less sagging. The sheets of mesh may be placed together or inserted separately in different tissue planes. The mesh is usually covered with a portion of the fibrous hernial flap (Figure 12.32). The reader is referred to an equine surgery textbook for a complete description of prosthetic reconstruction of an abdominal hernia with a

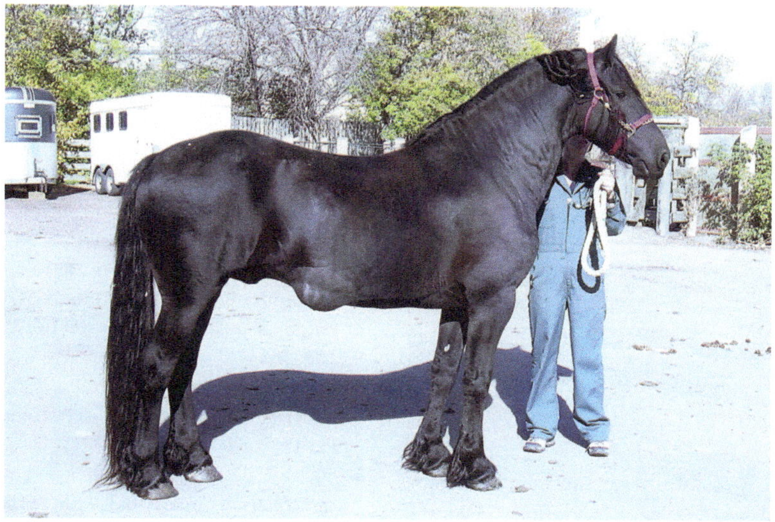

Figure 12.31 Chronic ventral hernia caused by landing on a sharp fencepost 2 years earlier.

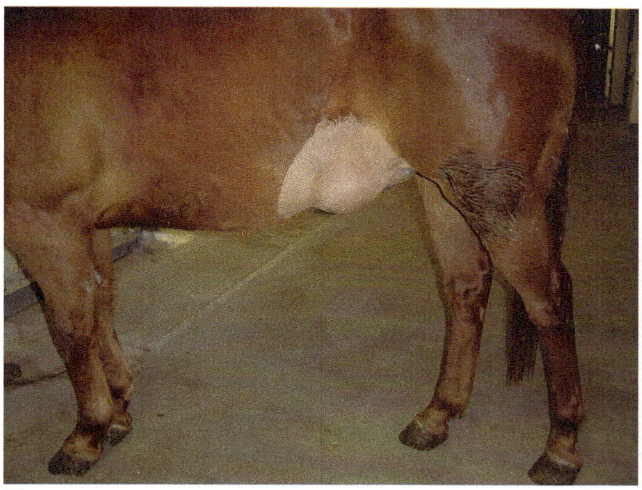

(a)

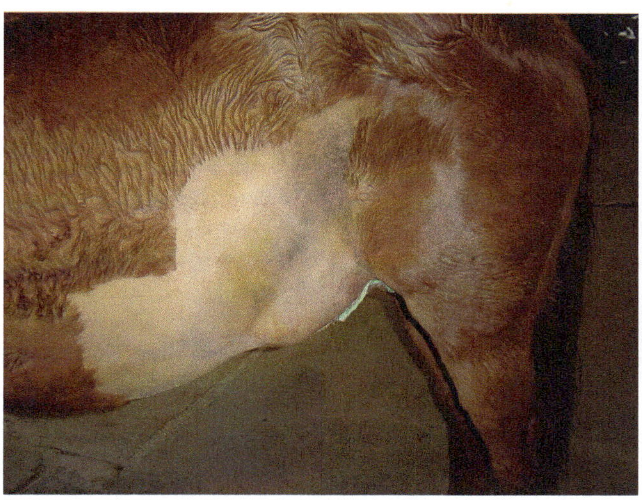

(b)

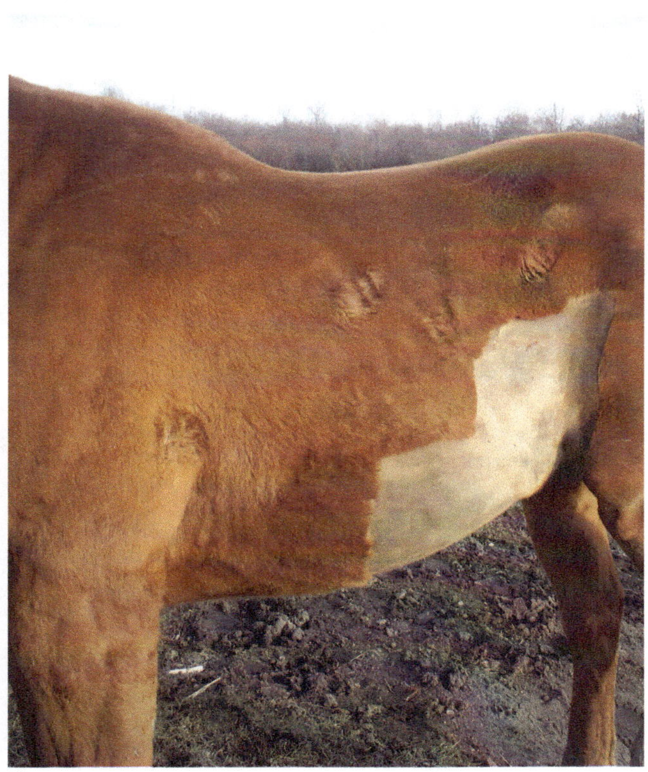

(c)

Figure 12.32 A rupture of the ventral aspect of the body wall of 3 months' duration. **(a)** The appearance was typical of that of other hernias in this region. The hernia was associated with a 13-cm diameter defect in the abdominal wall located 8 cm cranial to the superficial inguinal ring. The swelling resulted from herniation of intestine into the subcutaneous space. **(b)** Appearance of the abdomen on the first postoperative day after repair using two layers of mesh. The swelling was associated with formation of a seroma in the dead space, which could not be closed with sutures or compressed with bandaging. This seroma reabsorbed spontaneously and was not drained. Initially, the postoperative swelling is often almost as big as the swelling prior to surgery. **(c)** Appearance of the abdomen 4 months after the repair. The angle of the photograph is slightly different, but shows that the seroma has resorbed, and the cosmetic appearance is excellent.

synthetic mesh. Prognosis for return to full use and a cosmetic result is excellent, with proper treatment.

What to avoid

- Never perform centesis of a swelling that might be the result of an abdominal hernia.
- Do not attempt repair of a recently acquired abdominal hernia, unless the skin is disrupted.

Conclusion

Most horses may be treated successfully for the many types of wounds that can be found on the neck and body. Wound management may be prolonged, labor intensive, and costly, but often the horse can return to normal use or engage in a reasonable level of activity.

References

1. Carmichael SW. The tangled web of Langer's lines. *Clin Anat* 2014; **27**: 162.
2. Woollen N, DeBowes RM, Leiplod HW, *et al.* A comparison of four types of therapy for the treatment of full-thickness skin wounds of the horse. *Proc Am Assoc Eq Pract* 1987; 569.
3. Barber SM. Second intention wound healing in the horse: the effect of bandages and topical corticosteroids. *Proc Am Assoc Eq Pract* 1989; 107.
4. Barber SM. Diseases of the guttural pouches. In: Colohan PT, Merritt AM, Moore JN, Mayhew IG (eds). *Equine Medicine and Surgery*, 5th edn. Mosby: Philadelphia, 1999: 500.
5. Hare WCD. Equine respiratory system. In: Getty R (ed). *Sisson and Grossman's the Anatomy of Domestic Animals*, 5th edn. WB Saunders: Philadelphia, 1975: 512.
6. Shappell KK, Stick JA, Derksen FJ, *et al.* Permanent tracheostomy in equidae: 47 cases (1981–1986). *J Am Vet Med Assoc* 1988; **192**: 939.
7. McClure SR, Taylor TS, Honnas CM, *et al.* Permanent tracheostomy in standing horses: technique and results. *Vet Surg* 1995; **24**: 231.
8. Chesen AB, Rakestraw PC. Indications for and short and long-term outcome of permanent tracheostomy performed in standing horses: 82 cases (1995–2005). *J Am Vet Med Assoc* 2008; **232**: 1352.
9. Tate LP, Koch DB, Sembrat RF, *et al.* Tracheal reconstruction by resection and end-to-end anastomosis in the horse. *J Am Vet Med Assoc* 1981; **178**: 253.
10. Sisson S. Equine digestive system: esophagus. In: Getty R (ed). *Sisson and Grossman's the Anatomy of Domestic Animals*, 5th edn. WB Saunders: Philadelphia, 1975: 475.
11. Stick JA. Esophagus. In: Auer JA, Stick JA (eds). *Equine Surgery*, 4th edn. Elsevier Saunders: St Louis, 2012: 367.
12. Craig DR, Shivy DR, Pankowski RL, *et al.* Esophageal disorders in 61 horses: results of non-surgical and surgical management. *Vet Surg* 1989; **18**: 432.
13. Peacock EE. Esophagus. In: Peacock EE (ed). *Wound Repair*, 3rd edn. WB Saunders: Philadelphia 1984: 451.
14. Stick JA, Krehbiel JD, Kunze DJ, *et al.* Esophageal healing in the pony: comparison of sutured vs non-sutured esophagotomy. *Am J Vet Res* 1981; **42**: 1506.
15. Todhunter RJ, Stick JA, Slocombe RF. Comparison of three feeding techniques after esophageal mucosal resection and anastomosis in the horse. *Cornell Vet* 1986; **76**: 16.
16. Todhunter RJ, Stick JA, Trotter GW, *et al.* Medical management of esophageal stricture in seven horses. *J Am Vet Med Assoc* 1984; **185**: 784.
17. Stick JA, Slocombe RF, Derksen FJ, *et al.* Esophagostomy in the pony: comparison of surgical techniques and form of feed. *Am J Vet Res* 1983; **44**: 2123.
18. Stick JA, Derksen FJ, Scott EA. Equine cervical esophagostomy: complications associated with duration and location of feeding tubes. *Am J Vet Res* 1981; **42**: 727.
19. Read EK, Barber SM, Wilson DG, *et al.* Oesophageal rupture in a Quarter Horse mare: unique features of liquid enteral hyperalimentation and fistula management. *Equine Vet Educ* 2002; **14**: 126.
20. Gideon L. Esophageal anastomosis in two foals. *J Am Vet Med Assoc* 1984; **184**: 1146.
21. Knottenbelt DC, Harrison LJ, Peacock PJ. Conservative treatment of oesophageal stricture in 5 foals. *Vet Rec* 1992; **131**: 27.
22. Hoffer RE, Barber SM, Kallfelz FA, *et al.* Esophageal patch grafting as a treatment for esophageal stricture in a horse. *J Am Vet Med Assoc* 1977; **171**: 350.
23. Wilmink JM, Stolk PW, vanWeeren PR, *et al.* Differences in second-intention healing between horses and ponies: macroscopic aspects. *Equine Vet J* 1999; **31**: 53.
24. Rhinelander FW, Wilson JW. Blood supply to developing, mature and healing bone: compendium of blood supply in normal and healing mature long bones. In: Sumner-Smith G (ed). *Bone in Clinical Orthopaedics*, 1st edn. W B Saunders: Toronto, 1982: 145.
25. Chanavez M. Anatomy and histophysiology of the periosteum: quantification of the periosteal blood supply to the adjacent bone with 85Sr and gamma spectrometry. *J Oral Implantol* 1995; **21**: 214.
26. Bhandari M, Anthony D, Schemitsch EH. The efficacy of low-pressure lavage with different irrigating solutions to remove adherent bacteria from bone. *J Bone Joint Surg* 2001; **83**: 412.
27. Boy MG, Sweeney CR. Pneumothorax in horses: 40 cases (1980–1997). *J Am Vet Med Assoc* 2000; **216**: 1955.
28. Joswig A, Hardy J. Axillary wounds in horses and the development of subcutaneous emphysema, pneumomediastinum, and pneumothorax. *Equine Vet Educ* 2013; **25**: 139S
29. Sprayberry KA, Barrett EJ. Thoracic trauma in horses. *Vet Clinics N Am Equine* 2015; **17**: 199.
30. Bailey JV. Principles of and plastic and reconstructive surgery. In: Auer JA, Stick JA (eds). *Equine Surgery*, 4th edn. Elsevier Saunders: St Louis, 2012: 271.
31. Redding WR. Ultrasound, evaluation of foreign bodies. In: Baxter GM (ed). *Adams and Stashak's Lameness in Horses*, 6th edn. Wiley Blackwell: Oxford, 2011: 373.
32. Plumb DC. Penicillin. In: Plumb DC (ed). *Plumb's Veterinary Drug Handbook*, 8th edn. Wiley Blackwell: Ames, 2015: 825.
33. Lofmark S, Edlund C, Nord C. Metronidazole is still the drug of choice for treatment of anaerobic infections. *Clin Infect Dis* 2010; **50**: 516.

34. Richardson DW, Ahern BJ. Synovial and osseous infections. In: Auer JA, Stick JA (eds). *Equine Surgery*, 4th edn. Elsevier Saunders: St Louis, 2012: 1189.
35. Lugo J. Thoracic diseases. In: Auer JA, Stick JA (eds). *Equine Surgery*, 4th edn. Elsevier Saunders: St Louis, 2012: 650.
36. Stone WC, Trostle SS, Gerros TC. Use of a primary muscle pedicle flap to repair a caudal thoracic wound in a horse. *J Am Vet Med Assoc* 1994; **205**: 828.
37. Stick JA. Management of sinus tracts and fistula. In: Auer JA, Stick JA (eds). *Equine Surgery*, 4th edn. Elsevier Saunders: St Louis, 2012: 324.
38. Azizi S, Hashemi-Asl SM, Torabi E. Early herniorraphy of large traumatic abdominal wounds in horses and mules. *Equine Vet J* 2016; **48**: 434.
39. Scott EA. Repair of incisional hernias in the horse. *J Am Vet Med Assoc* 1979; **175**: 1203.
40. Tulleners EP, Fretz PB. Prosthetic repair of abdominal wall defects in horses and food animals. *J Am Vet Med Assoc* 1983; **182**: 258.
41. Adams SB, Fessler JF. Mesh repair of large body wall defects: In: Adams SB, Fessler JF (eds). *Atlas of Equine Surgery*. WB Saunders: Philadelphia, 2000: 401.

CHAPTER 13
Management of Wounds of the Distal Extremities

Jim Schumacher, DVM, MS, Diplomate ACVS, MRCVS and Ted S. Stashak, DVM, MS, Diplomate ACVS

Chapter Contents

Summary

Wounds of the distal aspect of the limb of horses are common and account for more than 60% of all wounds. These wounds are often more problematic than wounds located elsewhere because of their proximity to the ground, making them more likely to become contaminated and then infected, and because skin in the distal portion of the limb is poorly vascularized compared to skin located elsewhere on the horse's body. A wound to the distal aspect of the limb is much more likely to involve a vital structure and, if allowed to heal by second intention, to develop exuberant granulation tissue (EGT). The greatest difference in the rate of healing of wounds involving the body and those involving the distal aspect of the limb can be attributed to the greater contribution of contraction to the healing of wounds on the body.

Introduction

Although there may be geographic differences in terms of type and incidence of wounds encountered, wounds of the distal aspect of the limb (i.e., up to and including the carpus and tarsus) of horses are quite common and account for more than 60% of all wounds.[1] Geographic differences in types of wounds encountered relate to how the horse is confined (e.g., paddock or pasture – barbed wire fences versus board, pipe, or plastic fences, etc. – or a stall and run) and the manner in which the horse is used (e.g., Western performance versus hunter/jumper).

Sharp objects, such as sheet metal, broken glass, exposed nails or bolts, and barbed wire, are responsible for most lacerations and avulsion injuries, but serious wounds can be caused by smooth, high-tensile wire or by rope. Protruding objects, such as stubs of wood projecting from tree trunks or logs, or nails and

Equine Wound Management, Third Edition. Edited by Christine Theoret and Jim Schumacher.

Companion website: www.wiley.com/go/theoret/wound

bolts protruding from fences, buildings, or trailers, are often the cause of penetrating wounds. If the penetrating object becomes embedded within tissue, a foreign-body reaction develops, usually resulting in a persistently or intermittently draining tract.

The injury may be sustained by running into, brushing against, kicking at, or stepping on an object, or by becoming entangled in barbed or smooth wire or a rope (Figure 13.1). Horses that jump fences may sustain blunt trauma resulting in an abrasion or a penetrating wound, often on the dorsal surface of the pastern. Blunt trauma to the dorsal surface of the carpus can occasionally cause a substantial hematoma or hygroma (Figure 13.2). Penetrating wounds from jumping injuries often occur just proximal to the coronet on the hindlimb or at the distal end of the antebrachium, and, often, a splinter of wood becomes embedded in soft tissue (Figure 13.3). Horses that

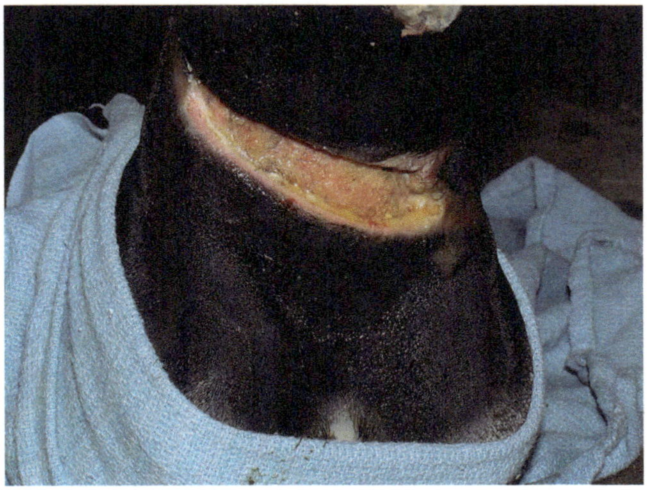

Figure 13.1 A full-thickness wound to the plantar surface of the pastern caused by a rope.

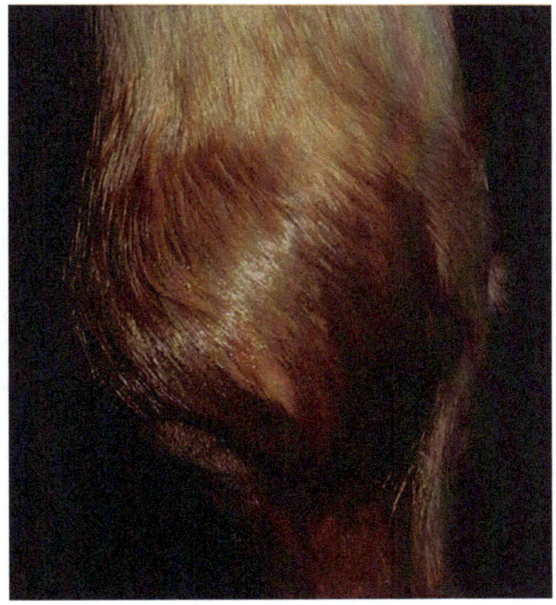

Figure 13.2 A hygroma unresponsive to medical treatment, on the dorsal surface of the carpus.

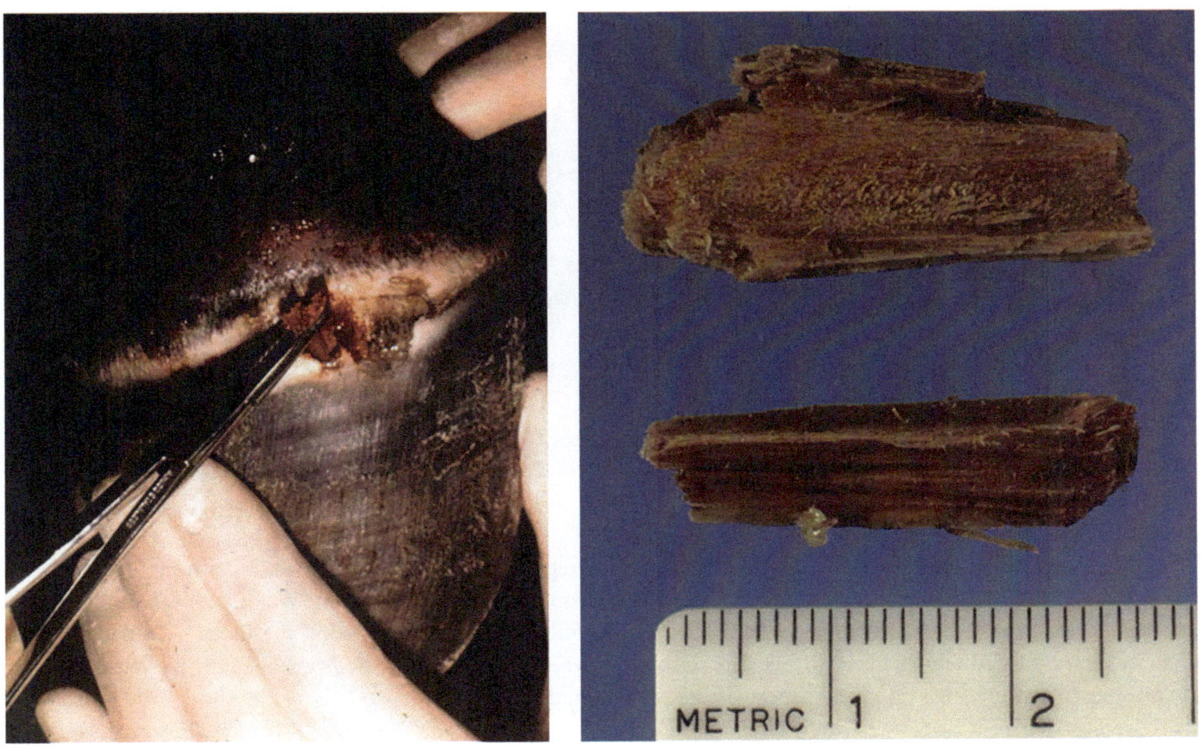

(a) (b)

Figure 13.3 A case of persistent drainage from a wound at the coronary band. **(a)** Splinter of wood being removed. **(b)** Wood splinter after removal.

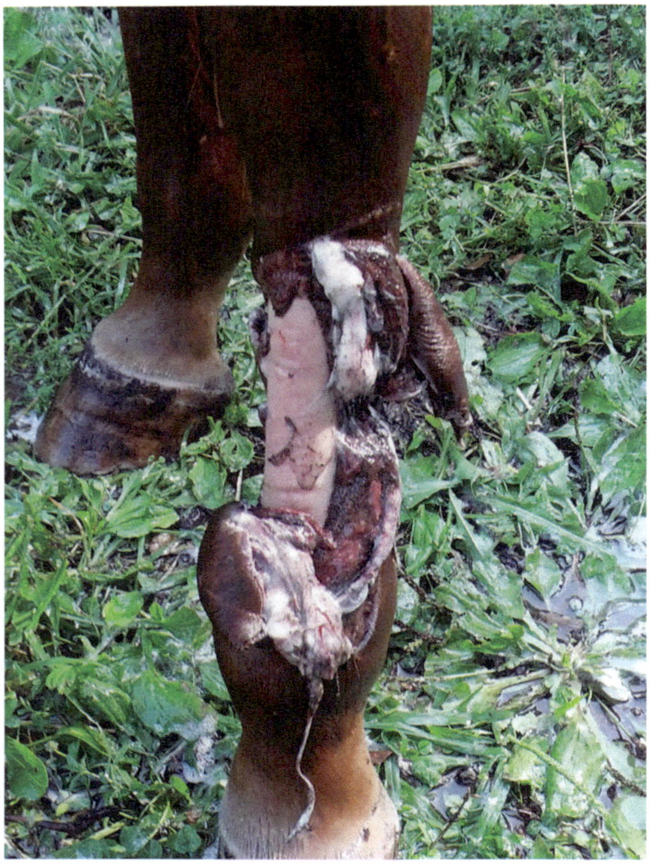

Figure 13.4 A degloving wound to the left hind limb. The metatarsal bone and the flexor tendons were exposed. Courtesy of Dr. Jon Koella.

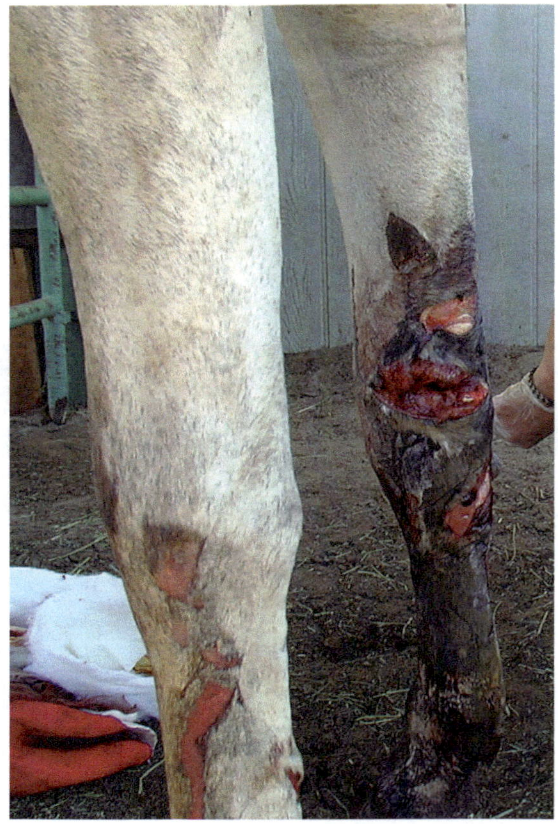

Figure 13.5 Acute laceration of the palmar carpal region that extended into the carpal canal.

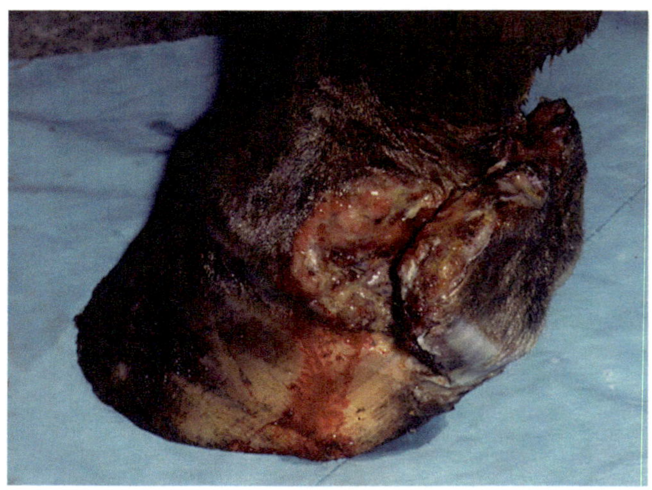

Figure 13.6 Chronically infected heel bulb laceration.

become entangled in barbed wire may sustain a serious wound, such as a degloving injury, which is particularly common in the metacarpal or metatarsal region (Figure 13.4), or a laceration that extends into a synovial cavity (Figure 13.5) or through a heel bulb (Figure 13.6). The extensor or flexor tendons may also be injured. For more information regarding injuries to tendons and their sheaths, see Chapter 17.

Wounds involving the distal aspect of the limb are often more problematic than wounds located elsewhere because their close proximity to the ground makes them more likely to become contaminated, and because skin in the distal portion of the limb is less vascular than skin located elsewhere. A wound to the distal aspect of the limb is much more likely to involve a vital structure because the distal aspect of the limb is populated by a high number of synovial structures, ligaments, and tendons.

Wounds involving the distal aspect of the limb are often more difficult to suture than are wounds of similar size on the body or proximal aspect of a limb because skin surrounding a wound on the distal aspect of the limb is more difficult to mobilize. Sutured wounds in this area are also more likely to dehisce. Second-intention healing of a wound on the distal aspect of the limb proceeds more slowly than it does in a wound proximal to the carpus and tarsus, because an unsutured wound in the distal aspect of the limb expands more after injury and has a longer preparatory phase of healing and a slower rate and earlier cessation of wound contraction.[2] Wounds of the distal aspect of the limb increase in size during the first 11–16 days after trauma, whereas those on the body change little in size.[2–4] Although one study showed that wounds of the distal aspect of the limb of horses epithelialized more slowly than did wounds on the thorax or flank,[2] an unpublished study demonstrated little difference between the rate of epithelialization of experimentally created, full-thickness, 7–9 cm^2 wounds on the distal aspect of the limb and the rate of epithelialization of similar wounds on the buttocks.[5] In that study, epithelialization progressed over metatarsal wounds at a rate of 0.48 mm/week and over wounds on the buttocks at a rate of 0.62 mm/week between the 3rd and the 7th weeks of healing.

The greatest difference in the rate of healing of wounds involving the body and those involving the distal limb is the greater contribution of contraction to the healing of wounds on the body.[6] Wounds that heal by contraction produce a more cosmetic outcome than those that heal by epithelialization because, with contraction, all layers of skin, including cutaneous adnexa (i.e., hair follicles, sebaceous and sweat glands), are carried centripetally (i.e., toward the center). The final appearance of wounds left to heal by second intention on the body or proximal aspect of the limbs is, therefore, much more cosmetic than the appearance of those of similar size on the distal aspect of a limb (Figure 13.7).

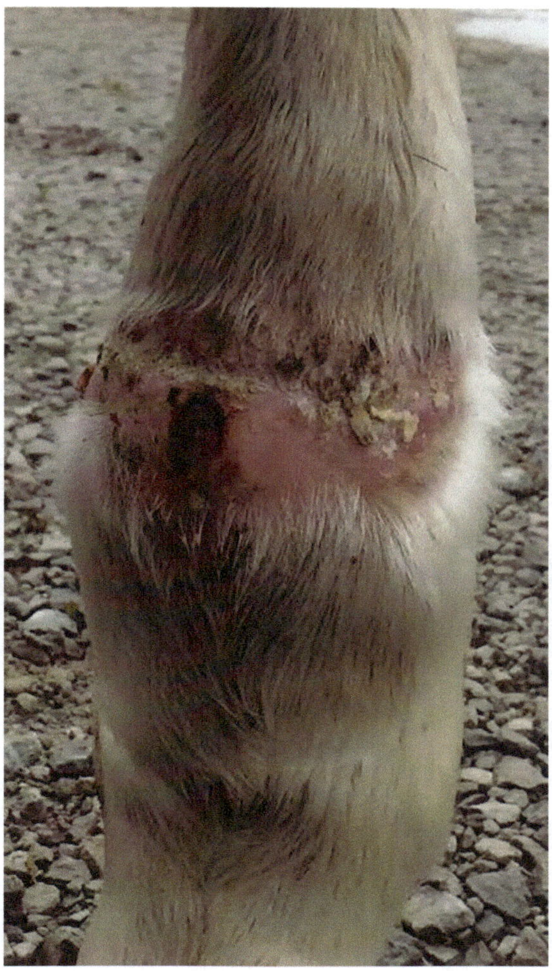

Figure 13.7 Wounds that heal to a large degree by epithelialization are less cosmetic than wounds that heal primarily by contraction because the epithelial scar is devoid of adnexa.

Horses have a greater propensity to develop EGT within a wound than do other domesticated animals, and a wound healing by second intention on the distal aspect of the limb is much more likely to develop EGT than is a similar wound proximal to the carpus and tarsus. Other factors, besides location, that promote exuberant production of granulation tissue in wounds of horses include chronic inflammation, motion, bandages, and casts.[7,8] More information regarding treatment for EGT can be found in Chapter 15.

A wound to the distal aspect of the limb should be meticulously examined after it has been properly prepared, as outlined in Chapter 4, so that damage to a vital structure is not overlooked. A wound that appears to be relatively innocuous (Figure 13.8) may be accompanied by damage to one or more vital structures deep within it, or it may contain a foreign body. Horses with an acute injury to the distal aspect of the limb involving a synovial structure often show little or no lameness, giving the owner and the attending veterinarian a false sense of security about the horse's prognosis for uncomplicated recovery. Lameness becomes apparent when intrasynovial pressure and concentration of inflammatory products increase. Ultrasonographic examination of the wounded region may provide the first evidence of synovial sepsis and/or identify a foreign body (see Figure 12.25c). Early ultrasonographic evidence of sepsis includes the presence of excess fluid, fibrin, or cells within the synovial fluid (Figure 13.9). Ultrasound may also be useful to guide collection of synovial fluid for cytologic analyses and for bacterial culture. Air introduced into the

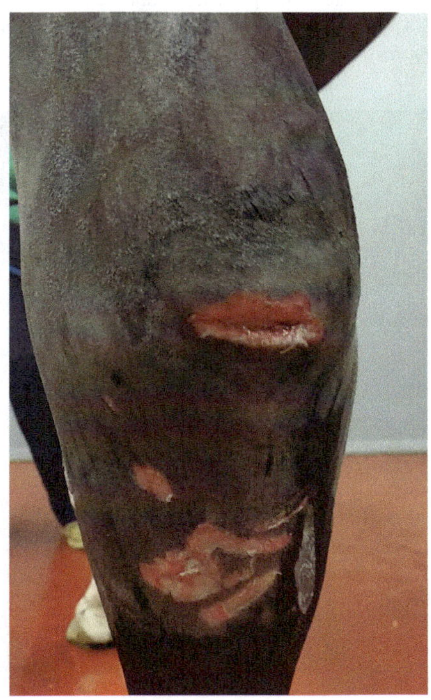

Figure 13.8 A harmless appearing wound over the *tuber calcis* that entered the calcaneal bursa, resulting in sepsis of that synovial structure. Courtesy of Dr. Blake Everett.

wound from breach of tissue, however, may limit the effectiveness of ultrasonographic examination if the wound is acute. Generally, primary closure is indicated for an acute, clean wound in which a vital structure has not been penetrated. For contaminated or contused wounds, delayed primary closure or delayed secondary closure is often selected. The decision to close the wound primarily or to delay closure – primary or secondary – or to allow it to heal by second intention can be made only after considering many factors (see Chapter 8 for more information regarding approaches to wound closure and Chapter 10 for more information regarding reconstructive surgical techniques, such as skin mobilization).

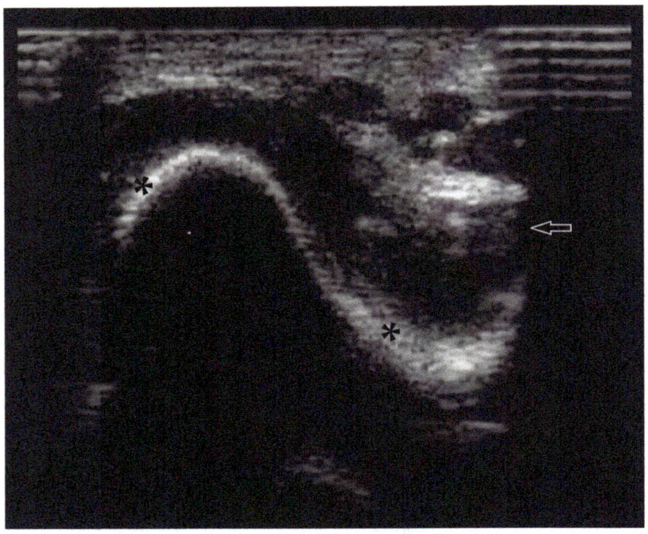

Figure 13.9 This ultrasonographic image of a tarsocrural joint shows evidence of sepsis, including the presence of fibrin and cells within the synovial fluid. The asterisks lie on the talus, and the arrow points to fibrin within the tarsocrural joint.

Heavily contaminated or infected wounds and those that are so large that they cannot be closed with sutures must heal by second intention. Without proper care, however, these wounds often develop EGT, leading to an unsightly epithelial scar that is susceptible to re-injury (Figure 13.10) or to a fibrous granuloma (see Figure 15.12). The reader is referred to Chapter 15 for discussion of EGT. See Chapter 18 if the wound is so large that skin grafting must be considered.

For purposes of discussion, this chapter has been separated into wounds (both open and closed) located from the fetlock to the carpus or tarsus, wounds of the pastern, avulsion injuries to the hoof capsule, and penetrating wounds to the hoof. A wound to a synovial cavity and treatment of horses with an avulsion injury accompanied by exposed bone and the presence of bone sequestra are not discussed in depth in this chapter. For more information, see Chapter 16, which covers treatment of horses with wounds involving synovial structures, and Chapter 14, which covers degloving injuries and bone sequestra.

What to do

- Suture wounds on the distal aspect of the limb, whenever possible, to avoid the development of EGT, protracted healing, and formation of an unsightly scar.

Tip

- A wound near a synovial structure should be examined meticulously to determine if the wound communicates with the synovial structure. Preventing a contaminated synovial structure from becoming infected is far easier than trying to resolve infection of that structure.

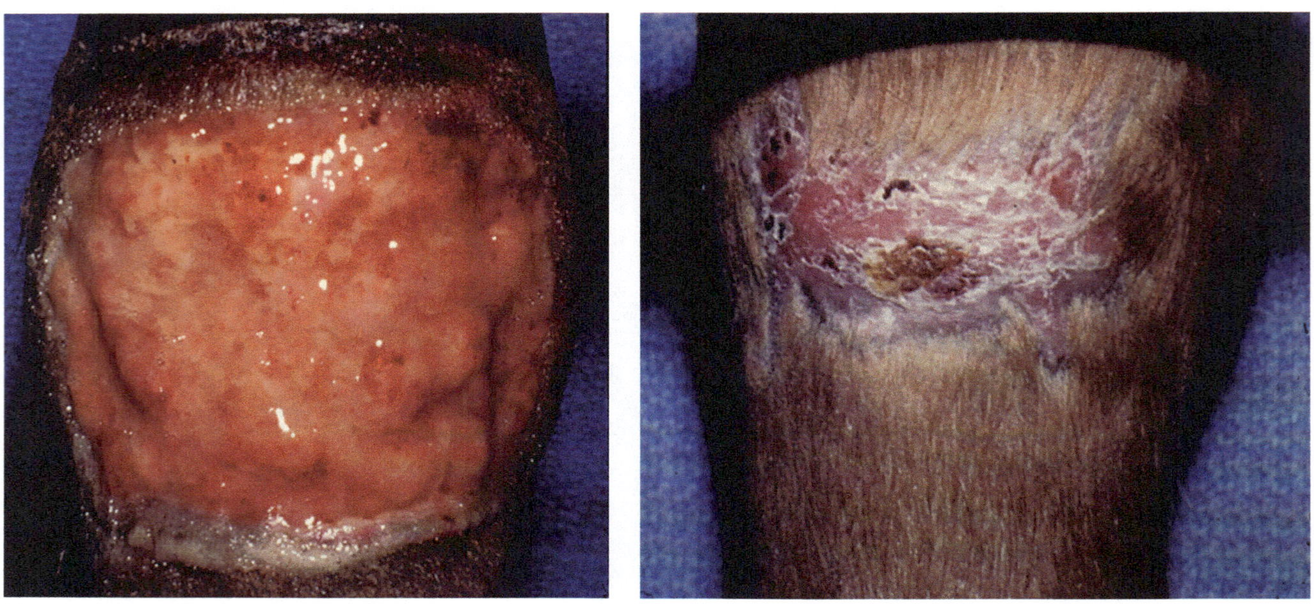

(a) (b)

Figure 13.10 A wound that healed with an unsightly epithelial scar is susceptible to re-injury. **(a)** A rectangular-shaped wound over the dorsal fetlock. **(b)** Healing after 75 days resulted in an unsightly epithelial scar susceptible to re-injury.

Wound categories

Wounds may be categorized as open (i.e., full thickness) or closed (i.e., partial thickness). Open wounds are those in which the entire thickness of the skin has been separated. They include incisions, which are wounds produced by a sharp object, either intentionally with a scalpel or accidentally by glass or sheet metal, for example. The skin edge of an incision is cut cleanly, resulting in little damage to underlying tissue. The victim experiences little pain. Lacerations are the most common type of open wound and are characterized by an irregular cutaneous margin and extensive damage to underlying tissue. They are accompanied by bruising, which results in considerable pain. A laceration accompanied by loss of tissue is termed an avulsion. A puncture is another type of open wound and is produced by a sharp object that perforates tissue. The perforating object may carry dirt, manure, or other debris into the depths of the wound and may enter a synovial cavity. Puncture wounds are easily trivialized because their size belies their severity.

Closed wounds are those that do not involve the entire thickness of skin; they include abrasions and contusions. An abrasion is an injury to the superficial layers of the skin caused by friction and is characterized by oozing of serum and only a small amount of hemorrhage. Exposure of many nerve endings results in considerable pain to the victim. A rope burn is an example of an abrasion. A contusion is a closed wound characterized by bleeding and destruction of tissue within and beneath undivided skin (see Figure 10.27).

Wounds involving the fetlock, metacarpus/metatarsus, and/or carpus/tarsus

Causes

Wounds involving the fetlock, metacarpus or metatarsus, and carpus or tarsus, are commonly inflicted by barbed wire or other metal objects. The hindlimb appears to be more susceptible than the forelimb to wounding in these regions. The soft tissues of the dorsal surface of the carpus are particularly prone to contusions and punctures, which are often incurred when the carpus strikes a fence or stall door, and these closed injuries and punctures often involve one of the many synovial structures found in the carpal region (see Figure 16.6a). Occasionally, a wire laceration or a puncture to the palmar surface of the antebrachium or carpus enters the synovial sheath of the carpal canal (Figure 13.5).

Closed injuries

The most common type of closed injury to the distal portion of the limb is the carpal hygroma, which appears as a fluid-filled swelling over the dorsal surface of the carpus. Its usual cause is blunt force to the dorsum of the carpus or antebrachium, such as that which might occur when the horse jumps a fence or hits the stall door with a forelimb. A carpal hygroma forms from accumulation of fluid in an adventitious bursa in the subcutaneous tissue, usually from a subcutaneous hematoma that develops into a seroma.[9] A hygroma often resembles an abnormal accumulation of fluid in the tendon sheath of an extensor muscle, making the two conditions sometimes difficult to differentiate.

Diagnosis

A carpal hygroma appears as a cyst-like, spherical, fluctuant swelling containing serous fluid (Figure 13.2). Its spherical appearance helps distinguish a hygroma from a longitudinally oriented, distended sheath of the tendon of an extensor muscle (i.e., the extensor *carpi radialis* muscle or the common digital extensor muscle) and from a horizontally oriented, distended carpal joint (i.e., the antebrachiocarpal joint).

Carpal flexion may be restricted if the hygroma is large. Palpation of the swelling does not usually cause the horse to show signs of discomfort, unless the hygroma is infected, and usually the horse is lame only if the hygroma interferes mechanically with the gait or is infected. Although a carpal hygroma can typically be differentiated from a swollen sheath of an extensor tendon or a distended carpal joint by inspection and palpation, ultrasonographic examination or contrast radiographic examination of the hygroma provides definitive diagnosis.

Treatment

The affected horse can usually be treated successfully by centesis and drainage of the hygroma, application of a pressure bandage, and confinement. A corticosteroid injected into the cavity of the hygroma at the time of drainage may be helpful in preventing reformation of fluid. If the hygroma fails to resolve in this manner, it can be drained through a distally located stab incision, through which the lining of the cavity is removed, by using a large curette, with the horse standing, or by using an arthroscopically guided, motorized synovial resector, with the horse anesthetized. A Penrose drain inserted through the stab incision ensures that it remains open until production of fluid has subsided (Figure 13.11a). The limb is bandaged and held in extension with a splint for several weeks (Figure 13.11b). If the hygroma fails to resolve with these treatments, the capsule can be excised with the horse anesthetized. After surgery, the limb is held in extension with a cast or splint for several weeks, after which a pressure bandage is applied for an additional 1–2 weeks. The horse can begin walking exercise after about 1 month.

Prognosis

If the horse is chronically affected, treatment may not restore full range of carpal motion due to the presence of fibrosis. The owner should be warned that surgical treatment may worsen the condition if healing is disturbed by motion or infection.

> **What to do**
>
> - Most carpal hygromas can be resolved by draining the hygroma, instilling a corticosteroid into its lumen, and applying a pressure bandage to the carpus.

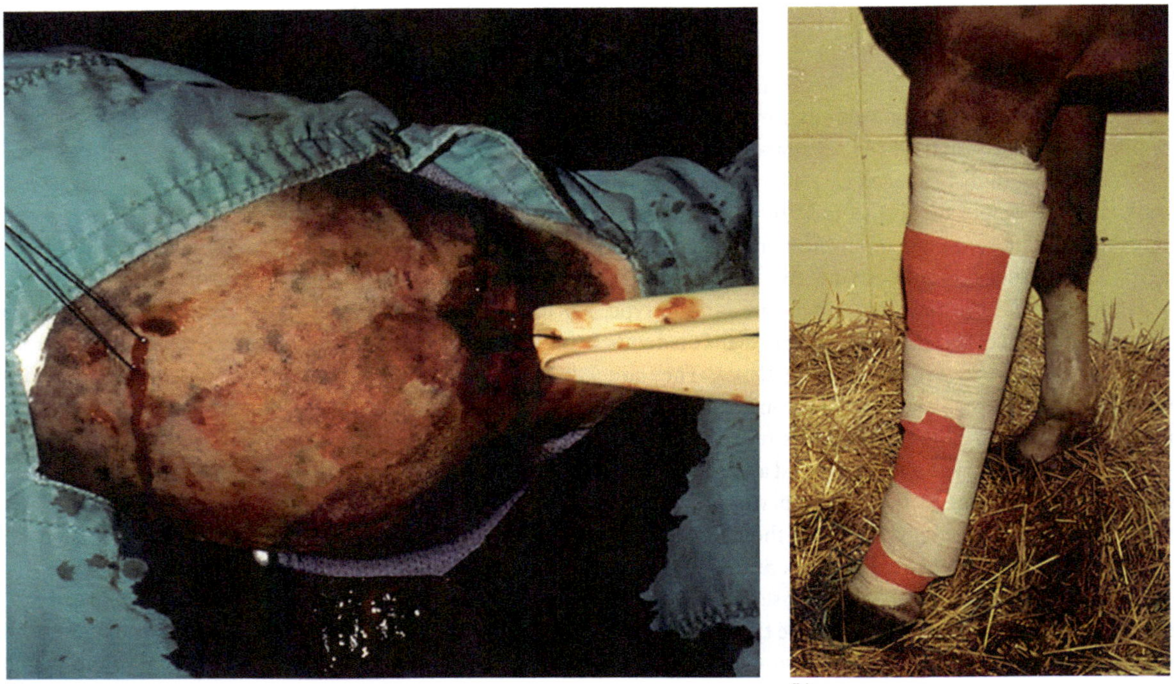

(a) (b)

Figure 13.11 Same horse as in Figure 13.2, at surgery. **(a)** A Penrose drain is inserted through the stab incision at the distal extent of the hygroma. The drain ensures that the incision remains open until production of fluid has subsided, usually within 7–10 days. **(b)** The limb is bandaged and held in extension with a splint for several weeks.

- The limb should be bandaged and held in extension, with a cast or a splint, for several weeks after a hygroma has been incised and its lining curetted, or after a hygroma has been excised.

Tip

- A carpal hygroma can be differentiated from a distended carpal joint or a distended extensor tendon sheath by examining the swelling ultrasonographically or by contrast radiography.

Open (full-thickness) injuries

Diagnosis

The carpus, tarsus, metacarpus, or metatarsus may suffer a degloving injury, which is a type of injury in which an extensive segment of skin and underlying tissue is lacerated, thereby exposing bone and often tendons. A large portion of the lacerated segment of skin is often devoid of vascular supply. The injury may result from a circumferential laceration accompanied by detachment of skin from the limb (Figure 13.4) or from an avulsion that is accompanied by such an extensive loss of tissue that the wound cannot heal by second intention alone (see Figure 5.4).

Contraction of large wounds over the flexor surface of a joint often results in contracture of the associated joint and distortion of the limb in people, dogs, and cats.[10,11] Wound contraction in horses, however, does not cause contracture and should be considered beneficial because it accelerates wound healing and decreases the size of the epithelial scar. Wounds healed by contraction are more cosmetic than those healed by epithelialization.

Wounds to the carpus, metacarpus, tarsus, or metatarsus frequently involve one or more of the many tendons, tendon sheaths, bursae, or joint capsules found in these regions (Figures 13.5, 13.8, 13.12). Breach of a synovial structure can be confirmed by injecting sterile fluid into the synovial cavity suspected of being penetrated, at a site remote from the wound, and observing it egress from the wound (see Figure 4.4). Synovial fluid aspirated from a synovial structure suspected of being penetrated can be analyzed to determine if the synovial structure is infected. Bacteria are not commonly seen during cytologic examination of synovial fluid from an infected synovial structure, and consequently, infection is usually determined by identifying an elevated concentration of neutrophils and protein in fluid aspirated from the cavity. Bacterial infection of a synovial structure can be definitively diagnosed by identifying bacteria within the cells present in synovial fluid, by bacterial culture, or by polymerase chain reaction (PCR).[12] For more information, see Chapter 16, which discusses lacerations associated with synovial structures.

Injury to the calcaneus and associated soft-tissue structures is common because the calcaneus is prominent and has little soft-tissue protection. Injury to the point of the hock, or calcaneal tuber, is frequently associated with lameness, swelling of surrounding soft tissues, periosteal new bone production and lysis of the calcaneal tuber, and infection of the calcaneal bursa (Figure 16.6b).[13] Injury to the distomedial enlargement of the calcaneus, or *sustentaculum tali*, is frequently associated with lameness, swelling of surrounding soft tissues, periosteal new

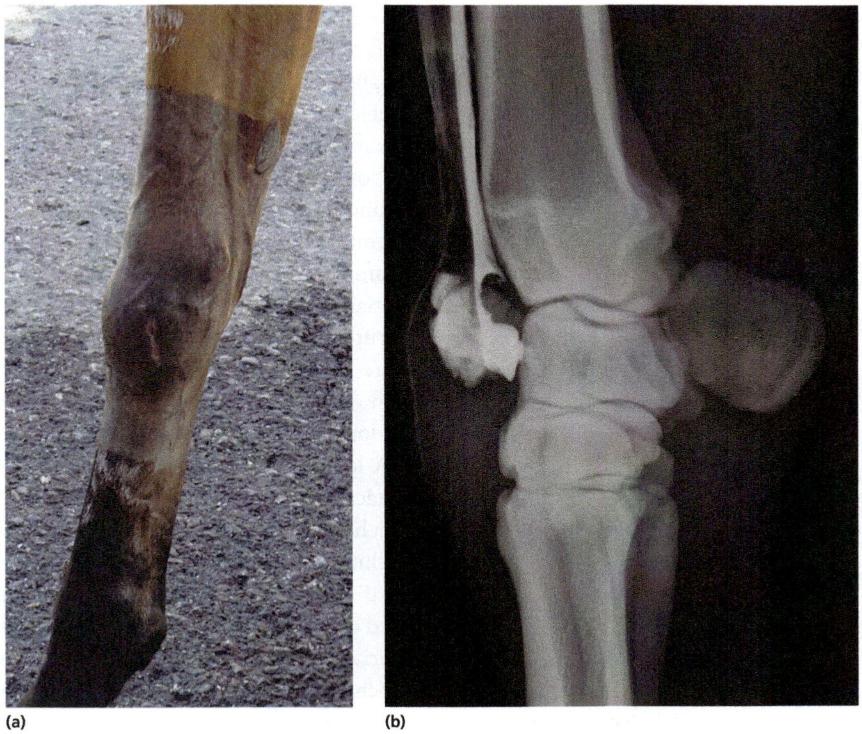

Figure 13.12 This horse suffered a puncture wound to the tendon sheath of the *extensor carpi radialis* muscle. **(a)** Appearance of the carpus and antebrachium. **(b)** Penetration of this synovial structure was confirmed by instilling a radiocontrast medium into the tendon sheath. Courtesy of Dr. Albert Sole.

bone production and lysis of the *sustentaculum tali*, effusion of the tarsal sheath, and damage to the deep digital flexor tendon (sometimes referred to as the lateral digital flexor tendon, which is the principal tendon of the deep digital flexor muscle at this level).[14,15] The tendon of the medial digital flexor muscle (medial head of the deep digital flexor muscle, sometime called the long digital flexor muscle) passes plantar to the medial collateral ligament joining the deep digital flexor tendon distal to the tarsometatarsal joint. A flexed, proximoplantar-to-distoplantar tangential (skyline) radiographic projection of the calcaneus is helpful in identifying lesions of the calcaneal tuber and *sustentaculum tali.* Sepsis of the calcaneal bursa or tarsal sheath is determined by analyzing synovial fluid obtained by centesis, and ultrasonographic examination is used to identify damage to the deep digital flexor tendon.

The extensor tendons are frequently involved in lacerations located in the carpal, tarsal, metacarpal, or metatarsal regions because they are located superficially in these regions. When the tendon of the *extensor carpi radialis* muscle is lacerated, the horse is still able to extend the distal aspect of the limb owing to the action of the common and lateral digital extensor muscles, but the carpus overflexes because resistance to the action of the flexor muscles is diminished.[16] Transection of the tendon of the common digital extensor muscle above or below the carpus seems to have no long-lasting detrimental effect on gait because the actions of the *extensor carpi radialis* and lateral digital extensor muscles and the extensor branches of the suspensory ligament compensate for the loss of action of this muscle.[17] Transection or rupture of the *peroneus tertius* tendon on the dorsal surface of the hock allows this joint to move independently of the stifle as a result of disruption of the reciprocal apparatus (Figure 13.13).

Laceration of an extensor tendon is often associated with a large avulsion wound on the dorsal surface of the metacarpus/metatarsus (Figure 13.4, Figure 13.14).[16] Extensor tendons of the hindlimb are lacerated far more frequently than are those of the forelimb,[18] and the tendon of the long digital extensor muscle is lacerated more frequently than is the tendon of the lateral digital extensor muscle, although, frequently, both tendons are lacerated. Because the primary function of the extensor tendons of the distal aspect of the limb is to extend the digit during locomotion, rather than to support weight, laceration of one or more of the extensor tendons does not alter the conformation of the limb but may result instead in an inability of the horse to extend the toe, causing the fetlock to knuckle during locomotion.

In contrast, the conformation of the limb is altered when a flexor tendon of the distal aspect of the limb is severed. The digit hyperextends when one or both flexor tendons have been severed. If only the superficial digital flexor tendon has been severed, the metacarpo-/metatarsophalangeal joint hyperextends, causing the fetlock to drop when weight is borne on the limb. Severance of the deep digital flexor tendon, coupled with severance of the superficial digital flexor tendon, causes the distal interphalangeal joint to also hyperextend, causing the toe to elevate upon weight bearing. If both flexor tendons and

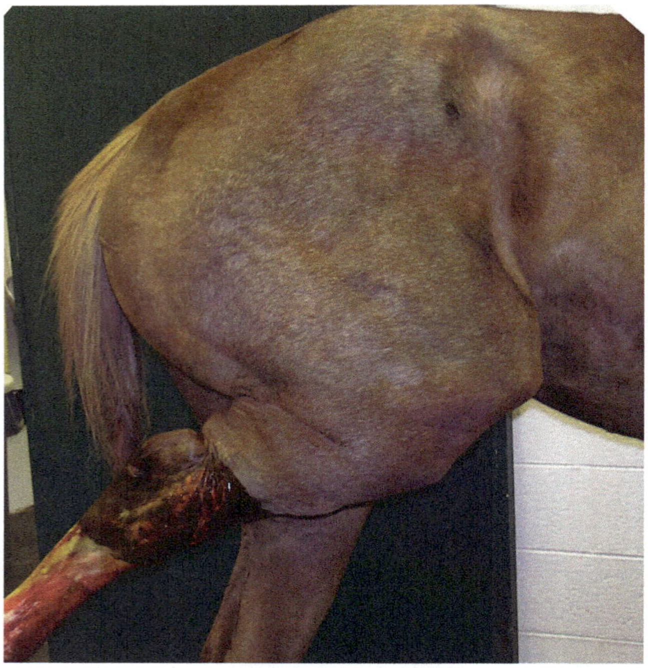

Figure 13.13 This horse sustained an avulsion injury to the dorsal surface of the hock that was complicated by laceration of the tendon of the *peroneus tertius*. Note that the hock is extended while the stifle is flexed.

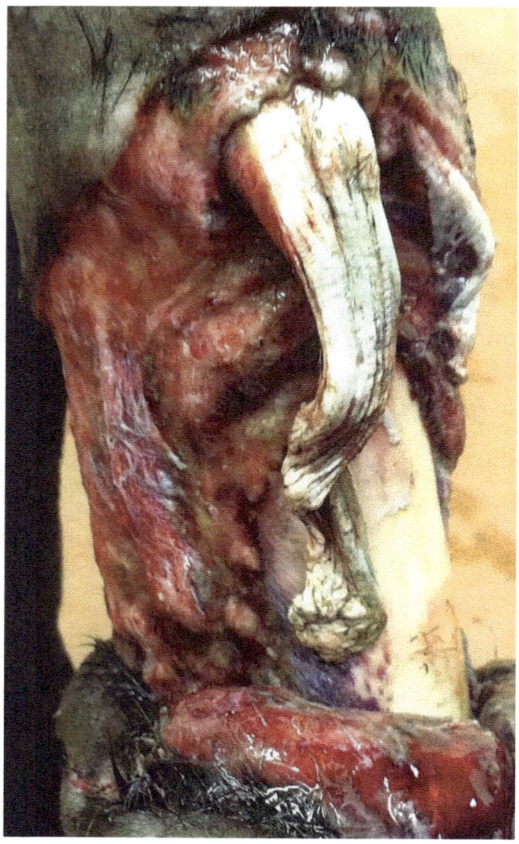

Figure 13.14 Large, degloving wounds on the dorsal surface of the metacarpus/metatarsus often are associated with laceration of the long and lateral digital extensor tendons. Courtesy of Dr. Michael Caruso.

the suspensory ligament have been severed, the palmar/plantar surface of the fetlock contacts the ground when the horse bears weight on the limb, and the solar surface of the foot fails to contact the ground. Whereas laceration of an extensor tendon is often associated with a large wound, laceration of a flexor tendon is typically associated with a small wound. The cutaneous wound may be slightly remote from the tendinous wound if the laceration occurred while the limb was flexed. Ultrasonographic examination of the flexor tendons may be necessary to detect partial disruption of a digital flexor tendon because partial disruption results in no postural changes. See Chapter 17 for more information about diagnosis and treatment of horses with lacerations associated with tendons, paratenons, and tendon sheaths.

A laceration to the dorsal, lateral, or medial surface of the metacarpus/metatarsus often exposes a large area of bone, which is often devoid of periosteum (Figure 13.15). The extreme thickness of the dorsal portion of the cortex of the diaphysis of the third metacarpal/metatarsal bone may predispose the outer third of this bone to develop a sequestrum, because trauma may deprive the bone of its periosteal blood supply leaving it dependent on medullary vessels traversing the cortex.

Occasionally, a foreign body becomes embedded within the soft tissues on the palmar or plantar surface of the metacarpal or metatarsal region. Although a foreign object may sometimes be identified by inserting a probe into the wound's tract, ultrasonographic examination or plain or contrast radiographic examination of the affected region is usually required to identify the foreign object (Figure 4.3).

Treatment

Sutured wounds of the carpus, tarsus, metacarpus, metatarsus, and fetlock are prone to dehisce because wounds in these regions rapidly become contaminated due to their proximity to the ground and because their blood supply is often attenuated from the tension exerted on the skin when closing the wound. Wounds of the fetlock, carpus, and tarsus are especially prone to dehisce because of tension caused by motion upon joint flexion/extension. The risk of dehiscence caused by infection can be diminished by properly preparing the wound or by using delayed primary or delayed secondary closure. See Chapters 4 and 8 for detailed accounts of techniques used to prepare wounds for suturing.

Wounds of the carpus, tarsus, metacarpus, metatarsus, and fetlock are often difficult to suture without tension because tissues in these regions are difficult to mobilize and because these regions are highly mobile or contain highly mobile structures (e.g., tendons). Dehiscence of wounds sutured under tension and excessive expansion of unsutured wounds can best be prevented by immobilizing the distal portion of the limb with a cast or with a splint applied over a bandage. Immobilizing the distal portion of a limb with a distal limb cast or a splint may be helpful in preventing dehiscence of a sutured wound in a mobile region, such as the fetlock, especially if the wound is perpendicular or

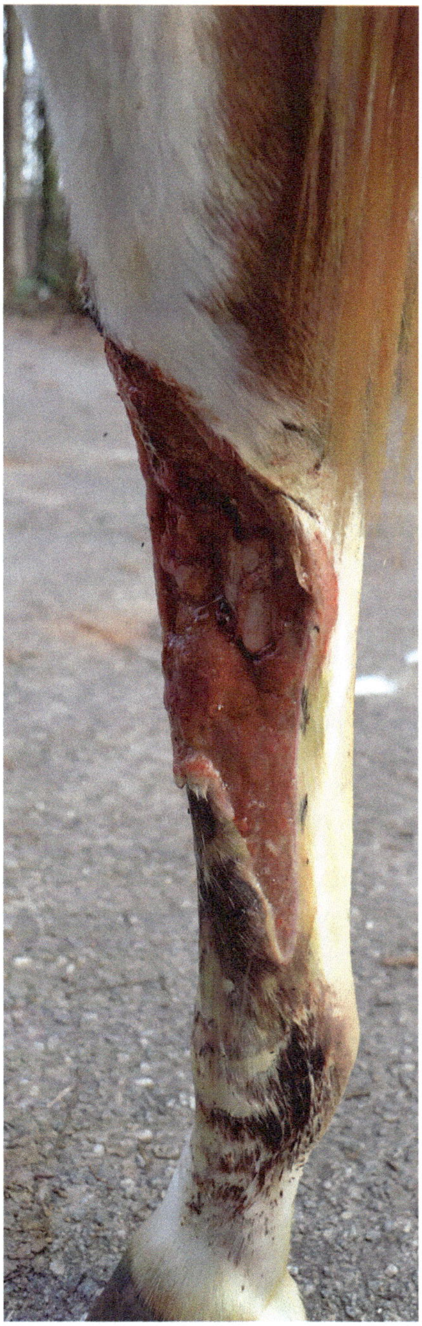

Figure 13.15 Laceration to the lateral surface of the metacarpus exposed a large area of bone. The upper layer of bone devoid of periosteum is ischemic and is likely to form a sequestrum.

oblique to the limb's long axis. Enclosing a lacerated tarsus in a cast is difficult because of the reciprocal apparatus of the hindlimb, but application of a full-limb cast or a bandage and splint to a hind imb may sometimes be indicated. For more information regarding techniques for casting and bandage splinting, see Chapter 7.

The length of time during which the distal aspect of the limb is immobilized depends on the amount of tension exerted on the wound during closure. Wounds with a good blood supply that are sutured with minimal tension are immobilized for only 10–14 days, whereas wounds sutured under great tension or those with a blood supply marginal enough to delay healing should be immobilized for 17–21 days. A limb with a wound left to heal by second intention may require a considerably longer period of immobilization (e.g., several months), especially if an extensor or flexor tendon has been lacerated.

Wounds closed under tension, especially those that have been excessively undermined, may dehisce because stretching the skin beyond its limits of maximal extensibility may obstruct blood flow through the dermal blood vessels, causing the sutured margin of the wound to necrose.[19] Techniques most commonly used to avoid excessive tension on the sutured laceration include: undermining of the skin adjacent to the wound; presuturing the wound; applying tension sutures, such as walking sutures or horizontal mattress, vertical mattress, or far–near tension sutures; and creating relaxing incisions.[20–23] For information regarding techniques used to relieve skin tension, see Chapter 10. If the wound cannot be closed completely, as much of the wound as possible should be sutured to prevent the margin of the wound from retracting. Preventing retraction improves the cosmetic outcome and speeds healing.

Treatment of injury to the calcaneus and associated soft-tissue structures may entail excising infected bone, endoscopically irrigating the tarsal sheath or calcaneal bursa, and administering antimicrobial therapy systemically and/or by regional limb perfusion. Excising the portion of the deep digital flexor tendon within the tarsal sheath may be necessary to resolve infection of the tarsal sheath if this tendon is infected.[14] The reader is referred to Chapter 16 for more information regarding treatment of infected synovial cavities.

Movement of an intact or severed or partially severed flexor or extensor tendon within a wound on a metacarpus or metatarsus often results in the formation of two separate granulation beds, one on the tendon and the other on tissue surrounding the tendon (see Figure 17.18). Granulation tissue provides myofibroblasts that normally span the wound, causing it to contract, but the presence of two separate granulation beds prevents myofibroblasts from spanning the wound. When movement of the tendon is restricted by immobilizing the limb, the granulation beds rapidly become confluent, resulting in prompt contraction of the wound.

Horses with an infected wound containing a foreign body or a bone sequestrum are usually presented with an intermittently or persistently draining tract within the wound. The wound fails to heal until the foreign object or sequestrum is removed.[24] A foreign object or sequestrum provides a nidus for bacterial growth, and its presence can cause infection when only a small quantity of bacteria contaminates the wound. For more information on the management of infected wounds, see Chapter 19. Treatment for a bone sequestrum is discussed in Chapter 14.

A degloving wound can be managed by primary closure or by delayed primary or secondary closure when no skin has been lost, provided that the lacerated skin has sufficient blood supply to sustain its survival. Often, a degloving wound has such an extensive loss of skin that the wound can be healed only by second intention or by applying a free skin graft to the wound (Figure 13.15). The reader is referred to Chapter 18 for more information about skin grafting. A degloving injury may, rarely, be accompanied by vascular damage to the limb so severe that the hoof capsule loses its laminar attachments (Figure 13.16). See Chapter 14 for more information about the treatment of degloving injuries

Prognosis

When treated properly, a horse with a wound of the fetlock, metacarpus, metatarsus, carpus, or tarsus that does not extend into a supporting structure or synovial cavity has a good prognosis for an excellent cosmetic outcome and soundness. Treatment is difficult when a synovial cavity, tendon, or bone becomes infected, and the outcome is often disappointing. Horses that have incurred damage to a synovial structure have a guarded prognosis for return to soundness.[25,26]

The nature of the injury affects outcome. For example, cutaneous incisions, whether created accidentally or purposely, result in minimal trauma and negligible contamination. Lacerations caused by impact, whether clean or heavily contaminated, are more susceptible to infection than are incisional wounds, and they tend to heal poorly because of injury to the blood supply. Sutured wounds parallel to the long axis of the limb are more likely to heal without complication than are sutured wounds transverse to the long axis of the limb. Sutured wounds aligned obliquely or transversely to the long axis of the limb are best protected from distractive forces by immobilizing the injured region in a bandage splint or a cast and commonly dehisce when protected by a bandage alone.

A deep wound to the dorsal surface of the metacarpal or metatarsal region is not usually career ending, even if extensor tendons are injured, because extensor function is usually restored if the distal portion of the affected limb is immobilized for 4–6 weeks with a cast or splint. Damage to the tendon of the lateral digital extensor muscle of the hindlimb, however, sometimes causes the horse to develop stringhalt in the affected limb when the tendon becomes immobile from fibrous adhesions that develop during healing. Because extensor tendons do not support weight, a decrease in their mechanical strength does not adversely affect the outcome of the horse. A wound to the palmar/plantar surface of the metacarpal/metatarsal region, however, is frequently career ending or even life threatening if one or both flexor tendons, suspensory ligament, or digital flexor tendon sheath are lacerated.

In one study, 75% of horses with wounds of the hock involving only the calcaneal bursa survived, but if the calcaneal tuber of the calcaneus was also infected, only 44% of survived.[27] Another study examining the treatment and outcome of 10 horses with a wound of the hock resulting in infection of the *sustentaculum tali* of the calcaneus, with or without infection of the tarsal sheath, found that of nine horses for which long-term follow-up was available, seven became sound.[14] The authors of that report

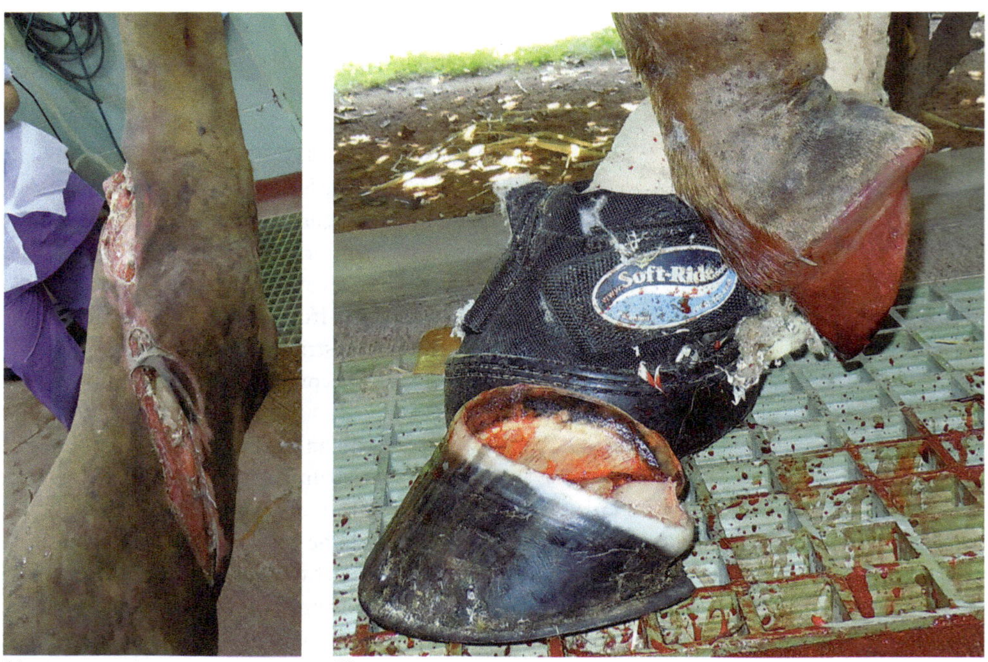

(a) (b)

Figure 13.16 (**a,b**) This horse suffered a degloving injury to the medial and dorsal surface of the metatarsus that so severely impaired the vascular supply to the foot that the hoof capsule was lost. The horse is in dorsal recumbency on a surgery table. Courtesy of Dr. Gal Kelmer.

concluded that horses with osteomyelitis of the *sustentaculum tali*, with or without concomitant infection of the tarsal sheath, can have an excellent to good outcome and may return to their previous use after surgical debridement of affected tissues and lavage of the tarsal sheath. They also observed that resection of the deep (lateral) digital flexor tendon, however, should be regarded as a salvage procedure, because athletic use after this procedure is unpredictable.

Infected wounds containing a foreign body or an osseous sequestrum generally heal without complication after the object or sequestrum has been removed. Antimicrobial therapy administered parenterally may temporarily decrease swelling and discharge from the wound,[28] but antimicrobial therapy alone is an ineffective treatment for a horse with a foreign object or sequestrum embedded in a wound, because drugs fail to contact bacteria harbored by the foreign object or sequestrum. Organic foreign objects, such as pieces of wood, have a greater tendency to potentiate infection and provoke a greater inflammatory response, resulting in more discharge of exudate, than do non-organic foreign objects, such as pieces of glass or metal. Bacterial culture of exudate from a draining sinus is not helpful in determining the organism associated with the foreign object because secondary pathogens rapidly colonize a draining sinus.

An avulsion injury to the carpus is particularly devastating because the success of sheet grafting a wound over the dorsum of the carpus is often compromised due to the movement the graft must withstand in this region (Figure 13.17). The carpus must be completely immobilized in a full-limb or sleeve cast for the graft to be accepted. After the graft has been accepted and after the limb is no longer immobilized, the graft and granulation tissue beneath the graft may split transversely along the dorsal surface of the antebrachiocarpal and middle carpal joints, sometimes opening the sheath of the tendon of the *extensor carpi radialis* muscle.

What to do

- Laceration or puncture of a synovial structure may be confirmed or excluded by injecting sterile fluid into the synovial cavity at a site remote from the wound. Exit of fluid from the wound indicates that the synovial structure has been penetrated.
- Applying a distal limb cast or a bandage and splint to the a limb is often helpful in preventing a sutured wound on the fetlock from dehiscing, especially if the wound is perpendicular or oblique to the limb's long axis.
- Wounds that drain intermittently or persistently should be examined for the presence of a foreign body or bone sequestrum.

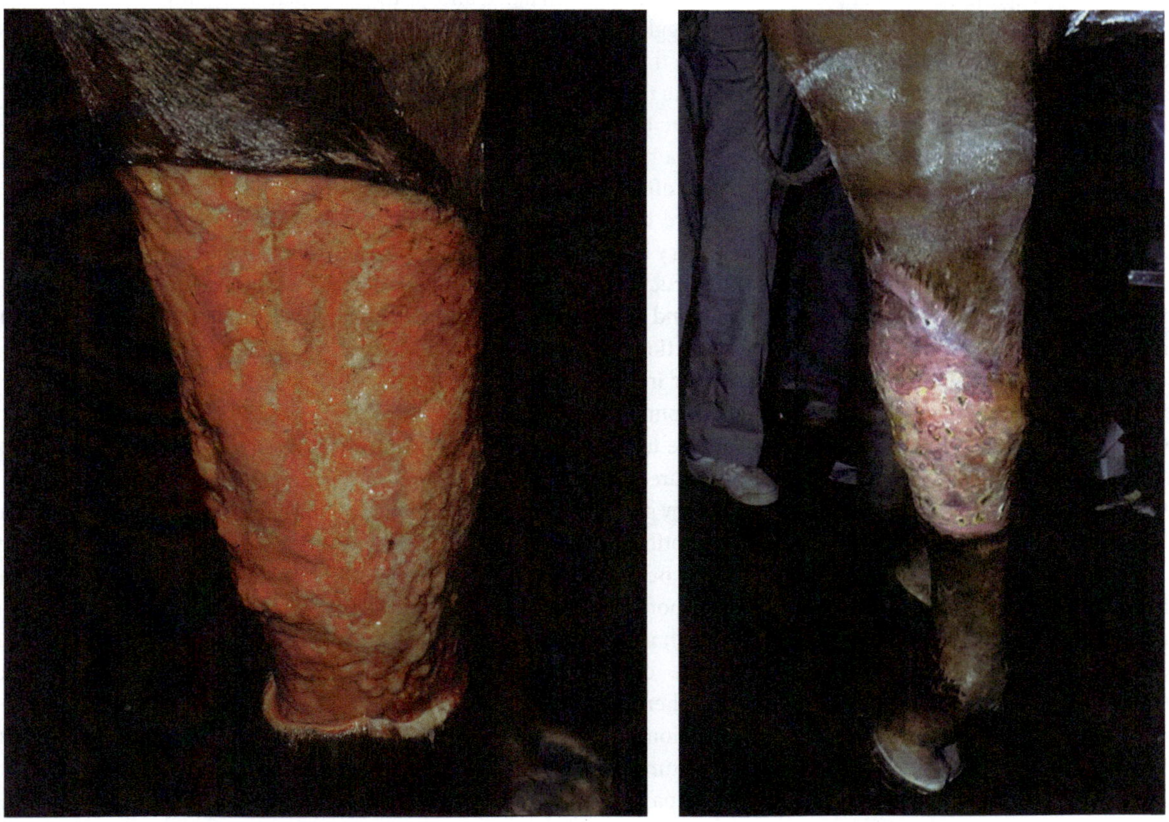

(a) (b)

Figure 13.17 This horse suffered an extensive avulsion injury to the carpus. **(a)** Granulation tissue fills the wound. **(b)** The wound was covered with a free, split-thickness, meshed skin graft. A large portion of the graft was accepted.

> **Tips**
>
> - The most useful test to determine if a synovial structure is infected is cytologic examination of fluid aseptically aspirated from the structure.
> - Bacterial infection of a synovial structure is definitively diagnosed by observing intracellular bacteria during cytologic examination or by culturing bacteria from the synovial fluid, but the sensitivity of these two methods of diagnosis of infection is low.
> - Healing of a fresh wound that cannot be closed completely may be speeded by suturing as much of the wound as possible to prevent the margin of the wound from retracting.
> - Damage to an extensor tendon does not usually end the horse's athletic career because extensor function is usually regained if the digit is immobilized, or partially immobilized, in extension, for 4–6 weeks.

Wounds involving the pastern

Causes

The pastern is particularly susceptible to trauma because of its proximity to the ground. Lacerations of the pastern are commonly inflicted by barbed wire or other metal objects (Figure 13.6; see Figure 4.2a), and occasionally, the pastern is injured when it becomes entrapped between immovable objects, such as the rails of a cattle guard or a wall and stall door. An injury caused by entrapment of the pastern is often accompanied by vascular trauma leading to ischemic necrosis of soft tissue and infection. The longer the horse is entrapped and the more it struggles to free itself, the greater the vascular injury. Occasionally, a rope encircling the pastern causes a rope burn severe enough to result in loss of a partial- or full-thickness portion of skin (Figure 13.1).

The coronary band of a hindlimb sometimes incurs a penetrating wound when the horse jumps a barrier, and often a splinter of wood is embedded within the wound (Figure 13.3). Lacerations of the pastern frequently involve the coronary band and variable portions of the hoof capsule, as well as structures deep to the hoof wall. Lacerations to the coronary band may result in permanent defects in the hoof wall (see the section on laceration and avulsion wounds of the hoof capsule later in this chapter). A wound on the pastern quickly becomes contaminated with manure and dirt because the pastern is close to the ground. A laceration incurred while the horse is at pasture may go unrecognized for days because it is hidden from view by grass.

The heel bulb is the region of the pastern most susceptible to injury. A heel bulb laceration, especially one caused by barbed wire, often extends in an arc from the quarter of the hoof wall to the depression between the heel bulbs (Figure 4.2a); occasionally, the arc extends from one quarter to the other (Figure 13.6). In either case, the wound often gapes when the horse bears weight on the limb. The deeper the laceration, the greater is the likelihood that one or more critical structures in the pastern or foot may be damaged. Lacerations of the pastern that course deep to the hoof wall may involve one or more collateral ligaments, the capsule of the proximal or distal interphalangeal joint, the deep digital flexor tendon and its digital flexor tendon sheath, a collateral cartilage of the distal phalanx, and/or the navicular bone and its bursa and ligaments (Figure 13.18, Figure 13.19; see Figure 16.6c). Occasionally, a laceration of the pastern is accompanied by fracture of the middle or distal phalanx.

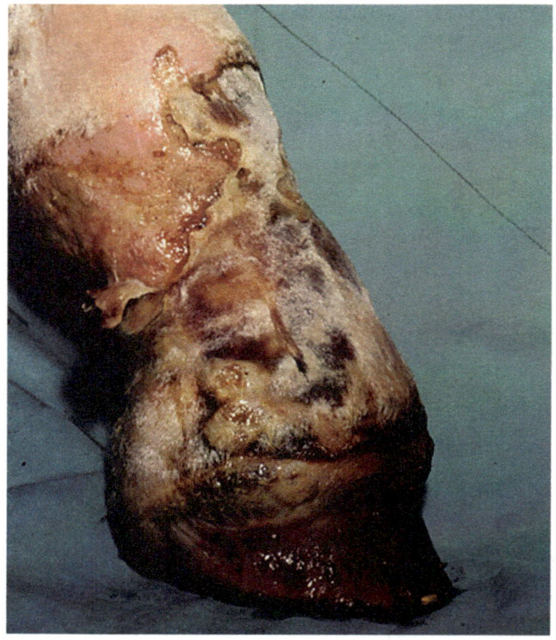

Figure 13.18 Vascular injury to the pastern that resulted from the limb becoming caught between the rails of a cattle guard. The hoof wall sloughed 2 weeks following the injury.

Rope burns are found most commonly on a pastern, usually that of a hindlimb, and result most commonly from entanglement of the limb in a rope while the horse is picketed. A rope burn is a combination of abrasion and thermal damage caused by friction. A rope burn may be superficial partial-thickness (first-degree burn) or deep partial-thickness (second-degree burn), or it may extend through all layers of the skin (full-thickness or third-degree burn) (Figure 13.1).

Diagnosis

Physical examination

A horse with a pastern wound is frequently lame, but the degree of lameness depends on the duration of the injury and the structures involved and whether or not the wound has become infected. Generally, the deeper the laceration, the greater the lameness, but lameness may be attenuated if a digital nerve has been severed. Even if a vital structure is not involved, the horse may be reluctant to fully bear weight on the injured limb, especially if the wound is infected.

Laceration of the digital artery and vein causes severe hemorrhage, sometimes resulting in cardiovascular shock. To avoid exacerbating hypotension caused by severe hemorrhage, the horse's cardiovascular status should be assessed prior to administering a sedative or tranquilizer to facilitate examination. Administration of a phenothiazine-derivative tranquilizer, in

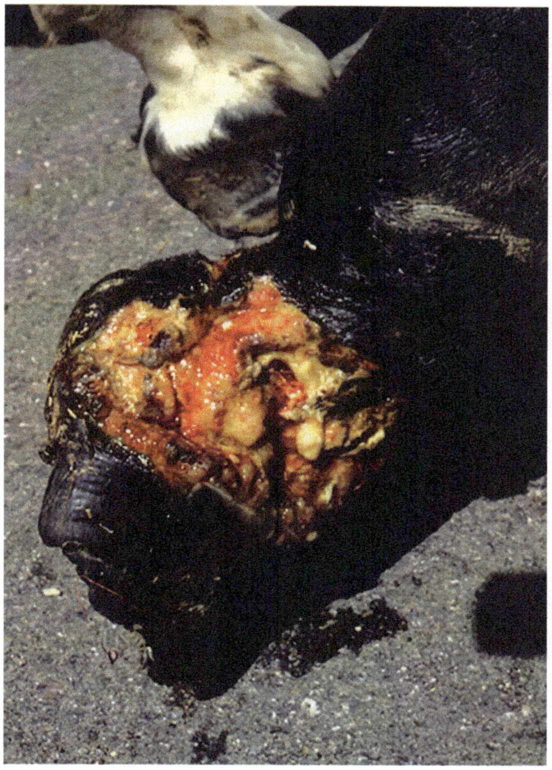

Figure 13.19 An extensive laceration of the pastern that entered the proximal and distal interphalangeal joints, transected the lateral collateral ligaments of both joints, and lacerated the collateral cartilage of the distal phalanx, as well as the coronary band.

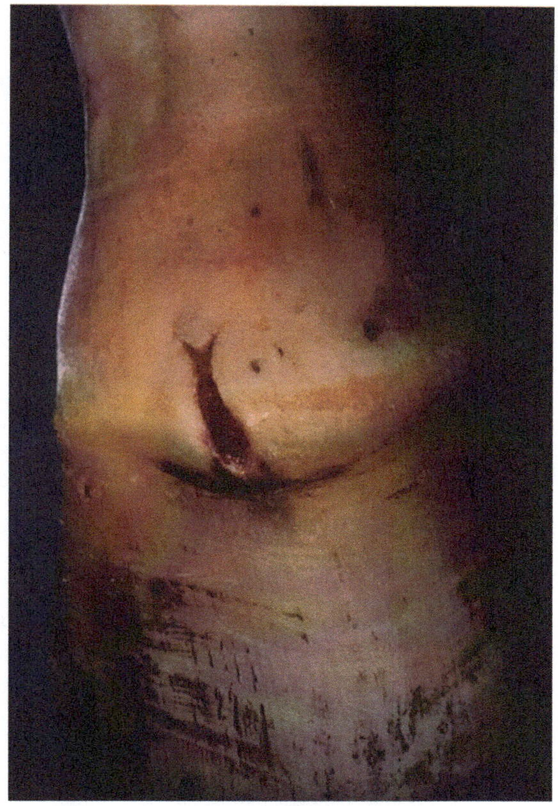

Figure 13.20 Wound to the coronary band that extended into the dorsal proximal pouch of the distal interphalangeal joint.

particular, should be avoided because it may result in severe hypotension if the horse is hypovolemic. Hemorrhage from the digital vessels can usually be controlled by applying a pressure bandage for 1 or 2 hours, but if the wound requires immediate examination, the digital vessels are best ligated. Anesthetizing the ipsilateral palmar/plantar digital nerve at the level of the proximal sesamoid bones may facilitate ligation by preventing pain caused by inadvertently disturbing the digital nerve, which courses next to the digital vessels. The blood supply to the foot is maintained if one of the arteries remains intact because of the terminal arch of the digital arteries.[29]

Damage to deep structures may be difficult to recognize visually, and, if suspected, the wound should be carefully palpated. To discriminatively inspect an acute laceration, the wound should be carefully palpated after the hair has been clipped and the wound irrigated with an antiseptic solution. A dilute solution of povidone–iodine [0.1% (1 mL of the 10% concentrate/L)] may be safer than a dilute solution of chlorhexidine diacetate [0.05% (25 mL of the 2% concentrate/975 mL]) for irrigation of any laceration that might involve a synovial structure because a solution of chlorhexidine diacetate can damage synovial structures. Indeed, one study examining the effects of lavaging the tarsocrural joint of horses with a solution of chlorhexidine diacetate found that a 0.05% solution caused synovial ulceration, inflammation, and deposition of fibrin.[30]

Devitalized tissue should be excised, and gross contaminants removed using irrigation/cleansing. After donning sterile gloves, the depths of the wound are palpated to detect damage to deeper structures. Discerning damage to structures deep in the wound using digital palpation may be difficult if granulation tissue has already formed. For a more complete discussion of the approaches used for examining wounds, see Chapter 4.

Laxity and instability of the middle or distal interphalangeal joint indicate disruption of a collateral ligament, and a sucking noise may indicate that the proximal or distal interphalangeal joint has been opened. A puncture wound of the coronary band may, deceptively, appear unimportant, but it should be inspected closely for the presence of wood splinters (Figure 13.3). A laceration or puncture to the dorsal aspect of the coronary band may involve the dorsal pouch of the distal interphalangeal joint, which extends proximad to the hoof capsule on the dorsal surface of the pastern (Figure 13.20).

The distal interphalangeal joint is the synovial structure most commonly involved in lacerations of the heel bulbs.[25] If the laceration extends completely through the collateral cartilage of the distal phalanx, the distal interphalangeal joint is likely to be breached because the collateral cartilage adjoins the capsule of this joint (Figure 13.21). If articular cartilage can be palpated or if synovial fluid is seen, penetration of a joint capsule is certain. Discerning penetration of the digital flexor tendon sheath may

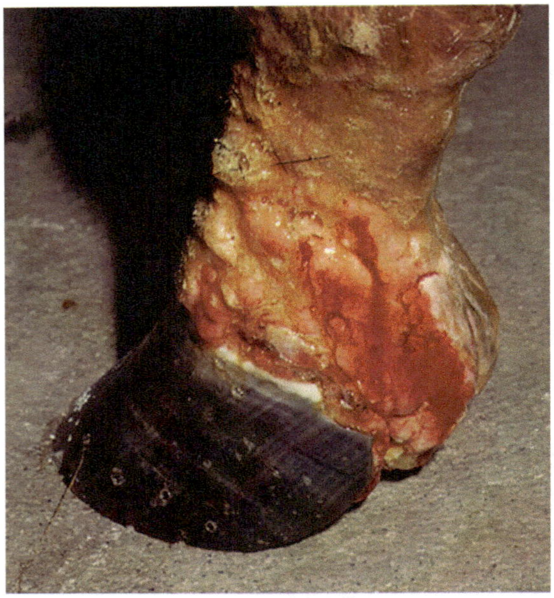

Figure 13.21 Extensive laceration of the pastern that extended through the collateral cartilage of the distal phalanx into the distal interphalangeal joint.

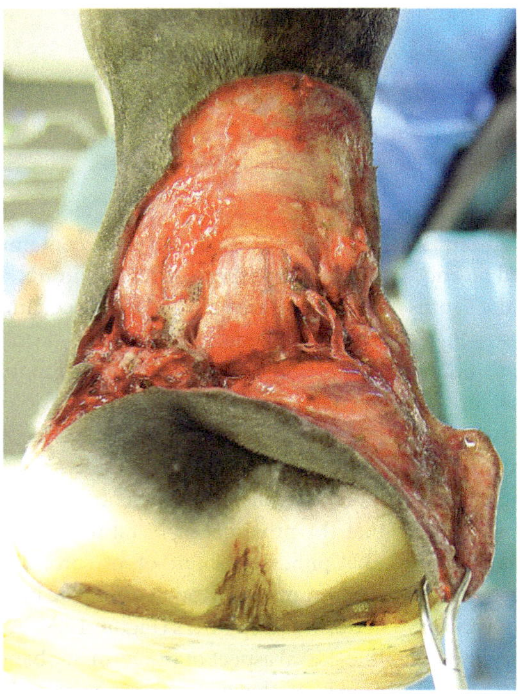

Figure 13.22 This wound over the palmar surface of the pastern entered the digital flexor tendon sheath, which lies superficially in this region.

be more difficult, but if a laceration in the deep digital flexor tendon can be palpated, penetration of the sheath is certain. A laceration over the palmar/plantar surface of the pastern is highly likely to have entered the digital flexor tendon sheath, which lies superficially in this region (Figure 13.22).

Determining the depth of a partial-thickness rope burn of the pastern may be difficult because swelling of the remaining skin

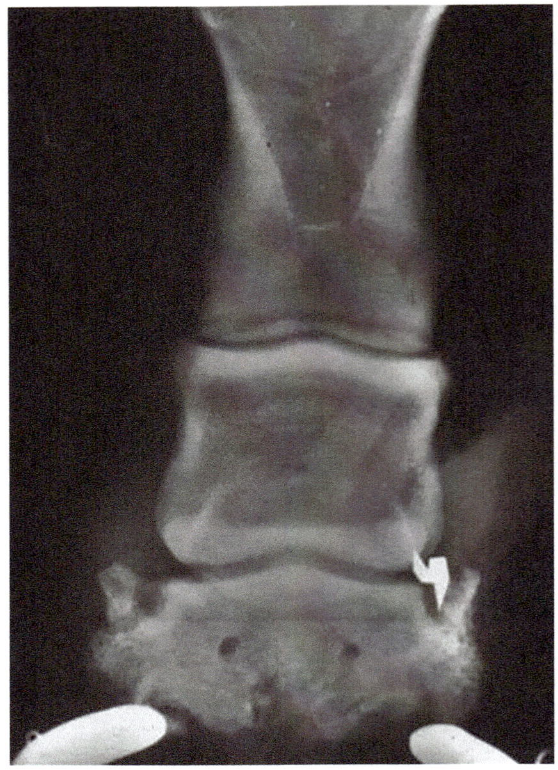

Figure 13.23 Radiographic examination of a deep wound to the pastern region might reveal the presence of a foreign body deep within the wound. This barb was not identified by visual or digital inspection of the wound.

may confound estimates of tissue loss. Superficial partial-thickness rope burns epithelialize within 3 weeks, and piliation at the site of injury is good. Deep partial-thickness rope burns may take months to heal, and the site may remain scarred and hairless. A full-thickness rope burn of the palmar/plantar surface of the pastern may breach the digital flexor tendon sheath resulting in unremitting lameness and failure of the wound to heal (Figure 13.1).

Imaging

The lacerated region should be examined radiographically to help ascertain the status of the bones and joints and to determine whether a radiopaque foreign body is present (Figure 13.23). The proximity of the laceration to critical structures, such as the navicular apparatus, can be determined by examining radiographs of the pastern and foot taken after inserting a sterile probe into the depths of the wound. If a laceration of a collateral ligament of the distal interphalangeal joint is suspected, the region can be examined radiographically with the collateral ligament of the lacerated side stressed to determine if the bones of the joint are shifted abnormally relative to each other. To obtain a stress radiograph of the distal interphalangeal joint, mediolateral force is applied to the joint as the region is radiographed, to determine if the middle and distal phalanges shift abnormally relative to one another. Force can be applied by standing the horse on a small block of wood placed beneath the side of the hoof contralateral to the wound.

A contrast study may be helpful if penetration of a synovial structure is suspected but cannot be confirmed by digital palpation. Air in the wound inhibits accurate ultrasonograph examination of the injured pastern, but, occasionally, ultrasonography may be valuable in detecting damage to ligaments or tendons or the presence of a foreign body. Doppler imaging may assist in determining the integrity of the vascular supply to the region. The structures involved in the laceration can sometimes be appreciated only when the wound is explored and debrided while the horse is anesthetized.

Treatment

Suturing a laceration in the pastern region and applying a distal limb cast (i.e., one that encompasses the foot and extends to the carpus or tarsus) or a phalangeal cast (i.e., foot–pastern, or slipper cast) usually provides the best cosmetic and functional outcomes. An acute laceration may be sutured without delay if the laceration is clean, tissue damage is minimal, and no synovial structure has been penetrated. In this case, systemic administration of an antimicrobial drug is often not necessary, but administration of a non-steroidal, anti-inflammatory drug (NSAID) may be indicated to reduce pain and inflammation.

Closure of an acute wound and application of a cast should be delayed for 2–3 days after injury if the exposed tissue is grossly contaminated or severely traumatized but should be performed before granulation tissue develops (i.e., delayed primary closure). The horse is best treated by second-intention healing or by delayed secondary closure of the wound (closure delayed until granulation tissue has formed) if presented after the wound appears infected (Figure 13.6).

To prepare a contaminated or infected wound for suturing, hair surrounding the wound is removed with clippers. Sterile, water-soluble lubricating gel or sterile gauze soaked in physiologic saline solution (authors' preference) can be inserted into the wound to prevent clipped hair from falling into it. Skin surrounding the wound should be cleansed with an antiseptic scrub or skin cleanser containing surfactant(s), but application of either to the wound itself should be avoided because the detergent, which is a surfactant, is cytotoxic and increases the wound's susceptibility to infection.[31,32] The use of hydrogen peroxide to irrigate the wound should also be avoided because, at its usual 3% concentration, it is cytotoxic and only weakly bactericidal.[32] The use of a dilute antiseptic solution [e.g., povidone iodine 0.1–0.2% (authors' preference)] or chlorhexidine (0.05%) using irrigation delivered at 10–12 psi is preferred. Various commercial wound cleansers can be used as an alternative – see Table 5.1 for more information. The wound is debrided; an antimicrobial solution, cream, or ointment is applied topically to the cleansed/irrigated wound to reduce the concentration of microorganisms within it; and the wound is bandaged. If the wound is infected and exudative or if it is difficult to debride, a debriding dressing may be applied and changed daily for several days – the reader is referred to Chapter 6 for more information regarding wound dressings. The bandage is usually changed daily or every other day to assess healing after application of the debriding dressing is discontinued. When the bandage is changed, the wound and surrounding skin and hoof wall are cleansed, and, if necessary, the wound is again debrided. This treatment is continued until the wound no longer requires debridement and appears healthy enough to heal by delayed primary closure.

The horse should receive broad-spectrum, antimicrobial therapy systemically, but if a synovial structure has been penetrated, antimicrobial therapy should also be delivered intrasynovially or by regional limb perfusion. When a synovial structure has been penetrated, the horse should receive antimicrobial therapy only after a sample of synovial fluid has been obtained for bacterial culture and sensitivity testing of bacterial isolates. The type of antimicrobial drugs administered should be adjusted, if necessary, according to the results of sensitivity testing of bacteria isolated by culture. The duration of systemic administration of antimicrobial therapy is dictated by the horse's response to therapy. Administration of a NSAID to reduce pain and inflammation is usually indicated. When a synovial structure has been penetrated, closure of the wound and application of a cast should be delayed for several days, even if the wound is clean. Heavily contaminated or badly damaged tissue surrounding the open synovial structure should be debrided, and synovial lavage should be executed through a needle or cannula inserted at a site remote to the wound, using 3–6 L of sterile, isotonic saline solution or a balanced electrolyte solution. Using arthroscopic equipment to lavage an infected synovial structure not only ensures thorough lavage but also allows the structure to be examined directly, aiding in predicting prognosis (see Figure 16.3). After the wound has been debrided and the synovial structure lavaged, the wound is protected under a sterile bandage, and the horse is confined to a dry area.

To aid resolution of synovial infection, an appropriate antimicrobial drug should be delivered to the infected tissue in a concentration greater than the minimum inhibitory concentration. Although broad-spectrum antimicrobial therapy should be administered systemically, vascular injury and thrombosis may limit delivery of drugs to the wound. Regional limb perfusion circumvents these limitations by delivering the antimicrobial drug, under pressure through the venous system, in a high concentration. For more information, see Chapter 16, which covers treatment of horses with a wound involving a synovial structure.

The wound is ready for delayed primary closure when it appears clean and contains little exudate, or it is ready for delayed secondary closure when healthy, pink, granulation tissue fills the wound (Figure 13.24a). If the horse remains or becomes severely lame, the wound should be reassessed to determine whether vital structures have been damaged. Provided that the horse is docile and the wound is uncomplicated, the wound can be sutured with the horse sedated after desensitizing the pastern and foot using regional anesthesia, but in most cases, the wound is best sutured with the horse anesthetized. The hoof should be cleansed and trimmed, especially if a

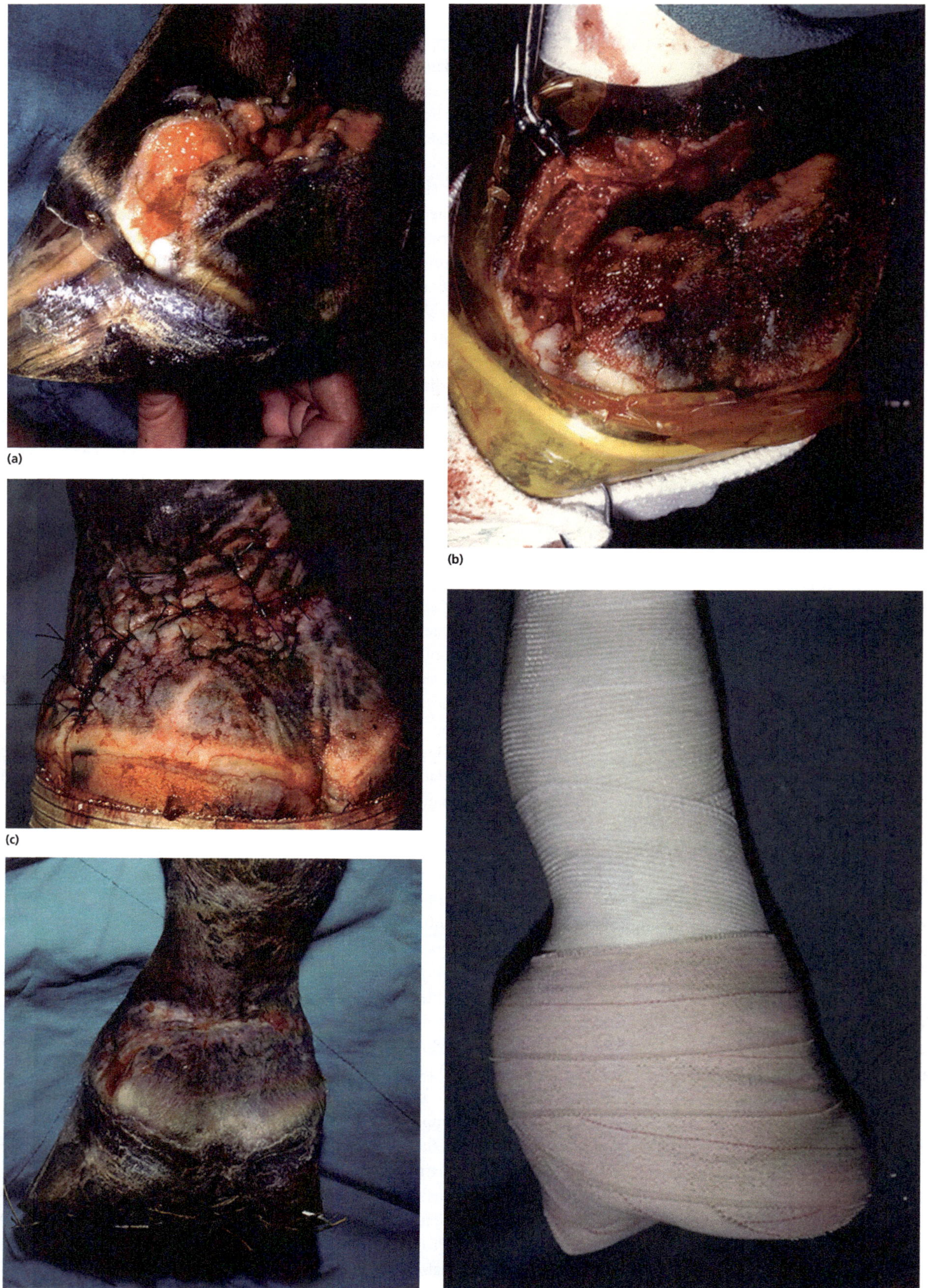

(a) (b) (c) (e) (d)

Figure 13.24 Same wound as in Figure 13.6, following 5 days of treatment. (**a**) Healthy, pink, granulation tissue fills the wound, indicating that it is ready for delayed secondary closure. (**b**) Excessive granulation tissue has been excised from the wound. (**c**) A combination of vertical mattress tension and simple interrupted sutures were used to close this wound. (**d**) A distal limb cast. (**e**) Excellent healing was observed when the cast was removed after 2 weeks.

cast is to be applied, either before or after the horse is anesthetized. Lightly rasping the hoof wall distal to the wounded region on the pastern reduces surface contamination. After the hoof has been scrubbed with antiseptic soap using a brush, a sterile glove is applied to the foot to protect the wound from contamination, and the wound is isolated with drapes. Applying a tourniquet proximal to the pastern may speed surgery by reducing hemorrhage and improving visibility.

Granulation tissue should be removed before the wound is sutured (Figure 13.24b) because doing so reduces the concentration of contaminating bacteria, exposes the depth of the wound for examination, and enhances mobility of the wound's margin for suturing. Care should be exercised to avoid damaging the digital vessels and unwounded portions of the coronary region while excising the granulation tissue.

The debrided wound is closed with size 0 or 1 sutures of monofilament nylon or polypropylene placed in a vertical mattress pattern (tension-relieving sutures) after which the skin edges are apposed with 2-0 monofilament nylon or polypropylene placed in either a simple interrupted or an interrupted vertical mattress pattern (Figure 13.24c). The edges of a wound on the coronary band should be aligned properly to prevent or minimize the development of a defect in the hoof capsule. Sutures placed through the coronary band do not impair formation of the hoof capsule distal to the laceration. Sutures can be placed through the lacerated hoof capsule, if necessary, to stabilize a wound that extends into the capsule. Thinning the wall with a rasp or burr and bandaging the foot with a wet dressing prior to surgery eases placement of sutures through the hoof wall (see the section on laceration and avulsion wounds of the hoof capsule, hereafter). The sutured wound is covered with a sterile, semi-occlusive dressing, which is maintained in position with sterile, elastic gauze. The distal portion of the limb, including the foot, is then enclosed within a bandage or cast (Figure 13.24d,e).

Protecting an unsutured wound in the pastern area with only a bandage results in a substantially longer time for the wound to heal and a poorer cosmetic outcome, especially if the laceration involves a heel bulb, than does immobilization of the foot and pastern within a cast (Figure 13.25). Protecting the wound with a bandage can be more costly than protecting it with a phalangeal cast, considering the quantity of bandage material that must be used over time. To minimize distractive forces on a sutured or unsutured laceration at a heel bulb, a cast that encompasses the foot and extends to the mid-pastern region is usually sufficient. To decrease distractive forces on a heel bulb wound that extends to the proximal third of the pastern, a cast that encompasses the foot and extends to the carpus or tarsus (i.e., a distal limb cast) may be necessary. Distal limb casts are more likely to cause cast sores than are phalangeal casts, which do not incorporate the fetlock region, a frequent site of sores caused by a distal limb cast.

The cast enhances healing of a laceration to the pastern by protecting the wound from the environment, limiting movement of

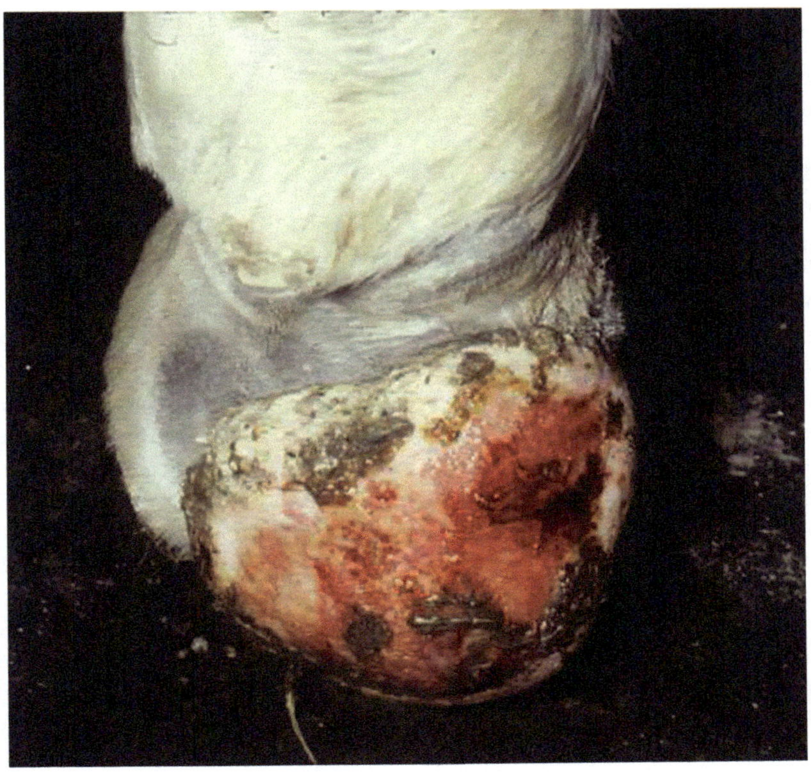

Figure 13.25 Failure to immobilize the distal portion of the limb of a horse that has incurred a heel bulb laceration is likely to result in movement, which in turn leads to production of EGT.

the wound's edges, relieving tension on the wound, and providing a moist environment for epithelialization. The time at which the cast is removed depends on the amount of tension required to close the wound or the deficit of tissue that must heal by second intention. The greater the tension on the sutured wound or the larger the deficit of tissue, the longer the cast should be maintained. Leaving the cast in place for 14–21 days is usually sufficient to facilitate healing of most wounds to the pastern.

Treatment of a horse with a recently acquired rope burn involves cleansing the wound, administering local and systemic anti-inflammatory drug therapy, and bandaging. Hair is clipped from the area in preparation for cleansing/irrigation. Skin surrounding the wound should be cleansed with an antiseptic soap, but application of soap to the wound itself should be avoided for the aforementioned reasons.

An ointment can be applied to the wound for its effect as an emollient, and a topical anti-inflammatory drug, such as dimethyl sulfoxide (DMSO) or diclofenac sodium (1%) cream (Surpass™, Idexx Laboratories), should be applied liberally to the edematous tissues surrounding the wound (but not to the wound itself). The wounded pastern is protected with a bandage between treatments to prevent the wound from becoming contaminated and desiccated, and damaged by excessive movement. The bandage should extend to the carpus or tarsus to prevent the limb from swelling and to minimize movement of the wound. The horse should receive a NSAID to attenuate pain and decrease swelling.

Prognosis

With proper treatment, a horse with a pastern laceration not involving a supporting structure or extending into a synovial structure has a good prognosis for a satisfactory cosmetic outcome and return to soundness. In a study of 101 horses that had incurred a heel bulb laceration, the laceration of 17 horses involved a synovial structure.[25] Of the 61 horses for which follow-up information was available, 94% (48 of 51) of horses, in which the laceration did not involve a synovial structure, were able to return to their intended use. Treatment was more problematic, and the results were poorer, when a synovial structure was involved. Only 30% of horses (3 of 10 for which follow-up information was available) in which the laceration involved a synovial structure were able to return to their intended use. Contrasting with the results of that study are the results of a more recent study of 49 horses with a wound of the pastern and foot region that were managed with a phalangeal cast.[33] In that study, 89.5% of the horses returned to soundness and had a good cosmetic outcome, regardless of whether or not a synovial structure was involved.

The prognosis for soundness is poor if the wound is accompanied by subluxation of the distal or proximal interphalangeal joint because osteoarthritis of the affected joint is likely to develop. Infection of a collateral cartilage may result in lameness and development of one or more chronic draining sinuses at the coronary band (i.e., quittor). To prevent infection of a collateral cartilage, discolored portions of cartilage should be excised when the wound is debrided. Formation of a painful neuroma after nerve transection rarely may cause lameness necessitating excision of the neuroma.

Healing of a deep, partial- or full-thickness rope burn is usually protracted, and the wound often heals with a blemish that resembles a keloid. The degree of dermal destruction governs the time required for complete healing. The deeper the destruction into the dermis, the fewer the adnexa remaining to provide keratinocytes for epithelialization, and the longer the time for healing. Full-thickness rope burns to the palmar/plantar surface of the pastern may require skin grafting.

What to do

- Lacerations of the pastern that course deep to the hoof wall should be inspected closely to determine if the distal interphalangeal joint, navicular bursa, or digital flexor tendon sheath have been penetrated. The flexor tendons should be inspected for damage. Penetration of the digital flexor tendon sheath is certain if the deep digital flexor tendon is lacerated.
- Immobilizing a lacerated pastern with a phalangeal or distal limb cast provides the best cosmetic and functional outcome, especially if the laceration involves a heel bulb.

What to avoid

- Skin surrounding a wound should be cleaned with an antiseptic soap, but soap should not be applied to the wound itself.

Tips

- Before ligating a severed digital vessel with the horse standing, the ipsilateral palmar digital nerve should be anesthetized to avoid a reaction from the horse that would undoubtedly occur if the palmar digital nerve was inadvertently grasped with a hemostat, along with the severed digital vessel.
- Accurate alignment of the coronary band using sutures is necessary to prevent a defect from developing in the hoof wall.

Lacerations and avulsion wounds of the hoof capsule

Anatomy and healing of the foot

The old adage, "no hoof, no horse," indicates the importance of the hoof and our need to fully understand the mechanisms governing repair of the tissues contained within this specialized anatomic structure. The hoof wall, or *stratum corneum*, is of epidermal origin and is usually divided into a *stratum externum*, which is a thin, superficial layer of horn that extends a variable distance from the periople, a *stratum medium*, which is thick and highly keratinized, and a softer *stratum internum*, which consists of the primary and secondary epidermal laminae (PEL and SEL, respectively). The *stratum medium* is composed of horn tubules that grow from the *stratum germinativum* of the coronary epidermis that surrounds the coronary papillae. The coronary corium and perioplic corium, both of dermal origin, and the coronary epidermis comprise the coronary band. The underlying modified subcutis, or coronary cushion, is often considered part of the coronary band. The lamellar corium, also of dermal origin, overlies the periosteum of the distal phalanx and is tightly interlocked with the epidermal laminae of the hoof. In cases of avulsion, the *stratum germinativum* of the epidermal laminae usually remains adhered to the dermal laminae of the lamellar corium, thus sparing the living cells responsible for the rapid epithelialization and keratinization often seen in the wound bed.[34] The lamellar basement membrane, left intact, is used as a template for proliferating epidermal cells.[35]

The distad growth of the hoof wall (10 mm per month) results from the differences between the PEL and the SEL of the *stratum internum* in their ability to keratinize. Cells of the PEL progressively keratinize while moving distally with the tubules of the *stratum medium*. The basal cells of the SEL, on the other hand, adhere to the dermal laminae of the lamellar corium and do not keratinize. A continuous cycle of breaking and reforming links between the two populations of cells ensures the maintenance of a very strong attachment of the hoof wall to the parietal surface of the distal phalanx, while allowing slow distal growth of the horn tubules.[36] Hoof wall renewal time for Thoroughbred foals (120–165 days) is approximately twice as fast as that of adults (270–365 days).[37] Upon reaching the solar surface of the hoof, the keratinized cells of the epidermal laminae form the junction between the hoof wall and the sole. This zone of softer and whiter horn is commonly termed the white line (Figure 13.26).

Specific biomechanical properties of the equine foot affect not only the pattern of injury but also repair. Any injury of sufficient force to invade the resistant *stratum corneum* usually results in a full-thickness wound. Full-thickness hoof wounds are rare, but when they occur, the rigidity of the *stratum corneum* usually prevents the wound margins from gaping, encourages fracture, as opposed to tearing, of the hoof capsule, and causes the tissues to completely avulse from the underlying structures, rather than to just lacerate.[39] Lacerations, tears, and partial-thickness wounds are more common at the coronary band and at the heel where the hoof wall is thinner and less rigid.

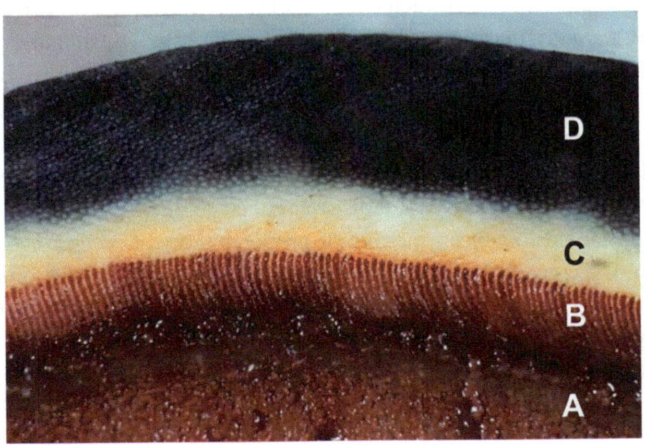

Figure 13.26 Cross-section of the hoof at the level of the white line. A: distal phalanx; B: interdigitation of dermal and epidermal laminae; C: white line; D: hoof wall. The keratinized cells of the epidermal laminae form a junction between the hoof wall and the sole made of softer and white horn and commonly called the "white line." Source: Celeste and Szoke 2005.[38] Reproduced with permission of Elsevier.

Wounds affecting tissues distal to the coronary band are contained within the rigid *stratum corneum* so that swelling during the inflammatory phase is impossible. Furthermore, the rigid nature of the hoof may prevent adequate drainage of exudate and spontaneous elimination of foreign bodies and necrotic tissues, leading to subsolar formation of an abscess and/or infection of deeper, underlying structures. Hoof wounds do not contract,[40] and they epithelialize differently than skin wounds. A full-thickness hoof wound involving the frog or sole usually evolves similarly to a full-thickness skin wound, with homogenous epithelial coverage coming from surrounding epithelium and by re-establishment of epithelial strata by local epithelial proliferation. In a full-thickness wound involving the hoof wall, epithelium is re-established by progressive growth of the hoof wall from the coronary band distally rather than by local epithelial proliferation. In some hoof wounds, however, and especially those involving the coronary band, the epithelial margins may be of one or more origins. In these cases, the final appearance and structure of the healed wound reflects the nature and source of epithelium that migrated to fill the defect.[39] Thus, full-thickness wounds involving the skin of the coronary band, healing by second intention, often heal with the formation of horny spurs and/or persistent defects in the hoof wall.

Causes

Laceration or avulsion of a portion of the hoof capsule is a relatively uncommon injury that is most often caused by kicking at or stepping on a sharp object, but may occasionally occur when the foot becomes entrapped between two immovable objects. The injury may result in permanent lameness, and in some cases, may necessitate euthanasia of the horse. A portion of the hoof capsule may be totally avulsed, or it may be partially avulsed so that it remains attached, to some degree, usually at the coronary band (Figure 13.27). Rarely, the hoof capsule is completely avulsed after the foot becomes entrapped momentarily between fixed objects during exercise.[41] An avulsion may involve critical structures deep to the hoof capsule, such as the distal phalanx or distal interphalangeal joint (Figure 13.28).

Complications that may arise following injury to the hoof capsule include infection of exposed laminae, fracture or partial loss of the distal phalanx (Figure 13.28c), and infection of the distal interphalangeal joint or digital flexor tendon sheath (see Wounds involving the pastern, discussed earlier). Even in the absence of these complications, the horse may remain lame after the wound heals, simply because of the quantity of hoof capsule that has been lost.

Diagnosis

Clinical signs

The degree of lameness varies with the duration, extent, and location of the injury to the hoof capsule. Because of its close proximity to the ground, a wound in the hoof capsule quickly becomes contaminated with manure and dirt, and if the horse is

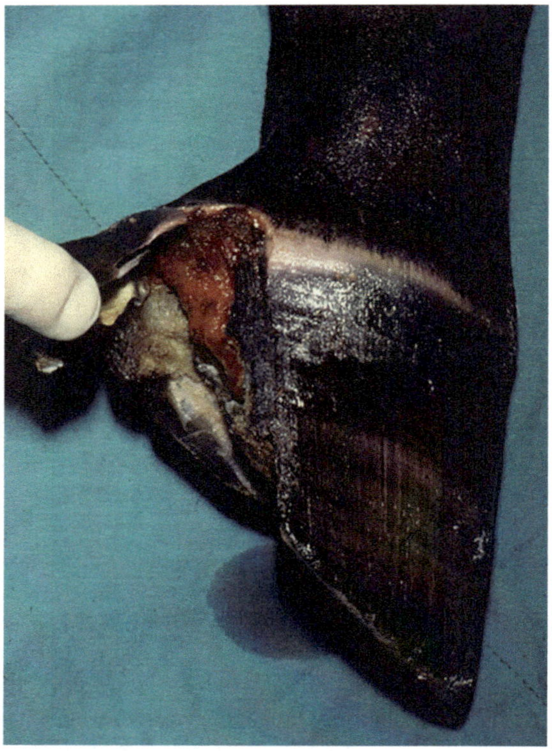

Figure 13.27 A partially avulsed portion of the hoof remains attached only at the coronary band.

not treated appropriately and promptly, contamination results in infection. Migration of infection may cause surrounding epidermal and dermal laminae to separate (Figure 13.29). The horse may be severely lame if vital structures deep to the hoof capsule are involved in the injury.

The presence of a horny spur at the distal extent of the pastern region, typically growing at a right or oblique angle to the pastern and sometimes accompanied by abnormal growth of hoof distal to it, is an indication that the horse suffered partial avulsion of a portion of the hoof capsule and coronary band (Figure 13.30). Although the wound may be healed, the horse may frequently traumatize the avulsed and displaced portion of the coronary band, causing it to bleed. Palpating the horny spur, and particularly pushing it proximad, usually causes the horse to show signs of discomfort.

Horses with an acute injury to the hoof wall that does not involve critical structures deep to the wall are usually only slightly to moderately lame, but palpation of the wound may cause the horse to show signs of considerable pain and may render the horse temporarily non-weight-bearing. Horses with extensive injury to the hoof capsule may refuse to bear weight on the affected limb. Lameness eventually subsides if the wound heals without complication. If lameness persists, the wound should be examined physically and radiographically for evidence of a complication, such as a fracture of the distal phalanx or perforation of the capsule of the distal interphalangeal joint. An acute avulsion injury of the hoof capsule is obvious, but the involvement of deeper structures may be difficult to discern. A horse that has had a complete avulsion of the hoof capsule should receive a venogram to evaluate the blood flow to the foot.[41]

Before embarking on a careful examination of the wound, the wound and surrounding area should be cleansed. The hair should be clipped from a broad area surrounding the wound, and the hoof wall distal and adjacent to the wound should be rasped lightly to remove superficial contaminants. Only portions of the hoof wall that are attached firmly to the underlying dermal laminae should be rasped, to avoid tearing laminar attachments. Skin surrounding the wound should be cleansed with an antiseptic soap, while avoiding direct contact of the soap with the wounded tissues.

The wound should be irrigated with a dilute antiseptic solution [e.g., povidone iodine (0.1–0.2%) or chlorhexidine diacetate (0.05%)] delivered at 8–12 psi. The use of a solution of chlorhexidine for irrigation should be avoided if laceration to the capsule of the distal interphalangeal joint or the digital flexor tendon sheath is suspected because this solution may damage synovial structures.[30] For more information regarding the techniques of wound cleansing and irrigation, see Chapter 4. The wound should be palpated only after donning sterile gloves. Manipulating the hoof and phalanges while palpating the wound may help to identify the extent of laminar separation, an open synovial structure, a fracture, or a lacerated supporting structure, such as a collateral ligament or the deep digital flexor tendon.

Because fracture of the distal or middle phalanx may accompany a laceration to the hoof capsule, the foot should be examined radiographically after the wound has been examined grossly (Figure 13.28c). Contrast radiographic studies of synovial structures associated with the foot region may be helpful in identifying a communication between the wound and a synovial structure.

Because healing of a complete avulsion injury or an incomplete avulsion injury with loss of the hoof capsule relies on epithelialization and reformation of the corium, rather than contraction, healing usually is protracted (3–5 months); thus, treatment can be costly, particularly if the horse has suffered a large avulsion injury (Figure 13.28, Figure 13.29). The wound should, therefore, be assessed carefully so that the owner can be apprised of the expense of treatment and the horse's prognosis for soundness or survival. If the distal or proximal interphalangeal joint is damaged, for example, degenerative joint disease is likely to develop and lead to permanent lameness, in spite of proper treatment. Even after a wound is carefully examined, predicting the horse's final outcome may be difficult. If a large portion of germinal tissue has been lost, or if infection has become established in a critical structure, the horse's initial response to therapy must be evaluated before outcome can be predicted.

Treatment

The selection of restraint required for repair depends on the nature and extent of the injury. An acute laceration or avulsion injury to the coronary band or hoof capsule can usually be sutured with the horse sedated after the foot is desensitized

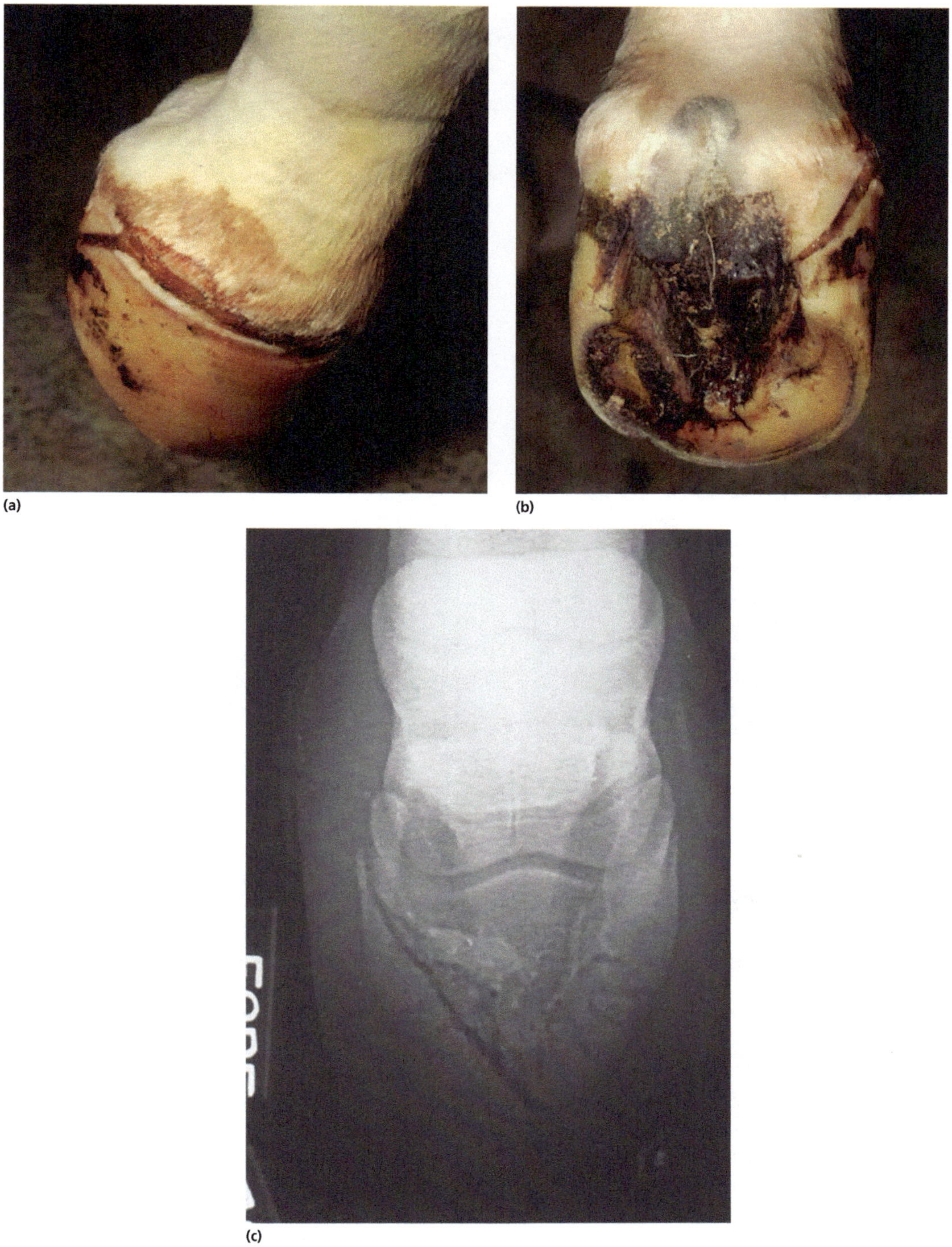

Figure 13.28 Extensive avulsion injury to the wall of a hoof. (**a**) Dorsal extent of the avulsion; note the separation at the coronary band. (**b**) The injury resulted in separation of the collateral sulcus of the frog. (**c**) Dorsoproximal–palmarodistal oblique view of the distal phalanx identifying a lateral solar margin fracture.

by administering regional anesthesia. The horse should be anesthetized if the laceration is extensive or involves the distal phalanx, a synovial cavity, or a supporting structure, such as a collateral ligament or the deep digital flexor tendon. The selection of treatment depends on whether the avulsion is partial or complete, whether the wound is fresh or chronic, and the extent of damage determined during exploration of the wound. If left to heal by second intention, a linear laceration to the coronary band usually results in a small defect in the hoof horn distal to the coronary band, whereas a partially avulsed segment of coronary band and hoof wall remains unstable, causing a large defect to develop in the hoof wall. If the partially avulsed segment is

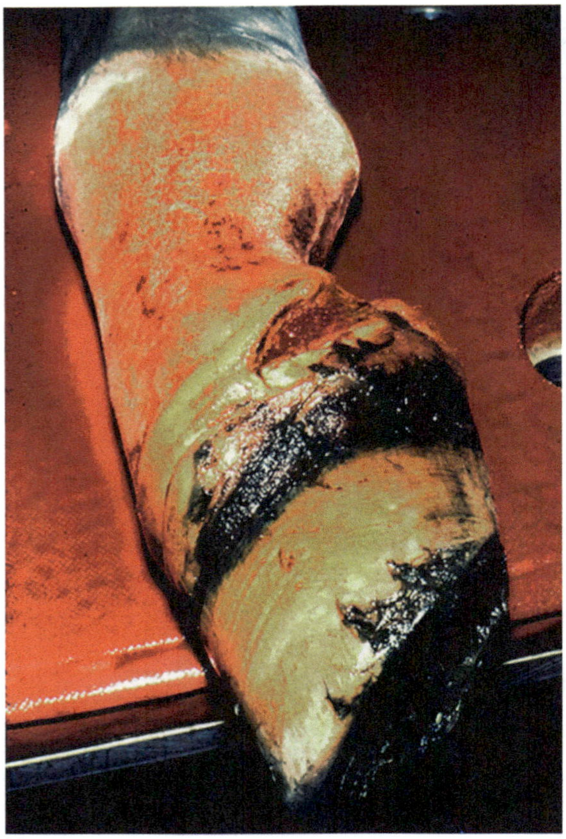

(a)

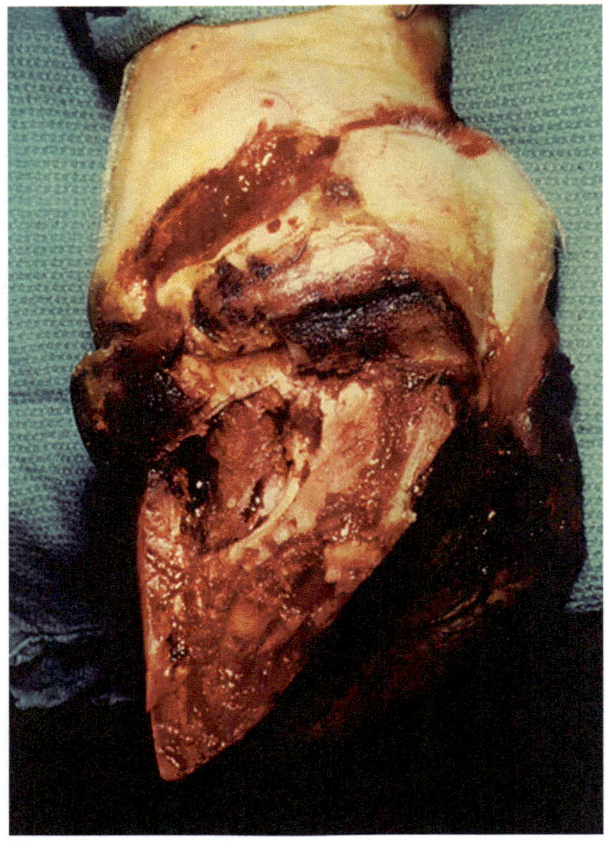

(b)

Figure 13.29 Migration of infection resulting from an injury caused surrounding epidermal and dermal laminae to separate. **(a)** At surgery. **(b)** After removal of the undermined hoof wall.

U-shaped and involves the coronary band, it can become displaced proximad, producing a horny spur on the pastern that is susceptible to additional trauma (Figure 13.30).

To prepare the horse for surgery, the hoof capsule surrounding the wound should be rasped to remove contaminants, and the foot trimmed, if these procedures were not performed when the wound was initially evaluated. The wound and surrounding area should be cleansed as described previously, and the wound should be isolated with sterile drapes.

When suturing a partially avulsed segment of hoof and coronary band, a tourniquet is placed proximal to the foot to aid visibility by limiting hemorrhage. One of two methods can be used to repair the avulsion: the hoof wall distal to the laceration in the coronary band can be retained and stabilized, or the avulsed hoof wall can be removed. For either method, the coronary band is carefully sutured, and the hoof is protected in a phalangeal cast.

Using the first method, the hoof wall adjacent to the defect, as well as the partially avulsed segment of hoof wall, can be thinned with a motorized burr to ease placement of sutures through the hoof wall, and the defect in the hoof wall is debrided to provide a clean, vascular bed into which the partially avulsed segment of hoof is replaced. The thinned horn of the partially avulsed segment is sutured to the thinned hoof wall adjacent to the defect using size 0, 1, or 2 polypropylene or nylon suture placed in a simple interrupted or vertical mattress pattern (Figure 13.31). A partially avulsed segment of hoof can also be immobilized by anchoring several sheet metal screws [6.35–9.53 mm (¼ in to ⅜ in)] within the insensitive portion of the hoof on either side of the defect and lacing orthopedic wire across the segment and around the screw heads. The avulsed segment may also be held in place with a fiberglass patch attached to the hoof wall with screws.

Using the second method to repair the avulsion, the separated portion of hoof wall distal to the coronary band is removed, and the coronary band is carefully sutured, allowing healing distal to the coronary band to occur by second intention (Figure 13.32). A small, partially avulsed portion of the hoof wall, without involvement of the coronary band, can be excised; the foot is then protected by a bandage or a foot cast until the wound has healed (Figure 13.33).

If the avulsion injury is associated with a fracture of the distal phalanx, the avulsed portion of the hoof capsule and the fracture fragment, in most cases, must be removed (Figure 13.34). After removing the fracture fragment and avulsed portion of the hoof capsule, the foot is covered with an impermeable bandage. For more information on bandaging the foot, see Chapter 7.

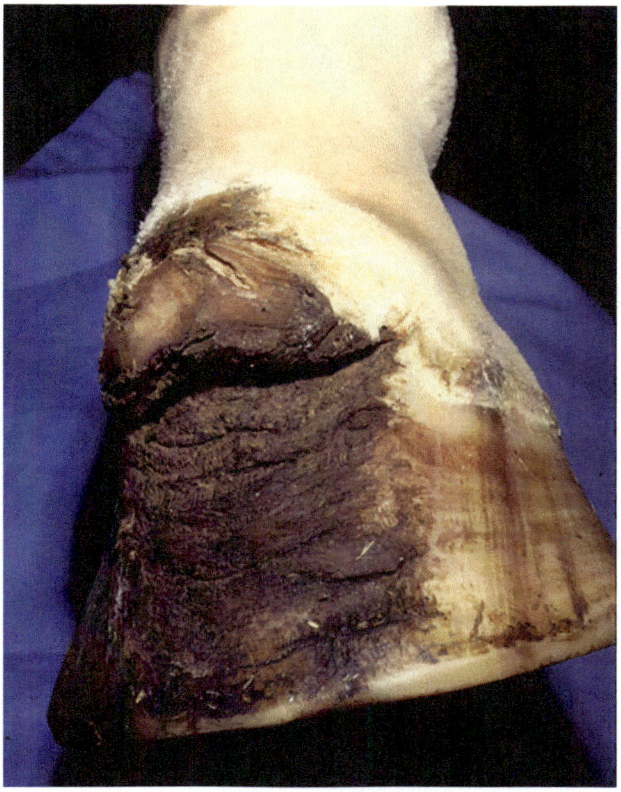

Figure 13.30 Partial avulsion of the dorsal hoof wall may cause lameness, and pushing the spur proximad often causes the horse to show signs of pain. This large partial avulsion of the dorsal hoof wall, in another horse, resulted in a horn spur growing at a right angle to the pastern and abnormal growth of the hoof distal to the spur. This horse had suffered partial avulsion of a portion of the hoof capsule and coronary band 1 year earlier. The horse was quite lame on the limb when the horn spur was not trimmed; the lameness would abate following trimming. Pushing the horn spur proximad caused the horse to show signs of discomfort.

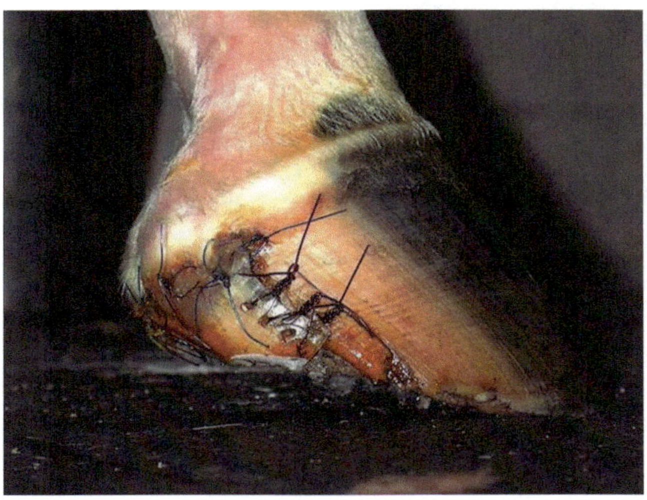

Figure 13.31 This laceration in the hoof capsule has been sutured.

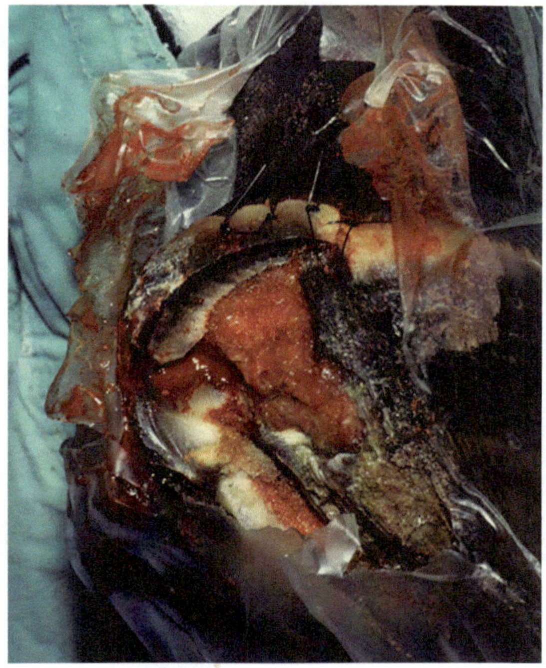

Figure 13.32 Same horse as in Figure 13.27 after excision of the avulsed hoof wall distal to the sutured coronary band.

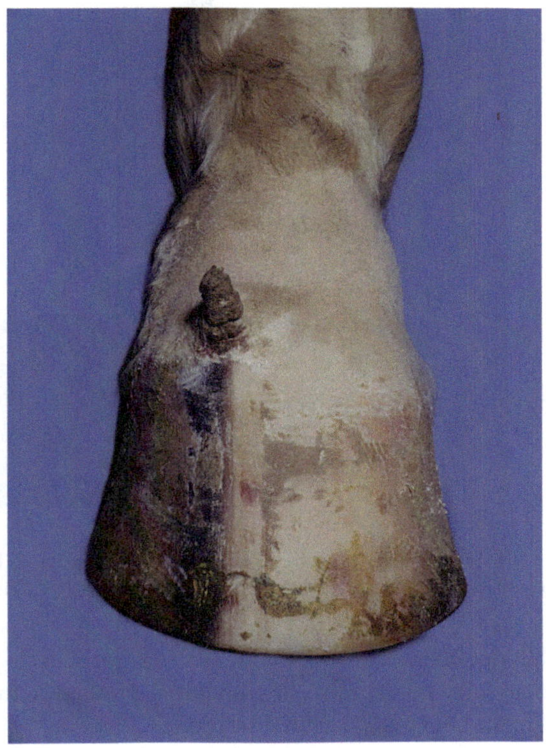

Figure 13.33 A small, partially avulsed portion of the dorsal hoof wall without involvement of the coronary band, such as this one, can be excised and the foot protected by a bandage.

In cases in which the wound resulting in proximal displacement of horny tissue is chronic, granulation tissue filling the defect in the hoof can be excised with a scalpel, and the horny spur produced by the displaced coronary band may be contoured and thinned with the burr until it fits into the defect in the hoof wall. The coronary band is sutured with size 0 polypropylene suture using a vertical mattress pattern (Figure 13.35). Accurate approximation of the coronary band is important to ensure that

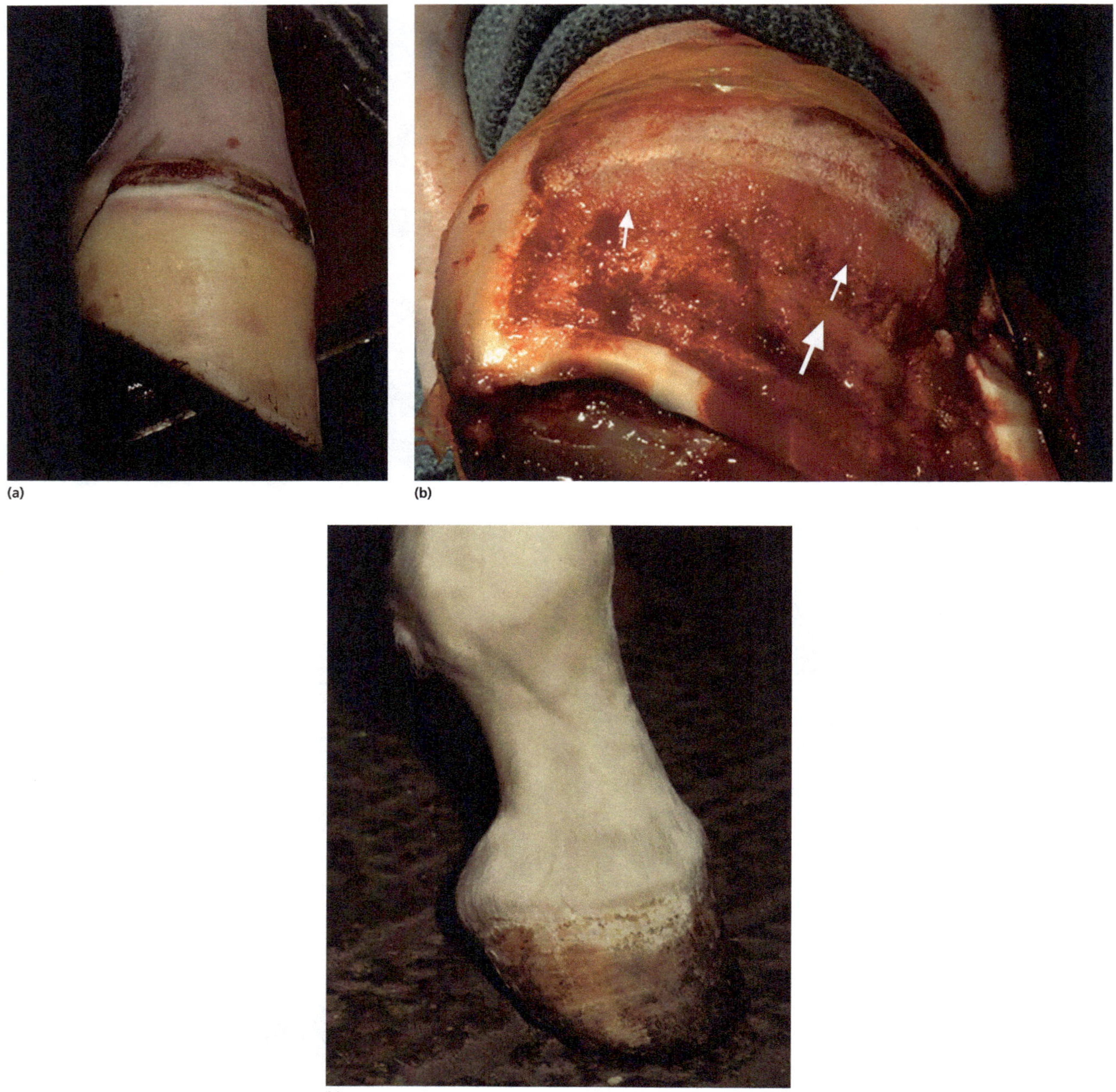

(a) (b) (c)

Figure 13.34 Same horse as in Figure 13.28. **(a)** The horse at surgery. **(b)** The avulsed hoof wall and fractured distal phalanx have been removed. Note the intact coronary papillae (small arrows) and the debrided border of the distal phalanx (large arrow). **(c)** The appearance of the foot 6 months after injury.

hoof produced by it conforms as much as possible to the direction of the hoof growth surrounding the wound so that a defect in the hoof wall does not develop.

If the proximally displaced section of coronary band and horn tissue cannot be replaced into the defect in the hoof wall, the horse is best treated by excising the germinal tissue that produces the horny spur. This is especially the case if the horse is lame because of the spur but becomes sound after the painful, horny spur is trimmed (Figure 13.36a–c). Dermal papillae at the coronary band should be spared as much as possible during excision of the germinal tissue. The resulting wound proximal to the coronary band is left to heal by second intention. If the wound is large, island grafts or a sheet graft can be applied to it to shorten the healing time (Figure 13.36d). See Chapter 18 for more information regarding skin grafting.

After surgery is complete, an antimicrobial dressing is applied to the wound. The foot should be immobilized within a phalangeal cast (Figure 13.37; see Figure 7.19), usually for at least 3 weeks, because in the absence of a cast, the rigidity of the hoof capsule, combined with the constant loading and unloading of the hoof, results in considerable movement at the wound.[42,43] When the cast is removed at 3–4 weeks, the coronary band should be healed, and

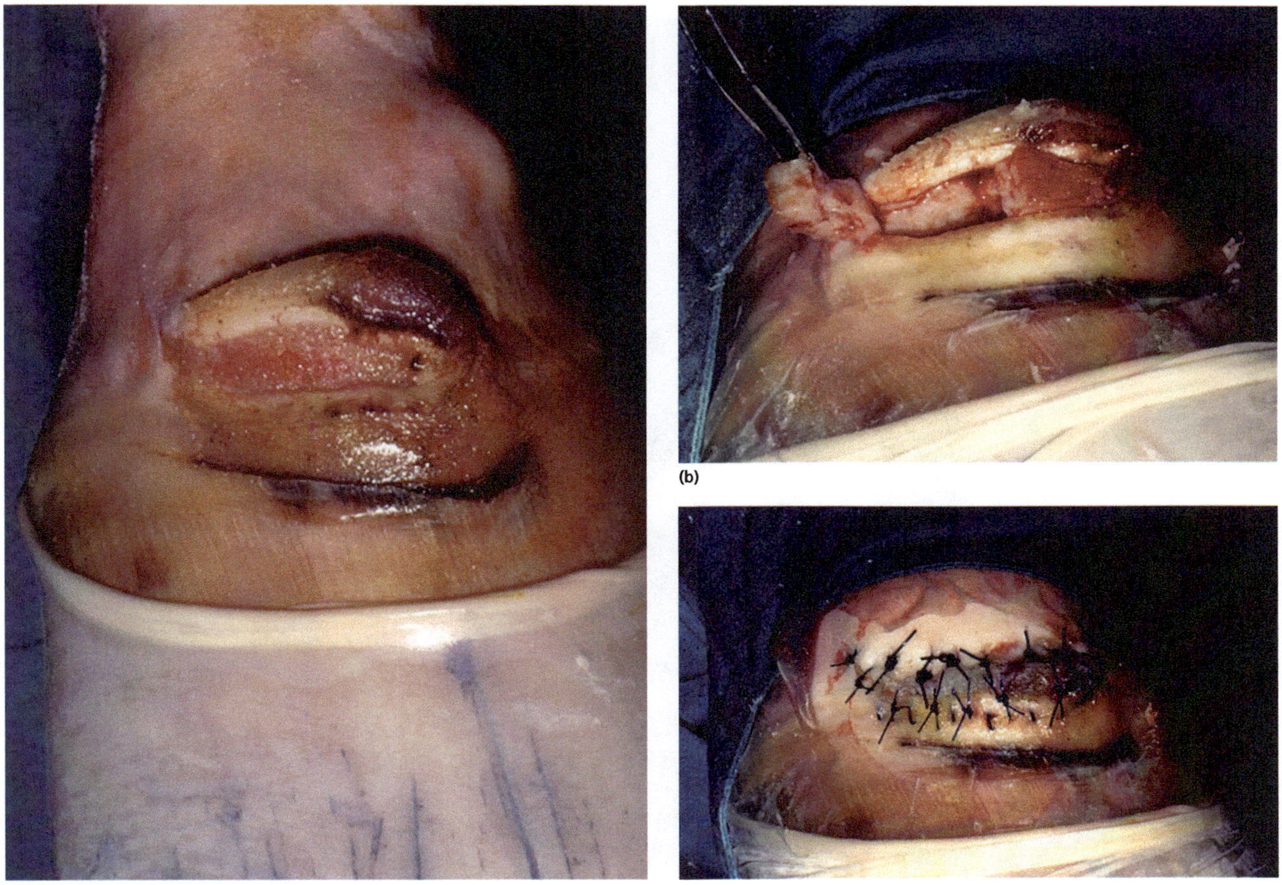

(a) (b) (c)

Figure 13.35 (**a**) The hoof wall has been prepared for surgery by removing the cornified *stratum externum* from the outer hoof wall. (**b**) Granulation tissue filling the defect in the hoof was excised with a scalpel. (**c**) The coronary band is sutured with size 0 polypropylene suture using a vertical mattress pattern. The foot was protected in a phalangeal cast for 3 weeks.

exposed laminae should be nearly cornified, obviating the need, in most cases, for continued protection of the wound. If only the hoof capsule has been lacerated, a cast that encompasses only the hoof capsule may be applied (Figure 13.38). A distal limb cast incorporating transfixation pins may be needed, for a prolonged period, to treat a horse that has sustained complete avulsion of the entire hoof capsule,[41] whereas a bandage is usually all that is needed after a small cornified spur in the pastern has been removed. Systemic administration of an antimicrobial drug after surgery is usually not necessary. If a large portion of the hoof capsule was lost, a full-support shoe (e.g., an egg-bar shoe combined with a heart-bar shoe, or an equine digital support system with a frog support pad and impression material) should be applied to the foot after the cast has been removed, and the region of the hoof wall distal to the defect should be removed (floated) to eliminate weight bearing on that portion of the hoof wall (Figure 13.39). Some roughening and thickening of the hoof wall distal to the defect may develop, in some cases, after healing,[42] but a hoof acrylic can be used to fill the cornified deficit in the hoof wall. Granulation tissue that forms in a defect in the hoof wall becomes cornified within about 4 weeks.

Prognosis

The time required for healing of an avulsion injury to the hoof and the horse's prognosis for soundness depend on the extent of the injury and the method of treatment, but most avulsion injuries heal without complication if the horse is treated correctly soon after the injury. Three to five months are usually needed for healing of a complete avulsion (Figure 13.36d), whereas incomplete avulsions that are reconstructed and sutured usually heal in 3–4 weeks. Even when healing is complete, soundness may not be regained for many months, and in some cases, up to 1 year. Partial loss of the distal phalanx, the digital cushion, or a collateral cartilage does not appear to be a serious detriment to soundness. Horses with a loss of up to one quarter of the distal phalanx can remain sound.[44] An avulsion injury that involves the coronary band may result in a permanent deformity of the hoof capsule (Figure 13.30).

Predicting the horse's outcome is difficult at the onset of treatment because recovery is a lengthy process. If a portion of the wound remains unhealed or if a draining tract appears, infection of a deep structure, such as a collateral cartilage, should be suspected.

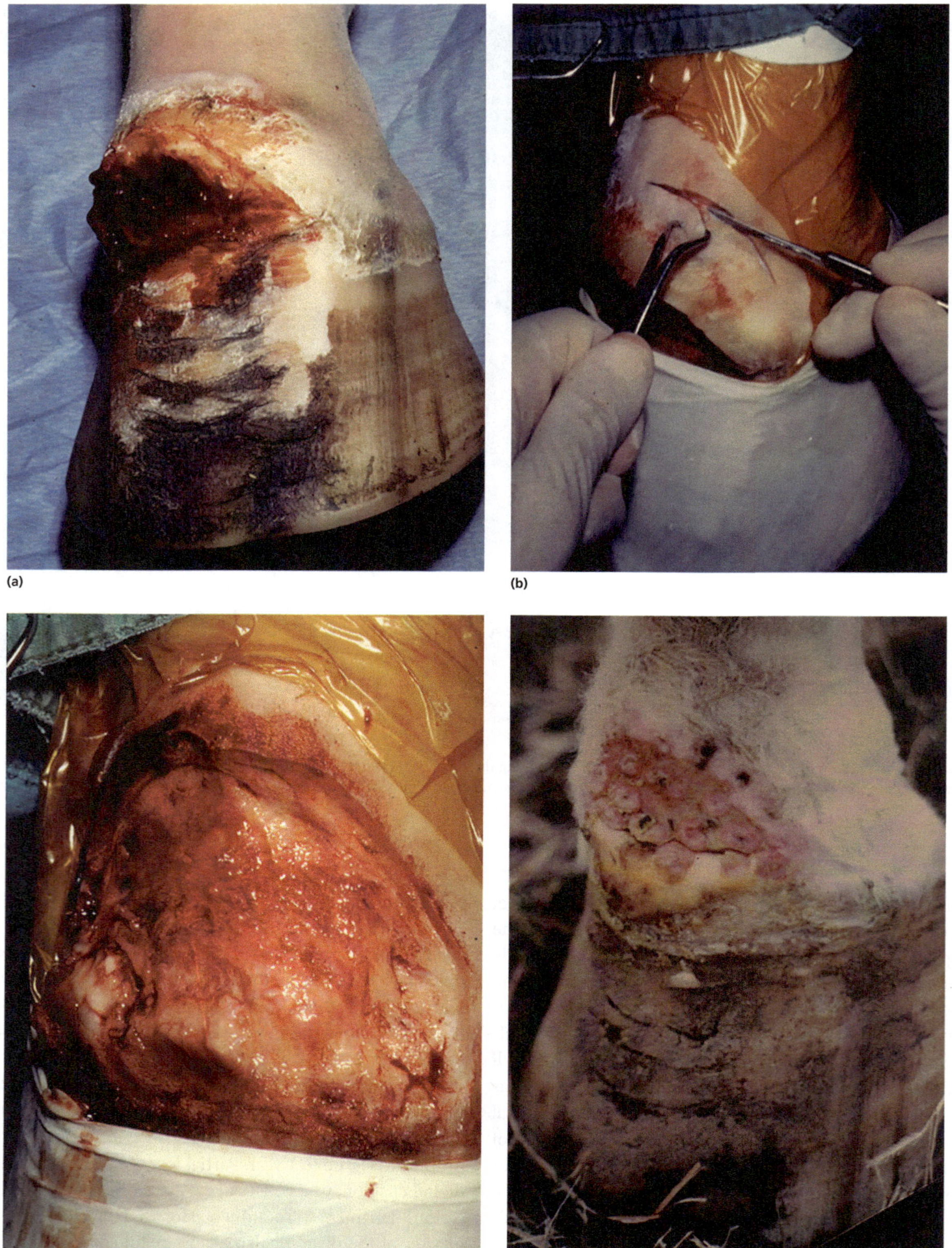

(a) (b) (c) (d)

Figure 13.36 Same horse as in Figure 13.30. **(a)** The horn spur was removed. **(b)** Germinal tissue was excised. Dermal papillae at the coronary band should be spared as much as possible during excision of the germinal tissue. **(c)** The wound bed after the germinal tissue was excised. The wound was bandaged and the horse was sent home with the recommendation that island grafts be inserted after a healthy bed of granulation tissue had developed. **(d)** The wound 4 weeks after surgery and 10 days after island skin grafting. This wound healed, and there was no evidence of regrowth of horn spur 1 year after surgery. The horse was free of lameness.

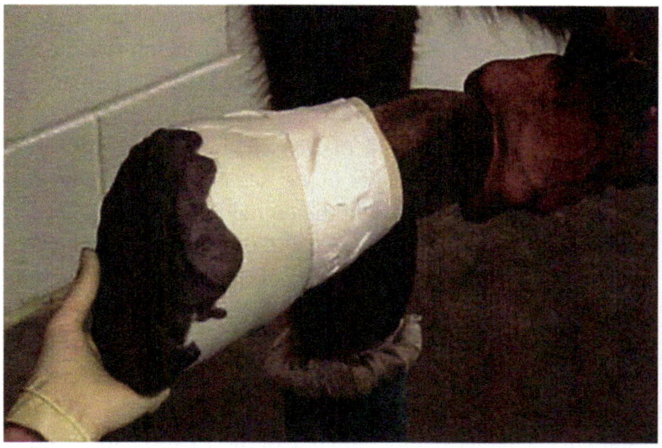

Figure 13.37 A phalangeal cast that encompasses the foot and a portion of the pastern.

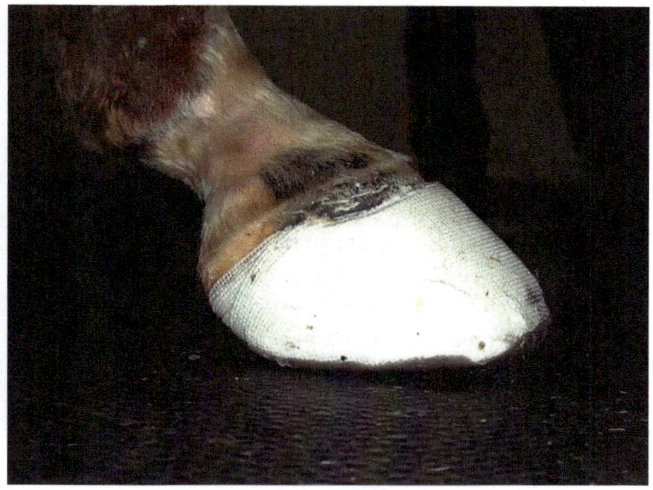

Figure 13.38 Same case as in Figure 13.31. A cast encompassing only the foot can be applied if just the hoof capsule has been lacerated.

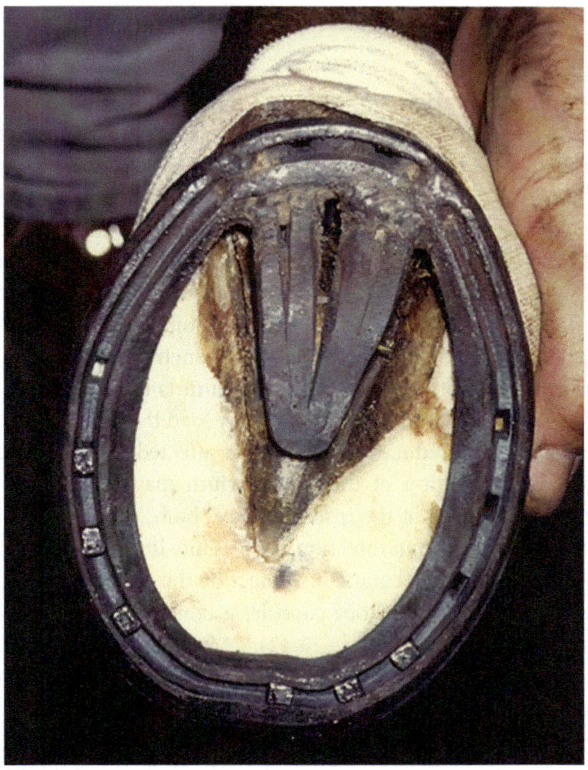

(a)

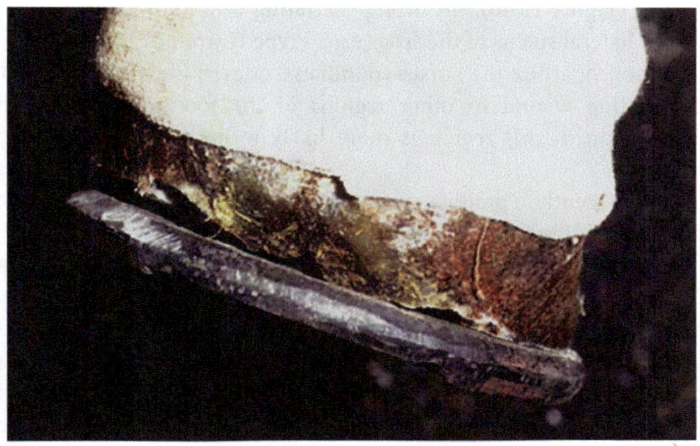

(b)

Figure 13.39 A complete support shoe is a combination of heart-bar and egg-bar shoes. (**a**) Solar view. (**b**) Side view. Note the quarter has been floated (does not contact the shoe) in the area beneath the avulsion injury.

Tips

- An avulsed segment of hoof wall can be reattached to the hoof wall with sutures. Thinning the avulsed segment and the site on the hoof wall to which it is being reattached, by using a motorized burr, aids inserting the suture needle through the hoof wall.
- An avulsed segment of hoof wall can also be anchored in position by lacing orthopedic wire across the segment and around the heads of 6.35–9.53 mm (¼ in to ⅜ in) sheet metal screws inserted into insensitive portions of the hoof on either side of the defect.
- An avulsed segment may be anchored in position with a fiberglass patch attached to the hoof wall with 6.35–9.53 mm (¼ in to ⅜ in) sheet metal screws.
- If a proximally displaced section of coronary band and horny tissue cannot be replaced into the defect in the hoof wall, the horse is best treated by excising the germinal tissue that produces the horny spur.
- A horse's prognosis for soundness after a portion of the distal phalanx has been lost is good, provided that no more than one quarter of the distal phalanx was lost.

Penetrating wounds to the foot

Causes

The foot may be penetrated when the horse steps on or strikes a sharp object [e.g., nail (most common), screw, or glass]. A wound that penetrates only horn (i.e., cornified epidermal tissue), of the sole or frog (*cuneus ungulae*), is considered to be superficial.[45] Wounds that penetrate the corium (i.e., dermis) are considered to be deep and can be categorized as one of three types, with each type affecting a particular region of the foot.[45] A type I deep puncture wound penetrates the solar corium, a type II wound penetrates the corium of the frog or one of its lateral sulci, and a type III wound penetrates the germinal epithelium of the coronary band.

Structures that can be damaged by deep penetration include the distal phalanx, distal interphalangeal joint, deep digital flexor tendon, digital flexor tendon sheath, or any part of the navicular apparatus (i.e., bursa, bone, and/or supporting ligaments) (Figure 13.40).[45] A deep penetrating wound to the frog or a collateral sulcus of the frog (e.g., a type II wound) is more likely to jeopardize the horse's soundness, or even life, than is a penetrating wound to other regions of the foot because a penetration in this region is more likely to enter a synovial structure.[46–49]

More recently, a grading system for severity of injury caused by a penetrating wound of the frog and collateral sulci has been suggested.[47] Grade 1 injury involves the superficial corium only (<2.5 cm); grade 2 injury involves the deeper corium (>2.5 cm) or digital cushion but not the distal phalanx; grade 3 injury involves the distal phalanx but not the synovial structures; and grade 4 injury involves a synovial structure (i.e., distal interphalangeal joint, navicular bursa, or digital flexor tendon sheath).

Multiple synovial structures may be damaged when an object penetrates the solar surface of the foot. For instance, an object having penetrated the navicular bursa may also penetrate the impar ligament (*ligamentum impar* or *lig. sesamoideum distale impar*), which separates the bursa from the distal interphalangeal joint, resulting in infection of the bursa and the distal interphalangeal joint. Or an object that has penetrated the navicular bursa may also penetrate one of the collateral sesamoidean ligaments (suspensory ligaments or *lig. sesamoidean collateralia*), which lie in close proximity to the digital flexor tendon sheath, resulting in infection of the bursa and the digital flexor tendon sheath.[49] One study found that 25% of the penetrating wounds communicating with the navicular bursa also communicated with another synovial cavity.[50] Another study found that 15 of 34 horses treated endoscopically for a penetrating injury to the navicular bursa had concurrent penetration of the adjacent distal interphalangeal joint, and one of the 15 also had penetration of the digital flexor tendon sheath.[51] Horses with a puncture wound in the caudal third or middle third (most common site) of the central region of the frog were twice as likely to suffer penetration of one or more synovial structures than were horses with a puncture wound in the cranial region of the frog.[47]

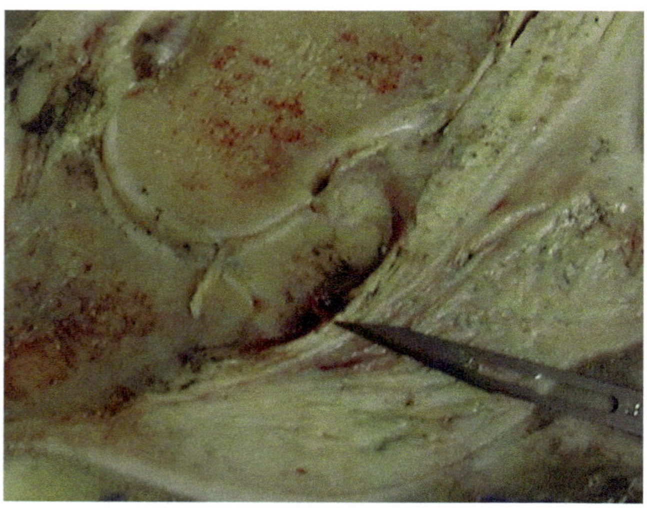

Figure 13.40 Sagittal section of a foot of a horse that incurred damage to the navicular bone when a nail entered the frog. The scalpel blade points to a necrotic area on the flexor surface of the navicular bone.

Diagnosis

Physical examination

Injury to the sensitive tissue of the foot that results in infection is generally accompanied by swelling proximal to the foot. The swelling is most commonly restricted to the coronary band, and in some cases, one heel bulb, but it may extend to the fetlock. The foot is often warmer than its contralateral counterpart, and the digital pulse is usually prominent, especially on the affected side of the foot. The digital flexor tendon sheath may be distended, even when it has not been penetrated.[52] A horse suffering from infection of the solar corium is usually moderately-to-severely lame, and the horse may load the affected foot asymmetrically to reduce pressure on the affected side. Exudate produced by infection of the solar corium may drain at the puncture site and/or at the ipsilateral heel bulb (Figure 13.41). Exudate produced by an infection in the white line may drain at the white line or at a cutaneous defect at the juncture of the coronary band and the hoof capsule, a condition sometimes referred to as "gravel" (Figure 13.42).[53] Migration of infection, caused by puncture of the sole may cause a substantial portion of the epidermal and dermal laminae to separate.

A hoof tester may be useful in localizing the site of puncture causing infection of the corium of the sole or at the white line (Figure 13.42a), but if the wound is chronic, a larger area of the foot may be so sensitive to pressure that localizing the site using hoof testers is difficult. If infection is caused by a shoe nail that was accidentally driven into the sensitive corium, careful application of the hoof tester over each nail hole, after the shoe has been removed, may cause exudate to ooze from the hole (Figure 13.42a).

A dark spot or defect in the sole should be explored to its depth to determine if it penetrates sensitive tissue. A previously unidentified puncture to the sole may become obvious after the foot is trimmed, whereas tracts left by penetration of the frog may be difficult to locate, even after the frog has been trimmed,

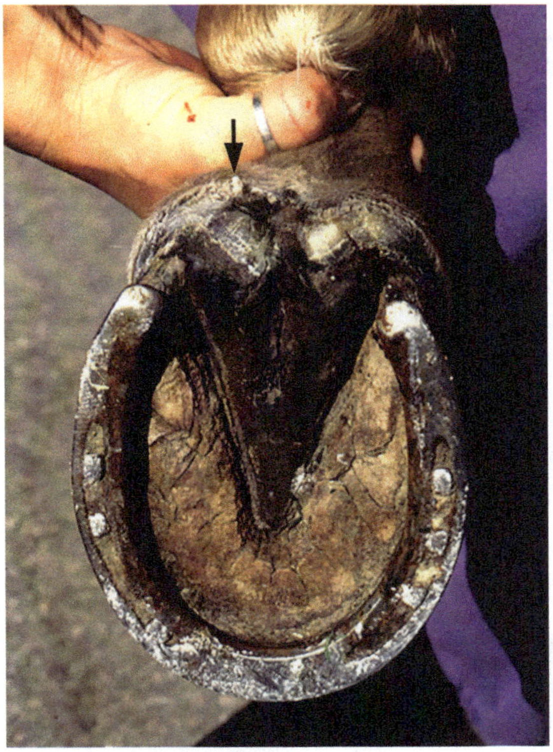

Figure 13.41 Exudate produced by infection of the solar corium caused swelling (black arrow) and drainage from the ipsilateral heel bulb.

because the soft horn of the frog collapses around the tract when the penetrating object is no longer present. After the foot is trimmed and desensitized, weight borne on the affected foot or application of a hoof tester to the site of infection may cause enough pressure on infected tissue to allow trapped exudate to emerge from the sole (Figure 13.43).[53]

The horse is usually severely lame if a synovial structure within the foot (e.g., the distal interphalangeal joint or navicular bursa) is infected. The absence of severe lameness, however, does not confirm that a synovial structure is not infected because a freely draining synovial structure does not develop pain-inducing pressure and because inflammatory products associated with infection are able to exit the wound.

Imaging

A foreign body found penetrating the hoof capsule should be left *in situ*, and the foot examined radiographically so that the object's depth and direction of penetration may be determined, provided that the foot can be examined radiographically without delay (Figure 13.44). If the foot cannot be immediately examined radiographically, the penetrating object should be removed to prevent more damage to the deep structures. The site of puncture should be marked, enabling it to be located at the time of radiographic examination so that a probe or radiographic contrast medium can be inserted into the tract (Figure 13.44b).

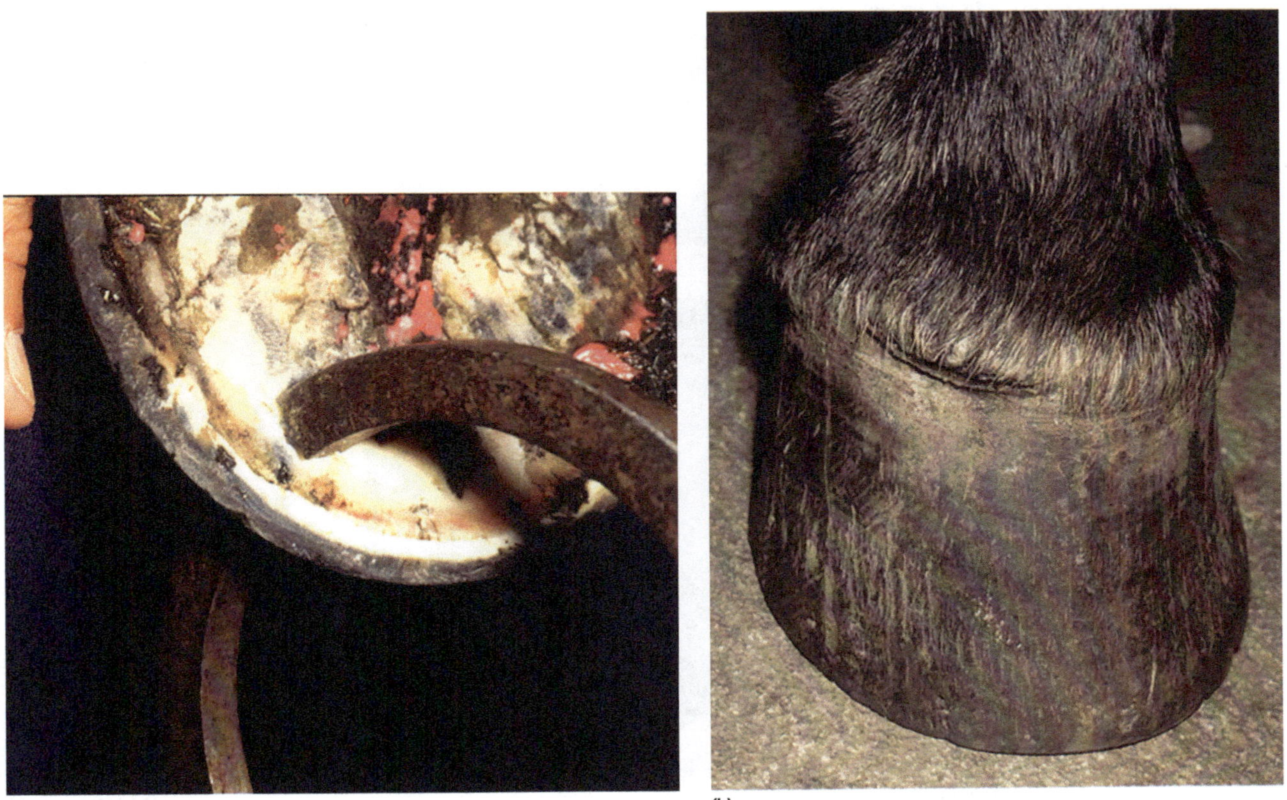

(a) (b)

Figure 13.42 Penetrating wound at the white line. (**a**) Exudate produced from infection of the white line may cause drainage from this structure. In this case hoof tester pressure caused the purulent material to exude from the puncture site. (**b**) Exudate produced by an infection in the white line has drained from this cutaneous defect at the juncture of the coronary band and the hoof capsule. This condition is sometimes referred to as "gravel."

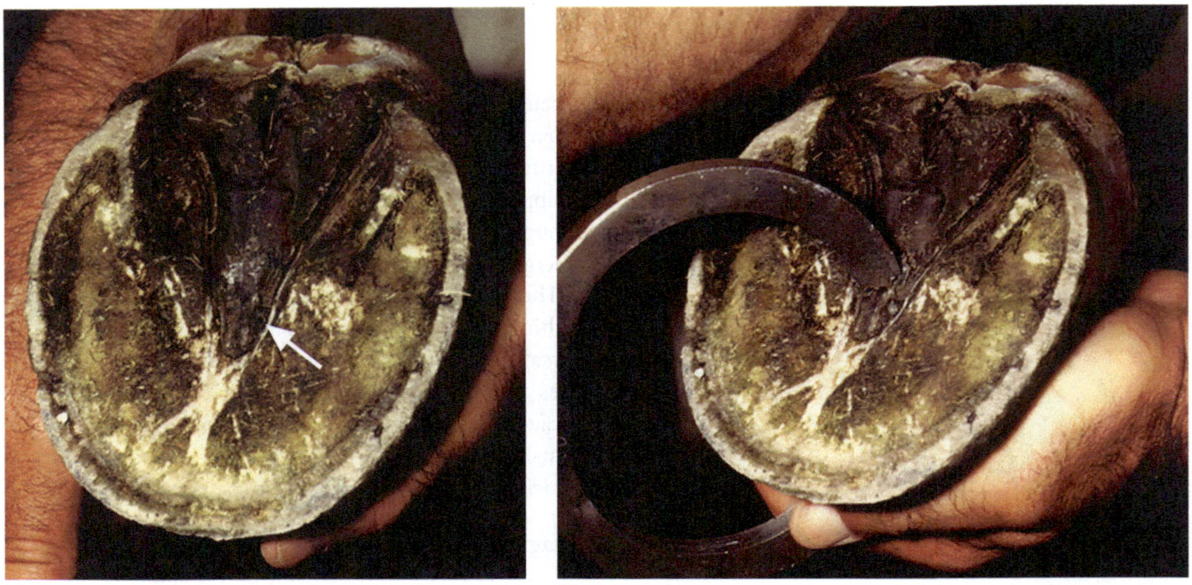

(a) (b)

Figure 13.43 **(a)** A small hole at the apex of the frog became evident after the foot was trimmed (arrow). **(b)** Hoof tester application caused enough pressure to elicit a painful response and also allowed trapped exudate to emerge from the frog.

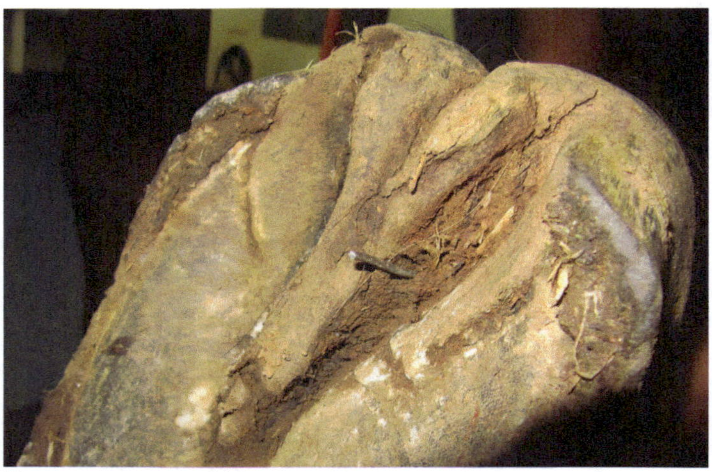

(a)

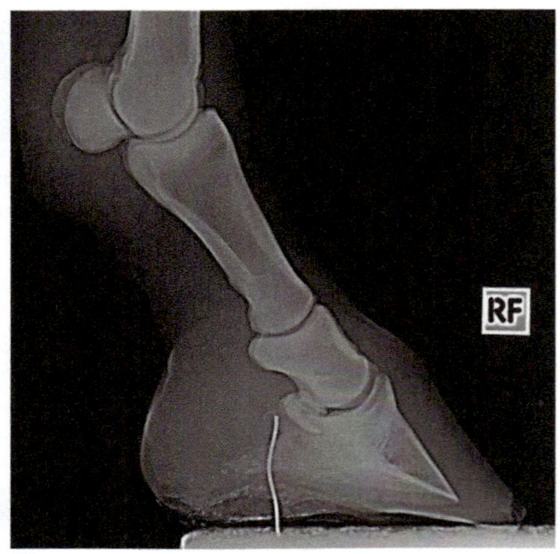

(b)

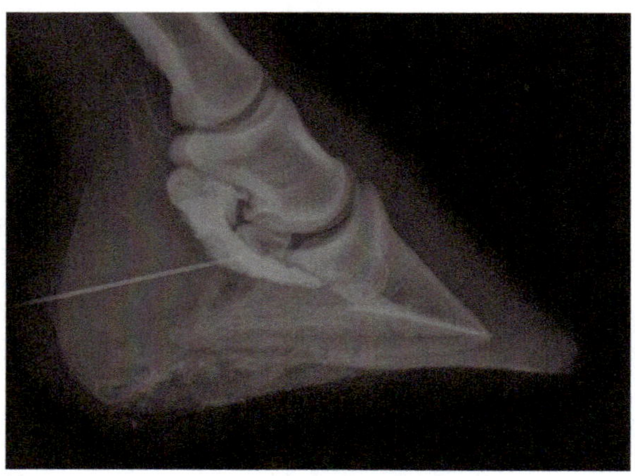

(c)

Figure 13.44 **(a)** A deep penetrating wound to the frog or a collateral sulcus of the frog (e.g., a type II wound). This type of wound to the foot is likely to involve a synovial structure. A foreign body penetrating the bearing surface of the foot should be left *in situ* until the foot can be examined radiographically to determine the proximity of the foreign body to critical structures. **(b)** A plain lateral to medial radiograph of the right foot with a probe inserted into the puncture wound confirmed the trajectory and location of the puncture wound. **(c)** Radiographic contrast medium injected into the navicular bursa. A dorso 65° proximal-palmarodistal oblique with the hoof on the radiographic plate would confirm the location of the probe. In this case, a latero-medial radiograph of the foot with contrast medium injected into the navicular bursa confirmed that the bursa did not communicate with the puncture wound. Courtesy of Dr. Albert Sole.

Non-metallic foreign bodies in the foot, such as wood or glass, may not be identifiable during radiographic evaluation. If the penetrating object has been removed, the direction and depth of the wound can sometimes be evaluated radiographically after inserting a blunt, flexible probe into the tract.[45,53] The probe should be inserted carefully because forceful introduction may damage healthy tissue. Insertion of the probe is often facilitated by anesthetizing the palmar/plantar digital nerves at the level of the proximal sesamoid bones (i.e., an abaxial sesamoid nerve block) to desensitize the foot. Two projections taken at right angles to one another should be obtained so that the spatial relationship of the foreign body or probe to critical structures can be assessed.

Penetration of a synovial structure can be confirmed by injecting a sterile, balanced electrolyte solution into the synovial cavity at a site remote from the wound and observing it egress from the wound (see Figure 4.4). If penetration of a synovial structure is suspected but cannot be confirmed using this method, the foot should be examined radiographically. In the acute phase, gas may be identified within a synovial cavity, thereby confirming penetration of that structure.[47] If gas is not seen, a radiopaque medium can be injected into the synovial structure with a hypodermic needle. Leakage of contrast medium from the synovial structure usually follows the penetrating tract, indicating that the synovial structure has been penetrated.

The navicular bursa can be entered most easily by inserting an 18- or 20-gauge, 8.9-cm (3.5-in), disposable spinal needle midway between the bulbs of the heel, immediately proximal to the hoof capsule, with the foot and pastern flexed.[33] The spinal needle is advanced along the sagittal plane of the foot toward the intersection between the sagittal plane and the long axis of the navicular bone, which is assumed to be midway between the most dorsal and the most palmar/plantar aspects of the coronary band, about 1 cm distal to the coronary band. The needle is advanced until its tip contacts bone. Fluid is seldom obtained regardless of whether the bursa has been damaged. The foot should be examined radiographically or ultrasonographically immediately before the bursa is injected with contrast medium to confirm that the tip of the needle is against the navicular bone.[54] An intact navicular bursa can be distended with 3–4 mL of fluid before marked resistance to injection is encountered. Radiologic identification of contrast medium within the bursa (Figure 13.44c) or observation of flow at the tip of the needle during injection and distension of the distal recess of the navicular bursa are evidence of a successful bursal injection,[54] and leakage of contrast medium from the bursa, other than from the site of centesis, indicates that the penetrating object has perforated the bursa.

The easiest method of entering the distal interphalangeal joint is to insert a 2.54-cm (1-in), 20- or 22-gauge hypodermic needle into the dorsal pouch of the joint (Figure 13.45a).[55] The needle is inserted into the dorsal pouch through the coronary band, on the dorsal midline, at the juncture of the hoof wall and skin, parallel to the bearing surface of the foot (i.e., the dorsal parallel approach) or perpendicular to the slope of the pastern (i.e., the dorsal inclined approach), until its point contacts the dorsal distal aspect of the middle phalanx. Synovial fluid usually

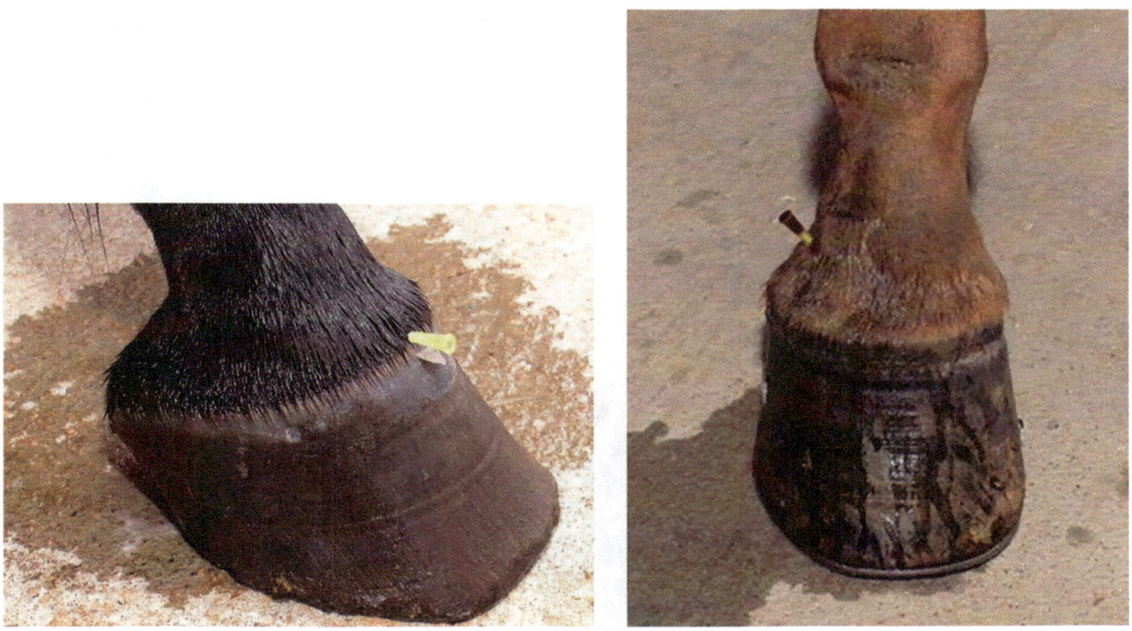

(a) (b)

Figure 13.45 Centesis of the distal interphalangeal joint. **(a)** Site for centesis in the dorsal pouch through the coronary band, on the dorsal midline, at the junction of the hoof wall and skin. The needle is inserted parallel to the bearing surface of the foot or perpendicular to the slope of the pastern until its point contacts the dorsal distal aspect of the middle phalanx. Synovial fluid usually appears in the needle hub. **(b)** Lateral approach to centesis of the joint by inserting the needle just proximal to the palpable, proximal edge of the collateral cartilage, approximately midway between the dorsal and palmar/plantar aspects of the middle phalanx.

appears in the needle hub. Centesis is most easily performed with the limb bearing weight (Figure 13.45a).

If a wound or infection precludes the use of the dorsal approach for centesis, the distal interphalangeal joint can be entered from the lateral aspect of the joint by inserting the needle just proximal to the palpable, proximal edge of the collateral cartilage, approximately midway between the dorsal and palmar/plantar aspects of the middle phalanx (Figure 13.45b).[56] The needle is angled downward toward the distal border of the hoof wall on the contralateral side of the hoof. The depth of penetration is less than 2.5 cm. The procedure is most easily performed with the foot flexed, but the navicular bursa or digital tendon sheath is less likely to be inadvertently entered if the horse is bearing weight on the foot.

A reliable method of centesis of the digital flexor tendon sheath is the palmar/plantar axial sesamoidean approach.[57] Using this approach, the needle is inserted through the palmar/plantar annular ligament of the fetlock. With the limb flexed, the needle is placed through the skin at the level of the midbody of the lateral proximal sesamoid bone 3 mm axial to the palpable palmar/plantar border of the lateral sesamoid bone and immediately axial to the palmar/plantar digital neurovascular bundle, and advanced though the palmar/plantar annular ligament. The needle is inserted in a transverse plane and advanced to a depth of about 1.5–2 cm at an angle to the sagittal plane, aiming toward the central intersesamoidean region. A recently described technique of centesis of the digital flexor tendon sheath is the basilar sesamoidean approach.[58] Using this approach, the limb is held in a mildly flexed position, and the needle is inserted into a depression created by the base of the lateral proximal sesamoid bone proximally and the lateral border of the superficial digital flexor tendon axially. The needle is directed lateromedially at a 45° angle to the transverse plane and distoproximally at a 45° angle to the dorsal plane. The needle enters the sheath at a depth of about 1 cm.

Before instilling contrast media into a synovial structure, fluid should be obtained, if possible, for cytologic examination and bacterial culture. Fluid is most reliably retrieved using the basilar sesamoidean approach. A markedly elevated white blood cell count and high concentration of protein in the fluid are suggestive of infection. For more information regarding laboratory findings associated with septic arthritis, see Chapter 16.

An alternative to injecting a synovial cavity with contrast material is to inject the contrast medium directly into a draining tract using a teat cannula or Foley catheter after which a radiograph is taken. Contrast medium entering a synovial structure confirms that it has been penetrated (Figure 13.46).[53] The downside to this approach is that contrast medium is injected into a synovial structure through a contaminated or infected site, but

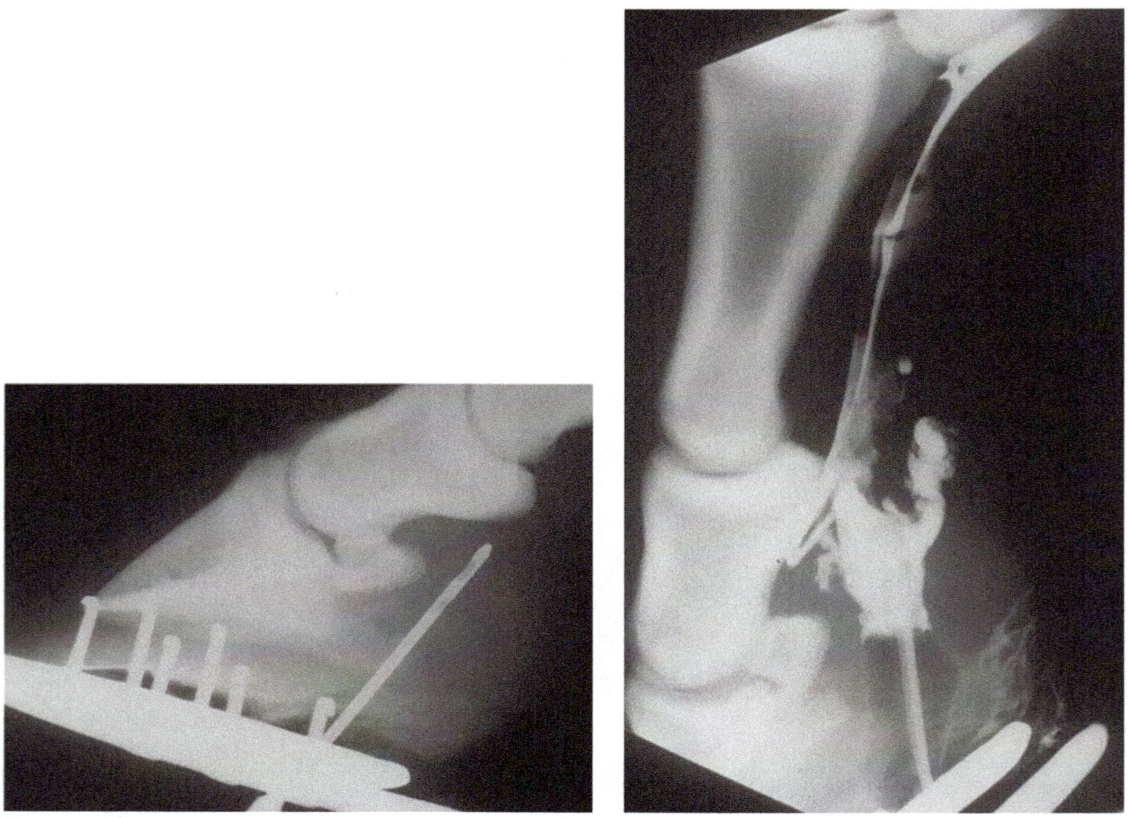

(a) (b)

Figure 13.46 A sharp piece of wood was found to have penetrated the palmar one-third of the frog in this horse. **(a)** A teat cannula is inserted in the tract. **(b)** Injection of contrast medium revealed that the puncture wound extended into the digital sheath.

this is less important than failing to recognize that the wound involves a synovial structure.

Confirmation of injury to the solar corium or distal phalanx from a penetrating wound, without evidence of a draining tract, may be obtained with radiographic examination. If the solar corium has been penetrated, gas may be seen between the sole and solar corium (Figure 13.47). Injury to the distal phalanx may appear on radiographic examination as a spherical lucency or as a sequestrum (Figure 13.48).

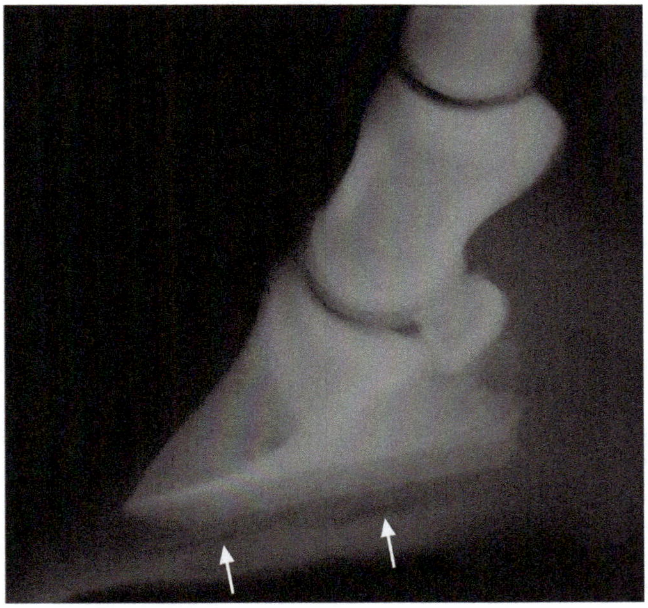

Figure 13.47 If the solar corium has been penetrated, gas (arrows) may be seen between it and the sole.

Although ultrasound, nuclear scintigraphy, and MRI have been used to identify a radiographically occult fracture or a foreign body (e.g., a piece of wood or glass) or to further elucidate the extent of the injury to the navicular apparatus and deep digital flexor tendon, the authors have rarely found the need to use these imaging modalities. Usually, lesions unrecognized radiographically can be identified during surgical exploration of the site of penetration, and appropriate surgical treatment can be instituted at the time of exploration.

Treatment

A horse with a superficial puncture wound to the sole or frog that has penetrated the keratinized horn should be treated by debriding contaminated and devitalized tissue from the puncture site, using a sharp knife, until healthy margins are obtained. This usually requires a modest degree of paring of the solar horn at the puncture site. The superficial margin of the wound should be beveled outward so that it does not close before the depth of the wound has healed (Figure 13.49). Lameness caused by a superficial puncture wound usually resolves quickly after a route for escape of exudate has been established, and, if debridement and drainage are adequate, the affected horse usually does not require systemically administered antimicrobial therapy. After irrigating the wound with a dilute antiseptic solution, the wound tract can be packed with antiseptic impregnated gauze (e.g., Kerlix AMD), to create a wicking effect. This approach is used until suppuration has ceased. The foot should be covered with a waterproof bandage until the granulation tissue that develops in the wound cornifies. If the defect is large, or if healing is protracted, a phalangeal cast or treatment (hospital) plate shoe can be applied to protect the sole (Figure 13.50). Although a phalangeal cast provides

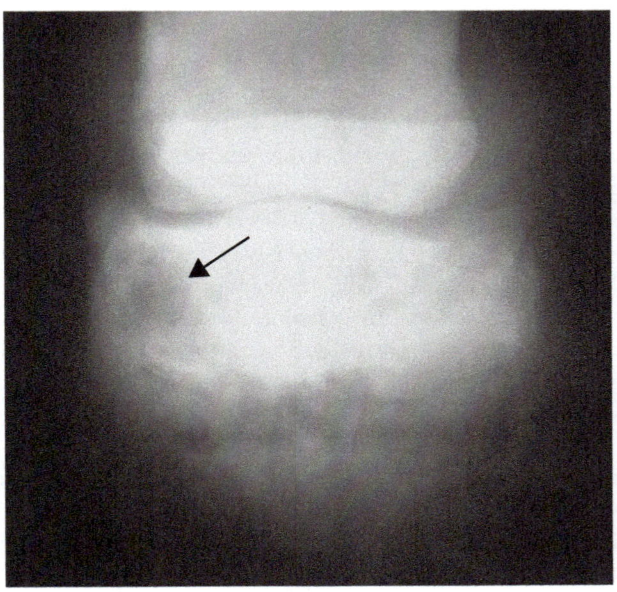

(a)

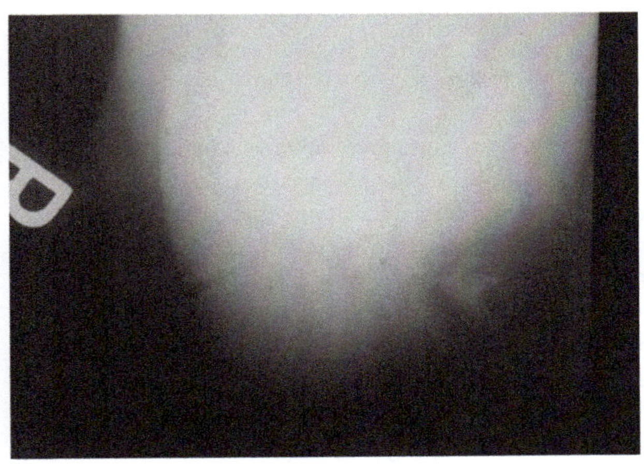

(b)

Figure 13.48 (a,b) Injury to the distal phalanx may appear on radiographic examination as a spherical lucency (arrow) or a sequestrum.

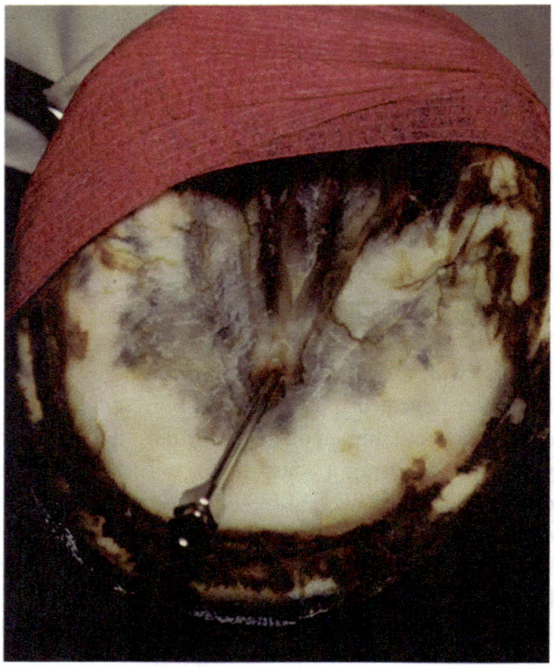
(a)

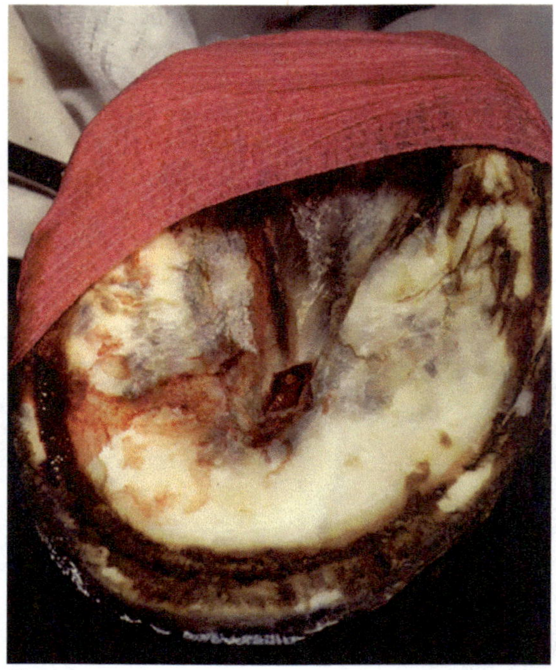
(b)

Figure 13.49 (**a**) Superficial puncture wound at the apex of the frog. (**b**) The superficial margin of the wound is beveled outward.

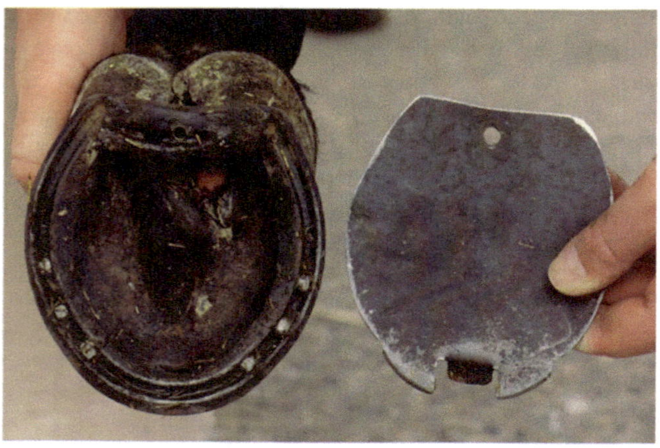

Figure 13.50 A treatment (hospital) plate shoe can be applied to protect the sole. The protection against environmental contamination provided by a plate shoe, however, is not as good as that provided by a foot cast.

better protection against environmental contamination than does a treatment plate shoe, it does not allow access to the wound for periodic examination and dressing changes. Consequently, if access to the healing site is needed, a treatment plate shoe, rather than a cast, should be applied.

Horses with penetration of the solar corium accompanied by septic osteitis, with or without a sequestrum, of the distal phalanx (Figure 13.48) should be treated by curettage of the infected portion of bone. Preparation of the foot for surgery should include paring to remove exfoliating horn/frog, cleaning, and bandaging with an antiseptic dressing. An Esmarch tourniquet (or Esmarch bandage) positioned proximal to the metacarpophalangeal/metatarsophalangeal joint facilitates surgery by improving visibility by minimizing hemorrhage during surgery and facilitates regional limb perfusion with an appropriate antimicrobial drug during or after surgery. The infected bone is accessed through the sole by sharply enlarging the penetrating wound or through a trephine hole created in the hoof wall adjacent to the infected portion of the phalanx. Horses are usually more comfortable after curettage if the distal phalanx is accessed through the hoof wall, rather than through the sole. Infected bone is soft and easily detached with a curette, whereas normal bone of the distal phalanx is hard and difficult to remove by curettage. The distal phalanx can be curetted with the horse standing after desensitizing the foot by anesthetizing the palmar/plantar digital nerves at the level of the proximal sesamoid bones (i.e., an abaxial sesamoid nerve block) or by anesthetizing the palmar/plantar nerves proximal to the digital flexor tendon sheath and the palmar metacarpal/plantar metatarsal nerves at the level of the distal end of the splint bones (i.e., a low four-point nerve block). Diseased bone should be submitted to a laboratory for bacterial culture and antimicrobial sensitivity testing of isolated bacteria. Culture of infected tissue usually produces growth of a variety of Gram-positive and Gram-negative bacteria, the most common being coliforms.[47]

Regional limb perfusion with a broad-spectrum antimicrobial drug, used alone or in conjunction with systemic administration of the drug(s), is indicated. For more information regarding the indications and techniques for regional limb perfusion, see Chapter 19. Horses with a deep puncture wound to the frog or one of its lateral sulci (i.e., a type II wound or a grade 4 injury) that enters the navicular bursa are best treated while anesthetized.

The extent of damage can be assessed, and diseased tissue removed after exposing the navicular bone by fenestrating the deep digital flexor tendon and opening the navicular bursa (i.e., a "street-nail" procedure) or by performing navicular bursoscopy. Applying a pneumatic or elastic tourniquet improves visibility during surgery by reducing hemorrhage and facilitates regional limb perfusion during or after surgery. The horse must be anesthetized for either procedure. With the "street-nail" procedure, a section of the frog, digital cushion, and deep digital flexor tendon are sharply excised to expose the flexor surface of the navicular bone (Figure 13.51). Discolored areas of the digital cushion and deep digital flexor tendon are sharply excised, and those on the flexor surface of the navicular bone are removed by curettage. Diseased tissue is submitted to a laboratory for bacterial culture and antimicrobial sensitivity testing of isolated bacteria. Communication between the distal interphalangeal joint and navicular bursa, through the impar ligament, can be determined by instilling sterile, isotonic saline solution, under pressure, into the distal interphalangeal joint, as described earlier. Exit of fluid through the navicular bursa is evidence of communication. Communication between the digital flexor tendon sheath and the navicular bursa, through one of the collateral sesamoidean ligaments, can be determined by instilling sterile, isotonic saline solution, under pressure, into the digital flexor tendon sheath, as described earlier.

The navicular bursa can also be examined, diseased tissue excised, and foreign material removed, using bursoscopy (Figure 13.52).[59] The arthroscope is inserted proximal to the lateral collateral cartilage on the abaxial border of the deep digital flexor tendon, axial to the digital neurovascular bundle. The digital flexor tendon sheath and the palmar/plantar pouch of the distal interphalangeal joint can also be examined through this portal. Instruments used to excise diseased tissue are introduced on the contralateral side of the pastern or, more commonly, through the wound on the solar surface of the foot. An endoscopic approach to examine the navicular bursa and bone and to treat disease encountered is less invasive and provides a more detailed examination of the bursa and its contents. Postoperative care of the horse is simpler, and the results are better, than when the horse is treated by using the street-nail procedure.[59] The distal interphalangeal joint and the digital flexor tendon sheath, if also affected, can be treated endoscopically at the same time. For a more complete discussion

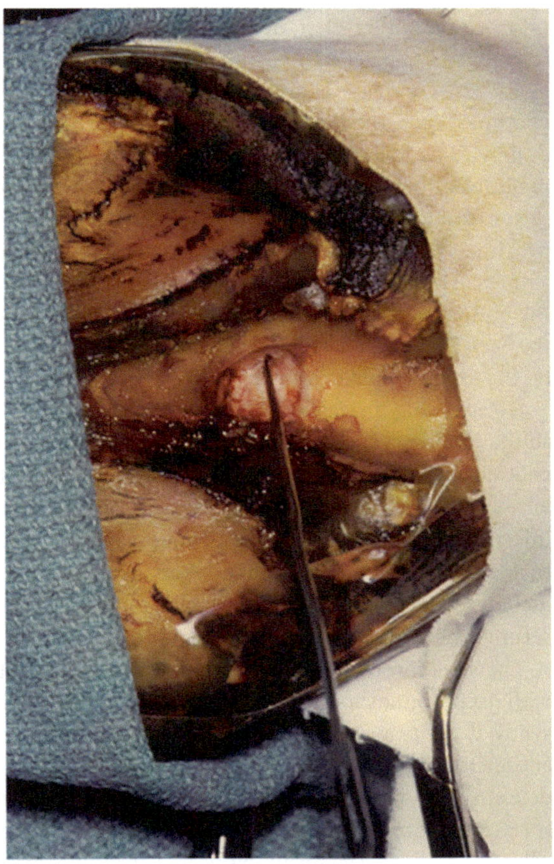

(a)

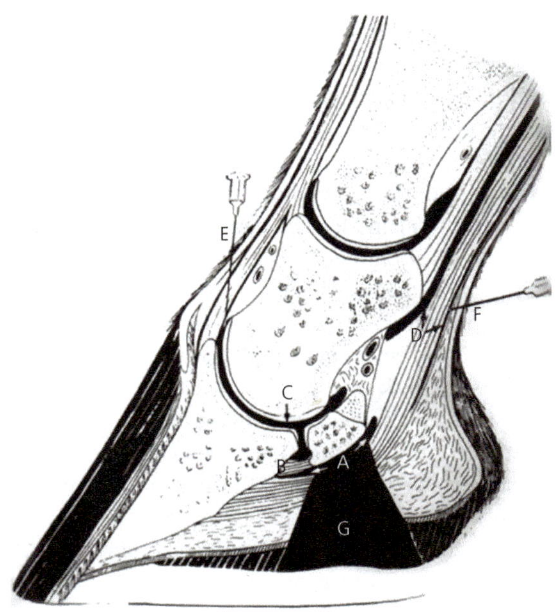

(b)

Figure 13.51 "Street-nail" procedure. (**a**) Sharp dissection of the frog exposes the digital cushion and the wound tract. Excision is continued through the deep digital flexor tendon to enter the navicular bursa. (**b**) Sagittal illustration defining the path of dissection through the frog to the navicular bone. A = navicular bursa; B = impar ligament; C = distal interphalangeal joint; D = digital flexor tendon sheath; E = needle in distal interphalangeal joint; F = needle in digital flexor tendon sheath; G = path of dissection through the frog to the navicular bone.

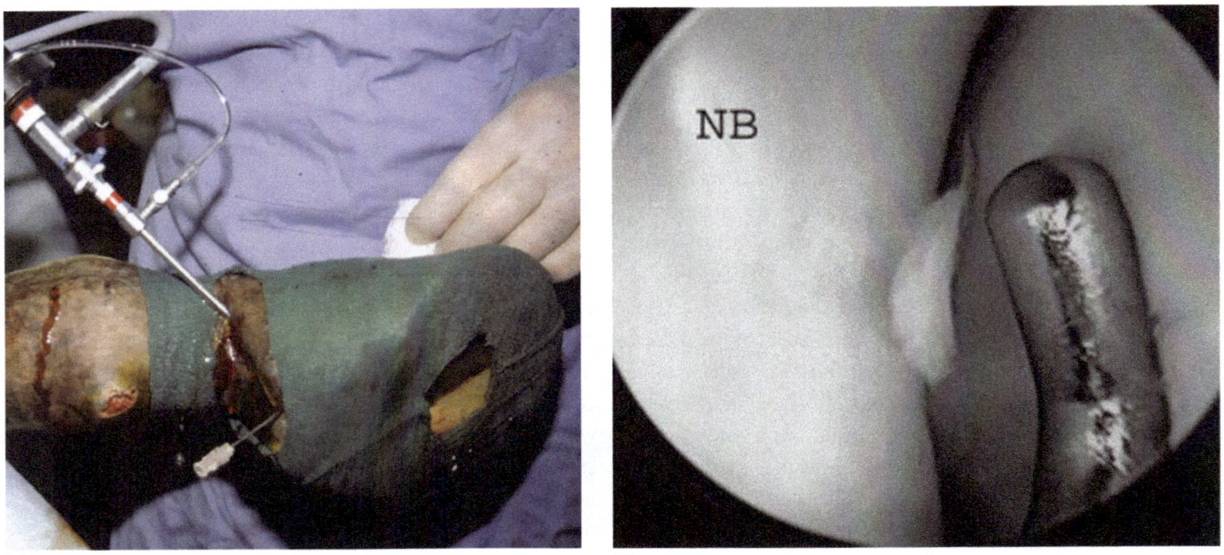

(a) (b)

Figure 13.52 **(a)** This photograph illustrates the approach to navicular bursoscopy. An arthroscope and cannula have been inserted into the navicular bursa. **(b)** Endoscopic view within the navicular bursa. Note the avulsed fibrocartilage, adjacent to the sagittal ridge (bottom), from the navicular bone (NB). The metal probe is covering the penetrating wound in the deep digital flexor tendon.

of the treatment of horses for septic arthritis see Chapter 16. After surgery, the foot is encased in a waterproof bandage until granulation tissue fills the wound. A treatment-plate shoe or a phalangeal cast may be applied after this time.

A less invasive method of debriding wounds that communicate with the navicular bursa by using medicinal maggots has been described.[50] Using this method, superficial damaged and necrotic tissue at the entrance of the tract is lightly and sharply debrided to enlarge the entrance for irrigation and drainage and to apply maggots. The deep digital flexor tendon and navicular bursa are not invaded during surgical debridement. Medicinal maggot therapy, using disinfected larvae of the common green bottle fly, *Lucilia sericata* (Monarch Labs in North America, Polymedics Bio Products in Belgium, BioMonde in the UK, Neocura in Germany, Japan Maggot Company in Japan, and the Department of Medical Entomology of the Westmead Hospital in Australia), is initiated on days 2 or 3 to remove necrotic tissue and bacteria from the tract and bursa. The larvae from one vial (~500–1000 larvae) are embedded in gauze, which is applied to the puncture site. A stack of dry, sterile 4×4 gauzes is gently bandaged over the larvae and wound, and the bottom of the foot is covered with a treatment plate. Gauzes are changed daily to remove discharge created by the maggots and the suppurating wound. Maggots become satiated in 5–7 days, at which time they are removed and replaced with a fresh batch of maggots.[50] The wound is dressed with maggots until all necrotic tissue is debrided and a healthy bed of granulation tissue is evident.[60] Maggots have a positive effect on wound healing by producing potent proteolytic enzymes that aid in debridement,[61] by destroying and digesting bacteria,[62] by producing antibacterial secretions,[62] by producing secretions that stimulate proliferation of fibroblasts,[63] and by breaking down biofilm.[64] For more information on maggot debridement therapy, the reader is referred to Chapter 22.

To assist irrigation and drainage and to allow maggots continued access to diseased tissue, a 0.64-mm (0.25-in) Penrose drain can be fed into the entrance of the wound and, using a malleable probe, directed just palmar/plantar to the deep digital flexor tendon. The drain emerges through a stab incision at the proximal extent of the heel where it is secured to the skin with sutures. The drain is removed after 10–14 days. Protection of the bottom of the foot with a treatment plate is continued, and the heels are elevated with a wedge or rail shoe to reduce tension on the deep digital flexor tendon.[50]

Determining if infection of the navicular bursa has resolved so that antimicrobial treatment or maggot therapy can be discontinued may be difficult. Obtaining fluid from the navicular bursa for cytologic examination and culture to determine if infection has resolved is difficult to impossible, but other criteria that can be used to determine when infection has resolved include amelioration of lameness and a marked decrease in the serum concentration of serum amyloid A.[65]

The selection of antimicrobial drugs administered to horses with deep wounds to the foot, with or without involvement of a synovial cavity or the distal phalanx, is guided by results of antimicrobial sensitivity testing of bacterial isolates. Until the definitive results are known, the horse should receive broad-spectrum antimicrobial therapy, such as a combination of penicillin or another β-lactam antibiotic and an aminoglycoside. The combination of penicillin and gentamicin is used most commonly. Regional limb perfusion with an antimicrobial drug is most often used in conjunction with systemic administration of an antimicrobial drug, but using regional limb perfusion alone may be just as effective.[66] The horse should receive analgesic therapy, usually with phenylbutazone or flunixin meglumine. Relieving pain in the affected foot decreases the likelihood of the contralateral limb developing laminitis. The horse should receive appropriate prophylaxis against tetanus. For some wounds of the foot, applying a cast to the injured digit after therapy has been discontinued, rather than a bandage or treatment plate shoe, increases the horse's comfort, in addition to simplifying care.

Prognosis

A horse lame because of a penetrating injury to the foot, such as a puncture wound to the solar corium, is likely to regain soundness if the injury does not involve a synovial structure or the distal phalanx, provided the horse is treated correctly, as outlined earlier.[49] Steckel *et al.* (1989) found that 95% of horses with a puncture through the sole returned to soundness,[49] and Kilcoyne *et al.* (2011) found that horses suffering a penetrating wound to the frog or collateral sulci of the foot had a good prognosis for return to soundness if the wound was superficial and the horse was treated within 48 hours.[47]

A horse with septic pedal osteitis, with or without a sequestrum of the distal phalanx, has a favorable prognosis for resolution of infection and return to soundness if the horse receives proper treatment, as outlined earlier.[44, 67–69] A meta-analysis of four studies of horses with a penetrating injury to a foot found that of 94 horses with septic pedal osteitis, only one died from causes directly related to the septic pedal bone, and 52 of 57 survivors returned to their previous level of performance.[48] Of the five horses that did not return to their previous level of performance, one was retired sound, and two were lame because of an unrelated problem.

Sepsis of the navicular bursa leads to serious sequelae, making it the most frequent reason for euthanizing a horse that has suffered a penetrating wound to the foot.[49] A horse with a puncture wound that extends into the navicular bursa has a more favorable prognosis for soundness and for survival if a hindlimb, rather than a forelimb, is affected, and if it receives surgical treatment within a week of the injury.[45, 49] In the authors' experience, a penetrating wound involving the navicular bursa and/or another synovial structure of the foot is a medical emergency since the earlier treatment is initiated, the better is the outcome. In one study, horses treated within 48 hours had a better prognosis than did horses treated more than 7 days after injury (81.6% vs 6.7% returned to soundness).[47] In one report of horses treated for septic navicular bursitis with a street-nail procedure, only 12 of 38 (31.6%) horses had a satisfactory outcome, and only four returned to athletic function.[45] Five were used as broodmares, three had no long-term follow-up, and 15 of 34 required additional wound debridement after the street-nail procedure, primarily due to necrosis of the deep digital flexor tendon. Steckel *et al.* (1989) found that only six of 19 horses treated with the street-nail procedure became sound.[49]

Prognosis for survival and return to soundness is better when horses with infection of the navicular bursa are treated by bursoscopy rather than with the street-nail procedure. In one study, 20 of 34 horses treated endoscopically returned to their pre-injury use, four were able to work at a lower level of performance, and two were useable after neurectomy of the palmar digital nerves.[51] The outcome of horses with infection of the navicular bursa that received maggot debridement therapy is encouraging. In a report of horses with chronic infection of the navicular bursa (i.e., >72 hours), the septic process resolved in 90% (18/20) of the horses after treatment, and 70% (14/20) of horses returned to their intended use or previous level of use with no complication.[50]

Systemic antimicrobial therapy alone is incapable of eliminating infection of the navicular bursa, distal interphalangeal joint, deep digital flexor tendon, and/or the digital flexor tendon sheath, and that associated with a sequestrum of the distal phalanx. The prognosis is markedly improved using a combination of surgery and broad-spectrum antimicrobial drugs administered systemically or by regional perfusion.[50] Chronic infection of one or more of the synovial structures of the foot, erosion of articular cartilage, septic osteitis, or fibrous adhesions between the deep digital flexor tendon and the navicular bone may be responsible for unremitting pain resulting in failure of the horse to return to soundness.[45] The navicular bone may suffer a pathologic fracture, or the deep digital flexor tendon may rupture, even after infection has resolved.

What to do

- If an object penetrating the frog must be removed before the foot can be examined radiographically, the site of penetration should be identified because the horn of the frog collapses around the tract after the penetrating object is removed, making the opening of the tract difficult to identify.

What to avoid

- Systemic antimicrobial therapy alone is incapable of eliminating infection of a synovial structure within the foot.

Tips

- Horses with a puncture wound in the caudal or middle third of the frog are far more likely to have suffered penetration of one or more synovial structures than are horses with a puncture wound in the cranial third of the frog.
- Infected bone of the distal phalanx should be removed by curettage. Horses are usually more comfortable if infected bone is accessed through the hoof wall, rather than through the sole.
- A horse that has suffered penetration of the navicular bursa by a foreign object can be treated by a street-nail procedure or by navicular bursoscopy. The results of the bursoscopic approach are generally better than the results achieved with the street-nail procedure, and the horse's aftercare is simpler.

Conclusion

The distal portion of the limb contains many critical synovial and supporting structures, injury to any one of which can result in permanent loss of function and even necessitate euthanasia of the horse for humane reasons. A horse with an injury to the distal portion of the limb that involves a critical structure may be able to return to full function when treated appropriately, but appropriate treatment requires early and accurate assessment of the wound. Identifying which structures have been damaged requires careful physical examination and various imaging techniques, and may necessitate surgical exploration of the wound.

References

1. Wilmink JM, van Herten J, van Weeren PR, *et al.* Retrospective study of primary intention healing and sequestrum formation in horses compared to ponies under clinical circumstances. *Equine Vet J* 2002; **34**: 270.
2. Jacobs KA, Leach DH, Fretz PB, *et al.* Comparative aspects of the healing of excisional wounds on the leg and body of horses. *Vet Surg* 1984; **13**: 83.
3. Bertone AL, Sullins KE, Stashak TS, *et al.* Effect of wound location and the use of topical collagen gel on exuberant granulation tissue formation and wound healing in the horse and pony. *Am J Vet Res* 1985; **46**: 1438.
4. Schumacher J, Brumbaugh GW, Honnas CM, *et al.* Kinetics of healing of grafted and non-grafted wounds on the distal portion of the forelimbs of horses. *Am J Vet Res* 1992; **53**: 1568.
5. Wilmink JM. Unpublished data on the rates of wound contraction and epithelialization in equids.
6. Wilmink JM, Stolk PW, Van Weeren PR, *et al.* Differences in second-intention wound healing between horses and ponies: macroscopic aspects. *Equine Vet J* 1999; **31**: 53.
7. Bertone AL. Management of exuberant granulation tissue. *Vet Clin N Am Equine Pract* 1989; **5**: 551.
8. Wilmink JM, Van Weeren PR. Treatment of exuberant granulation tissue. *Clin Tech Equine Pract* 2004; **3**: 141.
9. Garvican E, Clegg P. Clinical aspects of the equine carpal joints. *UK Vet* 2007 **12**: 1.
10. Rudolph R, Vande Berg J, Ehrlich HP. Wound contraction and scar contracture. In: Cohen IK, Diegelmann RF, Lindblad WJ (eds). *Wound Healing: Biochemical and Clinical Aspects*, 1st edn. WB Saunders: Philadelphia, 1992: 96.
11. Shin D, Minn KW. The effect of myofibroblasts on contracture of hypertrophic scar. *Plast Reconstr Surg* 2004; **113**: 633.
12. Elmas CR, Koenig JB, Bienzle D, *et al.* Evaluation of a broad range real-time polymerase chain reaction (RT-PCR) assay for the diagnosis of septic synovitis in horses. *Can J Vet Res* 2013; **77**: 211.
13. MacDonald MH, Honnas CM, Meagher DM. Osteomyelitis of the calcaneus in horses: 28 cases (1972–1987). *J Am Vet Med Assoc* 1989; **194**: 1317.
14. Hand DR, Watkins JP, Honnas CM, *et al.* Osteomyelitis of the *sustentaculum tali* in horses: 10 cases (1992–1998). *J Am Vet Med Assoc* 2001; **219**: 341.
15. Kainer RA, Fails AD. Functional anatomy of the equine musculoskeletal system. In: Baxter GM (eds). *Adams & Stashak's Lameness in Horses*, 6th edn. Wiley Blackwell: Oxford, UK, 2011: 44.
16. Baxter GM. Retrospective study of lower limb wounds involving tendons, tendon sheaths, or joints. *Proc Am Assoc Equine Pract* 1987; **33**: 715.
17. Booth TM, Abbot J, Clements A, *et al.* Treatment of septic common digital extensor tenosynovitis by complete resection in seven horses. *Vet Surg* 2004; **33**: 107.
18. Belknap JK, Baxter GM, Nickels FA. Extensor tendon lacerations in horses: 50 cases (1982–1988). *J Am Vet Med Assoc* 1993; **203**: 428.
19. Swaim SF. Management of skin tension in dermal surgery. *Compend Contin Edu Pract Vet* 1980; **2**: 758.
20. Bailey JV, Jacobs KA. The mesh expansion method of suturing wounds on the legs of horses. *Vet Surg* 1983; **12**: 78.
21. Bigbie RB, Shealy P, Moll D. Presuturing as an aid in the closure of skin defects created by surgical excision. *Proc Am Assoc Equine Pract* 1990; **36**: 613.
22. Liang M, Briggs P, Heckler FR, *et al.* Presuturing – a new technique for closing large skin defects: clinical and experimental studies. *Plast Reconstr Surg* 1988; **81**: 694.
23. Scardino M, Swaim SF, Henderson RA. Enhancing wound closure on the limbs. *Compend Contin Educ Pract Vet* 1996; **18**: 919.
24. Lawrence WT. Clinical management of nonhealing wounds. In: Cohen IK, Diegelmann RF, Lindblad WJ (eds). *Wound Healing: Biochemical and Clinical Aspects*, 1st edn. WB Saunders Co: Philadelphia, 1992: 541.
25. Janicek JC, Dabareiner RM, Honnas CM, *et al.* Heel bulb laceration in horses: 101 cases (1988–1994). *J Am Vet Med Assoc* 2005; **226**: 418.
26. Baxter GM. Management of wounds involving synovial structures in horses. *Clin Tech Equine Pract* 2004; **3**: 204.
27. Post EM, Singer ER, Clegg PD, *et al.* Retrospective study of 24 cases of septic calcaneal bursitis in the horse. *Equine Vet J* 2003; **35**: 662.
28. Clem MF, DeBowes RM, Yovich JV, *et al.* Osseous sequestration in the horse. A review of 68 cases. *Vet Surg* 1988; **17**: 2.
29. Céleste C, Szöke MO. Management of equine hoof injuries. *Vet Clin North Am Equine Pract* 2005; **21**: 167.
30. Wilson DG, Cooley AL, MacWilliams PS, *et al.* Effects of 0.05% chlorhexidine lavage on the tarsocrural joints of horses. *Vet Surg* 1994; **23**: 442.
31. Rani SA, Hoon R, Najafi RR, *et al.* The *in vitro* antimicrobial activity of wound and skin cleansers at nontoxic concentrations. *Adv Skin Wound Care* 2014; **27**: 65.
32. Rodeheaver G. Wound cleansing, wound irrigation, wound disinfection. In: Krasner D, Rodeheaver G, Sibbald G (eds). *Chronic Wound Care*, 3rd edn. HMP Communications: Wayne, 2001: 371.
33. Ketzner, KM, Stewart AA, Byron CR, *et al.* Wounds of the pastern and foot region managed with phalangeal casts: 50 cases in 49 horses (1995–2006). *Aust Vet J* 2009; **87**: 363.
34. Kainer R. Clinical anatomy of the equine foot. *Vet Clin North Am Equine Pract* 1989; **5**: 1.
35. Pollitt C, Daradka M. Hoof wall wound repair. *Equine Vet J* 2004; **36**: 210.
36. Leach D, Oliphant LW. Ultrastructure of the equine hoof wall secondary epidermal lamellae. *Am J Vet Res* 1983; **44**: 1561.
37. Curtis S, Martin J, Hobbs S. Hoof renewal time from birth of Thoroughbred foals. *The Vet J* 2014; **201**: 116.
38. Celeste C, Szoke M. Management of equine hoof injuries. *Vet Clin North Am Equine Pract* 2005; **21**: 167–190.
39. Parks A. Equine foot wounds: general principles of healing and treatment. *Proc Am Assoc Equine Pract* 1999; **45**: 180.
40. Fessler J. Hoof injuries. *Vet Clin North Am Equine Pract* 1989; **5**: 643.
41. de Gresti A, Zani DD, D'Arpe L, *et al.* A singular case of traumatic total hoof capsule avulsion. *Equine Vet Educ* 2008; **20**: 406.
42. Markel MD, Richardson GL, Peterson PR, *et al.* Surgical reconstruction of chronic coronary band avulsions in three horses. *J Am Vet Med Assoc* 1987; **190**: 687.

43. Riggs CM, Proudman CJ, Hughes I. Management of traumatic, partial hoof avulsion into two horses. *Equine Vet Edu* 1995, **7**: 140.
44. Gaughan, EM, Rendano VT, Ducharme NG. Surgical treatment of septic pedal osteitis in horses: nine cases (1980–1987). *J Am Vet Med Assoc* 1989; **195**: 1131.
45. Richardson GL, Pascoe JR, Meagher D. Puncture wounds of the foot in horses: diagnosis and treatment. *Compend Contin Educ Pract Vet* 1986; **8**: 379.
46. Honnas CM, Crabill MR, Mackie JT, *et al.* Use of autogenous cancellous bone grafting in the treatment of septic navicular bursitis and distal sesamoid osteomyelitis in horses. *J Am Vet Med Assoc* 1995; **206**: 1191.
47. Kilcoyne I, Dechant JE, Kass PH, *et al.* Penetrating injuries to the frog and collateral sulci of the foot in equids: 63 cases. *J Am Vet Med Assoc* 2011; **239**: 1104.
48. Smith MRW. Penetrating injuries of the foot. *Equine Vet Educ* 2013; **25**: 422.
49. Steckel RR, Fessler JF, Huston LC. Deep puncture wounds of the equine hoof: a review of 50 cases. *Proc Am Assoc Equine Pract* 1989; **35**: 167.
50. Bras RJ, Morrison S. A retrospective case series of 20 horses (2002–2009) sustaining puncture wounds to the navicular bursa with maggot debridement as an adjunctive treatment. *Proc Am Assoc Equine Pract* 2009; **55**: 241.
51. Wright IM. Arthroscopy of the navicular bursa as an alternative to street nail procedures. In: *Proceedings of the 39th ACVS Veterinary Symposium* 2004: 80.
52. DeBowes RM, Yovich JV. Penetrating wounds, abscesses, gravel, and bruising of the equine foot. *Vet Clin N Am Equine Pract* 1989; **5**: 179.
53. Stashak T. Penetrating wounds of the foot. In: Stashak T (ed). *Adam's Lameness in Horses*, 5th edn. Lippincott William and Wilkins: Philadelphia, 2002: 703.
54. Spriet M, David F, Rossier Y. Ultrasonographic control of navicular bursa injection. *Equine Vet J* 2004; **36**: 637.
55. Moyer W, Schumacher J, Schumacher J. *A Guide to Equine Joint Injections and Regional Anesthesia*, 4th edn. Veterinary Learning Systems: Yardly, PA, 2007.
56. Vazquez de Mercado R, Stover SM, Taylor KT, *et al.* Lateral approach for arthrocentesis of the distal interphalangeal joint in horses. *J Am Vet Med Assoc* 1998; **212**: 1413.
57. Hassel DM, Stover SM, Yarbrough TB, *et al.* Palmar-plantar axial sesamoidean approach to the digital flexor tendon sheath in horses. *J Am Vet Med Assoc* 2000; **217**: 1343.
58. Rocconi R, Sampson SN. Comparison of basilar and axial sesamoidean approaches for digital flexor tendon sheath synoviocentesis and injection in horses. *J Am Vet Med Assoc* 2013; **243**: 869.
59. Wright IM, Phillips TJ, Walmsley JP. Endoscopy of the navicular bursa: a new technique for the treatment of contaminated and septic bursae. *Equine Vet J* 1999; **31**: 5.
60. Morrison S. How to utilize sterile maggot debridement therapy for foot infections of the horse. *Proc Am Assoc Equine Pract* 2005; **51**: 461.
61. Lepage O, Doumbia, A, Perron-Lepage MF, *et al.* The use of maggot debridement therapy in 41 equids. *Equine Vet J Suppl* 2012; **43**: 120.
62. Daeschlein G, Mumcuoglu KY, Assadian O, *et al.* *In vitro* antibacterial activity of *Lucilia sericata* maggot secretions. *Skin Pharmacol Physiol* 2007; **20**: 112.
63. Prete PE. Growth effects of *Phaenicia sericata* larval extracts on fibroblasts: mechanism for wound healing by maggot therapy. *Life Sci* 1997; **60**: 505.
64. Cazander G, van de Veerdonk M, Vandenbroucke-Grauls C, *et al.* Maggot excretions inhibit biofilm formation on biomaterials. *Clin Orthop Relat Res* 2010; **468**: 2789.
65. Jacobsen S, Thomsen MH, Nanni S. Concentrations of serum amyloid A in serum and synovial fluid from healthy horses and horses with joint disease. *J Am Vet Med Assoc* 2006; **67**: 1738.
66. Kelmer G, Tatz AJ, Famini S, *et al.* Evaluation of regional limb perfusion with chloramphenicol using the saphenous or cephalic vein in standing horses. *J Vet Pharmacol Ther* 2015; **38**: 35.
67. Baird AN, Seahorn, TL, Morris EL. Equine distal phalangeal sequestration. *Vet Radiol* 1990; **31**: 210.
68. Cauvin ER, Munroe G. Septic osteitis of the distal phalanx: findings and surgical treatment in 18 cases. *Equine Vet J* 1998; **30**: 512.
69. Linford S, Embertson R, Bramlage L. Septic osteitis of the third phalanx: a review of 63 cases. *Proc Am Assoc Equine Pract* 1994; **40**: 103.

CHAPTER 14

Degloving Injuries of the Distal Aspect of the Limb

R. Reid Hanson, DVM, Diplomate ACVS and ACVECC and Jim Schumacher, DVM, MS, Diplomate ACVS, MRCVS

Chapter Contents

Summary

Degloving injury of the distal portion of the limb exposes bone due to avulsion of overlying skin and subcutaneous tissue and is one of the most challenging types of wounds on the distal portion of the limb to manage. Dressings that supply moisture to the wound assist in autolytic debridement and may prevent formation of a bone sequestrum by preventing exposed bone from becoming desiccated. Formation of healthy granulation tissue in a wound is essential for healing, and various methods have been used to speed formation of granulation tissue over exposed bone. Wounds with exposed bone are covered with granulation tissue earlier when the cortex of the exposed bone is fenestrated because granulation tissue forms directly from the sites of fenestration. A skin graft applied to exposed bone does not survive because the graft fails to revascularize, but skin grafts can be applied successfully to wounds that are vascular enough to produce granulation tissue. The possibility that a bone sequestrum has developed when a degloving injury exposes underlying bone must not be overlooked since a different approach must be used to manage this type of wound.

Introduction

Degloving injuries of the distal portion of the limb are a type of avulsion in which an extensive section of skin is torn from the underlying tissue, severing blood supply to all or a large portion of the skin.[1] They are characterized by extensive crushing or avulsion of soft tissue, exposure of bone, vascular compromise, and severe contamination, making second-intention healing or skin grafting the only options likely to enable successful wound management. The regions most susceptible to degloving injury are the metacarpus and metatarsus because they contain little soft tissue and are exposed to trauma more often than are other regions of the horse's body.

The degloving injury that damages the periosteum heals with difficulty because loss of periosteum delays the formation of granulation tissue over the exposed bone, which in turn, causes the wound to contract in a tardy fashion.[2] The time required by bone devoid of periosteum to become covered with a healthy, uniform bed of granulation tissue is much longer than that required by bone covered by periosteum, thus prolonging the proliferative phase of repair.[3]

Equine Wound Management, Third Edition. Edited by Christine Theoret and Jim Schumacher.

Companion website: www.wiley.com/go/theoret/wound

Healing may be accompanied by proliferation of the new bone, or the superficial layers of the cortex may die from desiccation and ischemia and form a sequestrum, a common cause of delayed healing of wounds on the distal portion of the limb of horses.[4] Encouraging rapid coverage of exposed bone with granulation tissue decreases healing time and prevents exposed bone from becoming desiccated, which in turn, protects against the formation of a sequestrum.

This chapter reviews the healing of wounds on the distal aspect of the limb and complications related to degloving injuries that expose bone.

Healing of degloving injuries on the distal aspect of the limb

Second-intention healing

Wounds on the distal aspect of the limb expand for approximately 11–15 days after wounding as the result of distractive forces applied across the wound during the inflammatory and debridement stages of healing.[5,6] Distractive forces are countered by myofibroblasts formed when granulation tissue develops within the wound. The surface area of wounds healing by second intention is reduced by contraction, brought about by the myofibroblasts in the granulation tissue, and by epithelialization.[7,8] The quicker a granulation bed forms, therefore, the faster the wound begins to contract (Figure 14.1).

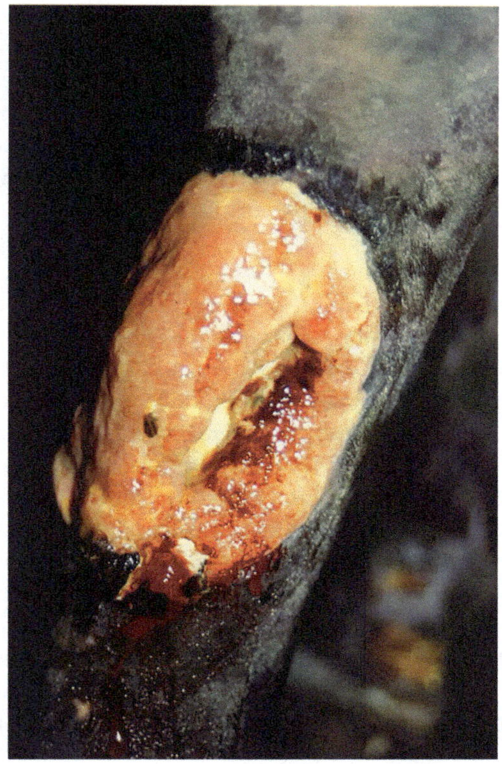

Figure 14.1 Cortical bone is exposed on the proximolateral surface of the third metatarsal bone and is visible in the depths of the wound in an area devoid of granulation tissue. Exposed bone is slow to be covered by granulation tissue, which in turn, impedes contraction.

Wounds on the distal aspect of the limb heal more slowly than those on the trunk because they have slower rates of epithelialization and contraction, and wounds on the distal aspect of the limb of horses heal more slowly than do wounds on the distal aspect of the limb of ponies because the latter contract more rapidly and to a greater extent than do the former.[8–10]

Comparison of histologic analyses of tissue samples from wounds of the distal portion of the limb of horses and of ponies shows that the inflammatory phase of healing is less intense and longer in the wounds of horses than in the wounds of ponies and that myofibroblasts within the wounds of horses are less organized than those within the wounds of ponies.[8,10] The higher concentration of transforming growth factor (TGF)-β in the wounded tissues of ponies may explain why the wounds of ponies have a more intense inflammatory response and contract to a greater degree than do the wounds of horses, because TGF-β induces fibroblasts in wounds to differentiate into contractile myofibroblasts.[11] The slower rate of epithelialization of wounds of the distal portion of the limb of horses, compared to that of similar wounds of ponies, has been attributed to inhibition of mitotic and migratory activity of keratinocytes by exuberant granulation tissue (EGT), which is much more likely to form in wounds of horses than in wounds of ponies (Figure 14.2).[10,12]

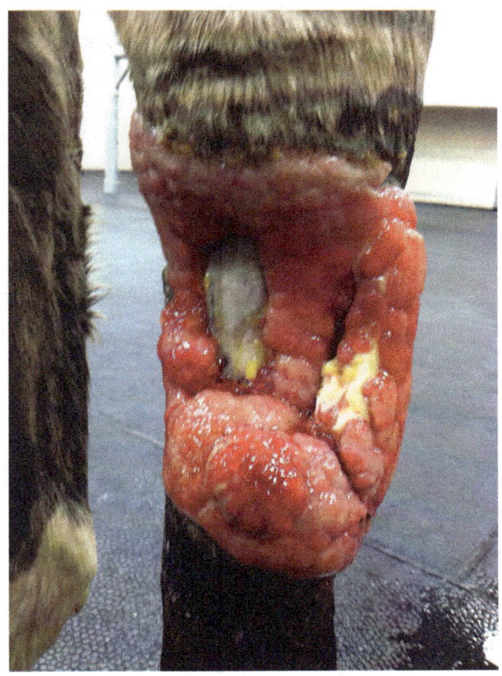

Figure 14.2 EGT in a wound located on the dorsal surface of the metatarsus. EGT decreases the rate of contraction and epithelialization by providing a physical barrier that impedes centripetal movement of the wound's margin and advancing epithelium.

Vascularity and granulation

The vascularity of a region directly influences its ability to produce granulation tissue.[4] Tissue with an abundant blood supply, such as muscle, can rapidly produce granulation tissue, whereas poorly vascularized tissue, such as bone, especially exposed bone, produces granulation tissue slowly, resulting in sluggish healing.[4] The total volume of a wound decreases rapidly as healthy granulation tissue develops.[8,13] When granulation tissue becomes exuberant, however, the wound may again expand as the wound edges are forced apart by the accumulation of new tissue.

Contraction

Contraction is the inward, or centripetal, movement of the wound's edge due to forces generated within the wound and is one of the major means whereby a wound heals by second intention. Fibroblasts and myofibroblasts are the major types of cells that contribute to contraction. Differentiation of fibroblasts into myofibroblasts is a complex process, regulated by at least one cytokine (i.e., TGF-β1) and a component of the extracellular matrix (the ED-A splice variant of cellular fibronectin). The myofibroblast is responsible for the remodeling of connective tissue during wound healing and fibrosis.[14] Reorganization of collagen by movement of fibroblasts causes the wound to contract by condensing or "piling up" the collagen into a smaller unit.[15,16] Peripheral skin, which is attached to the granulation tissue, is subsequently moved toward the center of the wound.

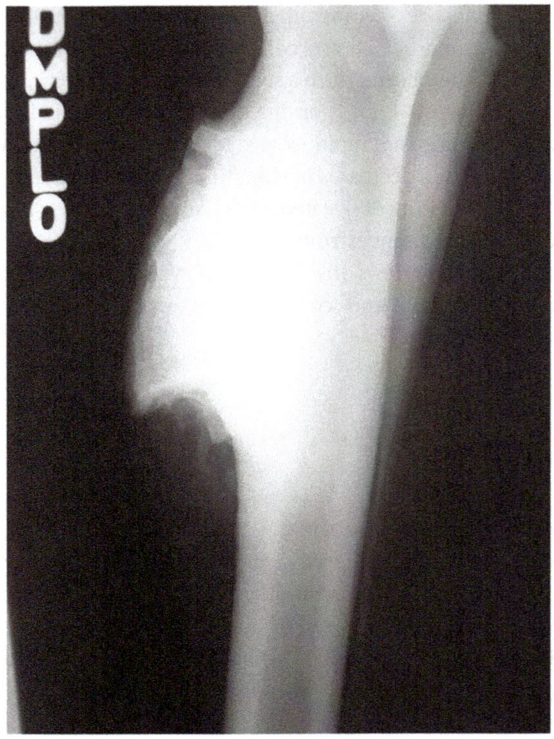

Figure 14.3 Injury to the periosteum may result in formation of new bone.

Healing of degloving injuries with exposed bone

Degloving injuries on the distal aspect of the limb that expose bone increase in size for 14–21 days. The presence of exposed bone delays healing by prolonging the inflammatory and repair phases of healing. Exposure of bone within a wound may delay healing directly, if the bone becomes infected, or indirectly, because the blood supply at its cortical surface is poor, impeding the formation of granulation tissue and contraction of the wound (Figures 14.1, 14.2). Indeed, healthy granulation tissue in the center of the wound is required to counteract the tensile forces exerted on the wound's margin by the surrounding skin during the inflammatory phase of healing.[7,12] Finally, exposed cortical bone is subject to desiccation of its superficial layers, which may result in superficial infectious osteitis and formation of a sequestrum.[2]

Periosteum

Periosteum is a well-vascularized osteogenic organ possessing two distinct layers, each of which contribute to wound repair. The outer fibrous layer contains fibroblasts, blood vessels, and fibers of Sharpey, and the inner cambium layer contains nerves, capillaries, osteoblasts, and mesenchymal stem cells (MSCs).[17] Periosteal vessels from the fibrous layer contribute to bone healing by nourishing the outer third of the diaphysis and by supplementing the epiphysio-metaphyseal vessels and the principal nutrient arteries found within the medullary cavity.[18] The cambium layer serves as a reservoir of undifferentiated pluripotent MSCs[19] and as a source of growth factors that play important roles in the healing and remodeling of the outer surface of damaged cortical bone.

Studies have shown that injured periosteum can regenerate cartilage and bone from its progenitor cells;[17,20] in horses, MSCs from the cambium layer were shown to differentiate directly into osteoblasts or into neochondrocytes that produce cartilage, later replaced by bone.[21]

A localized outgrowth of new bone beneath the periosteum, or an exostosis, results from the rapid formation of new or reactive bone, which is produced after progenitors of osteoblasts in the cambium layer are activated by avulsion, laceration, or blunt trauma.[22] Depending on its size and the inciting cause, an exostosis may persist or gradually be removed by remodeling.[23] Bone exposed in a wound on the distal portion of the limb (Figure 14.3) can develop an extensive amount of periosteal new bone, which can cause the wound to enlarge, and may result in an enlarged limb, even after the wound has healed.[8]

Formation of bone sequestra

A bone sequestrum may develop as a sequel to a degloving injury that exposes bone and injures the periosteum and is a common cause of delayed healing of wounds on the distal aspect of the limbs of horses.[2] A sequestrum can result from any insult that interrupts the blood supply to bone. Afferent vessels from the periosteum and medullary cavity provide capillaries that traverse the Haversian canals, which are connected by Volkmann canals, to provide blood to the compact portion of long bones. Outflow, or efferent flow, occurs at the periosteum and endosteum, so periosteal trauma can lead to local vascular stasis by reducing venous outflow.[4] The blood supply to the cortex of equine long bones is sensitive to trauma because the dense mineralized matrix of the cortex prevents rapid collateralization of vessels after injury.[24] Ischemia of the superficial layers of the cortex leads to necrosis of the affected area, and the necrotic bone incites an inflammatory response resulting in accumulation of exudate, which can lead to the formation of a draining tract in a wound that has otherwise healed.[3]

Periosteum may be avulsed from the bone at the time of injury, or infection or desiccation may cause the periosteum to separate from the bone.[25,26] Loss of periosteal blood supply leaves the bone dependent on endosteal vessels traversing the cortex, resulting in ischemic necrosis of the superficial portion of the cortex.[26,27] Superficial layers of cortical bone devoid of periosteum and exposed to the environment may become desiccated, compounding the effects of ischemia. Small areas of dead bone may be revascularized by microvessels in granulation tissue advancing superficial to the dead bone, or the bone may be revascularized by endosteal vessels of cortical bone deep to the dead bone.[28] Avascular cortical bone too thick to revascularize becomes sequestered by granulation tissue produced from viable bone. The body's attempts to extrude or absorb the dead bone result in a persistent sinus tract and excessive production of exudate. Ischemia caused by loss of periosteal blood supply alone, however, may not be sufficient to provoke formation of a sequestrum;[26] bacterial infection of the bone seems to be necessary as well, and ischemia of the bone induced by loss of the periosteum provides an ideal environment for colonization and multiplication of bacteria introduced into the wound from the injury. A sequestrum can delay healing by serving as a focus of continued inflammation and infection, thereby postponing the ensuing phases of repair.

Because the periosteum of young horses plays a greater role in cortical circulation, young horses may be more likely to form a sequestrum than are mature horses.[2,29] Moreover, mature horses are more likely than mature ponies to develop a sequestrum, perhaps because they are more likely to develop infection at the wound, a result of an inefficient inflammatory response and a reduced rate of formation of granulation tissue, and may have a slower onset and longer duration of the periosteal reaction.[8,30] In a retrospective study of 89 ponies and 422 horses with accidental wounds that had been sutured, ponies were found to have suffered less dehiscence and formed fewer sequestra than horses, even though conditions for first-intention healing of the ponies were less favorable (i.e., wounds were more severe, surgical debridement was less thorough, and systemic antibiotic therapy was administered less commonly).[30]

Radiographically, a sequestrum appears as a sclerotic segment of bone surrounded by a radiolucent zone of osteolysis (Figure 14.4).[26,27] The sequestrum and zone of osteolysis are surrounded by an envelope of sclerotic bone, termed an involucrum. The opening in the involucrum, through which exudate drains, is termed a cloaca. Extensive periosteal reaction is frequently observed on adjacent, normal bone. A triangular area of new bone that develops adjacent to the cortex from elevation of the periosteum ("Codman triangle") is sometimes observed at the proximal and distal extents of the involucrum.[26] The bone sequestrum contains no new periosteal bone, which aids in its identification.

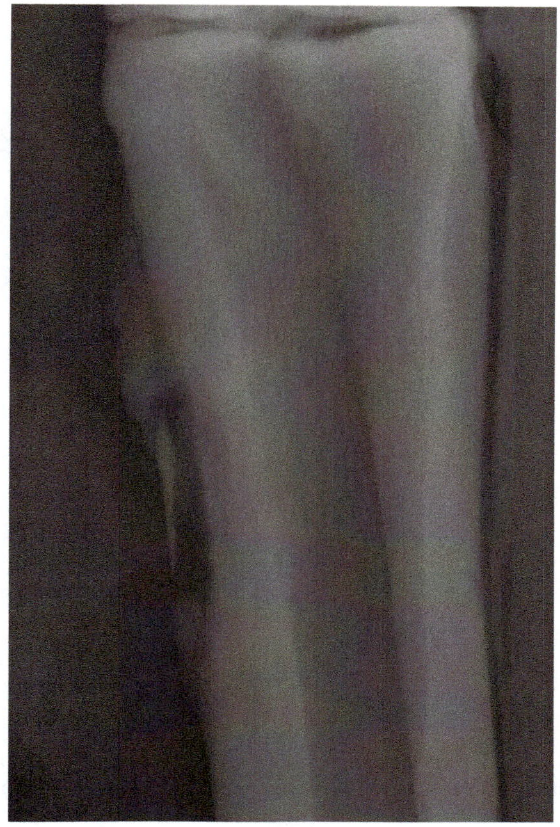

Figure 14.4 A sequestrum is seen radiographically as a sclerotic segment of bone surrounded by a radiolucent zone of osteolysis.

Exposed bone beneath a fresh wound should be examined radiographically about 10–14 days after injury to determine if a bone sequestrum is developing. Radiographic signs of a sequestrum cannot be detected for at least 7 days after injury but are usually evident within several weeks of injury (Figure 14.4).[26,27] An early radiographic sign that a sequestrum is forming, often seen 10–12 days after injury, is the presence of one or more radiolucent lines within the outer third of the cortex.[26,27] During subsequent radiographic examination, these fine radiolucent lines may be seen to have enlarged and coalesced into one radiolucent band separating viable and non-viable bone.[26] These early radiographic signs of formation of a sequestration sometimes vanish, and the sequestrum fails to form.

Methods used to stimulate the production of granulation tissue to cover exposed bone

Large degloving injuries with exposed bone must granulate to heal. Without granulation tissue to cover the exposed bone, the wound cannot contract, epithelium cannot migrate, and a free skin graft cannot be accepted. Therefore, formation of

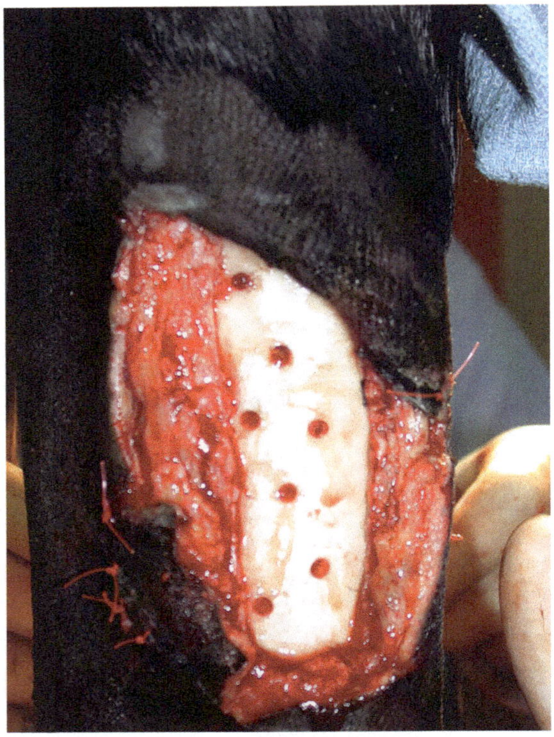

Figure 14.5 Cortical fenestration of the dorsal surface of the third metatarsal bone in a diamond-shape pattern produced using a 3.2-mm drill. The cortical fenestration allows granulation tissue to form rapidly over the associated exposed bone.

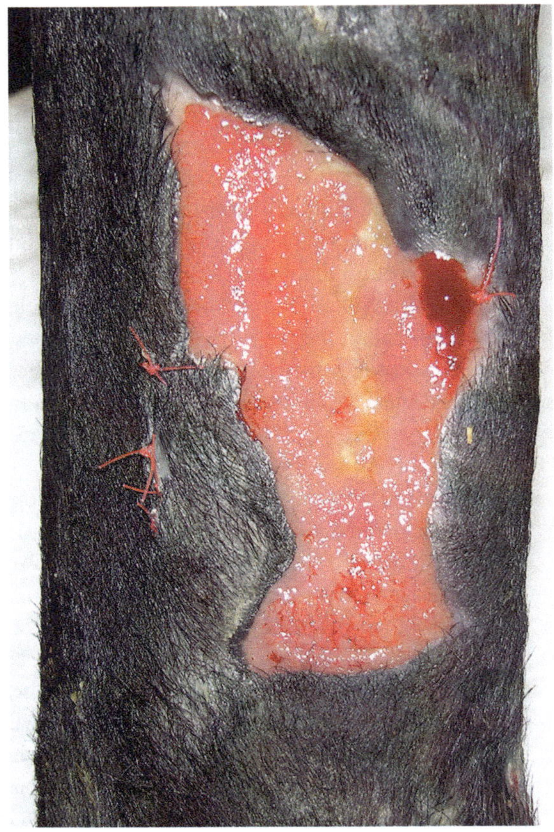

Figure 14.6 Same wound as in Figure 14.5. Granulation tissue has formed at the sites of cortical fenestration in a 14-day-old degloving injury to the dorsal surface of the metacarpus. Fenestrating the cortex of wounds with more than 36 cm^2 of exposed bone speeds formation of granulation tissue within the wound.

granulation tissue in the wound should be encouraged, at least initially. Granulation tissue plays an important role in second-intention healing by shielding underlying tissues from infection and trauma and by providing a moist surface for epithelialization. The delay in healing that occurs when bone is exposed has prompted searches for effective methods to promote coverage of exposed bone with granulation tissue, in people and in companion animals. Even though trauma to the distal aspect of the limb of horses is frequently associated with the presence of exposed bone, methods of stimulating coverage of exposed bone of horses have been poorly investigated. Exposed bone of horses, humans, and dogs has been fenestrated, curetted, or abraded with a file to promote formation of granulation tissue to enhance second-intention healing or to provide a vascular bed for skin grafting.[7,31,32]

Trauma, thermal injury, or oncologic surgery of the head of people often results in exposed bone of the cranium.[31,32] In these cases, to hasten coverage of exposed bone with granulation tissue, the outer cortex of the exposed portion of the cranium is often fenestrated with a drill, burr, or laser to expose the medullary cavity from which granulation tissue can emerge.[31,32] Likewise, the exposed cortex of long bones of people has been fenestrated with a drill to promote formation of granulation tissue.[31] The fenestrations may promote healing by allowing osteogenic factors from the medullary cavity access to the wound, or the fenestrations may enhance healing of bone and soft tissues by a non-specific response known as "the regional acceleratory phenomenon," whereby the rate of remodeling in the region of a bony defect exceeds normal.[33] Cortical fenestration (Figure 14.5), especially when combined with hydrogel dressings to provide moisture to the wound, may accelerate coverage of exposed bone of horses with granulation tissue.[7]

In one study, drilling 1.6-mm diameter holes through the cortex of the exposed second metacarpal bone in experimentally created wounds of dogs produced a greater amount of blood clot than did curetting the bone. Drilling the second metacarpal bone resulted in clots that protected the exposed bone from desiccation, and the early ingrowth of fibroblasts and capillaries from the surface of the bone and surrounding tissue into the clot sped formation of granulation tissue.[34]

Exposed bone in experimentally created wounds on the distal aspect of the limb of horses became covered with granulation tissue earlier after undergoing cortical fenestration with a 3.2-mm drill bit than did exposed bone in control wounds that did not undergo cortical fenestration because granulation tissue formed at the sites of cortical fenestration (Figure 14.6).[7] When the area of exposed bone was small (i.e., less than 6 × 6 cm), the contribution of the granulation tissue growing directly from the sites of cortical fenestration to overall coverage of the wound was not significant.[7] Cortical fenestration of exposed bone in wounds may be even more beneficial if fenestration is combined with other methods of promoting formation of granulation tissue.[7]

Autologous platelet-rich plasma (PRP) has been used with increasing frequency to treat horses for a variety of soft-tissue and bony defects. Application of PRP gel to experimentally created wounds of horses accelerated the formation of granulation tissue and epithelial differentiation and formation of dermal collagen that was better organized than that found in similar wounds not treated with PRP.[35] However, a different study found that topical application of autologous PRP to small granulating wounds on the limbs of horses did not accelerate healing, improve the quality of repair, or prevent the development of EGT.[36] The authors of this study suggested that treatment with PRP may be better suited for wounds characterized by massive loss of tissue or chronic wounds in need of a fresh source of mediators to accelerate healing.[36] The reader is referred to Chapter 22 for more information about the use of PRP for wound healing.

> **Tip**
>
> - Horses with a large or chronic wound may benefit from application of autologous PRP to the wound.

Management of degloving injuries

Wound evaluation and preparation

Using aseptic techniques to cleanse and bandage a wound containing exposed bone is important because exposed bone is susceptible to infection. In one study, the concentration of *S. aureus* adhered to the periosteum of equine bone was less than that adhered to cortical bone, cut cortical bone, and the endosteal surface of bone, indicating the necessity for meticulous cleansing of wounds with exposed and damaged bone.[37]

The hair of the skin surrounding the wound should be clipped, and the wound should be irrigated with sterile isotonic saline solution to which an antiseptic (e.g., 0.05% chlorhexidine or 0.1–0.2% povidone–iodine) has been added, using irrigation pressures between 8 and 15 psi.[12] After it is irrigated, the wound should be explored digitally, after donning sterile gloves, to establish the extent of injury and the degree of periosteal damage. Adjacent synovial structures, tendons, and ligaments should be evaluated carefully to determine if they are involved in the injury. The wound should also be examined carefully for the presence of bony fragments or foreign bodies. For a more in-depth discussion of wound preparation, see Chapter 4.

Distortion of bone underlying a wound suggests that the bone has been fractured, and horses with an open fracture of the distal aspect of the limb have a poor or guarded prognosis for survival. In these cases, radiographic examination of the injured region is indicated to assess osseous damage. The limb need only be bandaged if no fracture is observed, but a splint should be incorporated into the bandage when there is the possibility that a tendon has been lacerated or a synovial structure invaded. For more information regarding splinting, see Chapter 7.

Surgical management

Surgical debridement remains the technique of choice for removing devitalized tissues and tissues heavily contaminated by dirt and bacteria. Small, relatively clean wounds may be debrided with the horse standing after desensitizing the wound using local or, preferably, regional anesthesia. Large, heavily contaminated/infected wounds are often best debrided with the horse anesthetized. The wound is sharply debrided until only apparently healthy tissue remains (Figure 14.7). See Chapters 4 and 8 for more information regarding preparation of a wound to reduce the likelihood of infection.

If a flap of skin remains attached to a wound in which bone is exposed, the flap, or at least a portion it, can often be apposed to surrounding skin, using monofilament suture, to cover all or a portion of the exposed bone.[12] That portion of the wound that cannot be covered by the skin flap is allowed to heal by second intention. Because the loss of periosteum may cause ischemia of the outer third of the cortex, superficial ostectomy to remove ischemic bone, performed at the time of wound debridement, may prevent a sequestrum from forming or at least minimize its extent. A shallow portion of exposed bone can be excised with an osteotome,[38] a bone rasp, or an air drill until punctate hemorrhage or a yellow, serum-like fluid begins to exude from the cortex. Hemorrhage exudes if the horse's bone is immature, and serum-like fluid exudes if the horse's bone is mature. Granulation tissue grows directly from viable, exposed bone; therefore, exposing fresh, bleeding bone speeds proliferation of granulation tissue from the bone.[39] If the uncovered area of bone is larger than 36 cm^2, fenestrating its cortex, using a 3.2-mm drill bit, to facilitate the formation of granulation tissue may be useful.[7] Drilling small holes in exposed bone promotes healing by allowing osteogenic factors from the medullary cavity access to the wound.[40] The holes should be placed in a diamond-shaped pattern, so that they are equidistant from each other, and should be separated from one another by 12–15 mm to avoid substantially weakening the bone.[7] The cortex can be rasped in areas where drilling the full thickness of the cortex is contraindicated, such as in wounds where hairline fractures of the cortical bone are observed.

Because bacterial infection of the bone contributes to the formation of a sequestrum, efforts should be made to prevent exposed bone from becoming infected.[25,41] To prevent septic osteitis, the horse should receive parenteral, broad-spectrum, antimicrobial therapy soon after injury. Regional limb perfusion with an antimicrobial drug, used alone or in conjunction with systemic administration of an antimicrobial drug, may be indicated. A hydrogel dressing should be applied to the exposed bone to prevent desiccation, and the wounded portion of the

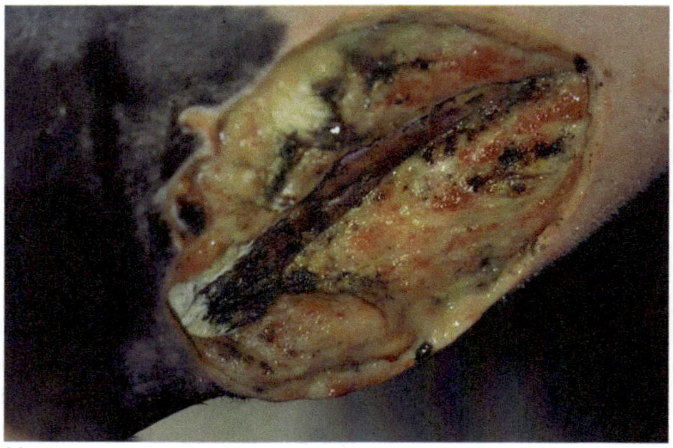

(a)

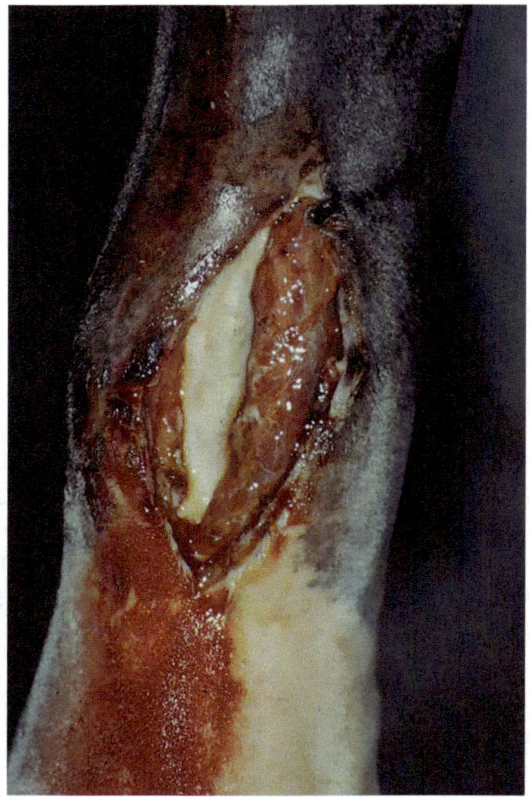

(b)

Figure 14.7 (**a**) Contaminated degloving wound with exposed bone on the distolateral surface of the metatarsus. Dry, necrotic tissue and debris are present within the wound. (**b**) Wound after surgical debridement, which is the technique of choice for removing devitalized tissues. Proper debridement removes tissues heavily contaminated with dirt and bacteria. The wound was sharply debrided until only healthy tissue remained.

limb should be bandaged to protect it from contamination and to absorb exudate. Non-steroidal anti-inflammatory drugs (NSAIDs) have been reported to have an adverse effect on the incidence of infection by negatively affecting migration of leukocytes, so they should be used only when indicated to relieve swelling and pain.[42,43]

Removing the sequestrum is the most effective treatment, but occasionally a sequestrum is shed spontaneously (Figure 14.8), and, rarely, a small sequestrum may be resorbed. Resorption of the sequestrum is hampered because osteoclasts are unable to migrate to the avascular sequestrum. The horse may respond initially to parenterally administered antimicrobial therapy with a decrease in swelling and discharge of exudate from the wound,[2] but treating an affected horse with antimicrobial therapy alone is ineffective because the lack of blood supply to the sequestrum isolates bacteria harbored by the sequestrum from antimicrobial drugs. Culture of exudate from the draining sinus, or even from around the sequestrum, is unlikely to be helpful in determining the organism(s) involved in formation of a sequestrum because secondary pathogens rapidly colonize an open wound or sinus.

Often, a sequestrum can be removed easily with the horse standing, provided that at least one edge of the sequestrum is not covered with granulation tissue (Figure 14.9). A sequestrum covered by tissue or embedded within the marrow cavity

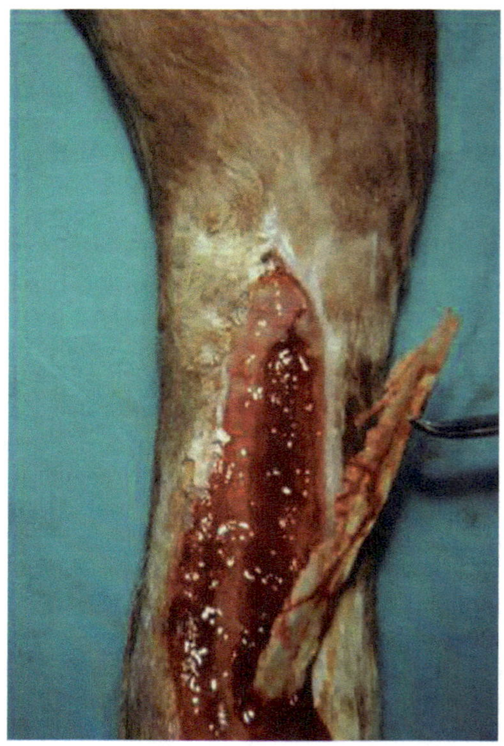

Figure 14.8 This figure illustrates extrusion of a bone sequestrum from a granulating wound.

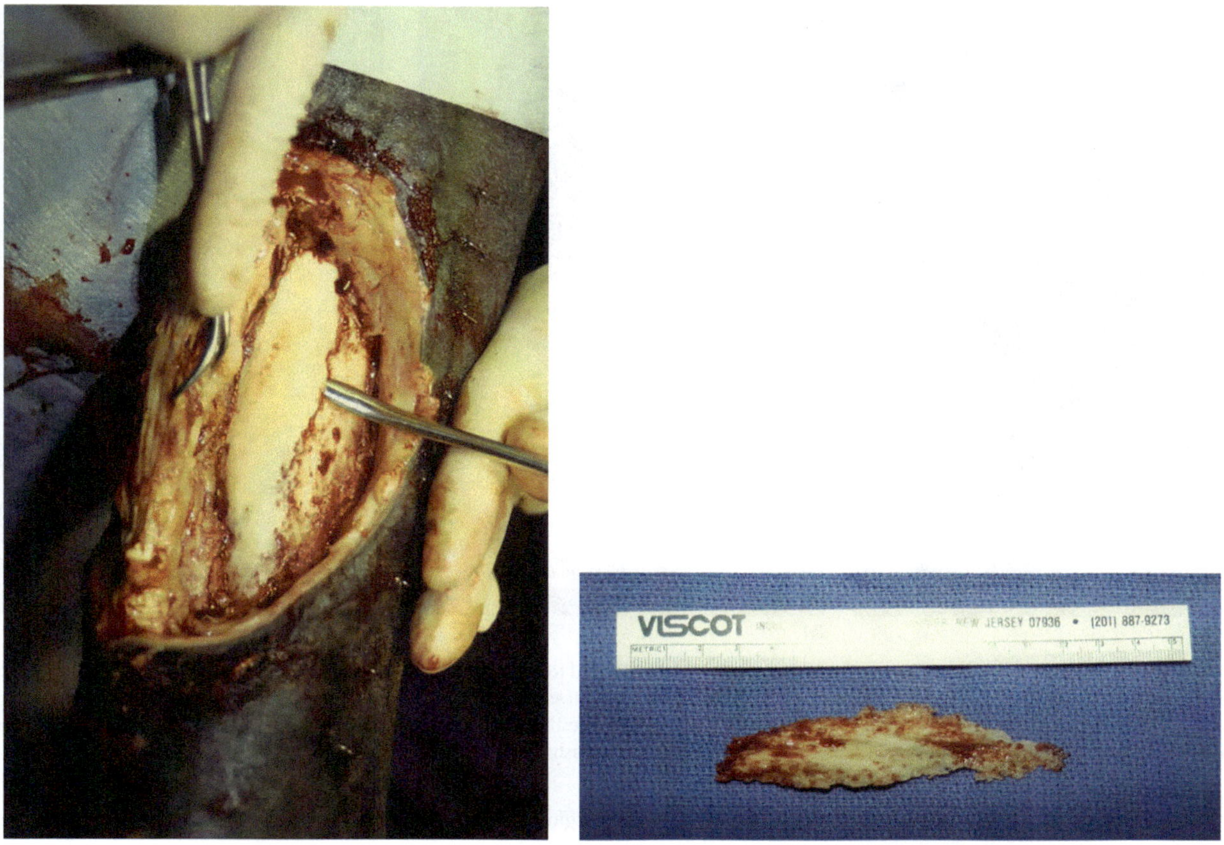

(a) (b)

Figure 14.9 **(a)** The sequestrum was removed with the horse standing, after sedation and desensitizing the surgical site with local anesthetic solution. A periosteal elevator was used to elevate the sequestrum from its involucrum. **(b)** Excised bone sequestrum.

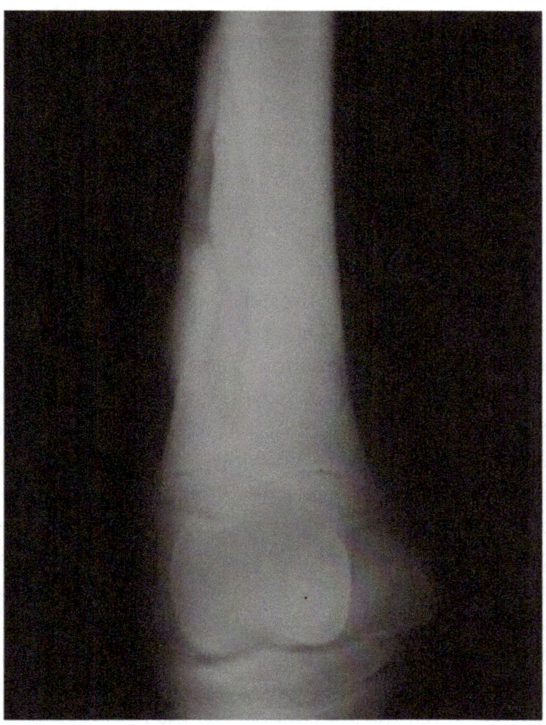

Figure 14.10 Radiograph identifying a large sequestrum embedded in bone.

is best removed with the horse anesthetized (Figure 14.10). The sequestrum should be removed as soon as its separation from viable bone becomes radiographically apparent. A large sequestrum embedded within the marrow cavity may have to be divided to remove it through the cloaca (Figure 14.11). In these cases, a cast should be applied to the limb prior to recovering the horse from anesthesia to reduce stress concentration at the cloaca, thereby decreasing the risk of a complete fracture.

Primary closure of the wound may be possible if the wound from which the sequestrum was removed is small,[29] but if a large amount of soft tissue was avulsed, the wound must heal by second intention or by skin grafting. Broad-spectrum, perioperative antimicrobial treatment should be administered before surgery if primary closure is planned. At surgery, the sequestrum is removed, and the membrane lining the involucrum is excised by curettage. Curettage is continued until punctate hemorrhage or serum-like fluid from the underlying cortical bone is observed. The curetted involucrum is irrigated with a dilute antiseptic solution, after which new sterile gloves are donned, and a new set of sterile instruments is used to close the wound. Proliferative bone, if present, can be removed prior to closing the wound (Figure 14.12).

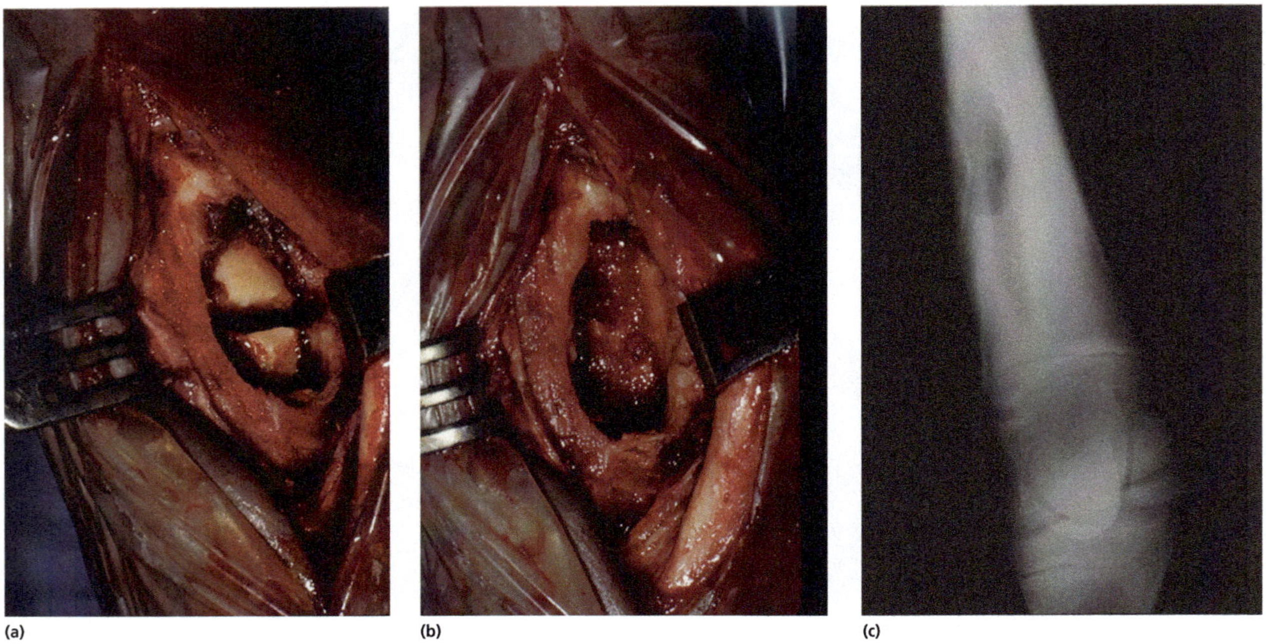

Figure 14.11 Same horse as in Figure 14.10. (**a**) The large sequestrum was divided to remove it through the cloaca. (**b**) View through the cloaca of the involucrum prior to debridement of its lining of granulation tissue. (**c**) Postoperative radiograph documents removal of the sequestrum seen in Figure 14.10. A limb cast should be applied prior to recovering the horse from anesthesia to reduce stress concentration at the cloaca, thereby decreasing the risk of a complete fracture of the third metacarpal bone. Courtesy of Dr. T. Stashak.

Tips

- An effort should be made to prevent exposed bone from becoming infected because bacterial infection of the bone contributes to the formation of a sequestrum.
- Removing the ischemic, outer portion of an exposed segment of bone with a bone rasp or an osteotome may prevent a sequestrum from forming.
- Horses are more likely than ponies to develop a bone sequestrum.
- A sequestrum is most easily identified radiographically about 14 days or more after the bone has been exposed.

What to do

- Wounds containing an area of exposed bone larger than 36 cm^2 may granulate more quickly if the full-thickness of the exposed cortex is fenestrated by using a 3.2-mm drill bit.
- Fenestrate the exposed cortex, using a diamond pattern. The holes should be separated from each other by 12–15 mm to avoid substantially weakening the bone.
- Cortical fenestration does not speed coverage of exposed bone by granulation tissue when the area of exposed bone is smaller than 36 cm^2.

Antimicrobial therapy

A broad-spectrum antimicrobial drug should be administered systemically or by intravenous regional perfusion of the limb if the degloving injury is severely contaminated, if a synovial cavity has been penetrated, or if bone is exposed (Figure 14.13). Treating a horse for infection of a synovial structure by systemic administration of an antimicrobial drug is usually insufficient to resolve infection.

One study evaluating the concentration and pharmacokinetics of amikacin in synovial fluid after intraosseous or intravenous regional limb perfusion found that each technique of administering amikacin produced mean peak concentrations of amikacin in the tarsocrural joint ranging from 5–50 times that of peak serum concentrations required for therapeutic efficacy.[44] A NSAID may be administered to the wounded horse, but administration should be judicious because administrating a NSAID during the inflammatory phase of healing may inhibit healing. The use of a NSAID may be justified, however, for humane reasons and to promote weight-bearing on the wounded limb to decrease the risk of laminitis developing on the supporting limb. The reader is referred to Chapter 4 for more information about administering NSAIDs to wounded horses.

Antibiotic-impregnated beads of polymethylmethacrylate (PMMA) or plaster of Paris (POP) have been used to deliver a high concentration of one or more antimicrobial drugs locally (see Figure 19.8). Approximately 80% of gentamicin was released from POP beads during the first 48 hours in an *in vitro* model, whereas 63% of gentamicin and 79% of metronidazole were released from PMMA during the first 24 hours in the same *in vitro* model.[45,46] Elution of the antibiotic was directly related to the amount of antibiotic incorporated into the PMMA or POP beads. Gentamicin-impregnated POP beads inhibited the growth of *E. coli in vitro* during the 14-day period of the study. Gentamicin- and metronidazole-impregnated PMMA beads, sterilized by ethylene oxide and stored at room temperature, retained their bactericidal activity for up to 2 months, and stored gentamicin-impregnated POP beads retained their bactericidal activity for up to 5 months. For more information about the preparation and use of antibiotic beads, see Chapter 19.

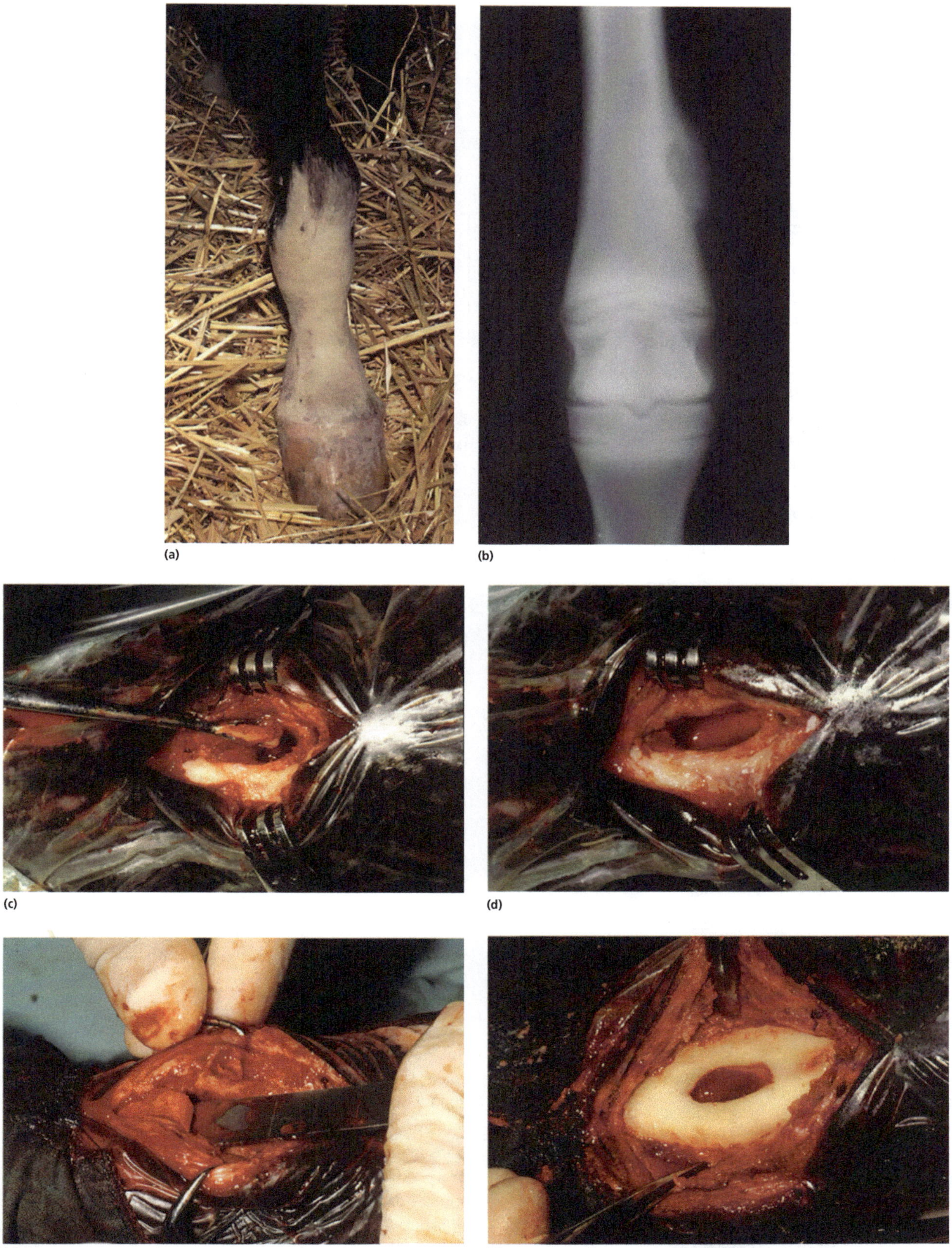

Figure 14.12 (**a**) Swelling on the lateral distal third of the left metacarpus in a yearling. Exudate drained from a tract located in the center of the swelling. (**b**) Radiographic evidence of a sequestrum. (**c**) The sequestrum was removed at surgery. (**d**) After sequestrectomy and curettage of the granulation tissue lining the involucrum, the wound was irrigated with a dilute antiseptic solution. Gloves and instruments were discarded and new ones were used to extend the incision in the skin overlying the proliferative bone. (**e**) Proliferative bone being removed with an osteotome. (**f**) Proliferative bone removed. Sharp periostectomy over the proliferative bone was performed with a #15 Bard Parker scalpel blade, after which a drain was inserted and the wound sutured. A pressure bandage was applied. The drain was removed 24 hours later. Courtesy of Dr. T. Stashak.

Antimicrobial therapy, whether administered systemically, by regional limb perfusion, or by implanting antibiotic beads, may be effective in the short-term management of wounds, but it should not be used as a substitute for thorough and meticulous debridement. For more information regarding the treatment of horses with a wound involving a synovial structure, see Chapter 16, and for more information regarding treatment of horses with an infected wound, see Chapter 19.

Wound dressings and topical agents used to promote healing

Until granulation tissue has begun to form, the wound should be covered with a hydrogel dressing to prevent it from becoming desiccated. Hydrogels are a three-dimensional network of hydrophilic polymers, the water content of which is 90–95%, made from gelatin or a polysaccharide cross-linked with a polymer. Hydrogel dressings are available as sheets or gels. The reader is referred to Table 6.2 for a selection of commercially available hydrogel dressings. These dressings have a soothing and cooling effect, protect the wound from contamination, assist in autolytic debridement, dissolve eschar and necrotic tissue by donating fluid to the wound, and reduce swelling.[47,48] These properties of hydrogel dressings encourage early formation of healthy granulation tissue. A hydrogel dressing should not be applied to the wound if the wound is infected or heavily exudative, or if the skin surrounding the wound is macerated because the dressings do not have a large absorptive capacity.[47] Hydrogels are indicated for treatment of clean, fresh wounds during the inflammatory phase of wound healing. They are particularly suited for dry or necrotic wounds and for fresh, painful wounds.

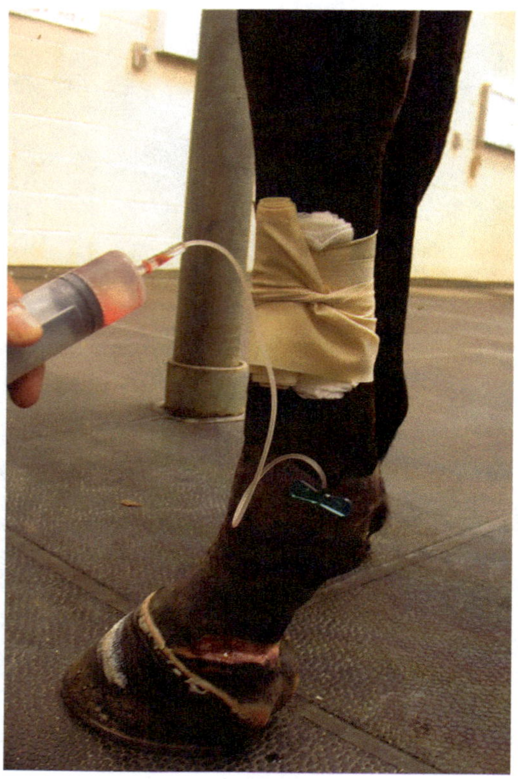

Figure 14.13 Intravenous regional limb perfusion of the left forelimb. Intravenous regional limb perfusion can provide concentrations of antibiotic 5–50 times the peak serum concentrations recommended for therapeutic efficacy.

Tips

- Apply a hydrogel dressing to a relatively clean wound to enhance autolytic debridement and to rehydrate dehydrated tissue.
- A hydrogel should not be applied to an infected wound, a heavily exudative wound, or a wound in which the surrounding skin is macerated.

Management of wound contamination in degloving injuries

Dressings

Dressings effective at debridement and reducing the concentration of bacteria in a wound can be used to accelerate the transition of a wound from heavily contaminated to clean. A fine-threaded and wide-meshed, woven, cotton gauze dressing or an antiseptic gauze dressing (the reader is referred to Table 6.4 for a selection of commercially available antimicrobial dressings) is most commonly applied, in a wet-to-dry fashion, when fluid in the wound has a high viscosity or when the wound's surface is dehydrated and scabs have formed. Dressings effective in debridement are also excellent for packing deeply contaminated wounds associated with the body or the proximal aspect of a limb. As the dressing dries, it adheres, by fibrin, to debris on the wound's surface. Removing the dressing, especially when it is completely dry, can cause pain to the horse; moreover, healthy tissue and cells, such as epithelial cells and fibroblasts, can be removed because this mode of debridement is non-selective. To prevent pain, the dressing can be moistened to encourage it to detach from the tissues to which it is adhered. Usually one to three applications of a wet-to-dry dressing, during the inflammatory phase of healing, are all that is needed to effectively debride most wounds.

Alginate dressings (the reader is referred to Table 6.2 for a selection of commercially available alginate dressings) are useful for dressing wounds characterized by substantial loss of tissue, such as degloving injuries. Alginate dressings can absorb 20–30 times their weight in fluid, so are useful for dressing moderately to heavily exudative wounds, as the wound transitions from the debridement/inflammatory phase to the repair/proliferative phase of healing.[49] Alginate dressings should be applied only to heavily exudative wounds because they require moisture to function properly.[49] They are not indicated for dressing dry wounds with sloughing or hard necrotic tissue. See Chapter 6 for more information regarding wound dressings. Interestingly, a study in human patients with a soft-tissue defect exposing bone showed that alginate dressings resulted in good coverage of bone with high-quality granulation tissue.[50]

Tip

- Alginate dressings can absorb 20–30 times their weight in fluid and are useful for moderately to heavily exudative wounds.

What to do

- Do not apply alginate dressings to non-exudative wounds.

Antimicrobial agents

In later stages of healing, when granulation tissue has formed within the wound, topical application of an antimicrobial agent is likely to be more effective than systemic administration of an antibiotic.[51] For wounds colonized with bacteria that can counter healing, and especially those in which bacteria have formed a biofilm, the use of an antimicrobial dressing is warranted.[52] If the wound is exudative, an antiseptic, such as povidone–iodine ointment, or an antibiotic, such as silver sulfadiazine, may be applied to the wound. Although nitrofurazone ointment is effective against Gram-positive and Gram-negative organisms, it has little effect against *Pseudomonas* spp., and, moreover, it has been shown to decrease the rate of epithelialization of clean wounds in pigs.[53] The authors, therefore, do not advocate its use in the management of wounds in horses. Silver sulfadiazine has a wide antimicrobial spectrum that includes *Pseudomonas* spp. and fungi.[54] Organisms resistant to silver are rarely encountered, suggesting that genes that impart resistance to silver are difficult to transfer and to be maintained by other bacteria.[55] The reader is referred to Chapters 5 and 6 for more information regarding topical wound-care products and wound dressings.

Honey reduces inflammation, debrides necrotic tissue, reduces edema, maintains a moist environment, and promotes angiogenesis, formation of granulation tissue, and epithelialization by stimulating the release of anti-inflammatory agents and growth factors from monocytes.[56–58] Whether honey affects other cell types, particularly endothelial cells and fibroblasts, involved in wound healing is not known. Honey can be incorporated into a sterile hydrogel dressing to make its application to wounds easier.[59] For more information on honey dressings, the reader is referred to Chapters 6 and 22.

Gentamicin sulfate has a narrow antimicrobial spectrum but is effective in eliminating infection when applied to wounds populated with Gram-negative bacteria, such as *Pseudomonas aeruginosa*. However, a 0.1% solution of gentamicin, in an oil-in-water cream base, applied to wounds on dogs, was shown to slow epithelialization and contraction.[60] Cefazolin is an effective antimicrobial against Gram-positive and some Gram-negative organisms that can be applied topically to treat wound infections.[60] The powder form of cefazolin provides an appropriate concentration of the antibiotic at the wound for a longer period than does the solution.[60] For more information regarding topical wound-care products and wound dressings, see Chapters 5 and 6.

Tip

- To facilitate the application of honey to a wound, the honey can be incorporated into a sterile hydrogel dressing.

What to do

- Neither povidone–iodine ointment nor an antibiotic ointment should be applied to a wound concurrently with honey, sugar, a silver-coated dressing, or an antimicrobial gauze dressing, because the polyethylene glycol base present in these ointments may interfere with the efficacy of the products.[53]

General care

A NSAID may be administered once or twice daily, for its analgesic effect, to a horse that has recently incurred a degloving injury, but administration should be discontinued as soon as possible to avoid dampening the inflammatory response, which is important for healing. Alternate-day bandage changes, using a hydrogel dressing, are continued until the wound is covered by healthy granulation tissue. If the wound is highly exudative or heavily contaminated, an alginate dressing is applied, and the bandage changed daily for as long as the wound is exudative. After granulation tissue has formed, a non-adherent, semi-occlusive foam dressing can be applied. This dressing absorbs exudate and keeps the wound's surface moist, thereby promoting epithelial migration. Protecting the wound from contamination with a bandage can be dispensed with if bandaging becomes financially difficult for the owner, provided that the horse is housed in a clean environment. Indeed, a healthy bed of granulation tissue provides resistance to infection and can be trimmed periodically, if need be, to allow unimpeded epithelialization (Figure 14.14).

Immobilization of the wound

Bandaging

Bandages applied to the distal aspect of the limb of horses are usually composed of a primary, a secondary, and a tertiary layer. The primary layer, or dressing, should be selected according to the condition of the wound and its phase of repair. The dressing is normally secured to the wound with conforming gauze, which is applied circumferentially around the limb. The secondary layer, which pads the wound, is frequently composed of cast padding or rolled cotton. The tertiary layer functions to hold the primary and secondary layers in place, provides pressure, and keeps the inner layers protected from the environment. This layer is usually composed of adhesive or self-adhesive elastic tape. The tertiary layer should be porous to air, yet waterproof. The tertiary layer is applied in a distal-to-proximal direction, with constant pressure applied during each revolution of the tape around the limb. The most proximal and distal extents of the secondary layer (i.e., cotton pad) are not covered by the tertiary layer, to avoid creating pressure points that may affect circulation to the skin at these sites. As a final step, the proximal and distal ends of the bandage are covered with adhesive, elastic

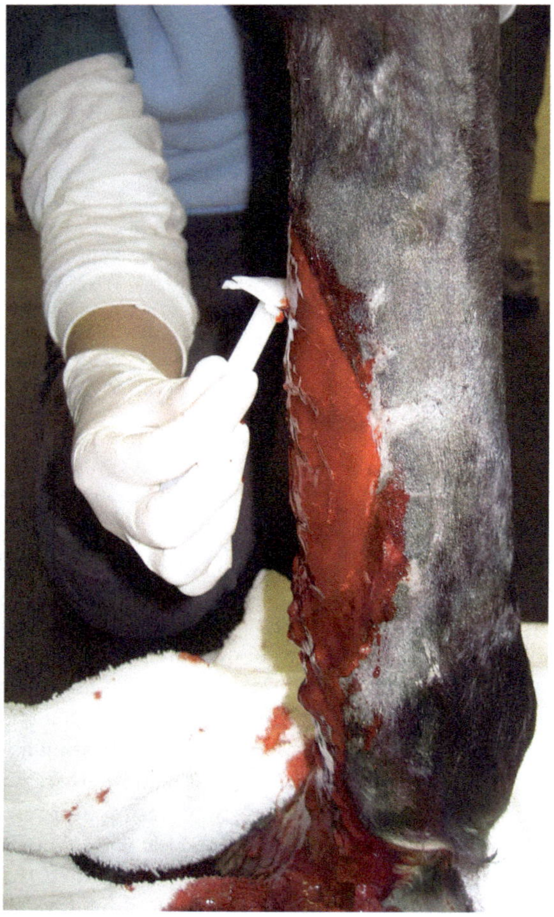

Figure 14.14 Completely granulated wound on the dorsomedial surface of the third metatarsal bone. Surgical resection of EGT, as was done in this case, is a simple and effective method used to control EGT. Shaving the wound bed in a distal to proximal direction facilitates identification of the wound's margin during debridement.

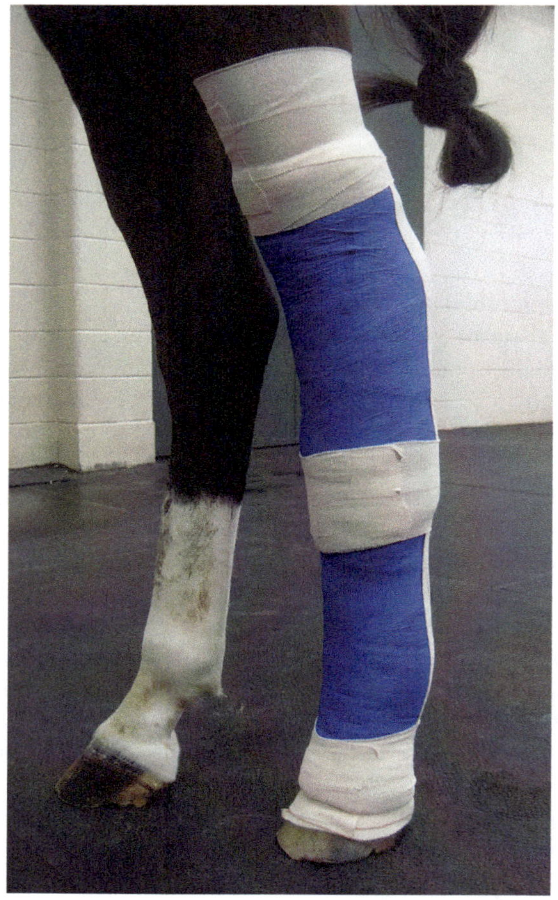

Figure 14.15 Pressure bandage with absorptive alginate dressing assists in debridement, absorbs exudate, provides protection from contamination, and reduces swelling of the limb.

tape that adheres to the third layer and to the skin to prevent debris from becoming interposed between the skin and the bandage (Figure 14.15).

Bandaging methods

The hock is difficult to bandage because of its conformation and the combination of forces that allow flexion and extension (i.e., the reciprocal apparatus). Horses are reluctant to accept any restriction to movement of the hock and frequently disrupt the bandage by flexing the hock exaggeratedly. Excessive pressure over the point of the hock (calcaneal tuberosity) and the Achilles tendon should be avoided when applying the primary and secondary layers of bandage. Two rolled bandages or thick sanitary pads can be placed in the hollows on each side of the gaskin cranial to the Achilles tendon to prevent the tertiary layer from exerting pressure directly on the tendon. The tertiary layer is applied in a figure-of-eight fashion, with circumferential wraps starting distal to the hock and continuing proximally with the crossover-points of the figure-of-eight wrap at the dorsum of the hock. Applying a length of 10-cm wide, low-stretch adhesive tape (Elastikon™, Johnson & Johnson, Inc.) longitudinally along the plantar surface of the tertiary layer and incorporating it at the proximal and distal ends of the bandage with the adhesive, elastic tape used to prevent debris from becoming interposed between the skin and the bandage assists in preventing the bandage from slipping distally (see Figures 7.5 and 7.6).

In addition, the author applies a thick cotton bandage to the distal aspect of the limb, from the coronary band to the proximal aspect of the metatarsus (see Figure 7.7), to prevent the bandage from slipping distally and to decrease the range of motion of the fetlock, thereby restricting movement of the hock. A rigid bandage or splint applied to the distal aspect of the limb with the fetlock partially flexed greatly decreases the range of motion of the hock, thereby increasing longevity of the bandage. For more information regarding application of bandages and techniques of splinting, see Chapter 7.

Casting

A limb with a degloving wound over a joint and/or tendon may require immobilization in a cast to avoid movement that disrupts healing. Frequently, the hock or carpus suffers a complex degloving injury involving the dorsal or palmar/plantar surface or both. The wound should be bandaged for a few days prior to applying a cast so that it can be debrided, if necessary, and to encourage dissipation of edema, thereby ensuring a better-fitting cast. Even though a cast provides an ideal environment for formation of granulation tissue, reduced motion provided by the cast tends to minimize the formation of EGT. The wounded limb should be maintained in a cast until a healthy bed of granulation tissue has developed. Generally, casts over wounds involving a joint and or tendon should be changed every 3–10 days but the interval between cast changes depends on the degree of exudation of the wound and the wound's location. A skin graft can be applied to the wound before the cast is applied to the limb or after the cast has been removed. For more information regarding application of a cast, see Chapter 7.

Skin grafting

A goal of managing a degloving wound on the distal aspect of the limb is to provide the most efficient, cost-effective treatment, which may entail application of a skin graft.[61,62] A skin graft can be applied to a fresh wound with a blood supply sufficient to support the graft or to a granulating wound, provided that the granulation tissue is healthy and not heavily populated with bacteria.[61,62] Skin grafts applied to exposed bone do not survive because the graft cannot be vascularized from exposed bone. Therefore, the wound can be grafted successfully only after the exposed bone is covered with granulation tissue. The granulation tissue bed to be grafted must be red to pink, smooth, and free of defects.[9,34] For more information regarding the methods used for skin grafting, see Chapter 18.

Tip

- Skin grafts can be applied to well-vascularized fresh wounds or to wounds with a clean, healthy-appearing bed of granulation tissue. Full-thickness sheet grafts may be applied to a fresh wound, whereas a partial-thickness sheet graft or island grafts (pinch, punch, or tunnel grafts) are more suitable for granulating wounds.

What to do

- Do not apply skin grafts to an unhealthy bed of granulation tissue.

Management of bone sequestra

Clinical signs most often produced by a sequestrum include soft-tissue swelling over the affected bone, palpation of which may cause the horse to show signs of discomfort, a mild lameness in the affected limb, and a draining tract found in the granulation tissue or in the epithelial scar of a wound that appears to have otherwise healed.[2] A probe introduced into the tract may strike bone, and occasionally, a sequestrum may be visible in the depths of a defect in the granulation tissue. Clinical signs either fail to resolve or only temporarily resolve when the horse receives anti-inflammatory and antimicrobial therapy.[2] Bone sequestration must be differentiated from other causes of chronic drainage from a sinus within the wound, such as the presence of a foreign body or communication of the wound with a synovial structure.

Wounds containing sequestered bone produce a large quantity of purulent exudate, form unhealthy granulation tissue, and contract and epithelialize poorly (Figure 14.16). Bacterial infection of bone, in addition to loss of the bone's periosteum, appears to be an important requisite for formation of a sequestrum, so measures to prevent infection, such as instituting perfusion of the wounded portion of the limb with an antibiotic, are key.[26,37]

What to do

- Radiograph the site of the wound to check for bone sequestration if bone remains uncovered by granulation tissue 2–4 weeks after injury or if exudate discharging from the wound increases in volume or becomes more purulent.

Tips

- Exposure of cortical bone does not always lead to formation of a sequestrum.
- Anticipate development of a sequestrum in a wound on the distal aspect of the limb if the bone has been traumatized.
- Suspect the presence of a sequestrum if purulent exudate is seen discharging from a wound, especially if the granulation tissue forming around the edges of the wound appears to be unhealthy.
- Lack of discoloration of exposed bone is not a reliable indicator that bone has not separated and sequestered.

A bony sequestrum must be eliminated, by autolytic debridement or by surgical removal, for the wound to heal. Waiting until the sequestrum has detached completely from the parent bone eases surgery. The sequestrum is removed by excising the overlying granulation tissue, and the involucrum is curetted to eliminate infected tissue. Many sequestra can be removed with the horse sedated and standing after administering regional anesthesia (Figure 14.9), although general anesthesia may be required if performing surgery with the horse conscious is dangerous or if the wound is close to a synovial structure. The horse should be recovered from general anesthesia, after the sequestrum is removed, with a rigid splint applied to the bandaged limb to avoid fracture at the site from which the sequestrum was removed.[63] The wounded site should be examined radiographically 2–3 weeks later to confirm healing of the involucrum.

Conclusion

Healing of a wound in which bone is exposed relies on the same cellular and humoral elements that contribute to healing of more superficial wounds, but the presence of exposed bone in wounds may directly and indirectly delay healing. Regardless of the methods used to manage wounds over exposed bone, the wound must fill with healthy granulation tissue before it

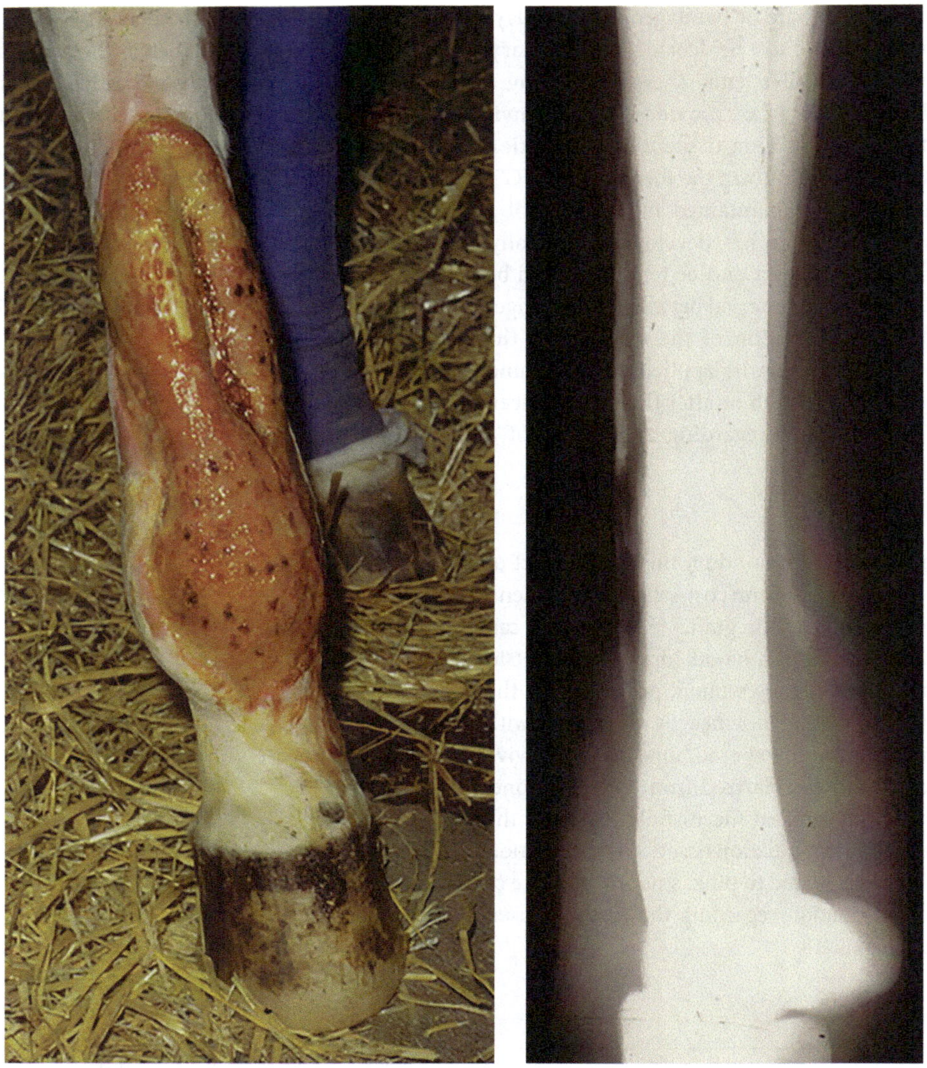

(a) (b)

Figure 14.16 **(a)** Degloving injury of 3 months' duration involving the dorsal surface of the metatarsus. Note the linear defect in the granulation tissue from which exudate drained. The appearance of the granulation tissue was unhealthy, and contraction of the wound was stalled. These signs suggested the presence of an underlying bone sequestrum. The dark spots in the granulation tissue, particularly overlying the fetlock region, are pinch grafts that have been accepted. **(b)** Lateral radiograph revealing a linear sequestrum with an involucrum along the dorsal surface of the third metatarsal bone. Courtesy of Dr. T. Stashak.

can heal. Special attention must be paid to identify or rule out the presence of a bone sequestrum when a degloving injury to the distal limb has exposed underlying bone because healing cannot proceed normally until the sequestrum is resolved.

References

1. Latifi R, El-Hennawy H, El-Menyar A, *et al.* The therapeutic challenges of degloving soft tissue injuries. *J Emerg Trauma Shock* 2014; **7**: 228.
2. Clem MF, DeBowes RM, Yovich JV, *et al.* Osseous sequestration in the horse: a review of 68 cases. *Vet Surg* 1988; **17**: 2.
3. Elce Y. Degloving injuries in horses: initial treatment. *Compend Contin Educ* 2011; **33**: E1.
4. Gift LJ, DeBowes RM. Wounds associated with osseous sequestration and penetrating foreign bodies. *Vet Clin N Am Equine Pract* 1989; **5**: 695.
5. Jacobs KA, Leach DH, Fretz PB, *et al.* Comparative aspects of the healing of excisional wounds on the leg and body of horses. *Vet Surg* 1984; **13**: 83.
6. Schumacher J, Brumbaugh GW, Honnas CM, *et al.* Kinetics of healing of grafted and non-grafted wounds on the distal portion of the forelimbs of horses. *Am J Vet Res* 1992; **53**: 1568.
7. Johnson R. The effects of cortical fenestration on second intention healing of wounds over exposed bone of the distal aspect of the limb of horses. (Masters thesis). Auburn, AL: Auburn University 2000.
8. Wilmink JM, Stolk PW, van Weeren PR, *et al.* Differences in second-intention wound healing between horses and ponies: macroscopic aspects. *Equine Vet J* 1999; **31**: 53.

9. Bertone AL, Sullins KE, Stashak TS, *et al.* Effect of wound location and the use of topical collagen gel on exuberant granulation tissue formation and wound healing in the horse and pony. *Am J Vet Res* 1985; **46**: 1438.
10. Wilmink JM, van Weeren PR, Stolk PW, *et al.* Differences in second-intention wound healing between horses and ponies: histological aspects. *Equine Vet J* 1999; **31**: 61.
11. van den Boom R, Wilmink JM, O'Kane S, *et al.* Transforming growth factor-β levels during second intention healing are related to the different course of wound contraction in horses and ponies. *Wound Repair Regen* 2002; **10**: 188.
12. Schumacher J, Stashak TS. Management of wounds of the distal extremities. In: Stashak TS, Theoret CL (eds). *Equine Wound Management*, 2nd edn. Wiley Blackwell: Ames IA, 2008: 375.
13. Ford TS, Schumacher J, Brumbaugh GW, *et al.* Effects of split-thickness and full-thickness skin grafts on secondary graft contraction in horses. *Am J Vet Res* 1992; **53**: 1572.
14. Desmoulière A, Chaponnier C, Gabbiani G. Tissue repair, contraction and the myofibroblast. *Wound Repair Regen* 2005; **13**: 7.
15. Ehrlich HP, Keefer KA, Roland L, *et al.* Vanadate and the absence of myofibroblasts in wound contraction. *Arch Surg* 1999; **134**: 494.
16. Rudolph R, Vandeberg J, Ehrlich H. Wound contraction and scar contracture. In: Cohen K, Diegelmann R, Lindblad W (eds). *Wound Healing: Biochemical and Clinical Aspects*, 1st edn. Saunders: Philadelphia, 1992: 96.
17. Malizos KN, Papatheodorou LK. The healing potential of the periosteum. *Injury* 2005; **36**: S13.
18. Glowacki J. Angiogenesis in fracture repair. *Clin Orthop Relat Res* 1998; **355**: S82.
19. Nakahara H, Bruder SP, Goldberg VM, *et al. In vivo* osteochondrogenic potential of cultured cells derived from periosteum. *Clin Orthop* 1990; **259**: 223.
20. Scott-Savage P, Hall BK. Differentiative ability of the tibial periosteum for the embryonic chick. *Acta Anat* 1980; **106**: 129.
21. Vachon A, McIlwraith CW, Trotter GW, *et al.* Neochondrogenesis in free intra-articular, periosteal, and perichondrial autografts in horses. *Am J Vet Res* 1989; **50**: 1787.
22. Alfieri KA, Forsberg JA, Potter BK. Blast injuries and heterotopic ossification. *Bone Joint Res* 2012; **1**: 174.
23. Thompson K. Bones and joints. In: Maxie MG (ed). *Jubb, Kennedy and Palmer's Pathology of Domestic Animals*, 5th edn. Saunders Elsevier: Philadelphia, 2007: 21.
24. Lopez MJ, Markel MD. Bone biology and fracture healing. In: Auer J, Stick J (eds). *Equine Surgery*, 4th edn. Saunders Elsevier: St. Louis, 2006: 1025.
25. Jann HW, Peyton LC, Fackelman GE. The pathogenesis and treatment of traumatically induced sequestra in horses. *Compend Contin Educ Pract Vet* 1987; **9**: 182.
26. Moens Y, Verschooten F, De Moor A, *et al.* Bone sequestration as a consequence of limb wounds in the horse. *Vet Radiol* 1980; **21**: 40.
27. Butler JA, Colles CM, Dyson SJ, *et al.* The metacarpus and metatarsus. *Clinical Radiology of the Horse*, 2nd edn. Blackwell Publishing: Oxford, 1993.
28. Brown PW. The fate of exposed bone. *Am J Surg* 1979; **137**: 464.
29. Caron JP, Barber SM, Doige CE, *et al.* The radiographic and histologic appearance of controlled surgical manipulation of the equine periosteum. *Vet Surg* 1987; **16**: 13.
30. Wilmink JM, van Herten J, van Weeren PR, *et al.* Retrospective study of primary intention healing and sequestra formation in horses compared to ponies under clinical circumstances. *Equine Vet J* 2002; **34**; 270.
31. Latenser J, Snow SN, Mohs FE, *et al.* Power drills to fenestrate exposed bone to stimulate wound healing. *J Dermatol Surg Oncol* 1991; **17**: 265.
32. Bailin PL, Wheeland RG. Carbon dioxide (CO_2) laser perforation of exposed cranial bone to stimulate granulation tissue. *Plast Reconstr Surg* 1985; **75**: 898.
33. Specht TE, Colahan PT. Osteostixis for incomplete cortical fracture of the third metacarpal bone: results in 11 horses. *Vet Surg* 1990; **19**: 34.
34. Lee AH, Swaim SF, Newton JC, *et al.* Wound healing over denuded bone. *J Am Anim Hosp Assoc* 1987; **23**: 75.
35. DeRossi R, Coelho AC, Mello GS, *et al.* Effects of platelet-rich plasma gel on skin healing in surgical wound in horses. *Acta Cir Bras* 2009; **24**: 276.
36. Monteiro SO, Lepage OM, Theoret CL. Effects of platelet rich plasma on the repair of wounds on the distal aspect of the forelimb of horses. *Am J Vet Res* 2009; **70**: 277.
37. Bauer SM, Santschi EM, Fialkowski J, *et al.* Quantification of *staphylococcus aureus* adhesion to equine bone surfaces passivated with plasmalyte™ and hyperimmune plasma. *Vet Surg* 2004; **33**: 376.
38. Booth LC, Feeney DA. Superficial osteitis and sequestrum formation as a result of skin avulsion in the horse. *Vet Surg* 1982; **11**: 2.
39. Lees MF, Fretz PB, Bailey JV, *et al.* Second-intention wound healing. *Compend Contin Educ Pract Vet* 1989; **11**: 857.
40. Hanson R. Management of avulsion wounds with exposed bone. *Clin Tech Equine Pract* 2004; **3**: 188.
41. Wilmink JM, van Weeren PR. Differences in wound healing between horses and ponies: application of research results to the clinical approach of equine wounds. *Clin Tech Equine Pract* 2004; **3**: 123.
42. Fairweather M, Heit YI, Buie J, *et al.* Celecoxib inhibits early cutaneous wound healing. *J Surg Res* 2015; **194**: 717.
43. Kahn LH, Styrt BA. Necrotizing soft tissue infections reported with nonsteroidal anti-inflammatory drugs. *Ann Pharmacother* 1997; **31**: 1034.
44. Scheuch, BC, Van Hoogmoed LM, Wilson D, *et al.* Comparison of intraosseous or intravenous infusion for delivery of amikacin sulfate to the tibial tarsal joint of horses. *Am J Vet Res* 2002; **63**: 374.
45. Ramos JR, Howard RD, Pleasant RS, *et al.* Elution of metronidazole and gentamicin from polymethylmethacrylate beads. *Vet Surg* 2003; **32**: 251.
46. Santschi EM, McGarvey L. *In vitro* elution of gentamicin from plaster of Paris beads. *Vet Surg* 2003: **32**; 128.
47. Jones V, Milton T. When and how to use hydrogels. *Nurs Times* 2000; **96**: 3.
48. Campbell BG. Current concepts and materials in wound bandaging. *18th North American Veterinary Conference* 2004; January 18–23; Orlando, FL: 1217.
49. Chaby G, Senet P, Vaneau M, *et al.* Dressings for acute and chronic wounds – a systematic review. *Arch Dermatol* 2007; **143**: 1297.
50. von Lindern JJ, Niederhagen B, Appel T, *et al.* Treatment of soft tissue defects with exposed bone in the head and face region

with alginates and hydrocolloid dressings. *J Oral Maxillofac Surg* 2002; **60**: 1126.

51. Robson MC, Edstrom LE, Krizek TJ, *et al.* Efficacy of systemic antibiotics in treatments of granulating wounds. *J Surg Res* 1974; **16**: 299.
52. Best Practice Statement: The use of topical antiseptic/antimicrobial agents in wound management. *Wounds UK* 2011. http://www.wounds-uk.com/pdf/content_9969.pdf (accessed August 15, 2015).
53. Geronemus RG, Mertz PM, Eaglstein WH. Wound healing: the effects of topical antimicrobial agents. *Arch Dermatol* 1979; **115**: 1311.
54. Berry DB, Sullins KE. Effects of topical application of antimicrobials and bandaging on healing and granulation tissue formation in wounds of the distal aspect of the limbs in horses. *Am J Vet Res* 2003; **64**: 88.
55. Woodward M. Silver dressings in wound healing: what is the evidence? *Primary Intention* 2005; **13**: 153.
56. Kingsley A. The use of honey on the treatment of infected wounds: case studies. *Br J Nurs* 2001; **10**: S13.
57. Tonks AJ, Cooper RA, Jones KP, *et al.* Honey stimulates inflammatory cytokine production from monocytes. *Cytokine* 2003; **21**: 242.
58. Visavadia BG, Honeysett J, Danford MH. Manuka honey dressing: an effective treatment for chronic wound infections. *Br J Oral Maxillofac Surg* 2008; **46**: 55.
59. Yusof N, Hafiza AHA, Zohdi RM, *et al.* Development of honey hydrogel dressing for enhanced wound healing. *Radiat Phys Chem* 2007; **76**: 1767.
60. Swaim SF, Lee AH. Topical wound medications: a review. *J Am Vet Med Assoc* 1987; **190**: 188.
61. Schumacher J, Hanselka DV. Skin grafting of the horse. *Vet Clin N Am Equine Pract* 1989; **5**: 591.
62. Schumacher J. Skin grafting. In: Auer J, Stick J (eds). *Equine Surgery*, 4th edn. Saunders Elsevier: St. Louis, 2006: 285.
63. Knottenbelt DC. *Handbook of Equine Wound Management.* Saunders: London, 2003: 95.

CHAPTER 15

Exuberant Granulation Tissue

Christine Theoret, DMV, PhD, Diplomate ACVS and Jacintha M. Wilmink, DVM, PhD

Chapter Contents

Summary

The formation of exuberant granulation tissue (EGT) is a frequent complication of wounds healing by second intention on the limbs of horses. Among the large number of contributing factors, chronic inflammation is foremost and often goes unrecognized because of the mild signs it elicits. The stimulus for formation of EGT is reduced when prevention and treatment of chronic inflammation are combined with excision of the protruding granulation tissue. This approach allows a smooth transition from fibroplasia to wound contraction and epithelialization and usually obviates the recurrence of EGT.

The topical application of a corticosteroid, used in a precise and controlled manner, and the use of silicone sheet dressings, as well as skin grafting, are valuable in preventing the formation of EGT. In cases where EGT is already present, excision of the protruding granulation tissue is, currently, the treatment of choice.

Introduction

The development of exuberant granulation tissue (EGT) in the horse has long been an enigma. Several studies, performed during the past two decades, have focused on equine EGT with the aim to elucidate the mechanisms underlying this phenomenon and thereby develop targeted therapies. The findings and interpretations of these investigations have been united in this chapter. They complement one another and have shed light on the pathophysiology of one of the most common and frustrating complications disturbing the repair of limb wounds of horses. The etiology of EGT appears to be multifactorial, involving

Equine Wound Management, Third Edition. Edited by Christine Theoret and Jim Schumacher.

Companion website: www.wiley.com/go/theoret/wound

environmental, biochemical, immunologic, and genetic factors. Insights into the physiology/pathology, predisposing factors, prevention, and treatment of EGT are described and discussed herein.

Physiology and pathology

Fibroplasia and the development of exuberant granulation tissue

Fibroplasia, or the formation of granulation tissue, is an essential component of wound healing. Apart from the nuisance of becoming exuberant, granulation tissue has many important functions that change continuously during healing. It fills in the wound gap, forms a barrier against external contaminants, provides myofibroblasts for wound contraction, and forms the bed over which epithelial cells migrate.

Granulation tissue provides several types of cells with important functions during healing. *Endothelial cells* form capillaries and other blood vessels through which oxygen and nutrients are transported to sustain cellular metabolism and through which leukocytes can migrate into the wound. *Leukocytes* clear the wound of contaminating agents and debris. Furthermore, they recruit additional inflammatory and mesenchymal cells and initiate healing. *Fibroblasts* form the extracellular matrix (ECM) needed to support cellular division, growth, and migration. The composition of ECM gradually changes as it is remodeled through the simultaneous synthesis and degradation of its components. Ideally, granulation tissue ceases to grow as soon as the gap in the wound has filled, allowing contraction and epithelialization to ensue. In many wounds on the limbs of horses, however, granulation tissue continues to grow for an indefinite period, resulting in the formation of EGT.

EGT is typically irregular and unhealthy in appearance, with many grooves and clefts, and protrudes over the margin of the wound (Figure 15.1). Although seen often in limb wounds, it is seen rarely in body wounds. EGT is characterized by chronic inflammation and the remains of fibrin deposits that have not been cleared by the acute inflammatory response. Microscopically, the tissue has an immature, chaotic appearance due to its disorganized cellular population (Figure 15.2).[2,3] In wounds suffering from EGT, cellular proliferation remains active, wound contraction is delayed, and the protruding granulation tissue may physically impede epithelial migration and/or may inhibit the growth of keratinocytes.[2,4]

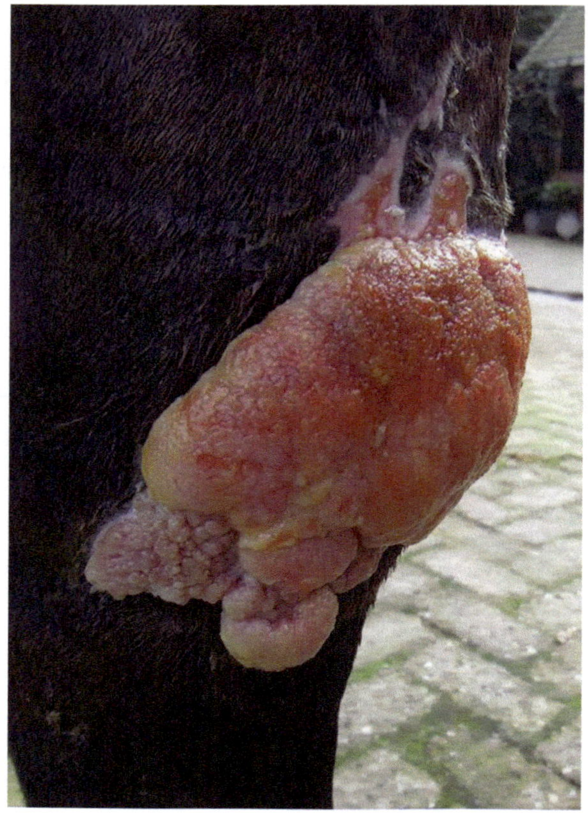

Figure 15.1 A wound on the dorsal surface of the tarsus showing the typical features of EGT: irregular surface riddled with grooves and clefts, protrusion over the wound margins, and purulent exudate.

Phenotype and function of fibroblasts

Phenotype and function of fibroblasts in normally healing wounds

The fibroblast, the major type of cell in granulation tissue and in EGT, changes its phenotype during healing. The phenotype and function of fibroblasts are closely related. When healing is uncomplicated, phenotypes reflect the various needs of the wound as healing progresses, and phenotypes succeed one another as the wound matures. Initially, fibroblasts have a migratory phenotype, allowing them to move from the surrounding tissues into the wound. Migration depends on chemoattractive agents released by platelets and macrophages at the wound's border in response to injury.[5] Once at its ultimate destination, the fibroblast changes its phenotype into a proliferative and synthesizing form. Consequently, the number of fibroblasts increases, and ECM is produced. The synthesis of ECM is stimulated by several cytokines, such as transforming growth factor beta (TGF-β), released either by inflammatory cells or by the fibroblasts themselves.[6,7] Thereafter, fibroblasts can differentiate into myofibroblasts, a phenotype that contains smooth muscle actin filaments and can pull the margin of the wound centripetally via the contractile force exerted by these filaments.[8] Differentiation of fibroblasts into myofibroblasts and the generation of contractile forces are also stimulated by TGF-β, but both are inhibited by many other mediators produced in a chronically inflamed environment. After contraction ceases, fibroblasts and myofibroblasts disappear from the wound by apoptosis (i.e. cellular fragmentation followed by phagocytosis by macrophages and activated fibroblasts), and the cellularity of the repair tissue diminishes.[9,10] Apoptosis, a form of non-inflammatory programmed cellular death, is thus critical to the transition from one phase of repair (proliferation and contrac-

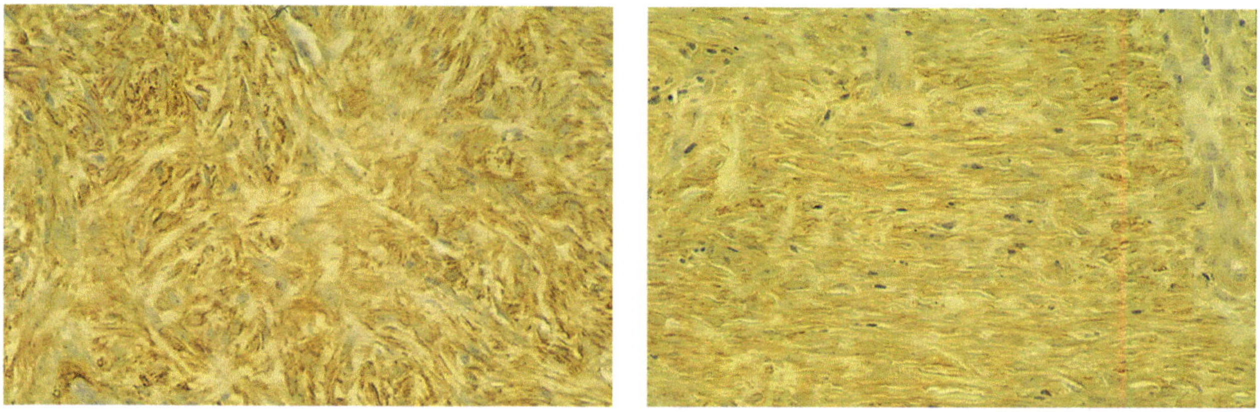

(a) (b)

Figure 15.2 **(a)** EGT, when viewed under a microscope, shows a high number of chaotically arranged cells and capillaries and looks very immature in contrast to **(b)** the regularly arranged cells and parallel capillaries of more differentiated and contracting granulation tissue. Smooth muscle actin staining. Source: Wilmink and van Weeren 2004.[1] Reprinted with permission of Elsevier.

tion) to the next (remodeling). Myofibroblasts may represent the terminal differentiation state of fibroblasts, after which apoptosis can occur.

Phenotype and function of fibroblasts in wounds with exuberant granulation tissue

The development of EGT in a wound coincides with a disordered succession of fibroblastic phenotypes. Specifically, the proliferative and synthesizing phenotypes predominate in EGT, while differentiation into contractile myofibroblasts is delayed.[3] This is consistent with the microscopic observation in limb wounds that persistent mitotic activity accompanies chaotically arranged myofibroblasts, a pattern not conducive to contraction,[2,3] as well as with the clinical observation that the presence of EGT is often coupled with poor contraction. Confirmation of this phenomenon was established *in vitro*, where the rate of proliferation of fibroblasts appeared inversely proportional to the capacity of fibroblasts for contraction because rapidly proliferating fibroblasts produced lower contractile forces (Figure 15.3).[11] Indeed, because myofibroblasts represent the terminal state of differentiation of fibroblasts, tardy progression to the contractile phenotype also implies that apoptosis will be impaired and high cellularity will be maintained, thereby favoring the development of EGT.

Because EGT occurs primarily in poorly contracting limb wounds, as opposed to efficiently contracting body wounds, investigators hypothesized that fibroblasts from diverse anatomical origins might possess different inherent characteristics accountable for the variable succession of phenotypes.[11,12] It was found, however, that the elevated mitotic activity in limb wounds is not based on innate differences in characteristics of growth between fibroblasts from limbs and those from the trunk because those of limb origin grow significantly more slowly than those of trunk origin when cultured *in vitro*.[11,12] Additionally, the inadequate contraction seen in limb wounds is not based on a weak inherent contractile capacity of fibroblasts

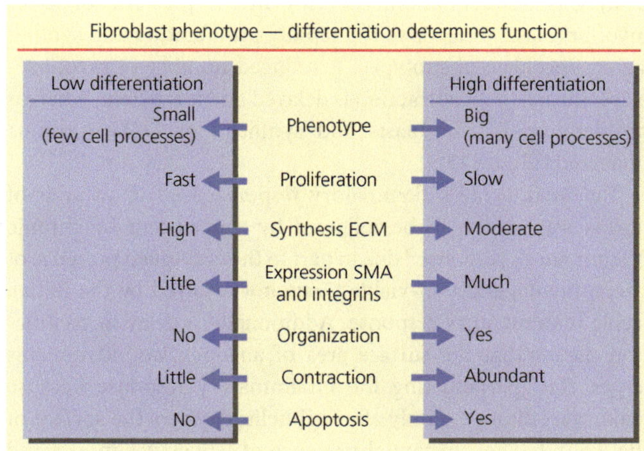

Figure 15.3 Fibroblast phenotype – differentiation determines function. Fibroblasts able to contract have different phenotypic features and are more differentiated than those exhibiting a proliferating phenotype.

from limbs; fibroblasts from limbs contract more than those from the trunk when cultured *in vitro*.[11]

In conclusion, the different phenotypes and functions attributed to fibroblasts from the limb or trunk, as well as the contrasting modes of repair characterizing limb and body wounds, are not based on distinct intrinsic cellular characteristics but, instead, must be the result of other factors. The extracellular environment's biochemical, molecular, and physical components govern the phenotype of the fibroblast, whereas the phenotype determines the fibroblast's response to environmental signals.[8]

Factors affecting the formation of exuberant granulation tissue

Although the exact causes of development of EGT during wound repair in the horse have yet to be established, research has revealed a number of factors that may contribute to this condition. Some of these factors cannot be controlled or can be only partially controlled, whereas others can be prevented or eliminated.

Physiologic factors

Inflammatory response

An inefficient inflammatory response to injury may influence the phenotype and function of fibroblasts and thereby play an important role in the development of EGT in limb wounds of horses (Figure 15.3). After trauma, the acute inflammatory response in limb wounds of horses is weaker during the first 3 weeks than that of limb wounds of ponies, and the concentration of TGF-β in limb wounds of horses is lower during the first 10 days than that in limb wounds of ponies.[3,13,14] TGF-β1 not only stimulates production of ECM but also favors the differentiation of fibroblasts into myofibroblasts, thereby encouraging wound contraction. An inferior initial concentration of TGF-β may delay this differentiation, resulting in the presence of fewer myofibroblasts in favor of the rapidly proliferating and synthesizing fibroblast phenotypes. A reduced number of myofibroblasts means that contraction is delayed and inefficient, whereas proliferation of fibroblasts and synthesis of ECM continue unabated (Figure 15.3).

The weak acute inflammatory response seen in wounds of horses was shown to be followed by a persistent or chronic inflammatory response,[3] due in part to the continued presence of contaminants and non-viable tissue not resolved by the initial, feeble inflammatory response. Additionally, a delay in contraction means that the surface area of an open wound remains larger, thus perpetuating the inflammatory response because leukocytes disappear only after epithelium covers the surface of the wound. The substantial presence of leukocytes in exposed granulation tissue may explain up-regulated synthesis of cytokines in the absence of epithelium[15] and may lower oxygen tension in the wound as a result of the high oxygen consumption by these cells. Persistence of mediators, such as TGF-β, platelet-derived growth factor (PDGF), and fibroblast growth factor (FGF), induces fibrosis, whereas prostaglandin (PG)E_1, PGE_2, and interferon (IFN)γ inhibit contraction, while yet others, such as tumor necrosis factor (TNF)α, interleukin (IL)-1, and IL-6 do both (Figure 15.4).[16,17] Low oxygen tension additionally stimulates proliferation of fibroblasts and production of ECM.[18,19] The inflammation persisting in limb wounds of horses, therefore, likely enhances the formation of EGT and inhibits contraction, phenomena that are often seen simultaneously in the clinical setting. This hypothesis is substantiated by a recent study confirming that exacerbated and prolonged inflammation in healing wounds on the ears of rabbits favors the development of hypertrophic scarring.[20] Moreover, the observation that corticosteroids, potent anti-inflammatory drugs, control the formation of EGT in the wounds of horses adds further credence to this scenario.[21]

In summary, the combination of an inefficient, weak, acute inflammatory response and the ensuing chronic inflammation in

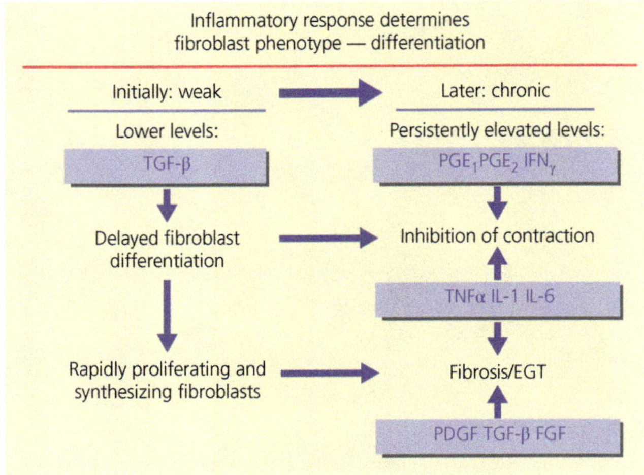

Figure 15.4 Fibroblast phenotype and differentiation is influenced by several cytokines present during the acute and chronic inflammatory response to wounding. Both the inefficient, weak acute inflammatory response and the ensuing chronic inflammation seen in limb wounds of horses delay the differentiation of fibroblasts into myofibroblasts, ultimately reducing wound contraction and favoring fibroblast proliferation.

limb wounds of horses delays the differentiation of fibroblasts into myofibroblasts, reducing wound contraction and favoring proliferation of fibroblasts and synthesis of proteins. This leads to a rapid increase in tissue volume by cellular proliferation, rather than a decrease in tissue volume by contraction (Figure 15.5). The chronic inflammation inherent to second-intention healing in limb wounds of horses, while often unrecognized clinically because of the mild accompanying signs, is no doubt a very important trigger for formation of EGT. The interaction between inflammation, subsequent formation of EGT, and lack of contraction establishes a vicious cycle because these physiologic phenomena stimulate one another.

Local cytokine profile

The aforementioned development of chronic inflammation in limb wounds of horses substantiates several studies documenting a fibrogenic-rich, local cytokine profile in limb wounds.[13,22–25] One of these cytokines, TGF-β1, stimulates migration and proliferation of fibroblasts and their production of ECM proteins, such as fibronectin and collagen,[6] while inhibiting the degradation of ECM.[25,26] It is thus noteworthy that the expression of TGF-β1 persists in limb wounds throughout the proliferative phase of repair, whereas it quickly returns to baseline values in body wounds after the initial inflammatory phase of healing.[13,22] Persistent production of TGF-β1 in limb wounds may partially be the work of the fibroblasts within the wound that also express more TGF-β receptors;[27,28] the signaling components are thus in place to stimulate cellular proliferation and encourage accumulation of components of ECM.

The persistent expression of TGF-β1 can be explained, at least in part, by various characteristics of limb wounds in horses, such as absence of epithelium, presence of tightly fixed

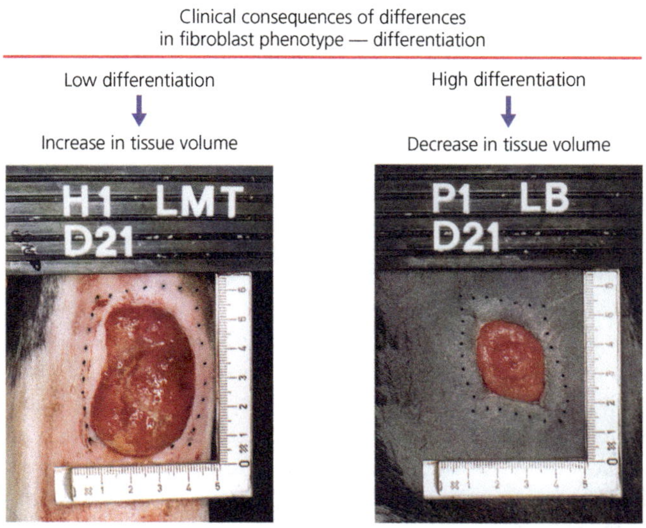

Figure 15.5 Experimental wounds initially of the same size, 21 days after creation on the limb of a horse (left) or on the buttock of a pony (right), which show the clinical consequences of differences in fibroblast phenotype and differentiation. Delayed differentiation of fibroblasts in limb wounds favors their proliferation but inhibits wound contraction, leading to an increase in tissue volume. In contrast, the faster differentiation of fibroblasts into myofibroblasts in buttock wounds of ponies, and the ensuing contraction, reduce tissue volume.

surrounding skin, as well as hypoxia of local tissue. Indeed, the synthesis of fibrogenic cytokines is up-regulated in the absence of an epithelial cover.[15] Persistent mechanical tension in a wound also plays a role, because mechanical unloading of fibroblasts is required to desensitize cytokine receptors, abrogating cytokine responsiveness and thereby favoring apoptosis.[29,30] Consequently, mechanical stress must be relieved for a wound to progress from granulation tissue to scar, by apoptosis.[29] Additionally, the secretion of TGF-β1 by fibroblasts is strongly stimulated by low oxygen tension.[19,31]

Collagen synthesis, deposition, and lysis

Investigators have assumed for some time that aberrant metabolism of collagen plays a key role in the formation of EGT. Theoretically, either abundant synthesis or impaired lysis may lead to excessive accumulation of collagen. The horse forms collagen speedily in response to wounding, indicating a prompt and excessive connective tissue response compared to the response of other species.[32] As described earlier, protracted expression of TGF-β1 in limb wounds may give rise to excessive formation of collagen and other proteins of the ECM.[13,23] Moreover, superior concentrations of type-I collagen and tissue inhibitors of metalloproteinase (TIMP)-1 mRNA have been measured in limb wounds compared to body wounds of horses at 1 and 4 weeks of healing.[24] Because TIMP-1 inhibits lysis of collagen, high concentrations present 4 weeks post wounding might favor accumulation of ECM. An imbalance between synthesis and degradation of collagen is likely correlated to the development of EGT, indicating that agents inhibiting collagen synthesis or stimulating the activity of MMPs, in particular collagenase, may represent therapeutic options. Indeed, the Food and Drug Administration approved intralesional collagenase for the treatment of Dupuytren's disease, a proliferative connective tissue disorder in humans;[33] moreover, this approach is currently under investigation for the management of keloid scarring in humans, a dermal fibroproliferative condition that resembles equine EGT.[34] Because an imbalance between synthesis and degradation of a single component of the ECM is unlikely to be the sole basis of formation of EGT, however, the effect of influencing only the metabolism of collagen might be limited.

Angiogenesis and wound oxygenation

Because low oxygen concentrations have been shown to stimulate the proliferation of fibroblasts and their synthesis of components of the ECM, it was postulated that local hypoxia within the granulation tissue of limb wounds of horses might contribute to the development of EGT. This hypothesis was verified via a series of experiments, the first of which mapped the expression of several genes and their corresponding proteins, selected from a larger pool[35–41] because of their known contribution to angiogenesis during wound healing.[42,43] Healing limb wounds of horses were found to be deficient in anti-angiogenic molecules, compared to body wounds, suggesting that the "control switch" to limit angiogenesis is defective in wounds on the limbs of horses. This coincides with the exacerbated angiogenesis observed clinically in limb wounds,[44] an important feature of EGT. Although the granulation tissue of limb wounds of horses is characterized by marked vascular regeneration, the lumens of these new microvessels are occluded significantly more than those of microvessels found in body wounds,[44] owing to hypertrophy of the lining endothelial cells.[45] This hypertrophy is also observed in keloid scars of humans,[46] which share numerous clinical and histopathologic features with equine EGT.[47,48]

Given this occlusion, the function of new blood vessels in healing wounds of horses was assessed by monitoring derivatives of cutaneous blood flow, namely the temperature of skin and wound[49] as well as transcutaneous oxygen saturation levels.[50] Cutaneous wound temperature, and by extension blood flow, was found to be significantly inferior in limb wounds compared to body wounds and even lower in limb wounds predisposed to the formation of EGT.[49] This data was corroborated using laser Doppler flowmetry.[51] Concomitantly, the degree of oxygen saturation in limb wounds of horses was found to be significantly inferior to that of body wounds during the early period of healing, indicating a temporary, relative state of hypoxia during the inflammatory phase of repair.[50] Likewise, metabolic disturbances were found, via microdialysis, confirming an inadequate supply of oxygen during healing of equine limb wounds that developed EGT.[51]

Because oxygen is required for bactericidal efficiency of leukocytes,[52,53] the relative hypoxia present acutely in limb wounds of horses may explain the feeble yet prolonged inflammatory response in these wounds thought to contribute to the development of EGT.[3] Moreover, hypoxia itself has been shown to up-regulate angiogenic and fibrogenic mediators,[54] thereby encouraging angiogenesis as well as the proliferation of fibroblasts and their synthesis of components of ECM, substantiating the relationship between the (low) oxygen saturation levels in a wound and the wound's propensity to become fibro-proliferative. These findings were confirmed in a study that showed that subjecting cultured equine dermal fibroblasts to hypoxia stimulated the fibroblasts to proliferate and to synthesize ECM while decreasing the turnover of ECM.[19] Interestingly, no behavioral differences in response to hypoxia were observed between fibroblasts originating from the body or the limb, implying that development of EGT does not depend on intrinsic properties of limb fibroblasts but rather on the local environment of the wound.

In view of these findings, one would assume that delivery of supplemental oxygen during the acute inflammatory phase of healing might protect against the development of EGT in limb wounds of horses. Hyberbaric oxygen therapy (HBOT) involves the inhalation of 100% oxygen within a pressurized chamber, which leads to increased tissue oxygen tensions (for more information on HBOT, the reader is referred to Chapter 19).[55] Topical oxygen therapy (TOT) involves increasing the supply of oxygen directly to the wound by placing an oxygen-filled bag, boot or extremity chamber around the limb or affected area. HBOT is used to manage wounds in humans but as yet, evidence of its efficacy, based on high-quality research, is lacking.[56] Preliminary evidence suggests that HBOT is not indicated for use in horses after full-thickness skin grafting of uncompromised, fresh, granulating wounds,[57] but this modality has not been evaluated in the management of other types of wounds in horses. Likewise, a preliminary study on the use of TOT in the management of experimental dermal wounds on the limbs of healthy horses also showed little effect on healing.[58]

Apoptosis

The elevated and persistent mitotic activity characterizing the granulation tissue of limb wounds may relate to deficient apoptosis. This assumption has been partially substantiated by the observation that the balance of apoptotic signals is skewed against apoptosis in limb compared to body wounds of horses.[44] High concentrations of TGF-β1 persisting in limb wounds[23] may play a role because this particular cytokine appears to have an anti-apoptotic effect on fibroblasts.[59,60] Furthermore, in addition to encouraging the synthesis of fibrogenic cytokines, the absence of an epithelial cover, as is characteristic of EGT, debilitates apoptosis because many signals that favor elimination of fibroblasts by this process are normally released by the keratinocyte.[61] Signals that bring about apoptosis also participate in decreasing deposition of collagen, not only by reducing numbers of fibroblasts but also by activating collagenase.[61]

If the signal to down-regulate the activity of fibroblasts and myofibroblasts is delayed beyond a specific point in time, then apoptosis is permanently impaired.[61] This may explain why wounds chronically affected with EGT are unlikely to resolve spontaneously; indeed, the impairment of apoptosis limits the elimination of unwanted cells and subsequent transition to the next phase of repair.

General clinical factors

Location of the wound

The likelihood that a wound will develop EGT depends on its anatomic location. Wounds of the body heal quickly and without the formation of EGT in contrast to limb wounds, which heal slowly and are prone to excessive fibroplasia. The exact location of the wound on the limb further influences healing and formation of EGT; wounds over the dorsal surface of the metacarpo/metatarsophalangeal joint (fetlock) heal more slowly than similar wounds located over the dorsal surface of the metacarpus/metatarsus.[62,63] Additionally, limb wounds located on the extensor and flexor surfaces of joints and the heel bulbs appear prone to the development of EGT. These clinical differences are assumed to relate to movement that tears the granulation tissue, inciting more inflammation and cellular proliferation (Figure 15.6). The movement of partially lacerated or frayed tendons may exert a similar influence. Indeed, restricting movement by applying a cast or splint can prevent repeated damage and reduce the formation of EGT in these wounds, despite the fact that the local environment created by the cast would normally favor the formation of EGT.[64]

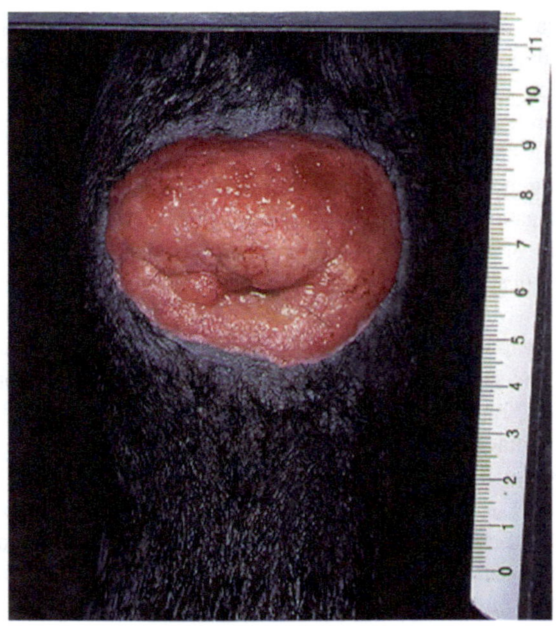

Figure 15.6 A 3-week-old wound at the dorsal surface of the fetlock joint. The groove in the granulation tissue is probably caused by tearing during flexion, which predisposes to EGT formation.

Another factor enhancing the formation of EGT in the distal aspect of the limb is the relative lack of tissue covering the underlying bone and, subsequently, a reduced vascular bed and relatively poor collateral circulation. Impairment of circulation from trauma results in lower oxygen tension in the healing wound, as addressed earlier, with the ensuing effects on proliferation of fibroblasts and synthesis of ECM.[31,54] Conversely, thick and well-vascularized musculature covers most structures of the trunk so that perfusion of a wound in this location is not usually substantially disturbed.

Breed

Formation of EGT is influenced by the breed, but not in an exclusive manner; both horses and ponies can develop EGT, although to differing extents.[2] Ponies form EGT with lesser frequency and quantity, and EGT of ponies tends to disappear spontaneously after the wound is left uncovered. In contrast, horses consistently form more EGT that does not disappear when left uncovered and must be excised. This variable breed predilection might be the confounding factor that explains the conflicting conclusions of past investigations of whether ponies heal with or without EGT.[21,62,64]

Factors related to inflammation and infection

Many factors in the wound can stimulate the overproduction of granulation tissue; most of them are related to inflammation and/or infection. A generalized wound infection may not lead to the formation of EGT but might arrest healing, resulting in an indolent wound. On the other hand, local infection related to the presence of bony sequestra, necrotic segments of tendons, ligaments or other tissue, and/or foreign bodies, triggers a chronic inflammatory response leading to the aforementioned cycle, especially when the condition is long-standing. Similarly, leukocytes are strongly attracted to wounds contaminated with dirt or bacteria, leading to chronic inflammation of the wound.

This emphasizes the importance of thoroughly examining a wound with EGT to identify or exclude factors related to inflammation and infection. If no specific causal factor is incriminated, the inherent chronic inflammatory response commonly occurring in limb wounds of horses may well be the trigger for the formation of EGT. This may, in fact, be the most common cause of EGT and often goes unrecognized because the signs of chronic inflammation may be limited to irregularity of the surface of the granulation bed accompanied by the presence of purulent exudate. These clinical signs, as well as culturing bacteria from the wound, do not indicate that a wound is infected. The wound usually improves dramatically, however, in response to reduction of the bioburden at the surface of the wound, in combination with a single local application of a corticosteroid, a fact substantiating the involvement of chronic inflammation in formation of EGT.

Specific clinical factors

Bandages and casts

Bandages used to cover wounds on the distal aspect of the limb are usually comprised of a primary layer (the dressing), a secondary layer that provides protection and support and can absorb excess exudate, and a tertiary layer that compresses and supports the other layers.[65] Full-thickness wounds on the distal aspect of the limb of horses have been shown to be more likely to develop EGT when covered with a bandage or cast than are similar wounds left unbandaged.[21,27,63–66] This effect is thought to result because bandaging or casting induce the following phenomena: (1) an increase in the oxygen gradient between deeper tissues and the surface of the wound, stimulating angiogenesis;[67] (2) a reduction in oxygen tension in the wound tissues, enhancing proliferation of fibroblasts;[18] and (3) the creation of a moist, warm, and acidic environment, favoring cellular migration and proliferation. Furthermore, some dressings can irritate the wound, evoking more inflammation, and can cause exudate to accumulate at the wound's surface. All these features prompt the formation of EGT.[62] In this respect, management practices can explain, at least partially, why EGT is more often seen in limb wounds because these wounds are usually bandaged whereas body wounds are not. Interestingly, body wounds, when bandaged, can also form EGT, albeit to a lesser degree. EGT would likely form more often in body wounds, if these wounds were routinely bandaged. In conclusion, management practices contribute to the effect of location on the formation of EGT.

The precise effect of bandages on the development of EGT is especially dependent on the type of dressing used. In general, the more occlusive the dressing, the higher is the incidence of EGT. Synthetic, occlusive dressings were shown to significantly stimulate the formation of EGT, thereby increasing the need to trim granulation tissue, compared to other less occlusive dressings.[68] This effect may be explained by an excessive accumulation of exudate beneath the occlusive dressing, which in turn, favors bacterial proliferation and encourages inflammation. Some dressings that are not occlusive by nature can nevertheless "seal" the wound because they insufficiently absorb exudate, causing it to accumulates at the wound's surface, thereby creating a barrier to diffusion. Likewise, the surface of wounds dressed with a non-occlusive dressing, such as gauze, may become occluded when exudate passing through the gauze into the secondary layer of the bandage causes the latter to become occlusive. Several topical wound-care products applied to the surface of a wound, particularly those of a fatty nature, may also cause occlusion.

Conversely, semi-occlusive dressings with a high absorptive capacity, such as foams, provide an environment for the wound that is less likely to induce the formation of EGT because exudate and bacteria are wicked away from the wound (the reader is referred to Chapter 6 for more information on wound dressings).

A notable exception to the general rule, "the more occlusive the dressing, the higher the incidence of EGT," pertains to an occlusive silicone gel sheet dressing (CicaCare®, Smith & Nephew) that was better able to prevent the formation of EGT in limb wounds of horses than was a permeable dressing (Melolite®, Smith & Nephew).[69] Silicone gel sheets are currently the gold standard dressing for managing excessive scarring of the skin in humans.[70,71] Although the mode of action of the silicone membrane is not entirely understood, the dressing has been shown, in people suffering from hypertrophic and keloid scars, to increase tissue temperature[72] and hydration,[73] thereby enhancing the activity of collagenase, which favors remodeling of ECM.[74]

Although bandages and casts can promote the formation of EGT, this does not preclude their use in managing wounds. To the contrary, bandages exert many positive influences on healing. They keep the wound clean and prevent contamination and irritation by environmental factors, such as dirt and straw, which induce inflammation. They facilitate administration of local wound therapies, stimulate more rapid formation of granulation tissue, which is initially required for healing, accelerate epithelialization by creating a moist environment, encourage the development of a more cosmetic scar,[64] reduce the risk for sarcoid transformation of the wound, and protect the wound from additional trauma. Additionally, casts restrict movement in highly mobile regions, thus reducing disruption of the healing process. All these functions limit the development of EGT. Bandages and casts are, therefore, an important component in the management of wounds healing by second intention, because the aim to support the overall healing process largely surpasses the need to prevent EGT.

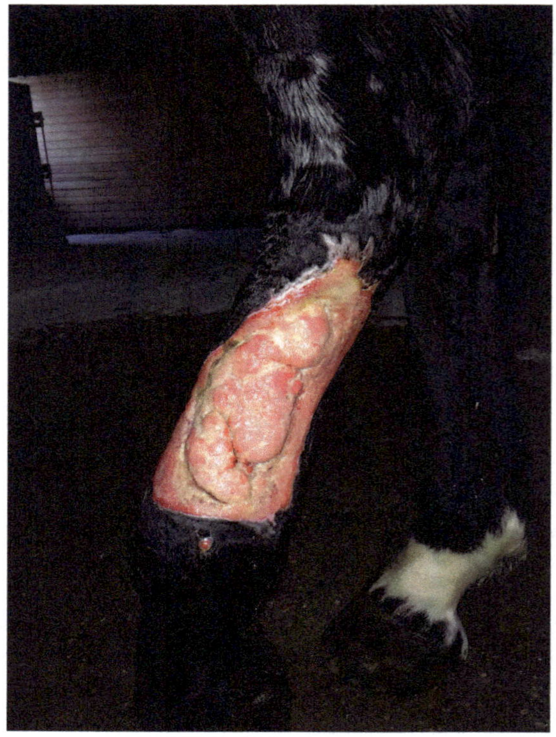

Figure 15.7 This wound, which initially exposed the metatarsal bone, was treated with disinfectant solutions (cleaned with Disifin solution – containing an N-chlorinated and N-deprotonated sulfonamide – followed by povidone-iodine spray 5%) for 2 months prior to the photo. The granulation tissue, which does not yet entirely fill the wound, is traversed by deep grooves and shows areas of necrotic tissue covered by purulent exudate. No bone sequestrum was visible radiographically. Although the disinfectants may have killed most bacteria in the wound, they are toxic to fibroblasts and could be responsible for the delayed formation of healthy granulation tissue.

Iatrogenic factors

The way in which a wound is managed in the early stages has a dramatic effect on the time required for healing, as well as on the formation of EGT. Application of non-physiologic materials, including powders and chemicals (e.g., antiseptics), as well as some antibiotics, may adversely affect wound healing (Figure 15.7). Additionally, application of caustic substances, including copper sulfate, nitric acid, acetic/malic acid mixtures, silver nitrate, triple dye, supersaturated potassium permanganate, sodium hypochlorite (Dakin's solution), lye, and many other home remedies, in an effort to prevent or treat EGT, seriously delays repair. These caustic agents induce necrosis not only of the granulation tissue but also of the migrating and proliferating epithelium.[62,75] Cryogenic surgery applied to granulating wounds similarly delays healing.[64] The resultant necrosis encourages a chronic inflammatory response and the release of many mediators that inhibit wound contraction and overstimulate cellular proliferation, as previously outlined. Healing by epithelialization and contraction is arrested, and the stimulus for formation of granulation tissue accrued, leading to a recurrence of EGT. Cautery of any type, therefore, delays healing and promotes more EGT. Although wounds treated in this way eventually heal, they are frequently characterized by unacceptable scarring.[75] The aforementioned problem is unfortunately still encountered in some equine practices, because many owners attempt to manage a wound themselves prior to consulting a veterinarian.

Differential diagnoses

EGT can be confused with tumors, especially sarcoids (Figure 15.8). An equine wound can transform into a sarcoid, a serious cause of failure of healing of a cutaneous wound (for more information the reader is referred to Chapter 21). Sarcoid transformation can occur at any wound, but the type of sarcoid that develops is highly dependent on the anatomic location of the wound. A sarcoid that forms in a wound on the distal aspect of the limb is invariably fibroblastic in nature, which explains why it is often confused with EGT. Horses with a sarcoid appear to be particularly prone to sarcoid transformation of wounds, as are horses in close contact with other horses bearing sarcoids. Transformation is also more likely to occur if the wound is left uncovered, especially in the summer when flies are abundant.

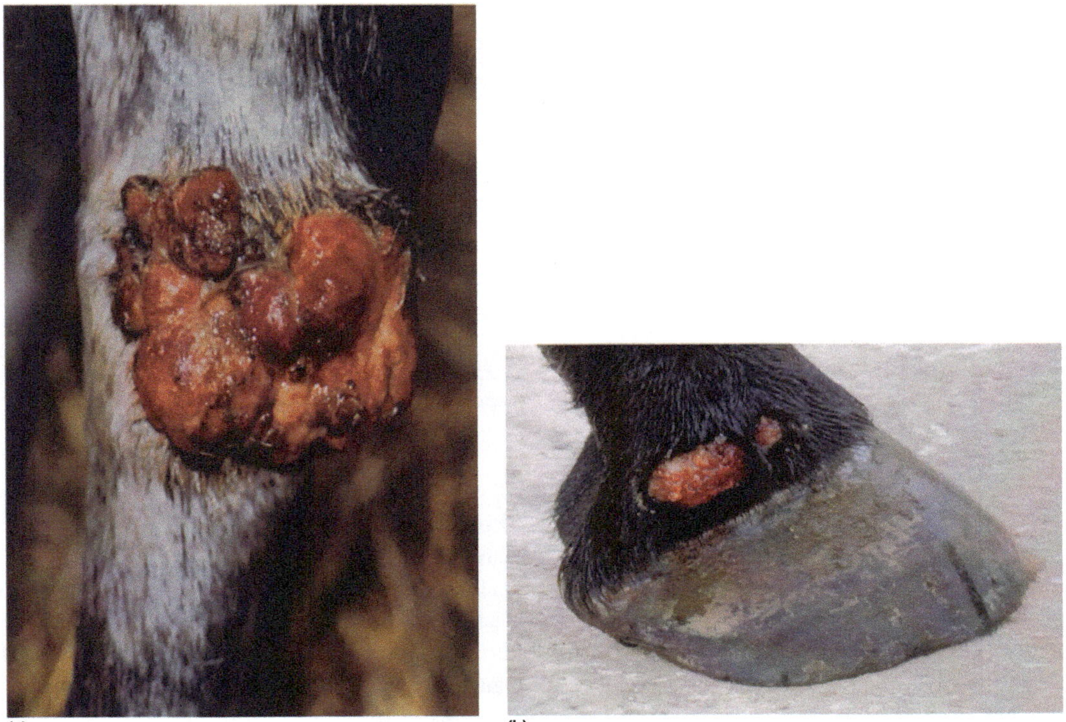

Figure 15.8 **(a)** A wound caused by a wire cut on the dorsal surface of the tarsus of a 5-year-old mare, which failed to heal. A harvested tissue sample allowed confirmation of pure sarcoid in the upper area and a mixture of sarcoid and EGT in the lower area of the wound. **(b)** Five-week-old wound in the pastern region of a gelding. The horse was admitted because the granulation tissue remained exuberant. Excised granulation tissue was examined histologically, enabling diagnosis of a pure fibroblastic sarcoid. Source: Wilmink and van Weeren 2004.[1] Reprinted with permission of Elsevier.

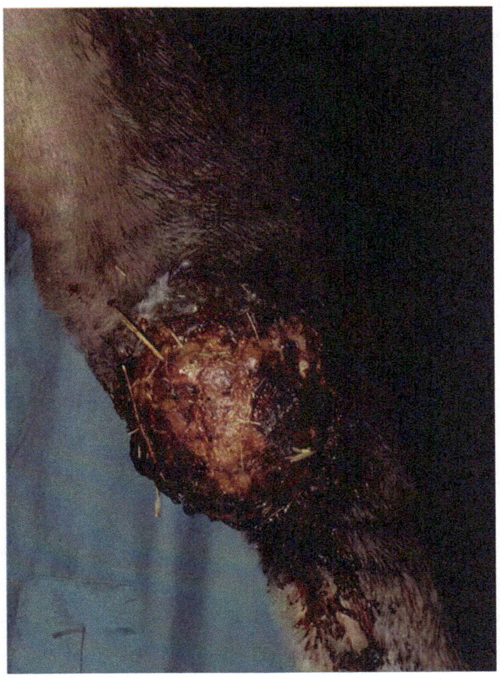

Figure 15.9 Wound on the dorsal surface of the tarsus that was treated for 6 months without resolution. Histologic examination of a tissue sample confirmed transformation to a squamous cell carcinoma. Courtesy of Dr. Ted Stashak.

Although uncommon, chronic granulating wounds can also transform into a squamous cell carcinoma (Figure 15.9). Conversely, some tumors, such as sarcoids, some hemangiomas, and squamous cell carcinomas, can develop independently of an apparent wound and adopt the appearance of granulation tissue.

If healing of a wound does not progress and tissue that appears to be EGT reappears regularly after being trimmed, excised tissue or a deep biopsy sample from the wound should be examined histologically, or a swab of the tissue should be examined using polymerase chain reaction (PCR),[76] to obtain a definitive diagnosis of sarcoid or other tumors. This is critical because the best practice for managing EGT is contraindicated in the management of sarcoids or other tumors.[75] For more information on the management of sarcoid transformation at wound sites, the reader is referred to Chapter 21.

Prevention of exuberant granulation tissue

Exclusion of factors related to inflammation and infection

The likelihood of a wound developing EGT can be reduced by excluding causal factors, particularly those that are related to inflammation and infection.

What to do

- Examine the wound for bony sequestra, necrotic segments of tendon or ligament, and foreign bodies, and eliminate these causes of inflammation.

What to avoid

- Avoid caustic compounds or other irritating substances.

Tip

- Use bandages (and splints or casts, where appropriate) to prevent additional contamination and trauma, protect exposed bone and tendons from desiccation and contamination, and reduce motion.

Use of bandages

Using pressure bandages to restrain excessive fibroplasia is counterproductive. These bandages may effectively suppress the swelling of young edematous granulation tissue but generally do not impair its formation.

The fact that bandaging limb wounds favors the development of EGT which, if not resected, delays healing, has led to the practice of controlling formation of EGT by omitting bandages after a wound has filled with granulation tissue. This approach was partly inspired by evidence that unbandaged wounds created experimentally in ponies healed faster and without EGT, although with more scarring, than did bandaged wounds in which healing was delayed by EGT.[64] Subsequent studies have determined that this approach may not be so straightforward. Unbandaged and bandaged experimental wounds on the limbs of horses healed in a similar amount of time when EGT that developed in the bandaged limbs was excised.[65,66]

Importantly, the magnitude of many clinically encountered wounds makes bandaging compulsory, in contrast to relatively harmless wounds created for experimental purposes that can be left unbandaged. In some situations, leaving a wound unbandaged after it is filled with granulation tissue is reasonable, for example when costs must be limited, when the horse is difficult to treat, or when the cosmetic outcome is unimportant. Leaving a limb wound unbandaged, however, may lead to increased swelling of the limb and arrested healing because of contamination and dessication.

In conclusion, the fact that bandages favor the formation of EGT, which can subsequently delay healing, must not be taken to mean that healing can be stimulated by omitting bandages. When managed correctly, EGT does not delay healing, and bandages provide more advantages than disadvantages. Moreover, the formation of EGT can be limited by selecting an appropriate wound dressing.

What to do

- Use bandages to prevent contamination and dessication of tissue.

What to avoid

- Avoid occlusion: i.e., occlusive dressings or topical products (except for silicone sheet dressings), collection of exudate on the wound due to infrequent bandage changes, wet padding (secondary layer of the bandage), and occlusive/plastic tapes as the tertiary layer of the bandage.

Tip

- Use a foam dressing as a primary layer, to absorb exudate and bacteria and thereby prevent occlusion.

Skin grafts

Skin grafts exert a significant inhibitory effect on the formation of EGT by controlling proliferation of endothelial cells and fibroblasts and by reducing the synthesis of components of ECM by fibroblasts. The inhibitory effect of grafts on fibroblasts may be regulated by a soluble epithelial-derived product that potentiates apoptosis of underlying cells.[61,77] A vascularized skin flap also favors apoptosis of fibroblasts and endothelial cells and rapid remodeling of the underlying granulation tissue.[78] This is likely the result of reduced expression of TGF-β1 along with increased degradation of the ECM due to an altered balance between MMPs and their inhibitor TIMP-1, as well as increased expression of inducible nitric oxide synthase (iNOS) generating free radicals that arrest the cell cycle and promote apoptosis.[78] Additionally, the ability of the graft to reduce the surface area of the wound, thereby attenuating inflammation, helps to control of the development of EGT. The reader is referred to Chapter 18 for more information on skin grafting in the horse.

Tip

- Skin grafts should be harvested from a site that normally heals well and in which contraction is prominent (e.g., the lateral cervical, abdominal, and pectoral regions).[75]

Treatment of exuberant granulation tissue

The treatment of EGT depends, to a certain extent, on the age of the wound and the nature of the granulation tissue. This section describes the situations most often encountered clinically.

Protruding young edematous granulation tissue

Young, edematous granulation tissue bulging just above the margin of the wound generally does not require special treatment. Swelling can usually be limited by moderate pressure exerted by

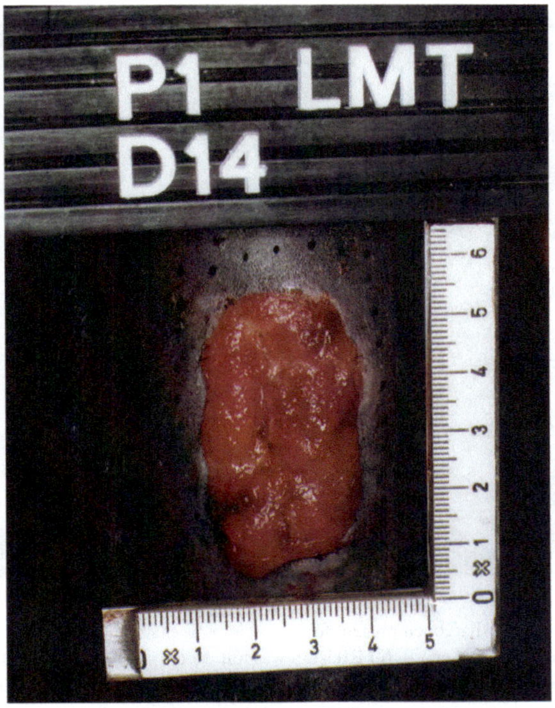

Figure 15.10 Example of a 2-week-old experimental wound created on the limb of a pony, showing edematous, protruding granulation tissue that does not yet qualify as EGT. Such increase of the swelling can be seen upon bandage change. Source: Wilmink and van Weeren 2004.[1] Reprinted with permission of Elsevier.

a bandage. Protrusion of the granulation tissue is noted when the bandage is removed, and increases when the wound is left uncovered for a short time (Figure 15.10). Frequently, the edematous swelling disappears when wound contraction begins. The tissue is classified as EGT when the protrusion feels firm and takes on a granular appearance. Firm tissue protruding over the margin of the wound should be treated.

Exuberant granulation tissue in general

Most limb wounds form some degree of EGT during healing. It is important to determine, by carefully examining the wound, if the periosteum was injured thereby exposing cortical bone or if a tendon or ligament was partially or completely severed. Bone sequestra, necrotic parts of tendons or ligaments, foreign bodies, or dirt can induce and perpetuate chronic inflammation that favors the development of EGT; these conditions, therefore, should be resolved.

What to do

- Probe any clefts that have formed within the new granulation tissue using flexible and rigid sterile probes to identify draining tracts. Complementary diagnostic modalities, such as radiographic or ultrasonographic examination, may be required.
- Radiographically examine underlying bone to rule out the possibility of a bone sequestrum when the injury has exposed cortical bone.

When the wound is located near or over a joint, movement is likely the reason EGT has formed. Immobilizing the wound, by applying a cast, can be helpful when the granulation tissue is freshly exuberant and appears healthy. When the wound is close to a synovial structure or when EGT is due to chronic inflammation that requires repeated treatment, a bandage splint is preferred to a cast (the reader is referred to Chapter 7 for more information on techniques of bandaging, splinting, and casting).

When no underlying inciting cause can be found, the most probable culprit for the formation of EGT is the inherent chronic inflammatory response characteristic of limb wounds of horses. Reducing surface contamination by thorough wound debridement and irrigation, followed by one topical application of corticosteroid, halts the aforementioned vicious cycle, allowing healing to ensue. The effect of a topically applied non-steroidal anti-inflammatory drug (NSAID) on chronic equine wounds is unknown, but topical application of a non-steroidal non-selective cyclooxygenase (COX) 1-2 inhibitor to experimental wounds of rabbits suffering chronic inflammation did not affect the number of leukocytes in the wounds and the NSAID delayed wound closure.[20]

In most cases, treatment of EGT is straightforward, and excision appears to be the best choice of treatment. Granulation tissue should be excised as soon as it protrudes above the wound's margin.[3] Excision can be performed with the horse standing, and desensitizing the wound is not necessary because granulation tissue is not innervated. The excess granulation tissue is excised as close to the adjacent skin level as possible while taking care to preserve the migrating epithelium at the wound's periphery. Excision should commence at the distal-most aspect of the wound and progress proximally so that hemorrhage does not obscure the surgical field. While a tourniquet may be applied above the wound in a sedated horse, it is rarely required to achieve the desired result. The goal of excision is to remove excess and non-viable tissue, as well as gross contaminants, which consequently, also eliminates a large number of leukocytes present in the superficial layer of the granulation tissue, thereby diminishing the stimulus for chronic inflammation. Dramatic improvement of the health of the wound's surface is usually achieved when excision is preceded by aseptic preparation of the skin around the wound and followed by sterile bandaging and a short period of topical antibacterial therapy to further reduce contamination (Figure 15.11). Indeed, repair gets a new impulse – contraction is "jump-started," and epithelialization proceeds. This said, repeated excisions may be required.

The use of silicone sheet dressings to prevent recurrence of EGT in horses has been validated.[69] The dressing should be applied after bleeding arising from excising EGT is controlled. The silicone sheet dressing should be maintained on the wound until contraction and epithelialization are underway, after which it may be replaced by a light foam dressing or maintained until healing is complete. The silicone dressing is reusable, which offsets its initial high cost.

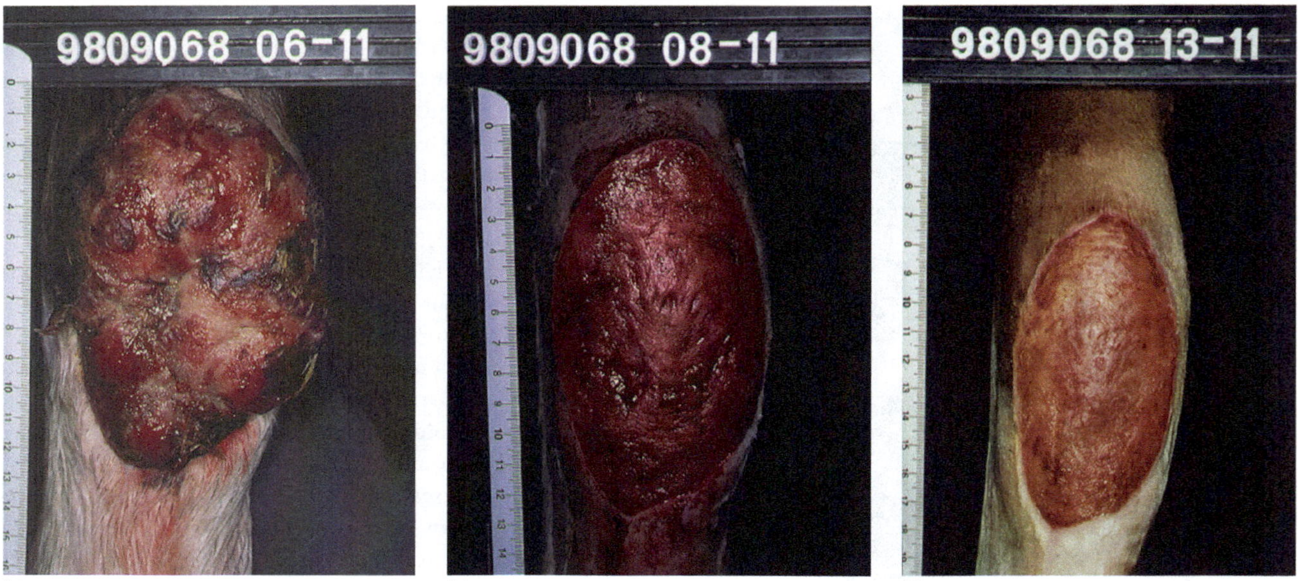

(a) (b) (c)

Figure 15.11 **(a)** Wound on the plantar surface of the metatarsus of a 3-year-old mare. EGT had been present for a couple of weeks and healing had ceased. **(b)** Two days after excision of EGT, dramatic improvement of the wound bed can be observed. **(c)** Excision was followed by a short-term course of topical antibacterial treatment supplemented with one topical application of corticosteroids the day before the picture was taken. Wound contraction has occurred and epithelialization has begun, thus diminishing the risk for recurrence of EGT. Source: Wilmink and van Weeren 2004.[1] Reprinted with permission of Elsevier.

Tip

- Washing a silicone sheet dressing gently under tap water with mild liquid detergent, as recommended by the manufacturer (Smith & Nephew), preserves the dressing's exceptional adherence to the wound's surface and allows it to be reused.

Topical application of a corticosteroid to arrest the formation of EGT remains controversial. Corticosteroids counter inflammation, and thus may be useful to control the chronic inflammatory response present in limb wounds of horses. Moreover, some corticosteroids may selectively attenuate the release of fibrogenic TGF-β1 and -β2 from monocytes and macrophages, counteracting proliferation of fibroblasts and formation of ECM.[79] This rationalizes the use of a corticosteroid in the treatment of newly formed EGT. Corticosteroids have been shown, however, to exert a negative influence on angiogenesis, contraction, and epithelialization thereby delaying wound healing.[80,81] A corticosteroid, therefore, if used, should be applied at the first signs of excessive fibroplasia but not repeatedly, so as to limit the negative influence exerted by the corticosteroid on healing.

A caustic agent or cryogenic surgery should not be used to treat EGT because these induce necrosis, stimulate chronic inflammation, damage the new epithelial border, and ultimately inhibit healing by promoting proliferation of the granulation tissue.

Recurrent exuberant granulation tissue

In some cases, in the absence of an apparent cause, EGT may recur in spite of repeat excisions and topical treatment to control chronic inflammation. This is seen more often when owners change the bandages. In these cases, the bandaging protocol should be critically assessed.

What to do

- Proceed with aseptic preparation of the skin surrounding the wound. Clean the wound using sterile isotonic saline solution and swabs, debride the wound using sterile instruments, apply antimicrobial dressings for 1–2 weeks to reduce surface contamination, and thereafter topically apply a single dose of a short-acting corticosteroid.

Tip

- Obtain a tissue sample for histologic examination in cases where tumor transformation of the wound is suspected.

Some horses mount a very strong and chronic inflammatory response at the site of a wound, often accompanied by periosteal new bone formation when the wound initially exposed bone. In such a case, resorting to repeated applications of a longer-acting corticosteroid, such as triamcinolone, may be appropriate to break the vicious cycle of "inflammation–proliferation."

Rarely, the only escape from recurrent EGT is to temporarily remove bandages in an effort to diminish the stimulus for fibroplasia. This option, however, may be considered unappealing from an esthetic perspective because such wounds are often large and particularly unattractive. Resuming bandaging of a large wound, after the wound is flat and contracting, is advantageous because bandaging provides a moist environment that encourages epithelialization. If exuberant-appearing granulation tissue recurs despite the aforementioned approach, the clinician should suspect tumor transformation of the wound.

What to do

- Obtain a tissue sample for histologic examination in cases where tumor transformation of the wound is suspected.

Exuberant granulation tissue after skin grafting

EGT may occur after skin grafting. In this case, excision is inadvisable because of the risk of damage to the newly grafted tissue. As soon as granulation tissue protrudes above the grafts, further development of EGT can be limited by intermittent topical application of a corticosteroid. Generally, after applying the corticosteroid topically only once or twice, epithelialization can be seen to progress from the grafts. The corticosteroid should not be applied too often because epithelialization from the graft margins will be disturbed. As soon as epithelialization progresses from the grafts, the development of EGT is naturally controlled.

Chronic exuberant granulation tissue

Horses having large lumps of chronic EGT are, unfortunately, known to most practitioners (Figure 15.12). Chronic EGT is usually very fibrous, is nourished by large blood vessels, and, in some cases, may be partially innervated. The impetus for healing of these wounds has disappeared and is unlikely to be recovered without intervention. Excising the EGT, followed by application of a skin graft is the best approach to get these wounds to heal at an optimum rate and with an acceptable outcome.[62] The wound can be debulked with the horse standing and sedated, but often debulking the wound with the horse anesthetized is more prudent because of the violent reaction that may be displayed when the EGT is excised, possibly because the tissue is partially reinnervated. Debulking with the horse anesthetized also allows for better control of hemorrhage and its possible systemic consequences. After excising the exuberant fibrous tissue, a pressure bandage is applied to control hemorrhage. Although excision can be followed immediately by skin grafting, in most cases, it is preferable to leave the wound ungrafted and bandaged for a few days until hemorrhage has abated and a new bed of granulation has begun to form (for more information on skin grafting, the reader is referred to Chapter 18).

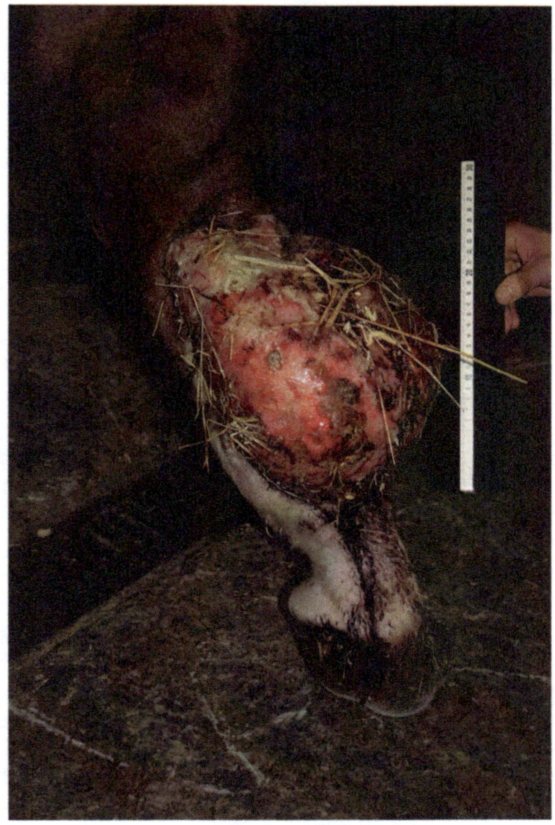

Figure 15.12 A wound with marked and chronic EGT. Treatment of such a wound is challenging. Excision of the EGT, followed by skin grafting, is the best approach.

Conclusion

The formation of EGT is a frequent complication in wounds healing by second intention on the limbs of horses. Among the large number of factors contributing to EGT, chronic inflammation is foremost and often goes unrecognized because of the mild accompanying signs. The stimulus for formation of EGT is reduced when prevention and treatment of chronic inflammation are combined with excision of the protruding granulation tissue. Transition from the fibroblastic phase of healing to the phases of contraction and epithelialization then occurs smoothly and usually obviates the recurrence of EGT.

Many approaches have been used to treat EGT, but the best therapy, at this time, remains excision of the protruding tissue. The limited and appropriate application of a corticosteroid and the use of silicone sheet dressings or skin grafting are useful to prevent EGT or its recurrence.

New methods of preventing the development of EGT are being sought through fundamental research in equine wound healing. Innovative, targeted therapies consisting of specialized interactive dressings combined with engineered reconstitution of tissues using cell-based therapy, scaffold-based therapy, and/or bioactive molecule-based therapy will likely someday be available (the reader is referred to Chapter 22 for more information on this topic).

References

1. Wilmink JM, van Weeren PR. Treatment of exuberant granulation tissue. *Clin Tech Equine Pract* 2004; **3**: 141.
2. Wilmink JM, Stolk PWT, van Weeren PR, *et al.* Differences in second-intention wound healing between horses and ponies: macroscopical aspects. *Equine Vet J* 1999; **31**: 53.
3. Wilmink JM, van Weeren PR, Stolk PWT, *et al.* Differences in second-intention wound healing between horses and ponies: histological aspects. *Equine Vet J* 1999; **31**: 61.
4. Shakespeare V, Shakespeare P. Effects of granulation-tissue-conditioned medium on the growth of human keratinocytes *in-vitro*. *Br J Plastic Surg* 1991; **44**: 219.
5. Moulin V. Growth factors in skin wound healing. *Eur J Cell Biol* 1995; **68**: 1.
6. Ignotz RA, Massague J. Transforming growth factor-β stimulates the expression of fibronectin and collagen and their incorporation into the extracellular matrix. *J Biol Chem* 1986; **261**: 4337.
7. Shah M, Revis D, Herrick S, *et al.* Role of elevated plasma transforming growth factor-beta1 levels in wound healing. *Am J Pathol* 1999; **154**: 1115.
8. Clark RAF. Regulation of fibroplasia in cutaneous wound repair. *Am J Med Sci* 1993; **306**: 42.
9. Stadelmann WK, Digenis AG, Tobin GR. Physiology and healing dynamics of chronic cutaneous wounds. *Am J Surg* 1998; **176**: 26.
10. Studzinski DM, Benjamins JA. Cyclic AMP differentiation of the oligodendroglial cell line N20.1 switches staurosporine-induced cell death from necrosis to apoptosis. *J Neurosci Res* 2001; **66**: 691.
11. Wilmink JM, Nederbragt H, van Weeren PR, *et al.* Differences in wound contraction between horses and ponies: the *in vitro* contraction capacity of fibroblasts. *Equine Vet J* 2001; **33**: 499.
12. Bacon Miller C, Wilson DA, Keegan KG, *et al.* Growth characteristics of fibroblasts isolated from the trunk and distal aspect of the limb of horses and ponies. *Vet Surg* 2000; **29**: 1.
13. Van Den Boom R, Wilmink JM, O'Kane S, *et al.* Transforming growth factor-β levels during second intention healing are related to the different course of wound contraction in horses and ponies. *Wound Repair Regen* 2002; **10**: 188.
14. Wilmink JM, Veenman JN, van den Boom R, *et al.* Differences in polymorphonucleocyte function and local inflammatory response between horses and ponies. *Equine Vet J* 2003; **35**: 561.
15. LePoole IC, Boyce ST. Keratinocytes suppress TGF-β1 expression by fibroblasts in cultured skin substitutes. *Br J Dermatol* 1999; **140**: 409.
16. Ehrlich HP, Wyler DJ. Fibroblast contraction of collagen lattices in vitro: inhibition by chronic inflammatory cell mediators. *J Cell Physiol* 1983; **116**: 345.
17. Kovacs EJ. Fibrogenic cytokines: the role of immune mediators in the development of scar tissue. *Immunol Today* 1991; **12**: 17.
18. Kirsner RS, Eaglstein WH. The wound healing process. *Dermatol Clin* 1993; **11**: 629.
19. Deschene K, Céleste C, Boerboom D, Theoret CL. Hypoxia regulates the expression of extracellular matrix associated proteins in equine dermal fibroblasts via HIF1. *J Dermatol Sci* 2012; **65**: 12.
20. Qian LW, Fourcaudot AB, Yamane K, *et al.* Exacerbated and prolonged inflammation impairs wound healing and increases scarring. *Wound Repair Regen* 2016; **24**: 26.
21. Barber SM. Second intention wound healing in the horse: the effect of bandages and topical corticosteroids. *Proc Am Ass Equine Practnrs* 1989; **35**: 107.
22. Cochrane CA. Models *in vivo* of wound healing in the horse and the role of growth factors. *Vet Dermatol* 1997; **8**: 259.
23. Theoret CL, Barber SM, Moyana TN, *et al.* Expression of transforming growth factor β_1, β_3, and basic fibroblast factor in full-thickness skin wounds of equine limbs and thorax. *Vet Surg* 2001; **30**: 269.
24. Schwartz AJ, Wilson DA, Keegan KG, *et al.* Factors regulating collagen synthesis and degradation during second-intention healing of wounds in the thoracic region and the distal aspect of the forelimb of horses. *Am J Vet Res* 2002; **63**: 1564.
25. Quaglino D, Nanney LB, Ditesheim JA, *et al.* Transforming growth factor-β stimulates wound healing and modulates extracellular matrix gene expression in pig skin: incisional wound model. *J Invest Dermatol* 1991; **97**: 34.
26. Sarrazy V, Billet F, Micallef L, *et al.* Mechanisms of pathological scarring: role of myofibroblasts and current developments. *Wound Repair Regen* 2011; **19**: S10.
27. Theoret CL, Barber SM, Moyana TN, *et al.* Preliminary observations on expression of transforming growth factors β1 and β3 in equine full-thickness skin wounds healing normally or with exuberant granulation tissue. *Vet Surg* 2002; **31**: 266.
28. De Martin I, Theoret CL. Spatial and temporal expression of types I and II receptors for transforming growth factor β in normal equine skin and dermal wounds. *Vet Surg* 2004; **33**: 70.
29. Grinnell F, Zhu M, Carlson MA, *et al.* Release of mechanical tension triggers apoptosis of human fibroblasts in a model of regressing granulation tissue. *Exp Cell Res* 1999; **248**: 608.
30. Suarez E, Syed F, Rasgado TA, *et al.* Skin equivalent tensional force alter keloid fibroblast behavior and phenotype. *Wound Repair Regen* 2014; **22**: 557.
31. Falanga V, Qian SW, Danielpour D *et al.* Hypoxia upregulates the synthesis of TGF-beta 1 by human dermal fibroblasts. *J Invest Dermatol* 1991; **97**: 634.
32. Chvapil M, Pfister T, Escalada S, *et al.* Dynamics of the healing of skin wounds in the horse as compared with the rat. *Exp Mol Pathol* 1979; **30**: 349.
33. http://www.fda.gov/NewsEvents/Newsroom/PressAnnouncements/ucm199736.htm (accessed February 10, 2015).
34. Bae-Harboe YS, Harboe-Schmidt JE, Graber E, Gilchrest BA. Collagenase followed by compression for the treatment of earlobe keloids. *Dermatol Surg* 2014; **40**: 519.
35. Lefebvre-Lavoie J, Lussier JG, Theoret CL. Profiling of differentially expressed genes in wound margin biopsies of horses using suppression subtractive hybridization. *Physiol Genomics* 2005; **22**: 157.
36. Ipiña Z, Lussier JG, Theoret CL. Nucleotide structure and expression of equine pigment epithelium-derived factor during repair of experimentally induced wounds in horses. *Am J Vet Res* 2009; **70**: 112.
37. Miragliotta V, Lefebvre-Lavoie J, Lussier JG, Theoret CL. OB-cadherin cloning and expression in a model of wound repair in horses. *Equine Vet J* 2008; **40**: 643.
38. Miragliotta V, Lefebvre-Lavoie J, Lussier JG, Theoret CL. Equine ANAXA2 and MMP1 expression analyses in an experimental model of normal and pathological wound repair. *J Dermatol Sci* 2008; **51**: 103.
39. Miragliotta V, Lussier JG, Theoret CL. Laminin receptor 1 is differentially expressed in thoracic and limb wounds in the horse. *Vet Dermatol* 2009; **20**: 27.

40. Miragliotta V, Raphäel K, Lussier JG, Theoret CL. Equine lumican (LUM) cDNA sequence and spatio-temporal expression in an experimental model of normal and pathological wound healing. *Vet Dermatol* 2009; **20**: 243.
41. Miragliotta V, Pirone A, Donadio E, *et al.* Osteopontin expression in healing wounds of horses and in human keloids. *Equine Vet J* 2016; **48**: 72.
42. Miragliotta V, Ipiña Z, Lefebvre-Lavoie J, *et al.* Equine CTNNB1 and PECAM1 nucleotide structure and expression analyses in an experimental model of normal and pathological wound repair. *BMC Physiol* 2008; **8**: 1.
43. Miragliotta V, Raphaël K, Ipiña Z, *et al.* Equine thrombospondin II and secreted protein acidic and cysteine-rich in a model of normal and pathological wound repair. *Physiol Genomics* 2009; **38**: 149.
44. Lepault E, Céleste C, Dore M, *et al.* Comparative study on microvascular occlusion and apoptosis in body and limb wounds in the horse. *Wound Repair Regen* 2005; **13**: 520.
45. Dubuc V, Lepault E, Theoret CL. Endothelial cell hypertrophy is associated with microvascular occlusion in limb wounds of horses. *Can J Vet Res* 2006; **70**: 206.
46. Kischer CW, Shetlar MR, Shetlar CL. Alteration of hypertrophic scars induced by mechanical pressure. *Arch Dermatol* 1975; **111**: 60.
47. Theoret CL, Wilmink JM. Aberrant wound healing in the horse: naturally occurring conditions reminiscent of those observed in man. *Wound Repair Regen* 2013; **21**: 365.
48. Theoret CL, Olutoye OO, Parnell LK, Hicks J. Equine exuberant granulation tissue and human keloids: a comparative histopathologic study. *Vet Surg* 2013; **42**: 783.
49. Céleste CJ, Deschesne K, Riley CB, Theoret CL. Skin temperature during cutaneous wound healing in an equine model of cutaneous fibroproliferative disorder: kinetics and anatomic-site differences. *Vet Surg* 2013; **42**: 147.
50. Céleste CJ, Deschene K, Riley CB, Theoret CL. Regional differences in wound oxygenation during normal healing in an equine model of cutaneous fibroproliferative disorder. *Wound Repair Regen* 2011; **19**: 89.
51. Sorensen MA, Petersen LJ, Bundgaard L, *et al.* Regional disturbances in blood flow and metabolism in equine limb wound healing with formation of exuberant granulation tissue. *Wound Repair Regen* 2014; **22**: 647.
52. Sen CK. Wound healing essentials: let there be oxygen. *Wound Repair Regen* 2009; **17**: 1.
53. McGovern NN, Cowburn AS, Porter L, *et al.* Hypoxia selectively inhibits respiratory burst activity and killing of *Staphylococcus aureus* in human neutrophils. *J Immunol* 2011; **186**: 453.
54. Falanga V, Zhou L, Yufit T. Low oxygen tension stimulates collagen synthesis and COLIA1 transcription through the action of TGF-beta1. *J Cell Physiol* 2002; **191**: 42.
55. Slovis N. Review of equine hyperbaric medicine. *J Equine Vet Sci* 2008; **28**: 760.
56. Eskes A, Vermeulen H, Lucas C, Ubbink DT. Hyperbaric oxygen therapy for treating acute surgical and traumatic wounds. *Cochrane Database Syst Rev* 2013; **12**: CD008059.
57. Holder TE, Schumacher J, Donnell RL, *et al.* Effects of hyperbaric oxygen on full-thickness meshed sheet skin grafts applied to fresh and granulating wounds in horses. *Am J Vet Res* 2008; **69**: 144.
58. Tracey AK, Alcott CJ, Schleining JA, *et al.* The effects of topical oxygen therapy on equine distal limb dermal wound healing. *Can Vet J* 2014; **55**: 1146.
59. Chodon T, Sugihara T, Igawa HH, *et al.* Keloid-derived fibroblasts are refractory to Fas-mediated apoptosis and neutralization of autocrine transforming growth factor-beta1 can abrogate this resistance. *Am J Pathol* 2000; **157**: 1661.
60. Zhao R, Yan Q, Huang H, *et al.* Transdermal siRNA-TGFβ1-337 patch for hypertrophic scar treatment. *Matrix Biol* 2013; **32**: 265.
61. Greenhalgh DG. The role of apoptosis in wound healing. *Int J Biochem Cell B* 1998; **30**: 1019.
62. Bertone AL. Management of exuberant granulation tissue. *Vet Clin N Am Equine Pract* 1989; **5**: 551.
63. Woollen N, RM DeBowes, Liepold HW, *et al.* A comparison of four types of therapy for the treatment of full thickness wounds of the horse. *Proc Am Ass Equine Practnrs* 1987; **33**: 569.
64. Fretz PB, Martin GS, Jacobs KA, *et al.* Treatment of exuberant granulation tissue in the horse: evaluation of four methods. *Vet Surg* 1983; **12**: 137.
65. Dart AJ, Perkins NR, Dart CM, *et al.* Effect of bandaging on second intention healing of wounds of the distal limb in horses. *Aust Vet J* 2009; **87**: 215.
66. Berry DB, Sullins KE. Effects of topical application of antimicrobials and bandaging on healing and granulation tissue formation in wounds of the distal aspect of the limbs in horses. *Am J Vet Res* 2003; **64**: 88.
67. Knighton DR, Silver IA, Hunt TK. Regulation of wound-healing angiogenesis. Effect of oxygen gradients and inspired oxygen concentration. *Surg* 1981; **90**: 262.
68. Howard RD, Stashak TS, Baxter GM. Evaluation of occlusive dressings for management of full-thickness excisional wounds on the distal portion of the limbs of horses. *Am J Vet Res* 1993; **54**: 2150.
69. Ducharme-Desjarlais M, Céleste CJ, Lepault E, Theoret CL. Effect of a silicone-containing dressing on exuberant granulation tissue formation and wound repair in horses. *Am J Vet Res* 2005; **66**: 1133.
70. Meaume S, Le Pillouer-Prost A, Richert B, *et al.* Management of scars: updated practical guidelines and use of silicones. *Eur J Dermatol* 2014; **24**: 435.
71. Monstrey S, Middelkoop E, Vranckx JJ, *et al.* Updated scar management practical guidelines: non-invasive and invasive measures. *J Plast Reconstr Aesthet Surg* 2014; **67**: 1017.
72. Musgrave MA, Umraw N, Fish JS, *et al.* The effect of silicone gel sheets on perfusion of hypertrophic burn scars. *J Burn Care Rehabil* 2002; **23**: 208.
73. Gilman TH. Silicone sheet for treatment and prevention of hypertrophic scar: a new proposal for the mechanism of efficacy. *Wound Repair Regen* 2003; **11**: 235.
74. Borgognoni L. Biological effects of silicone gel sheeting. *Wound Repair Regen* 2002; **10**: 118.
75. Knottenbelt DC. Skin grafting. In: Knottenbelt D (ed). *Handbook of Equine Wound Management*. WB Saunders Co: London, 2003: 79.
76. Martens A, De Moor A, Ducatelle R. PCR detection of bovine papilloma virus DNA in superficial swabs and scrapings from equine sarcoids. *Vet J* 2001; **161**: 280.

77. Desmoulière A, Redard M, Darby I, *et al.* Apoptosis mediates the decrease in cellularity during the transition between granulation tissue and scar. *Am J Pathol* 1995; **146**: 56.
78. Darby IA, Bisucci T, Pittet B, *et al.* Skin flap-induced regression of granulation tissue correlates with reduced growth factor and increased metalloproteinase expression. *J Pathol* 2002; **197**: 117.
79. Beer HD, Fässler R, Werner S. Glucocorticoid-regulated gene expression during cutaneous wound repair. *Vitam Horm* 2000; **59**: 217.
80. Hashimoto I, Nakanishi H, Shono Y, *et al.* Angiostatic effects of corticosteroid on wound healing of the rabbit ear. *J Med Invest* 2002; **49**: 61.
81. Kaufman KL, Mann FA, Kim DY, *et al.* Evaluation of the effects of topical zinc gluconate in wound healing. *Vet Surg* 2014; **43**: 972.

CHAPTER 16

Diagnosis and Management of Wounds Involving Synovial Structures

Kathryn A. Seabaugh, DVM, MS, Diplomate ACVS and ACVSMR and **Gary M. Baxter**, VMD, MS, Diplomate ACVS

Chapter Contents

Summary

Wounds in the horse frequently involve synovial structures. Prompt recognition of synovial involvement, and treatment, are important to prevent or resolve synovial infection. The primary goals of treatment are to remove bacteria, foreign material, and inflammatory mediators from the synovial structure, through the use of high-volume lavage and administration of broad-spectrum antimicrobial drugs. Methods of diagnosis and treatment of contaminated or infected synovial structures are detailed in this chapter.

Introduction

Horses frequently sustain injury. Forty percent of horse owners responding to a survey in the United Kingdom reported that their horse had suffered an injury within the previous 12 months.[1] Of those injuries, 54% were wounds.

Wounds of the limb are especially at risk of involving a synovial structure (joint, tendon sheath, or bursa). Wounds that communicate with a synovial cavity can result in synovial infection, which may lead to permanent disability. Septic synovitis can result in irreversible cartilaginous damage, capsular fibrosis,

Equine Wound Management, Third Edition. Edited by Christine Theoret and Jim Schumacher.

Companion website: www.wiley.com/go/theoret/wound

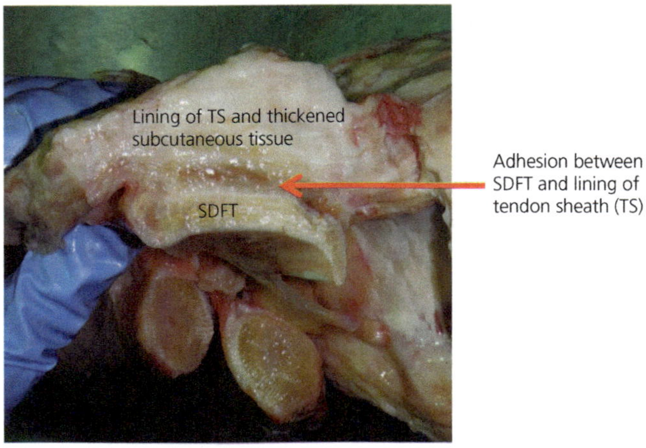

Figure 16.1 An adhesion is present between the superficial digital flexor tendon (SDFT) and the plantar surface of the digital flexor tendon sheath.

and intrathecal adhesions if the infection is not eliminated rapidly (Figure 16.1).[2] Early recognition of synovial involvement to prevent the development of infection, together with appropriate treatment, is the best protection against the negative consequences that often accompany these wounds.

Location of Injuries

Although any synovial structure of the horse might be breached by a laceration or a puncture, the synovial cavities of the distal aspect of the limb (i.e., distal to and including the carpus and tarsus) are most frequently wounded.[3–5] Synovial structures most often penetrated include the following: the digital flexor tendon sheath, the metacarpo/metatarsophalangeal joint, and the tarsal joints.[5–7] Although most injuries involve a single synovial structure, large wounds, particularly those of the foot, shoulder, and tarsal regions, may result in contamination of multiple synovial structures.

> **Tip**
>
> - Know the anatomy of the horse's limb. This allows quick identification of synovial structures that could be involved in the wound.

Synovial anatomy and physiology

Joints

Joints are closed, sterile spaces of variable size and shape located around opposing bony surfaces that enable the limb to flex and extend. The ends of bones within joints are covered with hyaline cartilage and are usually stabilized by a combination of collateral ligaments, a joint capsule, tendons, and muscle. The joint capsule is composed of an outer fibrous layer and an inner synovial membrane. The fibrous joint capsule is attached to bone and/or soft-tissue structures on the perimeter of the joint and serves to protect the joint cavity from injury. The synovial membrane is composed of intimal and subintimal layers that line the synovial capsule. The cells within the intimal layer are responsible for producing components of the synovial fluid, for absorbing products from the joint cavity, and for exchange of ions and molecules between blood and synovial fluid.[8] The subintimal layer contains the vascular supply and nerves to the joint.[8] Proper function of the synovial membrane is especially important for joints because the synovial fluid is vital for maintaining the health of the articular cartilage.

Synovial fluid contains lubricants (i.e., hyaluronan and lubricin) that ensure frictionless movement of opposing bone and/or soft tissue.[8,9] The close proximity of the fibrous layer of the joint capsule of many synovial cavities to the skin results in damage to the joint when the overlying skin is lacerated. Although a wound can penetrate the fibrous capsule without penetrating the inner synovial membrane, this situation is observed uncommonly in horses. Complications of joint infection in horses include damage to articular cartilage, leading to osteoarthritis and lameness, fibrosis of the joint capsule, resulting in reduced range of motion, and chronic osteomyelitis.[4]

Tendon sheaths and bursae

Tendon sheaths and bursae serve primarily to protect and promote the normal gliding motion of tendons. Bursae are located between a tendon and an adjacent bone in a high-motion area; examples are the navicular and the bicipital bursae. In contrast to joints, bone surfaces associated with bursae are covered with fibrocartilage, rather than hyaline cartilage. Tendon sheaths are located in areas of high motion, such as the palmar/plantar regions of metacarpo/metatarsophalangeal joints, and serve a function similar to that of bursae. Bursae, unlike tendon sheaths, do not completely surround the tendinous structure, and are located on one side of the tendon only, between the tendon and the underlying bony prominence.[10] Annular ligaments and retinaculi (adjacent to many sheaths and bursae) overlie the synovial cavity and form an inelastic canal through which the tendon glides.[11]

The inner synovial membrane and outer fibrous layer of tendon sheaths and bursae are anatomically similar to those of joint capsules. The primary anatomic difference is that most tendon sheaths and bursae have one or more annular ligaments and/or retinaculi that function to stabilize the tendon. Damage to these supporting structures can result in "subluxation" of the tendon from the synovial cavity, the most common subluxation being distraction of the superficial digital flexor tendon from the calcaneal bursa.[4,12]

The synovial fluid within a tendon sheath or bursa is similar to that within joints and possesses many of the same properties and functions. Lubrication within tendon sheaths and bursae is possibly even more critical to pain-free movement than is lubrication within joints due to the high mobility of the tendon within the tendon sheath or against the bursa.[11,13] Complications of infection of tendon sheaths and bursae include formation of adhesions within the sheath, septic and non-septic tendonitis, and osteomyelitis of the adjacent bone, leading to restricted movement and chronic lameness (Figure 16.2).

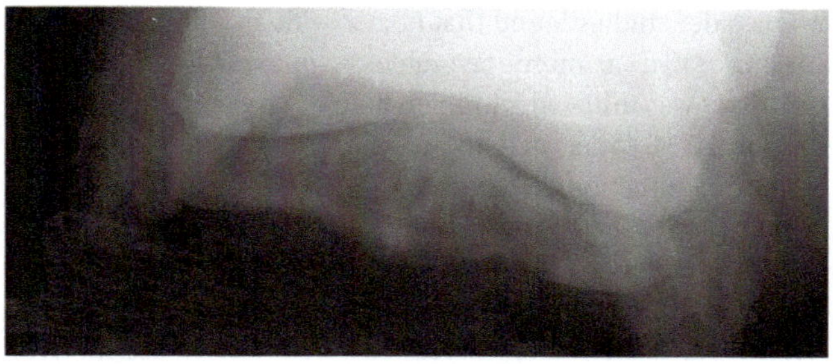

Figure 16.2 This skyline radiograph is from a horse that sustained a puncture wound to the foot approximately 6 weeks earlier. Severe lysis of the navicular bone is evident, consistent with chronic infection of the navicular bursa.

Pathogenesis of synovial infections

A laceration or puncture into synovial structures often introduces bacteria and contaminants (e.g., hair, dander, dirt) directly into the synovial space (Figure 16.3). Provided that appropriate treatment is performed early, infectious arthritis, tenosynovitis, or bursitis can be avoided.[3,4] Early diagnosis of and treatment for an open synovial structure is important to provide the best chance for the horse to return to pre-injury-level athletic performance.

The size of the bacterial inoculum required to produce a synovial infection varies according to: (1) the virulence of the bacteria; (2) the specific joint, tendon sheath, or bursa involved (i.e., size of the inoculum in relation to the size of the synovial cavity); (3) the severity of the concurrent soft-tissue trauma; (4) the immune response of the horse; and (5) whether or not foreign material is present.[14,15] Experimentally, 1.6×10^6 colony-forming units (CFU) of *Staphylococcus aureus* injected into the tarsocrural joint of normal horses caused synovial infection.[16] In another study, as few as 33 CFU of *S. aureus*, combined with polysulfated glycosaminoglycans (PSGAGs), inserted into the middle carpal joint of horses resulted in synovial infection.[17] The results of these studies indicate that a very small bacterial inoculum, under the right conditions, is capable of causing synovial infection.

Bacterial colonization of the synovial membrane incites an inflammatory response intended to re-sterilize the synovial structure.[18] The inflammatory cascade produces a multitude of cytokines, proteolytic enzymes, and other inflammatory mediators from a variety of cell types within the synovial cavity. These inflammatory mediators serve to increase vascular permeability within the synovium, attract neutrophils and monocytes to the synovial space, degrade hyaluronan within the synovial fluid, and promote the formation of fibrin.[18] Reactive oxygen metabolites and proteolytic enzymes derived from infiltrating neutrophils, chondrocytes, synoviocytes, monocytes, macrophages, and the bacteria may contribute to the degradation of hyaluronan and depletion of proteoglycans in the articular cartilage.[19,20] In one *in vitro* study, exposure of cartilage explants to *Escherichia coli* or *S. aureus* caused a 28% and 83% loss of glycosaminoglycan from cartilage, respectively, and induced death of chondrocytes within 48 hours of exposure.[21]

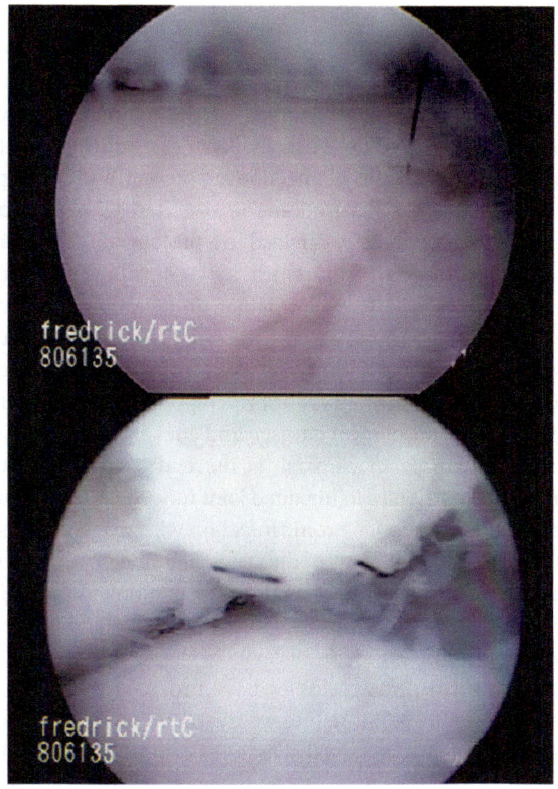

Figure 16.3 An arthroscopic view of the distal interphalangeal (coffin) joint that sustained a penetrating wound 24 hours earlier. Note the pieces of hair and debris within the joint. These foreign bodies could be identified only by endoscopic examination of the joint, and it is unlikely they could have been removed by lavage alone, without arthroscopic observation. Source: Baxter 2004.[4] Reproduced with permission of Elsevier.

Tip

- After bacteria within a closed synovial space overwhelm the natural defenses of the host, detrimental effects on cartilage, synovium, and other associated synovial structures ensue rapidly.

Synovial sepsis often results in the formation of a fibrinocellular clot, referred to as pannus, which is similar to the biofilm found on the surface of infected bone.[15] Pannus impedes effective treatment of synovial sepsis by protecting foreign debris and devitalized tissue, by serving as a bacterial growth medium, and by inhibiting delivery of drugs to the site of infection.[15] Although pannus is a term used primarily to describe what occurs within infected joints, a similar yet often more substantial deposition of fibrinous material often occurs within an infected tendon sheath or bursa. Fibrin is often abundant within an infected tendon sheath or bursa and should be removed because it may serve as a scaffold for the formation of fibrous tissue/adhesions within the structure.

Time to treatment

The longer the duration of the infection, the greater is the likelihood of permanent damage to the synovial structure. Alterations in synovial fluid usually occur early during infection, often before clinical signs of infection are present, and can impede function of the synovial membrane and interfere with nutrition of chondrocytes.[22] Chronicity can lead to a prolonged inflammatory response by the synovium, which may contribute to synovial hyperplasia and hypertrophy, vascular proliferation, thrombosis of synovial vessels, pannus, and fibrosis of the joint capsule.[15] Prolonged infection of a joint may lead to disease of the articular cartilage, resulting in the loss of proteoglycans and exposure of the cartilage to mechanical damage and enzymatic breakdown.[20] Irreversible damage to cartilage is the end stage of infectious arthritis and contributes to impaired joint function and permanent lameness (Figure 16.4). Chronic infection within a tendon sheath or bursa can lead to fibrosis of the synovial lining, tendonitis with superficial fraying of the tendon, formation of adhesions, development of fibrotic masses within the sheath, and osteomyelitis of bone within the synovial cavity.[4,11,13]

Multiple retrospective studies have provided mixed reports regarding the effect of timeliness of treatment on the outcome of horses with infected synovial structures caused by a wound.[23–28]

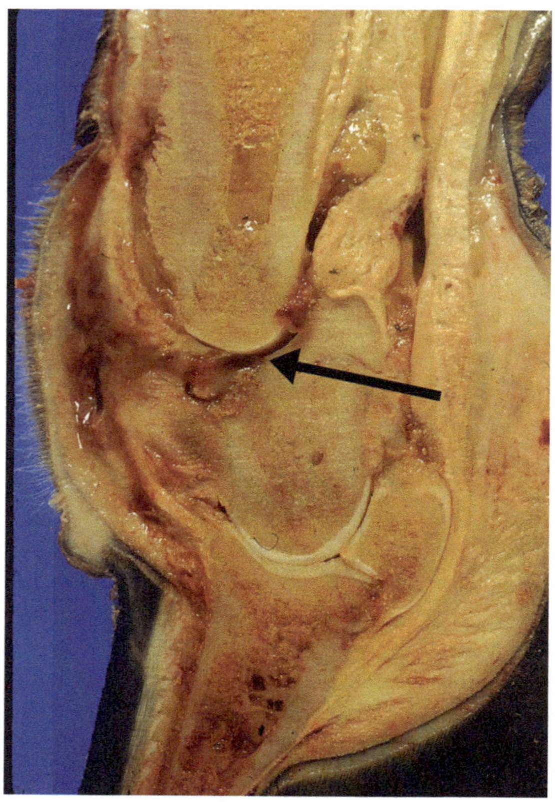

Figure 16.4 This postmortem sagittal section of the phalanges demonstrates the damage that can occur with chronic infection of the proximal interphalangeal joint secondary to a wound. The articular cartilage was completely lost from all joint surfaces, and bone within the middle phalanx was lysed (arrow).

A few older studies found that horses with an infected synovial structure had a more favorable response to treatment if treatment was initiated within 36 hours of injury.[27,28] Fraser and Bladon (2004) found that horses with a laceration involving the digital flexor tendon sheath were more likely to return to athletic function if the sheath was lavaged and debrided endoscopically within 36 hours of injury.[27] Gibson *et al.* (1989) reported a 65% incidence of survival when horses with an open joint were treated within 24 hours, whereas only 38.5% of horses survived when treatment was initiated more than 48 hours after injury.[28] Wereszka *et al.* (2007) found that horses with septic tenosynovitis were significantly more likely to survive if treated during the first day after clinical signs of synovial infection were first observed than were horses that did not receive treatment within 10 days after clinical signs of infection first appeared.[26] Promptness of treatment, however, did not seem to affect the incidence of survival of horses for which treatment was initiated between days 1 and 10 of observation of clinical signs of synovial infection. More recent reports have found no significant difference in the incidence of survival or the likelihood of return to function based on the time elapsed between the onset of clinical signs of synovial infection and initiation of treatment.[7,23,24,29] Although early treatment of horses with synovial infection is obviously desirable, the outcome for horses with delayed treatment of synovial sepsis may still be favorable.

Clinical findings

In most cases, a wound is the reason why a horse with a septic synovial structure is presented to a veterinarian. If the wound is fresh, the horse may be fully weight-bearing on the injured limb. A small wound may be missed until lameness or a swelling is observed (Figure 16.5). If the wound and synovial cavity continue to drain, lameness may be subtle, even when the

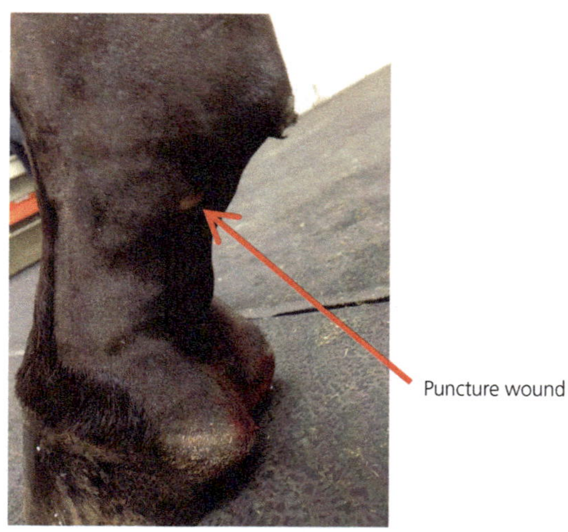

Figure 16.5 This horse was seen backing into a pitchfork 1 week prior. The small puncture wound was not identified until the area was clipped. The puncture communicated with the digital flexor tendon sheath.

wound is chronic. When infection becomes established within a closed synovial structure, however, lameness usually becomes severe.[30]

Wound assessment

Any wound near a synovial structure should be assumed to communicate with that synovial structure until disproven. The anatomic location of joints and tendon sheaths is well known, but some clinicians may not appreciate the magnitude of the various synovial pouches (Figure 16.6). For example, the palmar pouch of the metacarpophalangeal joint extends further distally on the proximal phalanx than most clinicians realize. The location of many bursae can be elusive, thwarting recognition of their involvement in a wound. Table 16.1 gives a list of bursae that could be involved in a wound.

Wounds near synovial structures must be cleaned thoroughly after the hair from the wound's edge has been clipped. After the wound is cleaned, it should be explored, once the clinician has donned sterile gloves, using caution to avoid carrying contamination deeper into the wound.[30] Proteinaceous fluid flowing from the edge of a wound often appears similar to synovial fluid; consequently, the presence of such fluid within a wound is not confirmation that the wound communicates with a synovial structure. Palpation or visual identification of the surface of a joint or tendon confirms that the wound communicates with a synovial structure. Contrast radiographic and/or ultrasonographic examinations may be necessary to assess the integrity of a synovial structure.

> **What to avoid**
>
> - While exploring a wound, do not inadvertently push debris further into it, especially if the wound could possibly communicate with a synovial structure.

If communication between a wound and a synovial structure cannot be determined by physical examination, further diagnostic tests may be necessary. Imaging of the region and cytologic evaluation of fluid obtained by synoviocentesis from synovial structures adjacent to the wound may provide additional clues as to whether a synovial structure has been breached.

Synoviocentesis

When performing synoviocentesis, the needle should be placed at a site remote from the wound to minimize the risk of iatrogenic contamination. When cellulitis is present, the risks of synoviocentesis should be weighed against its benefits. Cleaning the wound, bandaging the limb, and administering an antimicrobial drug for 24 hours prior to synoviocentesis may be advisable in some cases to reduce the risk of iatrogenically contaminating a

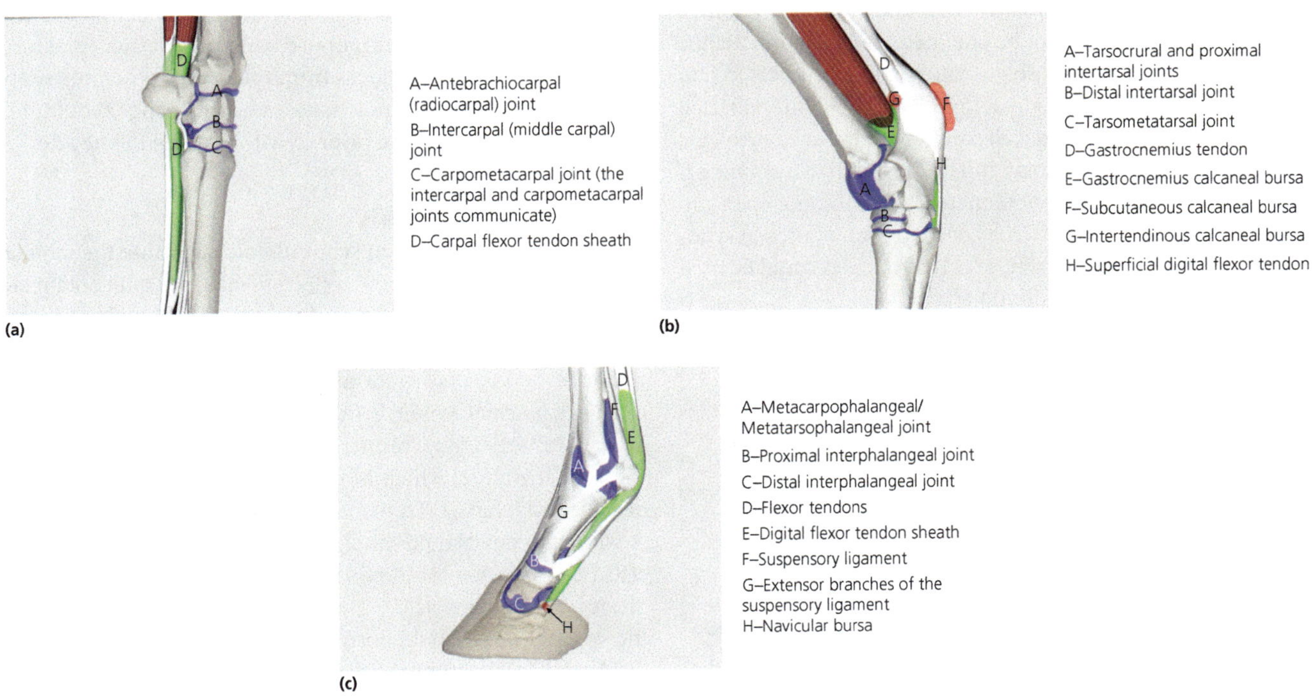

Figure 16.6 Important synovial structures associated with the carpus (a), tarsus (b), and distal aspect of the limb (c). Illustrations by Ray Wilhite.

Table 16.1 Bursae to consider when evaluating wounds in the horse. Bursae are located between the listed tendon/ligament and bone.

Name	Tendon/ligament	Bony structure	Further information
Cranial nuchal bursa	Nuchal ligament (funiculus)	Atlas (first cervical vertebra)	
Caudal nuchal bursa	Nuchal ligament (funiculus)	Axis (second cervical vertebra)	
Supraspinous bursa	Supraspinous ligament	Spinous process of thoracic vertebrae (~T3–T6)	
Subtendinous bursa of infraspinatous muscle	Infraspinatous muscle (tendon)	Greater tubercle of humerus	
Bicipital bursa	Biceps tendon	Intermediate tubercle and intertubercular groove of humerus	Also called intertubercular bursa
Subtendinous bursa of subscapularis muscle	Subscapularis muscle (tendon)	Lesser tubercle of humerus	
Subtendinous calcaneal bursa (SCB)	Superficial digital flexor tendon	Tuber calcaneus and gastrocnemius tendon	Also called intertendinous bursa Communicates with gastrocnemius bursa 50–100% of the time and the subcutaneous calcaneal bursa 39% of the time[31]
Gastrocnemius bursa (GB)	Gastrocnemius tendon	Proximal tuber calcaneus	
Navicular bursa	Deep digital flexor tendon	Navicular bone	
Subtendinous bursa of the deltoid muscle	Deltoid muscle	Deltoid tuberosity of the humerus	
Cunean bursa	Cunean tendon (from cranial tibial muscle)	Central and third tarsal bones, medial	
Trochanteric bursa	Medial gluteal muscle	Greater trochanter of the femur	

synovial structure. Synoviocentesis should be performed only after properly preparing the site and using aseptic technique.

Synovial fluid can be aspirated from most synovial structures, but if the wound and synovial cavity are open and draining, collecting fluid may be difficult. The presence of fibrin within the synovial structure may also complicate the collection of fluid. When a sample cannot be obtained, sterile isotonic saline solution or a balanced electrolyte solution can be injected into the joint to facilitate aspiration of fluid.[32] Although the collected sample is diluted, making cell counts inaccurate, cytologic examination of the sample may still be helpful in determining if the synovial structure is contaminated, and fluid obtained can be used for bacterial culture. The concentration of urea in synovial fluid mimics that in serum, so paired samples could be used to determine the degree of dilution.[33]

Tip

- When a synovial sample cannot be obtained, sterile isotonic saline solution or a balanced electrolyte solution can be injected into the joint to assist in aspirating fluid.

Synovial distension

After aspirating synovial fluid for bacterial culture and cytologic examination, the synovial structure should be distended with isotonic saline solution or a balanced electrolyte solution to determine if it communicates with the nearby wound. Fluid is injected into the synovial structure while the wound is observed for presence of fluid flowing from it (Figure 16.7). Communication between the synovial structure and the wound should be considered unlikely if fluid fails to flow from the wound when the synovial structure is pressurized. If the wound is in a high-motion area, the limb should be moved through an exaggerated range of motion to ascertain that fluid does not egress from the wound when the limb is placed in different positions. An antibiotic should be infused into the structure prior to withdrawing the needle.

Synovial fluid analysis

Elevation of total protein in synovial fluid can cause the sample of synovial fluid to clot if the collection vial does not contain an anticoagulant, therefore, synovial fluid should be collected into an ethylenediaminetetraacetic acid (EDTA) blood tube.[32] Inflamed or infected synovial fluid often contains red blood cells, but normal synovial fluid should contain few, if any.[32] Synoviocentesis may result in some hemorrhage into the synovial structure, which is another reason why fluid should be collected in an EDTA blood tube.

Normal synovial fluid should contain less than 1000 nucleated cells/μL, of which most should be mononuclear cells (i.e., macrophages and lymphocytes).[32] The concentration of total protein in the synovial fluid should normally be approximately 20–25% of the horse's concentration of plasma protein.[34] Generally, this concentration should be less than 2.0 g/dL. A differential cell count is also important for a complete assessment. Neutrophils

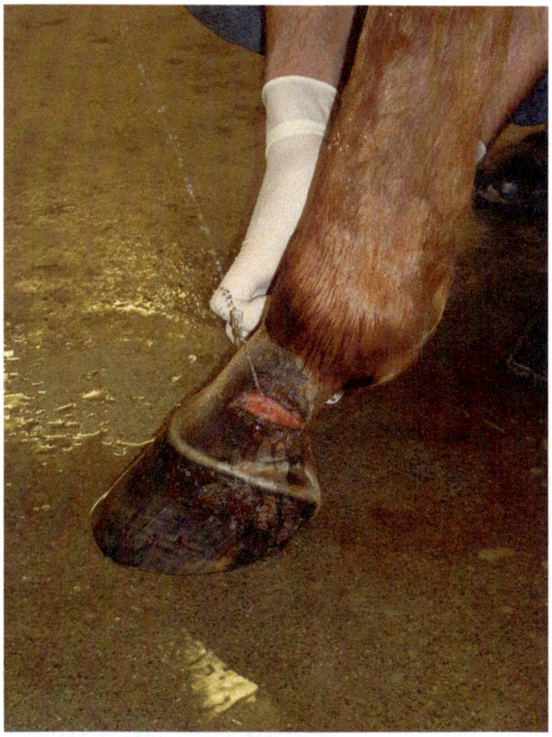

Figure 16.7 A needle was inserted into the proximal interphalangeal joint at a location distant from the wound. Isotonic saline solution instilled into the joint flowed from the wound.

should account for less than 10% of the cellular content.[32] Nucleated cell counts associated with non-septic osteoarthritis and traumatic synovitis are reported to be between 5000 and 10 000 cells/µL.[34]

Characteristics of synovial fluid consistent with synovial infection are reported to include a nucleated cell count greater than 30 000 cells/µL, of which more than 90% are neutrophils, and a concentration of total protein greater than 4.0 g/dL.[34] With experimentally induced septic arthritis, nucleated cell counts in the synovial fluid increased significantly within 8 hours, in one study, after the joints were inoculated with bacteria (range 23 000–37 000 cells/µL); by 12 hours, 80% of the infected joints had a white blood cell count greater than 50 000 cells/µL.[35] Substantial increases in nucleated cell counts were seen by 30 hours in another study, even after a corticosteroid had been administered into the joint.[22] In both of these studies, the most consistent findings indicating that a joint was infected were a concentration of neutrophils greater than 90% and a pH less than 6.9.[22,35] Total protein may be elevated in non-infectious inflammatory conditions, but it generally remains less than 4.0 g/dL.[32,34]

The concentration of total protein in an infected synovial structure has been used as a prognostic indicator.[23] A retrospective analysis found that the preoperative concentration of total protein in the synovial fluid could be used to predict survival after endoscopic treatment for synovial infection.[23] The cut-off value indicating that the horse was likely to survive was 5.5–6.0 g/dL.[23]

Bacterial culture

Bacteria are seen during cytologic examination of fluid obtained from an infected synovial structure in approximately 25% of cases.[5,32] Consequently, the "gold standard" for definitive diagnosis of septic arthritis is a positive bacterial culture. If contamination or infection of a synovial structure is suspected, synovial fluid aspirated from that structure should be placed into a dry, sterile tube (i.e., red top, or clot tube) for bacterial culture. When possible, synovial fluid should be placed into a blood culture enrichment medium. Using a blood culture enrichment medium resulted in 79% positive culture whereas other methods of culture resulted in 23–28% positive culture.[36] Although the primary benefit of a positive culture is to help direct antimicrobial therapy, a positive bacterial culture has also been reported to be a prognostic indicator. In one report, only 50% of horses with a positive culture from synovial fluid survived to discharge, whereas 71% of horses that did not have a positive culture survived.[6] In that report, culture of *S. aureus* was associated with a poor prognosis for return to function.[6] In another study, culture of *S. aureus* was associated with persistent infection.[24]

> **Tip**
>
> - Use blood culture enrichment medium, whenever possible, when submitting synovial fluid for bacterial culture.

Synovial infections associated with wounds are often polymicrobial.[5,37,38] A retrospective analysis of horses with septic arthritis or tenosynovitis found that the most common bacterial isolates associated with synovial sepsis due to a wound were Enterobacteriaceae, β-*Streptococcus*, non-hemolytic *Staphylococcus*, and hemolytic *Staphylococcus*.[5] Another study found that *S. aureus* was the isolate most frequently cultured from infected synovial structures. Thirty-three percent of infected synovial structures associated with a wound had a positive bacterial culture.[6]

Polymerase chain reaction

Although bacterial culture remains the "gold standard" for diagnosis of septic synovitis, results are frequently falsely negative (i.e., poor sensitivity). The use of polymerase chain reaction (PCR) has greatly improved the speed and accuracy of detecting bacteria in the synovial fluid of human patients.[39] Polymerase chain reaction identifies the presence of bacterial DNA within the synovial fluid sample. Elmas *et al.* (2013) reported the sensitivity and specificity of real-time PCR (RT-PCR) in detecting bacteria in infected synovial structures of horses to be 87% and 72%, respectively.[39] The turn-around time for test results was approximately 4 hours, which was much faster than the 24–48 hours required to obtain results of bacterial culture.[39] When possible, PCR should be used as a complement to bacterial culture.[40] In one study, the highest sensitivity (92%) for the detection of synovial infection was achieved when the results of incubating synovial fluid in blood culture medium and the results of PCR were combined.[41] Only a small volume of synovial fluid (200 μL) is required for PCR, which is helpful when only a small amount of synovial fluid can be collected. The sample should be collected in a blood tube containing EDTA and kept cool until the PCR can be performed.

Serum amyloid A

The concentration of serum amyloid A (SAA) within synovial fluid may be used as an indicator of septic synovitis. Serum amyloid A is an acute-phase protein produced primarily by the liver in response to inflammation and infection. It is also synthesized by synoviocytes in response to synovial inflammation and sepsis.[42] In one study, the concentration of SAA in synovial fluid was significantly higher in the synovial fluid of horses with suspected infectious synovitis than in that of healthy horses.[43] To the authors' knowledge, SAA concentration within synovial fluid is not routinely used clinically.

Imaging

Multiple imaging modalities can be used to determine if a wound and an adjacent synovial structure communicate.

Radiography

The region of a wound involving a synovial structure should be examined radiographically after obtaining a standard radiographic series of that region. Radiographs can be used to detect osseous injury, the presence of radiopaque foreign material, and, if the wound is chronic, osteomyelitis.[37] Radiography was found to be an important diagnostic tool in a study of horses with wounds that communicated with a synovial structure. In that study, joint involvement was identified radiographically in 80% of horses in which radiography was used.[28] Air present within the synovial structure adjacent to the wound confirms communication between the wound and the synovial structure, provided that the air has not been introduced by synoviocentesis. Care must be taken not to confuse subcutaneous air with intrasynovial air (Figure 16.8). Placement of a radiopaque probe into the wound may also be used to identify communication between a wound and a synovial structure (Figure 16.9).

Positive-contrast radiography using an iodinated solution can be used to demonstrate communication between a wound and an adjacent synovial structure and to outline radiolucent foreign material (Figure 16.10). A standard radiographic series of the wounded region should be obtained prior to infusing the contrast medium. After cleaning the wound, a teat cannula or catheter is inserted into the wound, sterile contrast medium is infused, and the region is radiographed (Figure 16.11). The contrast medium should be diluted with sterile isotonic saline solution to a concentration of 140 mg iodine/mL. Multiple radiographic views should be obtained to identify the boundaries of the tract of the wound outlined by the positive-contrast fistulogram.

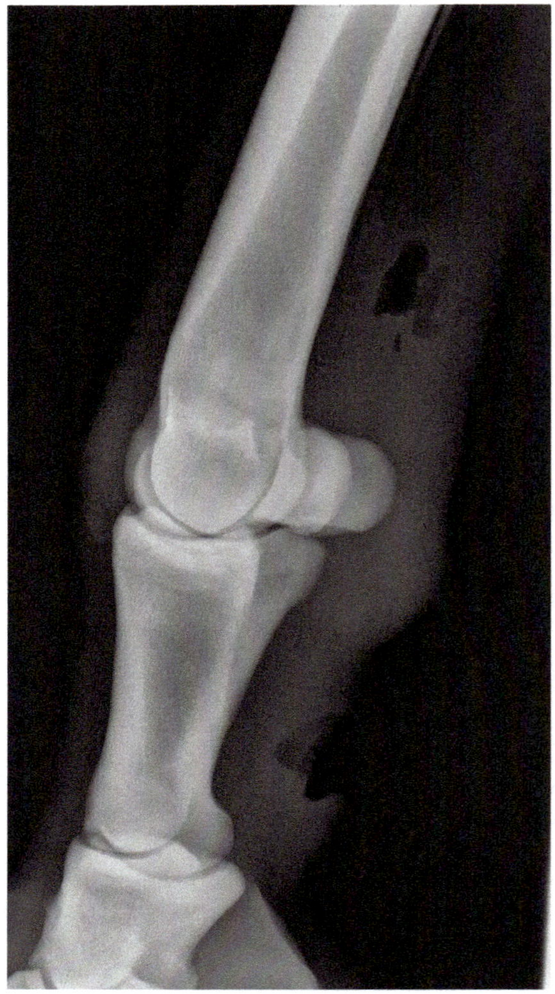

Figure 16.8 Laceration of the palmar pastern region introduced air into the digital flexor tendon sheath that can be visualized radiographically, thus confirming communication between the wound and the digital flexor tendon sheath.

The wounded area may require light bandaging, or the wound may need to be held closed, during injection, to prevent the contrast medium from exiting the wound. The radiographic identification of contrast medium within the synovial structure confirms communication. Contrast medium can also be injected directly into the synovial structure, at a site remote from the wound, in sufficient quantity to assess for exit of the medium from the wound (Figure 16.12). This technique is performed less commonly and should be performed using aseptic technique.

Ultrasonography

Ultrasonography can be used to assess the soft-tissue structures associated with the wound, to search for a foreign body, and to determine if the wound communicates with an adjacent synovial structure. The presence of air within the subcutaneous tissues, however, may impede the examination. To minimize the confounding effect of air, sterile lubricant can be applied liberally to allow sufficient contact between the probe and the

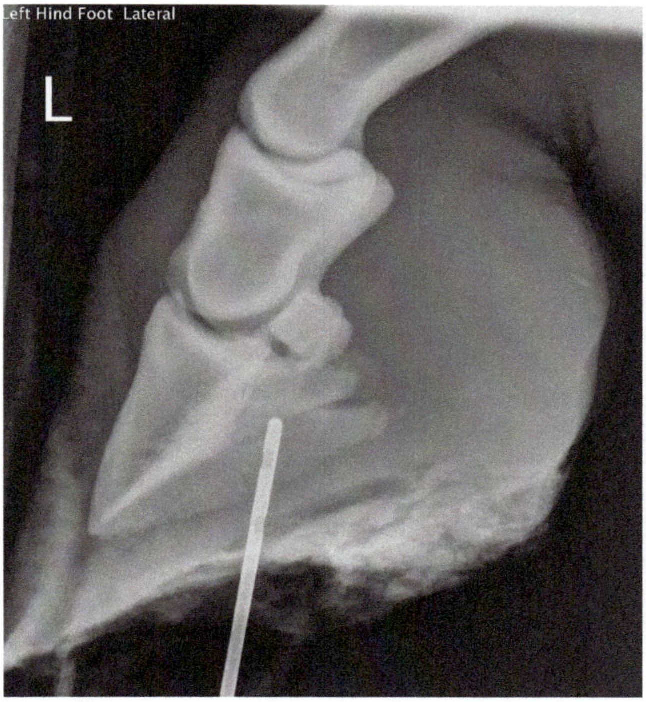

Figure 16.9 A metallic probe was inserted into the wound. The wound is radiographically examined to assess its depth. Multiple radiographic views are required.

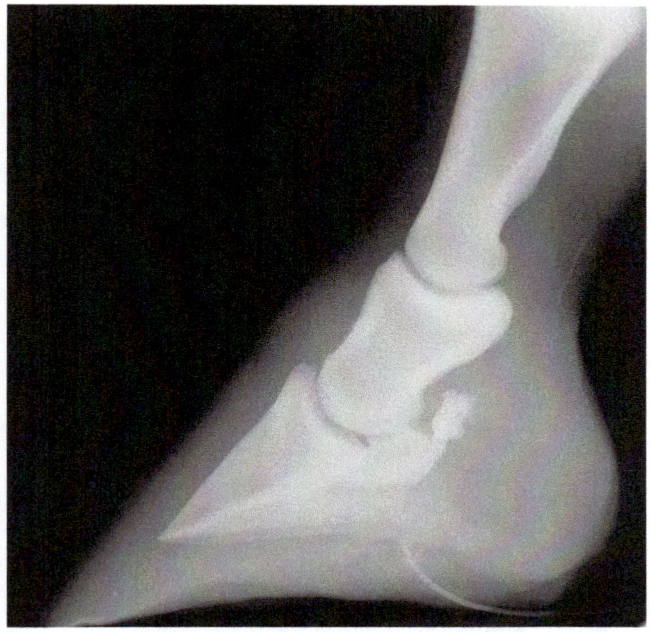

Figure 16.11 A flexible catheter was placed into a puncture wound in the sole of the hoof. Contrast medium was injected and can be seen filling the navicular bursa, confirming communication between the wound and the navicular bursa.

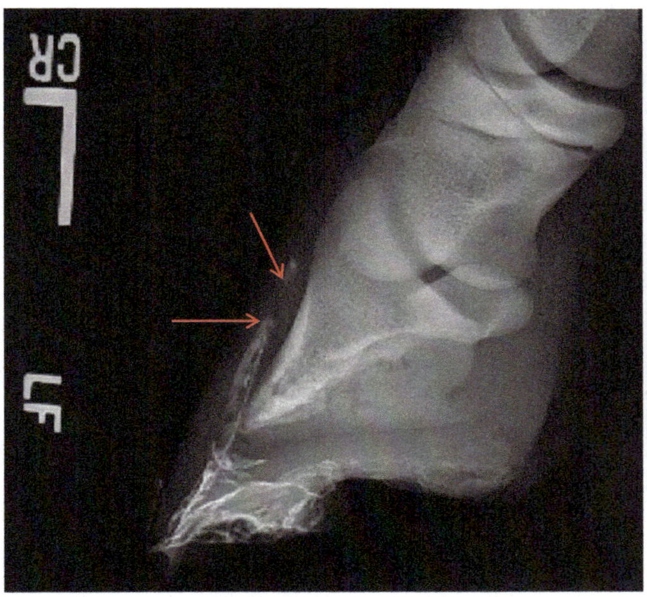

Figure 16.10 Contrast medium was injected into a chronic draining tract on the solar surface of the hoof. A filling defect (arrows) was identified. A piece of wood was later removed from the tract.

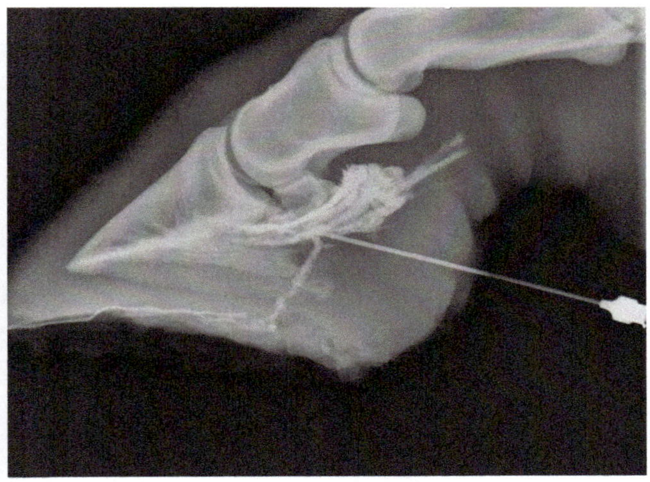

Figure 16.12 Contrast medium was injected, through a spinal needle, into the navicular bursa. Contrast medium is visible within the navicular bursa and flowing from the wound on the solar surface of the hoof. Courtesy of Dr. Randall Eggleston.

wound. A compression wrap applied to the wounded region of the limb for 24 hours prior to ultrasonography helps to reduce the amount of air within the subcutaneous tissues.

Synovial proliferation and capsular thickening visible during ultrasonographic examination of a synovial structure adjacent to a wound may raise suspicion that the synovial structure is infected. Beccati *et al.* (2015) found that when horses underwent an ultrasonographic examination of the wound more than 24 hours after they developed clinical signs consistent with synovial sepsis, ultrasonographic evidence of sepsis, such as marked synovial effusion, synovial thickening, and fibrinous loculations, was evident.[44] Tendons within injured tendon sheaths or bursae should be evaluated ultrasonographically. This may provide details regarding injury to the soft-tissue

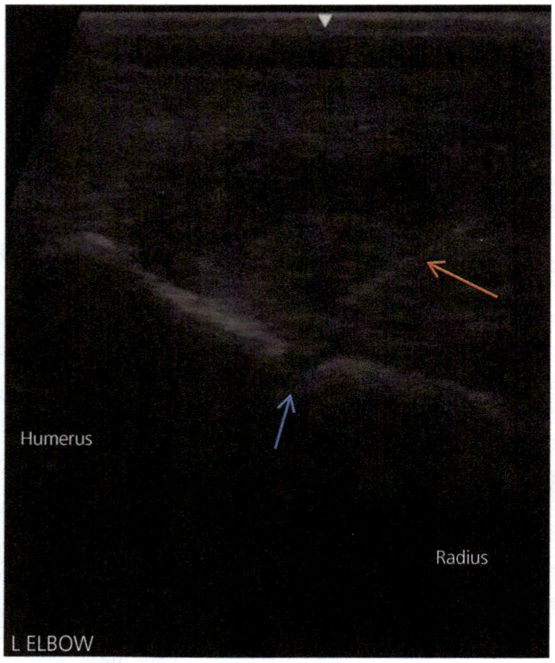

Red arrow–needle
Blue arrow–elbow joint space

Figure 16.13 The needle (red arrow) can be seen entering the humeroradial joint (blue arrow). This needle can be used to aspirate synovial fluid or deposit an antibiotic intrasynovially.

structures that could provide prognostic information. Moreover, ultrasound-guided needle placement is valuable when synoviocentesis is otherwise unsuccessful. Ultrasound can also be used to place needles into a synovial structure for lavage of that structure (Figure 16.13).[45]

Advanced imaging

Computed tomography (CT) and magnetic resonance imaging (MRI) can be extremely useful when synovial sepsis is suspected. These methods of imaging are often reserved for evaluating a chronically infected synovial cavity where response to therapy was not as expected, or for evaluating a synovial structure thought to contain a foreign body. Magnetic resonance imaging provides soft-tissue contrast and fluid-sensitive sequences superior to that provided by CT that can aid in detecting a nidus of infection, osteomyelitis, septic arthritis, a foreign body, or additional soft-tissue injury. Recent advances in MRI and CT allow for 3-D and multiplanar reconstructed images that may permit more precise surgical planning. Computed tomography also has the capability to create 3-D reconstructions for surgical planning.

Treatment

The main goal of treating horses with an infected synovial structure is to re-sterilize the synovial cavity as quickly as possible to minimize the negative consequences of synovial infection.[2,37] Synovial drainage/lavage and effective antibiotic therapy are usually necessary to eradicate bacteria from the synovial space.[2] Methods used for lavage/drainage include endoscopic lavage, through-and-through lavage, and intrasynovial continuous lavage. Antimicrobial therapy often includes a combination of systemic, regional, and intrasynovial administration of one or more antibiotics. Administration of a non-steroidal anti-inflammatory drug (NSAID) also plays a critical role in the treatment of horses with a wound involving a synovial structure. Dosages and indications for NSAIDs are covered in detail in Chapter 4 (Table 4.1).

Synovial lavage

Endoscopic lavage

Endoscopic lavage of an infected synovial structure is superior to through-and-through needle lavage or arthrotomy of the synovial structure because, using endoscopy, foreign material, fibrin, and devitalized tissue within the synovial cavity can be identified and removed.[23,46] Authors of a large retrospective study analyzing results of endoscopic lavage of 121 infected synovial structures reported that 90% of horses survived, and 81% returned to their pre-injury level of performance.[46] A more recent study found that 86% of horses with synovial infection survived to discharge after treatment that included endoscopic lavage.[23] High-volume endoscopic lavage allows maximum removal of inflammatory mediators from the synovial cavity.[23] In general, endoscopic lavage is most advantageous when the synovial structure has been infected longer than 24–48 hours. After this time, fibrinous material develops within the synovial structure, impeding through-and-through lavage by occluding needles and catheters. The ability to identify and remove foreign material during endoscopic lavage of an infected synovial structure can sometimes be "game changing" (Figure 16.14).[47]

> **Tip**
>
> - The endoscopic portals may be left open after surgery to permit continued drainage when the synovial structure is chronically infected or severely contaminated. Leaving the portals open also provides access to the synovial structure for repeated lavage through these sites with the horse standing.

Through-and-through lavage

Through-and-through lavage can be performed with the horse standing using large-bore needles (e.g., 14-gauge needles, Figure 16.15) or with the horse anesthetized using large cannulas or large-bore needles. Through-and-through lavage is best reserved for acutely and minimally contaminated synovial injuries.[37] It can also be used with the horse standing, in the days following endoscopic lavage. To place large cannulas, small incisions into the synovial structure are created. Two retrospective studies found no difference in outcome between horses with septic synovitis treated by endoscopic lavage and

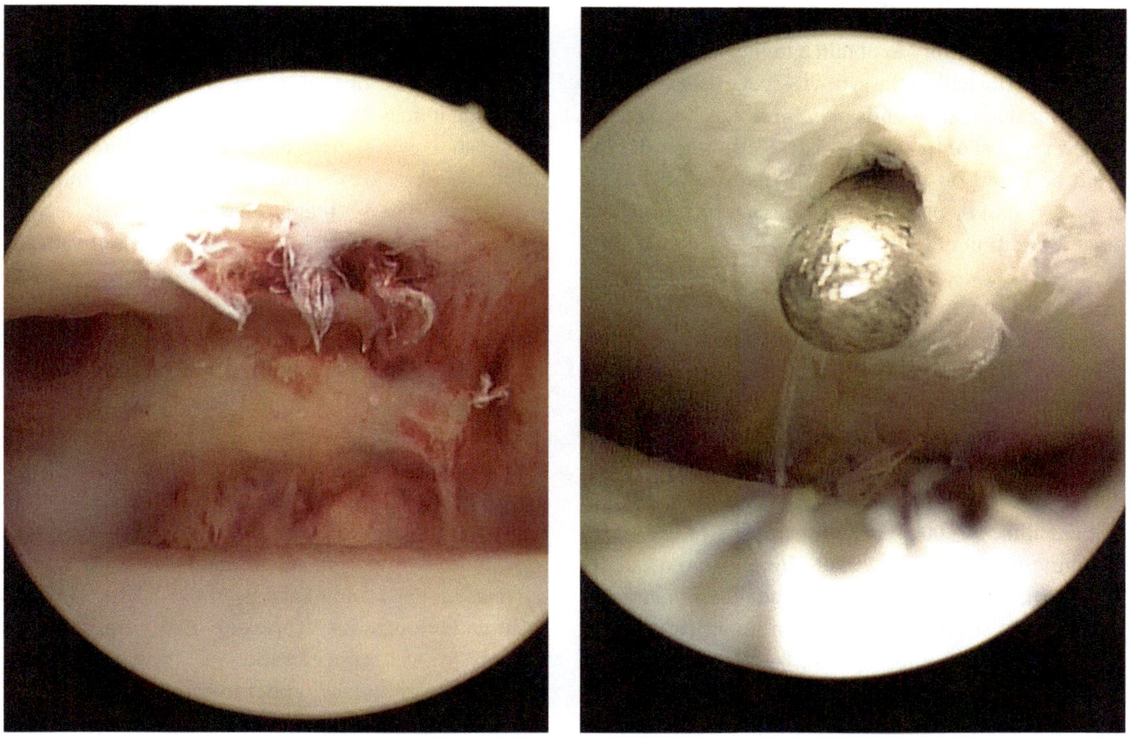

(a) (b)

Figure 16.14 **(a)** Navicular bursoscopy demonstrating focal inflammation and hemorrhage within the navicular bursa. **(b)** A probe has been inserted through the wound tract from the solar margin of the hoof, confirming communication with the navicular bursa.

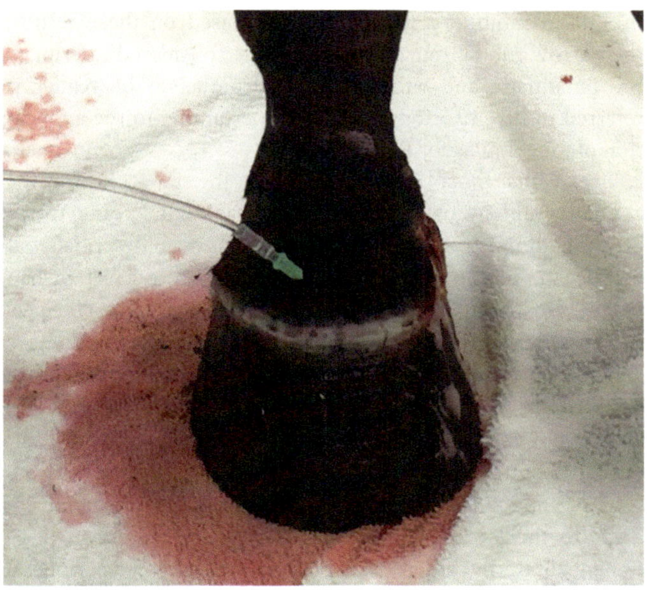

Figure 16.15 Through-and-through needle lavage of the distal interphalangeal joint with the horse standing. Multiple needles have been placed. The lavage fluid enters one needle and exits the joint through the remaining two needles and the wound.

those treated by through-and-through lavage.[7,26] Through-and-through lavage using three, 14-gauge needles, was found to be more effective than endoscopic lavage in removing microspheres from healthy tarsocrural joints (personal communication with Dr. Warren Beard, 2015). The disadvantages of through-and-through lavage include the inability to assess the articular cartilage, debride osseous lesions, and remove large pieces of fibrin or foreign material.

Intrasynovial continuous lavage

The use of an indwelling intrasynovial catheter for continuous lavage of a synovial structure has been reported.[7,48,49] This catheter can be placed through endoscopic portals at the conclusion of endoscopic lavage or through large cannulas at the conclusion of through-and-through lavage. An antibiotic may be infused through the indwelling catheters, and the synovial cavity can be lavaged daily or continuously [intrasynovial continuous lavage (ISCL)] through the catheter. In a recent report, though, horses with septic synovitis treated by ISCL (1–7 days) with sterile isotonic fluids had a worse prognosis for survival than did horses treated with methods other than ISCL.[7]

Wound closure

Ideally, acute wounds that involve synovial structures should be closed primarily after being irrigated and debrided appropriately.[30] Whether an infected synovial structure should be closed or left open to drain is debatable. Closing the wound traps bacteria within the synovial space, thereby increasing the risk of subsequent synovial infection, and lengthens the time of surgery. The wounded limb may require external coaptation to prevent the sutured wound from dehiscing. The advantages of closing the wound include quicker healing of the synovial defect and the wound itself and the ability to obtain a higher concentration of an antimicrobial drug within the synovial space using regional perfusion. Leaving synovial wounds open prolongs healing and increases the overall cost of treatment.[4] The decision to close the wound should be based on the amount of tissue available for closure, the presence of or potential for synovial infection, and the location and duration of injury.[30]

Antimicrobial therapy

Systemic administration of antimicrobial drugs

Systemic administration of antibiotics is the cornerstone of treatment for synovial sepsis. Due to the polymicrobial nature of most accidental wounds of horses, antimicrobial therapy should be broad spectrum. An antimicrobial drug commonly used to treat horses for infection of a synovial structure is penicillin [potassium penicillin, 22 000 U/kg, intravenously (IV), q 6 hours or procaine penicillin G, 22 000 U/kg, intramuscularly (IM), q 12 hours]. Administration of penicillin is generally combined with administration of gentamicin sulfate (6.6 mg/kg, IV, q 24 hours). Cefazolin sodium (11 mg/kg, IV, q 8 hours) or ceftiofur sodium (2.2 mg/kg, IV or IM, q 12 hours) may be administered alone or in combination with gentamicin. Amikacin sulfate (15–25 mg/kg, IV, q 24 hours) or enrofloxacin (5–7.5 mg/kg, IV, q 24 hours) can be used in place of gentamicin for treatment for Gram-negative bacterial infection. The use of enrofloxacin (and other quinolones) should be avoided in foals due to the risk of quinolone-induced arthropathy.[50,51] The combination of penicillin and amikacin is effective against most bacteria frequently isolated from infected synovial structures associated with a wound.[6,38] The reader is referred to Table 19.1 in Chapter 19 for more information about the common bacterial isolates obtained from wounds involving a synovial structure in horses and to Table 19.3 for information about *in vitro* antibiotic sensitivity patterns for the common equine pathogens. If culture results indicate that a single bacterial species is responsible for the infection, targeted therapy may be used, based on sensitivity testing.

Antibiotics should be administered parenterally for a minimum of 7–10 days. If, after that period, substantial clinical improvement is apparent, antimicrobial therapy may be switched to oral administration of an antibiotic for 2–4 weeks.[15,37,49] The reader is referred to Table 19.5 for guidelines regarding the duration of antibiotic therapy for specific types of wounds. Common orally administered antibiotics include trimethoprim–sulfadiazine (15–30 mg/kg, q 12 hours), minocycline (4 mg/kg, q 12 hours), doxycycline hyclate (10 mg/kg, q 12 hours), and compounded oral formulations of enrofloxacin (7.5 mg/kg, once daily) or chloramphenicol palmitate (44 mg/kg, q 6–8 hours). Orally administered minocycline (4 mg/kg) achieves a peak concentration in synovial fluid (0.33 µg/mL) lower than that achieved with orally administered doxycycline (10 mg/kg; 0.46 µg/mL) but high enough to inhibit growth of susceptible bacteria.[52,53]

Regional limb perfusion of antimicrobial drugs

Regional limb perfusion (RLP) is a method of providing a high concentration of one or more antibiotics to a localized area. Although it may be used alone, it is used most frequently in combination with systemically administered antimicrobial therapy. Kelmer *et al.* (2012) reported successful resolution of synovial infection of 14 horses that received systemic antimicrobial therapy only during the initial 24 hours after admission, after which time antimicrobial therapy was administered solely by multiple RLPs using an indwelling cephalic or saphenous venous catheter.[54]

Intravenous regional limb perfusion (IV-RLP) can be performed with the horse standing or anesthetized. A tourniquet is placed proximal to the wound and the infected synovial structure and proximal to a site accessible for venipuncture. A second tourniquet can be placed distal to the wound and infected synovial structure, if possible, to increase the concentration of the antibiotic at the site of infection (Box 19.5). Selection of the tourniquet is important. Pneumatic tourniquets and wide and narrow, rubber tubing have been used.[55] In one study, using a pneumatic tourniquet (pressure 420 mmHg) resulted in a greater synovial concentration of amikacin sulfate than did using a wide or narrow rubber tourniquet.[55] In contrast, another study found that using a wide rubber tourniquet (Esmarch bandage) resulted in a higher intrasynovial concentration of amikacin than did using a pneumatic tourniquet.[56] When a narrow rubber tourniquet (1 cm diameter) was used, the concentration of amikacin sulfate in the synovial fluid failed to rise above the minimum inhibitory concentration.[55] Based on these results, the narrow rubber tourniquet should be considered inferior to the pneumatic and wide rubber tourniquets. The reader is referred to Box 19.5 for information pertaining to the application of tourniquets for RLP.

The veins most commonly used for IV-RLP are the cephalic, saphenous, and palmar/plantar digital veins. Intra-arterial administration of the perfusate has been described, but because the endothelium of arteries is much more sensitive than that of veins, complications occur more frequently when the perfusate is delivered intra-arterially.[57] The site of venipuncture should be prepared for aseptic venipuncture. Clipping hair at the site is not necessary but may facilitate palpation of the vein and subsequent venipuncture. After the tourniquet has been positioned, a butterfly catheter is inserted into the prepared vein (Figure 16.16). The perfusate is injected into a peripheral vein distal to the tourniquet. After the tourniquet has been positioned, a butterfly catheter is inserted into the prepared peripheral vein, distal to the tourniquet, and the perfusate is injected into the vein. Nothing larger than a 20-gauge butterfly catheter should be used.

An indwelling, over-the-wire or over-the-needle, long-duration catheter may be used in the saphenous or cephalic vein if multiple IV-RLPs are anticipated.[54] The catheter must be cared for in a manner similar to that used to maintain any intravenous catheter, and the catheter must be positioned so that there is ample room to place a tourniquet proximal to it. In one study,

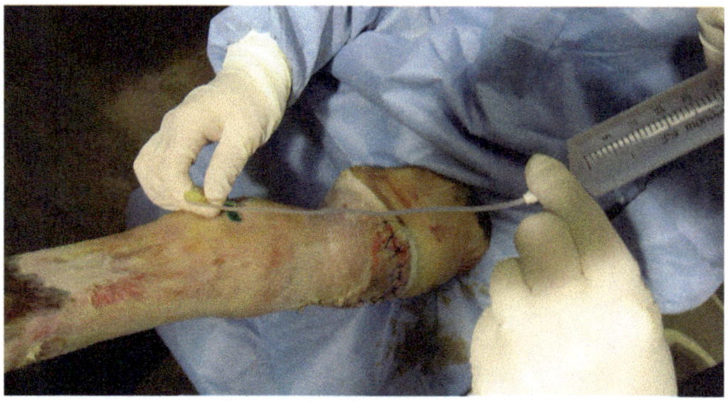

Figure 16.16 Regional limb perfusion with an antibiotic. A butterfly catheter was placed into the lateral plantar digital vein, and the perfusate is being injected. The tourniquet is proximal to the tarsus and not shown in the photograph.

phlebitis associated with the indwelling catheter occurred in 24% (11/45) of limbs.[54]

The volume of perfusate used is selected empirically because the ideal volume is unknown.[57] Volumes reported to be used depend on the site of injection and have ranged from 20 mL to 250 mL.[24,56,58,59] A small volume (10–30 mL) is used when the perfusate is injected into a digital vein, and a larger volume (30–60 mL) is used when the perfusate is injected into a more proximal vein, such as the saphenous or cephalic vein. A perfusate volume of 60 mL was consistently used in multiple publications.[24,56,58,59] Hyde *et al.* (2013) compared the effect of different volumes of perfusate injected into the lateral palmar digital vein (10, 30, and 60 mL) and found no significant difference in the antibiotic concentration achieved within the metacarpophalangeal joint, although a trend was seen for higher mean concentrations by using the 10-mL volume of perfusate.[58]

For more information on performing IV-RLP, see Box 19.3 in Chapter 19.

Antibiotics used for IV-RLP are listed in Table 16.2. Concentration-dependent antibiotics are preferred over time-dependent antibiotics because concentration-dependent antibiotics continue to provide antimicrobial activity as long as the concentration remains above the MIC for that bacterium. Amikacin is a popular antibiotic for IV-RLP because of its broad spectrum of antimicrobial activity, although, based on *in vitro* susceptibility testing, it is unlikely to be effective in treatment for streptococcal infection.[37,67] Parra-Sanchez *et al.* (2006) recommended using more than 250 mg amikacin in the perfusate because 250 mg amikacin in 60 mL perfusate did not achieve therapeutic antimicrobial concentrations in the interstitium, synovial fluid, or serum.[60] The synovial concentration of amikacin remained above the MIC for 24 hours after IV-RLP when the perfusate contained 1–2 g of amikacin.[68] Enrofloxacin (1.5 mg/kg per perfusion) should be used for RLP with caution because vasculitis has sometimes been observed after IV-RLP with this antibiotic.[60] Combining multiple antibiotics within the same IV-RLP should be done with caution. Studies have shown that more than one antibiotic in a perfusate

Table 16.2 Antimicrobials used for regional limb perfusion.

Antimicrobial	Dosage (500 kg horse)	References
Amikacin	250 mg–2 g	7, 54, 60
	5 mg/kg	61
Cefoxitine	1 g	54
Ceftiofur	1–2 g	62
Chloramphenicol	2 g (100 mL perfusate)	63
	1 g	54
Enrofloxacin	1 g	54
	1.5 mg/kg	60
Gentamicin	100 mg–1 g	7, 58, 64
	2.2 mg/kg (i.e., 1/3 of systemic dose)	58, 61
Imipenem	500 mg	54
Marbofloxacin	0.67 mg/kg (60 mL perfusate)	65
Ticarcillin	1.7 g	54
Vancomycin	300 mg	66
	1 g	54

resulted in lower synovial concentrations of each antibiotic than when those antibiotics were used alone.[59] Regional limb perfusion, using a concentration-dependent antibiotic, should be performed every 24–48 hours.

What to avoid

- Avoid combining multiple antibiotics in the perfusate when performing IV-RLP because the combination may decrease the synovial concentration of each antibiotic.

Tip

- Perform RLP every 24–48 hours when using a concentration-dependent antibiotic.

Complications associated with IV-RLP include thrombophlebitis, local swelling, hematoma, loss of venous definition due to repeated venipuncture, and cellulitis. The risk of complication is decreased by carefully preparing the site of venipuncture and closely monitoring the vein while infusing the perfusate. Sedating the horse minimizes movement during the infusion and reduces the risk of movement of the needle. Applying diclofenac sodium (Surpass®; Boehringer Ingelheim Vetmedica, Inc.) over the site of venipuncture helps to control local inflammation.[69]

Intraosseous perfusion of antimicrobial drugs

A high concentration of an antimicrobial drug within a synovial structure may also be achieved by using intraosseous regional limb perfusion (IO-RLP). Using this technique, the antimicrobial drug is administered into the medullary cavity of a bone proximal to the contaminated or infected synovial structure.[70–73] A cannulated cortical screw with a Luer-lock adapter welded to it is inserted through the cortex of the bone into the medullary cavity. The Luer-lock adapter allows for attachment of an extension set for the infusion of the perfusate. The screw may be placed with the horse anesthetized or standing.[71] An alternative method is to drill a 4.0-mm diameter hole into the bone through which the end of an extension set can be inserted directly into the medullary cavity without the need for a screw.

In one study, complications, though minor, occurred more frequently from IO-RLPs (33%) than from IV-RLPs (12%).[7] Complications associated with IO-RLP were screw-related (e.g., discharge of exudate around the screw, difficult injection, and loosening or breakage of the screw) whereas complications associated with IV-RLP were vein-related (e.g., hematoma, phlebitis, and thrombosis).[7] Intraosseous RLP using the metacarpus resulted in antibiotic concentrations in synovial structures and bones of the distal aspect of the limb that exceeded the reported MIC of common pathogens.[71] Intravenous RLP using the saphenous vein resulted in a greater concentration of amikacin sulfate within the tibiotarsal joint than did IO-RLP using the distal extremity of the tibia.[73] For more information on IO-RLP, the reader is referred to Box 19.4.

Intrasynovial administration of antimicrobial drugs

One or more antimicrobial drugs can be administered directly into the affected synovial structure. Intrasynovial administration guarantees a high concentration of the antibiotic in the synovial structure but requires repeated synoviocentesis. If intrasynovial injection cannot be performed, RLP has also been shown to lead to a high intrasynovial concentration of the perfused antibiotic when performed correctly and without complications, such as extravasation of the perfusate. If fluid must be obtained from the synovial structure for cytologic analysis and/or bacterial culture and antimicrobial sensitivity testing, the antibiotic should be injected directly into the synovial structure after fluid has been obtained by centesis. Antibiotics can also be administered intrasynovially through an indwelling catheter (Figure 16.17).[48] The indwelling catheter can also be used for repeated lavage of the synovial structure and is especially useful if extensive contamination is present. The use of a constant-rate infusion system for continuous intrasynovial antibiotic infusion has been described.[74,75] Constant-rate intrasynovial infusion of gentamicin (100 mg/mL), at 16 mL per day, into the tarsocrural joint had no significant negative effect on cartilage.[74]

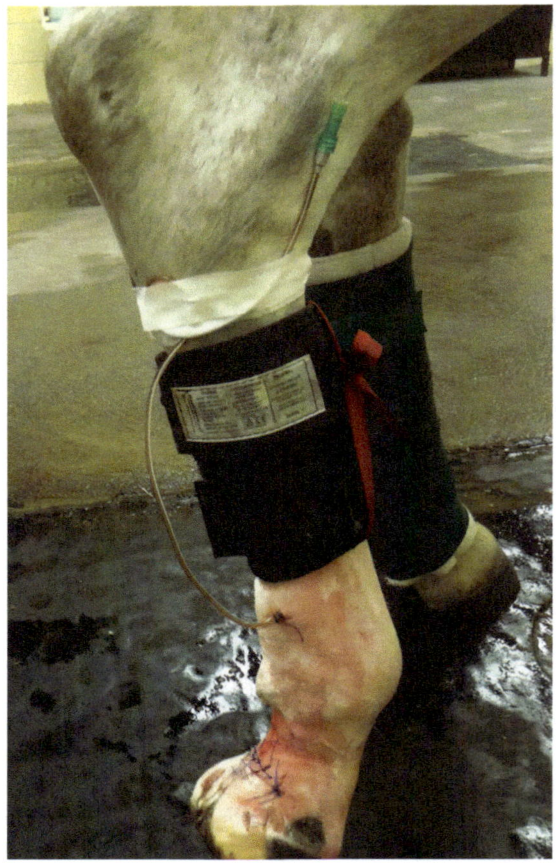

Figure 16.17 An intrasynovial catheter was placed into the digital flexor tendon sheath. This catheter can be used to inject antibiotics into the sheath or to perform repeated through-and-through lavages. A pneumatic tourniquet is also present because this horse was receiving a regional limb perfusion concurrently.

Complications

The most significant complication associated with treating horses with a synovial wound is the inability to resolve the infection and sterilize the synovial cavity. Continued infection damages the articular cartilage and subchondral bone in a joint, and can damage bone and tendon contained within an infected tendon sheath or bursa. In addition, the chronic inflammatory response contributes to fibrosis of the synovial capsule, leading to a reduced range of motion, the development of fibrous adhesions within the synovial space, and permanent enlargement of the affected area. In most cases, the wound can be managed successfully only if the synovial infection is resolved. Treatment, therefore, should be aimed primarily at resolving the synovial infection. The wound should be completely or partially closed whenever possible, and the limb immobilized when indicated. A synovial fistula may develop in a small percentage of synovial wounds left to heal by second intention due to the continuous flow of synovial fluid from the wound. Most eventually resolve with adequate immobilization, but occasionally, delayed surgical closure of the fistula is necessary. Immobilization of the limb should be considered for wounds located in areas of high motion, such as the dorsal surface of the metacarpo/metatarsophalangeal joint, the dorsal surface of the tarsus, or the palmar/plantar surface of the pastern or fetlock. The limb can be immobilized with a fiberglass cast, a bandage–cast, or a bandage and splint. Immobilization helps prevent dehiscence of a wound that has been completely or partially closed (Figure 16.18). For more information on bandaging and casting techniques, the reader is referred to Chapter 7.

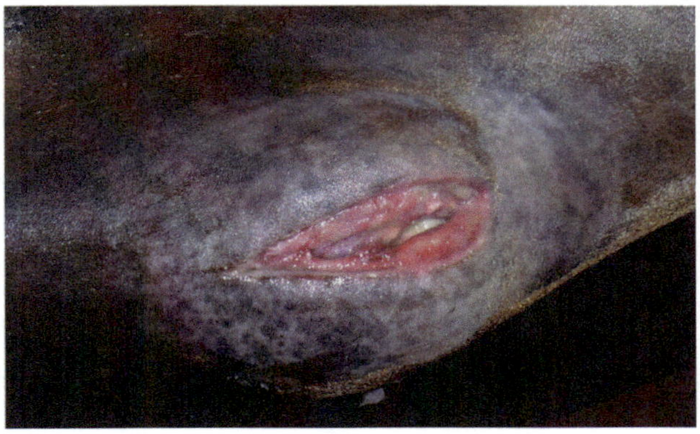

(a)

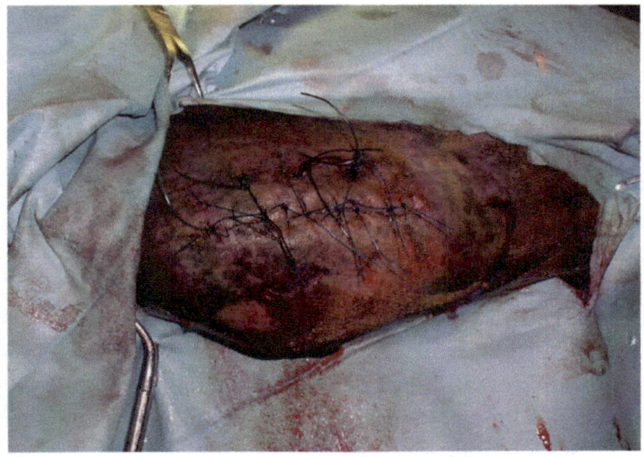

(b)

Figure 16.18 (**a**) This chronic laceration involved the lateral aspect of the calcaneal bursa. (**b**) The bursa was lavaged, and the wound was debrided and closed to prevent complications of healing associated with wounds located in areas of high motion. A bandage–sleeve cast was placed to immobilize the limb, and the wound healed with no complications.

Prognosis

Multiple reports have examined the outcome of horses with an infected synovial structure.[6,23–26] In one study, regardless of the technique of treatment, 84% of horses with infection of a synovial structure survived to discharge, and 54% returned to athletic function.[24] Factors associated with a favorable prognosis are treatment of the infected synovial structure within 36 hours of contamination[26–28] and administration of antimicrobial therapy prior to admission to the hospital.[7] Factors associated with a poor prognosis are a high intrasynovial concentration of total protein at the time of admission,[23] positive bacterial culture of synovial fluid,[6] and radiographic evidence of osteolysis.[48]

Special considerations

Tendon sheaths

Fraser *et al.* (2004) reported that the prognosis for a horse with an infected synovial structure is worse if multiple structures within the digital flexor tendon sheath are injured.[27] Horses with an infected digital flexor tendon sheath complicated by infection of the portion of the deep digital flexor tendon (DDFT) contained within it have been treated successfully by excising the infected portion of the DDFT.[76] Chronic tenosynovitis of the digital flexor tendon sheath may lead to infection of the proximal sesamoid bones, chronic infection of the tarsal sheath may lead to infection of the *sustentaculum tali*, and chronic infection of the calcaneal bursa may lead to infection of the *tuber calcaneus* (Figure 16.19).[77,78] Infection of bone and tendon within an infected synovial structure worsens the prognosis for survival and return to function.[24,48]

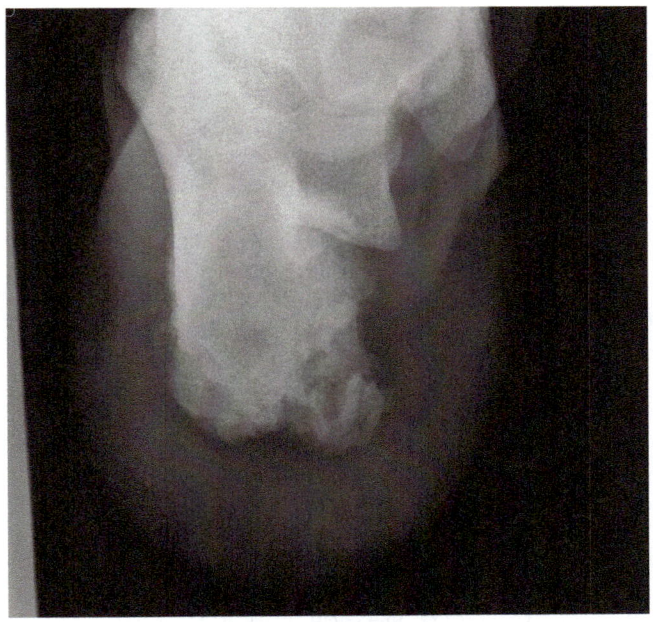

Figure 16.19 Severe osteomyelitis of the *tuber calcaneus*, due to chronic septic bursitis of the subcutaneous and intertendinous calcaneal bursae, is visible radiographically.

Bursae

Penetrating wounds to the frog or sole or deep lacerations of the heel bulb may result in infection of the navicular bursa. Horses with infection of the navicular bursa generally have a worse prognosis for survival and return to function than do horses with a wound involving another synovial structure. In a recent study, only 56% of horses survived to discharge after solar penetration of the navicular bursa, and only 36% returned to preinjury function.[25]

Conclusion

Wounds involving synovial structures (joints, tendon sheaths, or bursae) are common in horses, and synovial structures of the distal aspect of the limb are most commonly involved. Horses with an acute wound resulting in bacterial contamination of a synovial structure usually have a good outcome if treated promptly and properly. Horses with a chronic wound involving a synovial structure often have an established synovial infection and should be treated aggressively to resolve the infection.

Endoscopic lavage permits removal of foreign debris, contaminating or infecting bacteria, and inflammatory exudate. Through-and-through lavage may also be used successfully to treat horses for septic synovitis. Horses with an infected synovial structure associated with a wound should receive antimicrobial therapy administered systemically, intrasynovially, and/or by regional intravenous or intraosseous perfusion. Wounds that involve a synovial structure should be debrided and sutured whenever possible.

References

1. Owen KR, Singer ER, Clegg PD, *et al.* Identification of risk factors for traumatic injury in the general horse population of north-west England, Midlands and north Wales. *Equine Vet J* 2012; **44**: 143.
2. Schneider RK, Bramlage LR, Mecklenburg LM, *et al.* Open drainage, intra-articular and systemic antibiotics in the treatment of septic arthritis/tenosynovitis in horses. *Equine Vet J* 1992; **24**: 443.
3. Baxter G. Management of wounds. In: Colahan PT (ed). *Equine Medicine and Surgery* vol **II**. 2, 5th edn. Mosby: St Louis, 1999: 1808.
4. Baxter GM. Management of wounds involving synovial structures in horses. *Clin Tech Equine Pract* 2004; **3**: 204.
5. Schneider RK, Bramlage LR, Moore RM, *et al.* A retrospective study of 192 horses affected with septic arthritis/tenosynovitis. *Equine Vet J* 1992; **24**: 436.
6. Taylor AH, Mair TS, Smith LJ, Perkins JD. Bacterial culture of septic synovial structures of horses: does a positive bacterial culture influence prognosis? *Equine Vet J* 2010; **42**: 213.
7. Rubio-Martinez LM, Elmas CR, Black B, Monteith G. Clinical use of antimicrobial regional limb perfusion in horses: 174 cases (1999–2009). *J Am Vet Med Assoc* 2012; **241**: 1650.
8. Frisbie DD. Synovial joint biology and pathobiology. In: Auer JA, Stick JA (eds). *Equine Surgery*, 4th edn. Elsevier: St. Louis MO, 2012: 1096.
9. Todhunter RJ. Anatomy and physiology of synovial joints. In: McIlwraith CW, Trotter GW (eds). *Joint Disease in the Horse*. W.B. Saunders: Philadelphia, 1996.
10. Baxter GM. Management of bursitis. In: Auer JA, Stick JA (eds). *Equine Surgery*, 4th edn. Elsevier: St. Louis MO, 2012: 1148.
11. Janicek JC, Hunt RJ. Septic tarsal sheath tenosynovitis. *Comp: Equine Edn* 2006; **1**: 94.
12. Post EM, Singer ER, Clegg PD, *et al.* Retrospective study of 24 cases of septic calcaneal bursitis in the horse. *Equine Vet J* 2003; **35**: 662.
13. Frees KE, Lillich JD, Gaughan EM, DeBowes RM. Tenoscopic-assisted treatment of open digital flexor tendon sheath injuries in horses: 20 cases (1992–2001). *J Am Vet Med Assoc* 2002; **220**: 1823.
14. Goodrich LR. Osteomyelitis in horses. *Vet Clin North Am Equine Pract* 2006; **22**: 389.
15. Goodrich LR, Nixon AJ. Treatment options for osteomyelitis. *Equine Vet Educ* 2004; **16**: 267.
16. Bertone AL, McIlwraith CW, Jones RL, *et al.* Comparison of various treatments for experimentally induced equine infectious arthritis. *Am J Vet Res* 1987; **48**: 519.
17. Gustafson SB, McIlwraith CW, Jones RL. Comparison of the effect of polysulfated glycosaminoglycan, corticosteroids, and sodium hyaluronate in the potentiation of a subinfective dose of *Staphylococcus aureus* in the midcarpal joint of horses. *Am J Vet Res* 1989; **50**: 2014.
18. Bertone AL. Infectious arthritis. In: McIlwraith CW, Trotter GW (eds). *Joint Disease in the Horse*. W.B. Saunders: Philadelphia, 1996.
19. Spiers S, May SA, Harrison LJ, *et al.* Proteolytic enzymes in equine joints with infectious arthritis. *Equine Vet J* 1994; **26**: 48.
20. Hardy J, Bertone AL, Malemud CJ. Effect of synovial membrane infection in vitro on equine synoviocytes and chondrocytes. *Am J Vet Res* 1998; **59**: 293.
21. Smith RL, Merchant TC, Schurman DJ. *In vitro* cartilage degradation by *Escherichia coli* and *Staphylococcus aureus*. *Arthr Rheum* 1982; **25**: 441.
22. Tulamo RM, Bramlage LR, Gabel AA. The influence of corticosteroids on sequential clinical and synovial fluid parameters in joints with acute infectious arthritis in the horse. *Equine Vet J* 1989; **21**: 332.
23. Milner PI, Bardell DA, Warner L, *et al.* Factors associated with survival to hospital discharge following endoscopic treatment for synovial sepsis in 214 horses. *Equine Vet J* 2014; **46**: 701.
24. Walmsley EA, Anderson GA, Muurlink MA, *et al.* Retrospective investigation of prognostic indicators for adult horses with infection of a synovial structure. *Austr Vet J* 2011; **89**: 226.
25. Findley JA, Pinchbeck GL, Milner PI, *et al.* Outcome of horses with synovial structure involvement following solar foot penetrations in four UK veterinary hospitals: 95 cases. *Equine Vet J* 2014; **46**: 352.
26. Wereszka MM, White NA, 2nd, Furr MO. Factors associated with outcome following treatment of horses with septic tenosynovitis: 51 cases (1986–2003). *J Am Vet Med Assoc* 2007; **230**: 1195.
27. Fraser BS, Bladon BM. Tenoscopic surgery for treatment of lacerations of the digital flexor tendon sheath. *Equine Vet J* 2004; **36**: 528.
28. Gibson KT, McIlwraith CW, Turner AS *et al.* Open joint injuries in horses: 58 cases (1980–1986). *J Am Vet Med Assoc* 1989; **194**: 398.
29. Smith LJ, Mellor DJ, Marr CM, Mair TS. What is the likelihood that a horse treated for septic digital tenosynovitis will return to its previous level of athletic function? *Equine Vet J* 2006; **38**: 337.
30. Kraus BM. Lacerations involving synovial structures: initial treatment and novel therapy for infectious arthritis/tenosynovitis. *Clin Tech Equine Pract* 2006; **5**: 82.
31. Post EM, Singer ER, Clegg PD. An anatomic study of the calcaneal bursae in the horse. *Vet Surg* 2007; **36**: 3.
32. Steel CM. Equine synovial fluid analysis. *Vet Clin N Am Equine Pract* 2008; **24**: 437.

33. Gough MR, Munroe GA, Mayhew IG. Urea as a measure of dilution of equine synovial fluid. *Equine Vet J* 2002; **34**: 76.
34. Trotter GW, McIlwraith CW. Clinical features and diagnosis of equine joint disease. In: McIlwraith CW, Trotter GW (eds). *Joint Disease in the Horse*. W.B. Saunders: Philadelphia, 1996: 120.
35. Tulamo RM, Bramlage LR, Gabel AA. Sequential clinical and synovial fluid changes associated with acute infectious arthritis in the horse. *Equine Vet J* 1989; **21**: 325.
36. Dumoulin M, Pille F, van den Abeele AM, *et al.* Use of blood culture medium enrichment for synovial fluid culture in horses: a comparison of different culture methods. *Equine Vet J* 2010; **42**: 541.
37. Joyce J. Injury to synovial structures. *Vet Clin N Am Equine Pract* 2007; **23**: 103.
38. Moore RM, Schneider RK, Kowalski J, *et al.* Antimicrobial susceptibility of bacterial isolates from 233 horses with musculoskeletal infection during 1979–1989. *Equine Vet J* 1992; **24**: 450.
39. Elmas CR, Koenig JB, Bienzle D, *et al.* Evaluation of a broad range real-time polymerase chain reaction (RT-PCR) assay for the diagnosis of septic synovitis in horses. *Can J Vet Res* 2013; **77**: 211.
40. Fenollar F, Roux V, Stein A, *et al.* Analysis of 525 samples to determine the usefulness of PCR amplification and sequencing of the 16S rRNA gene for diagnosis of bone and joint infections. *J Clin Microbiol* 2006; **44**: 1018.
41. Pille F, Martens A, Schouls LM, *et al.* Broad range 16S rRNA gene PCR compared to bacterial culture to confirm presumed synovial infection in horses. *Vet J* 2007; **173**: 73.
42. Jacobsen S, Niewold TA, Halling-Thomsen M, *et al.* Serum amyloid A isoforms in serum and synovial fluid in horses with lipopolysaccharide-induced arthritis. *Vet Immunol Immunopathol* 2006; **110**: 325.
43. Jacobsen S, Thomsen MH, Nanni S. Concentrations of serum amyloid A in serum and synovial fluid from healthy horses and horses with joint disease. *Am J Vet Res* 2006; **67**: 1738.
44. Beccati F, Gialletti R, Passamonti F, *et al.* Ultrasonographic findings in 38 horses with septic arthritis/tenosynovitis. *Vet Radiol Ultrasound* 2015; **56**: 68.
45. Whitcomb MB, le Jeune SS, MacDonald MM, *et al.* Disorders of the infraspinatus tendon and bursa in three horses. *J Am Vet Med Assoc* 2006; **229**: 549.
46. Wright IM, Smith MR, Humphrey DJ, *et al.* Endoscopic surgery in the treatment of contaminated and infected synovial cavities. *Equine Vet J* 2003; **35**: 613.
47. Lescun TB. Orthopaedic infections; laboratory testing and response to therapy. *Equine Vet Educ* 2011; **23**: 127.
48. Stewart AA, Goodrich LR, Byron CR, *et al.* Antimicrobial delivery by intrasynovial catheterisation with systemic administration for equine synovial trauma and sepsis. *Austr Vet J* 2010; **88**: 115.
49. Ross MW, Orsini JA, Richardson DW, Martin BB. Closed suction drainage in the treatment of infectious arthritis of the equine tarsocrural joint. *Vet Surg* 1991; **20**: 21.
50. Bermingham EC, Papich MG, Vivrette SL. Pharmacokinetics of enrofloxacin administered intravenously and orally to foals. *Am J Vet Res* 2000; **61**: 706.
51. Vivrette S, Bostian A, Bermingham E, Papich M. Quinolone-induced arthropathy in neonatal foals. *Proc Am Assoc Equine Pract* 2001; **47**: 376.
52. Schnabel LV, Papich MG, Divers TJ, *et al.* Pharmacokinetics and distribution of minocycline in mature horses after oral administration of multiple doses and comparison with minimum inhibitory concentrations. *Equine Vet J* 2012; **44**: 453.
53. Bryant JE, Brown MP, Gronwall RR, Merritt KA. Study of intragastric administration of doxycycline: pharmacokinetics including body fluid, endometrial and minimum inhibitory concentrations. *Equine Vet J* 2000; **32**: 233.
54. Kelmer G, Tatz A, Bdolah-Abram T. Indwelling cephalic or saphenous vein catheter use for regional limb perfusion in 44 horses with synovial injury involving the distal aspect of the limb. *Vet Surg* 2012; **41**: 938.
55. Levine DG, Epstein KL, Ahern BJ, Richardson DW. Efficacy of three tourniquet types for intravenous antimicrobial regional limb perfusion in standing horses. *Vet Surg* 2010; **39**: 1021.
56. Alkabes SB, Adams SB, Moore GE, Alkabes KC. Comparison of two tourniquets and determination of amikacin sulfate concentrations after metacarpophalangeal joint lavage performed simultaneously with intravenous regional limb perfusion in horses. *Am J Vet Res* 2011; **72**: 613.
57. Rubio-Martinez LM, Lopez-Sanroman J, Cruz AM, *et al.* Evaluation of safety and pharmacokinetics of vancomycin after intraosseous regional limb perfusion and comparison of results with those obtained after intravenous regional limb perfusion in horses. *Am J Vet Res* 2006; **67**: 1701.
58. Hyde RM, Lynch TM, Clark CK, *et al.* The influence of perfusate volume on antimicrobial concentration in synovial fluid following intravenous regional limb perfusion in the standing horse. *Can Vet J* 2013; **54**: 363.
59. Zantingh AJ, Schwark WS, Fubini SL, Watts AE. Accumulation of amikacin in synovial fluid after regional limb perfusion of amikacin sulfate alone and in combination with ticarcillin/clavulanate in horses. *Vet Surg* 2014; **43**: 282.
60. Parra-Sanchez A, Lugo J, Boothe DM, *et al.* Pharmacokinetics and pharmacodynamics of enrofloxacin and a low dose of amikacin administered via regional intravenous limb perfusion in standing horses. *Am J Vet Res* 2006; **67**: 1687.
61. Beccar-Varela AM, Epstein KL, White CL. Effect of experimentally induced synovitis on amikacin concentrations after intravenous regional limb perfusion. *Vet Surg* 2011; **40**: 891.
62. Pille F, De Baere S, Ceelen L, *et al.* Synovial fluid and plasma concentrations of ceftiofur after regional intravenous perfusion in the horse. *Vet Surg* 2005; **34**: 610.
63. Kelmer G, Tatz AJ, Famini S, *et al.* Evaluation of regional limb perfusion with chloramphenicol using the saphenous or cephalic vein in standing horses. *J Vet Pharmacol Ther* 2015; **38**: 35.
64. Rubio-Martinez LM, Cruz AM. Antimicrobial regional limb perfusion in horses. *J Am Vet Med Assoc* 2006; **228**: 706, 655.
65. Lallemand E, Trencart P, Tahier C, *et al.* Pharmacokinetics, pharmacodynamics and local tolerance at injection site of marbofloxacin administered by regional intravenous limb perfusion in standing horses. *Vet Surg* 2013; **42**: 649.
66. Rubio-Martinez LM, Lopez-Sanroman J, Cruz AM, *et al.* Evaluation of safety and pharmacokinetics of vancomycin after intravenous regional limb perfusion in horses. *Am J Vet Res* 2005; **66**: 2107.
67. Theelen MJ, Wilson WD, Edman JM, *et al.* Temporal trends in in vitro antimicrobial susceptibility patterns of bacteria isolated from foals with sepsis: 1979–2010. *Equine Vet J* 2014; **46**: 161.

68. Kelmer G, Bell GC, Martin-Jimenez T, *et al.* Evaluation of regional limb perfusion with amikacin using the saphenous, cephalic, and palmar digital veins in standing horses. *J Vet Pharmacol Ther* 2013; **36**: 236.
69. Levine DG, Epstein KL, Neelis DA, Ross MW. Effect of topical application of 1% diclofenac sodium liposomal cream on inflammation in healthy horses undergoing intravenous regional limb perfusion with amikacin sulfate. *Am J Vet Res* 2009; **70**: 1323.
70. Keys GJ, Berry DB, Pleasant RS, *et al.* Vascular distribution of contrast medium during intraosseous regional perfusion of the distal portion of the equine forelimb. *Am J Vet Res* 2006; **67**: 1445.
71. Mattson S, Boure L, Pearce S, *et al.* Intraosseous gentamicin perfusion of the distal metacarpus in standing horses. *Vet Surg* 2004; **33**: 180.
72. Butt TD, Bailey JV, Dowling PM, Fretz PB. Comparison of 2 techniques for regional antibiotic delivery to the equine forelimb: intraosseous perfusion vs. intravenous perfusion. *Can Vet J* 2001; **42**: 617.
73. Scheuch BC, Van Hoogmoed LM, Wilson WD, *et al.* Comparison of intraosseous or intravenous infusion for delivery of amikacin sulfate to the tibiotarsal joint of horses. *Am J Vet Res* 2002; **63**: 374.
74. Lescun TB, Adams SB, Wu CC, *et al.* Effects of continuous intra-articular infusion of gentamicin on synovial membrane and articular cartilage in the tarsocrural joint of horses. *Am J Vet Res* 2002; **63**: 683.
75. Meagher DT, Latimer FG, Sutter WW, Saville WJ. Evaluation of a balloon constant rate infusion system for treatment of septic arthritis, septic tenosynovitis, and contaminated synovial wounds: 23 cases (2002–2005). *J Am Vet Med Assoc* 2006; **228**: 1930.
76. Marsh CA, Watkins JP, Schneider RK. Intrathecal deep digital flexor tenectomy for treatment of septic tendonitis/tenosynovitis in four horses. *Vet Surg* 2011; **40**: 284.
77. Hand DR, Watkins JP, Honnas CM, Kemper D. Osteomyelitis of the sustentaculum tali in horses: 10 cases (1992–1998). *J Am Vet Med Assoc* 2001; **219**: 341.
78. Santschi EM, Adams SB, Fessler JF, Widmer WR. Treatment of bacterial tarsal tenosynovitis and osteitis of the sustentaculum tali of the calcaneus in five horses. *Equine Vet J* 1997; **29**: 244.

CHAPTER 17

Tendon and Paratenon Lacerations

Linda A. Dahlgren, DVM, PhD, Diplomate ACVS

Chapter Contents

Summary

Due to their size and inability to ambulate on only three limbs, horses are uniquely dependent on the integrity of the structures supporting the distal aspect of the limb. Lacerations involving the tendons in this area represent a significant therapeutic challenge. Wounds are frequently associated with considerable soft-tissue trauma and require surgical debridement and primary closure or management by second-intention healing. Horses with a digital extensor tendon laceration can often be managed conservatively and have a good prognosis for return to athletic function, but when one or both digital flexor tendons have been transected, management is more complex. Tenorrhaphy to reduce gap formation and external coaptation to share loading may allow a more rapid return to function. This chapter describes the diagnosis and treatment of tendon lacerations in the horse and discusses the numerous associated factors that must be considered when managing wounds involving tendons.

Introduction

Tendons are highly specialized soft-tissue structures with unique anatomic features that make them critical to the athletic prowess of the horse. Because of the complex hierarchical organization of tendons and their essential role in locomotion, injuries to the tendons and ligaments of horses are a significant clinical problem. The supporting structures of the distal aspect of the limbs of horses are especially prone to injury because of their exposed location with respect to a variety of potentially damaging objects in the environment. The natural "flight" instinct of the horse in response to stimuli may lead not only to injury, but may exacerbate an injury as the horse attempts to flee a frightening situation. The result can be a devastating injury that sometimes leads to loss of function or necessitates euthanasia. Advances in veterinary medicine and surgery have led to more optimistic outcomes than historically described; despite these advances, however, tendon injuries still require a substantial commitment, on the part of the owner, to a protracted process of rehabilitation. This chapter reviews the basic anatomy and physiology of tendons, nuances of the basic principles of wound healing that pertain to tendons, and details relating to the management of tendon lacerations.

Tendon anatomy and function

Tendons are the fibrous extensions of muscles that connect muscle to bone, forming contractile units adapted to perform several specialized functions. By traversing the joints of the appendicular skeleton, tendons and their associated structures lend support to the limb by working with ligaments and joint capsules to maintain alignment of the bony column. More importantly, tendons function to translate muscle contraction into joint movement and enable highly efficient locomotion

Equine Wound Management, Third Edition. Edited by Christine Theoret and Jim Schumacher.

Companion website: www.wiley.com/go/theoret/wound

through the storage and release of elastic energy as the tendon lengthens under load and returns to its original length once unloaded. The impressive athletic ability of the horse is a remarkable example of this adaptation of form to function. The galloping horse must withstand extremes of force over endless repetition, resulting in maximal tendon stretch and return to rest. Maintenance of this finely tuned structural integrity of tendons was essential for survival when the horse was a prey animal and remains essential in the modern era where the horse is a domesticated athlete. Consequently, careful attention to the principles of wound management and tendon healing are paramount to a successful outcome after a tendon injury.

Tendons of the distal portion of the limb originate proximally, in the myotendinous junction, a transition zone between the muscle and tendon. The force generated by muscle contraction is transmitted, via the tendon, to its distal insertion(s) in the bone, resulting in joint movement. Distally, where the tendon inserts in the bone, lies a zone where tendon transitions to fibrocartilage, mineralized fibrocartilage, and finally bone. Between its origin and insertion, the tendon consists of tensile and compressive regions based on whether the tendon is oriented linearly or bends around a bony prominence. Injury may occur at any one of these tendinous segments, and injury to any segment presents a distinct set of challenges for the clinician. Knowledge of tendon anatomy and function and the ability to perform a thorough examination and arrive at a specific anatomical diagnosis provide the most accurate information so that the selected treatment results in the best possible outcome.

Tendon function is facilitated by a series of associated structures required to properly position and nourish the tendon and allow it to move in relation to surrounding tissues. As the tendon extends from muscle to bone, it spans a number of functionally distinct areas characterized by important adaptations. Tendon is surrounded by paratenon in regions of the limb proximal and distal to the joints where the tendon remains linear during locomotion (Figure 17.1). The paratenon is a layer of loose areolar tissue that allows the tendon to move independently beneath the skin and provides structural support for associated neurovascular structures.

The tendon itself is wrapped in a thin adherent layer of fibrous connective tissue called the epitenon that is contiguous with the progressively finer connective tissue organization within the tendon's parenchyma. The network of connective tissue extensions from the epitenon, termed endotenon, carries the blood vessels, lymphatics, and nerves into the core of the tendon. The endotenon encases small collagen bundles (fibrils), binding them together into the larger bundles (fascicles) that ultimately form the characteristic hierarchical organization of tendon. Encasement of collagen bundles by the endotenon keeps the collagen bundles in longitudinal organization while allowing them to slide relative to one another as the tendon stretches and relaxes. Organization of collagen fibrils and fibers parallel to the lines of tension along the long axis of the limb is reinforced by covalent crosslinks between the individual

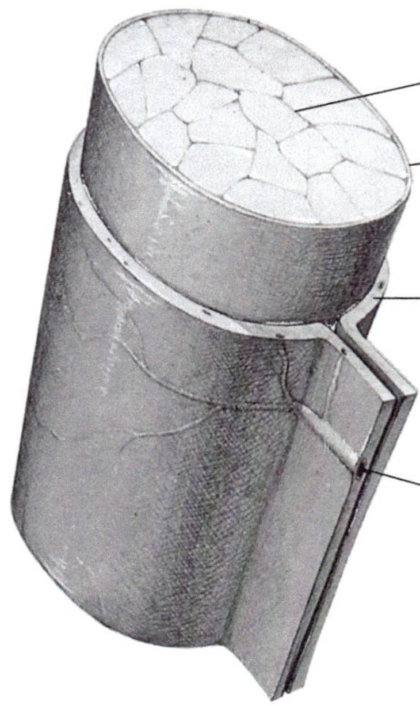

Figure 17.1 Longitudinal schematic of a tendon within the paratenon, as occurs between sheathed regions.

collagen fibers. It is this uniquely ordered arrangement that imparts very high tensile strength to the tendons and allows them to withstand the repetitive high loads they experience as the horse gallops.

As tendons pass over a joint or bony prominence, the increased friction and change of direction result in distinct structural adaptations endowing the tendon with the ability to withstand the increased compressive forces generated in these areas and thereby ensure anatomic integrity during locomotion. The paratenon in these regions is replaced by a fibrous synovial sheath that encases the tendon, bathing it in synovial fluid similar to that found in high-motion joints (Figure 17.2). The synovial sheath allows the tendon to glide smoothly as the joint flexes and extends and is composed of two layers: a fibrous support layer and an inner synovial membrane responsible for maintaining the health of the synovial environment (Figure 17.3). The inner synovial layer forms a contiguous layer lining the inside of the tendon sheath and the tendon. The mesotenon is a delicate sheet of connective tissue extending from the synovial membrane lining the sheath to the synovial membrane surrounding the tendon. It functions to carry the vascular supply to the tendon (Figure 17.4). Where movement or pressure is greatest, the mesotenon disappears entirely or is reduced to fine, thread-like soft-tissue structures called vincula that function to carry vascular supply to the tendon.[1] Proximally, the synovial membrane of the sheath contains a sickle-shaped fold of synovial membrane, which by its redundancy allows the tendon to move freely within its sheath (Figure 17.4).[1] Another structural adaptation critical to the maintenance of anatomic integrity as tendons span joints are fibrous bands called annular ligaments, or retinacula, that cross from medial to lateral, gently

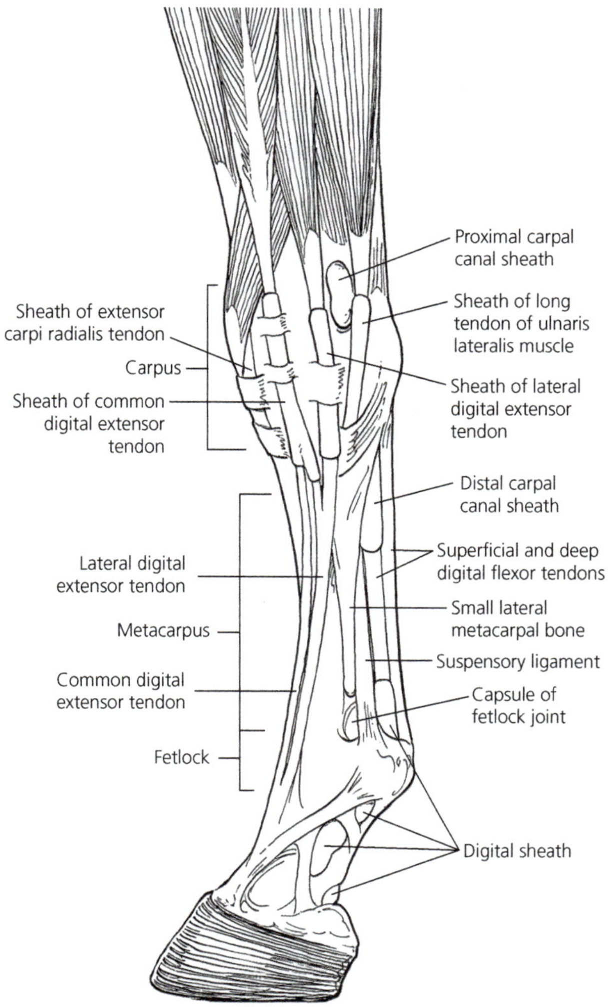

Figure 17.2 Lateral view of the forelimb showing individual sheaths that surround tendons where they cross points of friction such as joints or bony prominences.

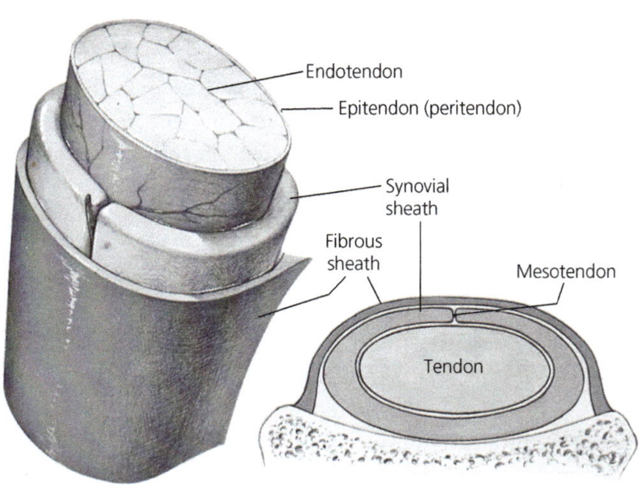

Figure 17.3 Longitudinal (left) and cross-sectional (right) views of a tendon within a synovial sheath.

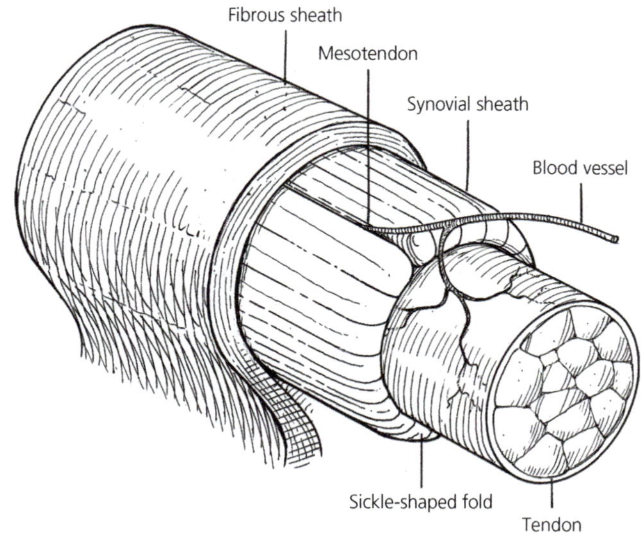

Figure 17.4 The proximal limits of the tendon sheath are characterized by a sickle-shaped fold of redundant synovial membrane that enables free movement of the tendon within the sheath as the tendon stretches and relaxes.

encircling the tendon and binding it against the bone, thereby preventing it from slipping off to the side.

Tendons receive their blood supply from four main sources. The proximal 25% of the tendon is nourished via the musculotendinous junction. The blood vessels that provide nutrition to the muscle via the endo-, epi-, and perimyseum continue to travel distally via the endo-, epi-, and paratenon to nourish the tendon. The distal 25% of the tendon receives its blood supply through its osseous insertions. Tendons receive an additional blood supply from surrounding soft tissue: the paratenon in unsheathed regions or the mesotenon or vincula in sheathed regions.[2,3] In sheathed regions, the tendon also receives nutrition via synovial diffusion. After a tendon has been injured, its vascular network is expanded dramatically as part of the healing process so that it can provide the critical cellular and paracrine signaling needed to direct the healing process.[4,5]

The tendon's extracellular matrix (ECM) is composed of fibrous elements (collagen and elastin) and amorphous ground substance (proteoglycans and structural glycoproteins), and is maintained by a small number of highly differentiated fibroblasts, or tenocytes, that are embedded within the connective tissue matrix. Mature tenocytes are characterized by an elongated cell body with multiple cytoplasmic extensions that reach between the surrounding collagen bundles and participate in cell-to-cell and cell-to-ECM interactions. These active communications are important in maintaining the homeostasis of the matrix and in transmitting load information that enables adaptation to training. Type I collagen, which makes up 80–86% of the dry weight of tendon, is the primary structural protein of tendon, and is largely responsible for the high tensile strength of tendon.[6] Elastin makes up as little as 1% of the dry weight of tendon but makes an important contribution to tendon's elastic properties.[7] Proteoglycans comprise less than 5% of the dry weight of tendon, but they play a central role in maintaining the viscoelastic properties of tendon. Proteoglycans perform the vital functions of regulating the water content of tendon, providing lubrication and spacing between fibrils, and imparting resilience and flexibility to the connective tissue matrix. They also play a role in the control of the diameter of collagen fibers and fibrillogenesis.[8–10] The specific type and amount of proteoglycan in tendon varies in response to the mechanical forces exerted on the anatomic segment and is an example of biologic adaptation to environment.[9–11] Regions under tension contain only small amounts of proteoglycan of small size (e.g., decorin, biglycan), whereas regions under compression contain larger amounts of proteoglycan of larger size (e.g., aggrecan and versican).[9]

The aforementioned unique macroscopic and microscopic adaptations of tendon are critical to normal locomotion. Should the tendon or its associated structures become damaged as a result of trauma or infection, debilitating lameness may ensue. An understanding of this relationship between structure and function can be exploited when treating horses with tendon injuries to make an accurate diagnosis and implement optimal treatment with the goals of returning the horse to athletic function.

Tendon healing

Because of the dense organization of collagen, sparse cellular population, and complex structural hierarchy, injuries to tendon present a therapeutic challenge. This is especially true in horses because of their large size and the resulting forces on their tendons, the risk of support limb laminitis, and the inability to prevent a horse from bearing weight on an injured limb during convalescence. Return to athletic function is hampered by the formation of scar tissue that lacks the viscoelastic properties and strength of normal tendon, resulting in a high incidence of re-injury.

Tendon undergoes the same general physiologic healing processes after injury, as do other soft tissues. The acute inflammatory and debridement phases may be prolonged in injured tendon because of the high content of collagen, which is resistant to proteolysis and slow to turnover.[12] Although the surrounding soft tissues may enter into the repair/proliferative phase of healing and form granulation tissue, the damaged collagen may still be undergoing debridement, extending the inflammatory phase beyond 10–14 days and well into the repair phase. The damaged collagen acts as a foreign body within the wound and delays healing. Healing of tendon is also slowed by the sparse blood supply to the tendon compared to that to some other tissues, such as muscle. The repair or proliferative phase of tendon healing begins at 3–4 days and lasts as long as necessary to produce adequate fibrovascular callous to stabilize the transected tendon ends; this is the first step critical to re-establishing the strength of tendon.

In tendon, the proliferative phase can last 21–45 days or longer. Even after the gap between the ends of the severed tendon is filled by a mass of collagenous scar tissue, the tensile strength of the tendon unit is low. To support the weight of the horse, the immature repair tissue must undergo the remodeling or maturation phase of tendon healing, which can last 6–12 months and is characterized by an increase in the tensile strength of the tendon and a decrease in the tissue's cellularity. As collagen is realigned along lines of tension, the content of type I collagen and the number of chemical crosslinks formed between the newly assembled collagen fibers rise. This brings about a gradual increase in tensile strength so that the injured tendon is able to withstand the forces required for standing and walking within a stall, without the need for external coaptation.

The nature of the cells that participate in the healing process remains a source of debate because few comprehensive studies have tracked the origin and migration of cells during healing of tendons. Tendon is not as inert a structure as was once thought. Healing is known to occur through extrinsic and intrinsic mechanisms.[13,14] Extrinsic healing occurs as fibroblasts migrate from the surrounding paratenon and/or tendon sheath into the injured area. The paratenon and tendon sheath represent a significant source of cells that contribute to the regenerative response, and for many years extrinsic healing was thought to be the sole mechanism whereby tendons underwent repair.

Tendons are now known to be capable of intrinsic repair, which occurs when tendon fibroblasts embedded within the ECM up-regulate their production of ECM components important to healing. Recent work suggests that progenitor cells embedded in the ECM may be activated in response to injury and thus contribute substantially to healing.[15,16] Another important source of cells for intrinsic repair is the endotenon. Following experimental injury, the endotenon becomes more prominent as a result of hypercellularity and neovascularization.[4,5] Big oval cells with large nuclei and nucleoli may represent progenitor cells that have migrated from the vasculature and/or have been quiescent within the endotenon and proliferate and differentiate in response to paracrine signals from the injured tissue. As knowledge of cell surface markers and cell tracking techniques increases, new studies may better define the cellular response that occurs within injured tendon. Although the extrinsic component of tendon healing is responsible for a robust cellular response, excessive scarring can result in the formation of adhesions between the tendon and the surrounding tissues past which the tendon must glide to function normally. This is especially important in the sheathed portions of the tendon where fibrous adhesions can significantly impair mobility, resulting in mechanical lameness and pain.

Diagnosis and treatment

Horses are prone to injuring themselves on a variety of objects found in their environment. Trauma can be self-inflicted while the horse is at play or being ridden, or it can be the result of actions by another horse. As is the case with any injured horse, the attending clinician must perform a thorough physical examination to determine the systemic status of the horse and the precise anatomic structures affected. This examination enables an accurate diagnosis, helps determine the prognosis and options for treatment, and helps the owner decide on how to manage the situation. If environmental factors do not allow for a complete physical examination at the time the horse is initially presented, a preliminary assessment must be made, and the horse must receive appropriate interim treatment prior to being transported to a referral center. The goals of initial first-aid are to immobilize the injured limb to prevent further damage to soft tissue or bone and to provide immediate life-saving treatment to stop hemorrhage and treat for shock.

Physical examination

What to do

- Perform a complete physical examination to evaluate for hypovolemic shock.
- Control hemorrhage.
- Immobilize the limb to prevent further damage.

What to avoid

- Avoid transportation without adequately stabilizing the injured limb.
- Avoid conservative management without fully assessing the structures involved.

The horse should be examined for signs of hypovolemic shock, which include rapid, thready pulse, pale mucous membranes, delayed capillary refill time, and skin tenting. The superficial location of the median artery in the forelimb, the dorsal metatarsal artery in the hindlimb, and the digital arteries in the distal aspect of the limb make them prone to transection. Hemorrhage can typically be controlled, at least temporarily, by the application of a pressure bandage to the wound until the wound can be fully assessed. Immobilizing the injured limb by using a Kimzey Leg Saver Splint (Kimzey, Inc.) (Figure 17.5) or a piece of PVC pipe incorporated into a heavy bandage and extending down to the ground (Figure 17.6) prevents a partially lacerated tendon from disrupting completely and protects neurovascular structures from additional trauma. Splints are placed either dorsally or on the palmar surface of the forelimb and on the plantar surface of the hindlimb (the reader is referred to Chapter 7 for more information on splints). When the horse is able to balance on the stabilized limb, it is more likely to remain calm, enabling the exam to be completed.

The injured horse may need to be sedated or otherwise restrained to complete the examination, always while keeping in mind the systemic state of the horse. Severe blood loss and associated hypovolemic shock dictate selection and dosage of a sedative or tranquilizer. It is important that the veterinarian, owner, and handlers be protected from harm and that the horse not suffer more injury to the damaged tendon. A severely lame horse, in pain, can be a challenge to handle, and care must be taken to thoroughly assess the situation.

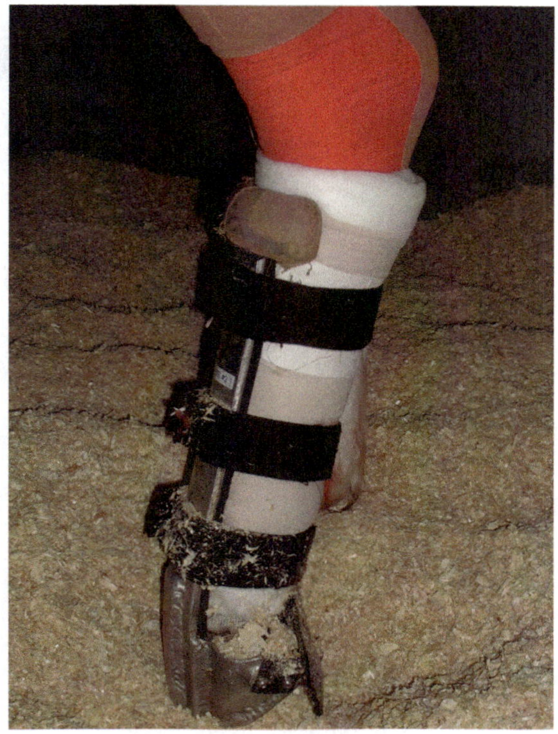

Figure 17.5 Kimzey Leg Saver (Kimzey, Inc.) applied to the hindlimb to provide support and prevent further tissue damage. Courtesy of Dr. Christophe Celeste.

Physical examination should begin with a basic assessment of the horse's temperature, pulse, respiratory rate, color of mucous membranes, and capillary refill time. The horse's history, including information as to the duration of the injury, the horse's vaccination status, and the use of any medications, should be recorded. The "big-picture" information, such as hemorrhage or evidence of prior hemorrhage, weight-bearing status, and pain level of the horse, as well as the horse's overall demeanor, can be useful in formulating an initial plan. It is critical that the entire horse be examined so as not to miss additional injuries that may affect prognosis.

Careful observation of how the horse is willing to use the limb provides key information. Is the horse able to weight bear when stationary and to lock the stay apparatus? Does the foot stay flat on the ground, or does the fetlock or hock drop when the horse bears weight on the affected limb? Is there an abnormal pattern of flexion and extension that suggests that the reciprocal apparatus is no longer intact? Is there a stable bony column to support the horse? Is there any evidence of fluid drainage suggesting that a synovial structure is open? An understanding of normal anatomy is important when examining the distal aspect of the limb specifically for laceration of a digital flexor tendon.

Observation as the horse bears weight or takes a careful step or two on the injured limb is one of the easiest ways to assess the integrity of the primary support structures, including the digital

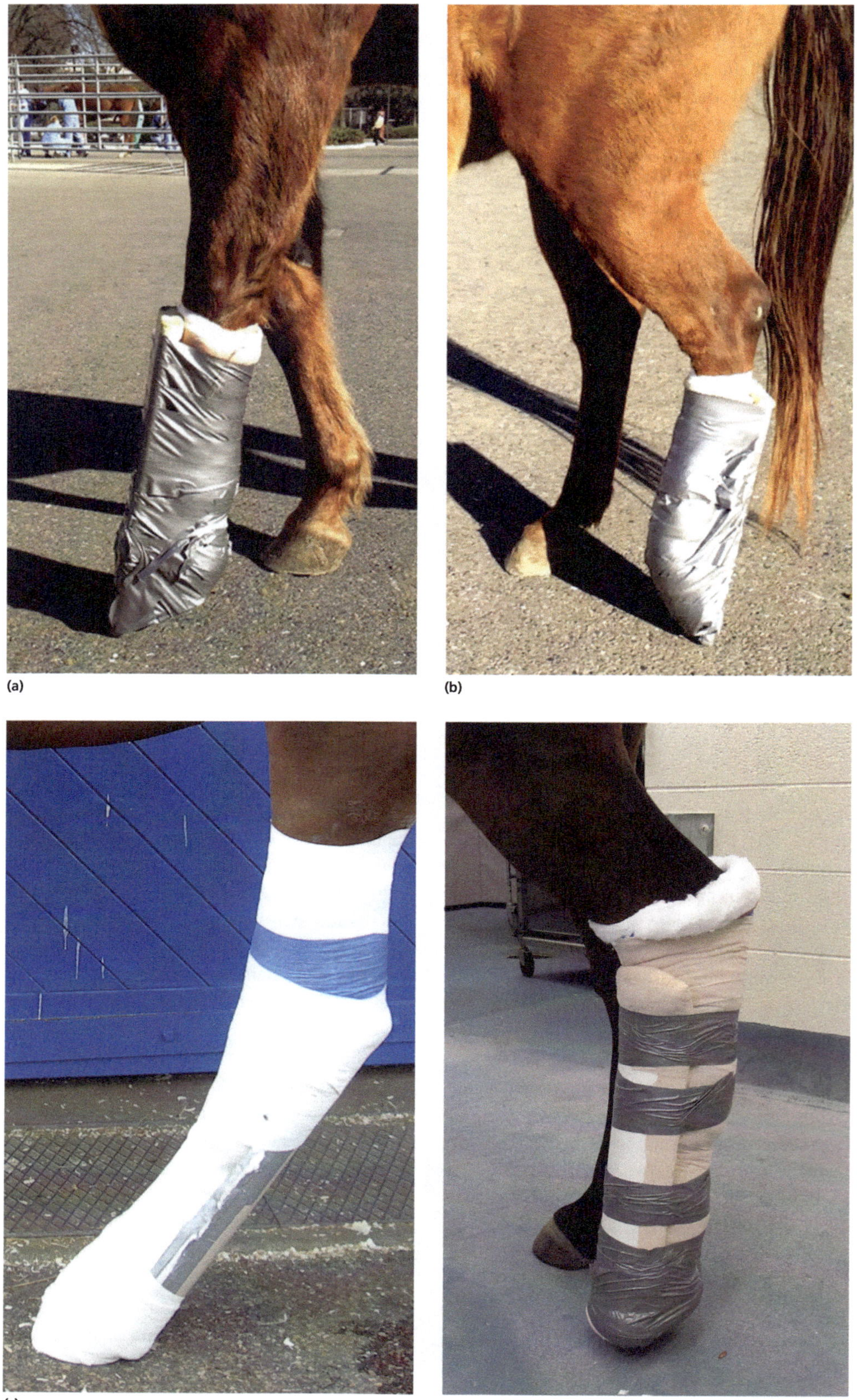

(a) (b) (c) (d)

Figure 17.6 PVC splint applied to achieve immobilization and support for transport to a referral facility. Splints are usually applied to the dorsal surface of the forelimb with the dorsal bone column straight **(a)**. For the hindlimb, splints are best placed on the plantar surface with the limb in partial flexion **(b)** or with the dorsal bone column straight **(c)**; however, dorsal splint placement can be useful if plantar placement is not possible **(d)**. Regardless of placement, the splint should extend to the ground and incorporate the foot for maximal stability. The flexed position **(b)** is indicated to relieve tension on the flexor tendons and prevent a partial flexor tendon tear from becoming complete. Courtesy of Dr. Larry Galuppo (a and b) and Dr. Olivier Lepage (c).

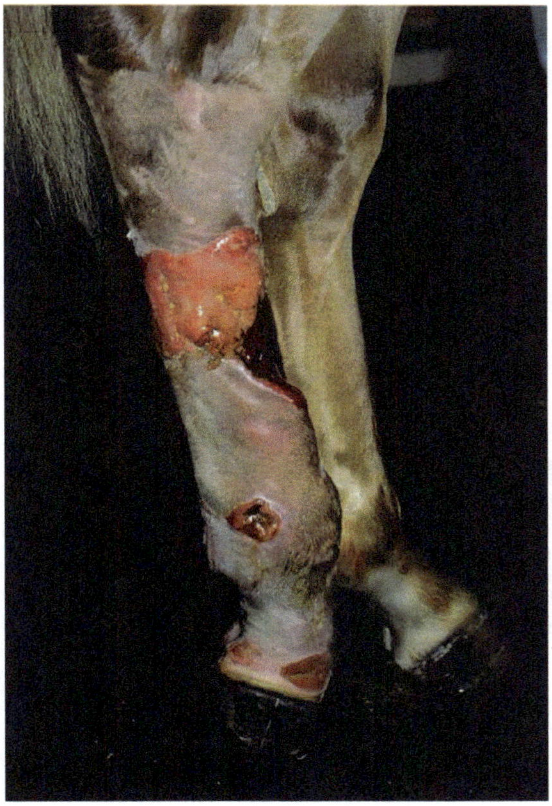

Figure 17.7 Knuckling of the right hind fetlock associated with transection of the long and lateral digital extensor tendons.

extensor and flexor tendons, suspensory ligament, and their associated structures (e.g., tendon sheath, digital annular ligament, neurovascular structures). Transection of the common digital extensor tendon of the forelimb, or both the lateral and long digital extensor tendons (or below where the two join) of the hindlimb, results in knuckling of the fetlock when the horse attempts to walk, because the horse has lost its ability to extend the toe as the limb is advanced (Figure 17.7). When the limb is manually placed in a normal weight-bearing position, a horse with a severed digital extensor tendon is able to bear weight on the limb without hyperextending the joints. Knuckling of the limb causes most horses to exhibit a substantial degree of anxiety, making restraint and stabilization with a splint an important aspect of treatment.

Transection of the tendons and ligaments on the palmar/plantar surface of the distal limb results in characteristic changes in joint position (Figure 17.8). Complete transection of the superficial digital flexor tendon (SDFT) at the metacarpal/metatarsal region or fetlock results in hyperextension of the metacarpo/metatarsophalangeal joint, characterized by "dropping" of the palmar/plantar aspect of the fetlock towards the ground (Figure 17.9). The toe remains on the ground. The pastern may subluxate dorsally after the SDFT is transected. A structure deep to the SDFT [e.g., the deep digital flexor tendon (DDFT) or suspensory ligament] may be injured in the absence of injury to a more superficial structure, such as the SDFT, but most lacerations involve the structures immediately

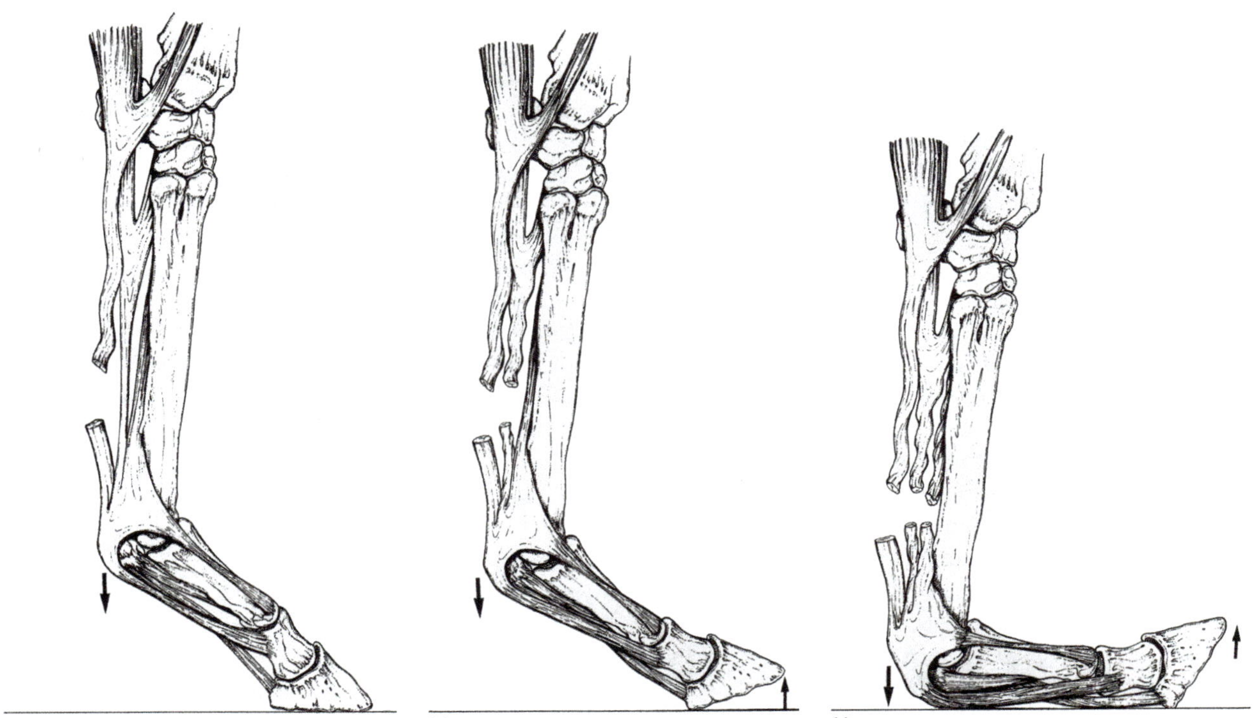

Figure 17.8 Schematic showing changes in joint position. **(a)** Transection of the superficial digital flexor tendon (SDFT) results in metacarpo/metatarsophalangeal hyperextension. **(b)** Transection of the SDFT and deep digital flexor tendon (DDFT) results in metacarpo/metatarsophalangeal hyperextension and toe elevation. **(c)** Transection of the SDFT, DDFT, and suspensory ligament results in complete loss of metacarpo/metatarsophalangeal support. Source: Watkins 1999.[17] Reproduced with permission of WB Saunders.

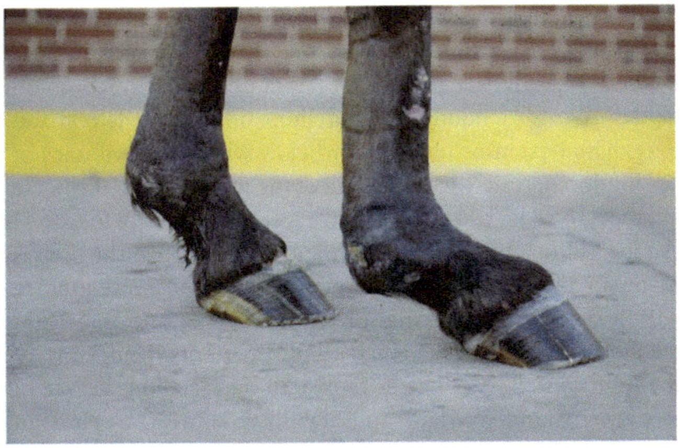

Figure 17.9 Example of mild hyperextension (fetlock drop) of the right metacarpophalangeal joint resulting from complete transection of the SDFT.

underlying the skin before they involve deeper ones. The distinctive clinical sign indicative of complete transection of the DDFT is elevation of the toe off the ground (Figure 17.10), resulting from loss of the tension band produced by insertion of the DDFT on the palmar/plantar surface of the distal phalanx. Transection of both the SDFT and the DDFT leads to hyperextension of the metacarpo/metatarsophalangeal and distal interphalangeal joints, as well as elevation of the toe off the ground (Figure 17.11). When the suspensory ligament, in addition to both of the digital flexor tendons, is transected, support to the palmar/plantar aspect of the limb is completely lost, and the palmar/plantar surface of the fetlock rests on the ground with the toe pointing up (Figure 17.12). Because the DDFT and its associated sheath are the only support structures present on the palmar/plantar surface of the pastern, injuries in this area typically affect only the DDFT. The clinical signs associated with partial transection of a digital flexor tendon vary depending on the percentage of remaining intact tendon and the location of the injury.

Careful palpation of the injury can be useful in confirming the information obtained by observing the stance assumed by the horse when it bears weight on the injured limb and in determining the extent of a partial laceration. Hair surrounding the wound should be clipped and the wound cleaned. Sterile gloves should be worn to prevent further contaminating wound, and for one's own protection against zoonotic infection. Many horses must be sedated and/or the region of the wound desensitized by regional or local anesthesia to ensure that the wound is examined thoroughly and safely. If the wound appears to be severe and clearly requires surgical repair, it can be assessed more thoroughly with the horse anesthetized. The potential risks associated with recovery from general anesthesia should be taken into account when deciding whether to anesthetize an injured horse for surgical treatment. External coaptation in the form a cast may be required to prevent more damage to injured structures while the horse recovers from general anesthesia. The systemic status of the horse must also be taken into consideration before general anesthesia is selected as the method of restraint; if the injury appears to be severe, however, the horse should be anesthetized so that the wound can be assessed thoroughly, irrigated, debrided, and repaired.

In addition to visually assessing the injury and palpating the wound, the limb, while being palpated, should be flexed and extended, to better assess the injury. The ends of a completely severed tendon may retract a substantial distance proximally and distally to the wound, making the severed ends difficult to see or palpate. Ultrasonographic examination may be useful in assessing the extent of soft-tissue injury; air trapped within the tissue planes of an open wound, however, creates artifacts that interfere with accurate sonographic examination. Nevertheless, use of ultrasound to assess vascular integrity in severe wounds remains an important adjunct to the rest of the examination. A horse with a completely disrupted or compromised blood supply has a grave prognosis for survival. Using radiography to rule out concurrent fracture is also warranted because the presence of bone involvement can impact the prognosis substantially.

General treatment considerations

Regardless of the structures involved, treatment of wounds involving a lacerated tendon is comprised of standard supportive care, including treatment of the horse for pain, dehydration, and/or hypovolemic shock, and of the wound for inflammation and contamination. Intravenous administration of fluids is indicated for horses suffering from hypovolemic shock resulting from hemorrhage or from dehydration resulting from decreased water consumption because of immobility and/or pain. In most cases, isotonic fluids, such as lactated Ringer's solution, are adequate and should be administered at a rate appropriate to the horse's needs. Administering plasma to treat for hypoproteinemia, or hypertonic saline solution or hetastarch to treat for hypovolemic shock, may be indicated in extreme circumstances. Additional nursing care specific to the horse's systemic status and individual needs should be considered. This might be as simple as treating other less severe wounds, or more intensive, such as providing sole and frog support and cold therapy to prevent support limb laminitis. When bandaging or casting limits the mobility of the horse, care must be taken to provide bedding that enables easy movement within the stall.

For many horses, conventional non-steroidal anti-inflammatory drug (NSAID) therapy may suffice to keep them comfortable. In these cases, phenylbutazone (2.2–4.4 mg/kg) or flunixin meglumine (0.5–1.0 mg/kg) given twice daily provide excellent anti-inflammatory and analgesic effects. Because most horses with a moderate or severe injury have an intravenous catheter in place for antibiotic therapy, the intravenous route is preferred for ease of administration and rapid, reliable effects.

Many horses with severe injuries may require analgesia beyond that provided by a NSAID, making it necessary to explore additional options to provide adequate analgesia. Administering

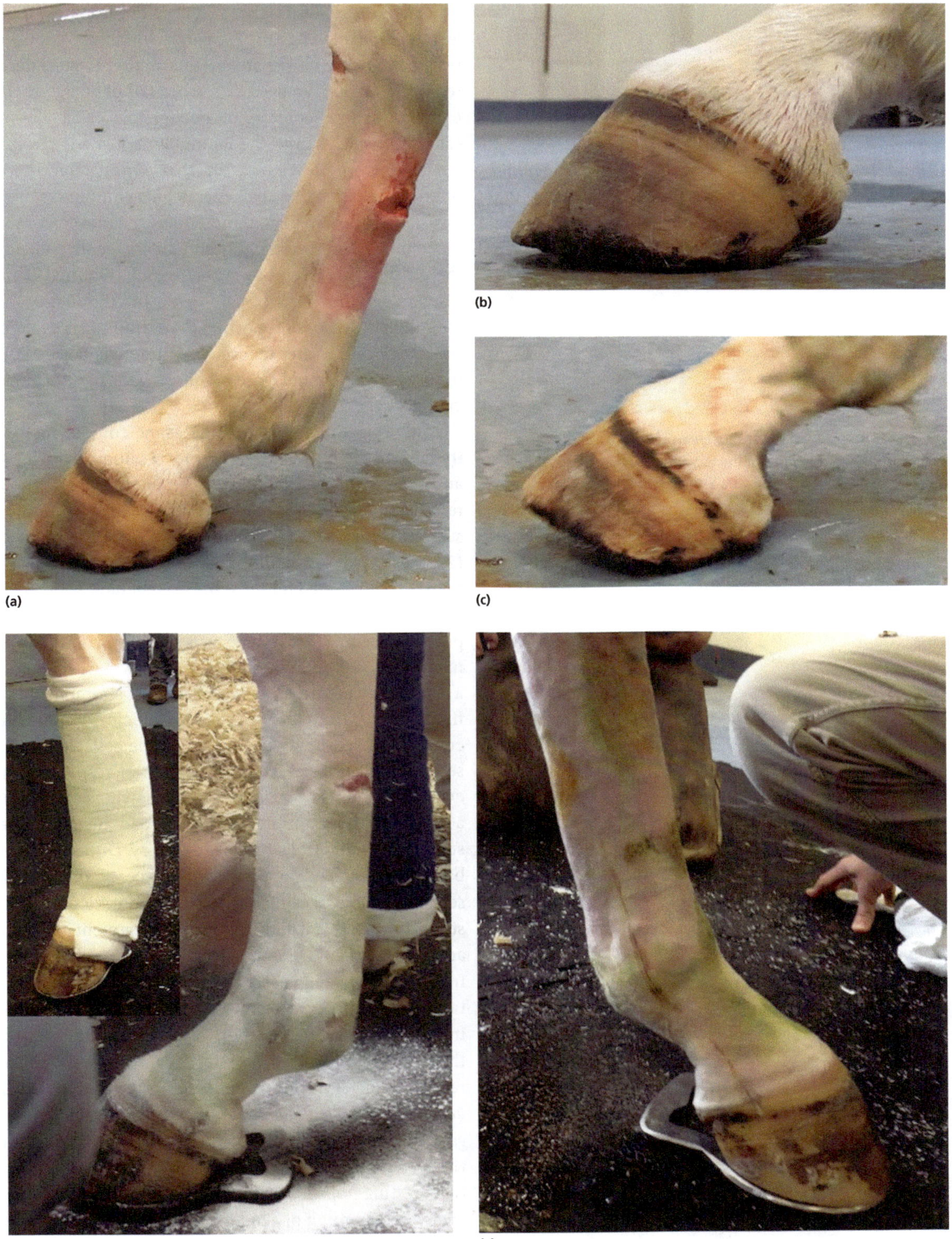

(a) (b) (c) (d) (e)

Figure 17.10 **(a)**–**(c)** Transection of the DDFT in the metatarsal region showing toe elevation but no fetlock hyperextension (shown approximately 2 weeks following injury). Note that the toe is only slightly elevated when the horse is partially weight bearing **(a, b)** but when weight bearing is increased the toe elevation becomes more exaggerated **(c)**. Because of the instability with increased weight bearing **(c)**, it was difficult to catch the image without motion artifact. **(d, e)** The same horse 2 weeks later when the fishtail shoe was applied at the time of cast removal showing how the shoe works to support the limb and prevent toe elevation. The cast was removed early at 2 weeks because the horse developed cast sores. In its place the fishtail shoe and a bandage cast **(d inset)** was applied for support and changed every 4 days for 4 weeks. Image **(d)** was taken after 4 days when the first bandage cast was changed. Courtesy of Drs. Mike Cissell and Elsa Ludwig.

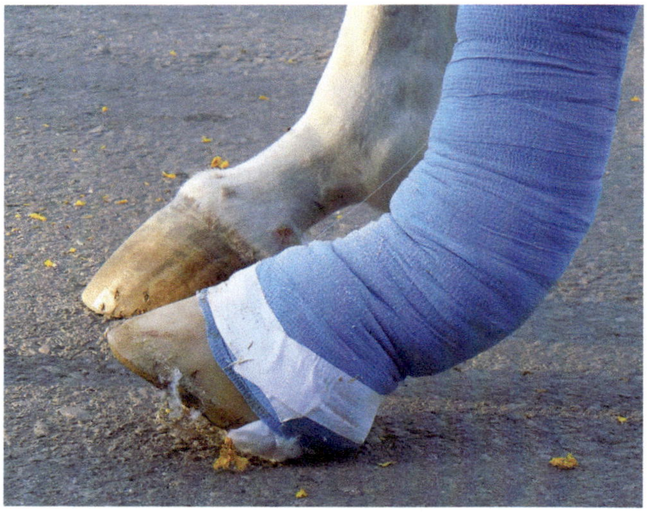

Figure 17.11 Hyperextension of the left metacarpophalangeal and distal interphalangeal joints and elevation of the toe off the ground associated with complete transection of both the SDFT and DDFT. Courtesy of Dr. Gal Kelmer.

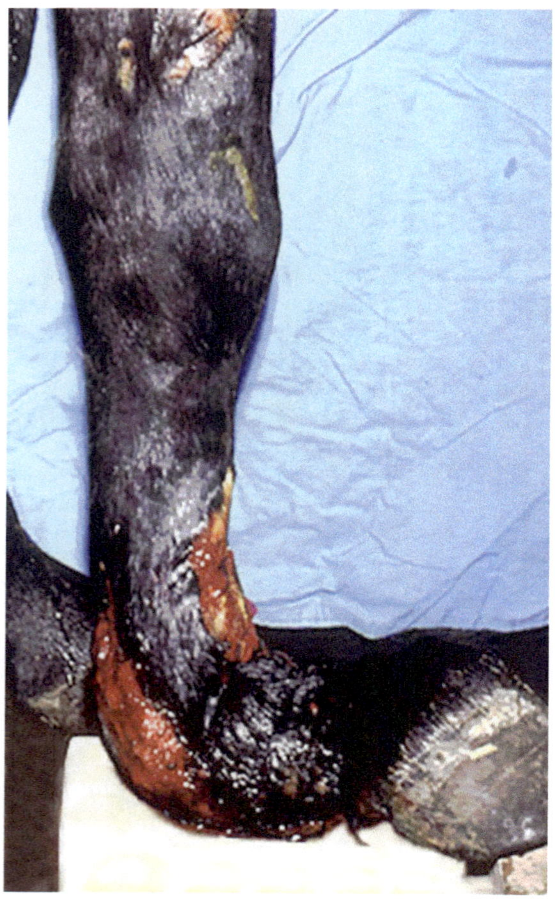

Figure 17.12 Complete loss of the palmar support structures occurs when the suspensory ligament and both digital flexor tendons are completely transected resulting in the fetlock resting on a block of wood and the toe pointing up. In this case, the toe elevation is less marked than normal because the extensor tendons were also transected.

an analgesic drug through a caudal epidural catheter is an excellent method of relieving pain in a hindlimb.[18–22] Continuous peripheral nerve blocks are another option to consider in cases requiring adjunct analgesia.[23,24] The goal of analgesic therapy is to make the horse comfortable enough to occasionally and modestly shift weight on to the injured limb just enough to prevent laminitis from developing in the contralateral limb. Other options for adjunctive analgesia include continuous intravenous infusion of lidocaine, ketamine, or butorphanol, fentanyl patches, morphine administered intramuscularly, and gabapentin;[25–27] these drugs, however, are generally only required if the horse displays extreme signs of pain or during the first 24–48 hours after injury. Because supporting limb laminitis is a major potential complication after tendon laceration, vigilance with respect to supportive care and close monitoring for signs of laminitis are crucial elements of nursing care.

Antibiotic therapy is an important component of wound therapy and is especially critical for wounds involving tendons and their associated structures. Antibiotics are often administered systemically and regionally. Broad-spectrum antibiotics, such as penicillin (22–44 000 IU/kg IV q 6 hours) or ceftiofur (2.2 mg/kg IV q 12 hours) and gentamicin (6.6 mg/kg IV q 24 hours) are indicated for most horses that have suffered a tendon laceration. Trimethoprim sulfa (30 mg/kg PO q 12 hours) may provide adequate coverage against most common contaminants, and its use may be sufficient if the wound does not involve a synovial structure. Whenever possible, a sample of (synovial) fluid or tissue from the wound for cytologic examination and/or culture and sensitivity testing should be collected to guide the selection of antibiotics. Based on lack of response to therapy, cytologic findings, or more appropriately, sensitivity testing, administering an antibiotic with a broad anaerobic spectrum, such as metronidazole, may be necessary. Duration of therapy is based subjectively on prior experience of the clinician, the severity, degree of contamination and duration of the wound, structures involved, and response to treatment. Antibiotics are administered intravenously as early as possible after tendon injury has been diagnosed; this is most likely to occur in consultation with a referral center with the aim to administer the initial dose prior to transport of the horse. Interim antibiotic therapy is an *empiric* drug selection, instituted while awaiting results of bacterial culture and antibiotic sensitivity testing. *For all severely infected wounds, rational antibiotic therapy must be guided by culture and sensitivity results.* Consequently, the referring veterinarian should collect a sample for culture and sensitivity testing *prior* to the initiation of interim antibiotic therapy and either submit it or send it along with the horse for testing at the referral hospital. The reader is referred to Chapter 16 for more information on the diagnosis and management of wounds involving synovial structures. Table 19.1 lists common bacterial isolates from various wounds in horses, and provides recommendations for interim systemic antibiotic therapy.

The large amount of tissue trauma and contamination in wounds involving a tendon result in a prolonged phase of debridement, which in turn, delays the formation of a healthy bed of granulation tissue. Antibiotic therapy should be administered for at least 3–5 days. Only for minimally contaminated wounds treated early (less than 3–6 hours after injury) would antibiotic therapy be maintained for as little as 3–5 days. Total duration of antibiotic therapy usually ranges from 7–28 days. A lengthy period of administration is most often associated with wounds involving a synovial structure and those with substantial contamination, a slow response to therapy, and/or persistent infection. For more information, refer to Table 19.5, which provides guidelines for duration of antibiotic therapy in specific types of wounds.

The increased use of regional antibiotic therapy in recent years has greatly improved the prognosis for horses with extensive tissue damage to a limb, with or without damage to a synovial structure. The antibiotic should be administered regionally and systemically for optimal results. Regional antibiotic delivery has the distinct advantage of achieving a much higher concentration of the antibiotic at the wound than can be achieved by systemic administration where high doses may be unacceptably expensive or cause detrimental side-effects. Additionally, a wider range of antibiotic options that can be delivered regionally enables the selection of an antibiotic with a susceptibility pattern or spectrum of activity different to that being administered systemically. A complete review of regional antibiotic delivery is beyond the scope of this chapter, but many excellent resources on the subject are available[28–30] and more information can be found in Chapter 19 of this book.

The choice of administering an antibiotic intravenously, intraosseously, intrasynovially, topically, or by sustained release from beads implanted at the wound is made on a case-by-case basis and depends on many factors, including the nature of the specific injury and the availability of a peripheral vein for delivery. Intravenous regional antibiotic delivery is a common choice because of general ease of administration and distribution to synovial structures and the surrounding soft tissues. Frequency of regional delivery depends on severity of contamination or infection, response to initial treatment, ease of delivery, and to some extent, prior experiences of the clinician. Although the literature contains various reports on the pharmacokinetics of regionally delivered antibiotics, the majority concern normal horses, and how these data may translate to horses with inflammation and possibly increased blood flow to the injured area is unknown. In many cases, therapy is administered by this route every other day, but frequency of administration can sometimes be reduced to every third day if the horse responds well to therapy.

In recent years, the use of regenerative therapies has gained popularity in veterinary medicine, especially in equine practice. Mesenchymal stem cells (MSC) are commonly delivered to the site of tendon and ligament injury caused by overuse, in the hope of stimulating a stronger healing response and reducing the incidence of re-injury. Sources of cells include bone marrow and adipose tissue. Additional biologic therapies, such as platelet rich plasma (PRP), concentrated bone marrow aspirate, autologous conditioned serum (irap® plus, Dechra Veterinary Products), and ECM (ACell *Vet*™, ACell, Inc.), have also been described for treating tendinitis and desmitis. Application of regenerative therapies in general wound healing is covered in Chapter 22 of this book. The use of regenerative therapies has not yet been described for adjunctive treatment of tendon and ligament lacerations, but theoretically, their beneficial effects would apply. Use of PRP gel (with or without MSC) or ECM at the site of tendon injury may provide a structural scaffold and bioactive proteins capable of contributing to a regenerative response. Judicious use of products shown to be safe for use in open wounds, especially those that can be produced for point-of-care application, may be beneficial.

Extensor tendon laceration

What to do

- Most extensor tendon lacerations do not require tenorrhaphy. Those over the fetlock are an exception and should be sutured.
- Splint the limb if the horse knuckles at the fetlock.

What to avoid

- Avoid closing a wound with severely traumatized tissue that cannot be adequately debrided.

Degloving wounds of the dorsal surface of the metacarpus/metatarsus are frequently accompanied by laceration of the associated extensor tendon(s) (Figure 17.13). Although the management of an extensor tendon transection can be challenging in the short term, these wounds typically heal by the formation of one large mass of scar tissue that incorporates the tendon and surrounding soft tissues. Despite the lack of mobility caused by this scar tissue, a good prognosis for return to athletic function can be expected. Treatment of wounds on the dorsal metacarpal/metatarsal surface should follow general principles of wound management first, with attention to the severed extensor tendon taken into consideration as a secondary factor in managing the wound. Careful attention to the potential for synovial involvement or sequestrum formation is critical in guiding therapeutic decisions. Whether or not to suture the lacerated tendon ends and/or to apply a half-limb cast is based more on the treatment the wound itself requires than on how the tendon should be treated. A lacerated extensor tendon generally does not require tenorrhaphy, unless the laceration is in the region of the fetlock, because a tendon lacerated at that site does not heal readily unless its ends are apposed. A recent report suggests that horses with combined laceration of the lateral and long digital extensors in the hindlimb may benefit from suturing the tendon to the periosteum on the dorsal surface of the third metatarsal bone.[31] Wounds with minimal soft-tissue damage and scant environmental bacteria and debris should be sutured. A degloving injury to the dorsal surface of the limb, however, is commonly associated with a high

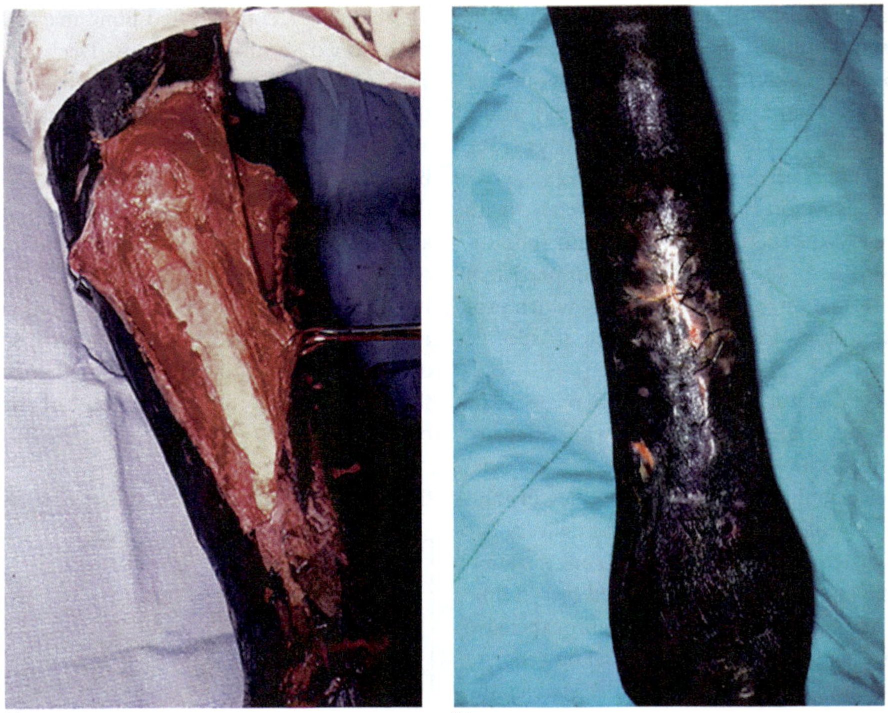

(a) (b)

Figure 17.13 **(a)** An extensive degloving wound over the dorsal metatarsus resulting in complete transection of the extensor tendons. **(b)** The same wound 2 weeks after wound revision, suturing, and cast application.

degree of tissue trauma and/or loss, maceration, and significant contamination. These severe wounds are best managed by partial closure, delayed primary closure, or second-intention healing. The reader is referred to Chapter 8 for more information on approaches to wound closure.

Expected outcome: If carefully managed, horses with a wound involving a digital extensor tendon have a good prognosis for return to athletic function and for good cosmesis. Approximately 70–80% of horses with a lacerated digital extensor tendon returned to soundness[32–35] and 50–60% of those horses performed at or above their previous level of performance.[32–34] No clear association has been identified between the prognosis for a horse with a laceration of a digital extensor tendon and factors such as duration of injury, tenorrhaphy, cast application, breach of a synovial structure, and whether the laceration to the tendon was partial or complete. One report suggests that the likelihood of a racehorse returning to its intended use after transection of the lateral and long digital extensor tendons may be lower than that for horses in the general population.[36] The decidedly lower likelihood of return to use for racing Thoroughbreds in this study (17%) may be biased by the high number of horses euthanized without treatment (41%) due to the extent of soft-tissue damage and vascular compromise.[36] Culture and perceptions of the Thoroughbred racing industry regarding the ability to race and/or greater emphasis on a business-based decision than is common among owners of sport or pleasure horses, may play a role in the poorer prognosis for racehorses. Racehorses, in two other reports, tended to have a poorer prognosis for return to their intended use after suffering a laceration to an extensor tendon.[32,34]

The treating clinician must weigh the advantages of irrigating, debriding, and repairing a wound with the horse anesthetized (e.g., ease and completeness of debridement and assessment of associated structures, arthroscopic lavage of an associated synovial structure, complete or partial primary closure, and cast application) against the disadvantages and/or risks associated with general anesthesia (e.g., cost, required expertise, risks of general anesthesia and recovery, and specific risks of complications related to anesthetic recovery in light of the injuries being treated). The decision of whether or not to anesthetize the horse must take into consideration available resources, training and expertise of the clinician, and the temperament and intended use of the horse. A successful, cosmetic outcome is, in most cases, a reasonable expectation with informed, attentive conservative management of lacerations involving a digital extensor tendon. In certain situations, synovial structures can be lavaged using ingress/egress needles with the horse standing. If the fetlock knuckles, a splint incorporated into a heavy support bandage may be required for the first 2–4 weeks of healing until enough peritendinous attachments develop to stabilize the wound and prevent the fetlock from knuckling (the reader is referred to Chapter 7 for more information on bandaging, splinting and casting).

Flexor tendon laceration

An important distinction must be made between lacerations involving a digital extensor tendon and those involving a digital flexor tendon. Although the principles of wound management generally apply equally to each, the management of flexor tendon injury must take into account several key differences when developing a treatment plan and providing a prognosis to an owner. The prognosis for lacerations of flexor tendons is substantially worse than that for extensor tendons. This is largely based on the high tensile forces that must be withstood by the flexor tendons during ambulation, as well as the critical gliding function of the flexor tendons as the fetlock goes through its range of motion. When a solid mass of collagen has filled the gap between the severed ends of a digital extensor tendon and collagen has reorganized enough to gain some tensile strength, the horse is able to extend the toe and avoid knuckling. Eventually, it can return to full performance. The same is not true for horses with a lacerated digital flexor tendon. Use of a heavy Robert Jones bandage or splint is typically adequate to stabilize an extensor tendon injury, and, despite gap formation, the horse can weight bear comfortably while the tendon heals. Conversely, when a flexor tendon is transected, external coaptation rarely provides sufficient support to allow the horse to bear weight comfortably. This leads to undue stress on the contralateral limb and/or the development of cast sores.

Expected outcome: The prognosis for soundness for a horse with a transected digital flexor tendon is poorer than that for a horse with a transected digital extensor tendon. The reported incidence of survival for horses with a transected digital flexor tendon exceeds 78%, whereas the incidence for return to previous function ranges from 18–55%.[34,37,38] While a lacerated extensor tendon most commonly does not require tenorrhaphy, the need to suture a transected flexor tendon is less clear. Although tenorrhaphy is not significantly associated with improved outcome in clinical cases,[34,37] suturing is generally recommended for transected flexor tendons,[34] based in part on experimental studies documenting significantly stronger repair with suturing than with cast immobilization alone.[39,40] Perceived advantages of tenorrhaphy include reduced gap formation, resulting in earlier union of the tendon ends, which in turn, results in earlier return of tensile strength and reduced formation of scar tissue. Reduction of scar tissue is especially important in sheathed regions of the tendon, to prevent the formation of adhesions. A horse with a partial tendon laceration may also benefit from tenorrhaphy to prevent worsening of the damage and to reduce gap formation. If greater than 75% of the diameter of the tendon is transected, tenorrhaphy is indicated; horses with a less extensive laceration (e.g., one involving 50–75% of the tendon), however, may also benefit from tenorrhaphy.

With the horse anesthetized, the wound is carefully and meticulously debrided with surgical instruments and by using a balanced polyionic solution, such as lactated Ringer's solution, delivered at ~10–15 psi (Figure 17.14). Dilute solutions of povidone–iodine (0.1–0.2%) or chlorhexidine (0.05%) may be used to irrigate the wound itself; however, use of even these dilute solutions should be avoided when lavaging an open synovial structure. Care should be taken to ensure that only the damaged and contaminated tissue is resected. The goal of debridement is to transform the contaminated wound into one suitable for tenorrhaphy and closure. Large vessels are ligated to achieve hemostasis. Synoviocentesis is performed, if required, to determine synovial involvement. While awaiting the results of cytologic examination of synovial fluid, the synovial cavity can be lavaged using needles or cannulas. To deliver a large volume of solution (typically lactated Ringer's solution without antiseptic) through the synovial cavity, arthroscopic cannulas should be used. Inserting an arthroscope through a cannula enables the surgeon to search for debris within the tendon sheath and allows for directed lavage to all recesses where bacteria may pool.

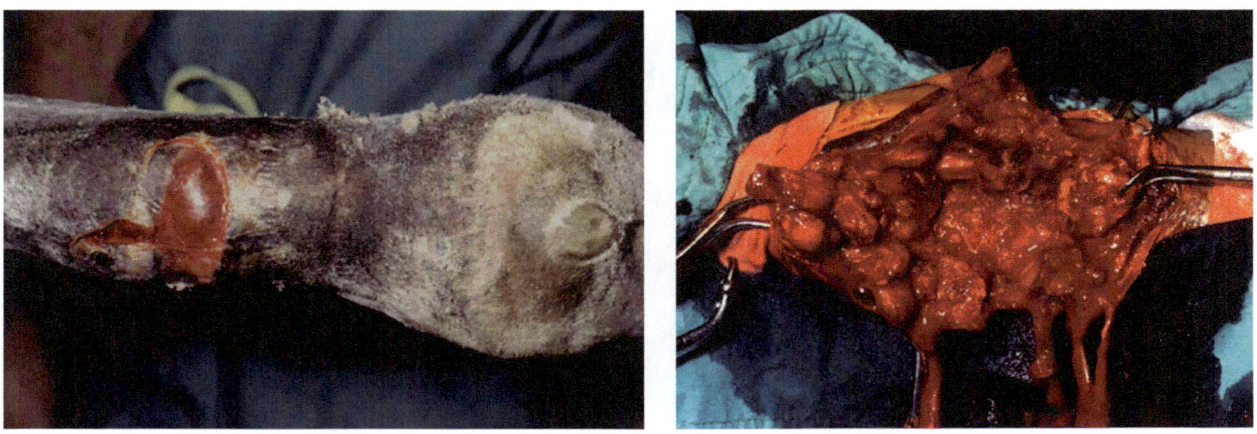

(a) (b)

Figure 17.14 **(a)** Severely contaminated/infected 4-day-old wound on the palmar surface of the metacarpus. **(b)** The same wound following extensive layered debridement. Both the SDFT and DDFT were completely transected, and the suspensory ligament was partially transected (<25%). Delayed tenorrhaphy was performed in this case.

When performing tenorrhaphy, one should remove only the minimum amount of tissue required to debride the tendon ends. This minimizes the gap between ends of the tendon and thus enables placement of the suture bites an adequate distance from the tendon ends (~1.5 cm) to allow for post-injury collagenolysis associated with the debridement phase of healing. A small horizontal laceration may require surgical extension of the skin wound proximally and distally, in a gentle curvilinear fashion, to allow access to the retracted ends of the tendon to achieve complete debridement and to place sutures. Placing the limb in hyperflexion helps minimize gap formation by relieving as much of the tension as possible while the tenorrhaphy sutures are tightened. The SDFT and DDFT should be sutured separately from one another, when both have been transected, to avoid adhesions forming between the two structures and subsequently preventing them from moving independently.

The selection of suture material and suture pattern for flexor tenorrhaphy is the subject of much debate and many experimental studies.[41–46] The ideal suture pattern should minimize gap formation, constriction of vascular supply, and adhesion formation while achieving a strong resistance to suture pull-through. Based on current studies, the three-loop pulley pattern (Figure 17.15), using size 2 polydioxanone suture, is the preferred approach to achieve these goals, is easy to place, and results in less exposed suture material. The triple locking loop pattern may be a suitable alternative, but the three-loop pulley pattern appears to result in less disruption of the vasculature and higher loads to failure than the triple locking loop pattern.[42,46,47] Recent studies have investigated the Savage suture pattern for tenorrhaphy because it provides higher loads to failure; concerns related to reduced perfusion to the encircled tendon bundles, however, make the Savage suture pattern unacceptable for clinical use at this time.[41,45,48]

Concurrent closure of the paratenon may aid in providing cells and vascular elements to strengthen the primary tenorrhaphy. Although some authors have, in the past, recommended the use of non-absorbable suture material, absorbable monofilament suture, such as polydioxanone, is preferred over nylon to reduce the incidence of adhesion formation and interference with the gliding of the tendon that may result from the permanent presence of suture material (i.e., a foreign body) in the healed tissues.

After tenorrhaphy, the wound is closed in a stepwise fashion according to standard principles. If the wound is sufficiently clean, it should be closed completely to protect the integrity of the tenorrhaphy and to achieve optimal cosmesis. Stepwise closure begins with suturing the damaged tendon sheath or paratenon. Closing the paratenon provides a barrier to infection between the tenorrhaphy and the superficial layers of the wound and brings the vascular and cellular elements of the paratenon in apposition, encouraging extrinsic repair. Closure of the subcutaneous tissues and skin provides further support for healing, prevents environmental contamination of the tenorrhaphy, and results in a more cosmetic outcome by preventing the formation of exuberant granulation tissue. Care should be taken to avoid over-tightening the skin sutures so that blood flow to the healing tissue is not impaired and to ensure complete apposition of the skin edges to achieve an efficient fibrin seal to protect the tenorrhaphy.

If the amount of trauma or degree of contamination preclude completely closing the wound, the wound can be partially closed, while allowing for ventral drainage. Whether placement of a drain is necessary to achieve drainage should be assessed. A fenestrated drain placed into a tendon sheath can be useful for continued lavage and/or antibiotic delivery (Figure 17.16a). A closed suction drain may be useful for evacuating the fluid contents of the sheath.[49] To install a fenestrated drain, the non-fenestrated portion is placed in the wound and advanced in a retrograde manner so that it exits a portal at the proximal extent of the digital flexor tendon sheath (Figure 17.16b). Alternatively,

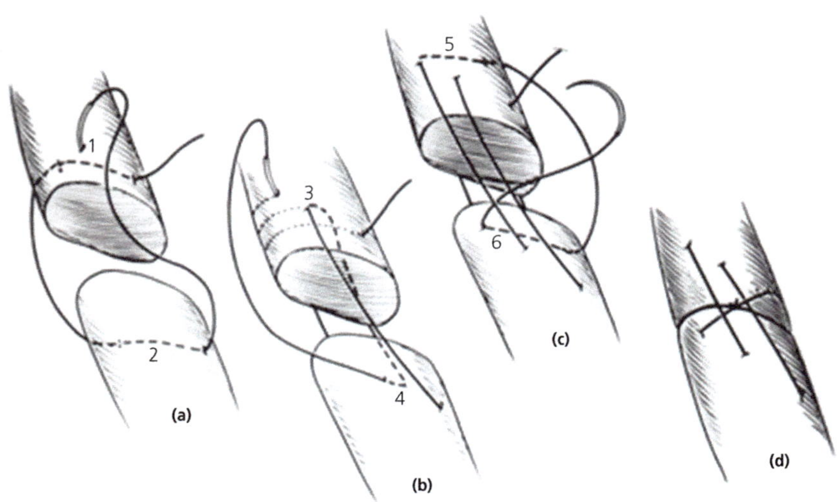

Figure 17.15 Placement of the three-loop pulley suture pattern.

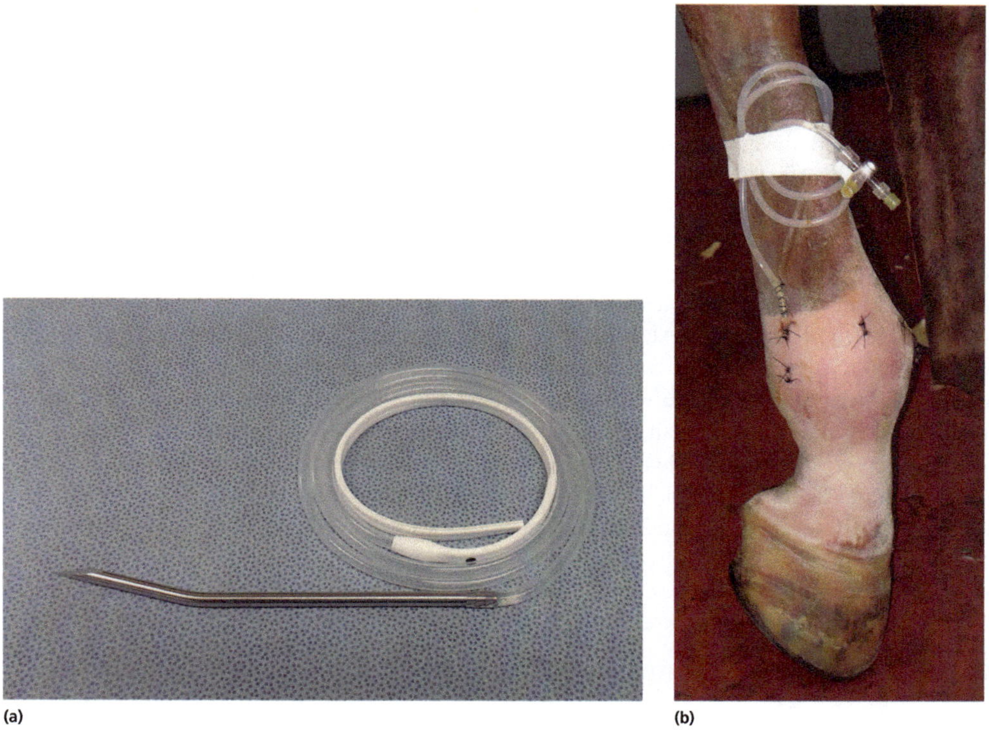

Figure 17.16 (a) Fenestrated drain used to lavage the digital synovial sheath. (b) Drain in place following surgery. The non-fenestrated portion of the irrigation tube exits through the proximal extent of the digital synovial sheath and is secured to the skin with the fenestrated portion remaining within the sheath.

the drain may be placed through the arthroscopic cannula and the cannula subsequently withdrawn over the top of the drain. The fenestrated portion of the drain remains within the sheath, and the non-fenestrated portion is secured to the skin with a suture. A Penrose drain may be used at the distal extent of the sheath, thereby establishing an ingress/egress system. If a drain system is used, the limb must be kept in a Kimzey splint, rather than a cast, for recovery from anesthesia and for access to the wound because a half-limb cast prevents access to the drain. The time at which the drain is removed after repair is based on clinical response to treatment and patency of the drain, but is generally 3–5 days. Drains should be used with caution because they can act as a foreign body and serve as an ingress portal for opportunistic bacteria.

Closure of wounds older than 6–12 hours, wounds that are severely contaminated, and wounds that contain a substantial amount of unhealthy tissue should be delayed for 4–6 days. During that time, the wound is debrided periodically, and the horse is given systemic and regional antibiotic therapy. The injured limb should be maintained in a Kimzey Leg Saver Splint or a heavily padded bandage with an incorporated PVC splint to protect the soft tissues from further damage. By 5–6 days, autolytic debridement along with repeated wound irrigation and bandage changes will have prepared the wound sufficiently for subsequent surgical debridement to achieve a clean wound suitable for tenorrhaphy and closure. Debridement and tenorrhaphy techniques are identical to those described earlier. Provision for ventral drainage and use of an ingress tube for lavage of the tendon sheath may still be indicated, depending on the degree of contamination and the health of the tissues at the time of closure. Complete closure is ideal and may be achievable after aggressive irrigation and regional antibiotic therapy in the days leading up to closure; however, even partial closure will generally result in a superior functional and cosmetic outcome.

Suture repair of flexor tendons of horses is insufficient, on its own, to prevent gap formation and to support weight bearing in the immediate postoperative period. External coaptation in the form of a cast or other rigid coaptation, such as a bandage along with a Kimzey or PVC splint, is necessary to protect the repair during recovery from anesthesia and to help share the load as the repaired tendon gains strength. The cast is commonly applied with the digit in slight flexion to reduce the load on the repaired tendon. The duration of casting after complete tendon transection is generally 6–8 weeks. The mean duration, in recent studies, was approximately 6 weeks.[34,37,50] This correlates with the amount of time required for the healing tendon to remodel sufficiently to support the weight of a horse of average size.[50] Half-limb casts are most commonly selected over full-limb casts for ease of application and management, increased patient mobility, and reduced expense. In the hindlimb, a full-limb cast is theoretically necessary to fully neutralize the reciprocal apparatus; in practice, however, a half-limb cast is generally effective and avoids complications, such as rupture of the *peroneus tertius*, femoral fracture, and coxofemoral luxation, that may occur when a full-limb cast is used. Horses should be confined to a stall during the convalescence period to reduce the forces on the repaired tendon and to reduce the risk of cast sores developing.

At the end of the casting period, the cast is removed with the horse standing so that general anesthesia and problems associated with recovery from it are avoided. After the limb is cleaned and skin sutures are removed, the limb is placed in a heavily padded support bandage for 3 weeks; the bandage is changed as required. A shoe with an extended heel is applied and maintained for several months to counteract hyperextension of the distal interphalangeal joint that occurs after transection of the DDFT (Figure 17.17). After an additional 6 weeks of stall confinement, short periods of hand walking can be initiated. The duration and frequency of walking is gradually increased during the next 2–3 months. A routine of strictly controlled exercise in hand is preferable to even small paddock turnout. Serial ultrasonographic examinations of the site of laceration and soundness evaluations form the basis for a decision on when to increase exercise from the walk to the trot, to the canter, and to return to full work. The total period of convalescence is typically 6–12 months, depending on the severity of the injury. Premature return to work increases the risk of injury to the repair tissue.

In summary, the current literature suggests a more favorable prognosis for transection of the digital flexor tendons than was previously believed. Although the number of structures involved is reported to have the most significant impact on outcome,[37] another study reported that horses that suffered laceration of both digital flexor tendons had an outcome similar to that of horses that suffered a laceration to a single digital flexor tendon.[34] Relatively small numbers of cases and many variables in how the horses were treated may explain this contradiction.

Another important factor to consider when predicting prognosis for horses with a completely or partially transected digital flexor tendon(s) is if the injury is within a synovial sheath, especially the digital synovial sheath. Horses with a tendon laceration occurring within the digital synovial sheath tend to have a

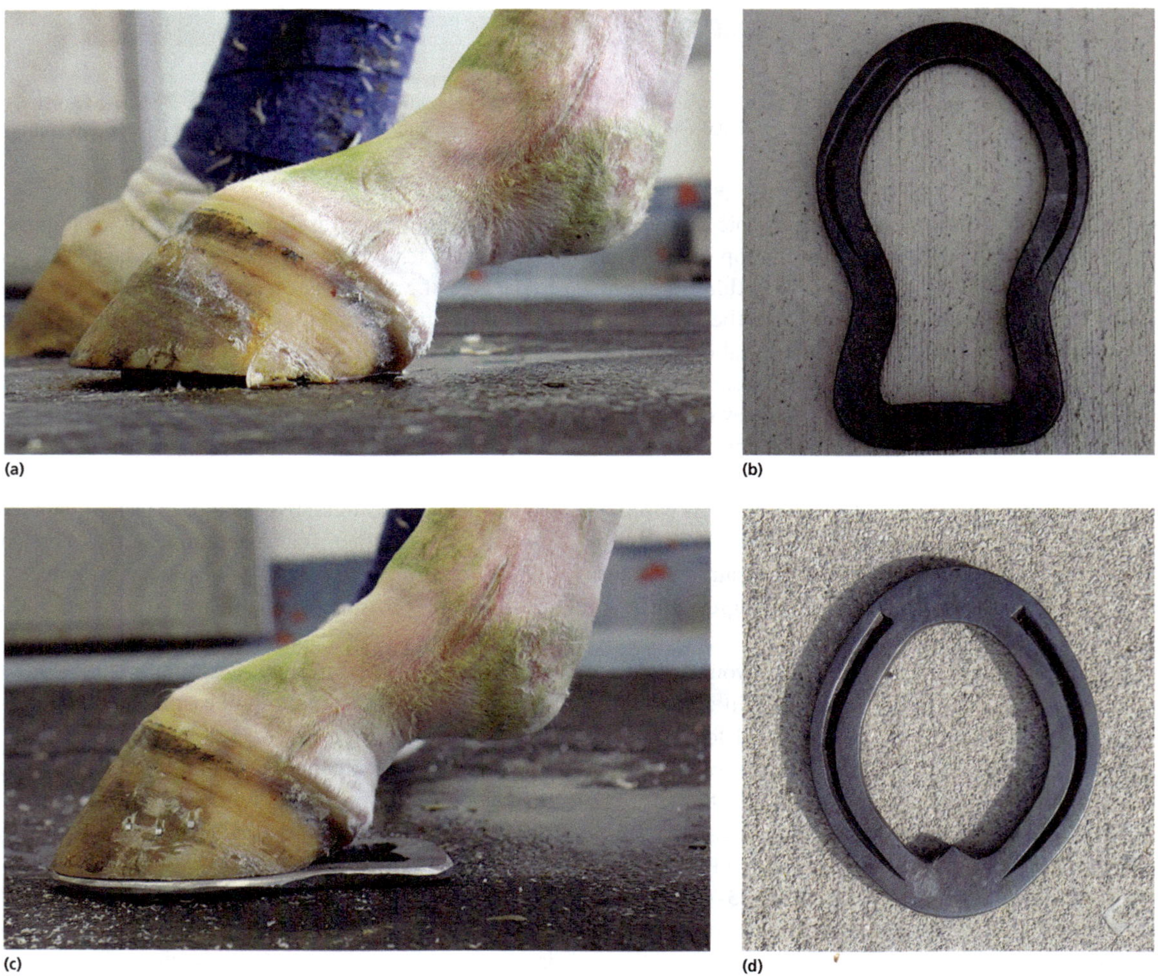

Figure 17.17 Photos showing before (a) and after (c) application of a fish-tail shoe (b) following cast removal to provide support after tenorrhaphy of the DDFT. A simple bar shoe (d) is an alternative if a fish-tail shoe is not available; however, its shorter lever will provide less support. Additional support with a heavy padded bandage is also indicated. Courtesy of Travis Burns, CJF, TE, AWCF (a–c), and Jamie Secoura, CJF (d).

more guarded prognosis for return to full athletic function than do horses that have a tendon laceration outside the sheath. This is because healing may be impaired within the synovial environment, because adhesions within the digital flexor tendon sheath may prevent normal gliding function, and because of the potential for complications resulting from persistent synovial infection. In contrast to the aforementioned commonly held clinical impression, however, a recent study found that synovial sheath involvement did not significantly negatively affect outcome.[37] Administration of hyaluronic acid into the tendon sheath or at the tenorrhaphy site may improve healing, prevent adhesion formation, and reduce inflammation within the tendon.[51–53]

What to do

- Carefully assess structures affected to provide the owner with a realistic prognosis; describe to the owner what will likely be involved in wound management.
- Perform tenorrhaphy if transection of a flexor tendon is complete.
- Provide robust external coaptation regardless of the need for tenorrhaphy.
- Consider regional antibiotic delivery in addition to systemic administration of antibiotics.

What to avoid

- Avoid delays in referral after administering first aid.

Paratenon laceration

Wounds involving the paratenon can be challenging to manage because of the constant motion that occurs as the flexor tendons stretch and relax. The result can be a non-healing wound characterized by the formation of concentric rings of granulation tissue (Figure 17.18). Granulation tissue associated with the skin, subcutaneous tissues, and the paratenon typically becomes exuberant around the wound's margin with an area of granulation tissue originating from the tendon itself. An oval area devoid of granulation tissue is present where differential movement occurs between the tissue layers. Treatment of this type of chronic wound involves excising the exuberant granulation tissue to the level of the surrounding skin and applying a heavy padded bandage and splint, or a bivalved cast, that is maintained until a strong bed of granulation tissue forms and the wound contracts adequately to become stable without crevices formed by motion between tissue planes. The problem can be prevented by restricting motion, either by applying a cast or by incorporating external coaptation into the bandage to minimize motion.

What to do

- Debulk exuberant granulation tissue if the wound is chronic.
- Immobilize the limb in a cast or a splint to prevent differential motion between the skin/subcutaneous tissue/paratenon and underlying tendon.

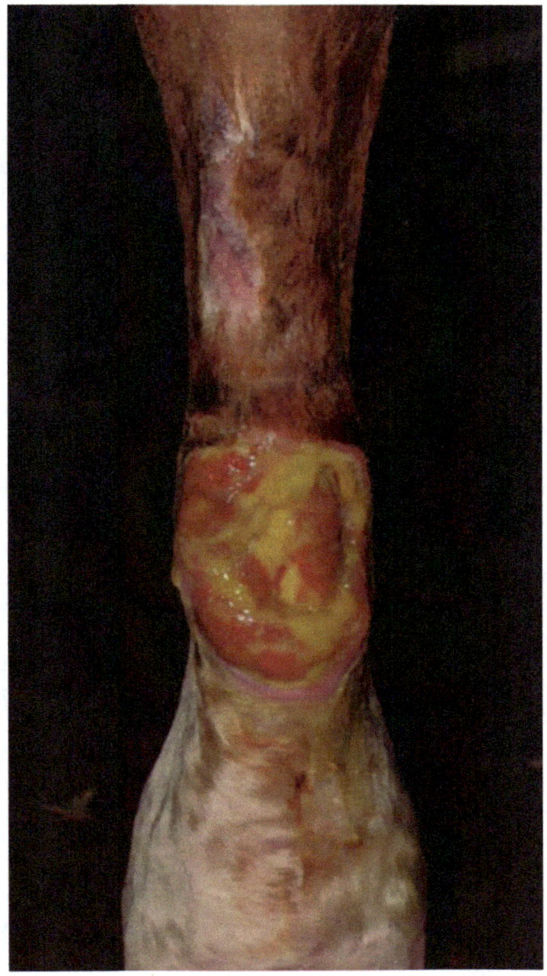

Figure 17.18 Granulating cast sore 3 weeks after the removal of a cast used to manage an open dorsal fetlock laceration. Concentric rings of granulation tissue have formed as a result of differential movement between the skin, subcutaneous tissues, paratenon, and the underlying tendon. A portion of the tendon is visible distally while the proximal portion of the tendon is covered by granulation tissue. The wound was managed by excising the exuberant granulation tissue, immobilizing the limb with a bandage splint, and skin grafting.

Conclusion

Overall, early aggressive treatment and suture repair of lacerated tendons, along with advancements in the management of infected wounds through the use of regional antibiotic delivery, may lead to a better outcome than previously attained. Treatment is not simple and requires a significant commitment of time and expense on the part of the owner to achieve a successful outcome. Potential complications include the formation of exuberant granulation tissue, dehiscence, sequestrum formation, septic arthritis or tenosynovitis, septic tendinitis, laminitis, cast sores, adhesion formation, and failure of tenorrhaphy. With careful attention to the daily details of wound management and nursing care, a successful outcome is nevertheless possible for horses suffering from lacerations of one or more extensor or flexor tendons.

References

1. St. Clair LE. General Myology. In: Getty R (ed). *Sisson and Grossman's The Anatomy of the Domestic Animals*, 5th edn. W.B. Saunders Company: Philadelphia, 1975: 39.
2. Kraus BL, Kirker-Head CA, Kraus KH, *et al.* Vascular supply of the tendon of the equine deep digital flexor muscle within the digital sheath. *Vet Surg* 1995; **24**: 102.
3. Kraus-Hansen AE, Fackelman GE, Becker C, *et al.* Preliminary studies on the vascular anatomy of the equine superficial digital flexor tendon. *Equine Vet J* 1992; **24**: 46.
4. Dahlgren LA, Mohammed HO, Nixon AJ. Temporal expression of growth factors and matrix molecules in healing tendon lesions. *J Orthop Res* 2005; **23**: 84.
5. Bosch G, Moleman M, Barneveld A, *et al.* The effect of platelet-rich plasma on the neovascularization of surgically created equine superficial digital flexor tendon lesions. *Scand J Med Sci Sports* 2011; **21**: 554.
6. Woo SLY, An KN, Arnoczky SP, *et al.* Anatomy, biology, and biomechanics of tendon, ligament, and meniscus. In: Simon S (ed). *Orthopaedic Basic Science*. The American Academy of Orthopaedic Surgeons: Rosemont, Illinois, 1994: 45.
7. Goodship AE, Birch HL, Wilson AM. The pathobiology and repair of tendon and ligament injury. *Vet Clin North Am Equine Pract* 1994; **10**: 323.
8. Birch HL, Bailey AJ, Goodship AE. Macroscopic 'degeneration' of equine superficial digital flexor tendon is accompanied by a change in extracellular matrix composition. *Equine Vet J* 1998; **30**: 534.
9. Vogel KG, Heinegard D. Characterization of proteoglycans from adult bovine tendon. *J Biol Chem* 1985; **260**: 9298.
10. Uldbjerg N, Danielsen CC. A study of the interaction in vitro between type I collagen and a small dermatan sulphate proteoglycan. *Biochem J* 1988; **251**: 643.
11. Vogel KG, Keller EJ, Lenhoff RJ, *et al.* Proteoglycan synthesis by fibroblast cultures initiated from regions of adult bovine tendon subjected to different mechanical forces. *Eur J Cell Biol* 1986; **41**: 102.
12. Cohen IK, Diegelmann RF, Lindblad WJ. *Wound Healing: Biochemical & Clinical Aspects*. W.B. Saunders Co: Philadelphia PA, 1992.
13. Fenwick SA, Hazleman BL, Riley GP. The vasculature and its role in the damaged and healing tendon. *Arthritis Res* 2002; **4**: 252.
14. Cadby JA, Buehler E, Godbout C, *et al.* Differences between the cell populations from the peritenon and the tendon core with regard to their potential implication in tendon repair. *PLoS One.* 2014; **9**: e92474.
15. Stewart AA, Barrett JG, Byron CR, *et al.* Comparison of equine tendon-, muscle-, and bone marrow-derived cells cultured on tendon matrix. *Am J Vet Res* 2009; **70**: 750.
16. Bi Y, Ehirchiou D, Kilts TM, *et al.* Identification of tendon stem/progenitor cells and the role of the extracellular matrix in their niche. *Nat Med* 2007; **13**: 1219.
17. Watkins JP. Tendon and ligament biology. In: Auer JA, Stick JA (eds). *Equine Surgery*, 2nd edn. WB Saunders: Philadelphia PA, 1999: 707.
18. Goodrich LR, Nixon AJ, Fubini SL, *et al.* Epidural morphine and detomidine decreases postoperative hindlimb lameness in horses after bilateral stifle arthroscopy. *Vet Surg* 2002; **31**: 232.
19. Derossi R, Medeiros U, Jr., de Almeida RG, *et al.* Meperidine prolongs lidocaine caudal epidural anaesthesia in the horse. *Vet J* 2008; **178**: 294.
20. Green EM, Cooper RC. Continuous caudal epidural anesthesia in the horse. *J Am Vet Med Assoc* 1984; **184**: 971.
21. Martin CA, Kerr CL, Pearce SG, *et al.* Outcome of epidural catheterization for delivery of analgesics in horses: 43 cases (1998–2001). *J Am Vet Med Assoc* 2003; **222**: 1394.
22. Valverde A, Little CB, Dyson DH, *et al.* Use of epidural morphine to relieve pain in a horse. *Can Vet J* 1990; **31**: 211.
23. Ilfeld BM. Continuous peripheral nerve blocks: a review of the published evidence. *Anesth Analg* 2011; **113**: 904.
24. Watts AE, Nixon AJ, Reesink HL, *et al.* Continuous peripheral neural blockade to alleviate signs of experimentally induced severe forelimb pain in horses. *J Am Vet Med Assoc* 2011; **238**: 1032.
25. Doherty TJ, Seddighi MR. Local anesthetics as pain therapy in horses. *Vet Clin North Am Equine Pract* 2010; **26**: 533.
26. Elfenbein JR, Robertson SA, MacKay RJ, *et al.* Systemic and antinociceptive effects of prolonged lidocaine, ketamine, and butorphanol infusions alone and in combination in healthy horses. *BMC Vet Res* 2014; **10** Suppl 1: S6.
27. Sanchez LC, Robertson SA. Pain control in horses: what do we really know? *Equine Vet J* 2014; **46**: 517.
28. Baxter GM. Management of wounds involving synovial structures in horses. *Clin Tech Equine Pract* 2004; **3**: 204.
29. Orsini JA, Elce Y, Kraus B. Management of severely infected wounds in the equine patient. *Clin Tech Equine Pract* 2004; **3**: 225.
30. Rubio-Martinez LM, Cruz AM. Antimicrobial regional limb perfusion in horses. *J Am Vet Med Assoc* 2006; **228**: 706.
31. Russell JW, Russell TM. A novel surgical technique for repair of combined lateral and long digital extensor tendon laceration in the equine hind limb. *Vet Surg* 2015; **44**: E17.
32. Mespoulhes-Riviere C, Martens A, Bogaert L, *et al.* Factors affecting outcome of extensor tendon lacerations in the distal limb of horses. A retrospective study of 156 cases (1994–2003). *Vet Comp Orthop Traumatol* 2008; **21**: 358.
33. Jansson N. Digital extensor tendon lacerations in horses: a retrospective evaluation of 22 cases. *J Equine Vet Sci* 1995; **15**: 537.
34. Foland JW, Trotter GW, Stashak TS, *et al.* Traumatic injuries involving tendons of the distal limbs in horses: a retrospective study of 55 cases. *Equine Vet J* 1991; **23**: 422.
35. Belknap JK, Baxter GM, Nickels FA. Extensor tendon lacerations in horses: 50 cases (1982–1988). *J Am Vet Med Assoc* 1993; **203**: 428.
36. Elliott CR, Vasey JR, Russell TM. Transection of the lateral and long digital extensor tendons in racehorses. *Aust Vet J* 2012; **90**: 20.
37. Jordana M, Wilderjans H, Boswell J, *et al.* Outcome after lacerations of the superficial and deep digital flexor tendons, suspensory ligament and/or distal sesamoidean ligaments in 106 horses. *Vet Surg* 2011; **40**: 277.
38. Taylor DS, Pascoe JR, Meagher DM, *et al.* Digital flexor tendon lacerations in horses: 50 cases (1975–1990). *J Am Vet Med Assoc* 1995; **206**: 342.
39. Bertone AL, Stashak TS, Smith FW, *et al.* A comparison of repair methods for gap healing in equine flexor tendon. *Vet Surg* 1990; **19**: 254.
40. Jann HW, Good JK, Morgan SJ, *et al.* Healing of transected equine superficial digital flexor tendons with and without tenorrhaphy. *Vet Surg* 1992; **21**: 40.
41. Everett E, Barrett JG, Morelli J, *et al.* Biomechanical testing of a novel suture pattern for repair of equine tendon lacerations. *Vet Surg* 2012; **41**: 278.

42. Adair HS, Gobel DO, Rohrback BW. In vitro comparison of the locking loop and the three loop pulley suture techniques in the repair of equine flexor tendons. *J Equine Vet Sci* 1989; **9**: 186.
43. Smith RL, Murphy DJ, Day RE, *et al.* An ex vivo biomechanical study comparing strength characteristics of a new technique with the three-loop pulley for equine tenorrhaphy. *Vet Surg* 2011; **40**: 768.
44. Easley KJ, Stashak TS, Smith FW, *et al.* Mechanical properties of four suture patterns for transected equine tendon repair. *Vet Surg* 1990; **19**: 102.
45. Barrett EJ, Munsterman AS, Hanson RR, *et al.* Biomechanical testing of a novel tendon implant device for the repair of equine flexor tendon lacerations. *Vet Surg* 2014; **43**: 685.
46. Jann HW, Stein LE, Good JK. Strength characteristics and failure modes of locking-loop and three-loop pulley suture patterns in equine tendons. *Vet Surg* 1990; **19**: 28.
47. Crowson CL, Jann HW, Stein LE, *et al.* Quantitative effect of tenorrhaphy on intrinsic vasculature of the equine superficial digital flexor tendon. *Am J Vet Res* 2004; **65**: 279.
48. Freeman KD, Barrett JG, Youngstrom DW, *et al.* Microangiographic comparison of the effects of 3 loop pulley and 6 strand savage tenorrhaphy techniques on equine superficial digital flexor tendon. *Vet Surg* 2015; **44**: 744.
49. Ross MW, Orsini JA, Richardson DW, *et al.* Closed suction drainage in the treatment of infectious arthritis of the equine tarsocrural joint. *Vet Surg* 1991; **20**: 21.
50. Bertone AL. Tendon lacerations. *Vet Clin North Am Equine Pract* 1995; **11**: 293.
51. Gaughan EM, Nixon AJ, Krook LP, *et al.* Effects of sodium hyaluronate on tendon healing and adhesion formation in horses. *Am J Vet Res* 1991; **52**: 764.
52. Abate M, Schiavone C, Salini V. The use of hyaluronic acid after tendon surgery and in tendinopathies. *Biomed Res Int* 2014; EPub:783632.
53. Sardari K, Nowrouzian I, Movaseghi A, *et al.* Experimental study of healing effect of sodium hyaluronate in deep digital flexor tendon injury in horses. *J Fac Vet Med, Univ Tehran* 2000; **55**: 1.

Webliography

- http://www.thehorse.com/articles/29034/tendon-lesions-in-horses-treatment-and-prognosis
- http://www.thehorse.com/articles/10619/equine-tendon-lacerations-part-2
- http://www.equilibriumproducts.com/equine_ailments/equine_digital_flexor_tendon_injuries/
- https://www.vetmed.vt.edu/emc/docs/WoundCare.pdf
- http://www.slideshare.net/blomenkampkj/digital-tendon-sheath-lacerations
- http://www.slideshare.net/dvmfun/equine-orthopedic-field-emergency?qid=0235a8b3-fb53-497b-bb15-1e33b4b9972b&v=default&b=&from_search=9

CHAPTER 18

Free Skin Grafting

Jim Schumacher, DVM, MS, Diplomate ACVS, MRCVS and Jacintha M. Wilmink, DVM, PhD

Chapter Contents

Summary

Skin grafting is indicated for full-thickness skin defects that cannot be closed using conventional suturing techniques or reconstructive surgical techniques and that require a long time to heal by contraction and epithelialization. This applies, in particular, to wounds at or below the carpus and hock because these wounds are incapable of significant contraction and because epithelialization of these wounds is slow and results in a fragile, unsightly scar. In those cases, grafting is less expensive than a lengthy period of bandaging. The most common type of skin graft applied to wounds of horses is the free skin graft. Techniques of free skin grafting include island grafting, sheet grafting, and Meek micrografting, which is a combination of sheet grafting and island grafting. Types of island grafts include pinch, punch, and tunnel grafts. Each type of free skin grafting has advantages and disadvantages, and the type selected, therefore, depends on the circumstances, such as the necessity for the best possible cosmesis, the size or location of the wound, available instrumentation, experience of the surgeon, and the horse owner's finances.

Introduction

Skin grafting should be considered for full-thickness skin defects that cannot be closed using conventional suturing techniques or reconstructive surgical techniques and that would require a long time to heal by contraction and epithelialization. This applies, in particular, to wounds at or distal to the carpus and hock because these wounds are capable of only limited contraction and because epithelialization of these wounds is slow and results in a fragile, unsightly scar (see Chapter 1). The purpose of this

Equine Wound Management, Third Edition. Edited by Christine Theoret and Jim Schumacher.

Companion website: www.wiley.com/go/theoret/wound

chapter is to describe the principles and various techniques of free skin grafting, the advantages and disadvantages of each technique, and the effects of grafts on the wound. Proper care of the wound, before and after grafting, is described so that failure of the graft can be avoided.

Classification of grafts

The two basic types of skin grafts are the pedicle skin graft and the free skin graft. A pedicle skin graft, or skin flap, is a full-thickness graft that remains joined by its vasculature to the donor site so that the graft does not depend on the vascularity from the recipient site to survive. Wounds healed with a pedicle graft have a good cosmetic appearance because the graft is composed of all layers of skin. Pedicle grafts are not as commonly applied to wounds of horses as they are to wounds of cats and dogs because mobilizing an adequate amount of skin on a horse to advance a pedicle graft is difficult.[1,2] An axial-pattern flap (i.e., a skin flap incorporating a direct cutaneous artery and vein into its base) can be transferred successfully to a wound at adjacent sites in humans and dogs,[3,4] or to a remote wound by using microsurgical techniques to anastomose the flap's vessels to local recipient vessels. Similar transfers in horses, using the circumflex iliac artery, have been unsuccessful, apparently because of reperfusion injury to the graft.[5,6]

A free skin graft is a section of skin that has been detached from its vascular supply and relocated to a wound at another site where it must create new vascular connections to the wound bed to survive. A free graft can be classified according to its source. The most common type is the autograft, or isograft, which is a graft relocated from one area to another on the same individual. An allograft, or homograft, is a graft transferred between two members of the same species, whereas a xenograft, or heterograft, is a graft transferred from a member of one species to a member of another. Although allografts and xenografts develop vascular connections to the recipient wound, the graft is eventually rejected because the host mounts an immune response against it.[7,8] An autograft is the most common and practical type of graft applied to wounds of horses because the host mounts no immune response to the graft. An allograft or xenograft is sometimes applied to a wound on a horse as a biologic dressing.[9–11]

Free skin grafts can also be classified as full-thickness or split-thickness. A full-thickness graft is composed of epidermis and the entire dermis, including adnexal structures, such as sweat glands and hair follicles, whereas a split-thickness graft is composed of epidermis but only a portion of the dermis. The thickness of split-thickness grafts can vary and is determined by the relative amount, rather than the absolute amount, of dermis included in the graft, because the thickness of the dermis varies between individuals and between regions on an individual.[12–14] The thickness of equine skin on the trunk and limbs varies widely (between 1 and 5 mm).[12] For example, the thickness of skin just proximal to the foot is about 5 mm, whereas the thickness of skin on the abdomen is between 1.5 and 2 mm (JW, personal observation).

Full- or split-thickness skin grafts are applied to the surface of wounds as sheet grafts or are embedded within the wound as island grafts. Each technique of grafting has its advantages and disadvantages, and the choice of technique depends on circumstances, such as the location and size of the wound, desired cosmetic appearance, available instrumentation, bias of the surgeon, and the financial resources of the horse's owner.

Requirements for graft acceptance

Nearly any type of tissue is capable of supporting a free graft, except bone devoid of periosteum, tendon devoid of paratenon, or cartilage devoid of perichondrium.[15–18] Tissues less likely to accept a free graft are adipose tissue, joint capsules, and ligaments. The presence of small avascular areas of tissue within a wound incapable of accepting a graft, such as tendon, may still be covered with a graft owing to the phenomenon of vascular bridging, whereby a portion of a graft overlying a small, avascular area of the wound is revascularized by capillaries from the vascularized portion of the graft.[17,19] Full-thickness grafts are more effective than split-thickness grafts at bridging avascular areas of the wound because they contain more dermis, which has superior collateral circulation.[19]

To accept a free graft, the wound must be vascularized and free of infection and necrotic tissue. Fresh wounds, created surgically or by accident, are the most capable of accepting a free graft because they are highly vascular and have not had time to become infected.[14,20,21] Granulating wounds may also accept grafts, though not as readily as can fresh wounds. An advantage of postponing grafting of a large fresh wound until fibroplasia is well under way is that contraction rapidly decreases the size of the wound after granulation tissue forms, allowing it to be covered by a smaller graft.

Physiologic events associated with graft acceptance

Revascularization

The graft is initially adhered to the wound by fibrin, produced by the wound, which binds to exposed collagen within the graft.[15,22–24] Vessels and fibroblasts from the wound invade the fibrin clot within 48 to 72 hours.

The graft is nourished initially by plasmatic imbibition, or plasmatic circulation, a process whereby transudate is imbibed passively, by capillary action, into the exposed lumen of the graft's vessels, much like fluid is absorbed into a sponge.[15,23,25] During the stage of plasmatic imbibition, which typically lasts about 48 hours, the graft has no blood supply of its own, and cells within the graft have depressed mitotic activity resulting from low oxygen tension. In this hypoxic state, metabolism

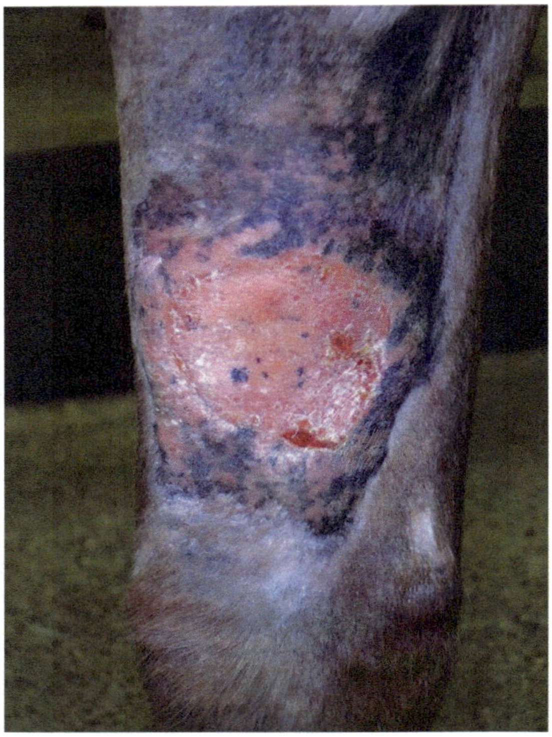

Figure 18.1 The entire epidermis of this graft has sloughed, exposing pale dermis beneath it. This dermis may resemble granulation tissue.

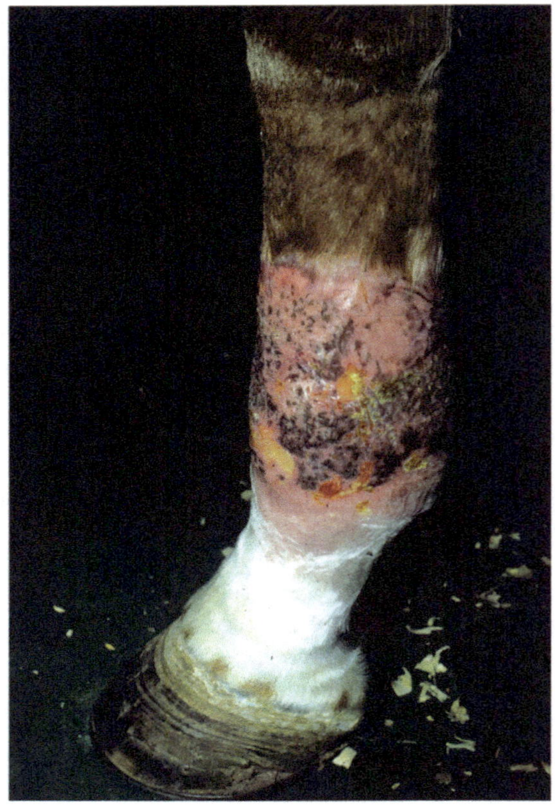

Figure 18.2 This split-thickness skin graft is beginning to pigment. Split-thickness grafts that have sloughed their epidermis are eventually epithelialized and usually begin to develop pigment by about 1 month after grafting.

becomes anaerobic, and metabolites accumulate. Thin grafts tolerate this ischemic phase better than do thick grafts. The graft becomes edematous and remains so until it revascularizes.

After the first 2 days, new capillaries from the wound cross the fibrin matrix to anastomose with capillaries in the graft, a process called inosculation,[15,22,25,26] which occurs mainly in the central region of the graft.[27] Following inosculation, new capillaries from the wound invade other vessels pre-existing within the graft and cut new vascular channels into its dermis, a process referred to as neovascularization. The graft revascularizes between the 4th and 5th day after being applied to the wound, and lymphatic circulation is re-established by 7 days, which resolves edema.[26] The graft can be considered accepted or to have "taken" when it has revascularized. The graft becomes firmly attached to the wound by the 10th day. Determining if a graft has been accepted can sometimes be difficult if the upper portion of the graft fails to vascularize and becomes desiccated. The desiccated tissue sloughs to reveal vascularized dermis (indicating that only the upper portion of the graft has failed to vascularize) or granulation tissue (indicating that the entire graft has failed to vascularize). Exposed dermis may closely resemble granulation tissue but can be differentiated from it by its paler color (Figure 18.1).

Graft regeneration

The epidermis of the graft becomes hyperplastic after grafting and may die and slough in some areas, exposing the pale dermis beneath it.[16,21] Epithelial cells migrating from the hair follicles and the eccrine glands within the dermis soon cover the dermis. Split-thickness skin grafts remain covered with flaky debris for several months, until the eccrine glands regenerate.[21] They usually regain pigmentation beginning about 1 month after grafting (Figure 18.2). Hair begins to appear between 4 and 6 weeks,[21] although it often grows abnormally long, perhaps because the origin of the graft is usually the trunk, where the local temperature is higher than that of the limbs and transfer of the graft to a cooler area (i.e., the distal portion of a limb) may stimulate hair growth.[13,28,29]

Nerves enter the base and margins of the graft and reconstruct the graft's pattern of innervation by following vacated neurolemmal sheaths.[30] Split-thickness grafts become re-innervated more rapidly but to a lesser extent than do full-thickness grafts.[15,30] Sensation to split-thickness grafts of humans usually returns between 7 and 9 weeks but is incomplete and patchy.[31] Humans sometimes develop hyperesthesia of the grafted wound,[16,30] and judging from incidents where horses have mutilated a healed, grafted wound, this may also occur in some horses.

Graft contraction and wound contraction

Recoil of elastin fibers within the deep layers of the dermis causes a graft to contract immediately after harvest.[32] This contraction is referred to as primary graft contraction. Full-thickness grafts contract more than do split-thickness grafts, and as the proportion of dermis within split-thickness grafts increases, so does the amount of primary contraction. The significance of primary contraction is minor for sheet grafts because it is reversed when the graft is stretched and attached to the wound's margin.

Contraction of the wound after the graft has been accepted is referred to as secondary graft contraction, which in reality, represents contraction of the grafted wound rather than of the graft itself. The extent of wound contraction after grafting depends on the relative thickness of the graft's dermis, the stage of healing of the recipient bed at the time of grafting, the percentage of area grafted, mechanical factors, and the species involved.

Contraction of granulating or fresh wounds of humans and rats that receive a full-thickness graft is less than that of those receiving a split-thickness graft, even when the full-thickness graft is thinner than the split-thickness graft (a spit-thickness graft removed from an area in which the skin is thick can be thicker than a full-thickness graft removed from an area in which the skin is thin). This indicates that the deep portion of the dermis may suppress formation or contraction of myofibroblasts in the granulation tissue.[33]

In contrast, contraction of experimentally created limb wounds of horses did not differ between wounds grafted with full-thickness skin and those grafted with split-thickness skin.[34] The stage of healing of these wounds, however, had an effect on contraction after grafting. Contraction was significantly less when fresh wounds were grafted than when granulating wounds were grafted, regardless of whether a split-thickness or full-thickness graft was applied.

Skin grafts are sometimes applied to wounds of humans to prevent wound contraction because contraction can result in contracture, or distortion, of parts of the body.[7,15] Conversely, skin grafts applied to granulating wounds of horses stimulate wound contraction rather than wound contracture,[35] particularly when Meek micrografts (see Island grafting later in this chapter) are used.[29] Contraction of wounds of horses should be considered beneficial because it accelerates wound closure and rarely results in contracture. The only contracture the authors have observed was around the proximal joints of a tail, from contraction of a wound near the tailhead.

Stimulation of wound contraction in horses after grafting may result from the presence of certain cytokines in the dermis of the graft, although these have not yet been identified. Both authors have noted that skin grafts applied to chronic, slow-healing wounds appear to speed contraction and epithelialization, even when the graft fails to be accepted. Healthy donor skin may stimulate healing of a chronic wound by supplying cytokines conducive to healing. Additionally and concomitantly, the reduction of chronic inflammation and, thus, the concentration of several contraction-inhibiting mediators (e.g., prostaglandin [PG]E_1, PGE_2, interferon [IFN]γ, tumor necrosis factor [TNF]α, interleukin [IL]-1, and IL-6) while the wound is being prepared for grafting, could increase the rate of contraction.[32] The superficial layer of exposed granulation tissue usually contains many leukocytes, which are not found beneath the leading edge of advancing epithelium. As the epithelium advances to cover the wound, the concentration of leukocytes in the granulation tissue decreases, and inflammation resolves. Reduction of the area of exposed granulation tissue, by grafts, is likely to have a similar effect on inflammation, which in turn accelerates contraction.

The influence of skin grafts on contraction may also depend on mechanical factors. Fixing a sheet graft to a wound under slight tension may influence the granulation tissue by partially relieving the mechanical stress exerted on it by tissue surrounding the wound. This, in turn, favors apoptosis of myofibroblasts, as suggested by *in vitro* studies of fibroblasts in collagen lattices.[36] The disappearance of myofibroblasts reduces contraction, however, and, although this is important in preventing contractures in humans, it is disadvantageous in horses, where wound contraction is beneficial. Whether fixation or certain characteristics of a sheet graft result in disappearance of myofibroblasts, and thus reduce contraction of equine wounds, is not known, but one author (JW) has the impression that wounds of horses contract less after receiving a split-thickness sheet graft than after receiving split-thickness island grafts (e.g., Meek micrografts).

In general, the responsiveness of equine wounds to dermal factors supplied by grafts is mainly determined by the age of the granulation tissue and, therefore, by the concentration and state of differentiation of the myofibroblasts.[34,37,38] Contraction is reduced when wounds are grafted soon after wounding when myofibroblasts are not yet present, and when grafting mature, fibrotic granulation tissue from which myofibroblasts have disappeared. Contraction is most obvious when wounds with healthy granulation tissue containing myofibroblasts are grafted.

Tip

- Skin grafts not only increase the rate of epithelialization, but also enhance wound contraction.

Causes of graft failure

Failure of skin grafts to be accepted can be caused by infection, inflammation, fluid accumulation beneath the graft, and motion.[13,16,24,25,29,32] Infection is reported to be the most common cause of failure in humans[39,40] and horses.[41]

Infection

Although the surface of granulation tissue has a resident bacterial population, abundant blood vessels and phagocytic cells within the tissue act as a barrier against bacterial invasion.[7,15,16,24,42,43] The wound becomes infected only when the tissue concentration of bacteria exceeds the ability of humoral and cellular defenses to destroy the microorganisms; this concentration is generally estimated to be 10^5 organisms per gram of tissue in a sutured wound or a wound covered with a graft. Skin graft survival is better correlated to the concentration of bacteria in the wound than to any other factor;[39,40] therefore, a wound should not be grafted if it is found, by quantitative bacterial analysis, to contain more than 10^5 bacteria per gram of tissue. Even though performing quantitative bacterial analysis of a wound before grafting would be useful in helping to determine if the wound is capable of accepting a graft, this type of analysis is impractical for most clinicians. The type of bacteria found in the wound also is an important consideration because, for some bacteria, the concentration necessary to infect a wound can be much less than 10^5 per gram of tissue.[24,42] β-hemolytic streptococci, in particular, produce proteolytic enzymes that catalyze the conversion of plasminogen to plasmin, which digests fibrin and degrades the graft's fibrinous attachment to the wound.[24,44] Pseudomonads also weaken the graft's fibrinous attachment by producing elastase, which specifically damages elastin in the graft's dermis, to which fibrin attaches.[24]

Inflammation

Although infection is reported to be the most common cause of graft failure in horses,[41] chronic inflammation, inherently present during second-intention healing of wounds on the distal aspect of limbs of horses, may be at least as important because it deteriorates the quality of the granulation bed and results in the production of moderate amounts of purulent exudate containing several detrimental enzymes, which negatively influence graft acceptance.[45,46] Grafts applied to wounds of horses may, therefore, be at greater risk of failure than grafts applied to wounds of other species. Wounds of ponies are less prone to chronic inflammation, and therefore may better accept a graft, though this has yet to be investigated.

Accumulation of fluid beneath the graft

Accumulation of fluid, such as blood, serum, or exudate, beneath a graft prevents fibrin from attaching the graft to the wound bed and obstructs vascularization of the graft.[17,25] Although a graft can survive for several days by imbibing nutrients from blood or serum, the graft perishes if capillaries from the wound are incapable of traversing the fluid to reach the graft within this time. To prevent the formation of a hematoma or seroma beneath it, the graft should be compressed firmly against the wound with a bandage, and meshing the graft before application allows escape of fluid that would otherwise accumulate (see Meshing sheet grafts later in this chapter).

Hemorrhage from a wound grafted with pinch or punch grafts may dislodge the grafts. Moderate hemorrhage, however, is not considered by the authors to be a big detriment to grafting when applying a meshed sheet graft or Meek micrografts. Hemorrhage ceases quickly after these grafts are applied, possibly because more donor skin is applied to the wound using these techniques, and therefore, more dermal factors from the grafts that stimulate hemostasis are provided. For this reason, the surface of the granulation tissue can be excised at the time of grafting, and by doing so, slightly protruding or poor quality tissue, bacteria, and leukocytes are removed. A fresh, clean surface is created to which the graft is rapidly attached by fibrin. Grafting to a severely hemorrhaging wound should be avoided. If severe hemorrhage is expected after excising exuberant granulation tissue (EGT), excision should be done well in advance of grafting. If hemostasis cannot be achieved at the time of surgery, the graft can be stored for later application (see Storing split-thickness sheet grafts later in this chapter).

Motion

To establish vascular connections, the graft must remain immobile. Shearing forces between the graft and the wound, caused by movement of the bandage, disrupt the fibrin seal, impairing plasmatic imbibition and revascularization. Shearing forces occur when the wound is located in a highly mobile region, such as over a joint, but can usually be prevented by application of a splint or cast. Open grafting (i.e., grafting without bandaging) is a technique sometimes used to avoid shear forces and is especially useful when grafting a wound located in a region difficult to bandage, such as the trunk (see Aftercare of the recipient site later in this chapter). Shearing forces that occur during dressing changes can be prevented by avoiding changing the bandages during the first week after grafting, using non-adherent dressings or foams, and by immobilizing the horse with sedation.

Fibrin glue has been used to encourage graft acceptance in humans by increasing the strength of the adhesive bond between the graft and the wound bed.[44] Fibrin glue enhances acceptance of skin grafts not only in this manner but also by providing hemostasis and enhancing phagocytosis. A trial using fibrin glue, made from equine fibrinogen, to attach autogenous, split-thickness skin grafts to experimentally created wounds on the dorsal surface of the metacarpi and metatarsi of horses, however, did not support its use to decrease the incidence of graft failure.[47] On the other hand, the authors' clinical experience is that intentionally provoking very slight hemorrhage from a wound before grafting provides fibrin, which promotes attachment of the graft.

Preparation of the wound

The wound must be properly prepared to optimize a graft's chances of survival. The most important factors to consider when evaluating a wound's readiness for grafting are its vascularity and whether it appears free of infection.[15] Grafting should be postponed if the vascularity of the wound seems inadequate to support a graft, if the wound appears to be infected or has an increased susceptibility to infection, or if the wound is chronically inflamed.[46]

Fresh tissue accepts a graft more readily than does granulation tissue, and new granulation tissue accepts a graft more readily than does mature granulation tissue, because vascularity diminishes as granulation tissue matures.[42] Consequently, fibrous, poorly vascularized granulation tissue should be excised to

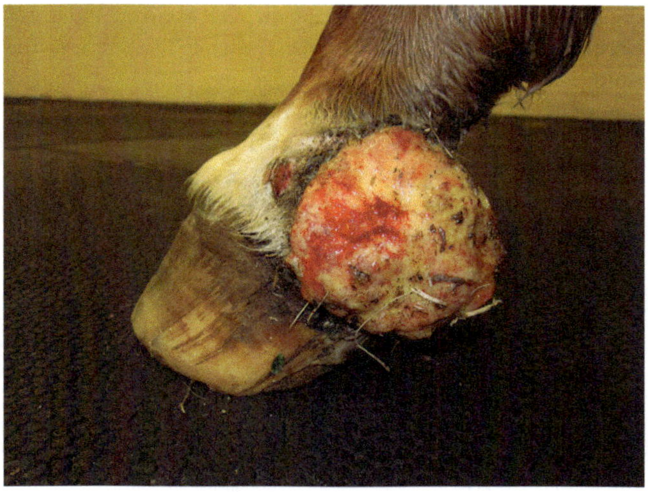

Figure 18.3 Some cutaneous neoplasms, such as this sarcoid on a pastern, resemble granulation tissue.

below the margin of the skin edge so that new, vascular granulation tissue can form prior to grafting.[13] Granulation tissue can usually be excised with the horse standing because granulation tissue has no innervation. When granulation tissue is allowed to proliferate for several days after wounding or after excision, the interval between application of the graft and the time at which it begins to vascularize (i.e., the phase of plasmatic imbibition) is reduced from about 48 to 24 hours, because sprouting capillaries capable of rapidly revascularizing the graft proliferate in the wound.[48] A wound should be examined thoroughly for infection or susceptibility to infection prior to grafting. A wound, particularly a slow-healing one or one with a draining tract, should be assessed for the presence of a foreign body and for evidence of damage to bone, ligaments, tendons, or synovial structures. Underlying bone should be examined radiographically for evidence of an osseous sequestrum or septic osteitis. Granulation tissue of slowly healing or non-healing wounds, particularly those that appear pruritic, should be examined histologically for the presence of larvae of the equine stomach worm, *Habronema*, or for a cutaneous neoplasm, such as a sarcoid or carcinoma, because these may resemble granulation tissue (Figure 18.3).

The bacterial status of a wound to be grafted is usually assessed qualitatively, rather than quantitatively. Quantifying the concentration of bacteria in a wound is time consuming and often impractical, and, moreover, the type of bacteria is often more important than the concentration of bacteria.[24] A wound is assumed to be infected if it shows signs of inflammation such as redness, swelling of the wound and surrounding area, and/or formation of exudate. Such wounds should not be grafted. Unfortunately, even wounds without signs of infection may contain a critical concentration of bacteria hindering acceptance of a skin graft.[40] A wound that is suspected of being infected can be cultured for bacteria, and isolates tested for susceptibility to antimicrobial drugs.

Infection is most often caused by *Streptococcus* or *Pseudomonas* spp. Resolving a streptococcal wound infection is usually relatively easy because this organism is nearly always susceptible to penicillin or other β-lactam antibiotics.[42,49,50] Occasionally, however, other bacteria in the wound secrete β-lactamase, which inactivates most β-lactam antibiotics. The efficacy of the β-lactam antibiotic against streptococci is maintained, however, if potassium clavulanate, or clavulanic acid, an inhibitor of β-lactamase, is administered concomitantly.[49] *Pseudomonas* infection, which is also highly detrimental to grafts, can be recognized by the characteristic bluish-green exudate and odor of grape juice produced by the bacteria. Pseudomonads are usually sensitive to silver sulfadiazine, aminoglycoside antibiotics, polymyxin-B sulfate, fusidinic acid, or mafenide acetate.[51] Using antimicrobial dressings or topical wound-care products whose activity is not based on antibiotics helps prevent the development of resistant bacteria in the wound, such as methicillin-resistant *Staphylococcus aureus* (MRSA) or *Pseudomonas* spp. (for more information on antimicrobial dressings, the reader is referred to Chapter 6; for more information on topical wound-care products, the reader is referred to Chapter 5).

Topical administration of an antimicrobial drug to an infected, granulating wound is usually more successful in resolving infection than is systemic administration of the same antimicrobial drug. Systemically administered antimicrobial drugs often fail to reach a therapeutic concentration within granulation tissue and at its surface, despite the good blood supply found in granulation tissue, because fibrin at the base of the granulation tissue prevents adequate penetration of the drug.[15,52] Wounds infected with streptococci may be treated with topically applied fusidinic acid cream, and wounds infected with *Pseudomonas* can usually be treated successfully with topically applied silver sulfadiazine.

Nevertheless, the most effective method of decreasing infection and/or chronic inflammation (i.e., the concentration of bacteria and leukocytes) is debridement. EGT can be excised to the level of or slightly below the margin of the surrounding skin, and for wounds containing granulation tissue that is not exuberant, the upper 2–3 mm of the surface should be excised.[29] Most bacteria, inflammatory cells, and debris are simultaneously removed, improving local wound conditions. EGT should be excised several days before grafting, and a pressure bandage should be applied to control hemorrhage. When excision is performed at least 24 hours in advance of grafting, the time provided is sufficient for the development of budding capillaries that subsequently vascularize the graft.[48] After excision, the bandage should be changed daily or every other day. The concentration of bacteria in the wound may be further reduced by topical application of a broad-spectrum antimicrobial drug or dressing (as described earlier), which simultaneously decreases the inflammatory response.

The chronic inflammation often present in wounds on limbs of horses can be further reduced with a single topical application of a corticosteroid, such as triamcinolone acetonide, 2 days

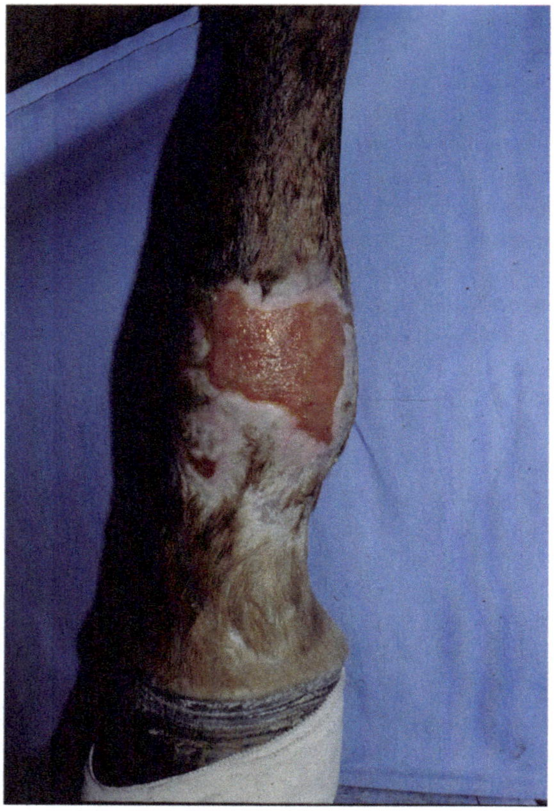

Figure 18.4 This granulating wound is firm, flat, vascular, and red, and is likely capable of accepting a free skin graft.

before surgery.[35] Reducing inflammation in this manner may improve graft acceptance. The potentially negative influence of the corticosteroid on angiogenesis is offset by reduction of the detrimental effect of inflammation on acceptance of the graft.

A granulating wound capable of accepting a free graft is firm, flat, vascular, and red, and contains no more than a few clefts. It should not bleed easily, and discharge from the wound should be slight and serosanguinous or only slightly purulent (Figure 18.4).[7] Adherence of a dressing to the wound bed by fibrin and the presence of advancing epithelium from the wound's margin are useful indicators that a wound is free of infection and receptive to grafting.

At the time of grafting, the recipient bed should be prepared by clipping or shaving the hair surrounding the wound, taking care to first cover the wound with moistened gauze sponges. The skin surrounding the wound can be cleansed with surgical soap, but the wound itself should be cleansed only by rinsing it with isotonic saline solution or a balanced electrolyte solution, because detergent found in surgical soap and disinfectants is cytotoxic, increases the wound's susceptibility to infection, and provokes more inflammation.[53] The surface of the wound can then be rubbed with a gauze sponge to remove fibrinous debris, or its most superficial layer can be excised (i.e., 2–3 mm). This excision is best done before the graft is harvested to allow time for the wound to cease hemorrhaging. Although slight hemorrhage caused by superficial excision enhances formation of fibrin, which enables the graft to adhere to the wound surface, too much hemorrhage may hinder revascularization of the graft. The wound should not be scraped because this damages the surface of the wound and makes it irregular.

What to do

- Graft acceptance can be enhanced by preparing the wound carefully before grafting. This entails reducing the wound's bacterial burden and reducing inflammation.

What to avoid

- Administering an antimicrobial drug systemically to resolve infection of a granulating wound is ineffective. An antimicrobial agent should be applied topically.

Tips

- Grafting to a fresh, non-contaminated wound is preferable to grafting to a granulating wound. Fresh tissue accepts a graft more readily than does granulation tissue, and new granulation tissue accepts a graft more readily than does mature granulation tissue.
- Fibrous or contaminated granulation tissue should be excised to below the margin of the wound 24–48 hours prior to grafting so that the graft can be applied to fresh granulation tissue.
- Applying an antibiotic topically can result in selection of resistant bacteria. Resistance by bacteria to most antimicrobial dressings, such as an antimicrobial dressing based on silver or polyhexamethylene biguanide HCl (PHMB), is rare, and therefore an antimicrobial dressing, rather than an antibiotic, should be used to dress the wound. Alternatively, an antibiotic can be alternated with an antimicrobial dressing.
- A β-lactam antibiotic applied to a wound to resolve streptococcal infection often loses its potency because other bacteria on the wound produce β-lactamase, which destroys the β-lactam antibiotic. By applying a preparation of the β-lactam antibiotic to which clavulanic acid has been added, the activity of the β-lactam antibiotic is preserved.

Preparation of the donor site

The area selected for harvesting a graft depends on the intended method of grafting and whether the graft is to be harvested with the horse standing or anesthetized. Because harvesting a graft, especially one of split-thickness, creates a blemish at the donor site, the site should be inconspicuous.

The donor site should be prepared for aseptic harvest. Hair can be removed from the donor site by clipping, shaving, or chemical depilation. Shaving or depilating the hair improves the performance of a power dermatome. The direction of hair growth should be marked so that it can be matched to that of the skin surrounding the wound to which it is grafted. After the donor site is prepared for surgery, it should be rinsed with water or isotonic saline solution to remove residues of surgical soap and disinfectant, which are detrimental to the graft and the recipient site.

Grafting techniques

Island grafting

Island grafts, sometimes referred to as implantation grafts or seed grafts, are small pieces of skin implanted either into or onto a wound.[54–56] The different types of island grafts applied to wounds of horses are punch grafts, pinch grafts, tunnel grafts, and modified Meek micrografts. Except for the Meek micrografts, island grafts are implanted into granulation tissue of horses, to prevent shearing forces between the dressing and the graft. Island grafts are used to increase the area of epidermis from which epithelialization can proceed.

Punch grafting

Punch grafts are full-thickness plugs of skin that are harvested and implanted into granulation tissue using skin biopsy punches. Punch grafts are harvested directly from the horse (Figure 18.5) or from a full-thickness piece of skin (Figure 18.6), usually excised from the cranial pectoral region.[57] Punch grafts harvested directly from the horse should be collected at a relatively inconspicuous site, such as the ventrolateral aspect of the abdomen, the perineum, or the portion of the neck that lies beneath the mane, because wounds created at the donor site heal with small scars.

Technique

The donor site is prepared as described earlier (see Preparation of the donor site) and desensitized by subcutaneous administration of local anesthetic solution, or if the perineum is the donor site, by administering caudal epidural anesthesia. Grafts should be harvested about 1 cm apart and in a symmetrical pattern in an effort to improve the cosmetic appearance of the donor site (Figure 18.5).[41] The small wounds created by the biopsy punch can be left unsutured to heal by second intention, but closing each wound with a staple or suture speeds healing and decreases scarring. Prior to implanting the grafts, subcutaneous tissue should be sharply excised from each graft to expose dermal vasculature and encourage plasmatic imbibition and inosculation.[54,58] This can be done after the plug has been excised or while the plug is still attached to the horse.[59]

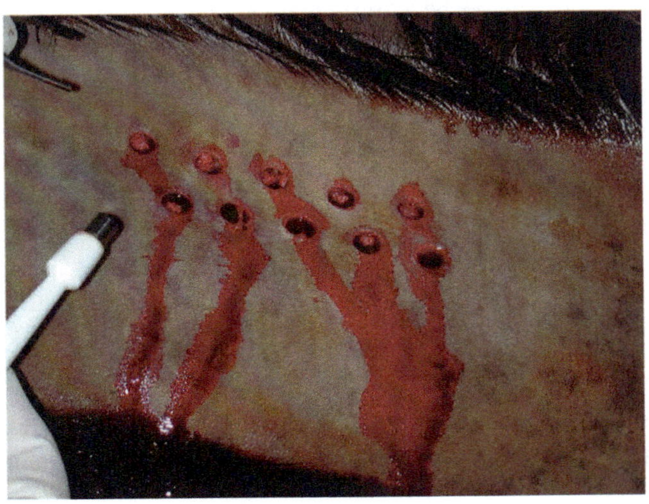

Figure 18.5 Punch grafts have been harvested directly from the neck of this horse.

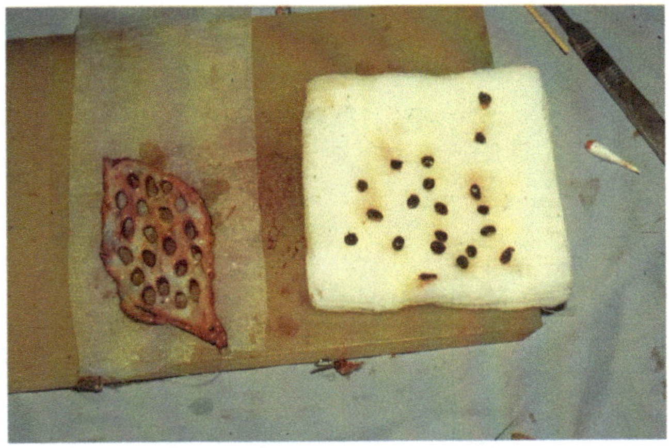

Figure 18.6 These punch grafts were harvested from a full-thickness section of skin excised from the cranial pectoral region. Subcutaneous tissue was sharply excised from the section of skin to expose the dermis prior to harvesting the grafts with a biopsy punch.

Because removing subcutaneous tissue from individual plugs of skin is tedious, some clinicians prefer to harvest punch grafts from a full-thickness section of skin from which the subcutaneous tissue has been removed (Figure 18.6). This section of skin is usually harvested from the pectoral region, where it is relatively thin and mobile.[57] A 10 × 4 cm section of skin provides a sufficient number of grafts to cover most wounds, and the resulting wound at the donor site can be sutured easily in one or two layers.[60] A tie-over bandage is sutured to the closed incision to decrease tension on the wound (Figure 18.7). The excised strip of skin is stretched and fixed, dermal side up, to a sterile piece of plastic, cardboard, or Styrofoam or to a polypropylene block or a sterile roll of elastic bandage, and subcutaneous tissue is sharply excised to expose the dermis (Figure 18.8). Plugs are cut from the skin with a 5–8-mm diameter skin biopsy punch. The grafts are covered with a sterile gauze sponge moistened with isotonic saline solution until they are implanted into the wound (Figure 18.6).

The recipient holes in the wound should be created before the grafts are harvested to ensure that hemorrhage has stopped before the grafts are implanted. The holes should be created in a symmetrical pattern, about 6 mm apart.[57] The depth of the recipient holes should correspond to the thickness of the grafts.[57] Creation of the holes should begin distally and proceed proximally so that the hemorrhage emanating from the holes does not obscure that portion of the wound that has not yet been perforated.[58] Inserting a cotton-tipped applicator into the holes prevents a blood clot from forming within and facilitates locating the holes for subsequent graft insertion.[60] One can

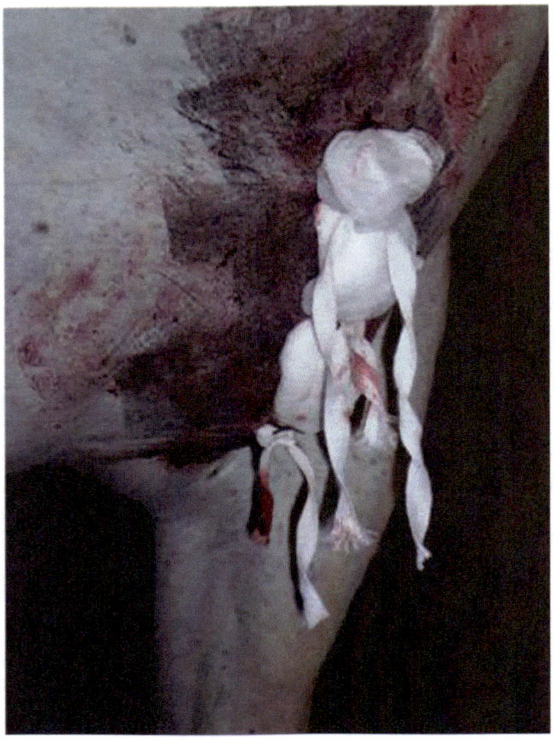

Figure 18.7 The wound created after excising a full-thickness section of skin from the chest is sutured in one or two layers, and a tie-over bandage is sutured to the closed incision to decrease tension on the wound.

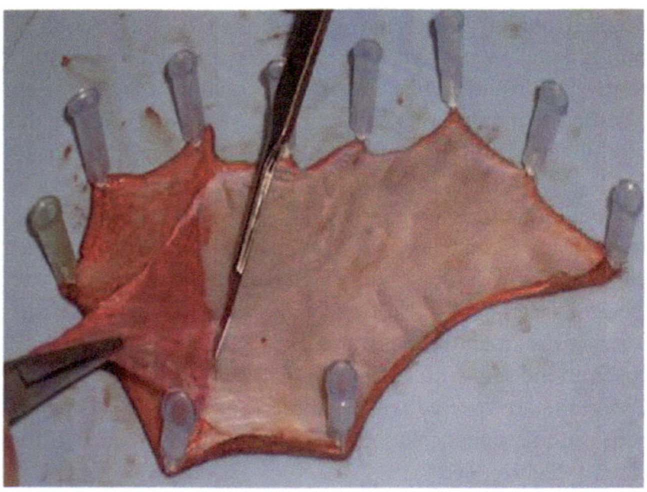

Figure 18.8 This section of skin has been stretched and fixed to a sterile piece of plastic. Subcutaneous tissue is being excised to expose the dermis.

ensure a hemorrhage-free wound for grafting by creating the recipient holes at least an hour in advance of implantation. In anticipation of primary graft contraction, the recipient holes should be created with a slightly smaller biopsy punch than that used to harvest the grafts. For example, if the grafts are harvested with a 6-mm diameter biopsy punch, the holes should be created with a 4-mm diameter biopsy punch. The holes should

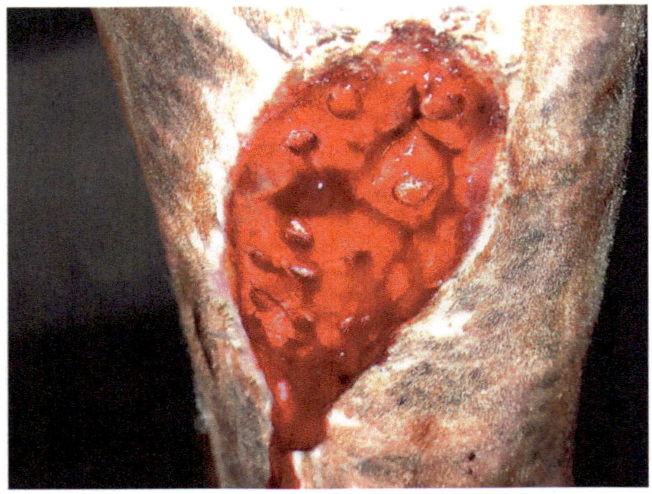

Figure 18.9 The recipient holes in this granulating wound have been filled with punch grafts.

be irrigated to remove blood clots before inserting the grafts. Each graft is inserted into a recipient hole (Figure 18.9), using a hemostat or tissue forceps, with the graft oriented according to the direction of its hair growth. The grafted wound is covered with a non-adherent dressing and then bandaged.

Acceptance and appearance

About 60–75% of the grafts can be expected to survive.[60] The superficial, pigmented portion of many of the grafts may slough between the 1st and 2nd week, exposing the pale, underlying dermis, which may be somewhat similar in appearance to surrounding granulation tissue. Difficulty in identifying many of the grafts and the presence of sloughed portions of graft on the primary dressing may cause the clinician to mistakenly assume that a large number of grafts have been lost. But by 3 weeks, the pale grafts can easily be recognized by the pink rim of migrating epithelium that surrounds them.[57] The time required for epithelium to fully cover the remaining wound is inversely proportional to the area of the wound covered with viable plugs. Wounds to which punch grafts have been applied heal with an epithelial scar from which emerge sparse tufts of long hair, which often grow in various directions. The cosmetic outcome can be improved by orienting the grafts during implantation according to the direction of their hair growth.

Advantages and disadvantages

Punch grafting requires little expertise and neither expensive nor sophisticated equipment, it may be performed with the horse standing. The grafts are often accepted into recipient wounds that are not suitable for sheet grafting, such as wounds in regions of high motion.[57] The grafts are independent of one another, and so, rejection of one graft has little or no effect on acceptance of other grafts. Punch grafting is usually reserved for small to moderate-sized wounds and for circumstances in which the cosmetic appearance of the healed wound is not important.

What to do

- The cosmetic appearance of a healed, punch-grafted wound is often poor. Implanting the grafts according to the direction of their hair growth improves the appearance of the healed wound.
- The likelihood of acceptance of punch grafts is increased if subcutaneous tissue is excised to expose the dermis of the graft.
- Some surgeons may find harvesting punch grafts from a full-thickness sheet of skin from which the subcutaneous tissue and fascia have been excised to be less tedious than harvesting punch grafts by excising these tissues from individual punch grafts harvested directly from the horse.
- A cotton-tipped applicator inserted into each recipient hole prevents a blood clot from forming within the hole and facilitates locating the hole for insertion of the graft.

Pinch grafting

Pinch grafts, sometime referred to as Reverdin grafts, are small disks of skin harvested by excising an elevated cone of skin, which are then implanted into pockets created in granulation tissue.[21,50,54–56,61] The perineum and the portion of the neck that lies beneath the mane are common donor sites for harvesting pinch grafts from horses because small scars created at these locations are relatively inconspicuous.

Technique

The donor site is prepared and desensitized as described for punch grafting. A cone of skin is tented with a tissue forceps, a hypodermic needle with a bent point, or a suture needle, and excised with a scalpel blade.[50,54–56,61] A disk of optimal size is about 3 mm in diameter.[55] A disk of this diameter is thin toward its periphery but nearly full thickness toward its center. The grafts are covered with a sterile gauze sponge moistened with isotonic saline solution until they are implanted.

As for punch grafting, implantation of pinch grafts should begin distally and proceed proximally so that the hemorrhage emanating from sites of implantation does not obscure the portion of the wound that has not yet been implanted. To implant a pinch graft, a #15 scalpel blade is stabbed into the granulation tissue at an acute angle to the wound to create a shallow pocket into which the pinch graft is inserted (Figure 18.10). The pockets are created about 3–5 mm apart.[55] The graft is placed on the wound, proximal to the pocket, with its epidermal side up. It is pushed into the pocket using a straight suture needle, hypodermic needle, mosquito hemostat, or, most conveniently, with the scalpel blade used to make the pocket. Orientating the pinches according to the direction of hair growth has little effect on the cosmetic outcome, because hair growth from pinch grafts is usually sparse. To speed implantation, three or more grafts may be placed on the wound, each several centimeters proximal to the proposed site of implantation. While the grafts remain adhered to the wound by surface tension, the surgeon creates a pocket distal to a graft and pushes the graft into it using the same scalpel blade that was used to create the pockets. This technique enables the surgeon to create and implant the pockets in quick succession, without looking away from the wound. Alternatively, each graft can be inserted into the granulation tissue, without making a pocket, using a curved mosquito hemostat. The graft is grasped in the midepidermal region and inserted obliquely, from proximal to distal, into the granulation tissue, after which the hemostat is opened to create more space for the graft. This technique is much quicker than making separate pockets using a scalpel blade (T. Stashak, personal communication).

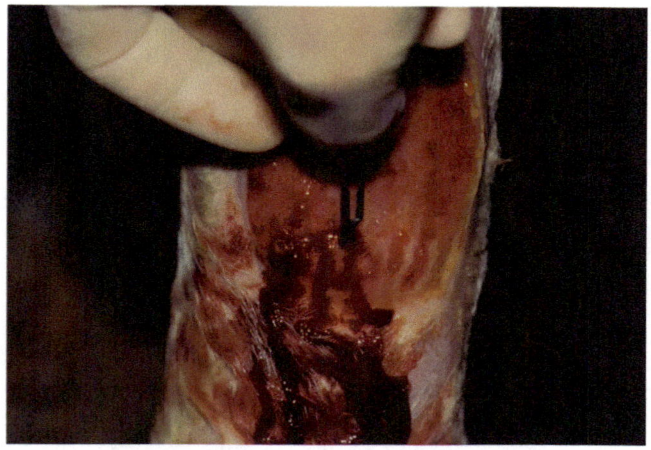

Figure 18.10 A shallow pocket, into which a pinch graft can be inserted, is created by stabbing a #15 scalpel blade into the granulation tissue at an acute angle.

The small, partial-thickness wounds created at the donor site can be left unsutured to heal by second intention, but closing each wound with a staple or suture speeds healing and may decrease scarring. The grafted wound is covered with a non-adherent dressing and then bandaged.

Acceptance and appearance

The grafts initially appear as dark spots on the wound. The thin layer of granulation tissue overlying each graft sloughs, usually between the 1st and 2nd week,[55] and, frequently, so does the superficial, pigmented portion of the graft. The exposed, pale dermis may be difficult to distinguish from surrounding granulation tissue, giving the impression that the entire graft has sloughed. By 3 weeks, however, grafts are surrounded by a pink rim of advancing epithelium, making them easily identified. Epithelium migrating from the wound's margin and from the periphery of each graft rapidly coalesces to cover the entire wound. Even when conditions for grafting are unfavorable, at least 50–75% of the grafts are usually accepted. The healed wound is covered by epithelium containing scattered islands of hair.

Advantages and disadvantages

Pinch grafting, like punch grafting, requires little expertise and is economical because only basic instruments are required and the procedure may be performed with the horse standing. Pinch grafts, like punch grafts, can survive in a granulation bed that is

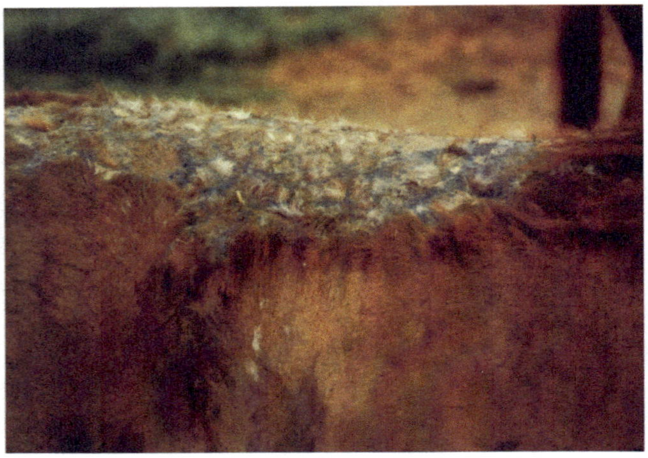

Figure 18.11 The wound on the back of this horse has healed with pinch grafts. The back is covered by an epithelial scar that contains scattered islands of hair.

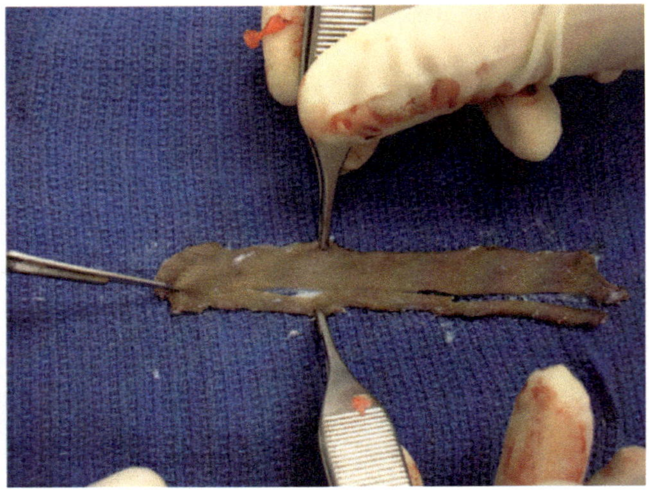

Figure 18.12 A full-thickness section of skin, harvested from the neck of a horse, is being divided into 2 mm wide strips for implantation in a granulating wound. Courtesy of Dr. P. Rakestraw.

not suitable for sheet grafting, such as a wound in an area of high motion.[54,62] Like punch grafts, pinch grafts are independent of one another, and therefore, rejection of one graft has no effect on acceptance of other grafts. Pinch grafting is tedious, however, and therefore is usually reserved for small wounds. The cosmetic appearance of a wound healed with pinch grafts is poor (Figure 18.11).

Tips

- Pinch grafts are most easily implanted when the diameter of the disk is about 3 mm.
- A pinch graft can be applied to the wound before creating the pocket into which it is to be inserted. The graft adheres to the wound by surface tension while the pocket is created. Using this technique, the surgeon can implant the graft without looking away from the wound.
- Spreading of epithelium from the grafts is usually not evident for about 3 weeks after grafting. Healing proceeds rapidly thereafter.
- The cosmetic appearance of a healed, pinch-grafted wound is poor.

Tunnel grafting

Tunnel grafts are narrow strips of skin implanted into tunnels created in granulation tissue.[2,63,64] Granulation tissue covering the grafts is removed days later, by which time the grafts have revascularized. Grafts may be split-thickness or full-thickness and can be harvested from a number of sites on the horse using a variety of techniques. They can be implanted with the horse standing or anesthetized.

Technique

Tunnel grafts can be harvested from the ventral region of the flank or from the neck or the pectoral region.[2,63,64] After aseptically preparing the donor site, linear wheals, 2–3 cm wide and slightly longer than the width of the wound to be grafted, are created along the longitudinal axis of the donor site by subcutaneously injecting isotonic saline solution when the graft is to be harvested with the horse anesthetized, or by injecting local anesthetic solution when the graft is to be harvested with the horse standing.

A long, straight Doyen intestinal forceps is applied to the base of each wheal, causing skin to protrude slightly above the jaws of the forceps.[2,63,64] The amount of skin that bulges above the jaws determines the width and thickness of the graft. Skin protruding above the jaws is excised with a scalpel blade. If the graft is split-thickness, the partial-thickness wound at the donor site heals by epithelialization. If the graft is full-thickness, the wound at the donor site should be closed. Subcutaneous tissue should be excised from full-thickness grafts to expose the dermal vasculature. Another option is to harvest an elliptical, 2–3 cm wide, full-thickness section of skin that is slightly longer than the width of the wound.[59] After excising subcutaneous tissue from the dermis, the section of skin is divided into 2–3 mm wide strips (Figure 18.12).

To implant a graft into the wound, the jaws of a long, narrow, rat-tooth, alligator forceps are inserted into granulation tissue at the edge of the wound and pushed through it at a depth of about 2–6 mm until they emerge at the opposite wound margin.[2,64] One end of the graft is grasped by the jaws of the forceps and pulled through the newly created tunnel, taking care to orient its epidermis toward the surface of the wound (Figure 18.13).

To permit easy entry and exit of the forceps, the graft should be implanted perpendicular to the long axis of the limb in granulation tissue that protrudes slightly above the margin of the skin.[64] The graft is implanted in two steps if the wound is too convex to be spanned by the alligator forceps, or if the forceps is too short to completely span the wound.[2,63,64] In either situation, the end of the forceps is inserted at the margin of the wound, pushed through the granulation tissue, and exited in

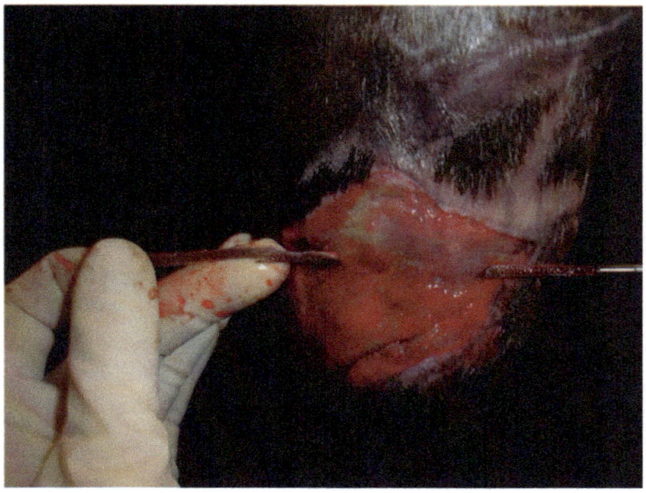

Figure 18.13 To implant a tunnel graft, one end of the graft is grasped by the jaws of an alligator forceps, which has been pushed through the granulation tissue at a depth of 5 mm or 6 mm, then dragged through the tunnel created by the forceps, with the epidermis facing the surface of the wound. Courtesy of Dr. P. Rakestraw.

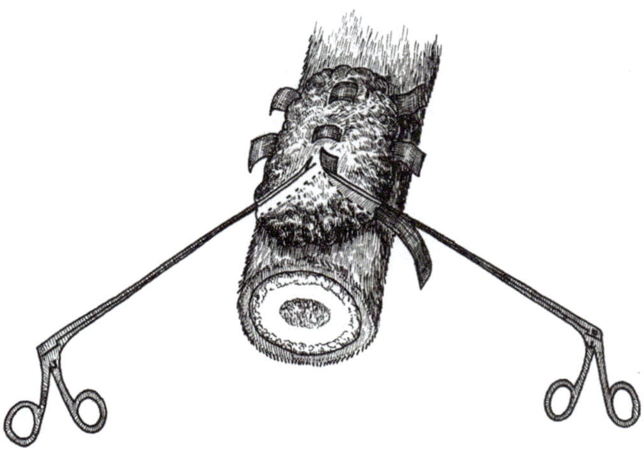

Figure 18.14 To implant a tunnel graft in a wound too convex to be spanned by alligator forceps, the forceps is inserted at the wound's margin and exited in the center of the wound. The graft is grasped by the jaws of the forceps and dragged back through the wound. The end of the forceps is re-inserted at the wound's opposite margin and exited close to the site of entry of the graft in the center of the wound. The end of the graft is grasped by the jaws of the forceps and pulled back through the wound. Courtesy of K. Abney.

the center of the wound. The graft is grasped by the jaws of the forceps and dragged back through the newly created tunnel. The end of the forceps is re-inserted into the granulation bed at the opposite side of the wound, pushed through the granulation tissue, and exited at or close to the site of exit of the graft in the center of the wound. The free end of the graft is grasped by the jaws of the forceps and pulled back through the second tunnel (Figure 18.14).

The protruding ends of the implanted grafts are fixed to the margin of the wound with a suture, staple, or cyanoacrylate glue, and the wound is covered with a non-adherent dressing and bandaged. Six to 10 days after being implanted, the grafts are exposed, with the horse sedated or anesthetized, by excising overlying granulation tissue.[2,63,64] This is done by carefully excising a V-shaped strip of granulation tissue over a small, malleable probe inserted into the tunnel superficial to the graft.

Acceptance and appearance

Complications of tunnel grafting include failure to locate buried grafts and inadvertent dislodging of a graft while attempting to expose it.[64] These difficulties can be avoided by exposing the grafts with the horse anesthetized or by applying a tourniquet proximal to the wound to enhance visibility by eliminating hemorrhage. We have found that when the strips of skin are inserted very superficially beneath the surface of the granulation tissue (~2 mm), the granulation tissue sloughs over the grafts within a week, obviating the need to expose the graft by surgical means. The healed wound is covered by pigmented epithelium that migrates from the margin of the wound and from the margin of each graft. Within this epithelium are diverging tufts of hair.

Advantages and disadvantages

Tunnel grafting is useful for grafting wounds located in regions of high motion, such as the dorsal surface of the hock, because the grafts are immobilized by overlying granulation tissue.[63,64] Like pinch and punch grafts, tunnel grafts are independent of one another, so rejection of one graft has no effect on acceptance of other grafts. Like other techniques of island grafting, tunnel grafting is economical because only basic instruments are required and because the procedure can often be performed with the horse standing. Tunnel grafting is limited to granulating wounds, however, and removing granulation tissue overlying the grafts is tedious, a disadvantage that can be avoided by implanting the grafts superficially so that overlying granulation tissue sloughs and need not be excised.

What to avoid

- Tunnel grafts can be inserted most easily perpendicular to the long axis of the limb. Inserting them parallel to the long axis of the limb is quite difficult.

Tips

- By using a narrow alligator forceps, tunnel grafts can be inserted superficially into the granulation bed, and if inserted at a depth of about 2 mm, the granulation tissue overlying the graft sloughs, obviating the need to remove overlying granulation tissue.
- The cosmetic appearance of a healed, tunnel-grafted wound is poor.

Modified Meek technique

The modified Meek technique is a combination of split-thickness sheet grafting and island grafting and has been evaluated in horses.[29] The technique entails creating split-thickness, 3 × 3-mm (9-mm²) islands of skin, referred to as micrografts. This technique, introduced in the 1990s as a method of grafting burn wounds of humans, has proved particularly suitable for grafting wounds of severely burned patients, who lack large donor sites, because greater expansion ratios can be achieved with these split-thickness micrografts than with meshed sheet grafts, and because all harvested skin can be used.[65] Moreover, Meek micrografts are more readily accepted than a meshed sheet graft by a wound of poor quality because micrografts are less susceptible to infection and inflammation.[65,66] These same advantages apply to wounds of horses.[29]

Technique

The Meek micrografting equipment consists of a cutting block, a frame, and a pneumatic or hand-driven motor. A 1.2-mm thick split-thickness graft is harvested from the abdomen or ventrolateral aspect of the thorax with the horse anesthetized (See Split-thickness sheet grafting later in this chapter). The graft is placed, dermal side down, on a 4.2 × 4.2-cm cork template then trimmed exactly to the size of the template. The cork template with graft is placed on a cork holder, which is placed in a cutting block (Figure 18.15), and the composite is passed through the motor-driven or hand-driven Meek micrograft machine where 13 circular knives cut the skin into 14 strips, each 3 mm wide (Figure 18.16). The machine cuts the skin, but not the cork. The cork holder is then rotated 90 degrees, replaced onto the cutting block, and again passed through the machine. The second passage produces 196 (14 × 14), 3 × 3-mm, split-thickness island grafts, or micrografts. Adhesive spray is applied to the epidermal layer of the grafts, and the grafts are glued to a pre-folded, pleated, polyamide gauze (i.e., plissé) (Figure 18.17) with a predetermined expansion ratio of 1:3, 1:4, 1:6, or 1:9. An expansion ratio of 1:3 is preferred for horses because availability of skin for harvesting a large split-thickness skin graft is usually not a problem, and with less expansion, more micrografts can be placed on the wound, resulting in faster healing and the best cosmetic outcome. The cork template is carefully removed, and the plissé is expanded in two directions, separating the 196 micrografts to a fixed distance. The supporting aluminum backing is peeled off the gauze, and

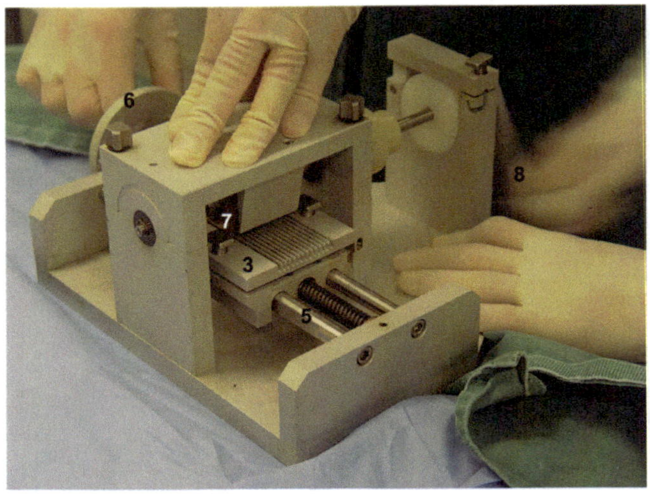

Figure 18.16 The cutting block (3) is placed on the guiding axes (5) of a Meek micrograft machine and moved by a hand wheel (6) under a bridge, where 13 circular knives (7) cut the skin into 14 strips, each 3 mm wide. A Meek micrograft machine is shown with a hand drive (8) instead of a pneumatic motor for turning the knives. Source: Wilmink 2006.[29] Reproduced with permission of John Wiley & Sons.

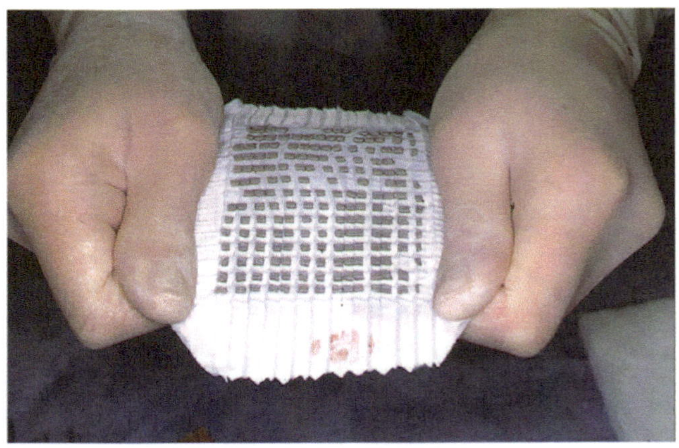

Figure 18.17 The epidermal side of the cut graft is sprayed with an adhesive and glued to the plissé, which is being unfolded in two directions to separate the micrografts. Source: Wilmink 2006.[29] Reproduced with permission of John Wiley & Sons.

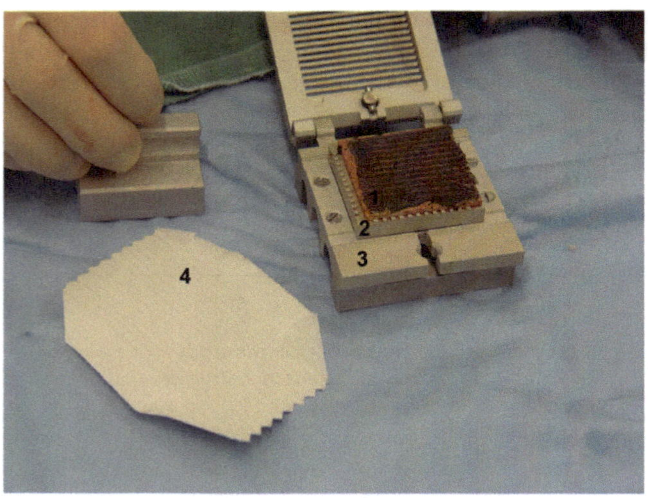

Figure 18.15 To create Meek micrografts, a split-thickness graft is placed on a 4.2-cm² cork template and trimmed exactly to the size of the template (1), placed on a square cork holder (2), and then placed in a cutting block (3). More to the left is a plissé 1:3 (4). Source: Wilmink 2006.[29] Reproduced with permission of John Wiley & Sons.

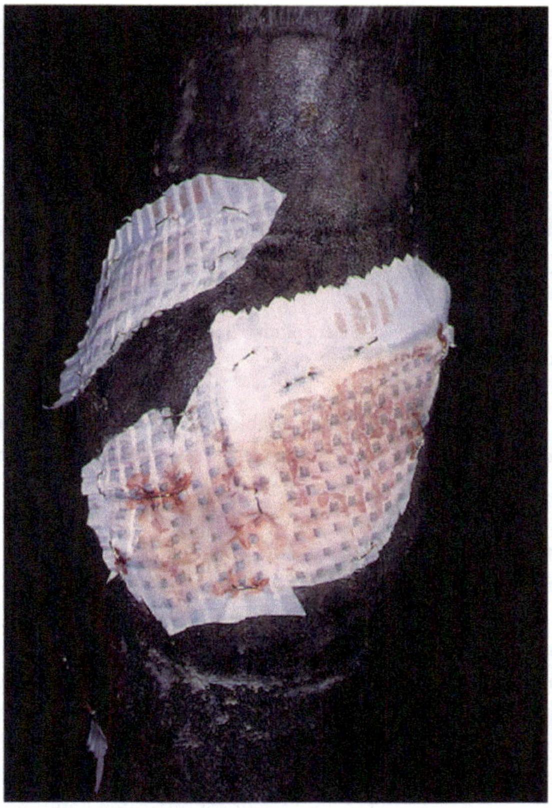

Figure 18.18 The expanded plissé is cut to the appropriate size and sutured or stapled to the wound. Source: Wilmink 2006.[29] Reproduced with permission of John Wiley & Sons.

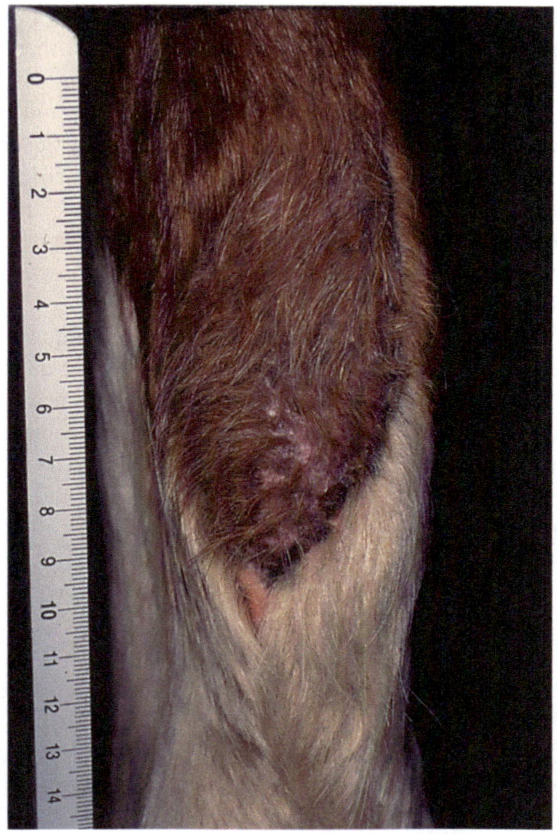

Figure 18.19 Wounds healed with Meek micrografts have regular though somewhat thinner than normal hair growth. Hairs usually grow longer than at the donor site or the area surrounding the wound.

the gauze trimmed to the appropriate size and sutured or stapled to the wound (Figure 18.18). The wound is protected with a bandage or a cast.

Acceptance and appearance

The acceptance of Meek micrografts is nearly 95% and is reported to be better than that achieved with any other type of skin grafting performed in horses.[29] The micrografts have an obvious effect on the granulation tissue, which can be seen when the bandage is changed or the cast is removed after 10 days.[29] Most wounds that were suffering from EGT and/or chronic inflammation before grafting appear flat, smooth, less inflamed, and the rates of contraction and epithelialization appear to have increased substantially.[29] These effects may result from the action of cytokines present in the dermis of the grafts. Although any type of graft that includes the dermis may have such an effect, dermal contact with the wound after Meek micrografting is greater than after the other types of island grafting because of the high number of islands and because the grafts are split-thickness. Micrografts up to 1.2 mm in thickness (i.e., almost full-thickness) can be applied closely together and uniformly in the same direction. The distance between the grafts diminishes as the wound contracts, which allows for rapid coverage of the wound largely by the micrografts. Most wounds that receive Meek micrografts are healed within a month, regardless of the wound's size and location.[29] Hair growth occurs from most of the grafts and is regular, though somewhat thinner and longer than normal, and hair color is the same as that at the donor site (Figure 18.19). In the second author's experience, the Meek micrografting technique provides consistent and reliable functional and cosmetic results due to the high percentage of acceptance of the micrografts, which are strong, uniformly oriented and have a high concentration of hair follicles.

Advantages and disadvantages

As with other techniques of island grafting, the Meek micrografting technique creates small islands of skin independent of one another, so that rejection of one or more grafts has no detrimental effect on acceptance of other grafts. In contrast, partial detachment of a sheet graft due to infection or movement may propagate into other areas of the graft, resulting in complete loss of the graft. Meek micrografts are, therefore, better accepted by poor-quality wounds than are sheet grafts. The micrografts tolerate the ischemic phase after grafting better than do meshed sheet grafts or other types of island grafts because of the relatively large surface area exposed for plasmatic imbibition and revascularization below and surrounding the micrografts.

For that reason, the micrografts can be made thicker than sheet grafts, while still preserving good acceptance, and, therefore, more hair follicles can be transferred to the donor site. The micrografts are better accepted than other types of island grafts because the granulation tissue is not incised to apply the grafts, obviating additional inflammation. Most Meek-micrografted wounds, when grafted using a plissé with a 1:3 expansion ratio, are healed within a month, because the grafts are applied in greater numbers than are grafts applied using other techniques of island grafting.[29]

A disadvantage of the Meek micrografting technique is that the horse must be anesthetized to harvest the split-thickness skin. Equipment to harvest the split-thickness skin and the micrografting machine are relatively expensive but comparable to that required for harvesting and meshing sheet grafts.

Sheet grafting

Full-thickness sheet grafting

> **Tips**
>
> - Grafting limb wounds of horses with Meek micrografts reduces healing time substantially and, therefore, saves the costs of a long period of bandaging. Meek micrografting a limb wound greater than 6 × 6 cm (36 cm^2) may, therefore, be more economical, despite the costs of surgery, than bandaging such a wound until it has healed by second intention.
> - Meek micrografts enhance wound contraction substantially, thus decreasing the final size of the scar.
> - The cosmetic appearance of a healed wound after being grafted with the Meek micrografting technique is good because numerous micrografts, containing hair follicles, can be applied in uniform direction and because the acceptance of these the micrografts is very good.

Technique

A full-thickness graft is usually harvested from the pectoral region, where the skin is relatively mobile,[60,67] with the horse sedated, after desensitizing the donor site with an anesthetic solution. The excised skin is stretched and fixed, dermal side up, to a sterile piece of cardboard, plastic, or Styrofoam, or to a polypropylene block or sterile roll of elastic bandage. Subcutaneous tissue on the undersurface of the graft obstructs plasmatic imbibition and inosculation and so must be sharply excised to expose the dermis and its vasculature (Figure 18.8).[25,62,67] Hair follicles in the dermis are visible when the subcutaneous tissue has been removed. Grafts are attached to the recipient site with staples or sutures (Figure 18.20). Attaching the graft to the recipient site with slight tension keeps the small dermal vessels open, thereby facilitating plasmatic imbibition and inosculation.[61] The donor site is sutured in two layers.

Acceptance and appearance

Full-thickness grafts are not as readily accepted as split-thickness grafts because of their greater requirement for nourishment and

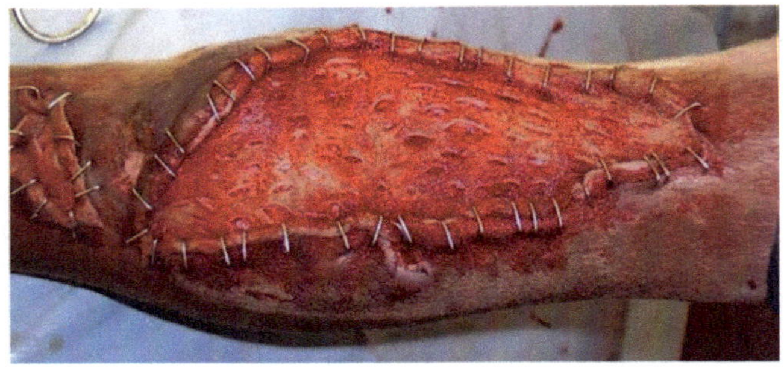

Figure 18.20 This meshed, sheet graft has been stapled to a wound on the dorsal surface of the fetlock.

fewer exposed blood vessels available for plasmatic imbibition or inosculation.[7,14,38,41,68] Circumstances at the recipient site, therefore, must be ideal for a full-thickness graft to be accepted. This type of grafting is usually reserved for fresh, uncontaminated wounds,[7,14,15,21,42] although a full-thickness skin graft can be applied successfully to healthy, new granulation tissue.[34]

Advantages and disadvantages

Wounds healed with a full-thickness skin graft have a superior cosmetic appearance and resist trauma better than those healed with a split-thickness sheet graft or with island grafts.[7,14,38,41,62] Full-thickness sheet grafts may be harvested and applied with the horse standing and in the absence of sophisticated equipment.

The horse's lack of redundant donor skin limits the practicality of full-thickness grafting to relatively small wounds, provided that the surgeon intends to suture the donor site after harvesting the graft. The largest graft that can usually be safely harvested from the cranial pectoral area is an ellipse not exceeding 8 cm at its widest point. The owner should be forewarned that the donor site might dehisce but be reassured that a wound in that region heals rapidly by contraction, leaving little epithelial scarring. A full-thickness graft can be meshed and expanded to cover a wound larger than the graft itself (see Meshing sheet grafts later in the chapter), but full-thickness skin of horses is too thick to be easily meshed using commercial meshgraft dermatomes. Unlike failure of one or more island grafts, which are independent of one another, failure of a portion of a full-thickness, may result in loss of the entire graft.

> **What to do**
>
> - The owner should be warned that the donor site of a full-thickness graft may dehisce but reassured that a dehisced wound in the pectoral region heals by second intention with little or no blemish.
>
> **Tips**
>
> - Full-thickness skin grafting is usually reserved for fresh wounds, but full-thickness grafts may also be accepted by granulating wounds, providing the granulation tissue is fresh and vascular.
> - The site from which a full-thickness graft is most easily harvested is the pectoral region.

Split-thickness sheet grafting

Instrumentation

A split-thickness graft is composed of epidermis and a portion of dermis. To harvest a split-thickness graft, the dermis is split using a power-driven dermatome, drum dermatome, or free-hand knife.

Power-driven dermatomes

A power-driven dermatome harvests a split-thickness skin graft with predictable depth and width using a rapidly oscillating blade, which is set in a housing and driven by an electric motor or gas turbine. Examples of commonly used power-driven dermatomes are the Stryker electric dermatome (Electric Dermatome, Stryker Electro-Surgical Unit, Orthopedic Frame Co.), Brown pneumatic or electric dermatome (Brown Dermatome, Zimmer), Padgett electric dermatome (Padgett Model B Dermatome, Padgett Instruments), and Humeca electric dermatome (Humeca Models D42 and D80, Humeca Instruments). A pneumatic dermatome generally provides a smoother harvest than does an electric dermatome of the same type because the cutting head of the pneumatic dermatome oscillates more rapidly.[25] Different types of power-driven dermatomes may vary in their ability to harvest skin smoothly, and some of the newer types of electric dermatomes may harvest skin as smoothly as do pneumatic dermatomes.

The Humeca dermatome is small and maneuverable and is powered by a rechargeable battery. It has a fixed width of either 42 mm or 80 mm, which can be reduced, if necessary, with clamps. The D42 model has the exact width required for harvesting skin to be used in the Meek micrograft machine. Thickness of cut can be adjusted from 0–1.2 mm; therefore, the dermatome is capable of harvesting thick split-thickness grafts that contain a large concentration of hair follicles. Unlike some power dermatomes, the Humeca dermatome is usually capable of easily harvesting skin from the ventral surface of the abdomen of horses. The ability of a power dermatome to split skin in compliant areas, such as the ventral surface of the abdomen, also depends on the skin's elasticity. Harvesting skin with a power dermatome presents similar challenges in humans, where harvesting the elastic skin of children is more difficult than harvesting the relatively inelastic skin of adults.

A power-driven dermatome allows harvesting of grafts of precise width and thickness, but the widest graft that can be harvested with many power dermatomes is only 80 mm, and the maximal thickness allowed by some is 1.2 mm, although thickness varies according to the amount of pressure applied to the dermatome. Most power-driven dermatomes have adjustable settings for thickness and width and can be operated with only a minimal amount of experience. Because power-driven dermatomes are expensive, they are generally found only at referral centers.

Drum dermatomes

The drum dermatome consists of a portion of a drum, which is coated with an adhesive, and a knife. A section of skin adheres to the drum as the drum is rolled across the skin, and the knife oscillates back and forth on a piston to precisely split the dermis at a predetermined thickness.

Using a drum dermatome, the surgeon can harvest a graft with the exact dimensions of the wound to be grafted by applying glue to an area on the drum that is identical to the dimensions of the wound, so that as the drum is rotated, only the adhered portion of skin is cut.[15] The drum dermatome requires no external power source and allows anyone to harvest a uniform section of skin with only minimal training.[14,15,25] The drum dermatome is not as expensive as a power-driven dermatome, although it is considerably more expensive than a free-hand dermatome. A major disadvantage of the drum dermatome for harvesting grafts from horses is that the length of the graft is limited by the circumference of the drum. An example of a drum dermatome is the Padgett Manual Dermatome (Z-PD-100R, Padgett Instruments, Inc.), which has a circumference of 31.9 cm.

Free-hand dermatomes

Large split-thickness grafts can be harvested with any one of a variety of free-hand dermatomes designed specifically for harvesting skin of humans. The Watson skin grafting knife (Watson Skin Grafting Knife, Padgett Instruments, Inc.) has an adjustable roller in front of a disposable blade and can harvest a graft 100 mm wide. Because the depth of cut is primarily controlled by the adjustable roller, only a moderate amount of practice is required to develop proficiency in harvesting uniform, split-thickness grafts with this knife. The position of the adjustable roller is controlled by a knob, marked with calibrations, at one end of the roller (Figure 18.21) and a lock at the other end (Figure 18.22). The thickness of graft corresponding to each calibration is learned by experience. The depth of cut depends not only on the distance of the roller from the blade, but also on the angle of incidence at which the knife is held, as well as the pressure applied to the knife while cutting.[42] By applying greater pressure to the knife or by increasing the knife's angle of incidence, the thickness of the graft can be increased without changing the position of the roller.

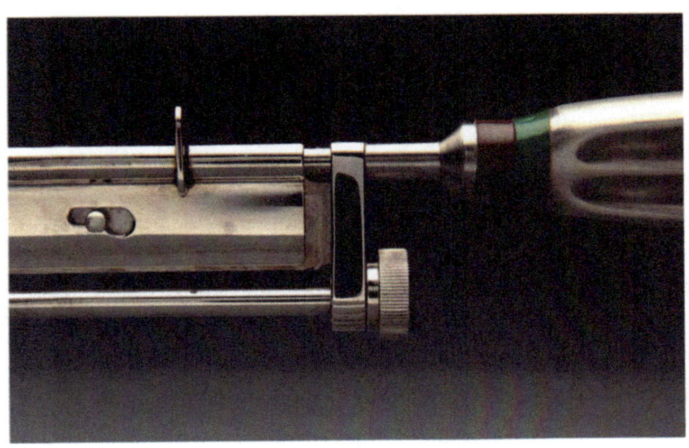

Figure 18.21 The position of the adjustable roller on the Watson skin graft dermatome is controlled by a knob marked with calibrations, at one end of the roller.

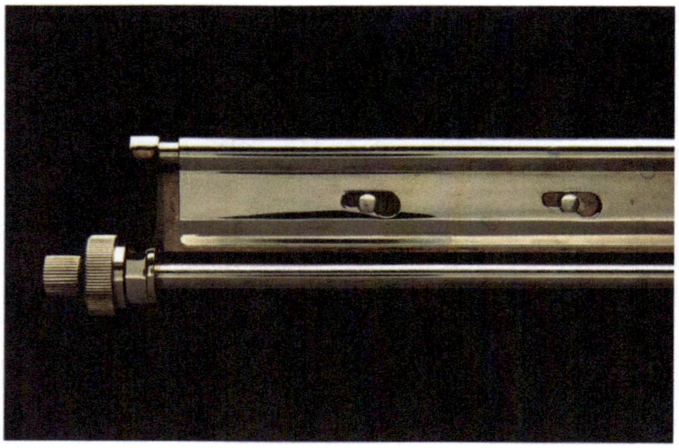

Figure 18.22 A knob located on one end of the knife locks the position of the roller.

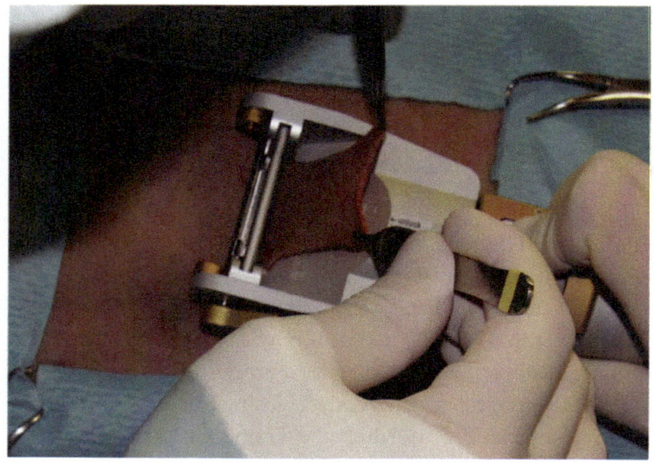

Figure 18.23 A graft is being harvested from the ventral aspect of the abdomen using a Humeca power dermatome, with the horse in lateral recumbency.

A free-hand knife is far less expensive than a power-driven dermatome, requires less maintenance, has fewer parts to malfunction, and can be easily transported. Skin can be harvested consistently from the ventral surface of the abdomen by using a free-hand knife, which is a difficult feat using some power-driven dermatomes. Wider grafts may be harvested with a free-hand knife than with most power-driven dermatomes.

Harvesting a split-thickness sheet graft

Harvesting a split-thickness graft leaves a large epithelial scar, and, therefore, cosmetic appearance should be considered when selecting a donor site. A split-thickness graft is usually harvested from a horse at the ventral surface of the abdomen or the ventrolateral surface of the thorax, caudal to the elbow.[1,28,29,67,69] The ventral surface of the abdomen is the least conspicuous site from which a split-thickness graft is easily harvested by using a free-hand knife, but harvesting skin with a power-driven dermatome, other than the Humeca dermatome, usually requires a firmer surface, such as the ventrolateral surface of the thorax.

To harvest skin from these sites, the horse is usually positioned in lateral recumbency (Figure 18.23), and the donor site is prepared for aseptic surgery. The mobile skin at the ventrolateral surface of the thorax can be stabilized by assistants who stretch it by hand or by using towel clamps (Figure 18.24). The donor site and the blade of the power dermatome or the free-hand knife are lubricated with isotonic saline solution or mineral oil to reduce friction. Mineral oil does not seem to adversely affect acceptance of the graft or its healing,[7,18] but it should not be used when harvesting a sheet for the Meek micrografting technique because the oil adversely affects adhesion of the micrografts to the plissé. Harvesting a split-thickness graft is quite painful to the horse, so the depth of anesthesia should be checked before beginning.

When harvesting with a power dermatome, the dermatome should be kept flat against the skin because tilting produces gouges at the donor site and an uneven graft.[18] Slight tension is applied, by an assistant, to the cut end of the graft during harvesting (Figure 18.23). When the graft is long enough, it is transected

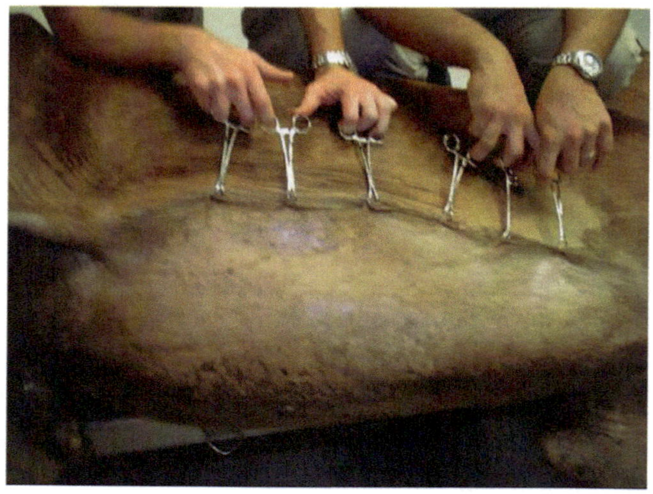

Figure 18.24 Stabilizing the skin with towel clamps is not usually necessary but may be somewhat helpful when harvesting skin from the ventral aspect of the abdomen.

by tilting the dermatome outward. When using a free-hand knife, the ventral portion of the abdomen must protrude over the edge of the table so that the surface of the table does not impair manipulation of the knife. Harvesting usually begins at the umbilicus and proceeds cranially. Depressing the abdomen inward with the non-dominant hand while harvesting with the dominant hand flattens the abdomen slightly, enabling a wider graft to be harvested. The knife is applied to the abdomen with moderate pressure at an angle of about 5°–10°, and the dermis is cut using a sawing motion, while concentrating on moving the blade up and down, rather than forward (Figure 18.25). This sawing motion causes the margin of the graft to assume an inconsequential saw-toothed appearance. An assistant should apply slight, uniform tension to the cut end of the graft during harvesting (Figure 18.25). The graft is transected by tilting the knife outward.

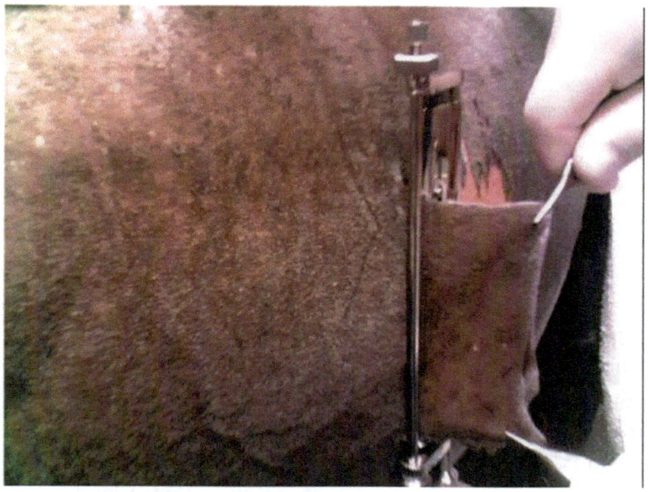

Figure 18.25 To harvest skin from the ventral aspect of the abdomen, the free-hand knife is pressed against the abdomen at an acute angle of about 5°–10° using moderate pressure, and the dermis is cut using a sawing motion. An assistant should apply tension to the cut end of the graft.

During harvesting, the surgeon should examine the graft and donor site to determine whether the graft is being harvested at the proper thickness. Thickness is judged by examining the graft for translucency and the donor site for the pattern of bleeding.[17,18] A shallow cut through the dermis severs many small vessels and creates a semi-transparent graft, whereas a deep cut severs fewer but larger vessels and creates a more opaque graft. When a power dermatome is used, the depth of the cut can be varied slightly by changing the pressure on the dermatome. If the depth must be changed substantially, the setting should be adjusted. When the free-hand knife is used, the depth of cut can be changed by repositioning the adjustable roller, changing the pressure applied to the knife, or changing the knife's angle of incidence. Harvesting a thin, split-thickness skin graft is much more difficult than harvesting a thick one. If the graft is to be meshed and expanded, it should be considerably longer than the recipient site because expansion shortens the graft.

Judging the depth at which a graft should be harvested is difficult because the dermis varies in thickness between horses and between donor sites.[13] Split-thickness grafts measuring between 0.63 mm and 0.76 mm in thickness, harvested from the ventral surface of the abdomen or thorax, have good durability and moderate to good hair coverage,[13,20] whereas split-thickness grafts of 0.5 mm or less, harvested from these same areas, lack durability and have sparse or no hair coverage.[20] Grafts with good hair coverage may, however, leave the donor site devoid of hair.

In cases of exceptionally large wounds, such as a burn wound that cover much of the back, a "two-layer" technique of harvesting split-thickness grafts may be useful. Using this technique, a thin split-thickness graft is harvested, after which a second split-thickness graft, composed only of dermis, is harvested from the same site. The recipient site is covered partly with the graft composed of both epidermis and a portion of the dermis and partly with the second graft composed solely of a portion of the dermis. This second graft contains no epidermis, but epithelialization proceeding from adnexa within the transplanted skin eventually resurfaces the dermis.[70] Another option for covering such large wounds is to use the Meek micrografting technique using plissés with an expansion ratio of 1:9 (see Modified Meek technique earlier in this chapter).

Tips

- Harvesting a split-thickness skin graft from the ventral surface of the abdomen, the most inconspicuous donor site on a horse, using a motorized dermatome other than the Humeca dermatome, can be difficult; a split-thickness graft can be easily harvested from the ventral surface of the abdomen with a free-hand knife.
- The most economical dermatome for harvesting a split-thickness sheet graft is a free-hand knife that uses disposable blades and has an adjustable roller to control the depth of the harvest. This dermatome is far less expensive than a motorized dermatome, and little experience is required to become proficient in its use.

Meshing sheet grafts

A split- or full-thickness sheet graft can be applied to a wound as a solid or meshed (i.e., fenestrated) sheet. The principal reason for meshing a sheet graft is expansion, so that the graft can uniformly cover a wound larger than itself.[1,13,15,17,25,67,71,72] Meshing a sheet graft also prevents collection of blood, serum, or exudate between the graft and the wound, thus improving the likelihood of graft adherence. Additionally, a meshed sheet graft conforms better to an irregular surface than a solid sheet graft, and, because it can expand, it has a greater tolerance to motion. Fibrin fills the fenestrations, increasing the graft's stability on the wound.[41] Meshing also enables a topically applied antimicrobial agent to contact a large portion of the wound.

A graft can be meshed manually with a scalpel blade or mechanically with a meshgraft dermatome. An example of a relatively inexpensive, commonly used meshgraft dermatome is the Padgett mechanical skin mesher (Mesh Skin Graft Expander, No. Z-PD-170, Padgett Instruments), which consists of staggered parallel rows of blades that fenestrate the graft, allowing it to be expanded to three times its original area. It accommodates grafts up to 110 mm wide but only up to 135 mm long, although a longer graft can be meshed in sections. The Zimmer mechanical skin mesher (Zimmer Meshgraft Dermatome, Zimmer) is more sophisticated and expensive but can create different patterns of fenestrations, depending on the carrier used, that allow the graft to be expanded to 1.5, three, six, or nine times its original area (Figure 18.26). The graft is placed dermal side down on a grooved plastic carrier, selected according to the amount of expansion desired, and the graft and carrier are advanced through the mesher by turning a hand crank. Grafts wider than 76 mm do not fit into a Zimmer mesher, but the length of

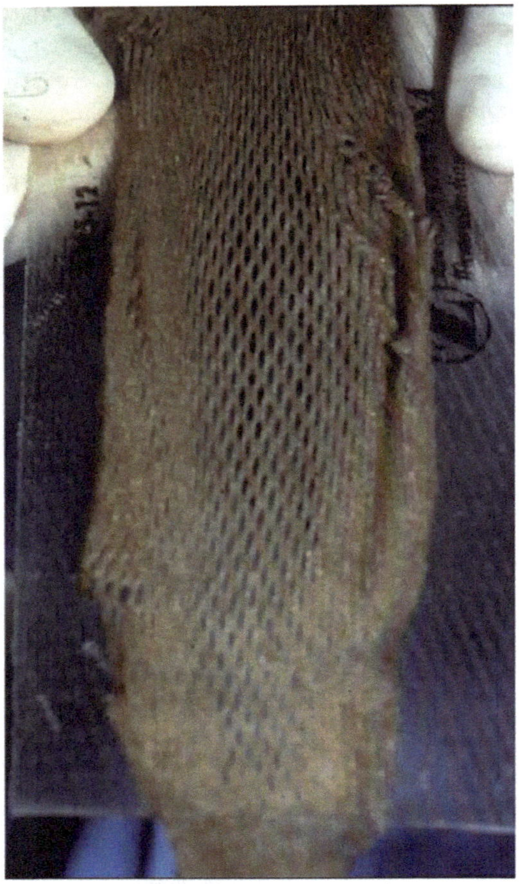

Figure 18.26 This split-thickness graft was meshed with a Zimmer meshgraft dermatome using a carrier that provided a 1:1.5 expansion ratio.

the graft to be fenestrated is unlimited because the graft can be placed on multiple carriers.

Full-thickness sheet grafts of horses, except those of foals, are difficult to mesh on commercial mechanical skin meshers and so must usually be meshed manually. To manually mesh a sheet graft, the graft is fixed to a cutting board, such as a sterile piece of cardboard or Styrofoam, and staggered, parallel rows of incisions are created in the graft. The more numerous and the longer the incisions, the greater is the expansion. Meshing a graft manually is tedious, especially if the graft is large or if it must be greatly expanded.

After a meshed graft is expanded, portions of the wound are exposed within the fenestrations. Greater expansion means more exposure of the wound and slower healing because the exposed portions must heal by contraction and epithelialization, whereas the portions covered by the meshed graft heal primarily. The exposed portions of the wound rapidly epithelialize, however, because meshing the graft provides an extensive border from which epithelial cells can migrate and proliferate.[1,28] The healed wound is eventually covered with a uniform pattern of diamond-shaped epithelial scars, which are more apparent if the graft was greatly expanded. These scars diminish in size as the grafted wound contracts.[1,14,28,42] When the wound is located on a limb, the size of epithelial scars can be minimized by applying the graft to the wound so that the fenestrations are parallel to the long axis of the limb.[28]

Tips

- Sheets grafts applied to wounds of horses are usually meshed so that the graft can uniformly cover a wound larger than itself. Meshing a sheet graft also prevents blood, serum, or exudate from collecting between the graft and the wound and allows a topically applied antimicrobial drug to contact the underlying wound.
- Meshing a full-thickness graft by using a commercial mechanical skin mesher is difficult; most full-thickness grafts must be meshed by hand.

Applying sheet grafts

The graft should be applied so that the direction of hair growth conforms to that of the surrounding skin. A graft harvested from the anesthetized horse can be sutured or stapled to the wound's margin while the horse is anesthetized. If the horse is standing, however, the margin of the wound must be desensitized, using local or regional anesthesia, prior to stapling or suturing the graft. To avoid the necessity of desensitizing the margin of the wound, the graft can be overlapped and glued to the wound's margin using cyanoacrylate glue (Super Glue, Loctite Co.). This is only possible, however, when ample skin has been harvested to permit overlap of the graft on to the skin surrounding the wound (Figure 18.27). The overlapped and glued portion of the graft eventually desiccates, sloughs, and separates without harming the rest of the graft as the underlying

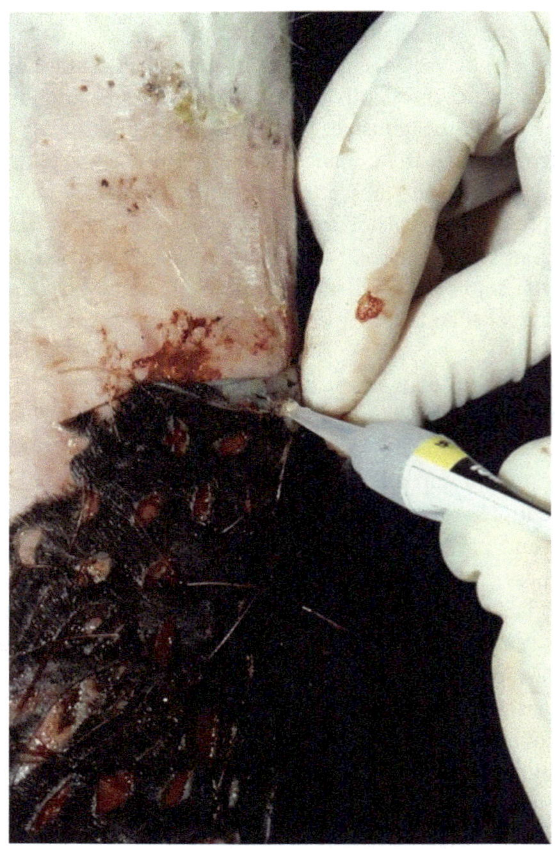

Figure 18.27 This graft is being attached in a standing horse by overlapping and gluing the margin of the graft to the margin of the wound.

epidermis desquamates. Applying the graft after the horse recovers from general anesthesia shortens the time of anesthesia and eliminates the possibility of damage to the graft that might occur during recovery.

A graft applied to a small wound in a non-mobile region need only be fixed to the wound's margin because fibrin firmly fixes the graft to the wound's surface within minutes of application.[14,21] A graft applied to a large wound or a wound in a region that is difficult to immobilize, such as the dorsum of a fetlock or hock, may be further secured to the wound with simple interrupted sutures placed through the fenestrations of the graft. The sutures are tightened sufficiently to secure the graft to the wound but not so tightly that they cut through granulation tissue. This can be done with the horse standing without anesthetizing underlying granulation tissue, because granulation tissue is not innervated. A fresh wound, however, must first be desensitized prior to suturing a graft to its base. Sutures can be removed after 1 week, when graft acceptance is certain.

A study comparing the outcome of autogenous split-thickness skin grafts attached to wounds of human patients with autogenous platelet-rich plasma (PRP) to the outcome of those attached with sutures, staples, or glue found that those patients whose grafts were attached by PRP required fewer changes of dressing, the grafts were less edematous, and discharge from the grafted wound was reduced.[73] Attaching grafts with PRP was thought to decrease graft edema by stimulating more rapid revascularization of the graft. Instantaneous adhesion of the graft to the wound prevented formation of a hematoma beneath the graft.

What to do

- A graft can be applied with the horse standing, without desensitizing the wound's margin, by fixing the edge of the graft to the margin of the wound with cyanoacrylate glue.
- Movement of the graft can be minimized by suturing it to the underlying wound via the placement of sutures through the fenestrations in the graft. This can be done with the horse standing if the graft is sutured to granulation tissue.

Acceptance and appearance of split-thickness sheet grafts

The thickness of the dermis of a split-thickness graft greatly influences the graft acceptance and the wound's healed appearance.[7,20,25,32,42,68,74] A graft that contains a large portion of dermis is more durable and imparts a better cosmetic appearance than one that contains a small portion of dermis. Conversely, a graft that contains a small portion of dermis is more likely to be accepted than one containing a large portion of dermis because a thin graft has reduced metabolic demands and more exposed cut vessels since blood vessels branch as they ascend the dermis. Because more vessels are exposed, plasmatic imbibition is better, and revascularization is faster. The acceptance of meshed sheet grafts has been reported to be 50–100%.[1]

The effect of hyperbaric oxygen therapy (HBOT) on grafts has been evaluated in various studies. HBOT improved survival of split-thickness grafts applied to wounds of people and of pedicle grafts and free grafts applied to wounds of rats.[75–77] HBOT, however, appeared detrimental to survival of grafts applied to experimentally created wounds of pigs,[78] and another study showed that daily, 1-hour administration of HBOT for 1 week decreased viability of full-thickness skin grafts applied to either fresh or granulating wounds of horses.[79] Although HBOT reduced graft edema, it negatively affected neovascularization, probably because it reduced the oxygen gradient between the wound and the graft. Tissue hypoxia is an important stimulus for neovascularization, which is essential for graft acceptance.

Advantages and disadvantages of split-thickness sheet grafts

The split-thickness sheet graft is more versatile than the full-thickness graft because it is more readily accepted and because it can be harvested in sheets large enough to cover wounds too large to be covered by a full-thickness graft.[7,42,68] The appearance and durability of a wound healed with a split-thickness skin graft, however, are poorer than those of a wound healed with a full-thickness skin graft. Its appearance and durability are comparable to those of a wound healed with Meek micrografts and better than those of a wound healed with other types of island grafts. Unlike failure of one or more island grafts, which are independent of one another, failure of a portion of a sheet graft, either split- or full-thickness, may result in loss of the entire graft. Harvesting a split-thickness graft is far less convenient and more expensive than harvesting a full-thickness graft or island grafts, because the horse must be anesthetized.

Tips

- Split-thickness grafts are accepted more readily than full-thickness grafts, and thin split-thickness grafts are accepted more readily than thick split-thickness grafts.
- Thin split-thickness skin grafts are more difficult to harvest, and a wound grafted with a thin split-thickness graft is less cosmetic than if the wound had been grafted with a thick split-thickness graft.
- The appearance of a wound grafted with a split-thickness sheet graft or Meek micrografts is superior to that of a wound grafted with punch, pinch, or tunnel grafts but inferior to the appearance of a wound grafted with a full-thickness skin graft.

Aftercare

Aftercare of the recipient site

The grafted wound is bandaged to protect the graft from the environment, to limit motion, to absorb exudate or transudate, and to exert pressure on the graft, thus preventing fluid from accumulating beneath it. The preferred primary layer is a sterile antimicrobial foam that absorbs exudate, along with bacteria and destructive enzymes, and limits bacterial growth (AMD foam, Covidien Animal Health/Kendall or Acticoat Moisture Control, Smith and Nephew). The dressing is secured to the wound with strips of adhesive tape, conforming rolled gauze, or, if the wound is located in a highly mobile region, with sutures or staples.[41]

The secondary layer of the bandage should be bulky to limit motion of the limb. If the grafted wound is located in a highly mobile region, a cast may be applied to completely immobilize the distal portion of the limb and thus eliminate shear forces acting between the bandage and the graft. If casting the limb is impractical, a splint or Robert Jones bandage may suffice. Grafted wounds over the dorsal surface of the hock can be immobilized effectively by applying a bandage–cast, a sleeve cast, or a splint (see Chapter 7).[59] A grafted wound in a less mobile region, such as the dorsal surface of the metacarpus or metatarsus, is usually immobilized sufficiently with a simple bandage. The bandage should not be changed for 7–9 days after grafting to avoid disturbing the fragile vascular and fibrinous attachments of the graft to the wound. By 5 days after grafting, fibrous and vascular attachments between the graft and the wound are secure enough that loss of graft from infection or motion becomes unlikely. A cast can be left in place for about 10 days. Great care should be taken during initial bandage changes to avoid disturbing the delicate fibrinous and vascular connections between the wound and the graft. Removing the primary dressing may be difficult if it is adhered to the wound. Tight adherence of the dressing to the wound indicates that the graft is also tightly adhered and that graft acceptance is proceeding unhindered by infection or motion. Saturating the primary dressing with isotonic saline solution may ease removal of the dressing, but if this proves difficult, the dressing should be left in place until the next scheduled bandage change. The dressing is most easily removed by grasping one end and pulling it parallel to the wound, while using the fingers of the other hand to prevent elevation of the graft. Pulling the dressing perpendicular to the wound tends to place excessive traction on the graft.

The bandage should be changed sooner and more frequently after grafting when infection with virulent bacteria, such as *Streptococcus* and *Pseudomonas* spp., is a common problem in the hospital, even though changing the bandage risks contamination of the wound and disruption of the graft's attachment. Changing the bandage allows removal of bacteria and destructive enzymes and allows application of an appropriate antimicrobial dressing or drug to the wound. Streptococci or pseudomonads can rapidly destroy a graft, so prompt recognition of infection, coupled with topical treatment, is necessary. Exudate from a grafted wound that appears infected should be cultured for bacterial growth, and antimicrobial susceptibility of isolates should be determined. While awaiting results, a broad-spectrum antimicrobial agent should be applied topically to the wound. This can be either an antimicrobial dressing based on silver (Acticoat Moisture Control, Smith and Nephew) or polyhexamethylene biguanide HCl (PHMB), (AMD foam, Covidien Animal Health/Kendall), or drugs such as ticarcillin with potassium clavulanate (Timentin, GlaxoSmithKline), effective against both β-hemolytic *Streptococcus* and *Pseudomonas* spp.[51] If the affected limb has been immobilized in a cast, and if the wound is at high

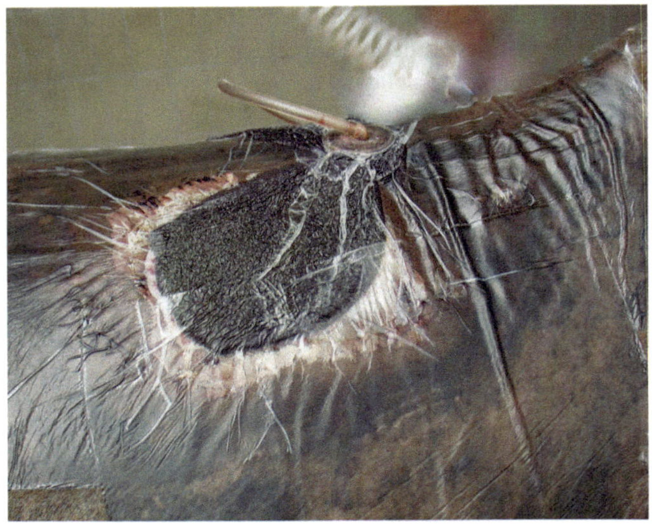

Figure 18.28 This Meek micrograft on the back of a horse was stabilized with negative pressure wound therapy. Courtesy of the Department of Equine Sciences, Utrecht University, the Netherlands.

risk of developing a streptococcal or pseudomonas infection, an antimicrobial foam dressing should be applied to the wound before casting, or a broad-spectrum antimicrobial drug should be applied to the wound at regular intervals through an infusion tube placed on the surface of the grafted wound and exited through the top of the cast.

Negative-pressure wound therapy, using open cell foam dressing to cover the wound, has been shown to increase the acceptance of free grafts applied to wounds of dogs,[80] cats,[81] and humans.[82,83] Using this therapy, the graft is firmly stabilized on the wound, shearing forces and accumulation of fluid are avoided, and edema in tissue surrounding the wound is reduced. Microstrain, the mechanical stretching of cells under negative pressure, causes cells to rapidly divide and proliferate,[84] and results in production of growth factors conducive to healing.[85] Although the use of negative pressure wound therapy in conjunction with free skin grafting of wounds of horses has not been reported, one of the authors (JW) has used this technique to good effect (Figure 18.28).

EGT sometimes proliferates through the fenestrations of an expanded meshed graft or in between island grafts, obscuring the grafts and retarding migration of epithelium. A corticosteroid applied to the grafted wound causes the EGT to regress, allowing epithelialization and contraction to proceed unhindered. Although a corticosteroid may reduce the rate of epithelialization, EGT exerts even more detrimental effects on this process.[13,86–89]

Ideally, a grafted wound should be protected by a bandage until it is completely epithelialized because bandaging produces conditions, such as warmth and moisture, conducive to epithelialization. If bandaging becomes impractical prior to complete epithelial coverage, however, small, non-epithelialized areas within the grafted wound can be allowed to heal beneath a scab, which soon develops when the wound is left exposed.

A grafted wound in a region difficult to bandage, such as the trunk, may be protected with a tie-over or stent bandage (see Chapter 7).[2,13,58] Movement of the wounded region does not create shear forces between the wound and the tie-over bandage because the latter is attached to the wound. Sometimes, such wounds are left unbandaged, a technique referred to as "open grafting," to eliminate shear forces that occur between a bandage and the graft.[14,25] Precautions must be taken, such as applying a neck cradle or tying the horse, to prevent the horse from disturbing the exposed graft.

Because some horses suffer from hyperesthesia at the grafted wound, tying a horse or applying a neck cradle may be prudent when bandaging is discontinued, to prevent the horse from damaging its grafted wound. Applying an ointment such as lanolin, cod-liver oil ointment, or petroleum jelly to the healed donor and recipient sites of a split-thickness graft may reduce scaling, which results from dysfunction of eccrine glands at these sites, and prevent the occurrence of small splits in the epithelium.[7]

What to do

- A cast or a bandage and splint may be applied to a limb to completely immobilize a grafted wound in a highly mobile region.

What to avoid

- Grafts are usually well accepted by 5 days after grafting. Changing the bandage before this time risks disrupting the fragile vascular attachments of the graft to the wound.

Tips

- Grafted wounds in areas difficult to bandage may be left unbandaged or covered with a tie-over bandage.
- The acceptance of a graft depends not only on the technique used but also relies strongly on the preparation and aftercare of the wound.

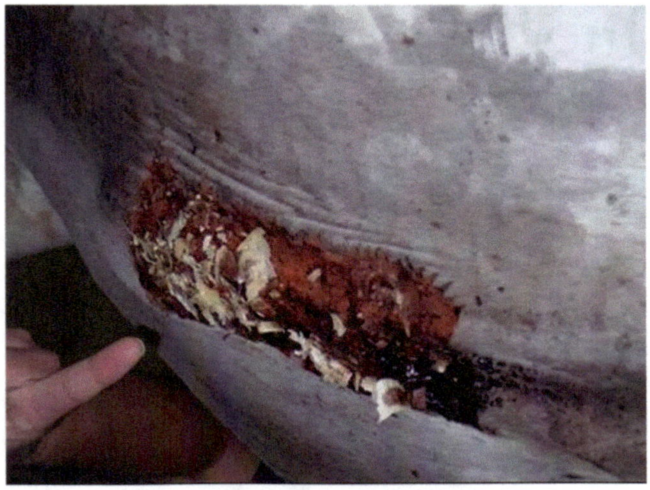

Figure 18.29 A scab at the donor site of a split-thickness graft is contaminated with bedding material. Removing the scab interferes with epithelialization and causes pain.

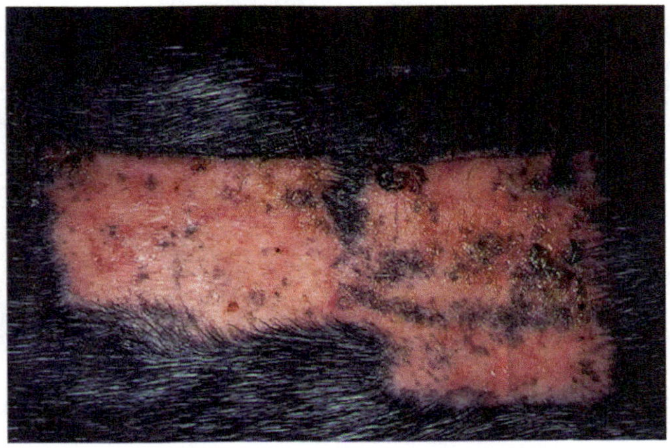

Figure 18.30 Harvesting a split-thickness graft leaves an unsightly scar at the donor site.

Aftercare of the donor site

The donor site of a split-thickness graft is similar to a deep abrasion and contains many exposed nerve fibers. To relieve pain, an analgesic drug, such as a NSAID, should be administered before the graft is harvested and for several days after surgery.

A scab of blood and fibrin, often containing bedding material, rapidly forms over the donor site of a split-thickness graft. Beneath this scab, proliferating epithelial cells from the margin of the wound and the remaining adnexa migrate to cover the surface of the site. A horse whose donor site is at the ventrolateral surface of the thorax may show signs of discomfort, such as a stilted gait, until the wound is covered with a scab. The scab that develops at the donor site of a split-thickness graft should not be removed, despite its contaminated appearance (Figure 18.29), because this interferes with epithelialization and is painful to the horse. A dressing applied to the donor site immediately after harvesting prevents the wound from desiccating and provides some relief from discomfort.

The donor site is covered by pink epithelium, usually within 1–3 weeks, but the time required for complete epithelialization depends on the depth at which the graft was harvested. Epithelium covers the donor site more quickly when a thin skin graft is harvested because skin adnexa, from which epithelium grows, are left in place.[15,20] Pigment soon appears in the new, pink epithelium, blackening the epithelial scar. The donor site heals with prominent epithelial scarring when a split-thickness graft thicker than 0.63 mm is harvested (Figure 18.30).[15,20]

One of the authors (JW) excises the remaining dermis from the donor site of a split-thickness graft, because this removes exposed nerve fibers, providing immediate pain relief (Figure 18.31a). The resulting full-thickness wound is closed after undermining the adjacent skin (Figure 18.31b). Relief incisions, or occasionally an H-plasty, may sometimes be required to close a wide wound. The sutured wound usually heals by

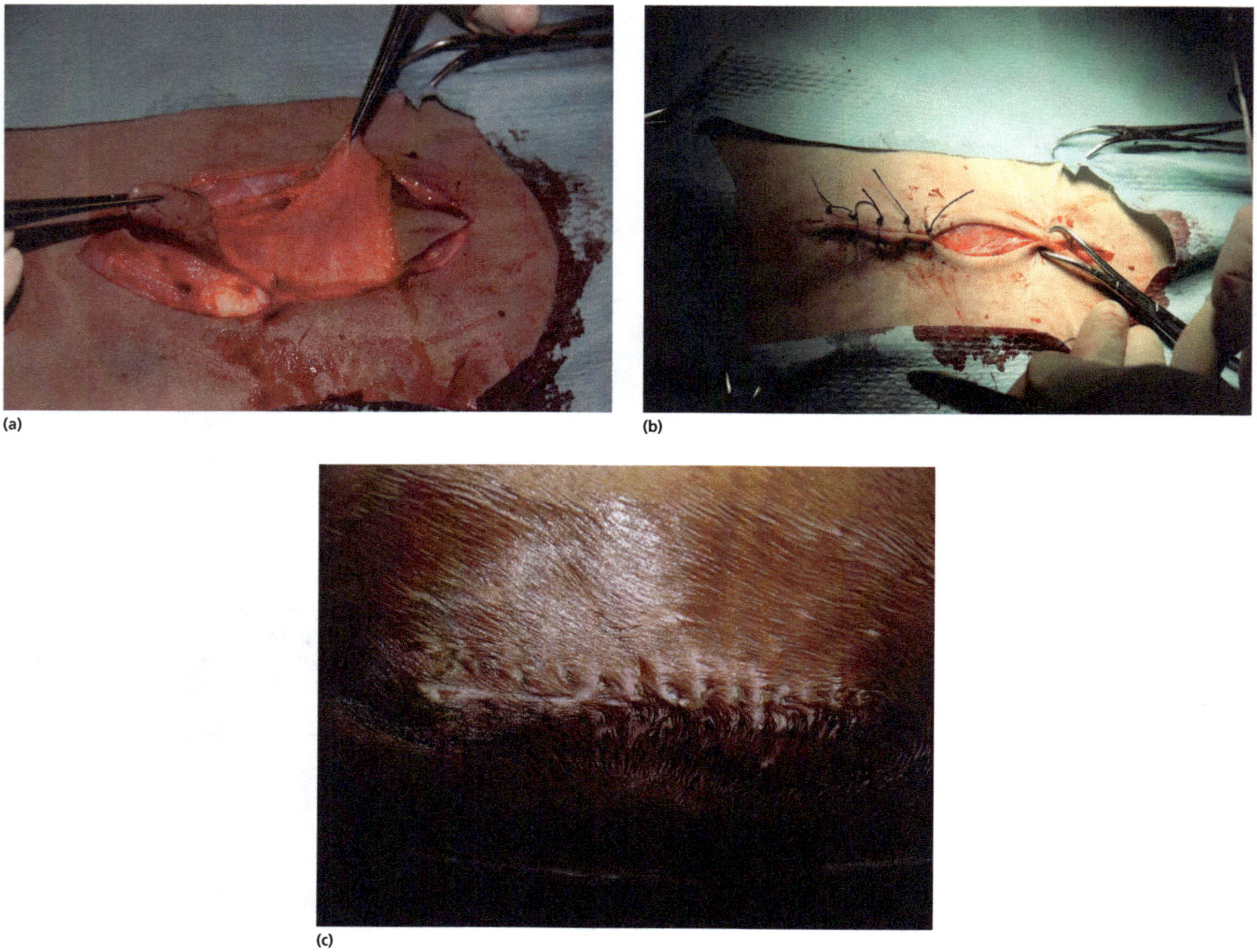

Figure 18.31 **(a)** Excising the remaining part of the dermis creates a full-thickness wound at the donor site of a split-thickness skin graft. The wound created at the donor site with a 42-mm wide Humeca dermatome can usually be closed primarily. **(b)** The donor site is sutured after undermining the wound margins. **(c)** Appearance of the healed donor site after excising the abrasion and suturing the full-thickness wound, just after the sutures have been removed.

primary intention (Figure 18.31c), but even if the wound dehisces or is left unsutured, it heals mainly by contraction because most donor sites are located on the body. The resulting scar is, therefore, always less obvious than that which would develop if the partial-thickness wound was not excised. Excising the deep abrasion at the donor site to create a full-thickness wound is, therefore, an effective method to relieve pain and reduce scarring after harvesting a split-thickness graft.

What to avoid

- The donor site of a split-thickness graft is very painful, so the scab that develops at the site should not be disturbed, even if it contains shavings or straw.

Tip

- Excising the dermis remaining at the donor site of a split-thickness graft relieves pain and allows the donor site to be closed primarily, preventing scarring.

Storing split-thickness sheet grafts

Storing sheet grafts is useful for several reasons. If more skin than is necessary to cover a wound is harvested, the surplus can be stored to cover defects created by a slough in the primary graft. A skin graft obtained at the same time a wound is created, such as when a cutaneous neoplasm is excised, can be stored for delayed grafting of that wound. Grafting can also be delayed to decrease the likelihood of a hematoma or seroma forming beneath the graft. A graft can be harvested for storage when a horse is anesthetized for treatment of a wound, such as removal of an osseous sequestrum or lavage of an open joint, and applied when the condition of the wound has improved enough to permit grafting.

A stored graft is more readily accepted than a fresh one because a stored graft undergoes anaerobic metabolism, which causes release of metabolites that encourage rapid vascularization of the graft.[90] A graft that has been stored for 24 hours or more is referred to as a "prepared graft," and by placing it on a "prepared wound" (see Preparation of the wound earlier in the chapter), the phase of plasmatic imbibition is decreased to less than 8 hours.[90] An unused stored graft may serve as a biologic dressing for a wound on another horse (see Use of allografts and xenografts later in the chapter).

Autografts and allografts can be stored successfully for several days in a refrigerator, wrapped in gauze swabs that have been soaked in isotonic saline solution or lactated Ringer's solution.[7,17,25] Skin can be stored in a refrigerator for even longer when placed in a tissue culture medium, such as McCoy's 5A medium, to which a small volume of serum has been added.[91–94] McCoy's 5A medium is a balanced electrolyte solution containing amino acids, vitamins, dextrose, and a pH indicator (phenol red). The concentration of serum in the storage medium should be between 10% and 33%.[95] A concentration of serum greater than 33% decreases the storage life of the graft by stimulating metabolic activity. Antigenic reaction of the graft to the serum is prevented by using pooled, homologous serum, the horse's own serum, or a commercially available, antibody-free equine serum (e.g., Gibco Laboratories, Inc).[92] To prepare a skin graft for storage, it is placed epidermis side down on a sterile gauze dressing. The gauze–graft composite is rolled up, with the gauze facing out (Figure 18.32), and placed in a sterile container with approximately 1–2.5 mL of the McCoy's 5A medium for each square centimeter of stored graft.[92,95] The stored graft should have access to air and, therefore, should not be placed in an airtight container.[91] The nutrient medium should be examined every few days for a color shift produced by a change in pH. A change in color from cherry-red to orange-yellow indicates that metabolites have accumulated to a dangerous concentration, necessitating immediate use of the graft or replacement of the medium. Only half of the storage medium should be replaced because complete replacement may be detrimental to the graft.[92] Skin from humans has been stored successfully in a nutrient medium at refrigeration temperature for 6–8 weeks,[91,92] and in raw honey, at 4 °C or room temperature, for up to 12 weeks.[96] Equine autografts stored for 3 weeks at 4 °C, in a solution composed of McCoy's 5A medium and horse serum, have been used to graft wounds, with consistently good results.[94] Allografts stored in this manner for up to 12 weeks have been successfully applied to wounds of horses by one of the authors (JS). This author also observed that an equine skin graft stored in honey appeared histologically healthier at 3 weeks than did a graft obtained from the same horse at the same time but stored in McCoy's 5A medium and serum (unpublished observation).

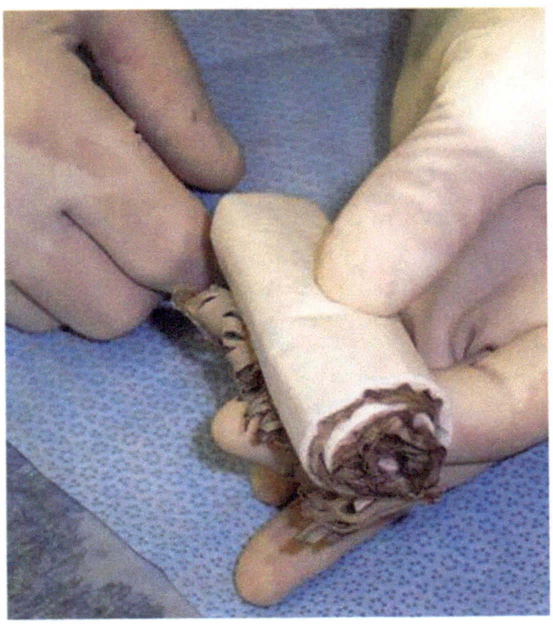

Figure 18.32 To prepare a skin graft for storage, the graft is placed on a sterile dressing with the epidermis against the dressing, and the dressing–graft composite is rolled up.

Tips

- Storing a graft for 24 hours or more decreases the time required for the graft to become vascularized once placed on a wound.
- Grafts may be stored in a refrigerator in isotonic saline solution or lactated Ringer's solution for several days without losing their viability or ability to be accepted.
- Grafts may be stored in a refrigerator, in honey, for up to 3 weeks without losing viability.
- Grafts may be stored in McCoy's 5A medium, to which the horse's serum has been added to make a 10% solution of serum, for over 3 weeks without losing viability or ability to be accepted.

Use of allografts and xenografts

Cutaneous allografts obtained from cadavers and xenografts obtained from pigs have been used extensively since the middle of the last century to temporarily dress large wounds on humans.[97,98] The use of xenografts arose because of the short supply of cadaveric allografts, but xenografts adhere poorly, allow higher bacterial counts in the wound, and cause a more intense immunologic rejection than do allografts.[8] Allografts and xenografts have been used infrequently in horses. Allografts, when used to dress small, experimentally created limb wounds of horses, showed no apparent advantages over non-biologic dressings in promoting healing.[11] Viable, cutaneous allografts can be harvested from refrigerated cadavers within 24 hours of death.[91] They seem to survive for at least 2 weeks after being applied to a wound on a horse, but duration of survival is often difficult to determine because even when the superficial layers of the graft seem desiccated, the deeper layers may still remain viable and firmly attached to the wound by fibrous and vascular connections.[11]

Cutaneous allografts or xenografts may be used to temporarily dress a wound when autografting is economically or physically impractical. A cutaneous allograft or xenograft applied to a wound on a human or horse stimulates angiogenesis and allows epithelialization to proceed rapidly beneath it, unimpeded by complications such as infection and the formation of EGT.[9–11,91,97,99]

An allograft or xenograft vascularizes before it is rejected, which further enhances its ability to defend the wound against infection.[8] Even a graft that is rejected before it can vascularize may protect the wound from bacterial infection, possibly by trapping bacteria in the fibrin that attaches the graft to the underlying wound.[9,10,15,24,43,100] Clinical trials have shown that cultured allogeneic and xenogeneic (from rats) epithelial cells applied to full-thickness wounds of rabbits have the potential to reconstitute epithelial defects,[101] and cultured keratinocytes have been shown to synthesize cytokines, such as epidermal growth factor and transforming growth factor alpha, conducive to healing.[102]

Tip

- Allografts may speed healing of slow-healing wounds.

Conclusion

Skin grafting should not be regarded as an option of last resort. It should be considered particularly useful for limb wounds that cannot be closed primarily because these wounds heal slowly and mainly by epithelialization, leading to a large epithelial scar. Although skin grafting may seem like an expensive method of therapy, it is often more economical to treat a horse with a large wound by grafting than by a lengthy period of bandaging. After grafting, the horse can be returned more quickly to function, the likelihood of persistent swelling of the wounded limb is diminished, and the scar is stronger, more functional, and more cosmetic. Grafting instruments, such as power dermatomes, meshgraft dermatomes, and Meek micrografting equipment are relatively expensive, but frequent use of these instruments warrants their purchase in a referral practice setting. Moreover, only a moderate amount of expertise is required to use these instruments. Full-thickness grafting and most types of island grafting require only common, basic surgical equipment and are thus accessible to most practitioners.

Small limb wounds can be easily grafted with pinch, punch, or tunnel grafts to speed healing when the cosmetic result is of no great concern. The use of full-thickness grafts can be considered for small wounds when the cosmetic result is important. Large limb wounds can be best grafted with split-thickness, meshed sheet grafts or Meek micrografts. Meek micrografts are well accepted, reduce healing time, and provide a better cosmetic appearance to the healed wound than do other types of island grafts. Full-thickness grafts are less suitable for large limb wounds because they are at greater risk of being rejected and because large, full-thickness grafts are less available. Grafting a wound on the trunk is necessary only when the wound is so large that wound contraction alone is insufficient for healing, resulting in a large area that must heal by epithelialization, or when the wound is in an area, such as the back, where the durability of healed tissue is important. Grafting these large wounds with pinch or punch grafts is often too tedious; therefore, applying a split-thickness meshed sheet graft or Meek micrograft may be a better option. Fixation is usually a problem for wounds on the trunk, and thus micrografts may be more suitable because they are less vulnerable to movement.

A split-thickness graft cannot easily be harvested from a standing horse. When a horse cannot be anesthetized, pinch, punch, tunnel, or full-thickness grafts are the only options. The selection of the type of graft also depends on the availability of equipment and the expertise of the surgeon.

References

1. Booth LC. Split-thickness autogenous skin transplantation in the horse. *J Am Vet Med Assoc* 1982; **180**: 754.
2. Wilson DG. Applications of skin grafting in large animals. *Probl Vet Med* 1990; **2**: 442.
3. Pavletic MM. Canine axial pattern flaps, using the omocervical, thoracodorsal, and deep circumflex iliac direct cutaneous arteries. *Am J Vet Res* 1981; **42**: 391.
4. Ma X, Li Y, Wang L, *et al.* Reconstruction of cervical scar contracture using axial thoracic flap based on the thoracic branch of the supraclavicular artery. *Ann Plast Surg* 2014; **73 Suppl** 1: S53.
5. Lees MJ, Bowen CV, Fretz PB, *et al.* Transfer of deep circumflex iliac flaps to the tarsus by microvascular anastomosis in the horse. *Vet Surg* 1989; **18**: 292.
6. Lees MJ, Fretz P, Bowen CV, *et al.* Experimental cutaneous free flap transfers in the horse. *Microsurgery* 1991; **12**: 130.
7. Bell R. *The Use of Skin Grafts*. Oxford University Press: New York, 1973.
8. May S. The effects of biological wound dressings on the healing process. *Clin Materials* 1991; **8**: 243.
9. Diehl M, Ersek RA. Porcine xenografts for treatment of skin defects in horses. *J Am Vet Med Assoc* 1980; **177**: 625.
10. Diehl M, Jeanmonod CA, Muller M, *et al.* Porcine skin as temporary covering of extensive skin defects in the horse. *Schweizer Archiv fur Tierheilkunde* 1979; **121**: 23.
11. Gomez JH, Schumacher J, Swaim S, *et al.* Effects of three biological dressings on healing of cutaneous wounds on the limbs of horses. *Can J Vet Res* 2004; **68**: 49.
12. Boyd CL. Equine skin autotransplants for wound healing. *J Am Vet Med Assoc* 1967; **151**: 1618.
13. Meagher DM, Adams OR. Split-thickness autologous skin transplantation in horses. *J Am Vet Med Assoc* 1971; **159**: 55.
14. Peacock E. *Wound Repair*, 3rd edn. WB Saunders: Philadelphia, 1984.
15. Argenta LC, Dingman RO. Skin grafting. In: Epstein E (ed). *Skin Surgery*. WB Saunders: Philadelphia, 1987: 129.
16. Flowers RS. Unexpected postoperative problems in skin grafting. *Surg Clin North Am* 1970; **50**: 439.
17. Rothstein AS. Skin grafting techniques. *J Am Podiatry Assoc* 1983; **73**: 79.
18. Rudolph R, Fisher JC, Ninnemann JL. *Skin Grafting*. Little, Brown and Co: Boston, 1979.
19. Gringrass PJ, Grabb WC, Gringrass RP. Skin graft survival on avascular defects. *Plast Reconstr Surg* 1975; **55**: 65.
20. Frankland AL. Autologous, split skin transplantation on the lower limbs of horses. *Vet Rec* 1979; **104**: 590.

21. Hogle RB, Kingrey W, Jensen EC. Skin grafting in the horse. *J Am Vet Med Assoc* 1959; **135**: 165.
22. Mir Y, Mir L. Biology of the skin graft. *Plast Reconstr Surg* 1951; **8**: 378.
23. Tavis MJ, Thornton JW, Harney JH, *et al*. Mechanism of skin graft adherence: collagen, elastin, and fibrin interactions. *Surg Forum* 1977; **28**: 522.
24. Teh B. Why do skin grafts fail? *Plast Reconstr Surg* 1979; **63**: 323.
25. Vistnes LM. Grafting of skin. *Surg Clin North Am* 1977; **57**: 939.
26. Converse JM, Smahel J, Ballantyne DL Jr, *et al*. Inosculation of vessels of skin graft and host bed: a fortuitous encounter. *Br J Plast Surg* 1975; **28**: 274.
27. O'Ceallaigh S, Herrick SE, Bluff JE, *et al*. Quantification of total and perfused blood vessels in murine skin autografts using a fluorescent double-labeling technique. *Plast Reconstr Surg* 2006; **117**: 140.
28. Hanselka DV. Use of autogenous meshgrafts in equine wound management. *J Am Vet Med Assoc* 1974; **164**: 35.
29. Wilmink JM, Van Den Boom R, Van Weeren PR, *et al*. The modified Meek technique as a novel method for skin grafting in horses: evaluation of acceptance, wound contraction and closure in chronic wounds. *Equine Vet J* 2006; **38**: 324.
30. Fitzgerald MJ, Martin F, Paletta FX. Innervation of skin grafts. *Surg Gynecol Obstet* 1967; **124**: 808.
31. Kernwein G. Recovery of sensation in split-thickness skin grafts. *Arch Surg* 1948; **56**: 459.
32. Rudolph R. Inhibition of myofibroblasts by skin grafts. *Plast Reconstr Surg* 1979; **63**: 473.
33. Hanson RR. Management of avulsion wounds with exposed bone. *Clin Tech Eq Pract* 2004; **3**: 188.
34. Ford TS, Schumacher J, Brumbaugh GW, *et al*. Effects of split-thickness and full-thickness skin grafts on secondary graft contraction in horses. *Am J Vet Res* 1992; **53**: 1572.
35. Wilmink JM, van Weeren PR. Treatment of exuberant granulation tissue. *Clin Tech Eq Pract* 2004; **3**: 141.
36. Grinnell F. Fibroblast biology in three-dimensional collagen matrices. *Trends Cell Biol* 2003; **13**: 264.
37. Bristol DG. Skin grafts and skin flaps in the horse. *Vet Clin North Am Equine Pract* 2005; **21**: 125.
38. French DA, Fretz PB. Treatment of equine leg wounds using skin grafts: thirty-five cases, 1975–1988. *Can Vet J* 1990; **31**: 761.
39. Krizek TJ, Robeson MC, Kho E. Bacterial growth and skin graft survival. *Surg Forum* 1967; **18**: 518.
40. Robson M, Krizek TJ. Predicting skin graft survival. *J Trauma* 1973; **13**: 213.
41. Booth L. Equine wound reconstruction using free skin grafting. *Calif Vet* 1991; **45**: 13.
42. Cason J. Skin grafting and diagnosis of depth of burn. In: Cason J (ed). *Treatment of Burns*. Chapman and Hall: London, 1981: 135.
43. Eade GG. The relationship between granulation tissue, bacteria, and skin grafts in burned patients. *Plast Reconstr Surg* 1958; **22**: 42.
44. Currie LJ, Sharpe JR, Martin R. The use of fibrin glue in skin grafts and tissue-engineered skin replacements: a review. *Plast Reconstr Surg* 2001; **108**: 1713.
45. Wilmink JM, Stolk PWT, van Weeren PR, *et al*. Differences in second-intention wound healing between horses and ponies: macroscopic aspects. *Equine Vet J* 1999; **31**: 53.
46. Wilmink JM, van Weeren PR, Stolk PWT, *et al*. Differences in second-intention wound healing between horses and ponies: histological aspects. *Equine Vet J* 1999; **31**: 61.
47. Schumacher J, Ford TS, Brumbaugh GW, *et al*. Viability of split-thickness skin grafts attached with fibrin glue. *Can J Vet Res* 1996; **60**: 158.
48. Smahel J. Free skin transplantation on a prepared bed. *Br J Plast Surg* 1971; **24**: 129.
49. Boon RJ, Beale AS. Response of *Streptococcus pyogenes* to therapy with amoxicillin or amoxicillin-clavulanic acid in a mouse model of mixed infection caused by *Staphylococcus aureus* and *Streptococcus pyogenes*. *Antimicrob Agents Chemother* 1987; **31**: 1204.
50. James J. Skin grafting in difficult situations. *Trop Doct* 1999; **29**: 41.
51. Moore R. Antimicrobial therapy in horses. In: Colahan P, Merritt AM, Moore JN, Mayhew IG (eds). *Equine Medicine and Surgery*, 5th edn. Mosby: St. Louis, 1999: 163.
52. Robson MC, Edstom LE, Krizek TJ. The efficacy of systemic antibiotics in the treatment of granulating wounds. *J Surg Res* 1974; **16**: 299.
53. Edlich RF, Schmolka IR, Prusak MP, *et al*. The molecular basis for toxicity of surfactants in surgical wounds. *J Surg Res* 1973; **14**: 277.
54. Davis JS. The use of small deep skin grafts. *J Am Med Assoc* 1914; **63**: 985.
55. Mackay-Smith MP, Marks D. A skin grafting technique for horses. *J Am Vet Med Assoc* 1968; **152**: 1633.
56. Oien RF, Hansen BU, Hakansson A. Pinch graft skin transplantation for leg ulcers in primary care. *J Wound Care* 2000; **9**: 217.
57. Boyd CL, Hanselka DV. A skin punch technique for equine skin grafting. *J Am Vet Med Assoc* 1971; **158**: 82.
58. Lindsay WA. Step-by-step instructions for equine skin grafting techniques. *Vet Med* 1988; **83**: 598.
59. Stashak TS. *Equine Wound Management*. Philadelphia: Lea and Febiger, 1991.
60. Stashak TS. Skin grafting in horses. *Vet Clin North Am Large Anim Pract* 1984; **6**: 215.
61. Davis JS, Trout HF. Origin and development of the blood supply of whole thickness skin grafts: an experimental study. *Ann Surg* 1925; **82**: 871.
62. Ross GE, Jr. Clinical canine skin grafting. *J Am Vet Med Assoc* 1968; **153**: 1759.
63. Bjorck GTK, Twisselman K. Tunnel skin grafting in the equine species. *Proc Am Assoc Equine Pract* 1971; **17**: 313.
64. Lees MJ, Andrews GC, Bailey JV, *et al*. Tunnel grafting of equine wounds. *Comp Cont Educ Pract Vet* 1989; **11**: 962.
65. Kreis RW, Mackie DP, Vloemans AWFP, *et al*. Expansion technique for skin grafts: comparison between mesh and Meek island (Sandwich) grafts. *Burns* 1994; **20**: S39.
66. Zermani RGC, Zarabini A, Trivisonno A. Micrografting in the treatment of severely burned patients. *Burns* 1997; **23**: 604.
67. Hanselka DV, Boyd CL. Use of mesh grafts in dogs and horses. *J Am Anim Hosp Assoc* 1976; **12**: 650.
68. Valencia IC, Falabella AF, Eaglstein WH. Skin grafting. *Dermatol Clin* 2000; **18**: 521.
69. Hanselka DV, Milne FJ. Inexpensive mesh grafting technique in the horse. *Proc Am Assoc Equine Pract* 1976; **21**: 191.
70. Kogan L, Govrin-Yehudain J. Vertical (two-layer) skin grafting: new reserves for autologic skin. *Ann Plast Surg* 2003; **50**: 514.
71. MacMillan BG. The use of mesh grafting in treating burns. *Surg Clin North Am* 1970; **50**: 1347.
72. Tobin GR. The compromised bed technique. An improved method for skin grafting problem wounds. *Surg Clin North Am* 1984; **64**: 653.

73. Waiker VP, Shivalingappa S. Comparison between conventional mechanical fixation and use of autologous platelet rich plasma (PRP) in wound beds prior to resurfacing with split thickness skin graft. *World J Plast Surg* 2015; **4**: 50.
74. Frankland AL, Morris PGD, Spreull JSA. Free, autologous, skin transplantation in the horse. *Vet Rec* 1976; **98**: 105.
75. Bowersox JC, Strauss MB, Hart GB. Clinical experience with hyperbaric oxygen therapy in the salvage of ischemic skin flaps and grafts. *J Hyperbaric Med* 1986; **1**: 141.
76. McFarland RM, Wermuth RE. The use of hyperbaric oxygen to prevent necrosis in experimental pedicle flaps and composite skin grafts. *Plast Reconstr Surg* 1966; **37**: 422.
77. Perrins DJD. Influence of hyperbaric oxygen on the survival of split skin grafts. *Lancet* 1967; **1**: 868.
78. Kalns JE, Dick EJ, Jr, Scruggs JP, *et al.* Hyperbaric oxygen treatment prevents up-regulation of angiogenesis following partial-thickness skin grafts in the pig. *Wound Repair Regen* 2003; **11**: 139.
79. Holder TE, Schumacher J, Donnell RL, *et al.* Effects of hyperbaric oxygen on full-thickness meshed sheet skin grafts applied to fresh and granulating wounds in horses. *Am J Vet Res* 2008; **69**: 144.
80. Stanley BJ, Pitt KA, Weder CD, *et al.* Effect of negative pressure wound therapy on healing of free full-thickness skin grafts in dogs. *Vet Surg* 2013; **42**: 518.
81. Nolff MC, Myer-Lindenberg A. Negative pressure wound therapy augmented full-thickness free skin grafting in the cat: outcome in 10 grafts transferred to six cats. *J Feline Med Surg* 2015; **17**: 1041.
82. Blume PA, Key JJ, Thakor P, *et al.* Retrospective evaluation of clinical outcomes in subjects with split-thickness skin graft: comparing V.A.C.® therapy and conventional therapy in foot and ankle reconstructive surgeries. *Int Wound J* 2010; **7**: 480.
83. Petkar KS, Dhanraj P, Kingsly PM, *et al.* A prospective randomized controlled trial comparing negative pressure dressing and conventional dressing methods on split-thickness skin grafts in burned patients. *Burns* 2011; **37**: 925.
84. Saxena V, Hwang CW, Huang S, *et al.* Vacuum-assisted closure: microdeformations of wounds and cell proliferation. *Plast Reconstr Surg* 2004; **114**: 1096.
85. McNulty AK, Schmidt M, Feeley T, *et al.* Effects of negative pressure wound therapy on cellular energetics in fibroblasts grown in a provisional wound (fibrin) matrix. *Wound Repair Regen* 2009; **17**: 192.
86. Kaufman, KL, Mann FA, Kim D, *et al.* Evaluation of the effects of topical zinc gluconate in wound healing. *Vet Surg* 2014; **43**: 972.
87. Baker BL, Whitaker WL. Interference with wound healing by the local action of adrenocorticoid steroids. *Endocrinol* 1950; **46**: 544.
88. Ehrlich HP, Hunt TK. The effects of cortisone and anabolic steroids on the tensile strength of healing wounds. *Ann Surg* 1969; **170**: 203.
89. Howes EL, Plotz CM, Blunt JW, *et al.* Retardation of wound healing by cortisone. *Surg* 1950; **28**: 177.
90. Smahel J. Preparation-phenomenon in a free skin graft. *Br J Plast Surg* 1971; **24**: 133.
91. Brown JB, Fryer MP, Zaydon TJ. A skin bank for postmortem homografts. *Surg Gynecol Obstet* 1955; **101**: 401.
92. Gresham RB, Perry VP, Thompson VK. Practical methods of short-term storage of homografts. *Arch Surg* 1963; **87**: 417.
93. Hurst LN, Brown DH, Murray KA. Prolonged life and improved quality for stored skin grafts. *Plast Reconstr Surg* 1984; **73**: 105.
94. Schumacher J, Chambers M, Hanselka DV, *et al.* Preservation of skin by refrigeration for autogenous grafting in the horse. *Vet Surg* 1987; **16**: 358.
95. Allgower M, Blocker TGJ. Viability of skin in relation to various methods of storage. *Texas Rep Bio Med J* 1952; **10**: 3.
96. Gupta M. Preservation of split-skin grafts in honey: a preliminary report. *Indian J Surg* 1977; **39**: 591.
97. Ambler J. Porcine xenografts to facilitate integumental wound healing. *Vet Rec* 1980; **106**: 437.
98. Marden DT. Use of pigskin to repair leg wounds in the horse. *Vet Med Small Anim Clin* 1974; **69**: 771.
99. O'Donoghue MN, Zarem HA. Stimulation of neovascularization—comparative efficacy of fresh and preserved skin grafts. *Plast Reconstr Surg* 1971; **48**: 474.
100. Burleson MD, Eiseman B. Mechanism of antibacterial effect of biological dressings. *Ann Surg* 1973; **177**: 181.
101. Hanifi N, Halim AS, Aleas CF, *et al.* Epidermal regeneration of cultured autograft, allograft, and xenograft keratinocytes transplanted on full-thickness wounds in rabbits. *Exp Clin Transplant* 2015; **13**: 273.
102. Beele H, Naeyaert JM, Goeteyn M, *et al.* Repeated cultured epidermal allografts in the treatment of chronic leg ulcers of various origins. *Dermatologica* 1991; **181**: 31.

CHAPTER 19

Management of Severely Infected Wounds

James A. Orsini, DVM, Diplomate ACVS, Yvonne A. Elce, DVM, Diplomate ACVS, and Beth Kraus, DVM, Diplomate ACVS

Chapter Contents

Summary

When managing serious wound infections in horses, it is important to consider the wound's entire ecology, including the source and extent of contamination, the presence of bacterial refugia (foreign bodies, surgical implants, devitalized tissue, inflammatory/necrotic debris, bacterial biofilms), the patient's immunocompetence, and tissue perfusion. In addition, the wound's pathogens and their antibiotic sensitivities must be identified. Culture-guided selection of antibiotic therapy and the use of local or regional modes of antibiotic delivery may be critical for success. By itself, antibiotic therapy may be insufficient to resolve bacterial infection in the presence of factors that contribute to the persistence or progression of infection and that otherwise delay wound healing.

Introduction

Wound infections usually are obvious clinically because they comprise the following readily identifiable elements:

1. signs of inflammation (swelling, heat, erythema, signs of pain during palpation, lameness or other dysfunction) that are excessive for the type, site, size, or age of the wound. In some cases, a systemic inflammatory response is also present (e.g., fever, malaise, inappetence, neutrophilia, hyperglobulinemia, elevated plasma fibrinogen or other acute-phase proteins);
2. purulent discharge, although its appearance may be delayed because of abscess formation or because the wound was closed primarily.

Any full-thickness disruption of the skin permits the entry of surface bacteria into the tissue(s) deep to the skin, which

Equine Wound Management, Third Edition. Edited by Christine Theoret and Jim Schumacher.

Companion website: www.wiley.com/go/theoret/wound

elicits an inflammatory response, but relatively few wounds become severely infected. Serious infections complicate wound management, so they are the focus of this chapter.

A wound infection should be considered severe or at least serious when it has evidently evaded or overwhelmed the body's defenses or when infection could have career-ending or life-threatening consequences. Examples include the following:

- infection that has persisted or progressed despite routine, empiric antibiotic therapy and wound care;
- infection that involves bone, a synovial structure (i.e., joint, tendon sheath, bursa), or a body cavity;
- infection that involves a surgical implant;
- infection that occurred subsequent to extensive trauma;
- infection accompanied by a systemic inflammatory response;
- presence of a mucoid film, which may represent a bacterial biofilm;
- presence of Gram-negative bacteria on cytologic examination or bacterial culture of wound exudate;
- multiple antibiotic resistance (to three or more drug classes) on *in vitro* antibiotic sensitivity testing.

Severely infected wounds are a particular challenge in this era of multiple antibiotic resistance in common bacterial pathogens. Examples include, but are by no means limited to, methicillin-resistant *Staphylococcus aureus* (MRSA)[1–5] and *Staphylococcus epidermidis* (MRSE),[6–9] vancomycin-resistant *Enterococcus* species (VRE),[10–14] heteroresistant vancomycin-intermediate *S. aureus* (hVISA),[15–18] penicillin-resistant *Actinobacillus* species,[19,20] aminoglycoside-resistant *Escherichia coli*,[21–24] and strains of *Pseudomonas aeruginosa* that are resistant to several commonly used antibiotics.[25,26] These multidrug-resistant strains are still relatively uncommon in equine practice, but their increase in prevalence and diversity – particularly in hospitalized patients (i.e., nosocomial infections) but also on-farm (i.e., community-acquired infections) – continues unabated[2–5,7–13,19–31] and spurs us to seek approaches to treatment that extend beyond a reliance on antibiotics.

Targeted antibiotic therapy directed by the results of bacterial culture and antibiotic sensitivity testing remains a cornerstone of effective management for severely infected wounds. Because of the character of these wounds, however, other factors beyond *in vitro* antibiotic sensitivity become crucial to a successful outcome. In this chapter, we briefly review several factors that may be involved in the development or persistence of severe wound infection and then discuss targeted approaches to treatment for each.

Origins of severe wound infections

A healthy body has the immunologic resources to deal with most instances of bacterial invasion, so in most wounds bacterial infection remains localized and is dealt with quickly and effectively by the patient, with or without the aid of veterinary treatment. Therefore, for a patient with a severe wound infection, effective treatment begins with a question: Why has this infection persisted and progressed?

Most severe wound infections are the result of at least one, and usually a combination, of the following factors:

Extensive contamination

Extensive contamination results in an overwhelming number of bacteria in the wound. Examples include the following.

- Fecal contamination – most likely to occur with wounds (including surgical wounds) involving the distal aspect of the limb and those that penetrate the abdomen or perineum, causing damage to intestine.
- Penetrating wounds to the oral cavity, pharynx, esophagus, or upper portion of the airway. Although these sites have a good blood supply, they also have an extensive population of resident microflora readily disseminated by mucous secretions.
- Environmental contamination – dirt, plant debris, or insect activity (e.g., flies) may introduce large numbers of bacteria into an open wound.

Although the site of the wound and the source of contamination are factors to consider when empirically choosing an antibiotic (discussed later), extensive contamination is less about the specific source and types of bacteria and more about the sheer numbers of bacteria invading the tissue and overwhelming the host's defenses.

Refugia

In this context, a refugium is any substance or circumstance that protects bacteria within the wound from the host's defenses and from effective concentrations of antibiotic drugs, thus enabling the infection to persist and perhaps to progress. Refugia commonly associated with persistent wound infections in horses include the following:

- foreign bodies – most often pieces of metal, wood, or other plant material (thorns, awns, etc.);
- surgical implants – metal plates, screws, pins, wire, surgical mesh, prostheses, embedded suture, etc;
- devitalized tissue – bone, muscle, tendon, ligament, fascia, or skin;
- inflammatory/necrotic debris – pockets or pools of free purulent material or an abscess;
- mucoid biofilms produced by the bacteria themselves.

Bacterial biofilms

The presence of bacterial biofilms in wounds is not a new phenomenon, but the importance of biofilms in the persistence and resistance of wound infections in animals has only lately come to light.[32,33] Bacterial biofilms are gel-like substances composed of an extracellular matrix of polysaccharides, proteins, glycolipids, bacterial DNA, water, the bacteria that secreted the matrix, and often other microbes that are taking advantage of the protected environment.[32–35]

Although a well-established biofilm may be discernible as a thin, slimy coating or sheen on an abiotic surface (e.g., orthopedic device or catheter),[35] the macroscopic identification of biofilms on biotic surfaces, particularly chronic wounds, is speculative and often based on a color induced by the overpopulating dominant sessile or planktonic aggregates of microbes. For example, *P. aeruginosa* produces a greenish pigment.[35] However, discoloration of the wound surface or dressing is not a reliable indicator of the presence of a specific pathogen nor of a biofilm. In fact, biofilms in wounds can only be recognized by microscopic techniques with appropriate staining methods.[35a]

The following dynamics are described for experimentally created bacterial biofilms that are similar to those found in wounds.[35] As discussed later, this timeline is a useful guide for the management of biofilm-infected wounds:

- Within minutes, free-living (planktonic) bacteria reversibly attach to an available surface (tissue, surgical implant, foreign body, etc.).
- Within 2–4 hours, biofilm-forming bacteria irreversibly attach to the surface (become sessile).
- Within 6–12 hours, an initial biofilm (slimy, extracellular polymeric substance around the bacterial microcolonies) has formed; it becomes increasingly well organized and tolerant of antiseptics and antibiotics.
- Within 2–4 days, the biofilm is mature; it is now highly resistant to adverse host and environmental influences, including biocides (chemical substances or biologic agents used to control potential pathogens), and it sheds bacteria singly and as microcolonies within fragments of biofilm that can colonize other areas.
- Within 24 hours of mechanical disruption, the mature biofilm reforms.

The biofilm provides a secure attachment for the bacteria and a moist, stable environment that protects against desiccation, deluge, and other adverse physical conditions.[34,35] It also protects the bacteria from the host's defenses and from potentially lethal concentrations of antibiotic drugs.[35,36]

Depending on the antibiotic, diffusion through the matrix may be impeded and/or the drug may be inactivated by chemical constituents of the matrix. In the presence of a mature biofilm, the minimum inhibitory concentration (MIC) of an antibiotic or disinfectant to which the wound pathogens are susceptible *in vitro* may be increased by as little as 2-fold and as much as 1000-fold.[32–39] Furthermore, bacteria within a biofilm alter their metabolism and gene expression in ways that promote their survival. These alterations include the formation of subpopulations that are metabolically inactive (quiescent) and thus relatively invulnerable to antibiotics at any concentration.[35,36,40] These quiescent or dormant bacteria within the biofilm are a source of persistent or recurrent infection.[32,33]

Even more problematic is the sharing of antibiotic resistance among bacteria within the biofilm. In a polymicrobial biofilm, antibiotic-binding or antibiotic-degrading substances secreted by bacteria that are resistant to a particular drug may also protect bacteria within the biofilm that are susceptible to that drug. In addition, antibiotic-resistance genes can sometimes be transferred from one bacterial species to another within the protected environment of the biofilm.[35,36]

Polymicrobial biofilms are documented to occur in various types of equine wounds (traumatic and surgical, acute and chronic).[41,42] Under experimental conditions, many different bacteria isolated from wounds or the normal skin of horses are capable of producing biofilms;[40,42] however, the conditions under which clinically relevant biofilms form in equine wounds require further study. In humans, problematic biofilms are most common in poorly perfused wounds, in malnourished patients, and in patients with co-morbidities that impair immune function, such as in those with diabetic ulcers or severe burns.[34–36]

This aspect of wound care is critical when dealing with a biofilm-infected wound. Even though many different wound pathogens are capable of producing a clinically relevant biofilm, most do not because tissue perfusion and bactericidal host defenses are adequate to prevent its establishment. So, when confronted with a biofilm-infected wound, the crucial question is not what, but why. When the factors that favor formation of a biofilm are identified, appropriate treatment can begin.

Immunocompromise

The patient's immunocompetence is of primary importance in preventing or resolving a wound infection. A number of conditions or circumstances may compromise the patient's ability to prevent or resolve bacterial infection, including the following:

- vulnerable age – especially neonatal foals (<2 weeks of age) and very old horses;
- antibody deficiency – failure of passive transfer of maternal antibodies (neonatal foals); congenital deficiencies of immunoglobulin production; loss of circulating antibodies through protein-losing enteropathy, nephropathy, or dermatopathy (e.g., extensive third-degree burns, large open wounds);
- malnutrition – of macronutrients (protein-calorie malnutrition) or micronutrients (e.g., deficiencies of a specific trace mineral, essential fatty acid, or amino acid);
- chronic physical or psychologic stress – intense athletic training, long-distance transport, competitive events, social isolation, sustained hypothermia (cold stress), hospitalization, etc;
- diseases affecting the pituitary–adrenal axis – notably, pituitary pars intermedia dysfunction (PPID), or equine Cushing's disease, which causes hypercortisolemia with or without hyperglycemia;*
- corticosteroid administration;
- sepsis (causes early hyperinflammation then severe immunosuppression); other concurrent systemic infection or debilitating systemic disease.

(*Hyperglycemia is a risk factor for wound infections and biofilm formation in human patients,[34] but there is little evidence that wound infections are more likely or more problematic in horses with hyperglycemia unrelated to PPID, possibly because hyperglycemia is an inconsistent feature of equine metabolic syndrome and because diabetes mellitus is relatively rare in horses.)

It is important to bear in mind that antibiotic therapy alone is inadequate in the face of an incompetent immune system. The administration of antibiotic drugs should be considered an adjunctive therapy, albeit a very important component of therapy for severely infected wounds.

Poor perfusion

An effective immune response to bacterial invasion relies not just on local tissue resources but also on the delivery of leukocytes and specific molecules (complement, antibodies, oxygen, nutrients, etc.) to the site of infection via the systemic circulation. Thus, any circumstance that limits optimal blood flow to, or at, the site of infection inevitably limits the host's immune response, as well as its ability to repair the wound, which renders the wound vulnerable to re-infection. Examples include the following:

- sustained hypovolemia or hypotension (e.g., endotoxemia, severe blood loss);
- thrombotic states (e.g., disseminated intravascular coagulation, vasculitis);
- extensive tissue trauma, particularly crushing, tearing, or strangulating injuries that result in local ischemia;
- fibrosis at or proximal to the site of infection;
- the presence of a foreign body, surgical implant, or devitalized tissue that impedes blood flow;
- pressure from an improperly applied bandage or cast, or from postural necessity (e.g., recumbency);
- severe local or regional edema (inflammatory or dependent).

Edema occurs so commonly with infected wounds that it is easily overlooked as an adverse factor in wound healing. Not only does severe edema cause the patient discomfort and negatively influence the client's perception of efficacy of treatment, it may impede perfusion of tissue in the wound by creating local interstitial pressures that exceed the perfusion pressure of the microvasculature.[43]

Antibiotic insensitivity

Antibiotic treatment may fail to resolve the infection for one or more of the following reasons:

- inherent antibiotic resistance – inappropriate choice of antibiotic drug for the pathogen(s) involved;
- acquired antibiotic resistance – such as methicillin resistance in *S. aureus*; unlike inherent resistance, acquired resistance is unpredictable;
- inappropriate antibiotic dosage, route, or duration of treatment – each may result in a subtherapeutic concentration of antibiotic drug at the site of infection, even when the pathogen is susceptible to the antibiotic *in vitro*;
- poor perfusion – it, too, may result in a subtherapeutic concentration of antibiotic at the site of infection, even when the choice and dosage of the antibiotic are appropriate;
- protection from inhibitory or lethal antibiotic concentrations by refugia, particularly purulent material, necrotic tissue, and bacterial biofilms.

This list illustrates the intersection and interdependence of pharmacology, physiology, pathology, and microbiology in clinical practice. Focusing primarily or exclusively on the pharmacologic aspect of treating complicated wounds, such as those discussed in this chapter, is likely to yield unsatisfactory results.

Empiric antibiotic therapy

Reliance on clinical experience alone to guide antibiotic therapy may result in the selection of antibiotic(s) to which the wound pathogens are not susceptible or for which therapeutic concentrations are not achieved at the site of infection. With wounds that are severely infected or at risk of becoming so, use of interim antibiotic therapy based on empiric choices can be crucial while awaiting results of culture and antibiotic sensitivity testing. An empiric choice, however, is little more than an educated guess. Because an incorrect choice of antibiotic drug may have disastrous consequences when treating a serious wound infection, empiric therapy must not take the place of specific therapy directed by bacterial culture and antibiotic sensitivity testing. This matter has become ever more important with the increasing prevalence and variety of multidrug-resistant strains of bacterial pathogens found in equine wounds.

Over-reliance on antibiotics

The usual response by clinicians to a severe, intractable wound infection is to change or add antibiotics, increase the antibiotic dosage(s), and/or add local or regional delivery to systemic administration of antibiotics – in other words, to continue to rely primarily on antibiotic therapy. Certainly, if culture and sensitivity results indicate that a change of drug is indicated or that a polymicrobial infection is present that necessitates the addition of a different class of antibiotic drug, then these measures must be implemented without delay. In addition, local and regional modes of antibiotic delivery have dramatically improved our ability to manage difficult infections in horses, such as septic arthritis and osteomyelitis.

In this era of multidrug resistance, however, when pharmacologic options may be unattractive or unavailable, the solution may be much more simple and direct, involving such measures as altering the physical environment within the wound to make it less hospitable to the bacteria. Here, our fundamental understanding of mammalian physiology and the basic biology of the invading bacteria may mean the difference between success and failure. The silver lining to this cloud, where we can no longer assume that every infection can be resolved simply with antibiotic therapy, is that we are forced back to basic principles of wound management, which we find still apply.

Targeted treatment approach

Identifying the factors involved in the persistence and progression of a wound infection allows us to formulate a targeted approach to treatment that optimizes the patient's defensive and reparative processes and the efficacy of the antibiotic drugs selected.

Extensive contamination

For wounds that remain contaminated with fecal matter or other material with a large bacterial load, the following dictum is useful: "The solution to pollution is dilution." Extravasation of serous fluid at the site of infection (as part of the inflammatory response) serves this purpose to some extent, but only if the fluid is allowed to drain from the wound. Furthermore, this natural process is limited in efficacy because it is restricted in volume. Hence, the following interventions are indicated.

Irrigation

Thoroughly irrigate the wound with sterile isotonic fluid until all visible contamination and purulent discharge have been removed.

What to do

- Use sterile 0.9% saline solution or a balanced electrolyte solution.
- Use copious quantities, as much as necessary, to thoroughly cleanse the wound.
- Use moderate delivery pressure (e.g., 30- or 60-ml syringe with an 18-gauge needle).
- Direct the fluid into every area of the wound.
- Repeat as necessary.

What to avoid

- Avoid using profoundly hypotonic fluid, such as tap water, other than to remove gross contamination.
- Avoid intense delivery pressures, as they may cause cellular damage, drive bacteria deeper into the tissues, and/or spray potentially infective material beyond the wound's margins (aerosolization).
- Avoid adding antiseptic agents to the irrigation fluid; they are unnecessary and unlikely to provide additional benefit to high-volume, pressurized irrigation.[44,45] Contact time is too brief, and some antiseptics (e.g., povidone–iodine) are inactivated by organic matter.

The goal of irrigation is simple: to substantially reduce bacterial numbers in the wound by physical expulsion of contaminated material, without causing more damage or deeper infection.

Debridement

Surgical debridement is another important component of managing wounds that contain heavily contaminated and compromised tissue.

What to do

- Debride all tissue that appears devitalized or irreparably damaged, such as necrotic skin, fascial tags, frayed tendon or ligament, soft and discolored bone, and bone fragments.
- Open the wound as much as necessary to allow thorough irrigation and debridement. Preserving healing/healed skin is of no value if the skin encloses infected tissue.
- Repeat irrigation to remove residual debrided tissue and cellular debris.
- Repeat debridement as necessary. This step is particularly important in a wound contaminated with a bacterial biofilm.

What to avoid

- Avoid removing more tissue than necessary. If in doubt, leave suspect tissue in place and re-evaluate the wound 24–48 hours later.

Tip

- Consider maggot debridement therapy as an alternative or adjunct therapy when complete surgical debridement would be difficult or impossible without damaging viable tissue. Maggot therapy may be particularly useful for debriding contaminated wounds with deep or multiple tracts, such as penetrating injuries to the foot or fistulous withers.[46,47] The reader is referred to Chapter 22 for more information on maggot debridement therapy.

Not only does debridement reduce bacterial numbers by removing heavily contaminated debris from the wound, it also enhances the effectiveness of irrigation by removing physical impediments to fluid flow. In addition, debridement aids subsequent drainage of inflammatory debris and infectious material from the wound.

Drainage

Discharge from severely infected wounds tends to be effusive and often purulent. This bacteria-laden, inflammatory exudate must have an egress for the immune system to control the infection and orchestrate wound repair. Thus, drainage is a key component of wound management, not just for extensively contaminated wounds but for every severely infected wound.

What to do

- Encourage gravity-assisted ("dependent") drainage from the most distal or ventral parts of the wound. Take advantage of the location, orientation, and shape of the wound where possible. If necessary, surgically create a drainage portal in the distal/ventral portion of the wound.
- When gas accumulates in the deeper tissue, the larger the egress, the better.
  - Wounds that act as one-way valves, such as deep wounds to the axilla or inguinal area, suck and trap air within the tissues, causing subcutaneous emphysema, which may become extensive.
  - Clostridial myonecrosis is often accompanied by extensive subcutaneous and intramuscular accumulation of gas, which may extend along fascial planes.
  - Both types of wounds are best left open, and enlarged if necessary, to prevent air from becoming trapped in the first instance and to facilitate treatment of the anaerobic infection in the second.
  - Intensive antibiotic therapy is also required when treating a horse for clostridial myonecrosis.

What to avoid

- Avoid opening the wound any more than is necessary to allow thorough irrigation, debridement, and continued drainage. In other words, limit exposing the interior of the wound to further contamination.

- For deep bone infections, thorough surgical debridement and irrigation are best performed with the horse anesthetized and followed by local implantation of an antibiotic-impregnated material (discussed later) and primary wound closure, leaving only a small gap for drainage.
  - Avoid prolonged use of Penrose drains and setons because they may suck or wick bacteria into the wound.

Tips

- Drainage may be further encouraged by controlled movement of the affected area and/or the horse. Specific techniques depend on the nature of the wound, the stage of healing, and the potential for harm with excessive or inappropriate movement.
- Massage and/or passive range-of-motion exercises may be appropriate for horses restricted to a stall. To avoid complications from passive or active movement, manual therapy is best directed by a physical therapist or veterinary rehabilitation therapist.
- Hand-grazing, hand-walking, or even limited turnout in a pen or small pasture may be appropriate for more ambulatory patients.
  - Avoid unattended turnout when wound dressings include bandages or leg wraps that may loosen and either leave the wound exposed or cause injury during unrestricted activity.

Movement may extend additional benefits by optimizing blood flow to, from, and within the wound; by limiting or preventing restrictive fibrosis; by preventing or resolving digestive and musculoskeletal problems associated with inactivity; by relieving the stress, social isolation, and boredom of confinement; and by improving the patient's physical and psychologic health and well-being. These aspects of nursing care are particularly important when the nature of the wound necessitates that the horse be confined to a stall for weeks or months.

Negative-pressure wound therapy

Drainage may also be achieved with negative-pressure wound therapy (NPWT), also known as vacuum-assisted closure. Subatmospheric pressure between −75 and −125 mmHg is applied to the wound using a small vacuum pump and an occlusive dressing (Figure 19.1). This technique speeds wound closure, evacuates inflammatory fluid and debris (including bacteria) from the wound, and improves microcirculation within the wound.[49,50] Originally developed for use in human medicine, NPWT is increasingly used in small-animal medicine for grossly contaminated or otherwise complicated wounds.[51–57] Improvements in the design of the dressing and in the size and portability of the pump make NPWT a good option for use in horses as well.[58] For more information on negative-pressure wound therapy, see Chapter 22.

Wound protection

The wound must be protected from additional contamination until the infection is under control. It may be protected by following these steps:

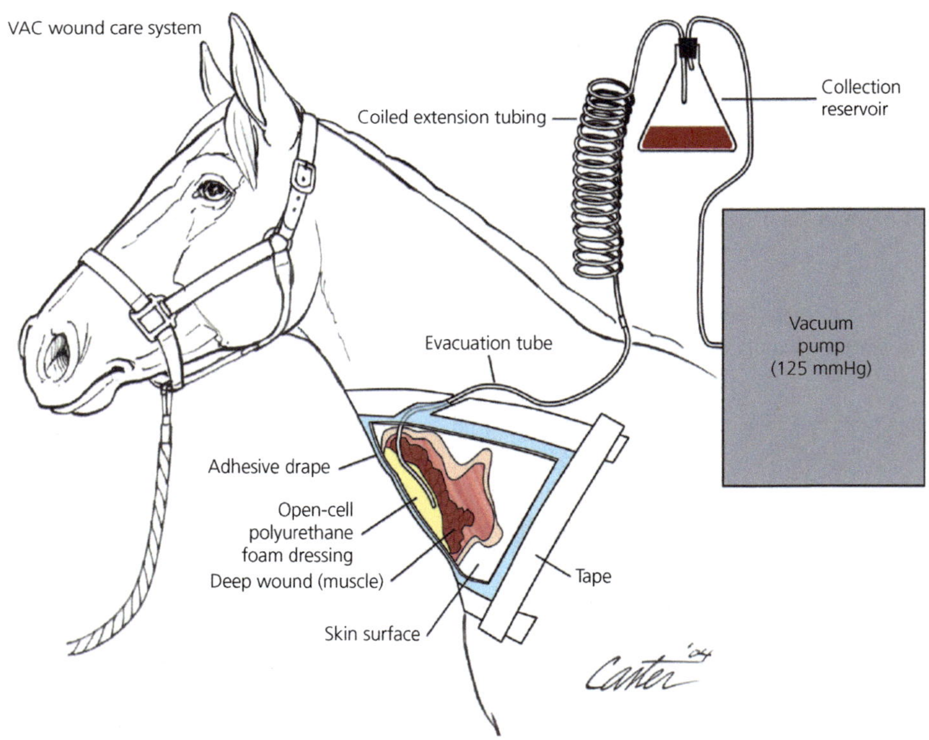

Figure 19.1 Vacuum-assisted closure. Source: Orsini 2004.[48] Reproduced with permission of Elsevier.

What to do

- Cover the wound with a sterile dressing and secure it as dictated by the location of the wound (bandage, adhesive tape, etc.)
- When maintaining a dressing is difficult or impossible, cover the wound with an antibiotic cream and apply fly repellant around the wound, as needed.
- Wounds with infections caused by obligate anaerobes, such as those that progress to clostridial myonecrosis, are best left uncovered.
- Maintain clean, dry bedding to prevent fecal contamination of the wound or dressings. Deeply bed the stall with clean wood shavings or straw, and keep the bedding free of manure and urine.
- Change the dressings and inspect the wound as often as necessary. The interval between dressing changes is dictated by the amount of drainage from the wound, the type of dressing, and how often the wound bed must be treated.

Daily treatment may initially be required for biofilm-infected wounds (discussed later). Daily dressing changes may also be needed for effusive wounds, such as those involving a synovial structure. A bandage that is wet all the way through to its outer surface may wick bacteria into the protected and nutrient-rich environment of the wound dressing. Similarly, a dressing moistened by water, urine, or fecal liquor no longer protects the wound and should be changed immediately.

On the one hand, frequently changing the dressing on an open wound can disrupt the granulation bed and the fragile neoepithelium, thereby impeding wound repair. On the other hand, persistent infection prevents effective wound repair. When treating any type of wound, a fine balance must be achieved between protecting the repair tissue and controlling infection, but when dealing with a severely infected wound, the latter is initially the most pressing concern.

What to avoid

- Avoid applying a caustic, desiccating, or other cytotoxic substance to the wound.
- Avoid uneven or excessive pressure on the wound from the bandage.
- Avoid zoonotic and reverse-zoonotic transmission of pathogens.
  - Communicate effectively with the nursing staff and encourage the practice of good hygiene.
  - Wear gloves or wash hands with soap and warm water *before and after* handling the wound or dressings.
  - Promptly dispose of all dressings and cleaning materials in the garbage or a biohazard container.

Not only do infected wounds in animals carry the potential for human infection (zoonosis), but humans can transmit pathogenic bacteria, such as *S. aureus*, *S. epidermidis*, and *E. coli* and other enterobacteria, to the animal patient (i.e., reverse zoonosis or "humanosis").[59]

Refugia

The presence of a bacterial refuge in an infected wound is not always obvious. When the convention is to focus on identifying the bacterial pathogens and determining their antibiotic susceptibility, the question of whether the chosen drug can reach the pathogen at a therapeutic concentration may not come up until the infection has failed to respond to antibiotic therapy. By this time, the infection and resulting inflammatory response may have caused considerable tissue damage, thereby creating a refuge in the form of devitalized tissue or a pool of purulent material, or the pathogens may have created their own refuge in the form of a biofilm.

The problem, and thus the solution, however, is not always so complicated. Sometimes identifying and removing a foreign body, problematic surgical implant, or sequestrum, or draining an abscess, are sufficient to tip the scales in favor of the host.

Foreign bodies

The presence of a non-surgically implanted foreign body within the wound can often be deduced from the cause of the wound (if known) and from the subsequent dynamics of the wound. For example, when a wound caused by collision with a wooden or metallic object fails to heal, despite standard wound care, and continues to drain purulent material from its depths, it likely houses a piece of wood or metal, or possibly a sequestrum of some kind, such as bone or devitalized connective tissue. Diagnostic imaging is indicated for such wounds.

What to do

- Use radiography when investigating wounds on a limb, head, neck, withers, or any other site amenable to radiograpic examination. *Note:* wood has a similar radiodensity to soft tissue, so unless it is outlined by air or another gas, a wooden foreign body is easily missed during routine radiographic examination. Contrast fistulographic examination may help to reveal the presence and location of the object in such cases.
- Alternatively or additionally, use ultrasonography to investigate a wound suspected of harboring a foreign body. Ultrasonography may be used to identify a foreign body in a wound on almost any part of the body, except when the foreign body is protected from view by bone or a gas-filled structure. The depth of penetration allowed by probes can limit the utility of ultrasound in deep wounds.
- Consider using computed tomography (CT) or magnetic resonance imaging (MRI), if available, when the results of radiographic and ultrasonographic examinations are negative yet a foreign body is strongly suspected.
- Digitally explore the wound, wearing sterile gloves (but see What to avoid), if the wound is at least finger-width and likely to be less than 8 cm deep. For smaller or deeper wounds, use a sterile hemostat to probe the wound.
- Surgically remove the foreign body, place it in a sterile container, and submit it for bacterial culture and antibiotic sensitivity testing of bacterial isolates. It is important to know if the foreign body harbors bacteria not identified by culturing the wounded tissue or the exudate.
- Thoroughly irrigate the wound, debride if necessary, ensure continued drainage, and protect the wound from additional contamination, as described earlier.
- Continue or initiate broad-spectrum antibiotic therapy while awaiting results of bacterial culture and antibiotic sensitivity testing (discussed later). Antibiotic therapy is not always indicated after removing a foreign body but is a wise precaution if the wound is severely infected.

- Check the horse's tetanus vaccination status and booster or administer tetanus antitoxin if needed. Tetanus prophylaxis is important with any wound, and particularly so for puncture wounds.
- Endoscopic exploration of an infected synovial structure may be necessary to identify and remove an intrasynovial foreign body.

What to avoid

- Avoid using MRI if the wound is likely to contain a metallic object.
- Avoid drawing surface bacteria deeper into the wound when digitally exploring the wound.
  - Before digitally exploring a wound, thoroughly clean the wound's margin and surrounding area using povidone–iodine or chlorhexidine surgical scrub, as for a sterile procedure.
  - Wear sterile gloves; rinse the gloves with sterile water/isotonic saline solution to remove surface talc before exploring the wound.

Surgical implants

Removal of a surgical implant may be indicated for some severely infected wounds. Surgical implants often loosen or otherwise fail at the site of infection. A loose implant no longer contributes to repair, and its repeated movement may cause tissue damage. In addition, surgical implants contribute to the infection if they harbor bacterial biofilms (discussed later). Even very smooth surfaces, such as metal bone plates and pins may become coated in a biofilm and thus become a site of persistent or recurrent infection. Biofilms can also form on embedded suture material.[60]

Furthermore, surgical inspection and, if indicated, removal of the implant provide the opportunity to directly examine and treat the site of infection. The wound can be irrigated, debrided, and drained during surgical inspection, the implant can be swabbed for culture and sensitivity testing, and, if needed, antibiotic-impregnated materials can be placed in the wound (discussed later). Submitting the implant or a sterile swab of its surface for bacterial culture and antibiotic sensitivity testing is essential. Confirming that the bacteria cultured from the implant are the same as those cultured from the wound's tissues or exudate is valuable; discovering that bacteria cultured from the implant are different is more valuable still, particularly if the wound is complicated by a biofilm.

Whether or not the implant should be replaced depends on the stage of healing, the quality of the remaining tissue after debridement, and whether an implant is still needed for structural support during healing. Structural defects of functional significance (e.g., complete fracture, large abdominal wall hernia) require some means of support, although external stabilization may be appropriate in some cases (e.g., external fixator and/or cast for a limb facture, belly band for an abdominal wall hernia). In making these decisions, access to the wound must be considered because the infection is not always resolved simply by removing the implant.

Subsequent wound care is similar to that described earlier for extensively contaminated wounds. Interim antibiotic therapy while awaiting results of culture and antibiotic sensitivity testing is discussed later. When an implant must remain in place or when debridement was necessarily incomplete, the various methods of local or regional antibiotic delivery, such as regional limb perfusion and insertion of antibiotic-impregnated implants, are particularly useful. These techniques are discussed later in the chapter.

What to do

- Remove the implant if it has loosened or failed and is likely to cause further damage.
- Remove the implant if it appears to be harboring a biofilm, provided that its removal (and replacement, if necessary) is unlikely to cause harm (see Biofilms on surgical implants, later).
- If in doubt about whether an implant should be removed, surgically explore the site and obtain samples for culture and antibiotic sensitivity testing, including samples from the surface(s) of the implant *in situ*. Consider using local or regional modes of antibiotic delivery if the implant must be left in place.
  - Remove the implant if indicated by the stage of healing and tissue quality after debridement, and if it is no longer needed for structural support.
  - Provide or continue wound care as described earlier for extensively contaminated wounds.
  - Start or continue interim broad-spectrum antibiotic therapy while awaiting results of culture and antibiotic sensitivity testing (discussed later).

What to avoid

- Avoid removing stable implants that are providing structural support when replacement may do more harm than good. Instead, use local/regional modes of antibiotic delivery, such as regional perfusion or antibiotic-impregnated implants, to control the infection to allow healing to proceed.

Sequestra

Devitalized tissue, whether skin, connective tissue, muscle, bone, or other tissue, may form a sequestrum, which acts as a bacterial refuge similar to a foreign body. Management, likewise, is similar to that for managing a wound containing a foreign body, but care should be taken to debride only the tissue that is devitalized. If the infection involves a structure, the loss of which the horse can accommodate, such as the common digital extensor tendon, complete surgical resection may be warranted if that structure is extensively contaminated or severely infected.[61]

Abscesses

An abscess can act as a bacterial refuge by protecting the bacteria from host defenses in its avascular and relatively hypoxic liquid or inspissated contents. Formation of an abscess creates conditions, such as low pH, that inactivate certain antibiotic drugs. Aminoglycosides, in particular, do not perform well in the presence of purulent exudate.[62] When the presence of an abscess is confirmed using diagnostic imaging and/or needle aspiration, the abscess should be surgically drained, if possible, and then debrided and irrigated as described for extensively contaminated wounds.

Bacterial biofilms

Bacterial biofilms present a particular therapeutic challenge. Not only do they protect the bacteria contained within them from the host's defenses and from antibiotics, they are also highly resistant to chemical damage. A mature biofilm is relatively impervious to common antiseptics, alcohols, acids, bleach, hydrogen peroxide, and other generators of oxygen radicals (e.g., ozone), unless these products are used at a concentration toxic to the host's cells.[36,37]

Plaque on dental enamel is a good example of a biofilm and a handy reminder of how quickly bacterial biofilms can form (and re-form) in a suitable environment and what is required to remove them. The biofilm on teeth must be physically degraded to expose the bacteria within to antibacterial substances, which then slow the re-formation of the biofilm. Antiseptic mouthwashes are of little and short-term benefit if they are not preceded by thorough brushing and flossing. Another essential element in treating biofilms is to remove the biofilm repeatedly (i.e., regular tooth brushing).

Ridding an infected wound of a biofilm requires the same basic approach as ridding the teeth of plaque (oral biofilm). The following is a step-by-step summary of what to do and what to avoid:[35–37,63]

Step 1. Physically degrade the biofilm.

- Vigorously debride the wound to remove purulent discharge, necrotic tissue, and any discernible biofilm, even if it causes minor bleeding. In fact, fresh blood contains antibacterial components that facilitate Step 2.
- Options for degrading the biofilm include the following:
  - drag a gauze swab (i.e., mildly abrasive material) across the surface of the wound;
  - use pulsed water-jet irrigation (e.g., Waterpik®; Water Pik, Inc.) to dislodge and rinse away the biofilm; this option is better than swabbing if the surface is very uneven;
  - use low-frequency ultrasonic debridement;*
  - draw the sharp* or blunt edge of a scalpel blade across the surface; this option is best suited to wounds with fairly even surfaces.

(*These are the most studied methods in human wound care.)

The goal is to remove as much of the biofilm and associated bacteria as possible and to expose the remaining bacteria to a biocide (Step 2). Surfactants, such as polyhexamethylene biguanide (polyhexanide or PHMB), may be useful adjuncts because they reduce the surface tension of the biofilm, which facilitates degradation and removal of the biofilm.

Gloves should be worn to protect against zoonotic and reverse-zoonotic infections. A surgical mask and protective eyewear should also be worn when using pulsed water-jet irrigation, particularly if the wound is known to be, or suspected to be, infected with MRSA or other multidrug-resistant bacteria.

Because this step may be uncomfortable for the patient, the horse should be sedated, and the wound desensitized by using local or regional anesthesia. The horse may need to be anesthetized, at least for the first debridement, if the wound is deep or extensive, or if the horse is uncooperative.

Step 2. Prevent or delay reconstitution of the biofilm.

- After the protective matrix has been removed or significantly degraded, most of the bacteria within the biofilm assume their "planktonic" antibacterial sensitivities.
- If current results of culture and sensitivity testing are available, use the most appropriate antibiotic(s), both topically and systemically. The efficacy of regional antibiotic delivery is also likely to be greatest immediately after the biofilm has been degraded.
- If sensitivity results are still pending, apply a broad-spectrum antibacterial cream,[36] such as povidone–iodine, chlorhexidine, 1% silver sulfadiazine,[63] or 1% hydrogen peroxide.[64]
- Honey is also documented to have some antibiofilm properties when applied topically.[65,66]

In most cases, bacteria found in biofilm are susceptible to a wide variety of biocides immediately after debridement, including ionic silver solutions[36,67] and ozone,[36,68–70] but the best choices may be those that have a residual effect by virtue of their adherent properties (e.g., gels, creams, honey). Antimicrobial dressings, such as silver-impregnated wound dressings, inhibit bacterial biofilms,[67,71–73] but, because their efficacy drops after the first 24 hours,[72] these dressings must be changed frequently. An added advantage to topically applied silver and other antimicrobial agents is that they increase the susceptibility of bacteria to antibiotic drugs, which may help counteract the antibiotic resistance acquired by bacteria in biofilms.[36,72]

Topical application of plasma (natural or hyperimmune) to the wound may also be useful because plasma inhibits bacterial adhesion and growth.[74–76] Platelet-rich plasma speeds wound healing, but the components of plasma other than platelets appear to provide plasma's bacteriostatic effect.[76] Whether or not antigen-specific equine hyperimmune plasma (see Immunocompromise, later) is superior to plain plasma for inhibiting the formation or re-formation of a biofilm remains to be determined, but an antigen-specific hyperimmune plasma might be of great benefit if the specific pathogen targeted by the hyperimmune plasma is present within the wound.

Other antibiofilm agents under investigation include lactoferrin, xylitol, ethylenediaminetetra-acetic acid (EDTA), RNA III inhibiting peptide, dispersin B (a bacterial glycoside hydrolase), gallium, acetylsalicylic acid, various phytochemicals, bacteriophages (antibacterial viruses), glucose oxidase, proteases, ultraviolet light, and low-voltage pulsed electric fields.[36,77,78]

Regardless of which methods are selected to degrade the biofilm, the biofilm bacteria should be targeted from above (topically) and below (systemically and/or regionally).

Step 3. Repeat steps 1 and 2 frequently and for as long as necessary.

- Mature biofilms can re-form in as little as 24 hours after debridement, so there is a narrow window of opportunity (at most, 72 hours) during which bactericidal drugs can have a substantial impact on the bacterial population within the wound.

- Repeat Steps 1 and 2 daily or every other day until the infection is well under control, as evidenced by a reduction in the signs of infection and the resumption of healing.

Most biofilms are microscopic, and bacterial culture of biofilm-protected inhabitants may be unrewarding,[35,41,42] so until a practical, stall-side test is available to identify the presence of a biofilm, clinical signs of persistent infection are the best guide. The wound should be reassessed frequently, and the method of debridement (Step 1) or inhibition (Step 2) should be changed if wound healing is not proceeding as expected.

Each step is equally important. Degrading the biofilm helps restore the susceptibility of the bacteria to antibacterial agents, but when a severely infected wound has a well-established or mature biofilm, one round of treatment to degrade the biofilm is insufficient. The wound must be treated daily, or at least every other day, using a combination approach (i.e., Steps 1 and 2) until the infection is resolved or is well on its way to complete resolution.[35–37,63]

This intensity of treatment disrupts the wound bed and interferes with repair of an uncomplicated wound, but wounds containing a bacterial biofilm are not simple or straightforward wounds, and many are chronic.[34] Wound repair cannot proceed normally in the presence of a bacterial biofilm, so the priority should be to degrade the biofilm and prevent it from reforming, and thereby resolve the infection. Thereafter, the intensity and invasiveness of treatment can be reduced and tailored to the rate and quality of wound repair.

The higher initial costs of this approach are counterbalanced by lower overall costs because chronic wounds are a considerable and protracted financial drain. In human patients with chronic wounds that are complicated by biofilms, frequently debriding the wound as part of a multifaceted approach to wound care shortens the duration of treatment and decreases the overall costs of treatment.[37]

Biofilms on surgical implants

Biofilms on unstable surgical implants are best resolved by removing the implant. Biofilms on surgical implants that are still performing the function for which they were applied (e.g., bone plate stabilizing a complete fracture) are more of a challenge, because there may be no indication for implant removal, other than removal of the biofilm, and good indications to leave the implant in place. In such cases, it may be best to anesthetize the horse, surgically expose the implant (or the infected portion thereof) and perform Steps 1 and 2 in a sterile surgical suite, and then pack the wound with an antibiotic-impregnated material[79] (discussed later).

Reminder: Biofilms in wounds are most likely to form and persist if the horse is immunocompromised and/or if perfusion of the wound is poor. These problems must be identified and addressed for treatment to be effective.

Immunocompromise

Typically, patients with severely infected wounds have already undergone initial systemic assessment and treatment. Even so, taking the following steps is wise:

What to do

- Review or further investigate the patient's signalment, history (including recent medications), findings during physical examination, and blood work.
- Repeat physical examination and/or blood work, as needed.
- Treat, if possible, any condition identified that may be compromising immune function. For example, a severely infected wound in a geriatric horse with PPID is unlikely to respond well to wound therapy until the PPID is controlled with pergolide.
- Consider topical application of plasma from a compatible donor.[74,75]
  - Fresh plasma from a healthy horse living on the same premises (and thus exposed to the same pathogens) is suitable.
  - Administering antigen-specific hyperimmune plasma may be of particular value when the pathogen causing the wound infection is known and a suitable hyperimmune product is available.
  - Commercially available equine plasma is available in the US from horses hyperimmunized against *E. coli*, *Salmonella* spp., *Streptococcus equi*, *Rhodococcus equi*, or *Clostridium* spp. (Lake Immunogenics, Inc.).
  - Supplemental plasma may also be administered intravenously.

What to avoid

- Avoid immunosuppressive therapies, such as systemic administration of a corticosteroid and cryotherapy (i.e., therapeutic hypothermia). Although both are highly effective anti-inflammatory therapies, they are also immunosuppressive.[80] If administration of a corticosteroid is necessary, such as for initial treatment of systemic inflammatory response syndrome, a short-acting corticosteroid (e.g., dexamethasone) should be used, and the course of treatment should be short (48 hours at most).

Supportive care

General supportive care is critical, particularly when specific treatment for the immunocompromised state is not possible.

What to do

- Maintain clean, dry bedding in a well-ventilated stall that is large enough for the horse to lie down and rise without risk of injury.
- Provide compatible company to prevent the stress of social isolation.
- Keep the area quiet and dark at night to encourage sleep.
- Feed a well-formulated diet that provides adequate protein, calories, and micronutrients, yet is low in simple carbohydrates (i.e., starch and sugars).[81] Base the diet on high-quality forages. When extra calories are needed, supplement the diet with fat (e.g., vegetable oils, rice bran).

What to avoid

- Small, cramped, poorly-ventilated stalls.
- Inadequate or dirty bedding. Failing to keep the stall deeply bedded and scrupulously clean is false economy.
- Isolated stalls that prevent the horse from seeing horses nearby.
- Constant light and activity in the barn.
- Diets high in grains and other soluble carbohydrates.

Poor perfusion

Blood flow is tightly regulated, so the extent to which it can be increased to a compromised area is limited. Nevertheless, severely infected wounds complicated by poor perfusion are difficult to manage unless impediments to optimal blood flow are identified and removed, if possible.

What to do

- Ensure good hydration and provide specific treatment for systemic disorders.
- Address blood loss, if substantial, that may have occurred at the time of injury.
- Remove impediments to blood flow within the wound, as described earlier. In particular, debride traumatized tissue that has been ischemic for longer than a few hours and is becoming, or is already, necrotic.
- Control edema.
  - Use a non-steroidal anti-inflammatory drug (NSAID) to help resolve vasculitis and inflammatory edema.
  - Use manual and movement therapy (see Drainage, earlier) to control dependent edema, which in turn improves blood flow.
  - Use a compression bandage where appropriate, applying the bandage from distal to proximal.
  - Consider using NPWT, if available (see Drainage, earlier).

What to avoid

- Avoid corticosteroid therapy and cryotherapy because both are immunosuppressive.
- Avoid creating excessive or focal pressure with bandages.

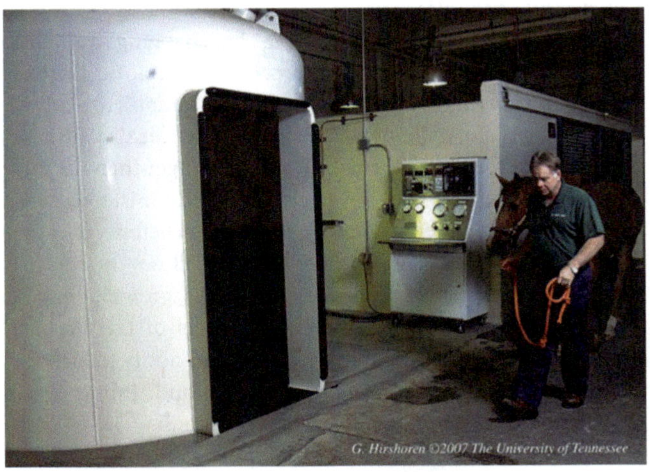

Figure 19.2 Hyperbaric oxygen chamber for horses. The hyperbaric chamber is used for wound healing therapy at the University of Tennessee College of Veterinary Medicine in Knoxville, Tennessee. Greg Hirshoren © 2007. The University of Tennessee.

Oxygen therapy

When blood flow cannot be improved, oxygen therapy may be a useful adjunct. Hyperbaric oxygen therapy (Figure 19.2) increases oxygen tension in the tissues, thereby facilitating all aerobic processes, both defensive and reparative, and it is potentially lethal to obligate anaerobes.[82,83] It may also stimulate the release of stem cells from the bone marrow into the peripheral blood.[84]

Ozone therapy and 1% hydrogen peroxide wound cream are two other oxygen therapies that may be useful. Ozone and hydrogen peroxide are oxygen donors, but their primary value in wound care may be as biocides because they increase the concentration of oxygen-derived free radicals within the wound, which supplements the bactericidal oxidative burst by neutrophils.[64,68–70,85,86] Medical ozone may be delivered topically or intravenously (dissolved in sterile isotonic saline solution). Topically applied ozone may be delivered in gaseous form (ozonized medical-grade oxygen), in solution (dissolved in water or isotonic saline solution), or as ozone-infused oil (e.g., ozone-infused vegetable oil).[69,70,85] However, in spite of preliminary evidence to the effect that ozone might control wound infection, in 2015 the United States Food and Drug Administration stated that for ozone to be effective as a germicide, it must be present in a concentration far greater than can be safely tolerated by man or other animals.[87]

Note: Oxygen radicals also cause oxidative damage to the patient's cell membranes, so overuse of ozone and hydrogen peroxide may be counterproductive.[69]

Antibiotic insensitivity

Antibiotic therapy may fail because of inherent or acquired bacterial resistance to the antibiotic(s), administration (dosage, route, or duration) that results in a subtherapeutic antibiotic concentration within the wound, poor perfusion of the wound, and/or the presence of one or more bacterial refugia within the wound. The latter two factors were discussed in previous sections. The following discussion focuses on antibiotic choices and routes of administration for optimal effectiveness.

Culture-guided antibiotic selection

Effective antibiotic therapy hinges on identifying the principal pathogens in the wound and determining or confirming their antibiotic sensitivities. It is essential to perform bacterial culture and antibiotic sensitivity testing when the wound is severely infected and to repeat these procedures if the wound has not responded to therapy as expected. Time and money spent on providing empiric antibiotic therapy may be wasted if culture and sensitivity testing are not already underway. Determining antibiotic sensitivity and resistance of the wound's pathogen(s) as soon as possible is crucial.

Conventional culture techniques are now known to identify only some of the bacterial genera and species that may be found in wounds, particularly in those containing biofilms.[41,42] Even when concerted efforts are made to sample the biofilm, bacteria in biofilm-mode, especially the metabolically inactive subpopulation, can be difficult to grow in culture. For this reason, rapid molecular methods of bacterial identification are being used increasingly to guide antibiotic therapy in human patients with chronic wounds.[35,36]

Although molecular methods of identifying pathogens are becoming more widely available in commercial veterinary microbiology laboratories, veterinarians are still left with the culture-based methods of determining antibiotic sensitivities. Thus, routine bacterial culture and antibiotic sensitivity testing remain essential components of managing severely infected wounds.

Ensuring reliable culture results

Obtaining results of bacterial culture and antibiotic sensitivity testing that reliably represent the principal wound pathogens hinges on three key steps. The following are step-by-step guidelines for what to do and what to avoid when sampling a wound for bacterial culture:

Step 1. Use strict aseptic techniques.

- Avoid contaminating the sample with commensal organisms from the surrounding skin and with opportunists that may be colonizing the superficial areas of the wound.
- For deep, narrow wounds, thoroughly cleanse the surrounding skin with surgical scrub, taking care to avoid exposing the wound to the scrub.
- For wound beds with a coating of purulent discharge or slough, irrigate the wound's surface with sterile isotonic fluid (no added antibiotic or antiseptic) to remove the more superficial material.
- Wear sterile gloves and use a sterile swab to collect the culture sample. Gloves also protect against zoonotic and reverse-zoonotic transmission of pathogens.
- Avoid contacting the skin margin or superficial areas of the wound with the swab; if necessary, gently part the wound's edges to insert the swab.

Step 2. Sample the surfaces and tissues where the pathogens are most likely to reside.

- Factor in the various types of refugia that may complicate the wound.
- Collect samples from the deepest recesses of the wound and sample multiple sites if the wound has multiple pockets, fissures, or layers.
- If the presence of a biofilm is suspected, draw the swab across the surface of the wound with enough pressure to collect a sample of the biofilm.
  - In the process, avoid causing hemorrhage, because blood contains antibacterial elements.
  - Superficial culture of a wound with a biofilm is likely to yield incomplete and potentially misleading results.
- Whenever possible, include tissue samples from the wound. For example, debride the wound and submit some of the debrided material.
  - Collecting fluid, such as purulent exudate, is easier and less invasive than collecting tissue, but tissue samples from the site of infection are more likely to yield reliable culture results.[41,42]
- For wounds involving (or suspected to involve) a synovial space, also aseptically collect a sample of synovial fluid, ideally using percutaneous aspiration at a site distant from the wound.
- Submit any other material removed from the wound, such as a foreign body, a surgical implant, or a sequestrum, to the laboratory for analysis.
- Submit all representative samples; it is false economy to submit only one sample when several different types of material (e.g., exudate, implant, tissue, biofilm) have been collected.

Step 3. Use the recommended laboratory submission procedures.

- Call the laboratory staff in advance to discuss the case and review appropriate collection materials, transport media, and shipping methods. The more the microbiologist knows about the case, the more help he or she can provide.
- For synovial fluid samples, use a blood culture medium and the appropriate sample-to-medium ratio, unless otherwise directed.
- Submit the samples as soon as possible. If there is to be a delay (e.g., over the weekend), either postpone sample collection until the next laboratory pick-up day or store the sample as advised by the laboratory staff (e.g., refrigerated, in the appropriate transport medium).
- Provide as much clinical information as possible and request cytologic examination, aerobic and anaerobic culture, and antibiotic sensitivity testing of bacterial isolates.
- Request quantitative antibiotic sensitivities, if they are available, that provide MICs for the drugs tested.
- If a fungal pathogen is suspected, discuss this possibility with the laboratory staff and request fungal cytology and culture.

Concurrent antibiotic use

Collect all samples before starting or changing antibiotic therapy. If the horse is already receiving antibiotic therapy, either suspend therapy or try to collect the samples for culture immediately before the next scheduled dose. Ideally, suspend therapy for a period that is at least 8 hours longer than the dosing interval; for example, for an antibiotic administered every 12 hours, suspend therapy for at least 20 hours before collecting samples for culture. This extended interval allows the residual bacteria to re-enter the log phase of active growth, making positive culture more likely. When time is of the essence, however, culture the wound immediately and notify the laboratory staff of the horse's antibiotic regimen and timing of the most recent dose in relation to sample collection.

Note: The goal is not simply to identify the pathogens that may be insensitive to the current antibiotic regimen, but to form as complete a picture as possible of the microbial ecology of the wound, in order to formulate an antibiotic regimen that addresses each pathogen and its sensitivities.

Interim antibiotic selection

With severely infected wounds, interim systemic therapy using an experience-guided (empiric) antibiotic selection can be critical to a successful outcome while awaiting results of culture and sensitivity testing. Table 19.1 lists the common bacteria isolated from various types of wounds in horses as a basis for empiric antibiotic choices that are most likely to be useful.[22,31,88–95]

Unless a specific pathogen with a well-established sensitivity pattern is strongly suspected (e.g., penicillin for clostridial myonecrosis), administering broad-spectrum antibiotic therapy is generally the best approach.

- A combination of penicillin G (crystalline or procaine penicillin) and gentamicin is widely used.

Table 19.1 Common bacterial isolates from various wounds in horses, and recommendations for interim systemic antibiotic therapy.

Tissue involved	Common genera	Therapeutic considerations
Skin (normal microflora)	Predominant: *Staphylococcus*, *Enterococcus*, *Bacillus*, *Micrococcus* Lesser: *Streptococcus*, *Streptomyces*, other non-enteric genera; *Corynebacterium pseudotuberculosis* (western US)	Environmental contamination, particularly with fecal matter, and human contact can alter the normal skin flora. These contaminants often play an important role in both traumatic and postoperative wound infections **Base empiric antibiotic selection on the deeper structures involved**, as detailed below
Wounds (in general)	Acute: *Staphylococcus*, *Aerococcus*, *Micrococcus*, *Alcaligenes*, *Bacillus*, *Propionibacterium*, *Acinetobacter*, *Clostridium* Chronic: *Pseudomonas* (*aeruginosa*), *Staphylococcus* (*epidermidis*, *aureus*), *Serratia*, *Enterococcus*, *Enterobacter*, *Proteus*	
Subcutis (cellulitis/ulcerative lymphangitis)	Most common: *Staphylococcus* Less common: *Streptococcus*, Gram-negative aerobes, anaerobes; *C. pseudotuberculosis* (western US)	Causal organisms are often resistant to penicillin, so use a cephalosporin + an aminoglycoside (e.g., ceftiofur + gentamicin/amikacin) Enrofloxacin alone is a reasonable alternative in adult horses For ulcerative lymphangitis in *C. pseudotuberculosis* endemic areas, consider a penicillin or a macrolide
Synovial structure (joint, tendon sheath, bursa)	Traumatic: Gram-negative enteric genera, *Streptococcus*, *Staphylococcus*, anaerobes; polymicrobial infection is common. Postoperative: *Staphylococcus*, *Streptococcus*, *Enterobacter*, other enteric genera, *Pseudomonas*	For either wound type: a cephalosporin + amikacin (or gentamicin) Enrofloxacin alone is a reasonable alternative in adult horses Add metronidazole for wounds on the distal aspect of the limb or otherwise likely to have fecal contamination (i.e., likely presence of obligate anaerobes)
Bone or physeal cartilage	Traumatic: *Enterobacter*, *Streptococcus*, *Staphylococcus*; in young foals, Gram-negative enteric genera Postoperative: *Streptococcus zooepidemicus*, *S. aureus*, other *Streptococcus* sp.	As for synovial structures
Distal aspect of the limb or foot	Polymicrobial infection that typically includes Gram-negative enteric genera and, with the foot, anaerobes such as *Bacteroides*	A cephalosporin (or penicillin) + an aminoglycoside + metronidazole (many *Bacteroides* sp. are resistant to penicillin and cephalosporins)
Respiratory tract (e.g., penetrating head, neck, or chest wounds)	Combinations of Gram-positive aerobes (especially *S. zooepidemicus*), Gram-negative aerobes (e.g., *Actinobacillus*, *Pasteurella*, enterobacteria), and anaerobes (e.g., *Bacteroides*, *Fusobacterium*, *Peptostreptococcus*)	A penicillin (penicillin G or ampicillin) + gentamicin Ceftiofur can be substituted for penicillin, and amikacin for gentamicin Add metronidazole if extensive tissue necrosis or dead space
Intestinal tract (e.g., penetrating abdominal or perineal wounds, open drainage for septic peritonitis)	If intestinal wall penetrated: Gram-negative enteric genera and anaerobes	Penicillin (penicillin G or ampicillin) + gentamicin + metronidazole Ceftiofur can be substituted for penicillin, and amikacin for gentamicin
Muscle	Common: skin microflora Gaseous myonecrosis: *Clostridium* Deep abscess: *C. pseudotuberculosis* (western US)	Penicillin (penicillin G or ampicillin) Add metronidazole for clostridial myonecrosis Add rifampin for *C. pseudotuberculosis*

Interim antibiotic therapy is an *empiric* drug selection, instituted while awaiting results of bacterial culture and antibiotic sensitivity testing. *For all severely infected wounds, rational antibiotic therapy must be guided by current culture and antibiotic sensitivity results.*
Enrofloxacin and other quinolones are not recommended for use in horses less than 12 months old.

- For some pathogens, penicillin G is best replaced with a synthetic penicillin (e.g., ampicillin) or a cephalosporin (e.g., ceftiofur, cefazolin, or cephalothin).
- Amikacin is sometimes a better choice than gentamicin.

Gram stain

Whenever possible, collect a separate swab or tissue sample from the wound and perform a Gram stain in-house or at a nearby veterinary clinic or human hospital (instructions for performing a Gram stain are provided in Box 19.1.) This simple procedure provides immediate information that can be useful in directing interim antibiotic therapy. Table 19.2 lists some key cytologic features of common equine wound pathogens, and Table 19.3 lists likely antibiotic sensitivities for each pathogen based on published studies of various equine populations in North America, Europe, Australia, and New Zealand during the past 25 years.[20,22,23,27–31,91,94–101]

Note: Antibiotic sensitivity patterns are quite variable and are always evolving. Sensitivity patterns vary among geographic regions and are heavily influenced by the extent of antibiotic use in the particular population of animals and their caretakers. Pathogens isolated from hospitalized horses or those on farms

Box 19.1 Performing a Gram stain

Overview

A fluid or tissue sample is smeared on a slide, heat-fixed, stained with crystal violet, fixed with iodine, then decolorized with acetone or alcohol, which removes the crystal violet from the Gram-negative cells. Finally, a red stain (safranin O or basic fuchsin) is applied to stain the Gram-negative cells. After Gram staining, Gram-positive bacteria are dark purple and Gram-negative bacteria are pinkish red under the microscope.

Materials

- Microscope that allows resolution up to 1,000×
- Glass microscope slides, coverslips, and microscopy oil
- Bunsen burner or cigarette lighter (i.e., an open flame)
- Gram-stain kit or separate bottles of crystal violet, Gram's iodine solution, acetone/ethanol, and either safranin O or basic fuchsin
- Gloves or tongs for handling slides during staining
- Water bottle or tap (note: staining of the sink is likely)

Steps

1. Make a thin smear of the fluid or tissue on a slide; air dry and then heat fix the sample by passing the slide over a gentle flame a few times. (Avoid overheating the slide, as it denatures the sample; the goal is simply to fix the cells to the slide.)
2. Add 5 drops of crystal violet to the sample; let stand for 1 minute. Briefly wash off the purple stain with a light stream of water and gently shake off the excess water. (Avoid strong water pressure, as it may wash off the sample as well.)
3. Add 5 drops of iodine solution to the sample; let stand for 30 seconds. Briefly wash off the iodine with water and gently shake off the excess.
4. Tilt the slide and wash the sample with acetone/ethanol until the purple color stops running (about 5 seconds). Be careful not to over-decolorize. *Immediately* wash the slide with water and then gently shake off the excess.
5. Add 5 drops of safranin O or basic fuchsin; let stand for 1 minute. Briefly wash off the red stain with water and gently shake off the excess.
6. Let the slide air dry or *gently* heat dry, then examine under the microscope at 400× and 1,000× (oil immersion).

Table 19.2 Cytologic features of common equine wound pathogens.

Pathogen	Cytologic features	Oxygen sensitivity*	Usual source
Gram-positive			
Clostridium sp.	Large, blunt-ended rods	Obligate anaerobe	Intestinal tract (feces)
Corynebacterium sp.	Unevenly Gram-positive; small, slender, pleomorphic rods that tend to clump to form odd linear shapes	Aerobe or facultative anaerobe	Soil; most common in the western US (including Midwest and Southwest)
Enterococcus sp.	Cocci are round or ovoid and are found in pairs or chains (similar to *Streptococcus* sp.)	Facultative anaerobe	Intestinal tract (feces)
Staphylococcus sp.	Darkly Gram-positive, round cocci that form clusters like bunches of grapes; may be found intracellularly	Facultative anaerobe	Skin and upper respiratory tract
Streptococcus sp.	Round or ovoid cocci, found in pairs or chains	Facultative anaerobe	Skin and upper respiratory tract
Gram-negative			
Actinobacillus sp.	Ovoid or rods (coccobacilli)	Facultative anaerobe	Intestinal tract (feces), environment
Enterobacter sp.	Rods	Facultative anaerobe	Intestinal tract (feces)
Escherichia coli, other enterobacteriaceae	Short rods; may be found intracellularly	Facultative anaerobe	Intestinal tract (feces)
Pasteurella sp.	Coccobacilli	Facultative anaerobe	Environment (other animals)
Pseudomonas aeruginosa	Coccobacilli	Aerobe or facultative anaerobe	Environment (soil, water, plant material); thrives in moist environments, including wet skin and wounds

* Facultative anaerobes can survive and even replicate under aerobic conditions, whereas obligate anaerobes cannot. Most wound pathogens are at least tolerant of oxygen in air and tissue fluids, and more so when protected by a biofilm, so these categorizations apply more to laboratory culture than to wound management.

where antibiotics are frequently used are more likely to show antibiotic resistance than are pathogens isolated from horses at premises on which antibiotic use is less common. Thus, these published antibiotic sensitivity patterns should be used as *a general guide only*, to aid in making rational choices for *interim* therapy, and never as a substitute for patient-specific, current results of bacterial culture and antibiotic sensitivity testing.

Options for treating multidrug-resistant bacteria

At the present time, two antibiotic drugs remain in the arsenal for multidrug-resistant bacteria: vancomycin and imipenem. Note, however, that bacterial resistance has been documented for both drugs, so they are by no means "silver bullets," and their use will not remain an option in veterinary or human medicine if they are used indiscriminately. Their use should therefore be reserved for situations in which results of culture and sensitivity testing clearly indicate sensitivity to the particular drug and absence of reasonable alternatives.

Vancomycin

Vancomycin is active against many Gram-positive bacteria, both aerobes and anaerobes, including MRSA and *Clostridium difficile*. Vancomycin, either alone or in combination with an aminoglycoside, is, therefore, an option for treating serious

Table 19.3 *In vitro* antibiotic sensitivity patterns for the pathogens listed in Table 19.2.

Pathogen	Likely sensitivity*	Notes
Gram-positive		
Clostridium sp.	Penicillins, metronidazole	1. Exposure to air or other oxygen source (hydrogen peroxide, ozone, hyperbaric oxygen therapy) facilitates antibiotic therapy and may be sufficient against this obligate anaerobe 2. Some clostridial isolates are resistant to metronidazole 3. Vancomycin is likely to be effective, but this drug should be reserved for **documented** multidrug-resistant, vancomycin-sensitive pathogens
Corynebacterium sp.	Penicillins, macrolides	Drainage is important for a successful outcome in cases with deep IM abscess, as antibiotic penetration of the dense abscess wall is poor
Enterococcus sp.	Penicillins, chloramphenicol	1. Ampicillin is more likely than penicillin G to be effective; cephalosporins are effective against few isolates 2. Gentamicin is likely to be effective against many** isolates, but amikacin is unlikely to be effective 3. Tetracyclines are likely to be effective against many** isolates 4. Vancomycin and imipenem are each likely to be effective, but these drugs should be reserved for **documented** multidrug-resistant, vancomycin- or imipenem-sensitive pathogens. Resistance to each of these drugs is documented for Enterococcus sp.
Staphylococcus sp.	Cephalosporins, enrofloxacin, aminoglycosides, chloramphenicol, rifampin	1. Amikacin is more likely than gentamicin to be effective, but susceptibility to amikacin in equine MRSA isolates is variable 2. Penicillins, macrolides, tetracyclines, and TMPS are each likely to be effective against many** isolates 3. Vancomycin is appropriate for **documented** cases of MRSA when other drugs are not suitable
Streptococcus sp.	Penicillins, cephalosporins, chloramphenicol	1. Gentamicin is likely to be effective against many** isolates; amikacin less so 2. Enrofloxacin, macrolides, tetracyclines, TMPS, and rifampin are each likely to be effective against many** isolates
Gram-negative		
Actinobacillus sp.	Cephalosporins, enrofloxacin, tetracyclines, TMPS, chloramphenicol	1. Penicillins are inconsistently effective; ampicillin may be more likely than penicillin G to be effective 2. Aminoglycosides and macrolides are each likely to be effective against many** isolates
Enterobacter sp.	Ceftiofur, enrofloxacin, aminoglycosides	1. Amikacin is more likely than gentamicin to be effective 2. Tetracyclines and TMPS may each be effective against many** isolates
E. coli, other enterobacteria	Enrofloxacin, aminoglycosides	1. Amikacin is more likely than gentamicin to be effective 2. Ceftiofur, ampicillin, tetracyclines, TMPS, and chloramphenicol may each be effective against many** isolates 3. Resistance to quinolones is documented for *Klebsiella pneumoniae*
Pasteurella sp.	1) Penicillins, cephalosporins, enrofloxacin, aminoglycosides, tetracyclines, TMPS, chloramphenicol	1. Ampicillin may be more likely than penicillin G to be effective 2. Gentamicin may be more likely than amikacin to be effective
P. aeruginosa	2) Amikacin	1. *P. aeruginosa* is resistant to most commonly used antibiotics in equine practice 2. Gentamicin and enrofloxacin are each likely to be effective against some isolates, as are carbenicillin, ticarcillin, and piperacillin 3. Imipenem use is appropriate for **documented** multidrug-resistant, imipenem-sensitive infections

* Sensitivity shown for at least 80% of clinical equine isolates in published studies; **sensitivity shown for 50–79% of clinical equine isolates.[22,27,91,94,99]
Abbreviations: IM, intramuscular; MRSA, methicillin-resistant *Staphylococcus aureus*; TMPS, trimethoprim–sulfonamide combinations.
Note: Enrofloxacin and other quinolones are not recommended for use in horses less than 12 months old.

infections caused by *Staphylococcus* sp. or *Enterococcus* sp. that are resistant to all other available options.[96]

The recommended systemic dosage in horses is 7.5 mg/kg q 8 hours, administered in isotonic saline solution by slow IV infusion over 30 minutes.[94] For infections confined to the distal aspect of the limb, vancomycin may be administered by regional perfusion, using either IV or intraosseous (IO) delivery. (Regional limb perfusion is discussed later.) A dose of 300 mg in 60 mL sterile isotonic saline solution appears well tolerated and achieves therapeutic concentrations in the synovial fluid and medullary sinusoidal plasma of the perfused area.[102–104] These regional modes of delivery help optimize the treatment of vancomycin-susceptible infections in the distal aspect of the limb while minimizing the cost of treatment, potential for toxicity, and development of bacterial resistance.

Imipenem

Imipenem-cilastatin is active against a wide range of Gram-positive and Gram-negative organisms, both aerobes and anaerobes, including multidrug-resistant enteric pathogens (*E. coli*, *Klebsiella* sp., *Salmonella* sp., etc.) and most strains of *P. aeruginosa* and *Bacteroides fragilis*. However, it is not effective against MRSA, and resistance is documented for some *Enterococcus* sp.[12,31]

The recommended systemic dosage in horses is 10–20 mg/kg by slow IV infusion, q 6–8 hours.[105] Intrasynovial administration is described in case studies, the dose ranging from 10 mg to 250 mg.[106] Imipenem may also be administered by IV regional perfusion. A dose of 500 mg in 100 mL sterile isotonic saline solution (5 mg/mL), delivered into the cephalic or saphenous vein, resulted in concentrations of imipenem in the metacarpo/metatarsophalangeal joint well above the MIC for most susceptible pathogens for approximately 6 hours.[107] Smaller volumes for perfusion (i.e., higher imipenem concentrations) have been described for IV regional perfusion,[106] but the safety of imipenem concentrations greater than 5 mg/mL has not been established.

Bacteriostats

Bacteriostatic antibiotics include tetracyclines, sulfonamides, trimethoprim–sulfonamide combinations, macrolides (e.g., erythromycin, azithromycin), and chloramphenicol. In general, severe wound infections are best treated with bactericidal drugs (e.g., penicillins, cephalosporins, aminoglycosides, quinolones [in adult horses], metronidazole, rifampin) rather than with bacteriostatic drugs.

These distinctions are, however, somewhat artificial, and they don't always reflect the drug's antibacterial activity in the patient. When laboratory results indicate sensitivity to a bacteriostat and resistance to most or all of the available bactericidal drugs, use of the bacteriostat should at least be considered. In combination with the physical measures discussed in this chapter that render the wound less hospitable to bacteria, inhibition of bacterial replication may be enough to tip the scales in favor of the host and thus resolve the infection, particularly when systemic administration is accompanied by local and/or regional antibiotic delivery.

These decisions must be made on a case-by-case basis. If persistence or progression of the wound infection would have career-ending or life-threatening consequences, then an appropriate bactericidal drug should be used, possibly even one of the reserved drugs (vancomycin or imipenem).

Local and regional antibiotic delivery

In most cases of severe wound infection, systemic parenteral antibiotic therapy is indicated, at least initially, particularly if there is evidence of a systemic inflammatory response. Local and/or regional delivery of the antibiotic(s) may also be needed, however, and in fact, may be pivotal to a successful outcome for deep-seated infections, wounds involving surgical implants that must remain in place, infections involving poorly perfused tissue, and biofilm-infected wounds. In some cases, these more targeted modes of antibiotic delivery may even obviate the need for systemic antibiotic therapy.

Local and regional routes of antibiotic delivery are summarized in Table 19.4 and include topical application, intrasynovial infusion (for wounds involving a synovial structure),[106,108] regional IV or intraosseous (IO) perfusion, for infections at or distal to the carpus/tarsus, (Figures 19.3, 19.4, 19.5, 19.6),[79,109–119]

Table 19.4 Local and regional routes of antibiotic delivery.

Route	Drugs and doses (adult horses)	Clinical notes
Topical	Silver (e.g., 1% silver sulfadiazine cream, silver-impregnated dressings), raw honey, 1% hydrogen peroxide cream, other antibacterial ointments and dressings Ozone therapy	Topical antibacterial therapy is particularly important in the treatment of biofilm-infected wounds, along with frequent debridement of the biofilm (see text)
Intrasynovial injection (joint space, tendon sheath, bursa)	Amikacin: 500–1000 mg Gentamicin: 150–500 mg Ceftiofur: 150 mg Cefazolin: 250–500 mg Na/K penicillin: 2 million–5 million units	Use strict aseptic technique to avoid further contamination even though injecting an antibiotic Administer the antibiotic intrasynovially after liberal lavage of the synovial space Constant-rate infusion of antibiotic is described for synovial infections in horses, but clinical response and long-term outcome appear comparable to intrasynovial injection[107]
Regional limb perfusion (IV or IO perfusion of carpus/tarsus or distal aspect of limb)	Amikacin: >250 mg, up to 2.5 g Gentamicin: 100–300 mg Na/K penicillin: 10 million–20 million units Ampicillin: 10 million–20 million units Ceftiofur: 2 g Enrofloxacin: 700 mg (1.5 mg/kg) Marbofloxacin: 300 mg (0.67 mg/kg)	Amikacin doses >250 mg are required to exceed the MIC in perfused tissues; the dose used is dictated by the size of the perfused area: 500–1000 mg for smaller areas (e.g., the digit via a palmar/plantar digital vein; the isolated carpus/tarsus); 2–2.5 g when perfusing the distal aspect of the limb via the cephalic/saphenous vein The size of the isolated area also dictates the perfusion volume (see Boxes 19.3 and 19.4), although higher drug doses in lower perfusion volumes are proving to be well tolerated and effective for some antibiotics (e.g., 500 mg gentamicin qs* 10 mL with sterile isotonic saline solution for perfusion of the distal aspect of the limb via a palmar digital vein)[116] Enrofloxacin may cause vasculitis even at the therapeutic dosage,[112] so reserve for documented enrofloxacin-sensitive infections with no other reasonable options. Marbofloxacin appears to be well tolerated[119]
Antibiotic-impregnated PMMA beads	Suitable drugs: Aminoglycosides (gentamicin, amikacin, tobramycin, streptomycin) Cephalosporins (cefazolin, ceftiofur) Penicillins Metronidazole Dosage: 1–4 g of antibiotic per 20 g of PMMA polymer (see Box 19.6)	When using more than one antibiotic, make a separate batch of PMMA beads for each drug Therapeutic concentrations may be sustained in the surrounding tissue for days or weeks, but bead removal may be required after treatment (see Box 19.7) Metronidazole may be mixed with hoof acrylic (Equilox, Equilox International) for polymicrobial infections of the foot

Abbreviations: IO, intraosseous; IV, intravenous; MIC, minimum inhibitory concentration; PMMA, polymethylmethacrylate.
* *quantum satis* (*qs*) – as much as needed

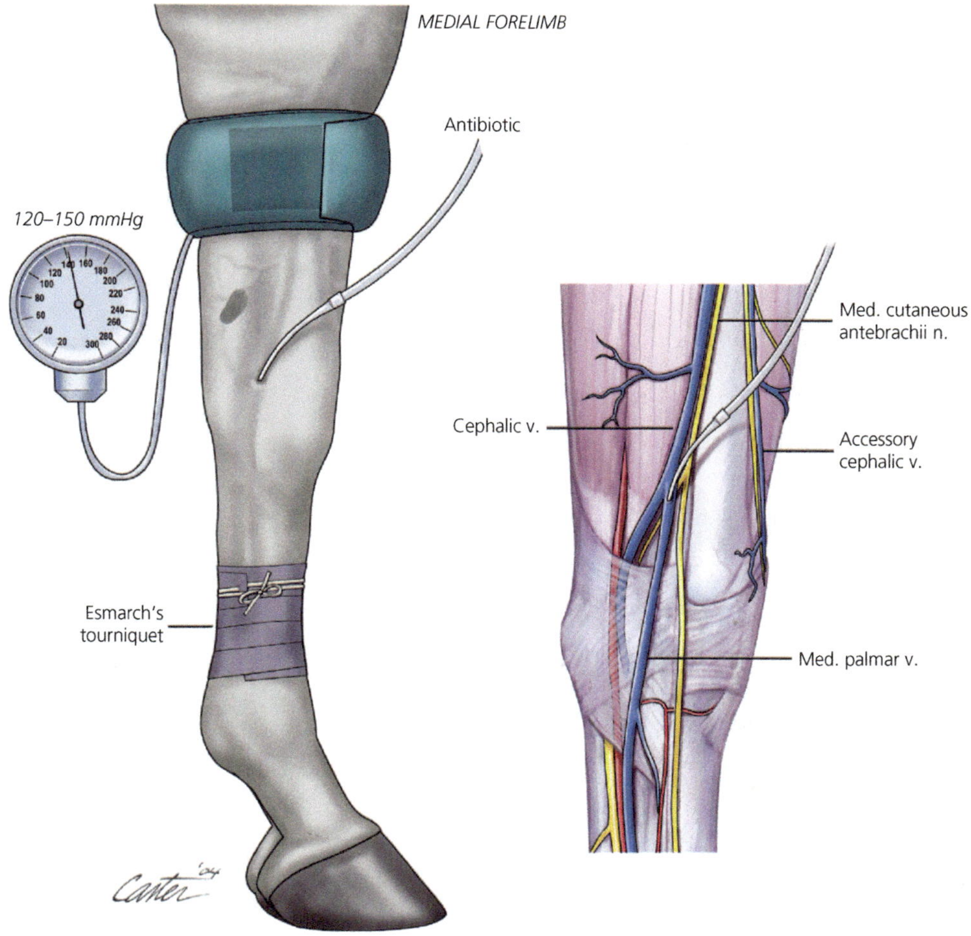

Figure 19.3 Intravenous regional perfusion for carpus. Source: Orsini 2004.[48] Reproduced with permission of Elsevier.

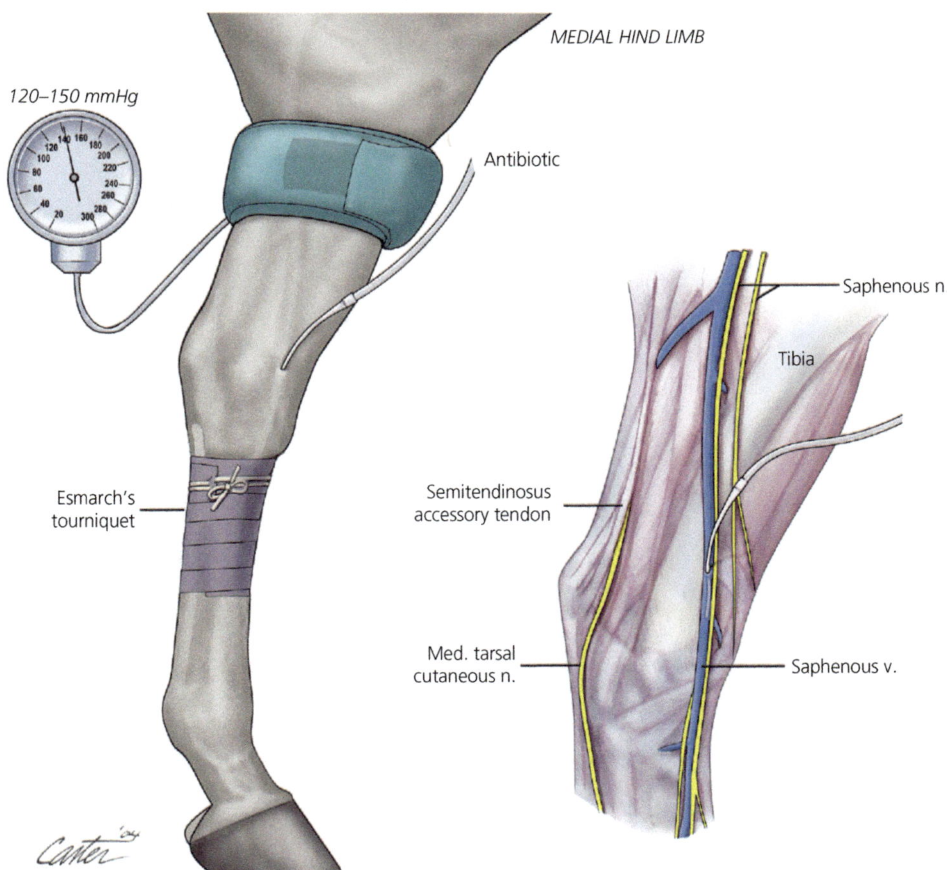

Figure 19.4 Intravenous regional perfusion for tarsus. Source: Orsini 2004.[48] Reproduced with permission of Elsevier.

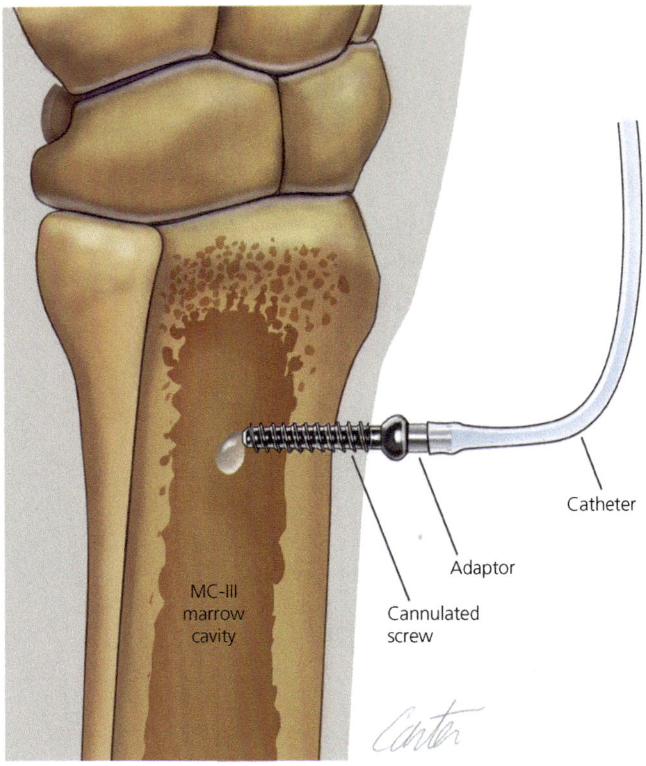

Figure 19.5 Intraosseous perfusion, metatarsus. Source: Orsini 2004.[48] Reproduced with permission of Elsevier.

and insertion of antibiotic-impregnated implants into the wound (Figures 19.7 and 19.8).[6,79,120–126] Regional perfusion is described in Box 19.2, and specific instructions are given in Boxes 19.3, 19.4, and 19.5. Making and using antibiotic-impregnated polymethylmethacrylate (PMMA) beads are described in Boxes 19.6 and 19.7.

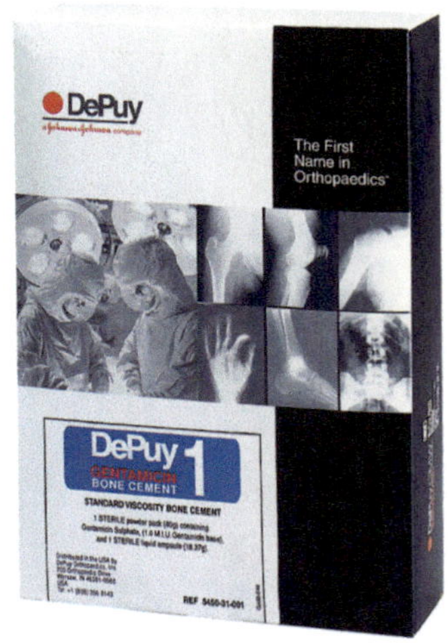

Figure 19.7 Bone cement with gentamicin. Courtesy of DePuy Orthopaedics, Inc.

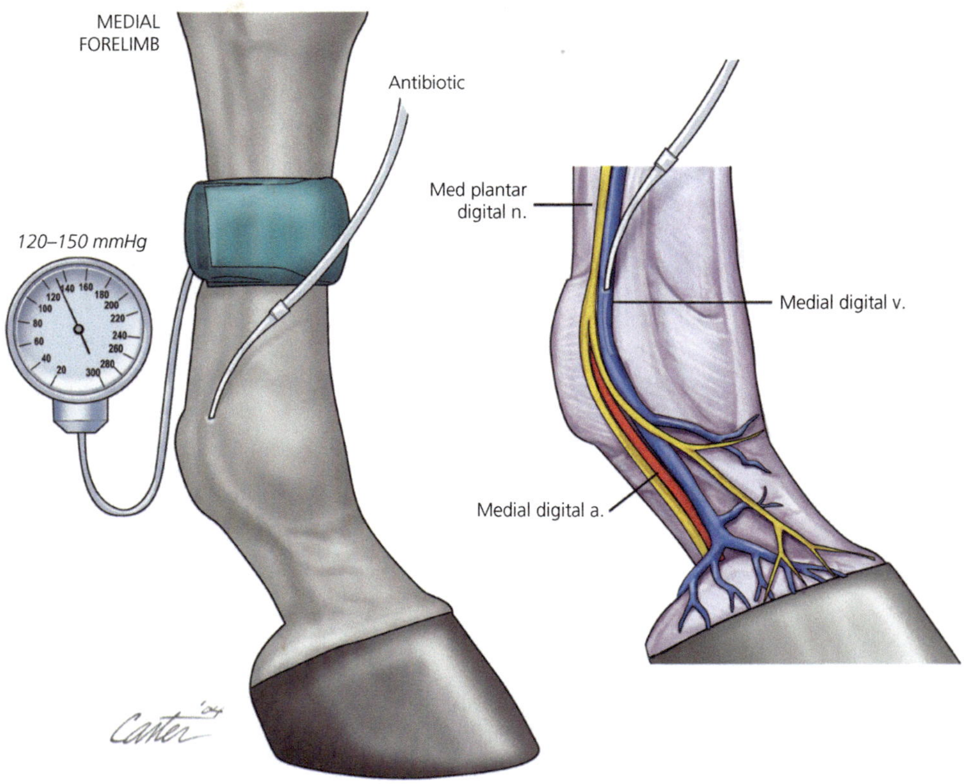

Figure 19.6 Intravenous regional perfusion for the metacarpo/metatarsophalangeal, proximal, and distal interphalangeal joints. Source: Orsini 2004.[48] Reproduced with permission of Elsevier.

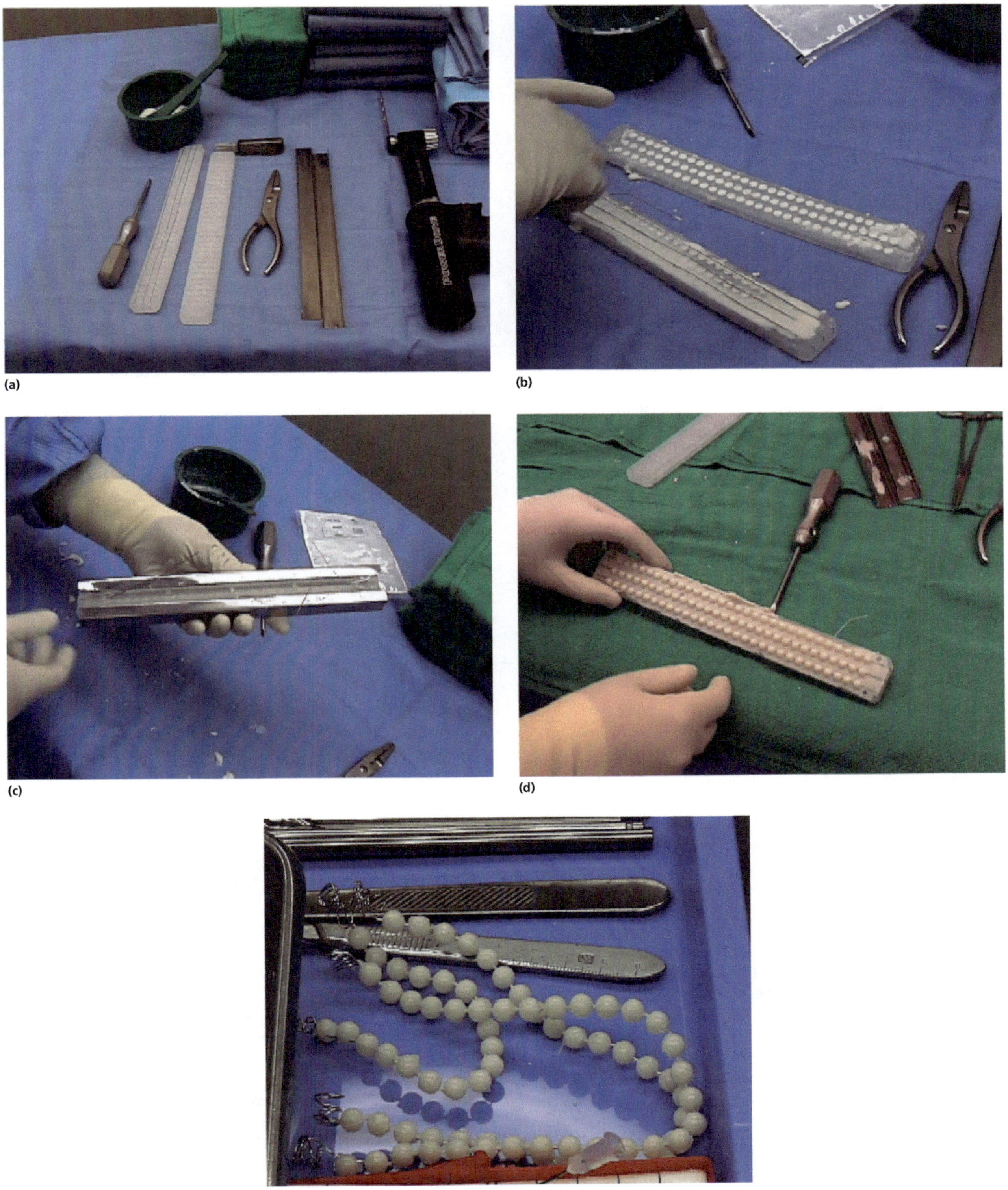

Figure 19.8 **(a–e)** Fabrication of antibiotic-impregnated PMMA beads. Courtesy of Schmidt AH, Tsukayama DT, Wickhind B, Midwest Orthopedic Research Foundation, Minneapolis.

Box 19.2 Regional limb perfusion with antibiotics

Overview

The antibiotic is delivered to the site of infection via the regional vasculature, using intravenous (IV) or intraosseous (IO) administration (see Boxes 19.3 and 19.4, respectively). Tourniquets confine the antibiotic to the perfused area for 30 minutes (see Box 19.5), thereby creating local concentrations of the antibiotic in tissues and fluids that greatly exceed those achieved with systemic administration. Thus, regional perfusion is most effective with concentration-dependent antibiotics, such as aminoglycosides, although it may also be effective with time-dependent antibiotics such as penicillins and cephalosporins (see Table 19.4 for drugs and dosages).

Advantages

- Uses a lower dose than does systemic therapy with the same drug, yet achieves a higher antibiotic concentration at the site of infection, so maximizes efficacy of treatment while minimizing the cost of the drug and the risks for toxicity and development of antibiotic resistance.
- Therapeutic concentrations can be achieved even in wounds with poorly perfused or necrotic tissue, as the drug diffuses down a concentration gradient from the vascular space to the interstitial space.
- For susceptible pathogens, a single treatment may be adequate (in concert with systemic antibiotic therapy).
- May be performed with the horse standing (although site preparation for IO perfusion may need to be performed with the horse anesthetized).
- Use of an indwelling catheter (IV) or cannula (IO) allows repeated perfusion with relative ease with the horse standing.
- Site options are not limited to the wound area: IV perfusion into the cephalic/saphenous vein may be used to treat infections of the distal aspect of the limb when swelling precludes use of a more proximal vein; and provided that a tourniquet effectively occludes venous outflow proximal to the wound, IV or IO perfusion may be performed either proximal or distal to the site of infection, depending on ease of access.

Disadvantages

- Both routes of administration are limited to wounds at or below the carpus/tarsus because a tourniquet must be applied proximal to the site.
- IV perfusion is difficult or impossible when soft-tissue swelling obscures the desired vein.
- There is potential for phlebitis and local tissue necrosis with IV perfusion, particularly when repeated or if perivascular leakage occurs.
- Preparation of the IO site may require that the horse be anesthetized, as it involves drilling a hole through cortical bone into the medullary cavity.
- There is limited residual effect (hours) after the tourniquet is removed (whereas antibiotic-impregnated implants may continuously deliver the drug for several days or weeks).

Box 19.3 Performing IV regional limb perfusion

Overview

An IV catheter is placed in the selected vein, and tourniquets are applied to isolate the site (see Box 19.5). The antibiotic, diluted in a suitable volume of sterile isotonic saline solution, is infused into the vein, and the tourniquets are left in place for 30 minutes; the tourniquets and catheter are then removed. An indwelling IV catheter may be used if repeated perfusion is anticipated.

Catheter and tourniquet sites

The smaller the perfused area, the smaller the drug dose and infusion volume needed to achieve a therapeutic antibiotic concentration at the site of infection. So, when placing the tourniquet(s), the goal is to isolate just the infected area and nearby vein. However, when swelling obscures the desired vein, more distant veins can be used (with larger infusion volumes and/or drug doses). Perfusion of the distal aspect of the limb may be achieved via a palmar/plantar digital vein or via the cephalic/saphenous vein, with a single tourniquet placed proximal to the wound and catheter site (metacarpus/metatarsus or distal aspect of the radius/tibia, respectively). Proximal to the pastern, the infection site may be isolated by placing a pair of tourniquets proximal and distal to the wound and site of catheterization.

Perfusion volumes

Common volumes used are 20–30 mL for perfusion of the digit via a digital vein, 60 mL for larger areas (carpus/tarsus, distal aspect of the limb), and up to 100 mL for distal limb perfusion via the cephalic/saphenous vein. However, lower perfusion volumes with higher drug doses may be equally effective. For example, perfusion of the distal aspect of the limb with 500 mg of gentamicin via a palmar digital vein (tourniquet at proximal aspect of the metacarpus) resulted in comparable gentamicin concentrations in the metacarpophalangeal joint for 10-mL, 30-mL, and 60-mL total perfusion volumes, with a trend for higher concentrations after the 10-mL perfusion volume.[117] Lower perfusion volumes may also reduce the risk of extravascular leakage and perivascular inflammation caused by high hydrostatic pressures associated with large volumes.

Materials

- Antibiotic dose (see Table 19.4), diluted in suitable volume of sterile 0.9% saline solution.
- Sedation, the drug(s) and dosage(s) dictated by the horse's temperament and severity of pain.
- Lidocaine, sufficient for perineural anesthesia (unless the procedure is performed with the horse anesthetized).
- Clippers, surgical scrub, isopropyl alcohol, roll cotton or gauze swabs for surgical skin preparation.
- Sterile gloves (optional, but recommended).
- Sterile IV catheter; use butterfly or short over-the-needle catheter for single treatment, use indwelling IV catheter for repeated treatment; select catheter gauge and length according to vein diameter and contour.
- Mini extension tube with stopcock or catheter cap, primed with perfusion solution.
- Adhesive tape or tissue glue for securing the catheter to the skin during the procedure (lasts at least 30 minutes).
- Tourniquet(s), one or two (see Box 19.5).
- Sterile dressing and bandage materials for light pressure wrap after catheter removal.

Steps

1. Sedate the horse and desensitize the catheter site and perfusion area with regional anesthesia. Perineural anesthesia (e.g., palmar nerve block for digital perfusion via a palmar digital vein) improves patient comfort and reduces movement during perfusion. A ring block may be used for areas with complex or deep innervation.
2. Clip and aseptically prepare the skin as for routine IV catheterization.
3. Insert the catheter into the vein (directed distally if possible), attach the extension tube, and fix the hub of the catheter to the skin with adhesive tape or a drop of glue.
4. Apply the tourniquet(s), as discussed in Box 19.5. (Steps 3 and 4 may be switched, but because the tourniquet must be removed after 30 minutes, and inserting and securing the catheter may take several minutes, it is best to place and secure the catheter before applying the tourniquet.)
5. Allow blood to flow freely from the extension tube until it slows to a drip, or aspirate an equal volume of blood as the infusion volume. (This step reduces hydrostatic pressure during infusion, which reduces the risk of extravascular leakage and perivascular inflammation.)
6. Slowly infuse the antibiotic solution over 1–2 minutes, then empty the extension line into the catheter with a small bolus of air to ensure that the entire drug dose is infused. (Avoid injecting air into the vein.)
7. After a total of 30 minutes, remove the tourniquet(s).
8. Unless using an indwelling catheter for repeated perfusion at a later time, remove the catheter, apply digital pressure over the venipuncture site for a few minutes, then cover with a sterile dressing and light pressure wrap. Aftercare for an indwelling catheter is the same as for IV catheterization at any other site.

Minor perivascular swelling may be present for 24–48 hours after catheter removal, but no other adverse effects are seen in most cases. Use of a topical NSAID (e.g., 1% diclofenac liposomal cream)[127] may be of value if an indwelling catheter was not placed and the site may need to be used again.

Box 19.4 Performing IO regional limb perfusion

Overview

Using regional or general anesthesia, a small hole is drilled percutaneously through the cortex of the bone with the largest and most accessible medullary cavity nearest the wound (e.g., distal aspect of tibia or proximal third of the metatarsus for IO perfusion of the tarsus). Choose a site that lies just under the skin, requiring little or no dissection to access. With tourniquets occluding blood flow proximally and distally, the antibiotic, diluted in sterile isotonic saline solution, is slowly infused into the medullary cavity, from where it is absorbed into the regional vasculature. The tourniquets are removed after 30 minutes. Perfusion may be repeated, if necessary, by seating a hollow bone screw in the hole and protecting the site with a catheter cap and sterile bandage between treatments.

Materials

- Antibiotic dose (see Table 19.4), diluted in 60 mL sterile isotonic saline solution.
- Sedation and lidocaine or other local anesthetic agent (unless the procedure is performed with the horse anesthetized); draw up enough lidocaine for regional anesthesia and an additional 2–3 mL for infusion into the medullary cavity.
- Clippers, surgical scrub, isopropyl alcohol, roll cotton or gauze swabs for surgical skin preparation.
- Sterile surgical gloves.
- Sterile scalpel, sterile hemostat (optional, but useful for keeping the skin incision open while the hole is drilled and the cannula is inserted).
- Power drill and sterile drill bit, size-appropriate for the cannula selected.
- Sterile cannula: bone marrow needle (single treatment) or hollow bone screw (multiple treatments); the catheter end of an IV extension set may be seated directly into the drill hole, but leakage is more likely to occur with this method.
- Mini extension tube with stopcock or catheter cap, primed with perfusion solution.
- Sterile catheter cap to occlude the injection port after infusion if a hollow bone screw is used.
- Suture material (optional; the incision may be left open to heal by second intention).
- Sterile dressing and bandage materials for protective wrap.
- Tourniquets, two (one each for proximal and distal to the infusion site).

Steps

1. Unless performed with the horse anesthetized, sedate the horse and desensitize the drill site using regional anesthesia (nerve or ring block, as appropriate).
2. Clip and aseptically prepare the skin as for a routine surgical procedure.
3. Wearing sterile gloves, make a 1 cm long incision through skin, subcutis, and periosteum over the infusion site, taking care to avoid other structures (nerves, vessels, tendons, etc.).
4. Drill a pilot hole through the bone cortex into the medullary cavity.
5. Insert the cannula such that it provides direct access to the medullary cavity; attach the extension tube.
6. Apply the tourniquets proximally and distally (see Box 19.5).
7. For standing horses, infuse 2–3 mL of local anesthetic solution into the medullary cavity; this step reduces discomfort caused by the increase in intramedullary pressure during infusion.
8. Slowly infuse the antibiotic solution into the medullary cavity over 10 minutes.
9. Remove the tourniquet 30 minutes after completing the infusion.
10. If planning to repeat IO infusion, cap the port in the bone screw and cover with a sterile dressing and protective bandage; otherwise, remove the cannula and either close the skin incision primarily or leave it open to heal by second intention. In either case, cover the site with a sterile dressing and light pressure wrap.

Localized soft-tissue swelling can be expected at the site for a few days after IO perfusion, as can a small amount of serosanguinous discharge when the incision is not closed primarily, but no treatment other than basic postsurgical wound care is needed.

Box 19.5 Applying tourniquets for regional limb perfusion

Overview

Whether using a single tourniquet proximal to the perfusion site or a pair of tourniquets placed proximally and distally to isolate the site, the tourniquet is applied firmly and then secured so that it occludes venous outflow for the duration of the procedure (30 minutes). A tourniquet that is applied too loosely or that loosens allows the antibiotic to exit the perfused area before the procedure is completed, defeating the purpose of achieving locally high antibiotic concentrations at the site of infection.

Materials

- Esmarch bandage or pneumatic tourniquet, one or two (depending on the site).[114,128]
- *Note:* narrow rubber tourniquets and elastic bandages are not suitable for this procedure.
- Adhesive tape or bandage (e.g., Elastikon®) to secure the Esmarch bandage after application.
  The ties or other fasteners on the Esmarch bandage are not reliable alone.

Notes

- Where possible, use a pair of tourniquets (proximal and distal) to isolate the wound and catheter/cannula site.
- The proximal tourniquet prevents escape of the antibiotic into the systemic circulation during perfusion.
- The distal tourniquet limits the volume of tissue being perfused, and thus dilution of the antibiotic in the extracellular fluid.
- For wounds at or distal to the metacarpo/metatarsophalangeal joint, use a single tourniquet placed proximal to the site.
- If using a palmar/plantar digital vein for IV perfusion, apply the tourniquet in the mid metacarpal/tarsal region.
- If having to use the cephalic/saphenous vein because of local swelling, apply the tourniquet to the distal aspect of the radius/tibia.
- If performing IO perfusion into the third metacarpal/metatarsal bone (MC/MT3), apply the tourniquet to the proximal metacarpal/metatarsal region (IO site in distal aspect of MC/MT3) or to the distal aspect of the radius/tibia (IO site in proximal aspect of MC/MT3).
- Leave the tourniquet(s) in place for no more than 30 minutes.
- Prepare the site, insert the catheter/cannula, and attach the extension tube before applying the tourniquets.
- Infuse the antibiotic solution immediately after applying and securing the tourniquets.

Box 19.6 Making antibiotic-impregnated PMMA beads

Overview

A suitable antibiotic is mixed with PMMA, which is then formed into small beads around a length of suture material. The beads are placed into the wound, where they steadily release the antibiotic into the surrounding fluid and tissue for several days or weeks. Locally high antibiotic concentrations are sustained in the wound, which may allow discontinuation of systemic antibiotic therapy. Antibiotic-impregnated PMMA beads are particularly useful for wounds that have a poor blood supply and for those containing surgical implants that must remain in place. They may also be useful for infected wounds in intractable patients that make other forms of antibiotic delivery and wound care difficult or impossible.

Materials

- Antibiotic dose (see Table 19.4), preferably in lyophilized form.
- PMMA kit (dry polymer and liquid monomer).
- Braided polyester suture material, size 0; use three strands (for easy implantation and removal of the beads).
- Bead mold that forms 6-mm diameter beads (optional, but recommended).
- Gloves.

Steps

1. Mix the antibiotic with the dry PMMA polymer at a rate of 1–4 g of antibiotic to 20 g of polymer. (If using more than one antibiotic for wound treatment, make a separate batch of beads for each antibiotic.)
2. Add the liquid monomer in a powder-to-liquid ratio of 2:1, and mix thoroughly for 1 minute.
3. If using a bead mold, lay the strands of suture material over one half of the mold, fill both halves of the mold with the PMMA mixture, close the mold, clamp it tightly, and allow the beads to harden for at least 10 minutes.
4. If not using a bead mold, hand-roll the PMMA into small beads as the material begins to set; make the beads an appropriate size and shape (spherical or cylindrical) for the wound and either form them around the suture material or create a hole through the center of the bead through which the suture may be threaded (like sinkers on fishing line); then put the beads aside to harden for at least 10 minutes.
5. Either use the beads immediately or store them in a sterile, airtight container away from direct light until needed.

Box 19.7 Using antibiotic-impregnated PMMA beads

Implanting and securing the beads

The size and number of antibiotic-impregnated PMMA beads implanted in a wound are determined by the dimensions of the wound. Unless the beads are being implanted while the horse is anesthetized, the horse is sedated and local or regional anesthesia is used as appropriate. The beads may be held in place by partially suturing the wound or by maintaining a sterile dressing over the wound.

Removing the beads

The PMMA beads do not biodegrade, so they may need to be removed after treatment, depending on the type of wound, ease of bead removal, and likelihood of them causing functional impairment if left in place. Removing the beads can be difficult after about 10 days because they become encapsulated by granulation or fibrous tissue as the wound heals. The beads may be left in place unless they are causing persistent drainage (foreign body reaction), are likely to interfere with future athletic function, or need to be replaced with fresh antibiotic-impregnated beads.

Note: Intrasynovial use is not advisable because it may cause synovial irritation and pain; but if used, the beads should be removed as soon as the infection is resolved, and at most in <10 days.

Note: Some authors correctly use "intramedullary" instead of "intraosseous" when describing regional perfusion into the medullary cavity; but to avoid confusion with abbreviations, we have chosen to use intraosseous (IO) instead of intramedullary (IM).

Duration of treatment

A final component of effective antibiotic therapy is duration of treatment, which is primarily dictated by the patient's response to therapy. The following criteria indicate a positive response:

- reduction and, ultimately, resolution of the signs of inflammation and purulent discharge;
- resolution of systemic signs of inflammation (note: absence of fever is not a reliable indicator of response to therapy for horses receiving NSAIDs);
- continued improvement in comfort and function;
- negative culture result;
- normal rate of wound healing.

According to the recent American College of Veterinary Internal Medicine concensus statement, "A common misconception is the need to complete a minimum duration of an antimicrobial drug to prevent the emergence of resistance. The Committee is aware of no foundation to this and antimicrobials should never be continued once there is clinical and microbiologic evidence that an infection has been eliminated or once an alternate diagnosis has been made, simply because of a perceived need for a minimum duration of administration."[129]

Response to treatment is dependent on many different factors and, therefore, can vary greatly among patients. Nevertheless, some useful generalizations can be made, as summarized in Table 19.5.

Wounds involving the gastrointestinal tract are particularly challenging for many reasons: the potential for formation of an abscess populated with anaerobes; the many recesses for bacterial sequestration, which make thorough lavage of the peritoneal cavity impossible in adult horses; the frequency with which multidrug-resistant Gram-negative aerobes are found in the equine intestine; and the necessity for parenteral antibiotic therapy to achieve effective concentrations of the antibiotic at the site of infection. For these reasons, systemic antibiotic therapy (parenteral initially) must be continued for weeks in most cases. Despite its limitations, peritoneal lavage and drainage are worthwhile, as much for removal of inflammatory cytokines and fibrin as for removal of bacteria. Active (closed-suction) abdominal lavage and drainage performed with the horse standing have been described.[130]

What to do

- Monitor the horse frequently (at least once daily initially) until the infection is resolved. A positive response should be seen within a few days, even though complete resolution may take much longer.
- Continue antibiotic therapy until signs of infection have resolved completely and wound healing is proceeding as expected.
- If improvement is not seen within 3 or 4 days of starting or changing treatment:
  - review the case; check that the antibiotic is being administered as directed;
  - repeat the physical examination and routine blood work;
  - further explore and debride the wound, as needed.
- Repeat bacterial culture and antibiotic sensitivity testing if, at any point, recovery is not proceeding as expected.
  - Reculture the wound if response to treatment is poor.
  - Reculture if signs of infection recur during therapy or after therapy has concluded.
  - Reculture during prolonged antibiotic therapy (weeks or months).
  - Reculture within a week of discontinuing antibiotic therapy if the infection was polymicrobial or it involved multidrug-resistant organisms.
- Adjust the treatment plan accordingly.

Table 19.5 Guidelines for duration of antibiotic therapy in specific types of wounds.

Tissue involved	Guidelines for antibiotic therapy
Wounds (general)	*Staphylococcus* sp. infections tend to be insidious in onset and incite a chronic inflammatory response, so therapy is typically required for weeks; base discontinuation of therapy on health of affected tissues and negative culture results *Streptococcus* sp. infections typically are more antibiotic sensitive, so treatment generally is shorter (10–14 days)
Synovial structure	Usually require treatment for weeks using a combination of methods: • Systemic, parenteral initially; depending on sensitivity results, may be switched to oral administration after substantial improvement is seen • Intrasynovial lavage and antibiotic infusion; repeated if needed • ± Regional perfusion (IV or IO) for wounds at or distal to the carpus/tarsus; repeated if needed
Bone or physeal cartilage	Usually require treatment for weeks or months using a combination of methods: • Systemic, parenteral initially; depending on sensitivity results, may be switched to oral administration after substantial improvement is seen • Regional perfusion (IV or IO) for wounds at or distal to the carpus/tarsus; repeated if needed • Antibiotic-impregnated PMMA beads; particularly important when complete debridement is not possible or when a surgical implant must remain • Repeated surgical debridement may also be needed
Respiratory tract	Often respond quickly, needing only a short course of treatment (5–10 days) When chest wounds are complicated by septic pleuritis, treatment for months may be required and must include pleural lavage and drainage
Intestinal tract	Systemic antibiotic therapy is needed for weeks in most cases (see text) Peritoneal lavage and drainage are also important with septic peritonitis
Muscle	Wounds typically respond very well, needing only a short course of treatment (5–10 days) Open drainage is easy at most sites and speeds resolution, particularly with IM abscesses Clostridial myonecrosis can rapidly cause severe systemic illness, but with aggressive surgical debridement and aeration, local and systemic antibiotic therapy usually is successful within days

Abbreviations: IM, intramuscular; IV, intravenous; IO, intraosseous; PMMA, polymethylmethacrylate.

What to avoid

- Avoid relying on results of the initial culture for the duration of treatment.
- Avoid staying with the present treatment plan when signs of infection are not resolving. Although patience is a virtue, monitor these wounds closely and be prepared to review and revise the treatment plan at any time.

Tip

Watch for signs of *laminitis* in the following situations:

- injury or infection that causes a non-weight-bearing lameness in one limb (creates high risk for laminitis in the contralateral supporting limb);
- infection accompanied by marked systemic inflammation (systemic inflammatory response syndrome, or SIRS).

Next step

After the infection is resolved, the various methods for enhancing wound healing discussed elsewhere in this book can be considered. Depending on availability and on the nature and location of the wound, these methods include delayed closure with sutures, NPWT, and topical application of growth factors, biomaterials/scaffolds, stem cells, and a skin graft.

References

1. Hartmann FA, Trostle SS, Klohnen AA. Isolation of methicillin-resistant *Staphylococcus aureus* from a postoperative wound infection in a horse. *J Am Vet Med Assoc* 1997; **211**: 590.
2. O'Mahony R, Abbott Y, Leonard FC, *et al.* Methicillin-resistant *Staphylococcus aureus* (MRSA) isolated from animals and veterinary personnel in Ireland. *Vet Microbiol* 2005; **109**: 285.
3. Bergström K, Bengtsson B, Nyman A, *et al.* Longitudinal study of horses for carriage of methicillin-resistant *Staphylococcus aureus* following wound infections. *Vet Microbiol* 2013; **163**: 388.
4. Schwaber MJ, Navon-Venezia S, Masarwa S, *et al.* Clonal transmission of a rare methicillin-resistant *Staphylococcus aureus* genotype between horses and staff at a veterinary teaching hospital. *Vet Microbiol* 2013; **162**: 907.
5. Vincze S, Stamm I, Kopp PA, *et al.* Alarming proportions of methicillin-resistant *Staphylococcus aureus* (MRSA) in wound samples from companion animals, Germany 2010–2012. *PLoS One* 2014; **9**: e85656.
6. Trostle SS, Peavey CL, King DS, *et al.* Treatment of methicillin-resistant *Staphylococcus epidermidis* infection following repair of an ulnar fracture and humeroradial joint luxation in a horse. *J Am Vet Med Assoc* 2001; **218**: 554.
7. Bagcigil FA, Moodley A, Baptiste KE, *et al.* Occurrence, species distribution, and antimicrobial resistance and clonality of methicillin- and erythromycin-resistant staphylococci in the nasal cavity of domestic animals. *Vet Microbiol* 2007; **121**: 307.
8. Corrente M, D'Abramo M, Latronico F, *et al.* Methicillin-resistant coagulase negative staphylococci isolated from horses. *New Microbiol* 2009; **32**: 311.
9. Kern A, Perreten V. Clinical and molecular features of methicillin-resistant, coagulase-negative staphylococci of pets and horses. *J Antimicrob Chemother* 2013; **68**: 1256.
10. de Niederhäusern S, Sabia C, Messi P, *et al.* VanA-type vancomycin-resistant enterococci in equine and swine rectal swabs and in human clinical samples. *Curr Microbiol* 2007; **55**: 240.
11. Lauková A, Simonová M, Strompfová V, *et al.* Potential of enterococci isolated from horses. *Anaerobe* 2008; **14**: 234.
12. Singh BR. Prevalence of vancomycin resistance and multiple drug resistance in enterococci in equids in North India. *J Infect Dev Ctries* 2009; **3**: 498.
13. Moura I, Radhouani H, Torres C, *et al.* Detection and genetic characterisation of vanA-containing Enterococcus strains in healthy Lusitano horses. *Equine Vet J* 2010; **42**: 181.
14. Gordoncillo MJ, Donabedian S, Bartlett PC, *et al.* Isolation and molecular characterization of vancomycin-resistant *Enterococcus faecium* from swine in Michigan, USA. *Zoonoses Public Health* 2013; **60**: 319.
15. Moellering RC Jr. The specter of glycopeptide resistance: current trends and future considerations. *Am J Med* 1998; **104**: 3S.
16. Sasidharan S, Prema B, Yoga LL. Antimicrobial drug resistance of *Staphylococcus aureus* in dairy products. *Asian Pac J Trop Biomed* 2011; **1**: 130.
17. Aminzadeh Z, Yadegarynia D, Fatemi A, *et al.* Vancomycin minimum inhibitory concentration for methicillin-resistant *Staphylococcus aureus* infections; is there difference in mortality between patients? *Jundishapur J Microbiol* 2014; **7**: e12831.
18. Koch G, Yepes A, Förstner KU, *et al.* Evolution of resistance to a last-resort antibiotic in *Staphylococcus aureus* via bacterial competition. *Cell* 2014; **158**: 1060.
19. Sternberg S, Greko C, Olsson-Liljequist B. Antimicrobial susceptibility of equine isolates of *Actinobacillus* spp. and identification of beta-lactamases in some strains. *Microb Drug Resist* 1999; **5**: 289.
20. Smith MA, Ross MW. Postoperative infection with *Actinobacillus* spp in horses: 10 cases (1995–2000). *J Am Vet Med Assoc* 2002; **221**: 1306.
21. Orsini JA, Benson CE, Spencer PA, *et al.* Resistance to gentamicin and amikacin of gram-negative organisms isolated from horses. *Am J Vet Res* 1989; **50**: 923.
22. Jack SS, Giguère S, Nguyen A. *In vitro* susceptibilities of *Rhodococcus equi* and other common equine pathogens to azithromycin, clarithromycin, and 20 other antimicrobials. *Antimicrob Agents Chemotherap* 2003; **47**: 1742.
23. Dunowska M, Morley PS, Traub-Dargatz JL, *et al.* Impact of hospitalization and antimicrobial drug administration on antimicrobial susceptibility patterns of commensal *Escherichia coli* isolated from the feces of horses. *J Am Vet Med Assoc* 2006; **228**: 1909.
24. Vo AT, van Duijkeren E, Fluit AC, *et al.* Characteristics of extended-spectrum cephalosporin-resistant *Escherichia coli* and *Klebsiella pneumoniae* isolates from horses. *Vet Microbiol* 2007; **124**: 248.
25. Hariharan H, McPhee L, Heaney S, *et al.* Antimicrobial drug susceptibility of clinical isolates of *Pseudomonas aeruginosa*. *Can Vet J* 1995; **36**: 166.
26. Sauer P, Andrew SE, Lassaline M, *et al.* Changes in antibiotic resistance in equine bacterial ulcerative keratitis (1991–2000): 65 horses. *Vet Ophthalmol* 2003; **6**: 309.
27. Peyrou M, Higgins R, Lavoie JP. Evolution of bacterial resistance to certain antibacterial agents in horses in a veterinary hospital. [Article in French] *Can Vet J* 2003; **44**: 978.
28. Schnellmann C, Gerber V, Rossano A, *et al.* Presence of new mecA and mph(C) variants conferring antibiotic resistance in Staphylococcus spp. isolated from the skin of horses before and after clinic admission. *J Clin Microbiol* 2006; **44**: 4444.

29. Williams A, Christley RM, McKane SA, *et al.* Antimicrobial resistance changes in enteric *Escherichia coli* of horses during hospitalisation: resistance profiling of isolates. *Vet J* 2013; **195**: 121.
30. Ewers C, Stamm I, Pfeifer Y, *et al.* Clonal spread of highly successful ST15-CTX-M-15 *Klebsiella pneumoniae* in companion animals and horses. *J Antimicrob Chemother* 2014; **69**: 2676.
31. Theelen MJ, Wilson WD, Edman JM, *et al.* Temporal trends in *in vitro* antimicrobial susceptibility patterns of bacteria isolated from foals with sepsis: 1979–2010. *Equine Vet J* 2014; **46**: 161.
32. Clutterbuck AL, Woods EJ, Knottenbelt DC, *et al.* Biofilms and their relevance to veterinary medicine. *Vet Microbiol* 2007; **121**: 1.
33. Jacques M, Aragon V, Tremblay YDN. Biofilm formation in bacterial pathogens of veterinary importance. *Anim Health Res Rev* 2010; **11**: 97.
34. Wolcott RD, Rhoads DD, Dowd SE. Biofilms and chronic wound inflammation. *J Wound Care* 2008; **17**: 333.
35. Philips PL, Wolcott RD, Fletcher J, *et al.* Biofilms made easy. *Wounds International* 2010; **1**: 1.
35a. Percival SL, Vuotto C, Donelli G, *et al.* Biofilms and wounds: an identification algorithm and potential treatment options. *Adv Wound Care* 2015; **4**: 389.
36. Rhoads DD, Wolcott RD, Percival SL. Biofilms in wounds: management strategies. *J Wound Care* 2008; **17**: 502.
37. Wolcott RD, Kennedy JP, Dowd SE. Regular debridement is the main tool for maintaining a healthy wound bed in most chronic wounds. *J Wound Care* 2009; **18**: 54.
38. Millward TA, Wilson M. The effect of chlorhexidine on *Streptococcus sanguis* biofilms. *Microbios* 1989; **58**: 155.
39. Voermans M, van Soest JM, van Duijkeren E, *et al.* Clinical efficacy of intravenous administration of marbofloxacin in a *Staphylococcus aureus* infection in tissue cages in ponies. *J Vet Pharmacol Ther* 2006; **29**: 555.
40. Yi L, Wang Y, Ma Z, *et al.* Biofilm formation of *Streptococcus equi* ssp. *zooepidemicus* and comparative proteomic analysis of biofilm and planktonic cells. *Curr Microbiol* 2014; **69**: 227.
41. Freeman K, Woods E, Welsby S, *et al.* Biofilm evidence and the microbial diversity of horse wounds. *Can J Microbiol* 2009; **55**: 197.
42. Westgate SJ, Percival SL, Knottenbelt DC, *et al.* Microbiology of equine wounds and evidence of bacterial biofilms. *Vet Microbiol* 2011; **150**: 152.
43. Bowering CK. Use of layered compression bandages in diabetic patients. Experience in patients with lower leg ulceration, peripheral edema, and features of venous and arterial disease. *Adv Wound Care* 1998; **11**: 129.
44. Petrisor B, Jeray K, Schemitsch E, *et al.* Fluid lavage in patients with open fracture wounds (FLOW): an international survey of 984 surgeons. *BMC Musculoskel Disord* 2008; **9**: 7.
45. FLOW Investigators, Petrisor B, Sun X, *et al.* Fluid lavage of open wounds (FLOW): a multicenter, blinded, factorial pilot trial comparing alternative irrigating solutions and pressures in patients with open fractures. *J Trauma* 2011; **71**: 596.
46. Bras R, Morrison S. Retrospective case series of 20 horses (2002–2009) sustaining puncture wounds to the navicular bursa with maggot debridement therapy as an adjunctive treatment. In: *Proceedings, 55th Annual Convention of the American Association of Equine Practitioners*. Las Vegas, NV, American Association of Equine Practitioners, 2009; **55**: 241.
47. Lepage OM, Doumbia A, Perron-Lepage MF, *et al.* The use of maggot debridement therapy in 41 equids. *Equine Vet J* Suppl 2012; **43**: 120.
48. Orsini JA, Elce Y, Kraus B. Management of severely infected wounds in the equine patient. *Clin Tech Equine Pract* 2004; **3**: 225.
49. Morykwas MJ, Argenta LC, Sheldon-Brown EI, *et al.* Vacuum-assisted closure: a new method for wound control and treatment: animal studies and basic foundation. *Ann Plast Surg* 1997; **38**: 553.
50. Argenta LC, Morykwas MJ. Vacuum-assisted closure: a new method for wound control and treatment: clinical experience. *Ann Plast Surg* 1997; **38**: 563.
51. Ben-Amotz R, Lanz OI, Miller JM, *et al.* The use of vacuum assisted closure therapy for the treatment of distal extremity wounds in 15 dogs. *Vet Surg* 2007; **36**: 684.
52. Demaria M, Stanley BJ, Hauptman JG, *et al.* Effects of negative pressure wound therapy on healing of open wounds in dogs. *Vet Surg* 2011; **40**: 658.
53. Buote NJ, Havig ME. The use of vacuum-assisted closure in the management of septic peritonitis in six dogs. *J Am Anim Hosp Assoc* 2012; **48**: 164.
54. Cioffi KM, Schmiedt CW, Cornell KK, *et al.* Retrospective evaluation of vacuum assisted peritoneal drainage for the treatment of septic peritonitis in dogs and cats: 8 cases (2003–2010). *J Vet Emerg Crit Care* 2012; **22**: 601.
55. Bertran J, Farrell M, Fitzpatrick N. Successful wound healing over exposed metal implants using vacuum-assisted wound closure in a dog. *J Small Anim Pract* 2013; **54**: 381.
56. Pitt KA, Stanley BJ. Negative pressure wound therapy: experience in 45 dogs. *Vet Surg* 2014; **43**: 380.
57. Nolff MC, Fehr M, Bolling A, *et al.* Negative pressure wound therapy, silver coated foam dressing and conventional bandages in open wound treatment in dogs. *Vet Comp Orthop Traumatol* 2015; **28**: 30.
58. Gemeinhardt KD, Molnar JA. Vacuum-assisted closure for management of a traumatic neck wound in a horse. *Equine Vet Educ* 2005; **17**: 27.
59. Morgan M. Methicillin-resistant *Staphylococcus aureus* and animals: zoonosis or humanosis? *J Antimicrob Chemother* 2008; **62**: 1181.
60. König L, Klopfleisch R, Kershaw O, *et al.* Prevalence of biofilms on surgical suture segments in wounds of dogs, cats, and horses. *Vet Pathol* 2015; **52**: 295.
61. Booth TM, Abbot J, Clements A, *et al.* Treatment of septic common digital extensor tenosynovitis by complete resection in seven horses. *Vet Surg* 2004; **33**: 107.
62. Vaudaux P, Waldvogel FA. Gentamicin inactivation in purulent exudates: role of cell lysis. *J Infect Dis* 1980; **142**: 586.
63. Seth AK, Geringer MR, Guriala AN, *et al.* Treatment of *Pseudomonas aeruginosa* biofilm-infected wounds with clinical wound care strategies: a quantitative study using an *in vivo* rabbit ear model. *Plast Reconstr Surg* 2012; **129**: 262e.
64. Tóth T, Broström H, Båverud V, *et al.* Evaluation of LHP® (1% hydrogen peroxide) cream versus petrolatum and untreated controls in open wounds in healthy horses: a randomized, blinded control study. *Acta Vet Scand* 2011; **53**: 45.
65. Bischofberger AS, Dart CM, Perkins NR, *et al.* The effect of short- and long-term treatment with manuka honey on second intention healing of contaminated and noncontaminated wounds on the distal aspect of the forelimbs in horses. *Vet Surg* 2013; **42**: 154.
66. Carnwath R, Graham EM, Reynolds K, *et al.* The antimicrobial activity of honey against common equine wound bacterial isolates. *Vet J* 2014; **199**: 110.

67. Adams AP, Santschi EM, Mellencamp MA. Antibacterial properties of a silver chloride-coated nylon wound dressing. *Vet Surg* 1999; **28**: 219.
68. Dmitrieva NA, Zyrianova NV, Grigor'ian AS, *et al.* Microflora dynamics in purulent skin wounds in rats after ozonized perftorane applications. [Article in Russian] *Stomatologiia* (Mosk) 2009; **88**: 14.
69. Elvis AM, Ekta JS. Ozone therapy: a clinical review. *J Nat Sci Biol Med* 2011; **2**: 66.
70. Al-Saadi H, Potapova I, Rochford ET, *et al.* Ozonated saline shows activity against planktonic and biofilm growing *Staphylococcus aureus in vitro*: a potential irrigant for infected wounds. *Int Wound J* 2015; Jan 14. doi: 10.1111/iwj.12412 [Epub ahead of print].
71. Woods EJ, Cochrane CA, Percival S. Prevalence of silver resistance genes in bacteria isolated from human and horse wounds. *Vet Microbiol* 2009; **138**: 325.
72. Kostenko V, Lyczak J, Turner K, *et al.* Impact of silver-containing wound dressings on bacterial biofilm viability and susceptibility to antibiotics during prolonged treatment. *Antimicrob Agents Chemother* 2010; **54**: 5120.
73. Stinner DJ, Waterman SM, Masini BD, *et al.* Silver dressings augment the ability of negative pressure wound therapy to reduce bacteria in a contaminated open fracture model. *J Traumatol* 2011; **71**: S147.
74. Felts AG, Grainger DW, Slunt JB. Locally delivered antibodies combined with systemic antibiotics confer synergistic protection against antibiotic-resistant burn wound infection. *J Trauma* 2000; **49**: 873.
75. Bauer SM, Santschi EM, Fialkowski J, *et al.* Quantification of *Staphylococcus aureus* adhesion to equine bone surfaces passivated with Plasmalyte and hyperimmune plasma. *Vet Surg* 2004; **33**: 376.
76. López C, Carmona JU, Giraldo CE, *et al.* Bacteriostatic effect of equine pure platelet-rich plasma and other blood products against methicillin-sensitive *Staphylococcus aureus*. An *in vitro* study. *Vet Comp Orthop Traumatol* 2014; **27**: 372.
77. Ammons MC, Copié V. Lactoferrin: a bioinspired, anti-biofilm therapeutic. *Biofouling* 2013; **29**: 443.
78. Seth AK, Geringer MR, Ngyen KT, *et al.* Bacteriophage therapy for *Staphylococcus aureus* biofilm-infected wounds: a new approach to chronic wound care. *Plast Reconstr Surg* 2013; **131**: 225.
79. Goodrich LR. Osteomyelitis in horses. *Vet Clin North Am Equine Pract* 2006; **22**: 389.
80. Polderman KH. Mechanisms of action, physiological effects, and complications of hypothermia. *Crit Care Med* 2009; **37**: S186.
81. Geor RJ. Nutritional considerations for the colic patient. In: *Proceedings, Focus Meeting of the American Association of Equine Practitioners*. Quebec, QC, American Association of Equine Practitioners, 2005: 1.
82. Slovis N. Review of equine hyperbaric medicine. *J Equine Vet Sci* 2008; **28**: 760.
83. Holder TE, Schumacher J, Donnell RL, *et al.* Effects of hyperbaric oxygen on full-thickness meshed sheet skin grafts applied to fresh and granulating wounds in horses. *Am J Vet Res* 2008; **69**: 144.
84. Dhar M, Neilsen N, Beatty K, *et al.* Equine peripheral blood-derived mesenchymal stem cells: isolation, identification, trilineage differentiation and effect of hyperbaric oxygen treatment. *Equine Vet J* 2012; **44**: 600.
85. Huang HJ, Yu B, Lin QR, *et al.* Effect of ozone water on the inflammation and repair of infected wounds. [Article in Chinese] *Nan Fang Yi Ke Da Xue Xue Bao* 2010; **30**: 515.
86. Gulmen S, Kurtoglu T, Meteoglu I, *et al.* Ozone therapy as an adjunct to vancomycin enhances bacterial elimination in methicillin-resistant *Staphylococcus aureus* mediastinitis. *J Surg Res* 2013; **185**: 64.
87. *Code of Federal Regulations, Title 21, Volume 8, section 801.415, United States Food & Drug Administration, April 1*, 2015. http://www.accessdata.fda.gov/scripts/cdrh/cfdocs/cfcfr/CFRSearch.cfm?fr=801.415 (accessed April 18, 2016)
88. Schneider RK, Bramlage LR, Moore RM, *et al.* A retrospective study of 192 horses affected with septic arthritis/tenosynovitis. *Equine Vet J* 1992; **24**: 436.
89. MacDonald DG, Morley PS, Bailey JV, *et al.* An examination of the occurrence of surgical wound infection following equine orthopaedic surgery (1981–1990). *Equine Vet J* 1994; **6**: 323.
90. Hague BA, Honnas CM, Simpson BR, *et al.* Evaluation of skin bacterial flora before and after aseptic arthrocentesis in horses. *Vet Surg* 1997; **26**: 121.
91. Wilson WD. Rational selection of antimicrobials for use in horses. In: *Proceedings, 47th Annual Convention of the American Association of Equine Practitioners*. San Diego, CA, American Association of Equine Practitioners, 2001; **47**: 75.
92. Zubrod CJ, Farnsworth KD, Oaks JL. Evaluation of arthrocentesis site bacterial flora before and after 4 methods of preparation in horses with and without evidence of skin contamination. *Vet Surg* 2004; **33**: 525.
93. Adam EN, Southwood LL. Primary and secondary limb cellulitis in horses: 44 cases (2000–2006). *J Am Vet Med Assoc* 2007; **231**: 1696.
94. Clark C, Greenwood S, Boison JO, *et al.* Bacterial isolates from equine infections in western Canada (1998–2003). *Can Vet J* 2008; **49**: 153.
95. Russell CM, Axon JE, Blishen A, *et al.* Blood culture isolates and antimicrobial sensitivities from 427 critically ill neonatal foals. *Aust Vet J* 2008; **86**: 266.
96. Orsini JA, Snooks-Parsons, C, Stine L, *et al.* Vancomycin for the treatment of methicillin-resistant staphylococcal and enterococcal infections in 15 horses. *Can J Vet Res* 2005; **69**: 278.
97. Magdesian KG, Dujowich M, Madigan JE, *et al.* Molecular characterization of *Clostridium difficile* isolates from horses in an intensive care unit and association of disease severity with strain type. *J Am Vet Med Assoc* 2006; **228**: 751.
98. Caron JP, Bolin CA, Hauptman JG, *et al.* Minimum inhibitory concentration and postantibiotic effect of amikacin for equine isolates of methicillin-resistant *Staphylococcus aureus in vitro*. *Vet Surg* 2009; **38**: 664.
99. Erol E, Locke SJ, Donahoe JK, *et al.* Beta-hemolytic *Streptococcus* spp. from horses: a retrospective study (2000–2010). *J Vet Diagn Invest* 2012; **24**: 142.
100. Herdan CL, Acke E, Dicken M, *et al.* Multi-drug-resistant *Enterococcus* spp. as a cause of non-responsive septic synovitis in three horses. *N Z Vet J* 2012; **60**: 297.
101. Davis HA, Stanton MB, Thungrat K, *et al.* Uterine bacterial isolates from mares and their resistance to antimicrobials: 8,296 cases (2003–2008). *J Am Vet Med Assoc* 2013; **242**: 977.
102. Rubio-Martinez LM, Lopez-Sanroman J, Cruz AM, *et al.* Evaluation of safety and pharmacokinetics of vancomycin after intravenous regional limb perfusion in horses. *Am J Vet Res* 2005; **66**: 2107.

103. Rubio-Martinez LM, Lopez-Sanroman J, Cruz AM, *et al.* Medullary plasma pharmacokinetics of vancomycin after intravenous and intraosseous perfusion of the proximal phalanx in horses. *Vet Surg* 2005; **34**: 618.
104. Rubio-Martínez LM, López-Sanromán J, Cruz AM, *et al.* Evaluation of safety and pharmacokinetics of vancomycin after intraosseous regional limb perfusion and comparison of results with those obtained after intravenous regional limb perfusion in horses. *Am J Vet Res* 2006; **67**: 1701.
105. Orsini JA, Moate PJ, Boston RC, *et al.* Pharmacokinetics of imipenem-cilastatin following intravenous administration in healthy adult horses. *J Vet Pharmacol Ther* 2005; **28**: 355.
106. Ribera T, Prades M, Costa C, *et al.* Intra-synovial imipenem therapy in 4 horses with severe septic arthritis or tenosynovitis non-responsive to conventional treatment. *J Latinoamer de Med Vet de Emerg y Cuidad Intens* 2014; **6**: 106.
107. Haziz E, Tatz A, Britzi M, *et al.* Evaluation of the pharmacokinetics of imipenem following regional limb perfusion using the saphenous and the cephalic veins in standing horses. In: *Proceedings, European College of Veterinary Surgeons Annual Scientific Meeting.* Rome, Italy. European College of Veterinary Surgeons, 2013; 132.
108. Meagher DT, Latimer FG, Sutter WW, *et al.* Evaluation of a balloon constant rate infusion system for treatment of septic arthritis, septic tenosynovitis, and contaminated synovial wounds: 23 cases (2002–2005). *J Am Vet Med Assoc* 2006; **228**: 1930.
109. Santschi EM, Adams SB, Murphey ED. How to perform equine intravenous digital perfusion. In: *Proceedings, 44th Annual Convention of the American Association of Equine Practitioners.* Baltimore, MD, American Association of Equine Practitioners 1998; **44**: 198.
110. Scheuch BC, Van Hoogmoed LM, Wilson WD, *et al.* Comparison of intraosseous or intravenous infusion for delivery of amikacin sulfate to the tibiotarsal joint of horses. *Am J Vet Res* 2002; **63**: 374.
111. Pille F, de Baere S, Ceelen L, *et al.* Synovial fluid and plasma concentrations of ceftiofur after regional intravenous perfusion in the horse. *Vet Surg* 2005; **34**: 610.
112. Parra-Sanchez A, Lugo J, Boothe DM, *et al.* Pharmacokinetics and pharmacodynamics of enrofloxacin and a low dose of amikacin administered via regional intravenous limb perfusion in standing horses. *Am J Vet Res* 2006; **67**: 1687.
113. Kelmer G, Catasus CT, Saxton AM, *et al.* Evaluation of indwelling intravenous catheters for the regional perfusion of the limbs of horses. *Vet Rec* 2009; **165**: 496.
114. Levine DG, Epstein KL, Ahern BJ, *et al.* Efficacy of three tourniquet types for intravenous antimicrobial regional limb perfusion in standing horses. *Vet Surg* 2010; **39**: 1021.
115. Kelmer G, Tatz A, Bdolah-Abram T. Indwelling cephalic or saphenous vein catheter use for regional limb perfusion in 44 horses with synovial injury involving the distal aspect of the limb. *Vet Surg* 2012; **41**: 938.
116. Rubio-Martínez LM, Elmas CR, Black B, *et al.* Clinical use of antimicrobial regional limb perfusion in horses: 174 cases (1999–2009). *J Am Vet Med Assoc* 2012; **241**: 1650.
117. Hyde RM, Lynch TM, Clark CK, *et al.* The influence of perfusate volume on antimicrobial concentration in synovial fluid following intravenous regional limb perfusion in the standing horse. *Can Vet J* 2013; **54**: 363.
118. Kelmer G, Bell GC, Martin-Jimenez T, *et al.* Evaluation of regional limb perfusion with amikacin using the saphenous, cephalic, and palmar digital veins in standing horses. *J Vet Pharmacol Ther* 2013; **36**: 236.
119. Lallemand E, Trencart P, Tahier C, *et al.* Pharmacokinetics, pharmacodynamics and local tolerance at injection site of marbofloxacin administered by regional intravenous limb perfusion in standing horses. *Vet Surg* 2013; **42**: 649.
120. Blackford JT, Latimer FG, Valk N. How to make and use antibiotic-impregnated poly(methylmethacrylate) beads to treat infected wounds in horses. In: *Proceedings, 43rd Annual Convention of the American Association of Equine Practitioners.* Phoenix, AZ, American Association of Equine Practitioners 1997; **43**: 145.
121. Holcombe SJ, Schneider RK, Bramlage LR, *et al.* Use of antibiotic-impregnated polymethylmethacrylate in horses with open or infected fractures or joints: 19 cases (1987–1995). *J Am Vet Med Assoc* 1997; **211**: 889.
122. Summerhays GE. Treatment of traumatically induced synovial sepsis in horses with gentamicin-impregnated collagen sponges. *Vet Rec* 2000; **147**: 184.
123. Booth TM, Butson RJ, Clegg PD, *et al.* Treatment of sepsis in the small tarsal joints of 11 horses with gentamicin-impregnated polymethylmethacrylate beads. *Vet Rec* 2001; **148**: 376.
124. Farnsworth KD, White NA II, Robertson J. The effect of implanting gentamicin-impregnated polymethylmethacrylate beads in the tarsocrural joint of the horse. *Vet Surg* 2001; **30**: 126.
125. Swalec Tobias KM, Schneider RK, Besser TE. Use of antimicrobial-impregnated polymethyl methacrylate. *J Am Vet Med Assoc* 1996; **208**: 841.
126. Ivester KM, Adams SB, Moore GE, *et al.* Gentamicin concentrations in synovial fluid obtained from the tarsocrural joints of horses after implantation of gentamicin-impregnated collagen sponges. *Am J Vet Res* 2006; **67**: 1519.
127. Levine DG, Epstein KL, Neelis DA, *et al.* Effect of topical application of 1% diclofenac sodium liposomal cream on inflammation in healthy horses undergoing intravenous regional limb perfusion with amikacin sulfate. *Am J Vet Res* 2009; **70**: 1323.
128. Alkabes SB, Adams SB, Moore GE, *et al.* Comparison of two tourniquets and determination of amikacin sulfate concentrations after metacarpophalangeal joint lavage performed simultaneously with intravenous regional limb perfusion in horses. *Am J Vet Res* 2011; **72**: 613.
129. Weese JS, Giguère S, Guardabassi L, *et al.* ACVIM concensus statement on therapeutic antimicrobial use in animals and antimicrobial resistance. *J Vet Intern Med* 2015; **29**: 487.
130. Nieto JE, Snyder JR, Vatistas NJ, *et al.* Use of an active intra-abdominal drain in 67 horses. *Vet Surg* 2003; **32**: 1.

CHAPTER 20

Treatment of Burn Injuries, Gunshot Wounds, and Dog-Bite Wounds

R. Reid Hanson, DVM, Diplomate ACVS, ACVECC and Amelia S. Munsterman, DVM, MS, Diplomate ACVS, ACVECC

Chapter Contents

Summary

Burns and dog-bite wounds can be superficial or extensive, involving muscle, bone, and vital organs. Bullet wounds may penetrate deeper tissues causing injury far from the point of entry. Burns that cover a large surface area result in substantial losses of fluids and electrolytes. Medications applied topically to burns should be easy to apply and should not interfere with healing.

Horses that have incurred a bullet wound may require antimicrobial therapy, due to the penetration of a viscus or a synovial structure. The bullet injures tissues directly in its path, and concussive forces injure tissue adjacent to the bullet's path. Dog-bite wounds are heavily contaminated and characterized by the presence of crushed, necrotic tissue. Damage to tissue caused by a bullet, a bite, or a burn progresses after injury, necessitating continuous re-evaluation of the wound.

Burn injuries

Introduction

Burns occur primarily from barn fires but may also result from contact with hot fluids; electrocution or lightning strike; friction, such as from a rope burn; radiation therapy; improper use of a cryogen; an electrosurgical accident; or a maliciously applied caustic agent, such as phenol or potassium hydroxide.[1,2] Horses are most commonly burned on the back and face.

Management of severe and extensive burns is difficult, expensive, and time consuming. The larger the surface area of the burn, the greater is the loss of fluids, electrolytes, and calories. Serious burns can rapidly result in severe shock, hypovolemia, and associated cardiovascular changes. The burned horse may also suffer from smoke inhalation or corneal ulceration.[1,2] Burns covering 50% or more of the body are usually fatal,

Equine Wound Management, Third Edition. Edited by Christine Theoret and Jim Schumacher.

Companion website: www.wiley.com/go/theoret/wound

although the depth of the burn also influences the horse's likelihood of survival. Because burns are often pruritic, a burned horse requires long-term close observation to ensure that it does not mutilate the wound. Burned horses are frequently disfigured or unable to return to full function. Prior to initiating treatment, therefore, the patient must be carefully examined, with particular attention paid to cardiovascular and pulmonary function, ocular structures, and the extent and depth of the burn. Cost of treatment and prognosis for survival and return to function should be discussed thoroughly with the owner before treatment is initiated.[1–4]

Classification of burn injuries

Burns are classified according to the depth of the injury.[1–3] First-degree burns involve only the most superficial layers of the epidermis. These burns are characterized by erythema, edema, and desquamation of the superficial layers of the skin. First-degree burns are painful because nerve endings are exposed. The germinal layer of the epidermis is spared, and the burn heals without complication (Figure 20.1).[4]

Second-degree burns involve the epidermis and may be superficial or deep. Superficial, second-degree burns involve the *stratum corneum*, *stratum granulosum*, and a few cells of the *stratum basale* (see Figure 1.2). Second-degree burns are painful because pain receptors remain intact. Because the basal layer of the epidermis (*stratum basale*) is largely uninjured, superficial second-degree burns heal rapidly, within 14–17 days, with minimal scarring (Figure 20.2).[5–7] Deep second-degree burns involve all layers of the epidermis, including the basal layer. These burns are characterized by erythema and edema at the epidermal–dermal junction, necrosis of the epidermis, accumulation of white blood cells at the base of the burn, and formation of eschar, a structure composed of exudate, collagen, and layers of dead skin resulting from destruction of the dermis. The only germinal cells spared are those within the ducts of sweat glands and hair follicles, which reside within the dermis. Deep, second-degree burns may heal within 3–4 weeks if care is taken to prevent progression of dermal ischemia that may lead to full-thickness necrosis, such as by reducing inflammation, removing tissue debris, and promoting a moist environment.[6,7] Deep second-degree burn wounds, unless grafted, usually heal with extensive scarring.[5]

Third-degree burns cause minimal or no pain because nerve fibers in the basal layer of skin are destroyed (Figure 20.3). Third-degree burns are characterized by loss of the epidermal and dermal components, including the adnexa, and range in color from white to black (Figure 20.4, Figure 20.5). They are accompanied by fluid loss and a marked cellular response at the wound's margin, formation of eschar, lack of pain, shock, local infection, and sometimes bacteremia and sepsis. Healing occurs by contraction and epithelialization from the wound's margin or by autografting. Fourth-degree burns involve all of the skin and underlying muscle, bone, ligaments, fat, and fascia (Figure 20.6).[6,7,9]

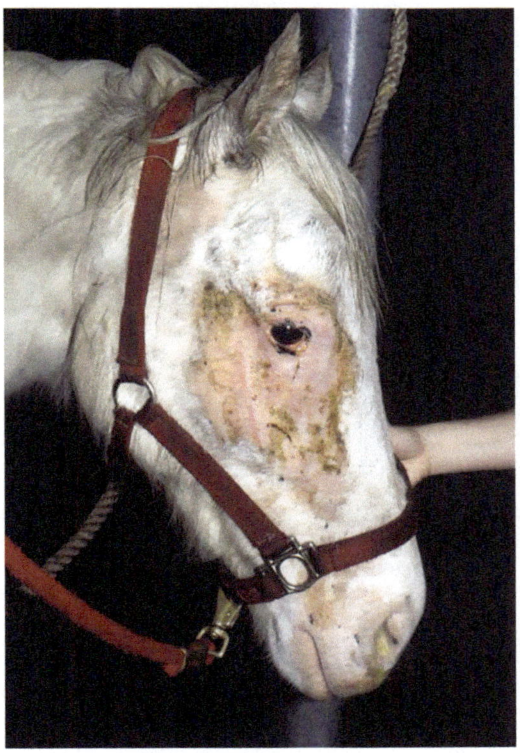

Figure 20.1 First-degree burn of the right facial and periocular regions. This type of burn involves only the most superficial layers of the epidermis. First-degree burns are painful and are characterized by erythema, edema, and desquamation of the superficial layers of the skin. The germinal layer of the epidermis is spared, and the burn heals without complication.

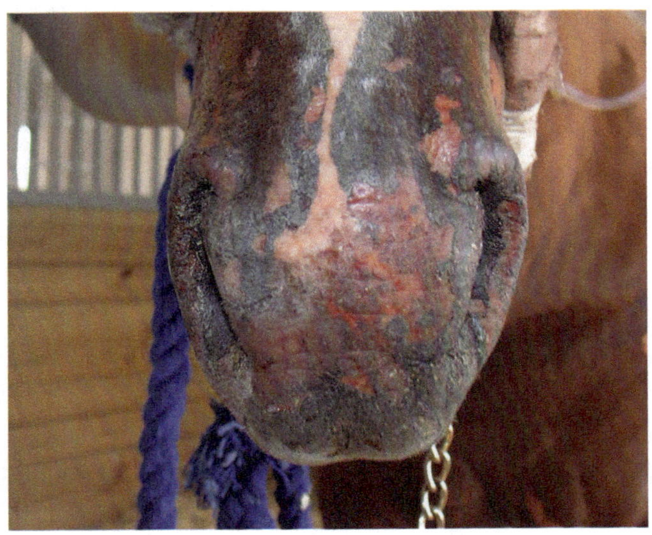

Figure 20.2 Superficial second-degree burn of the nose. Tactile and pain receptors remain intact. Because the basal layers of the epidermis are uninjured, superficial second-degree burns heal rapidly, within 14–17 days, with minimal scarring.

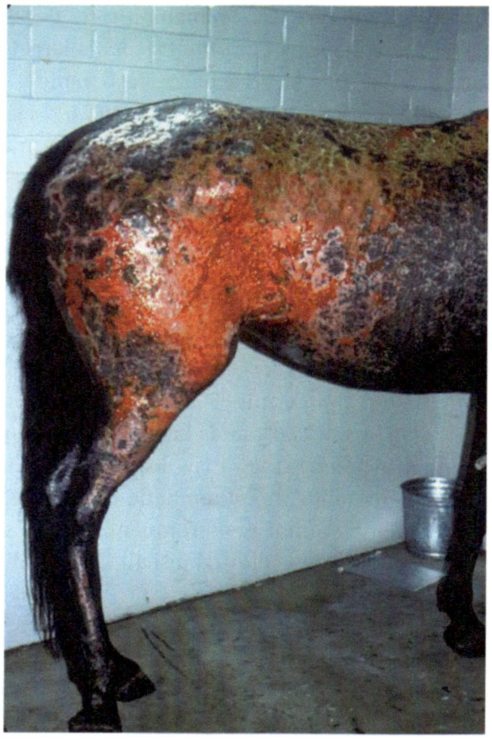

Figure 20.3 Deep second-degree burn of the right aspect of the back and right hind limb. Deep second-degree burns may heal within 3 to 4 weeks if care is taken to prevent dermal ischemia that may lead to full-thickness necrosis. Source: Hanson 2005.[8] Reproduced with permission of Elsevier.

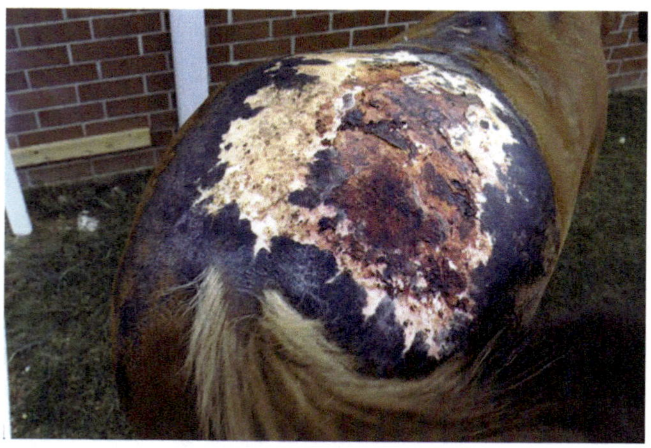

Figure 20.4 Third-degree burn of the left gluteal region incurred during a barn fire. The center of the burn is surrounded by deep and superficial second-degree burns of the flank.

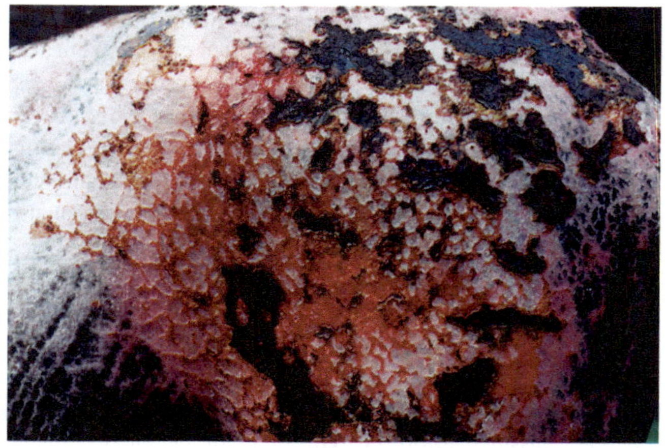

Figure 20.5 Deep second-degree and third-degree burns of the flank and hindquarters 3 weeks post injury.

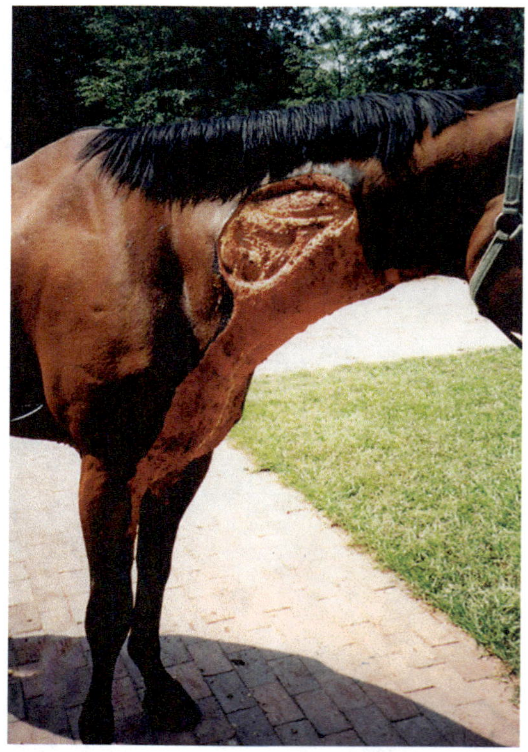

Figure 20.6 Fourth-degree burn of the right cervical region and pectoral area caused by an acid. Fourth-degree burns involve all layers of the skin and the underlying muscle, bone, ligaments, fat, and fascia.

Physical examination

The burned horse should receive a complete physical examination before the wound is evaluated. Only after the patient's condition is stable should the burn be assessed. The extent and severity of the burn should be determined. The *extent* of the burn refers to the size of the area exposed, whereas the *severity* is related to the depth of the wound, which in turn is related to the maximum temperature the tissue attains and the duration of overheating. Heat is slow to dissipate from a burn, often complicating accurate evaluation, early after injury, of the amount of tissue damaged. This explains why injury often extends beyond the original boundaries of the burn.[10]

Physical criteria used to evaluate a burn include erythema, edema, pain, blistering, the presence of an eschar, body temperature, cardiovascular status, and the presence of infection.[10]

In general, erythema, edema, and pain are favorable signs because they indicate that at least some superficial tissue is viable, but pain is not a reliable indicator of the wound's depth.[10] Often, time must elapse to allow tissue changes to progress before the extent and severity of the burn can be ascertained.

The burn may be characterized by erythema and the presence of vesicles and singed hair, and the horse may show signs of pain. The burned horse may exhibit blepharospasm, epiphora, or both, signifying corneal damage. Coughing may indicate that the horse suffers from smoke inhalation, and a fever signals a systemic response to injury. Increased heart and respiratory rates are often accompanied by discoloration of mucous membranes, indicative of poor cardiovascular function.

Prognosis in relation to the percentage of body surface area burned

The percentage of total body surface area involved in the burn usually correlates directly with mortality, whereas the depth of the burn determines morbidity.[6,7,9,11] In human patients, the "rule of 9" is used to estimate the total surface area that has been burned. This method allows prognosis to be estimated according to the extent of the burn. Each arm represents 9% of the body's surface area, each leg 18%, the head and neck 9%, and the thorax and abdomen each 18%.[4,6,7] Special care is taken to identify injury to major vessels of the legs and injury to the eyes, perineum, tendon sheaths, and/or joints.

Although specific guidelines do not exist for calculating the percentage of total surface area of the body of large animals that has been burned, euthanasia should be recommended for horses with deep second-degree or third-degree burns comprising 30% or more of the body's total surface area.[12,13] The availability of adequate facilities for treatment, cost of treatment, and pain experienced by a burned horse should be considered when deciding whether or not to recommend euthanasia. Because convalescence may take up to 2 years, euthanasia is often more humane than treatment.[14]

Treatment

Burn shock

Large volumes of fluid should be administered intravenously to combat burn shock. Fluid therapy is required to avoid circulatory collapse of human patients with burns exceeding 15% of their total body surface area.[15,16] Inadequate fluid resuscitation results in decreased renal and gastrointestinal perfusion, which can lead to gastrointestinal bacterial translocation and sepsis.[15–17]

A balanced electrolyte solution alone is generally administered unless analysis of serum electrolytes indicates that one or more specific electrolytes should be added to the solution. Isotonic fluids should be administered to the horse at a rate of 2–4 mL/kg for each percentage of surface area burned, but fluid resuscitation is best titrated to maintain stable and adequate blood pressure.[6,18] Patients suffering from inhalation injury, in addition to a burn, require 2 mL more fluid per percentage burn per kg than do those with burns alone to support adequate cardiac and urinary output.[7] An alternative to administering a balanced electrolyte solution is to administer hypertonic saline solution (4 mL/kg) at a rapid rate, intravenously, and to follow this with administration of isotonic fluids. Administration of hypertonic saline solution produces an osmotic gradient that promotes the flow of fluid from the extravascular space into the blood stream.[6]

If the horse has suffered pulmonary injury from smoke or heat inhalation, administration of a crystalloid fluid should be limited to the amount that normalizes circulatory volume and blood pressure. Continuing administration of fluids at the same rate after the resolution of shock leads to pulmonary edema, rather than to improvement in cardiovascular status. Administering 2–10 L of plasma provides albumin and antithrombin III to combat coagulopathies. The state of hydration, lung sounds, and cardiovascular status should be monitored carefully, while administering fluid therapy, by clinical assessment and by measuring packed cell volume (PCV) and total protein (TP).

Flunixin meglumine (0.25–1 mg/kg, IV, q 12–24 hours) and firocoxib, a COX-2 inhibitor (0.1 mg/kg, PO, q 24 hours), are effective analgesics for horses suffering pain from a burn. Pentoxyfylline (7.5–8.5 mg/kg, PO or IV, q 12 hours) may be administered to improve circulation by decreasing the viscosity of blood.

> **What to do**
>
> - Horses with burns exceeding 15% of the body's total surface area are likely to require fluid therapy.
> - When administering fluid therapy, use a balanced electrolyte solution unless assessment of serum electrolytes dictates otherwise.
> - Administer flunixin meglumine (0.25–1 mg/kg, IV, q 12–24 hours) or firocoxib (0.1 mg/kg, PO, q 24 hours).
> - Administer pentoxifylline (7.5–8.5 mg/kg, PO or IV, q 12 hours).
> - Carefully monitor the horse's hydration and cardiovascular status.

Pulmonary injury

The cornerstones of therapy for injury caused by smoke inhalation are to maintain a patent airway, to provide adequate oxygenation and ventilation, and to stabilize the cardiovascular system. Medical intervention and respiratory support are essential, even before the diagnosis of respiratory injury is confirmed. Insufflating the horse's lungs, nasally or through a temporary tracheostomy, with humidified 100% oxygen, counteracts the damaging effects of carbon monoxide and facilitates the clearance of carbon monoxide by decreasing its half-life in the blood. Oxygen should be insufflated at a rate of 15–20 L/min, and insufflation should be continued until the horse is able to autonomously maintain normal oxygenation, indicated by a respiratory rate of 12–20 breaths per minute. Humidification can prevent the airway from desiccating or becoming plugged with mucus.[6]

Nebulizing the lungs with N-acetyl cysteine and heparin, delivered in humidified oxygen, reduces the formation of pseudomembranous casts and aids in clearing secretions from the airway.[6,19,20] A horse suffering from respiratory distress and low arterial oxygen tension should receive a temporary tracheostomy through which large obstructive pseudomembranous tracheobronchial casts that may have formed can be removed.[21] Nebulizing the lungs with dimethylsulfoxide (DMSO) may decrease formation of fluid in the lungs, and nebulizing with the beta-adrenergic agonist albuterol may reduce bronchospasm.[19,20] Nebulizing with DMSO and heparin may protect against damage to the airway caused by smoke.[22–25] Administering DMSO (1 g/kg,) during the first 24 hours after injury may decrease pulmonary inflammation and edema. If pulmonary edema persists despite administration of DMSO, furosemide (1 mg/kg, IV or IM, q 12–24 hours) and dexamethasone (0.5 mg/kg, IV, one dose) should be administered.[17]

Systemic administration of antimicrobial drugs to a horse suffering from smoke inhalation is indicated only if the horse has a proven infection, which is more likely to be observed 2 to 3 days after smoke inhalation. Intramuscularly administered penicillin is effective against oral contaminants that colonize the airway.[22,26,27] If signs of respiratory disease worsen, a transtracheal aspirate should be submitted for bacterial culture and antimicrobial sensitivity testing of isolates, and the antimicrobial regimen adapted accordingly.[22,26,27]

A horse suspected to have incurred substantial smoke inhalation should be hospitalized. Therapy must be adjusted according to the clinical response and the results of serial blood gas analyses, complete blood counts, radiographic examination of the chest, endoscopic examination of the airways, and bacterial culture of a tracheal aspirate. Resolution of pulmonary injury depends on early and aggressive care, followed by frequent reassessment and adjustment of the therapy.[28]

What to do

- Auscultate the horse's thorax for evidence of pulmonary edema.
- Administer DMSO (1 g/kg, IV, within the first 24 hours) to decrease pulmonary edema and inflammation at the burn.
- If pulmonary edema persists after administering DMSO and furosemide, administer dexamethasone (0.5 mg/kg, IV), but only once.
- Transtracheal aspiration for cytologic interpretation, bacterial culture, and antimicrobial sensitivity of cultured isolates should be performed if the horse suffers from respiratory distress.
- Begin systemic antimicrobial therapy if the horse is suspected to be suffering from smoke inhalation (e.g., suspected because of burns to the face).
- Administer penicillin intramuscularly to prevent oral contaminants from colonizing the airway.
- Antibiotics with a broader spectrum of antimicrobial activity than that of penicillin should be administered if indicated by the results of Gram stain and/or antimicrobial sensitivity testing of bacterial isolates cultured from tracheal fluid.

Wound care

The hair surrounding a burn wound should be clipped, and the wound debrided of devitalized tissue.[9] The burned skin should be cooled using ice or a cold-water bath. The wound should be copiously irrigated with a sterile solution of 0.05% chlorhexidine digluconate.[11] A water-based cream or gel should be applied liberally to the burns to prevent loss of heat and moisture, to prevent bacterial invasion, and to loosen necrotic tissue and debris.

An effective and economical antibacterial water-based medication for treating burns is silver sulfadiazine (Silvadene, Par Pharmaceutical, Inc.) in a 1% water-miscible cream. This broad-spectrum antibacterial cream is capable of penetrating an eschar and is active against Gram-negative bacteria, especially *Pseudomonas*, and is effective against *S. aureus*, *E. coli*, *Proteus*, *Enterobacteriaceae*, and *C. albicans*.[29] It causes minimal pain when applied but must be applied twice daily because it is inactivated by tissue secretions.

Aloe vera, a gel derived from a yucca-like plant, is often applied to burns. It has antithromboxane and antiprostaglandin activities and is reported to relieve pain, decrease inflammation, stimulate cellular growth, and kill bacteria and fungi.[30,31] Aloe vera and silver sulfadiazine are good first choices in therapy for burns and are used extensively in human medicine. One study examining the effect of platelet-rich plasma (PRP) gel applied to deep second-degree burns of horses found that PRP gel increased the speed of repair of the extracellular matrix and its components but had the potential to cause excess fibrosis. Treatment with two applications of the PRP gel accelerated formation of the extracellular matrix during the first half of wound healing. The PRP gel possibly provided antibacterial activity in burn wounds, due to its inflammatory cytokine content, thereby preventing complications due to contamination.[32]

First-degree burns are generally not life-threatening, and thus, horses that have incurred a first-degree burn are managed simply, using topical therapy in the form of cool compresses, cold-water baths, and wound dressings to provide relief from pain. Pain can also be controlled by administering a nonsteroidal anti-inflammatory drug (NSAID) or narcotic.

What to do

- Immediately cool the burned areas with ice or cold water to draw heat from the tissues, thereby decreasing the likelihood of dermal necrosis.
- Apply water-soluble antibacterial creams, such as aloe vera or silver sulfadiazine cream, topically to the burn.

Second-degree burns are characterized by vesicles and blisters and are not life-threatening. Vesicles and blisters should be left intact for the first 24–36 hours after they form, because fluid within them provides protection from infection and because the presence of vesicles and blisters is less painful than the exposed burn. A topical wound-care product, such as silver sulfadiazine, should be applied to the burns before and after the eschar forms.[1,2,11]

What to do

- Manage the second-degree burn in the same manner as you would a superficial burn.
- Vesicles and blisters should be left intact, because fluid within them provides protection from infection, and because their presence is less painful than the exposed burn.

Third-degree (i.e., full-thickness) burns can be difficult to manage. The horse's condition should be stabilized as rapidly as possible prior to undertaking wound management. A third-degree burn may be managed with occlusive dressings (closed technique), application and removal of wet dressings (semi-open technique), allowing an eschar to form (exposed, or open technique), or excision and grafting.[6,7,10] The most effective and practical therapy for horses with a large burn is the open technique.[1,2,10]

Using the open technique, the wound is left exposed to the air to form its own biologic barrier, the eschar. Leaving the burn wound uncovered (i.e., open) is a method of treatment based on the principle that bacteria do not thrive on a dry surface. The eschar should be covered with an antibacterial agent twice daily. The eschar does not prevent bacterial contamination of the burn, loss of heat, or evaporation of water, and the depth of tissue destruction may be marginally increased as the wound dries. The wound does not contract while covered by the eschar. The eschar is sloughed by the activity of bacterial collagenase within 4 weeks.[33] The exposed bed then contracts. If the wound is too large to heal by contraction and epithelialization, the wound should be grafted.

Excising the eschar that results when a burn is left uncovered is not practical for horses if the burn is extensive because removing the eschar leaves the wound exposed to environmental contamination and may result in massive loss of fluids and heat. The goals of open therapy are to keep the wound dry and protected from self-mutilation.

Tips

- The burned horse should first be treated for shock and/or respiratory distress.
- The most effective and practical therapy for horses with a large burn is to leave the burn uncovered to form an eschar, which should be left undisturbed.
- Silver sulfadiazine should be applied liberally, twice daily, to the burn to prevent loss of heat and moisture prior to formation of the eschar, to protect the eschar once formed, to prevent bacterial invasion, and to loosen necrotic tissue and debris. Applying silver sulfadiazine causes the necrotic tissue to loosen slowly thereby preserving the healthy germinal layers of skin.

What to avoid

- The eschar should not be disrupted. It acts as a natural bandage until it eventually sloughs. Areas of the eschar or underlying wound that are fetid, however, should be surgically debrided.

Systemic administration of antibiotics does not favorably influence healing, fever, or mortality, and can encourage the emergence of resistant bacteria.[34–36] Circulation to the burn is often compromised, making systemically administered antibiotics unlikely to reach a therapeutic concentration at the wound.[37] Short-term antibiotic therapy, administered intravenously, may be indicated during the immediate post-burn period if a quantitative assay of a sample of the burn or a rapid-slide-dilution test indicates that the wound contains more than 100 000 bacteria/g of tissue.[34]

Nutritional requirements

The burned horse's nutritional intake should be assessed based on the horse's ability to maintain its weight. Nutritional support can include parenteral and enteral feeding, the latter being superior to the former.[20] Early enteral feeding not only decreases weight loss, but also maintains an intestinal barrier to bacterial invasion by minimizing mucosal atrophy. This reduces translocation of bacteria and toxins and the potential for sepsis.[20]

Gradually increasing the horse's intake of grain, adding fat in the form of 120–240 mL of vegetable oil daily, and offering free-choice alfalfa hay increases caloric intake. Stanozolol (0.55 mg/kg IM; Winstrol-V, Winthrop Laboratories) is an anabolic steroid that may help restore a positive nitrogen balance by improving appetite and promoting weight gain. It can be administered weekly for up to 4 weeks. If the horse suffers from smoke inhalation, the hay should be soaked in water and fed on the ground in a well-ventilated environment to minimize aspiration. If the horse's face has been burned, the hay should be soaked in water to ease mastication.[10]

Complications

Burn wounds are often pruritic, causing the horse to mutilate itself by rubbing, biting, and pawing.[2,10] The most intense pruritis usually occurs during the first weeks after injury, during the inflammatory phase of repair, when the eschar is sloughing. To prevent self-mutilation the horse with pruritic wounds should be cross-tied and/or sedated. Reserpine, used in the horse as a long-acting tranquilizer, may be effective in decreasing the horse's urge to scratch by breaking the itch–scratch cycle.

Other complications include habronemiasis, keloid-like fibroblastic proliferations, sarcoid transformation, and burn-induced carcinoma.[2,14] Hypertrophic scars, which are a common sequel to deep second-degree burns in horses, generally remodel to become more cosmetic within 1–2 years. Because scarred skin is hairless and often depigmented, its solar exposure should be limited. Chronic non-healing areas should be excised, and the wound autografted to prevent neoplastic transformation. Delayed healing, poor epithelialization, and complications of second-intention healing may prevent the horse from returning to its previous use.

Gunshot wounds

Introduction

Alhough gunshot injuries in horses are uncommon, a bullet may cause a wide range of severe injuries to various organs. A bullet produces a focal, penetrating wound; the entry wound is oval to circular, and its margins are clean. An exit wound is not always present. Close-range shotgun injuries completely destroy tissues in the path of the pellets.[38,39]

The wounding potential of a bullet is related to the following three factors: the energy of the missile on impact, the design of the bullet, and the characteristics of the tissues contacted by the bullet.[40] These variables directly affect the amount of damage transferred to the tissues from the bullet. Although describing the trauma based on the type of gun and the bullet's initial muzzle velocity is tempting, it is important to note that the speed at which the bullet leaves the gun is the maximum it reaches during flight. Multiple factors, including the shape of the projectile and the distance it travels before impact, can slow the speed and reduce the bullet's energy at impact. Objects the bullet encounters or passes through prior to striking the horse also affect the bullet's speed.

The type of tissue the bullet enters affects the distribution of the bullet's energy at impact.[40] Transfer of energy is directly related to the density of the tissue, and inversely related to the elasticity of the tissues involved. Examples of organs with low elasticity and high density include the liver, spleen, and bone, whereas organs with high elasticity and low density include muscle, skin, and lung. Tissues that deform easily but retain their form (i.e., elastic tissues) are less likely to absorb the energy from the projectile. Elastic organs that are filled with fluid, such as the gastrointestinal tract and heart, however, may be secondarily damaged by pressure waves that can expand thorough the fluid as the bullet passes through the tissue.

Classification of bullet injury

The trauma caused by the bullet induces two distinct types of injury.[40,41] The first is a crush injury, or *permanent cavity formation*, which is a direct injury to the tissue caused by impact of the bullet as it passes through the tissues. This injury can result from the bullet and its fragments, from other foreign bodies, such as dirt, hair, or pieces of tack, carried into the tissues by the bullet, and from shattered bone or tooth. The extent of the crush injury depends on the size and shape of the bullet and whether it is designed to fragment or deform on impact. Bullets that fragment or deform on impact cause more tissue damage than do those that do not. At high velocity, large-diameter projectiles can also cause blunt trauma, termed *temporary cavitation,* caused by lateral expansion of energy from the bullet's primary path.[41,42] This type of injury is more likely to occur in friable soft tissues with low elasticity, such as the liver or spleen, that expand to absorb the energy and are pushed beyond their breaking point.[43]

Treatment

The type of tissues involved is the most important factor in determining the severity of a bullet wound. The crushed tissues in the permanent cavity resulting from the bullet's path should not be expected to survive. The necessity for surgical debridement of the tissues in the bullet's path depends on the depth of the tract and the structures involved. The tissues outside of the bullet's path must also be assessed for injury caused by secondary cavitation. During the first 3 hours after injury, vessels in tissues surrounding the primary tract vasoconstrict, causing these tissues to appear non-viable.[44,45] After this time, hyperemia and hemorrhage from tissues previously thought non-viable may be noted. Initial debridement should, therefore, be conservative, to allow time for tissues to re-establish signs of viability.

Bullet wounds should be treated as contaminated and left open to allow for drainage and debridement of devitalized tissues. Broad-spectrum antimicrobial therapy effective against aerobic and anaerobic bacteria should be administered systemically, especially if the gastrointestinal tract was injured (See Chapter 19, Table 19.1 for recommendations for antimicrobial therapy). Results of bacterial culture performed immediately after injury are often not helpful due to contamination of the wound. Rather, exudate appearing in the wound after 3–5 days should be cultured for bacteria, and isolates should be tested for antimicrobial sensitivity. Removing the bullet is unnecessary, and dissection to remove it may cause further harm. It is unlikely that enough lead can leach from lead bullets into surrounding tissues to cause toxicity, and therefore, removing a lead bullet is rarely indicated for that reason alone.[46] A lead or copper pellet within a synovial structure, however, can cause inflammatory synovitis and, therefore, should be removed.[47] The pellet can be removed arthroscopically, but ultrasonographic guidance may be helpful in locating a pellet imbedded deeply within the synovium.

What to do

- A bullet wound should be treated as if it is contaminated. Establish drainage and manage a bullet wound as an open wound.
- The bullet tract should be irrigated thoroughly and debrided conservatively.
- Provide broad-spectrum antimicrobial coverage and tetanus prophylaxis.

What to avoid

- Do not close the wound.
- Avoid excessive debridement because the amount of devitalized tissue is easily overestimated.
- Do not remove a bullet or pellets unless they lie within a synovial structure.

Recommendations for the treatment of horses with a bullet injury to a specific anatomic region/structure

Head, neck, and spine

Cerebral or spinal penetration by a bullet is often fatal. Horses that survive an accidental shooting involving the central nervous system should be managed medically with antibiotics that penetrate the blood–brain barrier, analgesics, osmotic agents to combat edema, and an anti-inflammatory drug.[48–50] Systemic hypotension should be combated to preserve tissue perfusion and prevent the negative effects of hypotension on cerebral perfusion.[49] Although mannitol has an antioxidant effect and can reduce cerebral edema, it can also cause acute renal failure, and it may lose its osmotic effect with repeated doses.[50] Hypertonic saline solution may be more effective than mannitol as an osmotic agent and may also have an immunomodulatory effect.[51]

Gunshot wounds to the head and neck can lacerate large vessels, necessitating ligation or embolization of the lacerated vessels to stop severe hemorrhage. Injuries to the trachea and larynx should be assessed with radiography and endoscopy, but most horses suffering an injury to the trachea or larynx, are treated with conservative therapy.[52] The airway should be secured, if compromised, by inserting a nasotracheal tube or by performing a tracheostomy. For pharyngeal and esophageal wounds, surgical exploration and primary repair should be performed as soon as the horse is stable (see Chapter 12 for more information regarding the management of wounds involving the trachea and/or the esophagus).

Thorax

Horses that have suffered a gunshot wound to the thorax are likely to develop hemothorax, pneumothorax, or both. The source of hemorrhage may be from the primary wound external to the thoracic cavity or from a laceration to a thoracic vessel, pulmonary parenchyma, or an airway within the thorax.[53] The entrance and exit wounds should be sealed immediately with an airtight dressing, such as a self-adhesive, occlusive dressing or cellophane over a primary gauze dressing, and bandaged until patency of the airways and tissue oxygenation are assessed. The horse's vital signs should be assessed, and its thorax auscultated. Arterial blood gas analysis and measurement of serum lactate may be helpful. After the patient is stable, radiographic or ultrasonographic examination may localize the type and severity of the effusion and help determine the need for thoracentesis. If hemorrhage is the cause of the thoracic effusion, fluid resuscitation should be conservative to prevent exacerbation of hemorrhage. The goal of resuscitation is to maintain a mean blood pressure of 60 mmHg, a serum lactate less than 4 mmol/L, a blood pH above 7.25, and a serum creatinine less than 3 mmol/L.[54] If fluid resuscitation does not improve the horse's vital signs, the horse should receive a blood transfusion. If hemorrhage appears to be ongoing, an effort must be made to control the hemorrhage while the horse is receiving the transfusion. After the horse is stabilized, it can be successfully managed medically with minimal debridement, appropriate pain management, and antimicrobial therapy.[55,56]

Abdomen

Horses with an abdominal gunshot wound can be treated conservatively, in a manner similar to that used to treat horses with a thoracic gunshot wound, with fluid resuscitation, minimal wound debridement, abdominal lavage, and antimicrobial therapy.[42,57,58] The decision to explore the abdomen surgically should be based on adverse changes in the peritoneal fluid and abnormalities found during transrectal and transabdominal ultrasonographic examinations of the abdomen. Serosanguinous or suppurative effusions found to contain degenerative neutrophils, bacteria, or foreign material support the need for surgical intervention.[57–60] Although the bullet may not be recovered at surgery, injured intestines and other organs can be repaired, and the abdomen thoroughly lavaged. Antibiotic therapy should be continued for up to 7 days after a perforated viscus has been repaired, but the duration of treatment should be guided by results of repeat analysis of peripheral neutrophil counts and results of analysis of peritoneal fluid obtained by abdominocentesis. The course of antimicrobial therapy is extended if the horse develops septic peritonitis; antimicrobial treatment is guided by bacterial culture and antimicrobial sensitivity testing of isolates.

Musculoskeletal

Injuries to the skin and skeletal muscle are the most common reasons for which horses injured by a bullet are presented for medical assessment and treatment. Fortunately, the likelihood of survival is good; in one study, seven of eight horses injured by a bullet returned to their previous function.[61] When the bullet has struck the distal aspect of a limb, radiographs of the limb should be obtained to evaluate the extent of injury; MRI or CT may aid evaluation, but caution should be taken when using MRI if the bullets or pellets are numerous and are suspected to be composed of steel. The magnet forces encountered when using MRI can cause movement or heating of the metal or displacement of associated tissues.[47] Steel shot or a steel bullet is more likely to maintain its original shape on radiographs, whereas a lead pellet or bullet may be deformed.

The extent of injury is related to the force of the bullet on impact, and low-energy impact wounds are typically not associated with substantial damage or infection. Treatment by superficial debridement and irrigation of the wound's tract and application of a dressing appropriate to the affected region of the limb often suffices. The reader is referred to Chapter 7 for more information on bandaging techniques for wound management. The need for antibiotic therapy depends on the structures involved and the risk of infection. Antibiotic therapy should be selected according to results of bacterial culture and sensitivity testing of isolates. For high-energy impact wounds, more extensive debridement is required; debridement can be provided in stages over the course of treatment. In the acute phase, swelling of muscle and local edema may cause lactic acidosis resulting in compartment syndrome, which may require fascial fenestration.[39,45] As with any contaminated wound, only obviously devitalized tissue should be removed.

Involvement of a synovial structure can be confirmed by examining fluid obtained by synoviocentesis and by distending the synovial structure with sterile isotonic saline solution to determine if the synovial structure communicates with the wound. Contaminated synovial structures are best treated by endoscopic lavage or lavage using large-bore needles. Damage to intrasynovial bone or tendon, changes in the synovial fluid indicative of synovial infection 4–6 days after initiating therapy, and a positive microbial culture are negative prognostic indicators associated synovial infections.[47] For more information on the diagnosis and management of wounds involving synovial structures, the reader is referred to Chapter 16. Lead pellets identified within the synovial cavity should be removed to prevent synovitis and damage to articular cartilage.[47] Fractures associated with bullet wounds are beyond the scope of this review but should be treated as open and evaluated immediately for the possibility of repair.

Dog-bite wounds

Introduction

Bite wounds caused by dogs occur most commonly in small equids, such as foals, American miniature horses, ponies, and donkeys (Figure 20.7). Debilitated or geriatric horses, however, may also be victims of bite wounds, especially when a pack of dogs is involved. Injuries associated with bite wounds are usually multifocal and most commonly involve the limbs, perineum, and neck.[62] Due to the location of these wounds, joints, tendons, and major blood vessels are likely to be damaged.

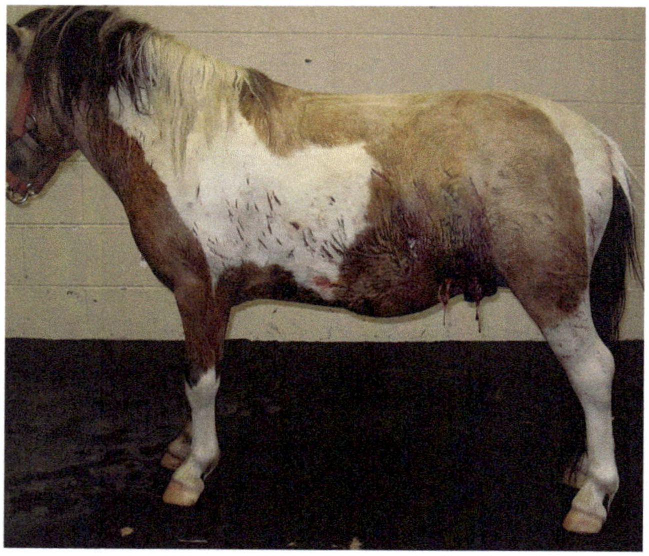

Figure 20.7 A 4-year-old American Miniature Horse stallion was presented after it was attacked by a pack of dogs. Over 80% of the body was wounded; the most severe wounds were on the abdomen, inguinal regions, perineum, and hindlimbs.

The configuration of dog bites is caused by shearing and compressive forces, resulting from the shape of the canine tooth and the strength of the musculature of the canine jaw.[63] Soft-tissue injuries incurred may include abrasions, avulsions, lacerations, and/or puncture wounds. In addition to causing trauma to the skin, dog bites frequently cause severe damage to deeper soft-tissue structures, including organs and vessels. This type of crush injury leads to ischemia and can result in a condition termed traumatic rhabdomyolysis.[64] Other consequences of crush injury include dysrhythmias, renal damage, acute respiratory distress syndrome, coagulopathies, and sepsis (Figure 20.8).

Treatment of shock

Initial examination of a horse with a bite wound should start with a thorough assessment of cardiovascular status. Substantial blood loss from vascular disruption often results in hypovolemic shock. In addition to loss of fluid from hemorrhage, distributive shock secondary to release of inflammatory mediators may result in up to 30% of total body water shifting into the damaged muscle.[65,66] Shock should be recognized early and combated aggressively by administering fluids intravenously before proceeding with a more detailed examination of the wounds.

What to do

- Fluid therapy must be administered to combat shock by using a balanced electrolyte solution at a bolus dose of 20 mL/kg of body weight, as rapidly as possible.

Tips

- The shock dose of 20 mL/kg can be administered up to three times, based on the response of the patient. Higher doses should be avoided to prevent fluid overload.
- Clinical signs of adequate resuscitation include urination, a decrease in heart rate, and improvements in color of the mucous membranes and mentation.
- Objective measures that indicate a positive response to fluid therapy include a serum lactate <4 mmol/L, blood pH >7.25, and a serum creatinine <3 mmol/L.

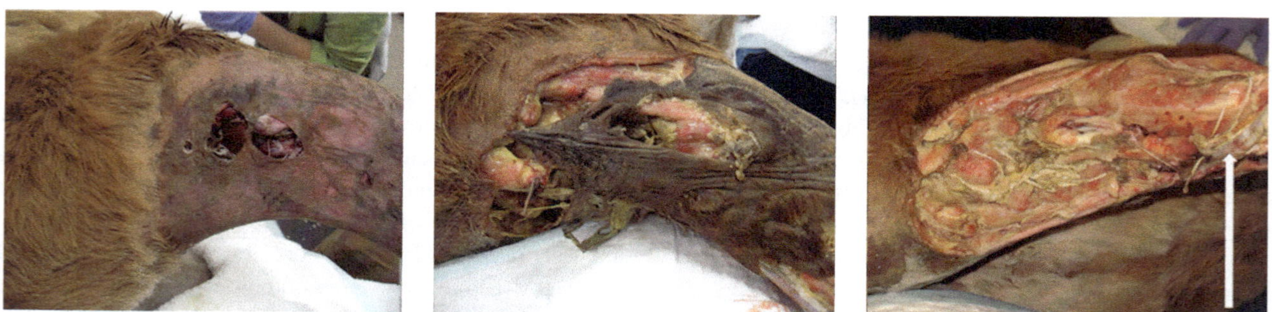

(a) (b) (c)

Figure 20.8 Dog-bite wound over the right stifle of a 5-week-old American Quarter Horse filly. (a) The wound was initially irrigated and packed with wet-to-dry bandages to assist autolytic debridement. (b) Over the next few days, the skin became necrotic due to the crushing caused by the dog bite. (c) By 1 week after injury, the majority of the *semimembranosus* and *semitendinosus* muscles was lost, and the *gastrocnemius* tendon had ruptured. Arrow points to the distal portion of what remains of the *gastrocnemius* tendon.

Assessment of injuries

The bite wounds should be examined, with the horse sedated, after administering appropriate fluid and analgesic therapy. Diagnostic tests used to evaluate the wound may include ultrasonographic and radiographic examinations, including radiographic contrast studies, and examination of fluid obtained by synoviocentesis or abdominocentesis. Assessment should include evaluation of cranial nerves if the head has been bitten and neurovascular structures if the limbs have been bitten. The horse's vaccination status regarding tetanus and rabies should be determined. Knowing if the dog is current on its rabies immunization helps when making decisions regarding vaccination and quarantine of the horse.

What to do

- Vaccinate the horse for rabies and determine the vaccination status of rabies of both animals involved (horse and dog).
- Contact the county health department or state department of public health regarding the need for and duration of quarantine for the dog and the horse.
- Keep a list of persons having come in contact with the horse if the horse is quarantined, to allow for post-exposure prophylaxis for humans if the horse develops signs of rabies.

Hematology and electrolytes

A complete blood count and serum biochemical analyses should be performed when the horse is initially presented. Although the hemogram may not indicate that the wound is infected, it provides a baseline for monitoring the horse. A hematocrit can also provide a baseline to evaluate blood loss, but the veterinarian should be aware that the packed cell volume may take 8–12 hours to stabilize after hemorrhage. Knowing the horse's concentration of serum electrolytes at the time it is examined initially is valuable so that hyperkalemia secondary to muscle damage can be identified. Muscle enzymes, notably creatine kinase, should be monitored at the time of admission and during repeat biochemical analyses, to determine the extent of myonecrosis. Knowing the horse's serum concentration of creatinine and urea nitrogen and the results of a urinalysis is helpful in determining if the horse has suffered renal damage from myoglobinuria or if the horse suffers from prerenal azotemia.

The horse can be treated for severe hyperkalemia caused by myonecrosis by administering sodium bicarbonate, insulin, or dextrose intravenously to increase transfer of potassium into the intracellular space. With extensive injuries, the size of the intracellular compartment may be reduced by the loss of tissue, causing potassium to remain in circulation. Studies have indicated that these therapies have minimal effect on shifting serum concentrations of potassium in foals, which normally have a smaller intracellular fluid compartment.[65] Other methods to lower a high serum concentration of potassium by excretion include administering a diuretic (e.g. mannitol, furosemide) and peritoneal dialysis.[67,68]

In addition to changes in the serum concentration of potassium, a low serum concentration of ionized calcium may be noted as calcium shifts from the extracellular space into the cytoplasm of the myocytes due to disruption of the cell membrane.[69] Deposition of calcium into muscle of horses with rhabdomyolysis has been noted, and this deposition can lead to more muscle damage through the activation of phospholipase and proteases.[65] Although calcium should be supplemented intravenously to maintain normal serum concentrations, excessive supplementation should be avoided to prevent deposition of calcium in the myocytes.

Coagulopathies

Hypercoagulation is associated with multi-organ failure caused by disseminated intravascular coagulation (DIC) and should be prevented or resolved by inhibiting deposition of fibrin and formation of microthombi.[70] Administering low-molecular-weight heparin, such as enoxaparin (0.35 mg/kg, SQ, daily for 3 days) , may prevent DIC and result in removal of thromboemboli already present within the microvasculature. Low-molecular-weight heparin inhibits coagulation factor Xa through binding with antithrombin.[71] It also inhibits the production of superoxide anion and reduces activity of granulocytes and migration of neutrophils.[71] Unlike unfractionated heparin, low-molecular-weight heparin does not cause red blood cells to agglutinate or lower the hematocrit in horses.[72] Platelet counts and clotting times are also not affected. Additional therapies for DIC include administration of fresh, whole blood and transfusion of plasma to provide clotting factors and platelets.

Rhabdomyolysis

Rhabdomyolysis is evidence of crush syndrome and may indicate the need for interventions to prevent renal damage. Fluid therapy is indicated for diuresis and to increase glomerular blood flow in the face of prerenal vasoconstriction caused by scavenging of nitric oxide by myoglobin. Administration of sodium bicarbonate may reduce formation of casts in the renal tubules by inhibiting the precipitation of myoglobin with Tamm-Horsfall proteins. After the horse is rehydrated, administration of mannitol (1–2 g/kg/day) may be useful in preventing renal damage because it is an osmotic diuretic and a free radical scavenger.[73] Because it is an osmotic agent, it helps to reduce edema associated with the traumatized tissue. Administration of bicarbonate and mannitol, however, has not been shown to provide any benefit for survival in humans.[74]

Treatment of bite wounds

Initial wound management includes appropriate irrigation of the wounds at a pressure of 10–15 psi, which can be achieved using a 19-gauge needle attached to 35-mL syringe. Approximately 30 mL of isotonic saline solution per square centimeter is adequate to irrigate most wounds.[75] Often, the viability of damaged tissues may be questionable, or the damaged tissue may be severely contaminated. In these cases, a wet-to-dry bandage,

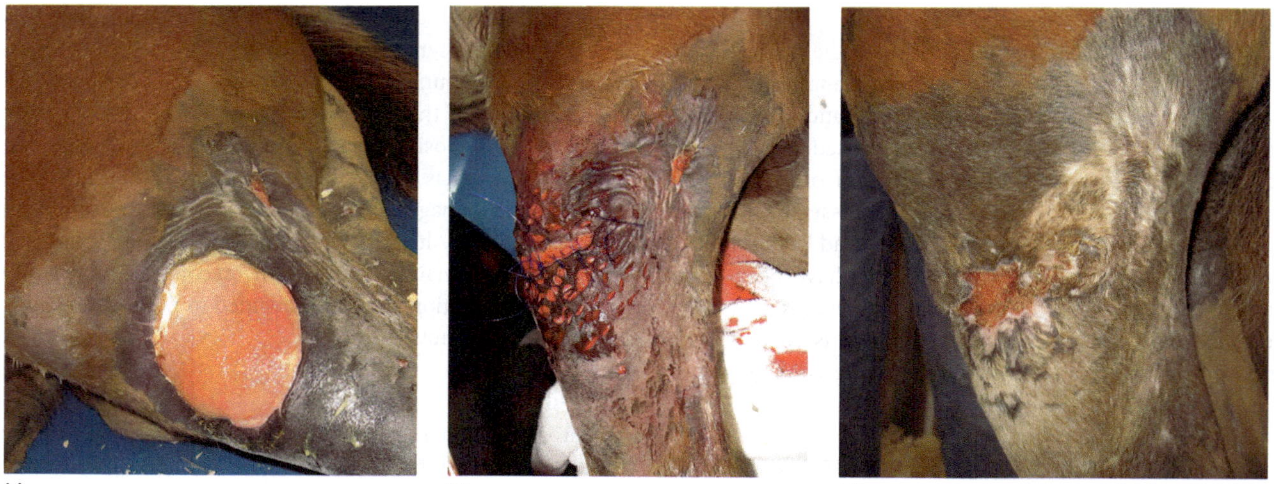

(a) (b) (c)

Figure 20.9 **(a)** Delayed primary closure of a wound on the left hindlimb of a 2-month-old Tennessee Walking Horse filly. Dressings composed of honey were used to combat contamination and to enhance the development of a healthy bed of granulation tissue. **(b)** The wound was sutured, but, to do so, skin surrounding the wound was meshed to relieve tension on the suture line. The limb was immobilized using a full-limb cast to reduce the tension on the sutured wound that would arise upon limb flexion. **(c)** The healed wound was cosmetically acceptable to the owner (right) but might have been improved with the use of skin grafting.

a hypertonic dressing, honey or sugar is helpful in removing debris and reducing edema. The wounds should be re-evaluated during the following days to determine if surgical debridement is needed. Puncture wounds, crush wounds, contaminated wounds, and wounds over joints or on extremities should be left open to heal by second intention or by delayed primary closure (Figure 20.9).[76] Delayed closure can be attempted after a wound appears to be healing without signs of infection (the reader is referred to Chapter 8 for more information regarding selection of approaches to wound closure).

What to do

- Dog-bite wounds are contaminated and, therefore, should be managed by second-intention healing or by delayed primary or secondary closure.
- Irrigate the wound thoroughly and make use of dressing-enhanced autolytic debridement.
- Recognize that crush injury results in substantial and continued necrosis in the days following the injury; continuous fluid therapy, therefore, may prevent renal damage and help to maintain electrolyte balance.

The administration of antibiotics to people suffering from a dog bite is controversial, and studies support their use only in bite wounds on an extremity.[76,77] Dog bites result in the inoculation of the wound with the dog's oral bacteria. Unlike dog bites inflicted on people, dog bites inflicted on horses are usually severely contaminated by the environment, either from the horse's struggle to escape, or from the time that elapses between the injury and its discovery by the horse's owner. The horse should, therefore, receive antibiotic therapy for at least 5 days, but the duration of antibiotic therapy should be extended if the bite is associated with severe edema, crushing of tissue, or synovial contamination or infection.[76,77] Signs of an infection, including erythema, swelling, and pain, clearly indicate that administration of antimicrobial drugs should be continued and adjusted as guided by bacterial culture and results of antimicrobial sensitivity testing of isolates. Regional limb or intraosseous perfusion with an antibiotic and intrasynovial instillation of an antibiotic are methods used to increase the concentration of an antibiotic in an infected synovial structure (the reader is referred to Chapter 16 for more information on the management of wounds involving a synovial structure).

Bite injuries to the thorax of the horse are uncommon, perhaps because the size of the horse's thorax in relation to the size of the average dog reduces the risk of severe thoracic injury, except for foals and American miniature horses. Radiographic and ultrasonographic examinations may be helpful in localizing thoracic and abdominal effusions and injuries. A horse with an axillary wound should be monitored closely for the development of subcutaneous emphysema, which can progress to pneumothorax or pneumomediastinum. To inhibit air from moving into the tissues, the wound can be packed with sterile gauze, and the wound temporarily occluded with a stent bandage or cellophane. The dressing and packing should be replaced every 24–48 hours until healthy granulation tissue has occluded the defect. To further reduce the likelihood of subcutaneous emphysema, the horse should be confined to a stall or cross-tied to minimize movement.[78]

To determine if a bite to the abdomen has penetrated the peritoneal cavity, the wound should be explored, and abdominal fluid, obtained by abdominocentesis, examined cytologically. Ultrasonographic examination of the abdomen and palpation of the viscera *per rectum* may be helpful in determining if the peritoneal cavity has been penetrated. If the injury has penetrated the peritoneum, the horse is best treated while anesthetized so that the wound can be better explored, debrided, and closed, and so that the abdomen can be thoroughly lavaged. If the wound has resulted in eventration, the exposed intestine should be irrigated with isotonic saline solution and replaced, and protected with a bandage or temporarily closed with sutures, or clamps until the horse can be anesthetized and the wound explored and repaired. If the viscera are severely contaminated, large-bore drains should be placed in the ventral aspect of the peritoneal cavity to allow repeated abdominal lavage after surgery. Large, partial defects in the abdominal wall should be left to heal by second intention.

Complications

Because many dog-bite wounds are managed by second-intention healing, exuberant granulation tissue (EGT) may form, especially if the wounds are on the distal aspect of a limb. Surgical resection is a simple method to control EGT, although EGT does have a tendency to recur so that resection may need to be repeated. The procedure can be performed with the horse standing because granulation tissue is not innervated. Strips of granulation tissue can be shaved from the wound in a distal to proximal direction to produce a flat surface level with or slightly below (~2 mm) the surrounding edge of the wound. The epithelial margin should be preserved to allow epithelium to continue to advance. Application of a pressure bandage is usually necessary to control hemorrhage after excising EGT.

An ointment or cream containing a corticosteroid may be applied topically to curb the early formation of EGT, thus facilitating epithelialization and contraction. A corticosteroid is generally applied at the earliest signs of formation of EGT, and application of the corticosteroid at one or two bandage changes is usually adequate to achieve the desired effect. Continued application may exert negative effects on angiogenesis, contraction, and epithelialization.[79] A corticosteroid should not be applied to an infected wound, because corticosteroids inhibit the inflammatory response required to eliminate microorganisms. The reader is referred to Chapter 15 for more information regarding the prevention and management of EGT.

A wound over a joint and/or tendon may require immobilization, in the form of a cast, because continued movement disrupts healing. The cast should be removed as soon as the wound no longer requires immobilization, to avoid the development of cast sores. Generally, a cast over a dog-bite wound should be changed every 3–10 days, but the frequency of cast change depends on the nature and location of the wound and the temperament of the horse. The reader is referred to Chapter 7 for more information regarding techniques of bandaging and casting for wound management.

Conclusion

Horses with serious burns can rapidly develop severe shock and hypovolemia with associated cardiovascular changes. The burned horse may also suffer from smoke inhalation and corneal ulceration.[1,2] Burns covering 50% or more of the body are usually fatal, although the depth of the burn also influences the likelihood of mortality. Because burn wounds are often pruritic, self-mutilation is common, and care must be taken to prevent the horse from mutilating itself. Burned horses are frequently disfigured and unable to return to their previous function. Before initiating treatment of a burned horse, the horse must be carefully examined to determine the extent and severity of the burn. Particular attention should be paid to cardiovascular and pulmonary function and to ocular structures. Cost of treatment and prognosis for survival or return to function should be discussed thoroughly with the owner.[1–4]

Damage caused by a bullet is non-specific, and the degree of injury depends on the energy imparted on impact and the types of tissues involved. The wound should be evaluated thoroughly to determine the organs and systems damaged. Removal of the bullet is necessary only if it lodges within a synovial structure. A bullet wound should be considered contaminated and should be treated as such. A bullet wound should be managed by second-intention healing, and the tract caused by the bullet should be frequently assessed for the presence of non-viable tissue.

Dog-bite wounds typically involve small equids, such as American miniature horses, ponies, and foals. Common sites of injury include the head, neck, limbs, and perineum. The crushing nature of the injury and inoculation of the wound with the dog's oral bacteria result in contamination and infection and gradually developing necrosis, requiring frequent reassessment and debridement of the wound. Loss of fluid and blood may be severe, necessitating emergency resuscitation. Continuous diuresis may be needed to treat rhabdomyolysis, often seen as a consequence of a crush injury. The status of vaccination against rabies of both the horse and the dog should be determined, and the state health department should be contacted for recommendations regarding vaccination and quarantine of the victim and its attacker.

Damage caused by a burn, a bullet, or a dog bite progresses after the initial injury and is characterized by necrosis and infection. A wound caused by a burn, a bullet, or a bite should be assessed repeatedly to identify organs involved and to allow for changes in the plan of wound management. These types of wounds often require extensive revision and skin grafting, and a good cosmetic and functional outcome may not be possible. Complications of these types of injuries, such as renal failure, pneumonia, and coagulopathy, may prove fatal to the horse.

References

1. Fubini SL. Burns. In: Robinson NE (ed). *Current Therapy in Equine Medicine*, 2nd edn. WB Saunders: Philadelphia, 1987: 639.
2. Fox SM, Cooper RC, Gilis JP, Groce AW. Management of a large thermal burn in a horse. *Comp Cont Educ Pract Vet* 1988; **10**: 88.
3. Baxter GM. Management of burns. In: Colahan P, Mayhew I, Merritt A, Moore J (eds). *Equine Medicine and Surgery*, 4th edn. American Veterinary Publication Inc: Goleta, 1991: 1843.

4. Warden GD. Outpatient care of thermal injuries. *Surg Clin North Am* 1987; **67**: 147.
5. Robson MC, Heggars JP. Pathophysiology of the burn wound. In: Carvajal H, Parks D (eds). *Burns in Children—Pediatric Burn Management*, 1st edn. Year Book Medical Publishers: St Louis, MO, 1988: 27.
6. Church D, Elsayed S, Reid O, *et al.* Burn wound infections. *Clin Microbiol Rev* 2006; **19**: 403.
7. Mosier MJ, Gibran NS. Surgical excision of the burn wound. *Clin Plast Surg* 2009; **36**: 617.
8. Hanson RR. Management of burn injuries. *Vet Clin North Am* 2005; **21**: 107.
9. Provost PJ. Thermal Injuries. In: Auer J, Stick J (eds). *Equine Surgery*, 2nd edn. WB Saunders: Philadelphia, 1999: 179.
10. Geiser D, Walker RD. Management of large animal thermal injuries. *Compend Cont Educ Pract* 1985; **7**: S69.
11. Fraser JF, Cuttle L, Kemp M, *et al.* Cytotoxicity of topical antimicrobial agents used in burn wounds in Australasia. *ANZ J Surg* 2004; **74**: 139.
12. Johnston DE. Burns: electrical, chemical and cold injuries. In: Slatter D (ed). *Textbook of Small Animal Surgery*, 1st edn. WB Saunders: Philadelphia, 1985: 516.
13. Fox SM, Goring RI, Probst CW. Management of thermal burn injuries, part II. *Compend Cont Educ Pract* 1986; **8**: S439.
14. Schumacher J, Watkins JP, Wilson JP, *et al.* Burn-induced neoplasia in two horses. *Equine Vet J* 1986; **18**: 410.
15. Deitch EA. Nutritional support of the burn patient. *Crit Care Clin* 1995; **11**: 735.
16. Herndon DN, Thompson PB, Linares HA, *et al.* Part I: incidence, mortality, pathogenesis and treatment of pulmonary injury. *J Burn Care Rehabil* 1986; **7**: 184.
17. Hanson RR, Gaughan EM, Grenager NS, *et al.* Burns, acute soft tissue swellings, pigeon fever, and fasciotomy. In: Orsini J, Divers T (eds). *Manual of Equine Emergencies*, 4th edn. WB Saunders: Philadelphia, 2014: 608.
18. Herndon DN, Curreri PW, Abston S, *et al.* Treatment of burns. *Cur Probl Surg* 1987; **24**: 347.
19. LaLonde C, Demling R, Brain J, *et al.* Smoke inhalation injury in sheep caused the particulate phase, not the gas phase. *J Appl Physiol* 1994; **77**: 15.
20. Nguyen TT, Gilpin DA, Meyer DA, *et al.* Current treatment of severely burned patients. *Ann Surg* 1996; **223**: 14.
21. Kemper T, Spier S, Barratt-Boyes SM, *et al.* Treatment of smoke inhalation in five horses. *J Am Vet Med Assoc* 1993; **202**: 91.
22. Muller MJ, Herndon DN. The challenge of burns. *Lancet* 1994; **343**: 216.
23. Brown M, Desai M, Traber LD, *et al.* Dimethylsulfoxide with heparin in the treatment of smoke inhalation injury. *J Burn Care Rehabil* 1988; **9**: 22.
24. Cox CS Jr, Zwischenberger JB, Traber DL, *et al.* Heparin improves oxygenation and minimizes barotrauma after severe smoke inhalation in an ovine model. *Surg Gynecol Obstet* 1993; **176**: 339.
25. Kimura R, Traber L, Herndon D, *et al.* Ibuprofen reduces the lung lymph flow changes associated with inhalation injury. *Circ Shock* 1988; **24**: 183.
26. Herndon DN, Barrow RE, Traber DL, *et al.* Extravascular lung water changes following smoke inhalation and massive burn injury. *Surg* 1987; **102**: 341.
27. Stevens DL, Bisno AL, Chambers HF, *et al.* Practice guidelines for the diagnosis and management of skin and soft-tissue infections. *Clin Infect Dis* 2005; **41**: 1373.
28. Mosier MJ, Gibran NS. Management of the patient with thermal injuries. *Trauma and Therm Inj* 2010; **7**: 1.
29. Pirnay JP, De Vos D, Cochez C, *et al.* Molecular epidemiology of *Pseudomonas aeruginosa* colonization in a burn unit: persistence of a multidrug-resistant clone and a silver sulfadiazine-resistant clone. *J Clin Microbiol* 2003; **41**: 1192.
30. Grindlay D, Reynolds T. The aloe vera phenomenon: a review of the properties and modern uses of the leaf parenchyma gel. *J Ethnopharmacol* 1986; **16**: 117.
31. Dat AD, Poon F, Pham KB, *et al.* Aloe vera for treating acute and chronic wounds. *Cochrane Database Syst Rev* 2012; **2**: 1.
32. Maciel FB, DeRossi R, Modolo TJ, *et al.* Scanning electron microscopy and microbiological evaluation of equine burn wound repair after platelet rich plasma gel treatment. *Burns* 2012; **38**: 1058.
33. Heimbach DM. Early burn excision and grafting. *Surg Clin North Am* 1987; **67**: 93.
34. Mozingo DW, McManus AT, Kim SH, *et al.* Incidence of bacteremia after burn wound manipulation in the early postburn period. *J Trauma* 1997; **42**: 10061.
35. Murphy KD, Lee JO, Herndon DN. Current pharmacotherapy for the treatment of severe burns. *Expert Opin Pharmacother* 2003; **4**: 369.
36. Barajas-Nava LA, López-Alcalde J, Roqué i Figuls M, *et al.* Antibiotic prophylaxis for preventing burn wound infection. *Cochrane Database Syst Rev* 2013; **6**: 1.
37. Durtschi MB, Orgain C, Counts GW, *et al.* A prospective study of prophylactic penicillin in acutely burned hospitalized patients. *J Trauma* 1982; **22**: 11.
38. Di Maio VJM. Gunshot wounds. In: *Practical Aspects of Firearms, Ballistics and Forensic Techniques*. CRC Press: Boca Raton, FL, 1998.
39. Rozen N, Dudkiewicz I. *Wound Ballistics and Tissue Damage*. Springer-Verlag: Heidelberg, 2011: **21**.
40. Gugula Z, Lindsey RW. Classification of gunshot injuries in civilians. *Clin Orthop Relat Res* 2003: **408**; 65.
41. Lichte P, Oberbeck R, Binnebosel M. A civilian perspective on ballistic trauma and gunshot injuries. *Scand J Trauma Resusc Emerg Med* 2010; **18**: 1.
42. Hollerman JJ, Fackler ML, Coldwell DM, *et al.* Gunshot wounds: 1. bullets, ballistics and mechanisms of injury. *Am J Roentgenol* 1990; **155**: 685.
43. Dodd, MJ. *Terminal Ballistics: a Text and Atlas of Gunshot Wounds*. CRC Press: Boca Raton FL, 2006.
44. Alexandropoulou CA, Panagiotopoulos EE. Wound ballistics: analysis of blunt and penetrating trauma mechanisms. *Health Sci J* 2012; **6**: 33.
45. Bartlett CS, Helfet DL, Hausman MR, *et al.* Ballistics and gunshot wounds: effects on musculoskeletal tissues. *J Am Acad Orthop Surg* 2000; **8**: 21.
46. Ordog GJ. Lead toxicity secondary to retained missiles. In: Ordog GJ (ed). *Management of Gunshot Wounds*. Elsevier: Amsterdam, 1988: 405.
47. Hollerman JJ. Gunshot wounds: 2. Radiology. *Am J Roentgenol* 1990; **155**: 691.
48. Feary DJ, Magdesian KG, Aleman MA, *et al.* Traumatic brain injury in horses: 34 cases (1994–2004). *Am J Vet Med Assoc* 2007; **231**: 259.

49. Chesnut RM, Marshall LF, Klauber MR, *et al.* The role of secondary brain injury in determining the outcome from severe head injury. *J Trauma* 1993; **34**: 216.
50. Shawkat H, Westwood M, Mortimer A. Mannitol: a review of its clinical uses. *Contin Educ Anaesth Crit Care Pain* 2012: **12** :82.
51. Kamel H, Navi B, Nakagawa K, *et al.* Hypertonic saline versus mannitol for the treatment of elevated intracranial pressure: a meta-analysis of randomized clinical trials. *Crit Care Med* 2011; **39**: 554.
52. Velmahos GC, Souter I, Degiannis E, *et al.* Selective surgical management in penetrating neck injuries. *Can J Surg* 1994; **37**: 487.
53. Sprayberry KA, Barrett EJ. Thoracic trauma in horses. *Vet Clin North Am Equine Pract* 2015; **31**: 199.
54. Magdesian KG, Fielding L, Rhodes DM, *et al.* Changes in central venous pressure and blood lactate concentration in response to acute blood loss in horses. *J Am Vet Med Assoc* 2006; **229**: 1458.
55. Bastos R, Baisden CE, Harker L, *et al.* Penetrating thoracic trauma. *Semin Thorac Cardiovasc Surg* 2008; **20**: 19.
56. Demetriades D, Velmahos GC. Penetrating injuries of the chest: indications for operation. *Scand J Surg* 2002; **91**: 41.
57. Como JJ, Bokhari F, Chiu WC, *et al.* Practice management guideline for selective nonoperative management of penetrating abdominal trauma. *J Trauma* 2010; **68**: 721.
58. Inaba K, Barmparas G, Foster A, *et al.* Selective nonoperative management of torso gunshot wounds. *J Trauma* 2010; **68**: 1301.
59. Biffl WL, Moore EE. Management guidelines for penetrating abdominal trauma. *Curr Opin Crit Care* 2010; **16**: 609.
60. Pryor JP, Reilly PM, Dabrowski GP, *et al.* Nonoperative management of abdominal gunshot wounds. *Ann Emerg Med* 2004; **43**: 344.
61. Vatistas NJ, Meagher DM, Gillis CL, *et al.* Gunshot injuries in horses: 22 cases (1971–1993). *J Am Vet Med Assoc* 1995; **207**: 1198.
62. Dukti SA, Southwood LL, Van Metre DC. Survival and factors affecting survival in small ruminants and camelids attacked by dogs: 62 cases (1994–2004). *J Vet Em Crit Care* 2007; **17**: 257.
63. Kannikeswaran N, Kamat D. Mammalian bites. *Clin Pediatr* 2009; **48**: 145.
64. Genthon A, Wilcox SR. Crush syndrome: a case report and review of the literature. *J Emerg Med* 2014; **46**: 313.
65. Perkins G, Valberg SJ, Madigan JM, *et al.* Electrolytes disturbances in foals with severe rhabdomyolysis. *J Vet Intern Med* 1998; **12**: 173.
66. Better OS. Traumatic rhabdomyolysis ("crush syndrome")-updated 1989. *Isr J Med Sci* 1989; **25**: 69.
67. Han JH, McKenzie HC. Intermittent peritoneal dialysis for the treatment of acute renal failure in two horses. *Equine Vet Educ* 2008; **20**: 256.
68. Kritchevsky JE, Stevens DL, Christopher J, *et al.* Peritoneal dialysis for presurgical management of ruptured bladder in a foal. *J Am Vet Med Assoc* 1984; **185**: 81.
69. Smith J, Greaves I. Crush injury and crush syndrome: a review. *J Trauma* 2003; **54**: S226.
70. Cotovio M, Monreal L, Navarro M, *et al.* Detection of fibrin deposits in tissues from horses with severe gastrointestinal disorders. *J Vet Intern Med* 2007; **21**: 308.
71. de la Rebière de Pouyade G, Grulke S, Detilleux J, *et al.* Evaluation of low-molecular-weight heparin for the prevention of equine laminitis after colic surgery. *J Vet Emerg Crit Care* 2009; **19**: 113.
72. Monreal L, Villatoro AJ, Monreal M, *et al.* Comparison of the effects of low-molecular-weight and unfractioned heparin in horses. *Am J Vet Res* 1995; **56**: 1281.
73. Sever MS, Vanholder R, Lameire N. Management of crush-related injuries after disasters. *New Engl J Med* 2006; **354**: 1052.
74. Brown CVR, Rhee P, Chan L, *et al.* Preventing renal failure in patients with rhabdomyolysis: do bicarbonate and mannitol make a difference? *J Trauma* 2004; **56**: 1191.
75. Brook I. Management of human and animal bite infection: an overview. *Curr Infect Dis Rep* 2009: **1**: 389.
76. Smith PF, Meadowcroft AM, May DB. Treating mammalian bite wounds. *J Clin Pharm Ther* 2000; **25**: 85.
77. Henton J, Jain A. Cochrane corner: antibiotic prophylaxis for mammalian bites (intervention review). *J Hand Surg Eur* 2012; **37**: 804.
78. Hendrix SM, Baxter GM. Management of complicated wounds. *Vet Clin North Am Equine Pract* 2005; **21**: 217.
79. Kaufman KL, Mann FA, Kim DY, *et al.* Evaluation of the effects of topical zinc gluconate in wound healing. *Vet Surg* 2014; **43**: 972.

CHAPTER 21

Sarcoid Transformation at Wound Sites

Derek C. Knottenbelt, OBE, BVM&S, DVMS, Dip ECEIM, MRCVS, **John Schumacher**, DVM, MS, Dip ACVIM, and **Ferenc Toth**, DVM, PhD, Dip ACVS

Chapter Contents

Summary

Equine sarcoids are likely caused by bovine papillomavirus. Sarcoid-affected horses are capable of transmitting the virus, often by flies, to other horses to cause development of sarcoids. Early signs that a sarcoid is developing within a wound are dehiscence, unhealthy appearance of granulation tissue, lack of wound contraction, and inability to control exuberant granulation tissue (EGT). Sarcoids in a wound are difficult to diagnose histologically because sarcoid tissue is often admixed with granulation tissue. Pathologists unfamiliar with the histologic appearance of sarcoids often misdiagnose the lesion. Recurrence of a sarcoid after simple surgical excision is common. Other treatments that may offer better success than excision include: cryotherapy; laser surgical excision; immunotherapy in the form of cell-wall extracts of mycobacteria or subcutaneous implantation of sarcoid tissue; repeated topical application of a cytotoxic drug, such as cisplatin, administered alone or in combination with electric-impulse therapy, the anti-mitotic drug, 5-fluorouracil, or an antiviral ointment, such as acyclovir or imiquimod; and radiation therapy. Sarcoid contamination of wounds can be prevented by covering wounds, if possible, and by fly control.

Introduction

Horses have been affected by sarcoids for centuries,[1] but the condition was first described by Jackson in 1936.[2] Sarcoids occur in all equine populations, with a prevalence varying between 0.6% and 12%.[3] This unique, benign fibroblastic tumor is, by far, the most prevalent skin neoplasm of horses. Analyses of records from veterinary diagnostic pathology laboratories showed that 24% of all tumor biopsy specimens and 46% of biopsy specimens obtained from cutaneous neoplasms contained tissue determined to be a sarcoid when examined histologically.[4,5] Other equidae, including donkeys, mules, and zebras, are also affected.[3] Conversely, the role of the sarcoid in failure of wound healing has only recently come to light.[6]

The equine sarcoid has the following six different clinical manifestations:

1. **Occult (flat) sarcoid**: the mildest and most superficial form is called the occult form. It is characterized by a vague (often circular) change in the color or density of the hair coat. The epidermis is thickened, and there is invariably at least one small nodule within the affected area.

Equine Wound Management, Third Edition. Edited by Christine Theoret and Jim Schumacher.

Companion website: www.wiley.com/go/theoret/wound

2. **Nodular sarcoid**: the nodular form is solid and often spherical. Lesions of this type can vary widely in size and number; some involve the dermis, whereas others are entirely subcutaneous.
3. **Verrucose sarcoid**: the verrucose form is "warty" in appearance and usually ill defined. The size can vary widely from limited zones to extensive plaques.
4. **Fibroblastic sarcoid**: the fibroblastic form is fleshy and exophytic in appearance and is usually exudative and infected. Lesions can be pedunculated or sessile with a broad base. The latter type is that most commonly involved in problems with healing and is often similar in appearance to EGT.
5. **Mixed sarcoid**: mixed sarcoids show characteristics of several of the other types and are relatively common, occurring spontaneously or in association with certain types of wounds.
6. **Malignant (malevolent) sarcoid**: the malignant form is a rare and very dangerous expanding invasive tumor. It can arise spontaneously and may also develop when a milder form (most often the fibroblastic type) is subjected to repeated trauma (including biopsy). Although this form is rare, it can develop in sarcoid-contaminated wounds, especially if repeated surgeries are performed (usually in response to excision of tissue presumed to be EGT).

Occult and nodular forms seldom complicate wound healing, except when these forms are subjected to incomplete surgical removal or are traumatized.

Etiopathogenesis

There is extensive evidence to indicate that equine sarcoids are caused by bovine papillomavirus 1 (BPV-1) and BPV-2, which are associated with transient, benign warts in their natural bovine host. Some investigators have speculated, however, that cattle-to-horse viral transmission does not result in development of sarcoids, because the majority of sarcoids evaluated harbored an equine-specific version of the BPV not found in cattle.[7] Conversely, stabling of sarcoid-affected horses with unaffected horses has been shown to result in the transmission of BPV and development of sarcoids.[8] Using polymerase chain reaction (PCR) techniques, viral DNA has been found in sarcoid tissue and in intact, normal skin of sarcoid-affected horses, but not in the skin of unaffected horses.[9] In one report, however, DNA of BPV was found in normal skin of horses unaffected with sarcoid but exposed to sarcoid-affected horses (i.e., latent infections).[10] Similarly, the proportion of horses having BPV DNA (73%) or BPV RNA (64%) identified in their skin samples was found to be the same in horses affected with sarcoids and in healthy horses living in contact with cattle having recently suffered BPV infection.[11] Furthermore, BPV DNA (30%) and BPV RNA (20%) were also detected in healthy, control horses. In a recent study, severity of disease, characterized by the number and growth rate of sarcoids, nevertheless, showed a highly significant correlation with intralesional viral load.[12] Altogether, these findings have implications concerning the diagnosis of sarcoids using PCR.

Some horses appear to be genetically predisposed to develop sarcoid. The incidence of sarcoids in Quarter Horses is nearly twice that of Thoroughbreds, and the incidence in Standardbreds is half that of Thoroughbreds.[10] Predisposition to sarcoids appears to be strongly associated with particular major histocompatibility complex (equine leukocyte antigen) haplotypes[13] and may be related to suppressed local immunity.[14]

Because sarcoids tend to develop in wounds, flies attracted to wounds may act as vectors of either viral particles or viral-infected fibroblasts. The infection can be transmitted from horse to horse or from one site to another on the same horse. Indirect transmission of BPV may also occur via tack or grooming equipment.[10]

Horses have a reputation for developing non-healing wounds, particularly those involving the distal aspect of the limb (carpus/tarsus and distally to these joints). The vast majority of equine wounds, however, heal if inhibitory factors, such as infection, movement, necrotic tissue, foreign body, etc., are removed. When a wound is affected by a sarcoid, however, the healing inevitably becomes suspended, often indefinitely. Sarcoid transformation of wounds is, therefore, a serious complication associated with cutaneous wounds in horses.[6]

Fibroblastic sarcoids and verrucose sarcoids are the usual types of sarcoid encountered as a complication of wound healing.[6,15–17] Sarcoids developing in wounds on the trunk tend to be verrucose and to remain superficial, whereas those on the limbs are likely to be the invasive, fibroblastic type.[3]

Transformation of a wound into a sarcoid often goes unrecognized, mainly because of the similar appearance of the sarcoid tissue to granulation tissue or a keloid/hypertrophic scar. Treatment of a wound affected by sarcoid transformation is difficult because consistently effective treatments are lacking. This chapter focuses primarily on the clinical features of sarcoid transformation and the challenges of treating those wounds in which sarcoid is identified.

Any type of wound is susceptible to transforming into a sarcoid, and even a small wound, such as a skin puncture at an injection site or caused by an insect bite, can be transformed into a non-healing, sarcoid-contaminated wound. Surgical wounds can easily be infected with BPV, either naturally or by iatrogenic transfer of BPV-infected tissue into the wound during surgery (e.g., a castration site).

The time required for a sarcoid to develop at a wound after infection is extremely variable. In some cases, the transformation is obvious early in healing, whereas for other wounds, transformation occurs much later, even long after the wound appears to have healed (e.g., months or years).

Sarcoid transformation within a wound can occur in the following ways:

- Injury (accidental or surgical) to sarcoid-affected skin. In this case, a sarcoid is wounded, and if the wound extends into normal skin adjacent to the tumor, the entire wound is susceptible to sarcoid tranformation (Figure 21.1).

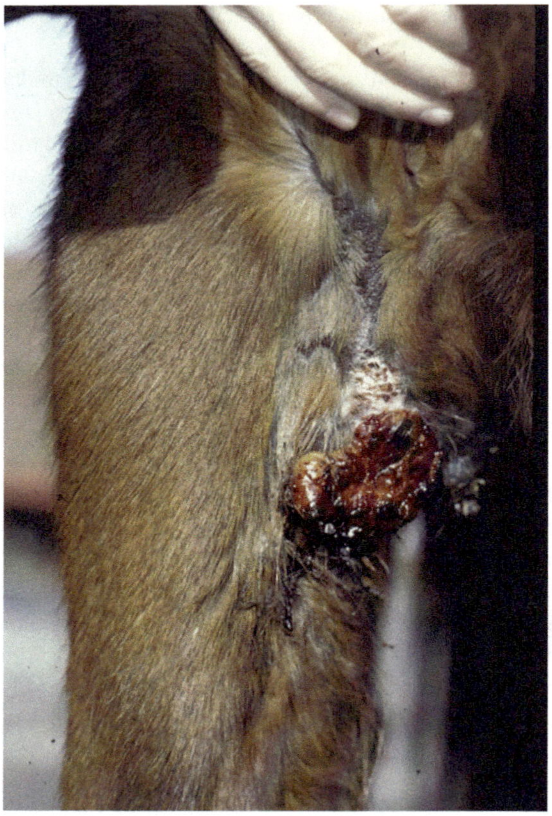

Figure 21.1 This horse sustained an accidental wire cut to its axilla over a site that was already affected by occult and verrucose sarcoid. The sarcoid had been quiescent for at least 4 years, but within weeks of the relatively trivial injury, the region had deteriorated badly into a deep and invasive fibroblastic lesion.

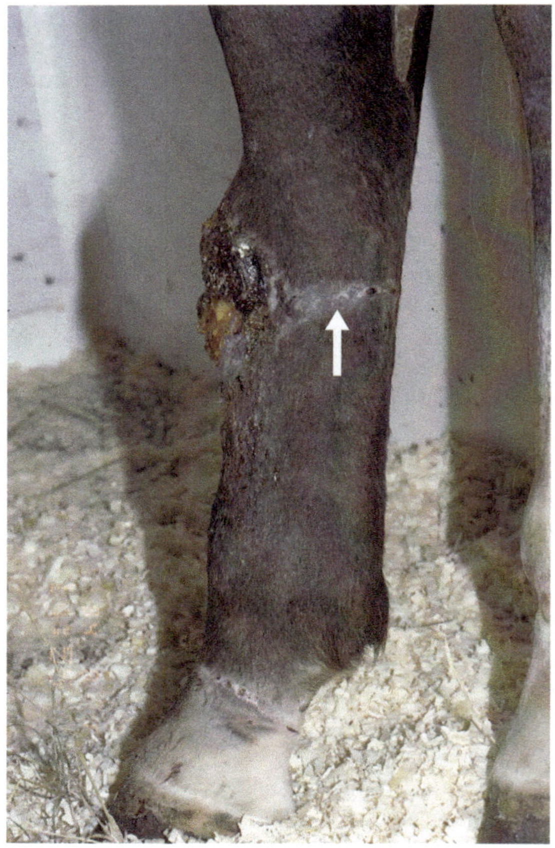

Figure 21.2 This circumferential laceration around the mid-cannon region healed remarkably well except for the area dorsally. The horse had several other occult and verrucose sarcoids on the medial thigh and axillary regions. Several attempts were made to excise the "granulation tissue" and graft the early "granulating" wound bed after each excision. Histologic examination of the granulation tissue obtained from each debridement later confirmed that the tissue was, in fact, almost pure fibroblastic sarcoid. Note the remarkably good healing that had taken place away from the sarcoid region (white arrow).

- Development of a sarcoid in a wound in normal skin when there are sarcoids at other sites (Figure 21.2). In this case, the virus or cells from the sarcoid are transmitted from the tumor into the wound. Cellular transfer from a sarcoid to a wound at another site can easily take place, and the "autograft" of cells results in a high probability of cellular survival in the wound. Vector transmission provides the only plausible explanation for this transfer because there is no evidence to support hematogenous dissemination of either sarcoid-transformed cells or virus or genomic particles of the virus.[18]
- Sarcoid transformation occurring at a wound when there are no sarcoids at other sites, but the host has contact with horses affected with sarcoids (Figure 21.3). In this situation, cells or particles of virus from the sarcoid of one horse are transferred into the wound of another horse, probably by a vector. Alternatively, the horse may have a latent infection of BPV, and epithelial damage activates the virus to cause formation of a sarcoid.
- A wounded horse is in contact with a fomite, such as tack or grooming equipment, containing the BPV.[10]
- Sarcoid can be transferred iatrogenically into a surgical site when surgical instruments (or even hypodermic needles) are used at a sarcoid site and then used for a surgical procedure at another site (Figure 21.4).
- Failure to remove all sarcoid cells during surgical excision of a sarcoid. In this case, residual sarcoid is responsible for recurrence. Rapid growth or transformation of the sarcoid is common under these circumstances, even after harvesting a sample from a sarcoid (Figure 21.5). The time required for recurrence is unpredictable. Wound dehiscence, failure of the wound to epithelialize, a lack of wound contraction, or any combination of these complications may indicate that the sarcoid has recurred.

Larger wounds may be more susceptible to the development of sarcoids than smaller wounds in the following situations: (1) when normal skin is wounded and sarcoids are present at other sites; (2) when normal skin is wounded, and the horse is in contact with horses that have sarcoids; or (3) when normal skin is wounded and the horse is in contact with a source of BPV (a vector or fomite). Small wounds, such as a wound created by

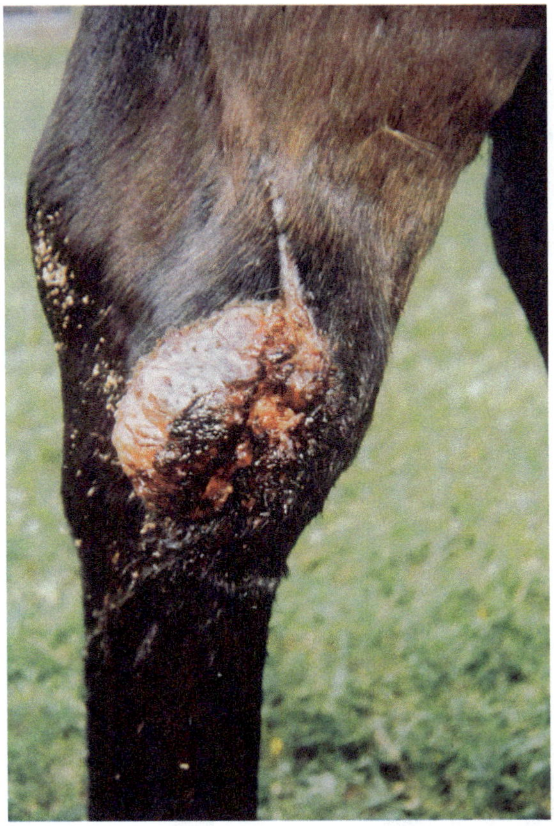

Figure 21.3 This horse sustained a deep laceration to the lateral surface of the hock. The wound healed along most of its length but was slow to close at the distal extent. The normal scar at the proximal extent of the wound can be appreciated. Two attempts were made to excise the "granulation tissue." Fortunately, the tissues from each excision had been retained in formalin solution, and when these were examined histologically, a mixture of sarcoid and infected granulation tissue was identified. The horse had no other sarcoids, and there were no cattle in the vicinity. Two other horses in the same field, however, had several small, ulcerated fibroblastic/nodular sarcoids and several verrucose lesions each.

a needle puncture (Figure 21.4), heal more quickly than large wounds, thereby decreasing the risk of prolonged exposure to vectors for transmission of virus or sarcoid cells. The proximity of a sarcoid to a wound can influence the likelihood of the wound undergoing sarcoid transformation (Figure 21.6), but this may depend on the feeding behavior of insects.

Flies have been implicated in the epidemiology of sarcoids; they may act as vectors for the BPV particles, but it seems far more likely that the sarcoid-transformed cell itself is transferred from a sarcoid to a wound (Figure 21.7). In this event, the location of the wound has an important bearing on the type of sarcoid that develops. Transfer of sarcoid cells to a wound on a limb

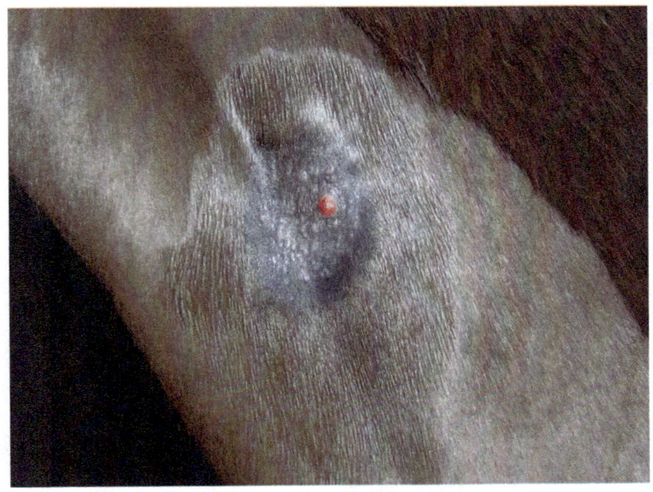

Figure 21.4 This verrucose sarcoid with occult skin changes in a roughly circular shape developed at the site of an intravenous injection. The needle used to infiltrate this site with local anesthetic solution prior to venipuncture had been used to infiltrate the site of a sarcoid prior to biopsy. The lesion developed over a period of 5 weeks; there was no evidence of a pre-existing sarcoid at this site.

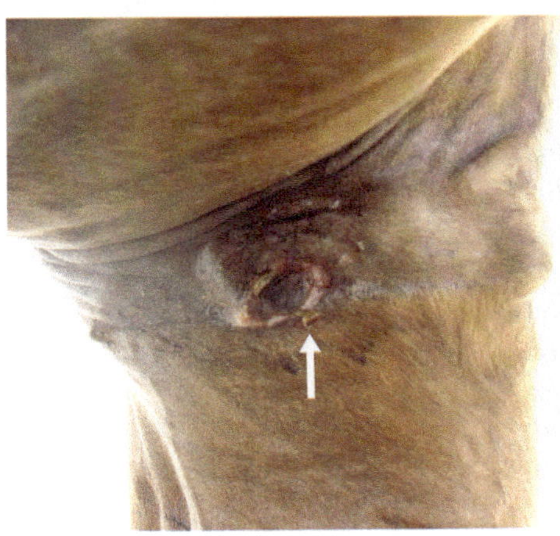

(a)

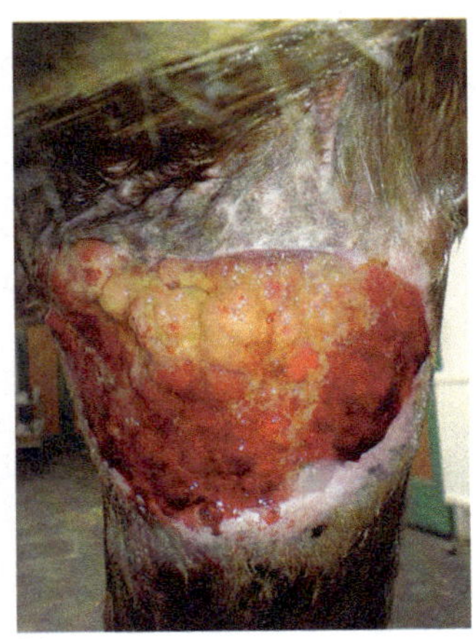

(b)

Figure 21.5 (**a**) This horse had been subjected to surgical excision of a sarcoid in the axillary area some 8 months prior. A second attempt was made to remove the lesion in the center of the scar (arrow). (**b**) Wound dehiscence and massive exacerbation developed during the ensuing months.

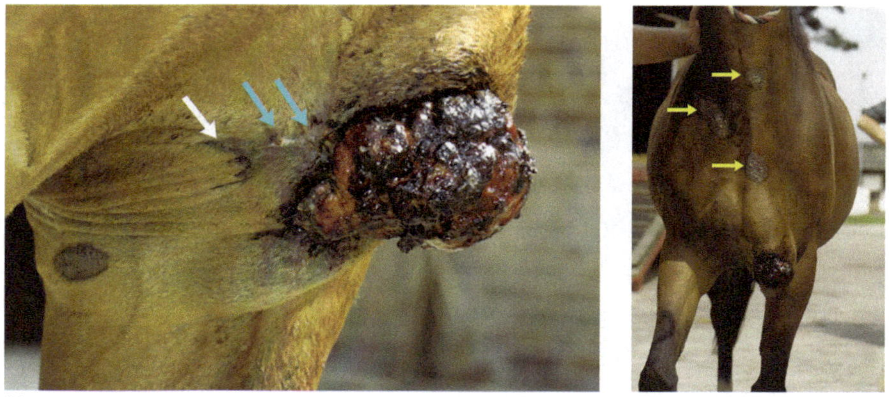

(a) (b)

Figure 21.6 **(a)** This pony sustained a wire laceration across the front of the left shoulder. The white arrow points to the scar. The wound appeared to heal well at first, but around 4 weeks post injury, an "EGT mass" developed at the most lateral extent of the wound. Several smaller fibroblastic growths developed along the wound shortly afterwards (blue arrows). **(b)** Clinical examination showed the main bulk to be very extensive subcutaneously and identified several occult and verrucose sarcoids in the adjacent regions (yellow arrows). Biopsy and histologic examination confirmed the main mass and the smaller ones to be pure sarcoid.

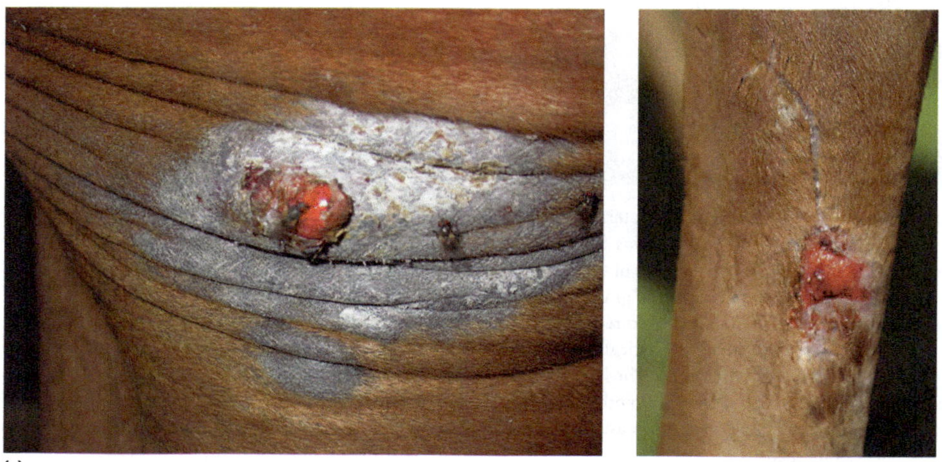

(a) (b)

Figure 21.7 **(a)** The sarcoid illustrates the preferential feeding pattern of certain species of fly for sarcoid tissue (note the flies present in the photo). **(b)** This horse sustained a minor injury to the medial surface of the metatarsal region that failed to heal in a localized area. Biopsy of the site was undertaken because of the presence of sarcoid at other sites, and subsequent histologic examination revealed almost pure features of sarcoid. Flies were noted by the owner to move between the fresh wound site and the sarcoid.

(e.g., elbow/stifle and distal regions) tends to induce formation of a fibroblastic sarcoid (Figure 21.8), whereas a wound on the body and neck more commonly develops into a verrucose sarcoid (Figure 21.9).[6,17]

Warm, still weather results in a large population of flies and far more fly activity on the horse. Flies frequently feed on sarcoids, especially if the sarcoids are ulcerated. Sarcoid cells seem to have a better chance of survival if they are transferred, by a fly, from a sarcoid near a wound than from a sarcoid remote from it (Figure 21.7).

When a sarcoid is diagnosed on the limb of a horse, a wound (ranging from a minor abrasion to a full-thickness laceration) very likely preceded the sarcoid; sarcoids rarely develop spontaneously on the limb distal to the femorotibial joint (stifle)/cubital joint (elbow) in the absence of cutaneous trauma.

Tip

- Preventing flies from contacting a wound decreases the likelihood that the wound will transform into a sarcoid.

Clinical aspects

A general medical history of the horse and a specific history of the wound should be obtained at the outset. Establishing if the horse has other sarcoids or has had sarcoids is important. Even if previous treatment for a sarcoid was successful, the horse is likely genetically prone to develop other sarcoids. The presence or history of sarcoids affecting in-contact horses is also important. Given the familial tendencies to develop sarcoids,[19] information

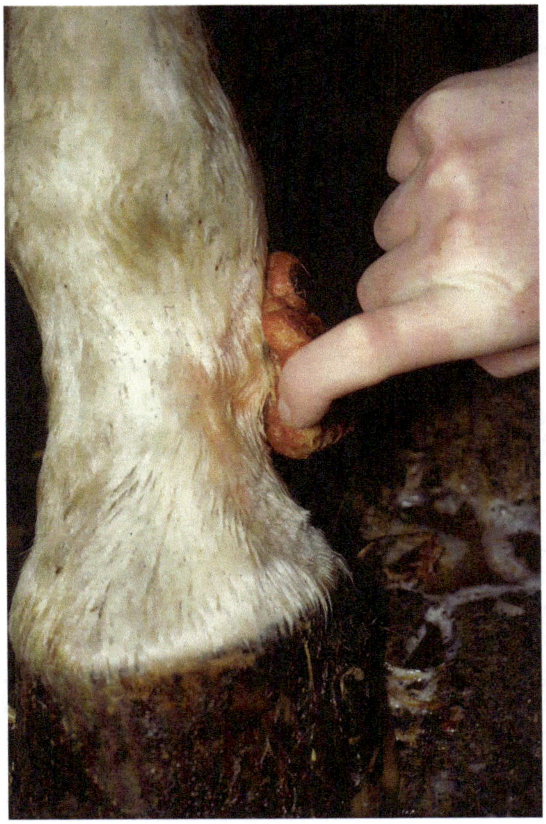

Figure 21.8 A pedunculated sarcoid developed at one of a number of small wire wounds that had occurred several months previously. The horse had several other superficial sarcoids on the head and axilla. Diagnosis was confirmed by biopsy and histologic examination.

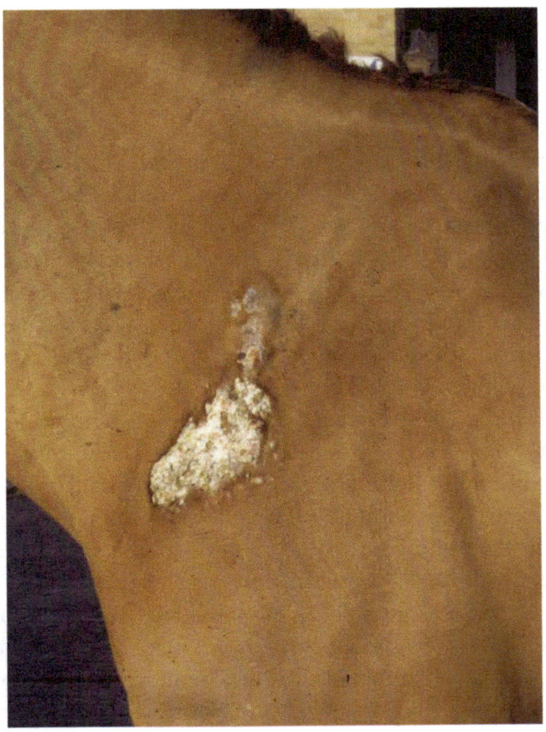

Figure 21.9 This horse sustained a large degloving wound on its shoulder, from a fall. The horse had several types of sarcoids at other sites. The wound appeared to heal reasonably well but was left with this verrucose area that was confirmed histologically as sarcoid.

concerning sarcoid history of related horses may be particularly important. Horses with sarcoids at other sites are far more likely to develop a sarcoid in a wound than are those without a sarcoid. Close contact of a wounded horse with a sarcoid-affected horse may be an important factor in contamination of a wound with sarcoid cells. Wounds occurring during summer (i.e., fly season) are far more likely to develop a sarcoid, and the longer the wound remains unhealed or uncovered, the greater is the opportunity for sarcoid transformation to take place (Figure 21.10).

A physical examination of the wound is important because factors that inhibit wound healing, such as infection, movement, impaired local blood supply, necrotic tissue, or foreign bodies, may also facilitate transformation of the wound into a sarcoid. When sarcoids are detected at other sites on the wounded horse, transformation of a wound into a sarcoid becomes likely.

Recognizing that a wound has transformed into a sarcoid

- A common feature of sarcoid-contaminated wounds is unexpected *early wound dehiscence*. Often, the wound dehisces within days of repair if the sutured wound was left uncovered and was attacked by flies. In the primary author's experience, dehiscence seems to be more likely if the horse has ulcerated sarcoids at other sites. Managing a wound by delayed primary closure or relying on second-intention healing may increase the opportunity for deposition of BPV-infected fibroblasts in the wound.
- Delay in healing or dehiscence of the sutured wound after surgical excision of a sarcoid usually indicates that sarcoid tissue remains in the wound, even if the wound eventually appears to heal by second intention. Recurrence of sarcoid at such sites can occur in days to years.[15] Laser surgery may reduce the risks of recurrence,[20,21] but simple removal of sarcoid tissue is often followed by recurrence, regardless of whether or not the wound was sutured or left to heal by second intention.
- Although the earliest signs of development of a sarcoid within a wound are subtle (wound dehiscence, unhealthy appearance of granulation tissue, or lack of wound contraction), later signs, such as an *inability to control EGT* by medical or surgical treatment, are far more obvious. A wound left to heal by second intention may expand, rather than contract and epithelialize, if contaminated with sarcoid (Figure 21.10). *The value of diagnostic pathology in cases in which granulation tissue is excised cannot be overstated*; if a sarcoid is detected, the approach to wound management must change dramatically.
- There are some anatomic differences in the clinical manifestations of sarcoids; for instance, limb wounds appear to have a greater tendency to develop fibroblastic sarcoids, either the type-1 (pedunculated) fibroblastic form or the type-2 (sessile) fibroblastic form (Figure 21.10). In contrast, the trunk and neck have a greater tendency to develop verrucose, or less commonly, occult (flat) forms of sarcoid (Figures 21.4 and 21.9). Fibroblastic or verrucose sarcoids can develop in wounds of the head. The anatomic differences associated with sarcoid types may be related to observations that limb wounds heal less by contraction than do wounds on the trunk, and that EGT is more likely to form in wounds of the distal aspect of the limb (carpus/tarsus and distally) than it is in wounds of the trunk. These regional differences in normal healing are attributed to local factors rather than to any particular differences in fibroblastic behavior,[22] and it seems likely that the same local factors influence the behavior of the sarcoid-transformed fibroblasts. The specific factors responsible for these anatomic differences with respect to sarcoid types are, however, far from clear.

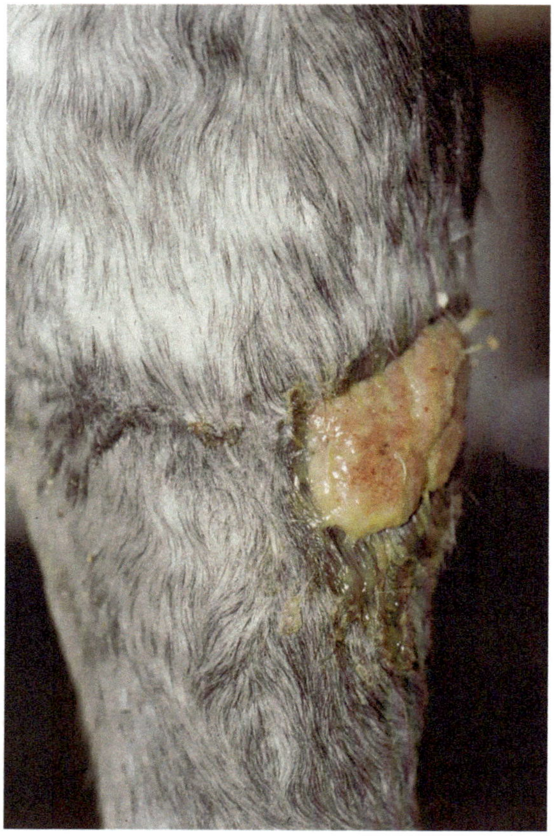

Figure 21.10 Most of this horizontal wire wound over the dorsal surface of the tarsus healed remarkably well with excellent wound care, despite a 3-day delay in seeking veterinary attention. The medial limit failed to heal over many months, however, and perhaps justifiably, suspecting the problem to be EGT, several vain attempts at surgical debridement and even an attempt at pinch grafting were performed. A biopsy sample of the wound was found to contain sarcoid. The lesion had a broad flat (sessile) base. The horse had no other sarcoids but several in-contact horses were affected.

Tip

- Delayed healing of an open wound or an inability to control granulation tissue should arouse suspicion that the wound has been contaminated with sarcoid.

Identification

Early stages of sarcoid transformation of a wound are often impossible to recognize. Granulation tissue and bacterial pyogranuloma can appear remarkably similar to a wound that is partially or exclusively sarcoid (Figure 21.11a-c). Likewise, a keloid or hypertrophic scar can easily be mistaken for a verrucose sarcoid and vice versa (Figure 21.11d,e).

Establishing whether or not a sarcoid is involved in a non-healing wound is important because the management of EGT and sarcoids is very different. Martens *et al.*[23] described a PCR method to identify sarcoid that is based on the presence of BPV DNA, collected by swabbing the suspected sarcoid lesion; this test may be particularly valuable for detecting sarcoid in non-healing wounds.[3] The test is unsuitable for detecting occult-type sarcoids,[23] however, and due to high prevalence of BPV DNA in normal equine skin, the test may result in a false-positive diagnosis.[3] Presence of any type of sarcoid lesion at other sites on the body should immediately alert the clinician to the possibility of sarcoid transformation in a non-healing wound.[24]

Differential diagnosis of sarcoid-contaminated wounds

The differential diagnosis of sarcoid transformation is complicated because there may be admixtures of granulation tissue, scar tissue, and infection within the wound. In some cases, sarcoid transformation is quite obvious to an experienced clinician. The majority of sarcoids in a wound, however, are difficult to diagnose. The differential diagnoses for equine sarcoids in wounds include the following:

- (exuberant) granulation tissue (Figure 21.11b);
- staphylococcal pyogranuloma (pseudomycetoma) (Figure 21.11c);
- oomycotic or fungal granuloma (e.g., *Pythium* spp., *Conidiobolus coronata*, etc.);
- foreign body granuloma;
- keloid scars, which can closely resemble verrucose sarcoids (Figure 21.11e).

Various features help to differentiate these clinical conditions (Table 21.1).

Pathology

Histologic examination of the tissues excised from a normal healing wound characteristically reveals organizing granulation tissue with a well-recognized parallel arrangement of new blood vessels (see Figure 1.7). The healing process whereby normal granulation tissue is formed has been outlined in Chapter 1, and certainly it is well recognized by pathologists. Although samples obtained from a chronic, granulating, non-healing wound may contain some possible causative factors (e.g., bacterial or fungal infection, foreign matter, necrotic tissue, etc.), the normal underlying structure of the granulating wound remains invariably recognizable.

The histologic appearance of sarcoids, both within a wound and at other sites, is well documented.[25] There is little difference in the histologic features of sarcoids in wounds and those arising *de novo* (i.e., without the history of a wound at the site), except where admixtures of sarcoid and granulation tissue are present within the wound. Histologic characteristics of a sarcoid include fibroblastic proliferation, with fibroblasts arranged in a whorling pattern (Figure 21.12). Random arrangement of fibroblasts is also common. The fibroblasts themselves can show anisocytosis (abnormal variations in cell size) and anisokaryosis (abnormal variation in nuclear size in the cells). The number of mitotic figures varies but usually is

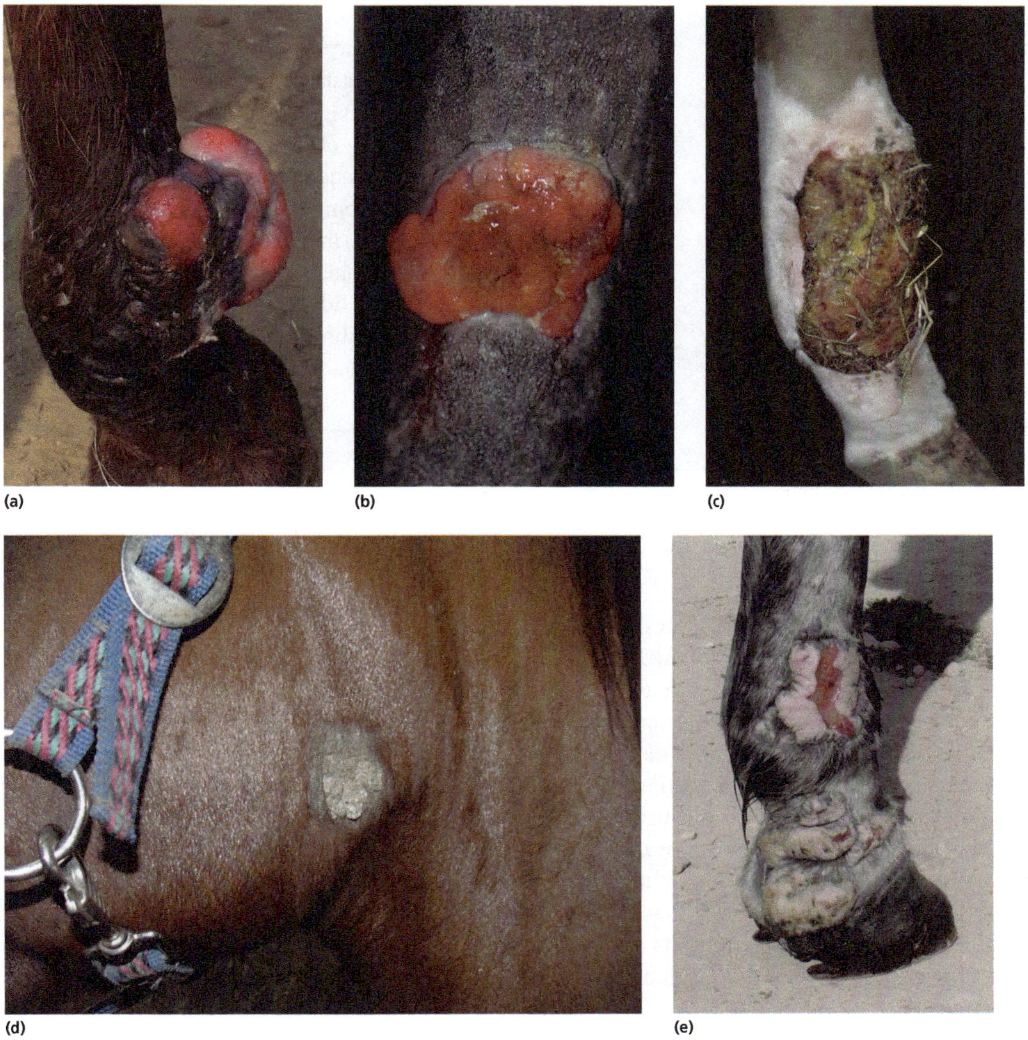

Figure 21.11 Clinical appearance of the more common primary changes occurring at wounds. Each example shown developed in a wound. **(a)** Fibroblastic sarcoid. **(b)** EGT. **(c)** Pseudomycetoma/pyogranuloma. **(d)** Verrucose sarcoid. **(e)** Keloid/hypertrophic scar.

Table 21.1 Main differentiating clinical features for sarcoid-affected wounds.

	Fibroblastic sarcoid	Granulation tissue	Pyogranuloma/ pseudomycetoma	Verrucose sarcoid	Keloid/hypertrophic scar
Appearance	Figure 21.11a	Figure 21.11b	Figure 21.11c	Figure 21.11d	Figure 21.11e
Keratinization	No	No	No	Yes	Yes
Proliferation	Yes	Yes	Yes	Possible	Yes
Ulceration	Yes	Yes	Yes	No	No
Vascularization	High	High	Moderate	Low	Low
Exudation	Yes	Yes	Yes/Low	No	No
Bacterial culture	Mixed commensals	Mixed pathogens/ commensals	Staphylococci	Commensals only	Commensals only

low or rare. The abundance and features of the extracellular matrix also vary.

The absence of overlying epithelium in tissues taken from an ulcerated sarcoid can complicate diagnosis. The first descriptions of the equine sarcoid were made by Jackson, who, in 1936, identified a variable epithelial component to the typical sarcoid.[2] Skilled pathologists usually have little difficulty in recognizing the full range of sarcoid types, even in the absence of epidermis. The diagnosis, however, depends heavily on the harvest of a truly representative sample of tissue, and this is often a major problem when sarcoid and granulation tissue are admixed.

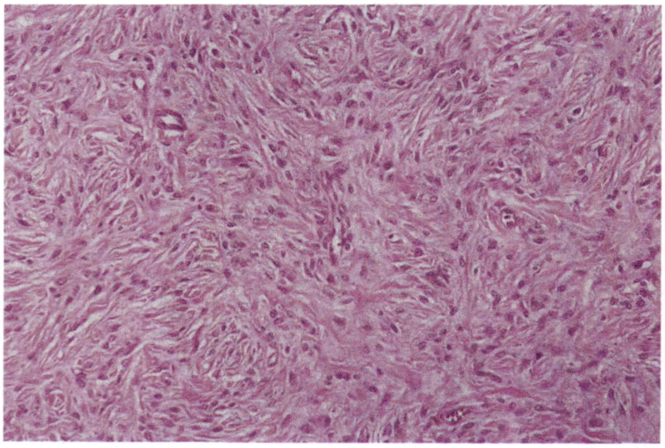

Figure 21.12 The histologic appearance of this equine sarcoid demonstrates the characteristic whorling patterns of the fibroblasts and the random/chaotic arrangements of the capillaries. There is little extracellular matrix, and the mitotic index is very low, despite a clinically rapid rate of growth.

Samples obtained by shaving off the surface of a granulating wound bed may show infected, ulcerated granulation tissue only. A far better representation of the true nature of the non-healing tissues is obtained when a core biopsy sample is taken from the depth of the tissue. Deep core biopsy samples may reveal sequential "layers" of sarcoid and granulation tissue or nests of sarcoid tumor cells. Sampling of only one tissue type or inappropriate histologic preparation of the sections may, therefore, be deceptive; a single small sample may show only sarcoid, only pyogranuloma, or only granulation tissue. Because treatment of a non-healing wound based on results of a single, small sample may be inappropriate, several deep biopsy samples using a wide biopsy punch (6–8 mm) should be harvested to maximize the chances of an accurate diagnosis.

Biopsy technique is important. The site should not be scrubbed or otherwise molested. Desensitizing the wound with local anesthetic solution is usually not necessary because both sarcoid and granulation tissue are free of nerve endings. If the wound must be desensitized, a regional nerve block, if possible to perform, is preferred to local infiltration of the site with an anesthetic solution, which may cause inflammation. A suspicious area of granulation tissue, such as a nodular region denser than surrounding tissue, should be sampled. When a preferred site for harvesting cannot be identified, several 6-mm to 8-mm biopsy punch samples should be taken from the central portion of the tissue, and each sample placed in an individual container of 10% formalin. Photographing the biopsy sites is useful so that the pathologist can see the appearance of tissue sampled. Samples taken from the skin margin are not usually diagnostic; moreover, taking samples from the margin is ill advised, because doing so encourages the tumor to extend further into normal skin. Small lesions may be subjected to excisional biopsy with the precautions outlined later in Treatment/management. Verrucose changes in wound sites are harvested in the same way, although for many of these samples, the skin edge can be included.

The value of histologic examination cannot be overstated because findings influence the therapy and the prognosis. The concurrent presence of a sarcoid and granulation tissue within a wound occurs with some frequency. Sarcoids inhibit healing, regardless of the amount of sarcoid tissue found in the wound. When "granulation tissue" is removed as a part of wound management, it should be submitted for histopathologic examination. Because of the variations in matrix type and staining characteristics of sarcoid tissue and inexperience of the pathologist, sarcoid tissue may be erroneously identified as fibroma, fibropapilloma, neurofibroma, neurofibrosarcoma, Schwannoma, low-grade fibrosarcoma, or spindle-cell tumors of various types.

> **Tip**
>
> - Confirming diagnosis of sarcoid histologically, as a cause of delayed wound healing, is important to determine appropriate therapy and offer prognosis. False-negative or erroneous histologic diagnosis is common, however, especially when tissue samples are read by a pathologist inexperienced in examining sarcoids.

Treatment/management

Clinical management of conventional sarcoids is a considerable challenge, and this challenge is increased substantially when the sarcoid is one that contaminates a wound. The existence of many suggested treatments for a sarcoid indicates that none are ideal. The options for treatment of wounds affected by sarcoid transformation are even less promising. Whatever method is employed, all sarcoid cells must be removed because residual cells replicate to create a new sarcoid that is often more aggressive than the initial sarcoid. Attempts to skin graft a sarcoid-affected wound are warranted only after surgical excision of sarcoid tissue has been ascertained to be complete.

The site of the sarcoid-contaminated wound has a major bearing on the choice of treatment, as well as the prognosis. Wounds of horses are often difficult to manage, and even more so when they are located on the distal aspect of the limb. It is not surprising then, that sarcoid-contaminated wounds of the limb are one of the most demanding therapeutic challenges in equine wound management. Currently available treatment options include the following:

- surgery – surgical excision, cryosurgery, laser surgery, and combinations of these surgical treatments;
- immunomodulatory therapy (i.e., using foreign/exogenous proteins, such as Bacillus Calmette-Guerin, Regressin®, Equimune®, etc.);
- topical or intralesional administration of cytotoxic/antimitotic/caustic chemicals;
- photodynamic therapy;
- radiation therapy;
- antiviral drugs.

> **Tip**
>
> - Before treatment of a sarcoid-transformed wound is started, the client should be appraised of the challenge of treatment and that multiple treatments using multiple methods of therapy may be necessary.

Surgery

Surgical methods, including various techniques of skin grafting, are commonly used to manage granulating wounds. Before embarking on any such procedure, the surgeon is strongly advised to closely examine the wound for sarcoid tissue, the presence of which invariably results in surgical failure (Figure 21.13). Nevertheless, resecting a spontaneously occurring sarcoid (i.e., not one that has contaminated a wound) and then applying a full-thickness or split-thickness skin graft to the wound created by the resection may be an effective treatment.[26]

Sharp surgery

Surgical excision alone of a sarcoid-transformed wound is usually unsuccessful, and recurrence of the tumor is very common for a number of reasons, including the following:

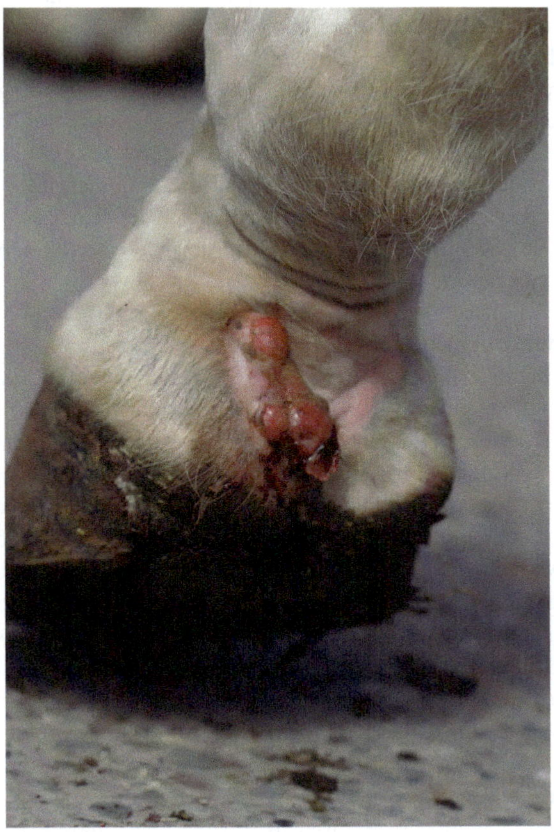

Figure 21.13 Multiple fibroblastic sarcoids developed at the site of a wire wound over the palmar pastern/heel bulb region. The injury had occurred some months previously; although part of the wound healed rapidly, this area had failed to heal. Pinch grafts were used after surgical debridement of the granulation tissue on three occasions but failed to help heal the wound. The horse had no other sarcoids and no contact with cattle.

- Anatomic limitations. Very often, insufficient skin is available, after excision, to close the wound without creating excessive tension on the sutures. Additionally, wounds on the distal aspect of the limb affected by a sarcoid are commonly over joints or tendons/ligaments, thus limiting the opportunity for complete excision with sarcoid-free margins. The surgeon can do little to overcome these anatomic limitations, although skin grafting of the operative site should be considered if a large margin of tissue surrounding the sarcoid-transformed wound is excised. The technique of pre-suturing or other techniques of skin expansion may be helpful in allowing removal of a large margin of skin. See Chapter 10 for a more information regarding techniques of skin expansion and Chapter 18 for more information regarding skin grafting. Pre-suturing involves placing sutures through skin near the margin of the lesion and then through skin at the margin of the other side of the lesion. When the suture is tightened, skin is stretched to cover the lesion. Chronic stretching (e.g., for 2–8 hours) causes the collagen fibers in skin adjacent to the lesion to relax. When the lesion is surgically removed, the previously stretched skin can be apposed with less tension, thereby decreasing the likelihood of dehiscence.
- Difficulty in defining a safe excisional margin that ensures removal of all sarcoid tissue, even when anatomic boundaries are not restrictive.
- Seeding of the operative site with sarcoid cells often occurs during its surgical removal. Covering the exposed, ulcerated sarcoid-contaminated tissue with a gauze swab or a plastic aerosol dressing is a wise precaution, as is the use of the "one cut, one blade" principle of "clean surgery." In this technique, each instrument is used only once and then laid aside. This applies to surgical blades, scissors, forceps, suture, and suture needles. This at least limits the risk of direct transfer of sarcoid cells across the wound. Laser surgery also reduces the risk of reseeding the sarcoid. An alternative method to avoid "rub-off" during surgical removal of an exposed, contaminated, ulcerated sarcoid is to remove it to just below the skin level using electrosurgery, after which the entire site is prepared for surgical excision with wide margins. "Clean surgery" techniques are fundamental to successful excision of a sarcoid.

Failure to remove every cell of the tumor leads to recurrence of the sarcoid along the wound's scar (Figure 21.14). Because discriminating between normal tissue and sarcoid during routine surgery is often impossible, a high risk of failure remains. A wide margin of excision can sometimes overcome this problem to some extent, but excessive removal of healthy tissues has the potential to delay or complicate healing. The use of the Mohs' surgical technique may allow for increased precision in obtaining clean margins after surgical excision of sarcoid-transformed wounds by confirming removal of all sarcoid tissue. This technique involves histologic examination of frozen sections of tissue from the margins of a tumor at the time of surgery, and it has been used successfully to remove a squamous cell carcinoma on the penis of a horse.[27]

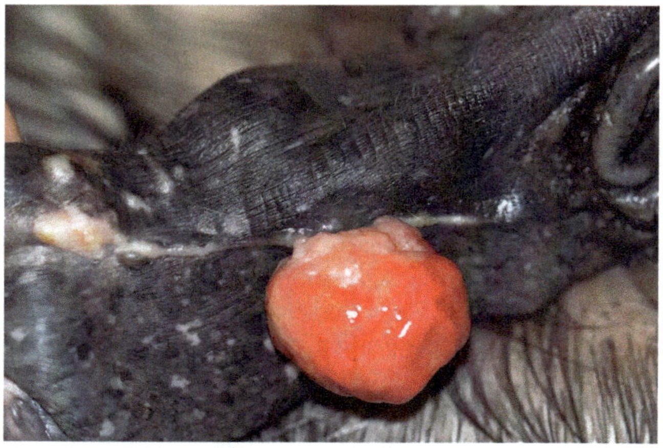

Figure 21.14 A nodular sarcoid was removed from the penile skin some 10 weeks previously with laser surgery. Most of the wound healed well, but this fibroblastic lesion developed in the wound's scar. The possibilities of "cell seeding" or residual "root" were considered. The laser surgery was repeated with good results.

Adjunctive measures are sometimes used to complement surgical excision; these involve cauterizing the wound bed by thermal cautery or using a cryogen after the combined sarcoid–granulation tissue has been excised. Although this technique may seem harsh and crude, the results are anecdotally reported to be acceptable and better than surgical excision alone; this probably reflects the importance of preventing deposition of viable sarcoid cells in the wound. Other adjunctive measures to surgery are described in subsequent sections.

Tip

- Surgical excision alone of a sarcoid-transformed wound is likely to be unsuccessful. Freezing or cauterizing the wound bed after surgical removal may decrease the incidence of recurrence of sarcoid.

Cryosurgery

Cryonecrosis, achieved by rapid freezing to temperatures below −40 °C[28] followed by slow thawing after each freeze (freeze–thaw cycle), has been widely used for many years in the management of sarcoids.[29] Determining the margin of the affected tissue and ensuring that the freeze extends to this point is always difficult, even when a well-defined sarcoid is present, let alone when sarcoid and granulation tissue are mixed. Cryonecrosis is not discriminatory: both normal and neoplastic tissues are destroyed, and extensive necrosis necessarily follows treatment. Given that necrosis is an undesirable feature of wound healing, poor overall results are typically achieved. The common necessity of repeated freezes adds to the shortcomings of this method.

Cryosurgery is sometimes used to destroy sarcoid cells potentially present in the wound after the sarcoid has been surgically debulked, on the premise that cryonecrosis is easier to achieve when the bulk of the abnormal tissue has been removed. Cryonecrois must be delayed after surgical debulking because a bloody field prevents an adequate freeze of tissue. In the authors' opinion, cryonecrosis has little to offer in the management of wounds contaminated with fibroblastic sarcoid.

Cryoantigen-induced regression of sarcoids at remote sites has been described,[30] but the primary author has not observed regression of remote sarcoids after cryosurgery, and to expect a benefit/cure of a sarcoid-contaminated wound after cryosurgical treatment of a remote sarcoid is unreasonable.

Laser surgery

Laser surgical excision/ablation is a reasonable technique for surgical removal of sarcoids because the wound margins are not seeded with sarcoid cells during the procedure.[31,32] Either CO_2 laser, YAG laser or diode laser can be used. Laser excision of granulation tissue alone has advantages over sharp surgery because of "die back" at the margin of the excision site because damaged cells along the margin are sloughed. Although "die back" may delay healing, laser excision/ablation is unlikely to substantially affect wound healing, whereas the effects of leaving residual sarcoid tissue within the wound bed are substantial. Apart from these advantages, the method has the same constraints as other surgical therapies, in that ascertaining that all sarcoid cells have been removed is impossible. Laser surgery used for treatment of "conventional" sarcoids is reported to carry a high chance of success.[32] A recent study examining the use of laser surgery for the resection of histologically confirmed sarcoids found that 83% of horses had no recurrence of sarcoid at the site of laser excision. Verrucose sarcoids and sarcoids located on the head or neck were more likely to recur.[21] The efficacy of lasers in treating sarcoid-transformed wounds is, however, not reported.

Hyperthermia

Reports describing the use of radiofrequency hyperthermia for treatment of sarcoids are scarce, making assessment of the efficacy of this treatment difficult. Sarcoids in three horses were reported to regress after being subjected to hyperthermia,[33] but in another report,[34] hyperthermia alone was not effective in treating sarcoids. For treatment of cancers in people, local hyperthermia has been shown to increase the effectiveness of chemotherapy or radiation therapy.[35] Resolution of sarcoids was observed in two horses treated with a combination of hyperthermia and iridium-192 interstitial radiation therapy.[34] Devices that deliver a local heat source are not readily available for use in horses, making hyperthermia an unlikely form of treatment for sarcoids.

Immunotherapy

Immunotherapy can be used to provoke the immune system into attacking sarcoid cells. Immunostimulants, such as cell-wall extracts of mycobacteria (Regressin-V, Bioniche Animal Health), *Propionibacterium acnes* (EqStim, Neogen Corp), or attenuated live *Mycobacterium bovis* (Bacillus Calmette–Guérin or BCG), have anti-tumoral activity and have been used to effectively treat horses for sarcoid.[36–38] The mechanism of action may be stimulation of cell-mediated immunity.[39] There are no reports that specifically describe the use of immunotherapy in the management of sarcoid-contaminated wounds. Intralesional or intravenous administration of *Propionibacterium acnes* once weekly for 6–8 weeks, however, is reported to result, in some cases, in tumor necrosis and slough,[40] indicating that this type of therapy may be beneficial in treating sarcoid-contaminated wounds. Local immunotherapy may be contraindicated for treatment of sarcoid-contaminated wounds on the limbs, distal to the elbow and stifle, because injection of BCG into sarcoids on the limb has been associated with severe edema and infection.[41,42] More recently, soluble extract of the oomycete, *Pythium insidiosum*, administered subcutaneously in eight to nine serial treatments has been successful in the treatment of some fibroblastic sarcoids. Resolution of sarcoids after administering *Pythium* proteins may be due to an enhanced immune response, more specifically the down-regulation of the Th_2 subset of cells and up-regulation of the Th_1 cells.

Imiquimod 5% cream (Aldara™, 3M Pharmaceuticals), a modifier of immune response with antiviral activity used to treat actinic keratosis, genital warts, and superficial basal cell carcinoma in people, has been used to treat sarcoids in horses.[43] The immune response created by imiquimod does not appear to be systemic. Application of imiquimod at sites where tissue is harvested for histologic examination may prevent the sarcoid from transforming into a more aggressive form.[40]

The sudden and complete spontaneous disappearance of sarcoids in up to 14% of affected horses is a recognized phenomenon;[44] this implies that an immunologic approach could be exploited. Because BPV is the accepted etiology of equine sarcoids, vaccination against this virus seems a reasonable approach to treatment, but no such vaccine is available. Stimulating immunity to cause regression of sarcoids by subcutaneous implantation of pencil eraser-sized pieces of sarcoid frozen in liquid nitrogen was reported to be highly effective (80%) in the treatment of 15 horses with a sarcoid.[45] Similar positive response to subcutaneous implantation of frozen sarcoid tissue was noted in a report of 18 horses.[46] In that report complications of this treatment were minor, such as mild swelling at the site of implantation and formation of an abscess in one horse. The first author, however, has observed this technique to be ineffective for treatment of sarcoids, more often than not. In recent years, *in vitro* studies of the biology of equine sarcoid have provided new insights into the pathogenesis of this disease; findings from these studies have provided routes of investigation for development of vaccines for treatment of sarcoids.[47,48]

Topical or intralesional cytotoxic/antimitotic/caustic chemicals

Topical chemotherapy

For many years, topical agents, such as inorganic (heavy) metal salts (arsenic, antimony and zinc salts, silver nitrate), plant extracts (such as extract of *Sanguineus canadensis*), often mixed with metal salts such as zinc chloride, and modern antimitotic compounds, such as 5-fluorouracil, and retinoids, such as tazarotene, have been used to treat sarcoids. Some of these topical agents, such as those used in combination at Liverpool University (in a compound named AW4-LUDES) may be effective in the treatment of some sarcoid-transformed wounds (Figure 21.15).

Nevertheless, most topically applied chemicals are not ideal for treatment of sarcoid-contaminated wounds because of their non-discriminatory, caustic, and necrotizing nature. If topical agents are to be applied, conventional surgical, laser surgical, or cryosurgical debulking of a large sarcoid-contaminated mass from a wound is helpful because debulking reduces the amount of the topical agent that must be applied and the depth to which the agent must penetrate to be effective.

The best approach when using a topical agent is to debulk the lesion by any suitable surgical means and then, after abatement of hemorrhage (usually after 24–36 hours), to apply a gentle but effective topical therapy, such as 5-fluorouracil 5% cream to the wound (twice daily for 7 days, then once daily for 7 days is an effective treatment in the primary author's experience). This relatively gentle approach allows the 5-fluorouracil cream to penetrate the wound and reduce the number of residual sarcoid cells.

Stronger caustic materials, such as copper sulfate, silver nitrate, and herbal extracts, such as XXTERRA® (Indian mud [*Sanguineus canadensis*/blood root extract] with zinc chloride, Larson Laboratories, Vetline Inc.), may be applied to debulked wounds, but the primary author does not recommend applying these caustic agents to sarcoids or sarcoid-contaminated wounds. Their efficacy is low, and some have a highly destructive nature; others simply exacerbate the condition. Topical application of AW4-LUDES, which is a combination of heavy metals, present in low concentrations, and 5-fluorouracil cream and natural oils, present in high concentrations, has been used for many years to treat sarcoids at Liverpool University with good results (Figure 21.15). Treatment with AW4-LUDES achieves a reasonable rate of success (around 58%).

> **Tip**
>
> - Avoid using caustic compounds, such as copper sulfate, silver nitrate, and blood root extract on sarcoid-contaminated wounds. The efficacy of these caustic compounds is low, and these compounds can exacerbate the condition.

Intralesional chemotherapy

Intralesional administration of an antimitotic or cytotoxic drug minimizes adverse systemic effects associated with chemotherapeutic agents normally delivered intravenously in large doses, while exposing tumor cells to high concentrations of the chemotherapeutic agent. Successful treatment of non-wound-related sarcoids using intralesional injection of stable emulsions of

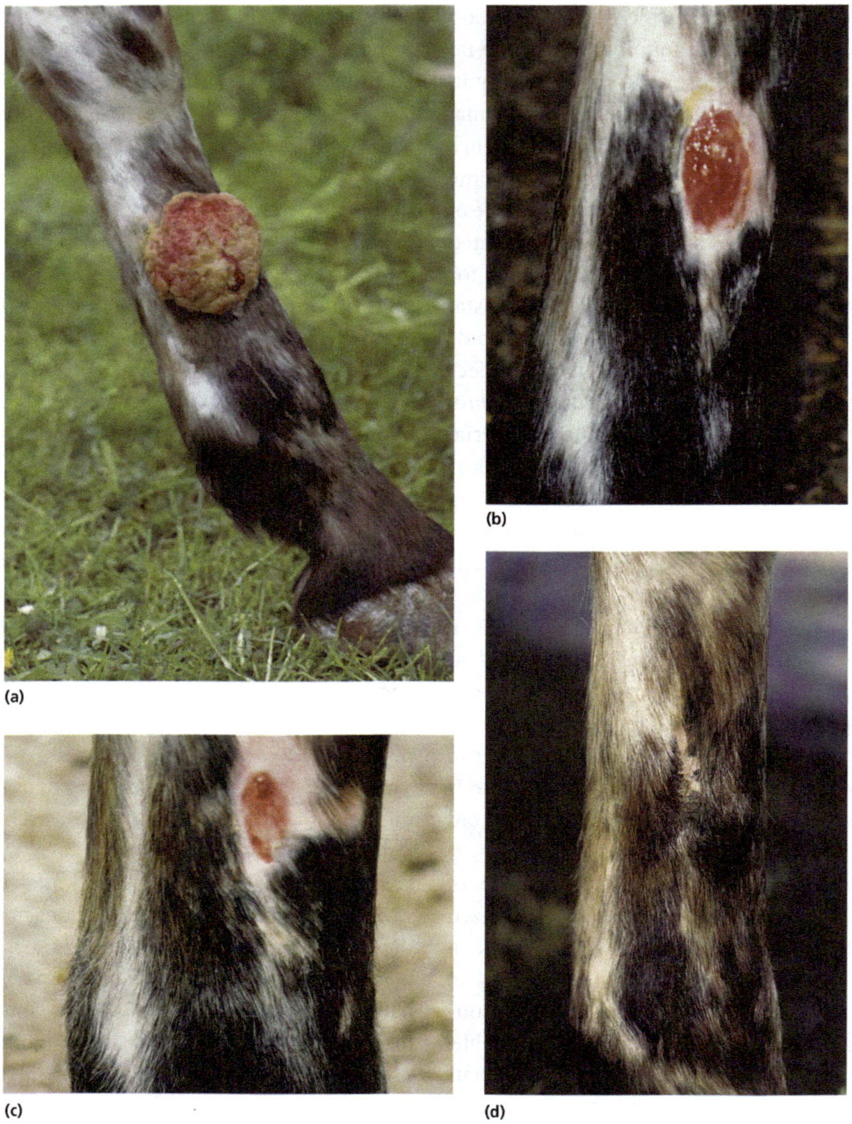

Figure 21.15 (a) This 8-year-old Appaloosa horse developed a fibroblastic sarcoid in a wound on the dorsolateral surface of the metacarpus. The lesion had a palpable and visible subcutaneous component. It was treated with the material known as AW4-LUDES. (b) The same horse, 6 weeks after treatment; (c) 8 weeks after treatment. (d) The outcome was highly satisfactory. No recurrence was reported at 4 years post treatment, and only a small pink scar was visible.

cisplatin at 1 mg/cm^3 in sesame oil[49] or implantation of slow-release cisplatin beads has been reported.[50] These drugs tend to be highly destructive to tissues and so may be less appropriate for treatment of sarcoid-contaminated wounds on the limbs and the face. Some sarcoids refractory to other treatments, however, can be managed economically using intralesional chemotherapy. Mitomycin-C (0.04% solution), an antibiotic with anti-tumoral activity, was found to be highly effective in causing complete regression of nodular or fibroblastic sarcoids, and had a low incidence of tumor recurrence, when administered intralesionally at 0.5–1.0 mL/cm^3 every 8 weeks until resolution of the tumor.[51]

Administration of electrical field pulses at the site of sarcoid injected with an aqueous solution of cisplatin (electrochemotherapy) markedly increases the concentration of cisplatin within tumoral cells. Electrochemotherapy recently was shown to be a highly effective treatment for sarcoids.[52] This mode of therapy involves saturating the sarcoid and surrounding skin with cisplatin, after which electric impulses are applied to the tumor. To apply electrochemotherapy, the horse usually must be anesthetized, and often multiple treatments are required (Figure 21.17). Considering the expense of the electropulsator and the requirement for repeated general anesthesia, the cost of this treatment is high.

The owners should be advised of the possible untoward effects that may occur when intralesional chemotherapy is used. Complete destruction of the sarcoid using intralesional chemotherapy necessarily involves some collateral damage, which makes sarcoid-contaminated wounds over vital structures, such as joints, synovial sheaths, nerves, blood vessels, tendons, and ligaments, particularly risky to treat in this manner.

> **Tip**
>
> - Administration of electrical field pulses at the site of sarcoid injected with an aqueous solution of cisplatin (electrochemotherapy) is likely to be effective for treatment of sarcoid.

Photodynamic therapy

Photodynamic therapy of sarcoids after injection with hypericin has been evaluated in non-wound-related sarcoids.[25] Although the tumor size is reduced, total resolution is difficult to achieve. Several other agents, for example, 5-aminolevulinic acid, can also be used topically and possibly systemically prior to exposing the site to an appropriate wavelength of light (usually ultraviolet). Chromophore materials, such as melanin, methylene blue, riboflavin, etc., also can be injected into the sarcoid prior to laser exposure or surgery to improve the rate of destruction of tumor cells.

In theory, photodynamic therapy is an attractive option for treatment of sarcoid-contaminated wounds given the rich blood supply to many wounds. No standardized approach is available yet, and calculating the correct amount of photodynamic agent and the amount of light required to resolve any particular lesion/type is difficult. Despite quite severe necrosis following photodynamic treatment, the eventual recurrence of sarcoid is common, often in higher proportion than granulation tissue. There are no reports of extensive clinical trials of this method as a means to treat sarcoid.

Radiation

Radiation therapy (interstitial or topical brachytherapy, or teletherapy) is the gold standard to which all other methods of treating sarcoids should be compared. Radiation therapy is highly effective but is limited by its availability and the high costs of all its forms of administration. Correctly applied, it is one of the best approaches to treat wounds contaminated with fibroblastic sarcoids on the distal aspect of the limb and other sensitive areas, such as the eyelid. The process of cellular damage with radiation begins with production of ionizations in tissue. With ionization, a positively charged atom and free electron are produced. This electron can directly damage the DNA and render a cell reproductively dead. The majority of the damage is, however, indirect. Indirect damage occurs through the production of free radicals produced by the interaction of the electron with water. High-energy free radicals damage DNA, thus preventing cellular growth and division. Thus, the effects of all forms of radiation are likely to be slow, and radiation treatment can take more than 12 months to be effective.

Radiation is not discriminatory, so physiologic processes of healing (e.g., fibroplasia, angiogenesis, and epithelialization) may be adversely affected, anatomic restrictions may prevent its use, and secondary complications may arise. Complications include synovial, articular, periosteal, and vascular damage in the immediate vicinity of the targeted tissue. Focused teletherapy minimizes these problems, of course, but defining the entire affected area to be radiated is a major challenge.

The cosmetic result of radiation therapy is usually excellent. Although there are no reports of comparative therapeutic studies involving wound-related sarcoids, in the primary author's experience, the outcome of treating sarcoids with radiation is excellent and better than that achieved with any other type of treatment. Owners should be advised, however, that the treatment is slow to deliver its maximum effect. Regrettably, few veterinary facilities have suitable radiotherapy equipment for use in horses.

Teletherapy

Radiation can be applied directly via teletherapy using gamma (electromagnetic) or beta (high-energy electrons) radiation delivered from a linear accelerator, either in a single beam or in a focused system of multiple low-level beams. Repeated treatment, with the horse anesthetized, is required in most circumstances, but effectively radiating a lesion on the distal aspect of a limb with the horse standing may be possible under strictly controlled conditions. Accurate dosimetry and fractionation are essential, and there is little information on the sensitivity of transformed fibroblasts to either form of radiation. The number of reports concerning teletherapy for treatment of sarcoids is insufficient to provide a definitive prognosis, but, where teletherapy can be applied, it is likely to be highly effective.

Brachytherapy

Brachytherapy involves the precise placement of short-range radiation-sources (radioisotopes) directly at the site of a tumor (as needles or seeds), allowing very high doses of localized radiation, yet reducing the probability of unnecessary damage to surrounding healthy tissues. Various forms of interstitial brachytherapy, including gold-198 in pellet form and the more common platinum-sheathed linear iridium-192 sources, have been used routinely to treat sarcoids,[34,53–56] and the methods are equally applicable to treatment of sarcoid-contaminated wounds. Accurate dosimetry is essential to achieve a good result without causing secondary/unwanted radiation damage to normal tissues. Probably the biggest hindrances are the logistics of the procedure and the cost, which is prohibitive in most circumstances. The limited size of the lesion that can be radiated in this way is also a major obstacle; this can be partially overcome through surgical debulking prior to irradiation. Despite its difficulties, brachytherapy provides an exceptionally good prognosis when compared to other methods of treating sarcoids. The primary author has found that more than 85% of sarcoids, including those at wounds, are resolved when brachytherapy is properly executed. Typical to all forms of radiation, the effects are slow to become apparent, and there may be episodes of secondary infection and waves of tissue necrosis. The surrounding area usually loses pigmentation, so the presence of a pink scar surrounded by white hairs is a common side-effect.

Topical brachytherapy using strontium-90 plaques or ruthenium patches is not applicable to wounds contaminated with sarcoid because beta emissions have poor penetration and, consequently, a correspondingly low efficacy. Furthermore, this particular technology is suitable only for extremely small areas, making it impractical.

Tip

- Although expensive, radiation therapy in the form of either teletherapy or interstitial brachytherapy is likely to be effective for treatment of a sarcoid-contaminated wound.

Antiviral therapy

Five percent acyclovir ointment, marketed as a treatment for cutaneous herpes viral infections in people, was reported to be highly effective as a topical treatment for flat sarcoids and as an adjunct therapy for debulked or excised sarcoids.[57] Topical application of 1% cidofovir cream used in humans to treat acyclovir-resistant herpes infection and other recalcitrant cutaneous viral infections was anecdotally reported to be efficacious in treatment of two horses for sarcoids.[58] Cidofovir may be cost-prohibitive for treating equine sarcoid, but acyclovir cream is more affordable, especially if the drug can be purchased from a compounding pharmacy. Because acyclovir cream appears to cause very little tissue irritation,[59] its use in wounds to prevent sarcoid transformation or in sarcoid-contaminated wounds is likely to be efficacious. The cream is applied daily to a sarcoid until resolution is complete, often within 2–6 months.[57]

Homeopathy/natural medicines

In the authors' experience, homeopathic or other alternative approaches, such as acupuncture and herbal remedies are consistently useless. Exacerbations and extensions are far more common than any resolutions. Many such attempts are borne out of a combination of client dissatisfaction (usually a result of weak efficacy of the chosen method of treatment and poor communication by the veterinarian with the owner) or some owners looking for an inexpensive treatment. Pure chemical applications (including inorganic arsenic salts and zinc chloride) and plant extracts with known biologic effects, such as bloodroot and aloe vera, may have an effect, but are unlikely to resolve the problem. Their use should be very carefully considered at the outset, and their effect closely monitored.

Summary of treatment

In conclusion, the treatment of sarcoid-transformed wounds is always likely to be problematic. Availability of particular treatments, cost, logistics, and client/owner compliance are just a few of the several factors to consider when designing a treatment regimen.

Verrucose lesions on the body are best treated by topical applications of a cytotoxic or antimitotic drug and/or wide surgical excision followed by focused antimitotic treatment of areas of regrowth or application of an antiviral cream, such as acyclovir. Fibroblastic lesions on the limbs produce a serious therapeutic challenge. The objective is to remove all abnormal sarcoid tissue and this must usually be done in stages. Surgical debulking (including laser surgery, cryosurgery, or hyperthermia) or photodynamic therapy followed by topical application of cytotoxic or antiviral medications is usually the preferred option if radiotherapy is unavailable. The difficulties are compounded by the invasive nature of many of these lesions and the need to destroy every sarcoid cell. In many cases, treatment has implications for underlying vital structures, including joints, tendons, nerves, blood vessels, and bone/periosteum.

Recent development of a murine model for BPV-1 protein-expressing equine sarcoid-like tumors is likely to provide an economical platform for the testing and development of novel therapeutic approaches.[60]

Prognosis

The pathologic behavior of the equine sarcoid makes it virtually impossible for a sarcoid-affected wound to heal. There is, however, a significant and important difference in the prognosis for wounds affected by sarcoid on the trunk and those on the limbs (Figure 21.16).

Normal accidental wounds on the limbs of horses have a somewhat unfair and largely unjustified reputation for non-healing; non-healing is principally due to the presence of complicating factors that tend to inhibit healing. Sarcoid transformation of the wound is possibly the most important of these factors simply because there are few reliably effective treatments.

Early dehiscence is a common feature of sarcoid-transformed wounds on limbs. Inhibition of epithelialization and wound contraction is also characteristic of the sarcoid-transformed wound. The prognosis for healing of a sarcoid-transformed wound on a limb is poor without treatment because normal healing is suspended. The otherwise poor prognosis is further worsened by the lack of efficacy of most currently available treatments. Either the treatment is effective in removing all sarcoid tissues but causes unacceptable damage to surrounding tissues, or the treatment is ineffective, resulting in return of the sarcoid, usually in a more aggressive form.

Conversely, because sarcoid-contaminated wounds on the trunk and neck tend to contract and tend to develop into verrucose lesions, and because the trunk is far more tolerant of skin loss, sarcoid-contaminated wounds in these anatomic regions have a reasonable prognosis for healing. Topical agents, such as AW4-LUDES, 5-fluorouracil cream, or even bloodroot and zinc chloride ointments, can be singularly effective in treating sarcoids on the neck and trunk, even though this may be a prolonged process requiring several courses of treatment. Often, wounds are amenable to repeated topical applications, so persistence can result in a cure, even though scarring often results.

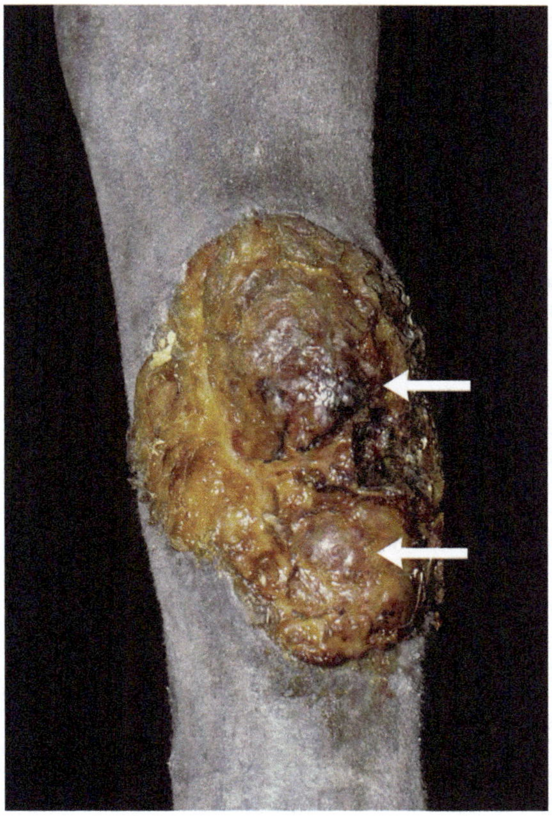

Figure 21.16 A small area of skin necrosis was caused by an overly tight bandage. The early stages of wound management included regular changes of dressing; after the eschar sloughed, the small wound was left open to heal. Within 4 weeks, the wound had deteriorated to this position. Because the horse had sarcoids elsewhere, tissue samples were harvested from the two major nodular areas (arrows). Shave biopsies performed at the surface of the lesion yielded infected granulation tissue with small areas suspicious of sarcoid. A deep central biopsy sample showed irregular areas of sarcoid and granulation tissue. Treatment proved impossible. Repeated attempts with both topical and surgical management simply resulted in exacerbation. The horse was euthanized.

Prevention

Prevention is a far better course of action than any current treatments for the sarcoid-transformed wound. Pre-emptive measures taken at the time of wounding have a profound limiting effect on the tendency toward sarcoid transformation within the wound. Immediately covering a wound and, in particular, prevention of fly contact, are vital measures. When treating a wound on a horse with a sarcoid, or where the wounded horse is in contact with other sarcoid-infected horses, the wound should remain protected until it has clearly healed to the point that flies are not attracted to the site. Fly populations can be reduced by using predator wasps, feed-through fly-control products, and composting manure. Fly repellants and petroleum jelly can be used to further restrict fly contact. Clearly, there is a far lower risk of a sarcoid developing at the site when these measures are implemented immediately after wounding. The longer wounds are left open and the greater the fly population, however, the greater is the risk of sarcoid transformation.

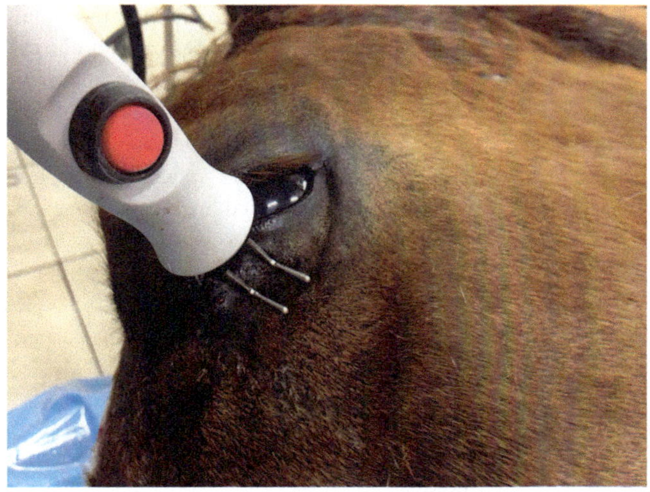

Figure 21.17 A nodular, periocular sarcoid was treated with two series of eight electric pulses using an electropulsator (ELECTROvet S13 LEROY biotech) in the anesthetized horse shortly after injecting the tumor as well as its margins with cisplatin, at a dose of 0.3 mg/cm^3. Courtesy of Dr. Fabien Relave.

Tip

- Controlling fly populations, by using predator wasps, feed-through fly-control products, and composting manure, and protecting wounds from contact with flies may decrease the incidence of sarcoid transformation of wounds.

Conclusion

The equine sarcoid is a skin disease with a disturbingly high number of suggested treatments,[53,61] implying that none is universally efficacious. Sarcoid-transformation in wounds has probably been, for many years, an unrecognized cause of failure of wounds to heal. The sarcoid-contaminated wound on a limb tends to develop a granulation tissue/fibrous tissue admixture that is often very difficult to differentiate clinically from normal granulation tissue. Most sarcoids that occur on the limb distal to the stifle/elbow are preceded by cutaneous injury and develop into the aggressive, fibroblastic type of sarcoid that is very difficult to treat. The combination of an aggressive tumor-transformed wound bed and anatomic restrictions makes predictions on cures ill advised. Transformation occurring in body wounds tends to result in a more distinct verrucose sarcoid, which is far more amenable to treatment.

Although the clinical appearance of EGT and pyogranuloma can be very similar to the appearance of the fibroblastic sarcoid, treatments for these conditions are very different. Treatment that is suitable for "proud flesh" (cutting back and grafting) usually serves only to aggravate sarcoid tissue.

Among the large number of publications on the treatment of sarcoids, little or no mention is made concerning the specific problem of treatment of sarcoid-transformed wounds; this may reflect the lack of appreciation of the problem. A delay in wound healing is a strong indicator of an "unrecognized" problem, which may be sarcoid contamination. Any tissues removed from a granulating wound should be submitted for histologic examination. When sarcoids are noted on the horse, or when the wound involves sarcoid-affected skin, a tissue sample of the wound should be harvested and examined histologically before beginning any therapy.

The need to explore novel ways to manage sarcoid-contaminated wounds is urgent; developing immunologic methods of management may possibly be the ultimate solution.

References

1. Erk N. A study of Kitab al-Hail wal-Baitar, written in the second half of the ninth century by Muhammed Ibn ahi Hizam. *Hist Vet* 1976; **1**: 101.
2. Jackson C. The incidence and pathology of tumours of domestic animals in South Africa. *Ondes J Vet Sci Anim Ind* 1936; **6**: 378.
3. Bogaert L, Martens A, Depoorter P, Gasthuys F. Equine sarcoids – part 1: clinical presentation and epidemiology. *Vlaams Diergeneeskundig Tijdschrift* 2008; **77**: 2.
4. Knowles EJ, Tremaine WH, Pearson GR, Mair TS. A database survey of equine tumours in the United Kingdom. *Equine Vet J* 2016; **48**: 280.
5. Schaffer PA, Wobeser B, Martin LE, *et al.* Cutaneous neoplastic lesions of equids in the central United States and Canada: 3,351 biopsy specimens from 3,272 equids (2000–2010). *J Am Vet Med Assoc* 2013; **242**: 99.
6. Knottenbelt DC. Sarcoid transformation at wound sites. In: Knottenbelt DC (ed). *Handbook of Equine Wound Management.* WB Saunders: London, 2003: 31.
7. Nasir L, Brandt S. Papillomavirus associated diseases of the horse. *Vet Microbiol* 2013; **167**: 159.
8. Nasir L, Campo MS. Bovine papillomaviruses: their role in the aetiology of cutaneous tumours of bovids and equids. *Vet Dermatol* 2008; **19**: 243.
9. Carr EA, Theon AP, Madewell BR, *et al.* Bovine papillomavirus DNA in neoplastic and nonneoplastic tissues obtained from horses with and without sarcoids in the western United States. *Am J Vet Res* 2001; **62**: 741.
10. Bogaert L, Martens A, De Baere C, Gasthuys F. Detection of bovine papillomavirus DNA on the normal skin and in the habitual surroundings of horses with and without equine sarcoids. *Res Vet Sci* 2005; **79**: 253.
11. Bogaert L, Martens A, Van Poucke M, *et al.* High prevalence of bovine papillomaviral DNA in the normal skin of equine sarcoid-affected and healthy horses. *Vet Microbiol* 2008; **129**: 58.
12. Haralambus R, Burgstaller J, Klukowska-Rotzler J, *et al.* Intralesional bovine papillomavirus DNA loads reflect severity of equine sarcoid disease. *Equine Vet J* 2010; **42**: 327.
13. Brostrom H, Fahlbrink E, Dubath ML, Lazary S. Association between equine leucocyte antigens (ELA) and equine sarcoid tumors in the population of Swedish halfbreds and some of their families. *Vet Immunol Immunopathol* 1988; **19**: 215.
14. Mahlmann K, Hamza E, Marti E, *et al.* Increased FOXP3 expression in tumour-associated tissues of horses affected with equine sarcoid disease. *Vet J* 2014; **202**: 516.
15. Broström H. *Equine sarcoids: a clinical, epidemiological and immunological study.* University of Uppsala, Stockholm, Sweden; 1995.
16. Cochrane CM. *An investigation into equine wound healing and sarcoid formation.* University of Liverpool, Liverpool, UK; 1996.
17. Knottenbelt DC. Equine wound management: are there significant differences in healing at different sites on the body? *Vet Dermatol* 1997; **4**: 273.
18. Nasir L, McFarlane ST, Torrontegui BO, Reid SW. Screening for bovine papillomavirus in peripheral blood cells of donkeys with and without sarcoids. *Res Vet Sci* 1997; **63**: 289.
19. Angelos J, Oppenheim Y, Rebhun W, *et al.* Evaluation of breed as a risk factor for sarcoid and uveitis in horses. *Anim Genet* 1988; **19**: 417.
20. Marti E, Lazary S, Antczak DF, Gerber H. Report of the first international workshop on equine sarcoid. *Equine Vet J* 1993; **25**: 397.
21. Compston PC, Turner T, Wylie CE, Payne RJ. Laser surgery as a treatment for histologically-confirmed sarcoids in the horse. *Equine Vet J* 2016; **48**: 451.
22. Wilmink JM, Nederbragt H, van Weeren PR, *et al.* Differences in wound contraction between horses and ponies: the in vitro contraction capacity of fibroblasts. *Equine Vet J* 2001; **33**: 499.
23. Martens A, De Moor A, Ducatelle R. PCR detection of bovine papilloma virus DNA in superficial swabs and scrapings from equine sarcoids. *Vet J* 2001; **161**: 280.
24. Knottenbelt DC. A suggested clinical classification of the equine sarcoid. *Clin Tech Eq Pract* 2005; **4**: 278.
25. Laursen BA. Behandling af equine sarcoider med krokirurgi. *Dansk Vet Tidskr* 1987; **70**: 97.
26. Toth F, Schumacher J, Castro F, Perkins J. Full-thickness skin grafting to cover equine wounds caused by laceration or tumor resection. *Vet Surg* 2010; **39**: 708.
27. Hazen PG, Berthold B, Turgeon KL, Nuovo G. Use of Mohs micrographically controlled surgery in the management of equine penile squamous cell carcinoma. *J Equine Vet Sci* 2009; **29**: 95.
28. Gage AA, Baust JM, Baust JG. Experimental cryosurgery investigations in vivo. *Cryobiology* 2009; **59**: 229.
29. Lane JG. The treatment of equine sarcoids by cryosurgery. *Equine Vet J* 1977; **9**: 127.
30. Vingerhoets M, Diehl M, Gerber H, *et al.* Traitement de la sarcoide equine au laser à gaz carbonique. *Schweiz Arch Tierheilkd* 1988; **130**: 113.
31. Carstanjen B, Jordan P, Lepage OM. Carbon dioxide laser as a surgical instrument for sarcoid therapy – a retrospective study on 60 cases. *Can Vet J* 1997; **38**: 773.
32. Flemming DD. BCG therapy for equine sarcoid. In: Robinson NE (ed). *Current Therapy in Equine Medicine.* WB Saunders: Philadelphia, 1983: 539.
33. Hoffmann KD, Kainer RA, Shideler RK. Radio-frequency current-induced hyperthermia for the treatment of equine sarcoid. *Equine Pract* 1983; **5**: 24.
34. Turrel JM, Stover SM, Gyorgyfalvy J. Iridium-192 interstitial brachytherapy of equine sarcoid. *Vet Radiol* 1985; **26**: 20.
35. Wust P, Hildebrandt B, Sreenivasa G, *et al.* Hyperthermia in combined treatment of cancer. *Lancet Oncol* 2002; **3**: 487.
36. Davies M. Bacillus Calmette-Guerin as an anti-tumor agent. The interaction with cells of the mammalian immune system. *Biochim Biophys Acta* 1982; **651**: 143.
37. Misdorp W, Klein WR, Ruitenberg EJ, *et al.* Clinico-pathological aspects of immunotherapy by intralesional injection of BCG cell walls or live BCG in bovine ocular squamous cell carcinoma. *Cancer Immunol Immunother* 1985; **20**: 223.

38. Owen RA, Jagger DW. Clinical observations on the use of BCG cell wall fraction for treatment of periocular and other equine sarcoids. *Vet Rec* 1987; **120**: 548.
39. Pascoe JR, Knottenbelt DC. *Manual of Equine Dermatology*. WB Saunders: London, 1999.
40. White SD, Yu AA (eds). Equine dermatology. II. Nodules, lumps, and bumps. 52nd Annual Convention of the American Association of Equine Practitioners; 2006; San Antonio, TX.
41. Klein WR, Bras GE, Misdorp W, *et al.* Equine sarcoid: BCG immunotherapy compared to cryosurgery in a prospective randomised clinical trial. *Cancer Immunol Immunother* 1986; **21**: 133.
42. Theon AP. Intralesional and topical chemotherapy and immunotherapy. *Vet Clin North Am Equine Pract* 1998; **14**: 659.
43. Nogueira SA, Torres SM, Malone ED, *et al.* Efficacy of imiquimod 5% cream in the treatment of equine sarcoids: a pilot study. *Vet Dermatol* 2006; **17**: 259.
44. Christen-Clottu O, Klocke P, Burger D, *et al.* Treatment of clinically diagnosed equine sarcoid with a mistletoe extract (*Viscum album austriacus*). *J Vet Intern Med* 2010; **24**: 1483.
45. Espy BMK (ed). How to treat equine sarcoids by autologous implantation. 54th Annual Convention of the American Association of Equine Practitioners; 2008; San Diego, CA.
46. Rothacker CC, Boyle AG, Levine DG. Autologous vaccination for the treatment of equine sarcoids: 18 cases (2009–2014). *Can Vet J* 2015; **56**: 709.
47. Ashrafi GH, Piuko K, Burden F, *et al.* Vaccination of sarcoid-bearing donkeys with chimeric virus-like particles of bovine papillomavirus type 1. *J Gen Virol* 2008; **89**: 148.
48. Mattil-Fritz S, Scharner D, Piuko K, *et al.* Immunotherapy of equine sarcoid: dose-escalation trial for the use of chimeric papillomavirus-like particles. *J Gen Virol* 2008; **89**: 138.
49. Theon AP. Cisplatin treatment for cutaneous tumours. In: Robinson NE (ed). *Current Therapy in Equine Medicine*, 4th edn. WB Saunders: Philadelphia, 1997: 372.
50. Hewes CA, Sullins KE. Use of cisplatin-containing biodegradable beads for treatment of cutaneous neoplasia in equidae: 59 cases (2000–2004). *J Am Vet Med Assoc* 2006; **229**: 1617.
51. McKane SA, Cooner RP (eds). A practical protocol for the clinical use of mytomycin-C in the treatment of sarcoids in horses. 6th Congress of the European College of Equine Internal Medicine; 2006; Le Touquet, France.
52. Tamzali Y, Borde L, Rols MP, *et al.* Successful treatment of equine sarcoids with cisplatin electrochemotherapy: a retrospective study of 48 cases. *Equine Vet J* 2012; **44**: 214.
53. Knottenbelt DC, Kelly DF. The diagnosis and treatment of periorbital sarcoid in the horse: 445 cases from 1974 to 1999. *Vet Ophthalmol* 2000; **3**: 169.
54. Theon AP, Pascoe JR. Iridium-192 interstitial brachytherapy for equine periocular tumours: treatment results and prognostic factors in 115 horses. *Equine Vet J* 1995; **27**: 117.
55. Wyn-Jones G. Treatment of periocular tumours of horses using radioactive gold-198 grains. *Equine Vet J* 1979; **11**: 3.
56. Wyn-Jones G. Treatment of equine cutaneous neoplasia by radiotherapy using iridium-192 linear sources. *Equine Vet J* 1983; **15**: 361.
57. Stadler S, Kainzbauer C, Haralambus R, *et al.* Successful treatment of equine sarcoids by topical aciclovir application. *Vet Rec* 2011; **168**: 187.
58. Scagliarini A, Bettini G, Savini F, *et al.* Treatment of equine sarcoids. *Vet Rec* 2012; **171**: 330.
59. Tucker WE, Jr. Preclinical toxicology profile of acyclovir: an overview. *Am J Med* 1982; **73**: 27.
60. Bogaert L, Woodham AW, Da Silva DM, *et al.* A novel murine model for evaluating bovine papillomavirus prophylactics/therapeutics for equine sarcoid-like tumors. *J Gen Virol* 2015; **96**: 2764.
61. Genetzky RM, Biwer RD, Myers RK. Equine sarcoid: causes, diagnosis and treatment. *Comp Cont Educ Pract Vet* 1983; **5**: 416.

CHAPTER 22

Innovative Adjunctive Approaches to Wound Management

Christine Theoret, DVM, PhD, Diplomate ACVS
With contributions from: Olivier Lepage – Maggot debridement therapy; Andrew Dart and Andrea Bischofberger – Honey; Bryden Stanley – Negative-pressure wound therapy; and Judith Koenig – Extra-corporeal shockwave therapy

Chapter Contents

Summary

This chapter focuses on some of the more promising adjunctive and novel therapies developed for or adapted to the horse, based on the specific underlying characteristics that govern wound repair in this species. The choice of topics covered in this chapter is based on the volume and quality of data published in the veterinary medical literature pertaining to each of these adjunctive approaches since the publication of the second edition of this textbook.

Introduction

Problems frequently develop during wound repair in horses and may lead to extensive scarring with adverse effects on cosmesis and on function, often by causing lameness. In addition to welfare concerns, defective healing represents an important economic burden to the equine industry because most horses are destined to an athletic career (the reader is referred to Chapter 1 for more information on the economic consequences of wounds in horses). Consequently, the search for innovative adjunctive approaches to accelerate and improve the quality of repair is paramount.

The choice of topics covered in this chapter is based on the volume and quality of data published in the veterinary medical literature pertaining to each of these adjunctive approaches since the publication of the second edition of this textbook.

Innovative adjunctive approaches

Although similar data are not available for the veterinary industry, the global market for wound care in humans is expected to reach US$18.3 billion by 2019, growing at a compound annual rate of 3.2% from 2014 when it totalled US$15.6 billion.[1] A particular niche within this market comprises advanced wound-care products, which include specialized dressings, bio-active wound-care products, such as skin substitutes, as well as therapeutic devices that use negative-pressure wound therapy or oxygen and hyperbaric oxygen equipment, to name a few. In 2013, the global market for advanced wound care had an estimated value of US$6.2 billion, having grown by 5% since 2012.[2]

In our quest to improve the success of wound management in horses, extrapolating the results of preclinical studies (in laboratory animals) and clinical trials (in humans) to equine

Equine Wound Management, Third Edition. Edited by Christine Theoret and Jim Schumacher.

Companion website: www.wiley.com/go/theoret/wound

patients is tempting. One must bear in mind, however, that due to the unique nature of wound healing in the horse (reviewed in Chapters 1, 2, and 15), therapies beneficial to other species may not be suitable to equids. Although providing innovations in wound management to the equine practitioner is crucial, many products available to veterinarians rely heavily on anecdotal evidence, and their true effectiveness has yet to be thoroughly evaluated. This chapter focuses on some of the more promising adjunctive and novel therapies developed for or adapted to the horse, based on the specific underlying characteristics that govern wound repair in this species.

A wound, when first examined, may be several hours old or perhaps a few weeks old. The different phases of repair should be recalled prior to designing the treatment regimen, keeping in mind that the approach must be dynamic. Indeed, accelerating and/or improving repair are not as simple as applying a single treatment to the wound and maintaining it for the duration of the healing process. A robust yet transitory inflammatory response to injury cleanses the wound in an effort to stave off infection. Moreover, inflammatory cells, along with the platelets that predominate during the coagulation phase, orchestrate the initiation and maintenance of the proliferative phase of repair through the release of cytokines and growth factors. Given that the inflammatory response to wounding is weak but protracted in horses and correlates with the development of chronic, indolent wounds and exuberant granulation tissue (EGT), normalizing the inflammatory response might enhance certain aspects of repair and prevent complications.[3]

One way to curtail the inflammatory phase is to debride the wound to demarcate non-viable tissue, particularly when necrosis, exposed cortical bone, or frayed tendons are present because non-viable tissue facilitates bacterial colonization. Conventional wound debridement involves irrigation and sharp resection. Although low-pressure irrigation fails to dislodge contaminants effectively, high-pressure irrigation might damage wounded tissues. Moreover, with sharp debridement, there is a risk of removing viable tissue or leaving necrotic tissue in the wound, especially when the margin between the two is ill defined.

Maggot debridement therapy (MDT)

An alternative method of wound debridement relies on the use of maggots. Maggots have been used to treat wounds for centuries,[4] and nowadays, larval therapy is generally categorized as a "biosurgical" therapy. Maggot debridement therapy (MDT) for human[5] and veterinary medical purposes[6] uses freshly emerged, germ-free larvae of the common green bottle fly, *Lucilia sericata*, produced by specialized centers. At the time of writing, these include Monarch Labs (North America), Polymedics Bio Products (Belgium), BioMonde (UK), Neocura (Germany), Japan Maggot Company (Japan), and the Department of Medical Entomology of the Westmead Hospital (NSW, Australia). The action of maggots on wound healing is attributed to debridement via the production of potent proteolytic enzymes,[7] up-regulation of the expression of genes involved in wound healing,[8] an antiseptic effect,[9] and an inhibitory effect on the formation of biofilm.[10] During the process of dissolving fibrin and necrotic tissue, maggots also destroy and digest bacteria, and the excretions/secretions of *L. sericata* possess significant antifungal properties.[11] In relation to the rising incidence of antibiotic resistance, the action of maggots against methicillin-resistant *Staphylococcus aureus* (MRSA) is of particular interest.[12]

Sterile maggots can be applied to a wound using a direct (free-range) or indirect (contained) contact method. With the direct contact method, maggots are applied on to the wound with a dressing fixed to the surrounding healthy tissue (Figure 22.1). After placing the maggots on to the

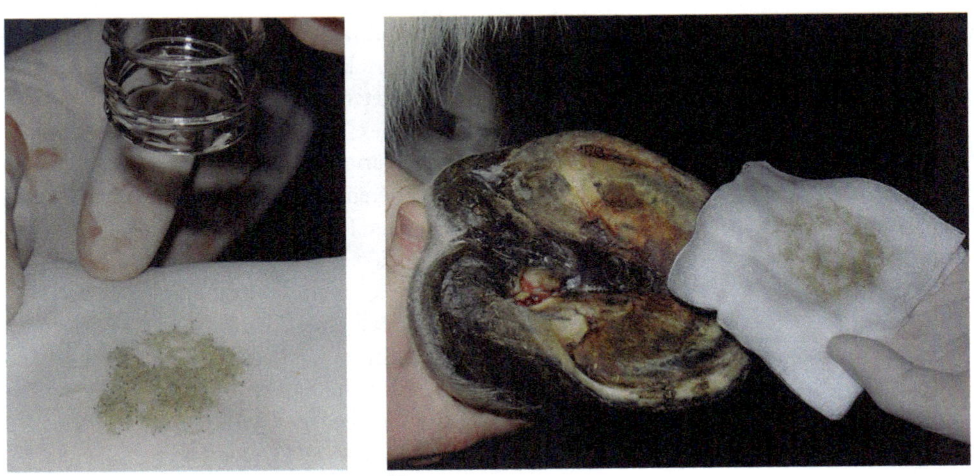

(a) (b)

Figure 22.1 Maggots used in the direct contact manner (free-range maggots). **(a)** Larvae being prepared for application in the direct contact manner. **(b)** Larvae are applied directly to a penetrating injury of the foot. Courtesy of Dr. O.M. Lepage.

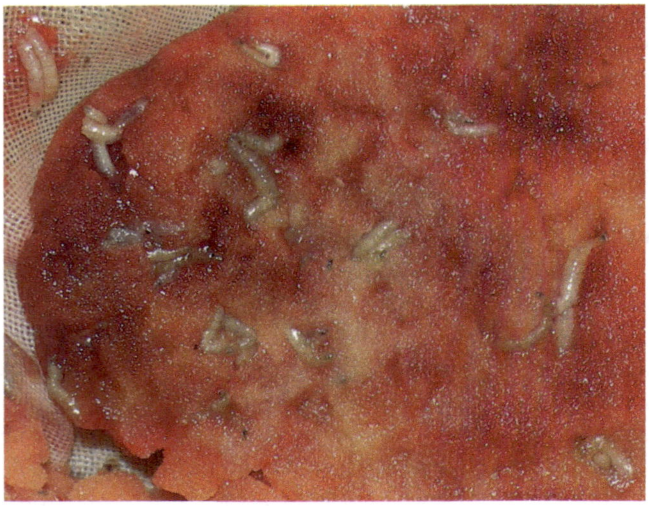

Figure 22.2 Maggots and pieces of foam within a closed polyester net to be used in the indirect contact (contained) method. Pieces of foam offer a physical environment to stimulate the activity and development of the maggots whilst assisting with management of exudate. Courtesy of Dr. O.M. Lepage.

wound, a nylon mesh is fixed to the dressing to confine the maggots within the wound and to prevent them from escaping. Using the indirect contact method, maggots are supplied within a closed polyester net filled with absorbent hydrophilic polyurethane foam (Figure 22.2).[13] Although the indirect contact method has obvious practical and esthetic advantages over free-ranging maggots, a study of 64 human patients with signs of gangrenous or necrotic tissue showed that a better outcome is achieved with the direct contact method of application than with the indirect contact method.[14] The authors of an equine study using MDT[15] reached a similar conclusion and considered the direct contact method superior. An additional benefit of free-range maggots is the reduced cost of therapy.

In horses, MDT is described as an alternative approach to the management of septic navicular bursitis, laminar necrosis associated with complicated laminitis,[16] and subsolar infection-associated osteomyelitis of the distal phalanx.[4] Maggot debridement therapy has also contributed towards a successful outcome in limb lacerations, including those leading to chronic non-healing wounds, in orthopedic infection free of bony sequestrae, in various soft-tissue abscesses, in supraspinous bursitis, and in dehiscence of the *linea alba* following exploratory celiotomy.[15] In a retrospective study of 41 equids treated with MDT, 38 had a favorable outcome less than 1 week after initiation of therapy. Lesions enrolled in this study were subacute or chronic and had been managed in diverse ways prior to receiving MDT.

When considering MDT, the practitioner should keep in mind that free drainage of exudate is required and that the maggots must have an adequate supply of oxygen.

What to do

- Leave draining tracts open and protect surrounding intact skin with a zinc paste.
- Institute MDT only after blood and/or exudate have been cleared from the wound to avoid drowning the maggots.

What to avoid

- Occlusive or film dressings must not be used because these may asphyxiate the maggots.

A preliminary surgical debridement usually precedes MDT, though this may not be necessary in the absence of foreign bodies and/or organic matter in the wound. In some cases, after 3–4 days of MDT, a second treatment is required to reach the desired degree of debridement, disinfection, and fibroplasia (i.e. healthy granulation tissue filling the wound). Orthopedic shoeing, stent bandaging, and non-occlusive sleeve bandaging, typical to MDT, are adapted for each type of wound and anatomic location[6,12] (Figure 22.3, Figure 22.4). Because maggots, after being applied to a wound, contain viable bacteria and continue excreting these, they are regarded as medical waste and must be disposed of after use according to local regulations.

In conclusion, based on clinical observations in equine medicine and a systematic review of MDT for chronically infected wounds and ulcers in humans,[17] MDT is recommended for use in horses to ensure debridement and disinfection and to enhance healing of subacute and chronic, non-healing wounds, when complete surgical debridement is difficult or impossible, and to enhance healing of obviously infected wounds.

Platelet concentrates

Although a robust inflammatory response is required for prompt initiation of the subsequent proliferative phase of healing, it is the products of the inflammatory cells, rather than the cells themselves, that mediate the desired effects. It is, therefore, tempting to be drawn to the promise of bioactive molecules, such as cytokines/growth factors released by inflammatory cells and/or platelets, as therapeutic tools.

Complex combinations of cytokines involved in wound healing variably stimulate migration, attachment, proliferation, and differentiation of endothelial cells, epithelial cells, and fibroblasts (the reader is referred to Chapter 1 for more information on cytokines). In spite of a drive, in the past two decades, to ascertain the therapeutic effects of purified forms of specific cytokines in the clinical management of non-healing wounds in humans, the overall conclusion of a recent critical analysis of the literature is that larger randomized controlled trials are needed to document side-effects and to confirm efficacy and long-term outcomes.[18]

The intricate mechanism of action of cytokines has yet to be fully elucidated. Because these molecules network both spatially and temporally amongst themselves and also with cells and the

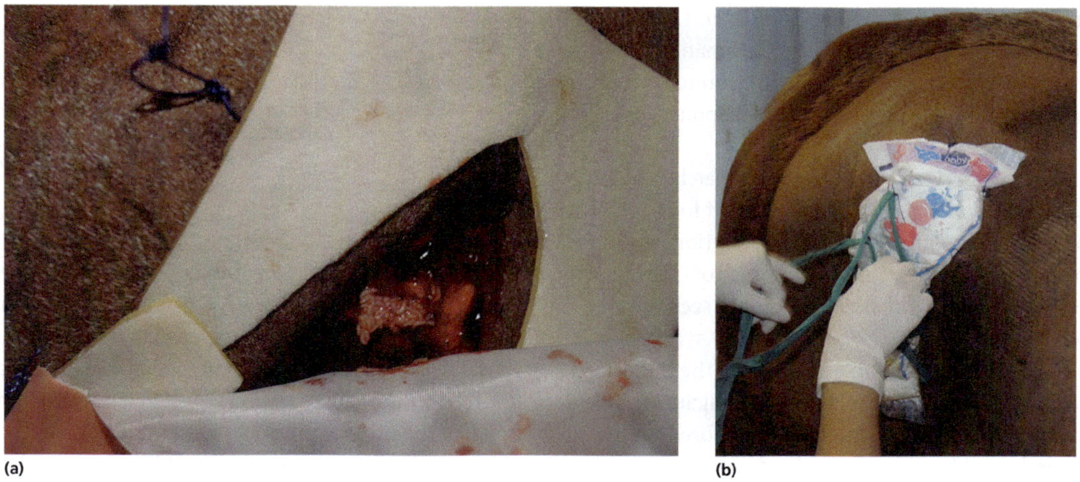

Figure 22.3 A chronic abscess has developed over the *tuber coxae* subsequent to a fracture leading to bony sequestration. (**a**) Maggots are placed in the cavity created by surgical debridement and removal of the bone sequestrum. (**b**) A stent bandage made from a baby diaper is sutured over a non-occlusive wound dressing. Courtesy of Dr. O.M. Lepage.

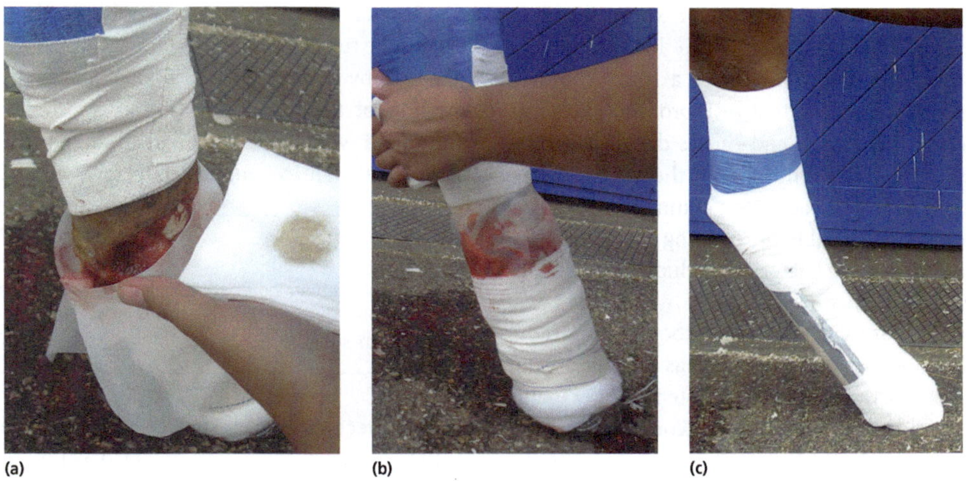

Figure 22.4 Use of MDT and application of a non-occlusive "sleeve bandage" in a horse with a wound on the distal aspect of the limb. (**a**) The net provided by the manufacturer is placed in a 360° bracelet and attached to the limb, distally, with an elastic adhesive bandage, before pouring on the maggots. (**b**) The net is then fixed to the limb, proximally, with an elastic adhesive bandage, to seal the treatment area. (**c**) A cotton pad is applied on top to absorb secretions, and a rigid prosthesis is added, if necessary. Courtesy of Dr. O.M. Lepage.

surrounding matrix, addition of an isolated cytokine might disturb the fine balance. Furthermore, the exogenous cytokine may not exert its anticipated impact because interaction with endogenous counterparts (e.g., degradative enzymes) could abrogate its *in vivo* effect. As such, expecting an individual molecule to enhance repair is illusory, particularly if it is not known whether a deficiency of this specific molecule is at the root of the problem. Instead, as is the case with dressings that must vary to suit the needs of each phase of repair, a dynamic "combination" therapy based on the use of a physiologically natural mixture of cytokines may be most appropriate.

With the aim to provide combination therapy, investigators have turned to "platelet concentrates," the preparation of which may be achieved using various methods, each leading to a specific product that differs from the others in its biologic effect and potential use. In an effort to dispel confusion and better discriminate between the therapeutic successes and failures reported in the literature, a classification scheme was recently proposed wherein platelet concentrates are grouped in four main categories: pure platelet-rich plasma (P-PRP), leukocyte-rich PRP (L-PRP), pure platelet-rich fibrin (P-PRF), and leukocyte-rich PRF (L-PRF).[19] In the latter two categories, activation of platelets and polymerization of fibrin are triggered artificially to generate a high-density fibrin clot that can serve as a biologic healing matrix by supporting cellular migration and release of cytokines. The true impact of leukocytes in platelet concentrates is unknown and remains the subject of controversy. Some authors recommend eliminating leukocytes, whereas others emphasize the need for leukocytes in platelet concentrates because of their anti-infectious and immunoregulatory activities, critical to repair.[19] The concern that L-PRP or L-PRF might induce negative effects (via activation of inflammation) does not apply to the management of acute open wounds of horses where stimulation of a robust inflammatory response is, in fact, desirable.[3]

Normal horse blood contains approximately 142 000 platelets/μL, a far weaker concentration than that found in other mammals, including humans.[20] The active secretion of proteins by platelet α-granules begins within 10 minutes of clotting, with more than 95% of the presynthesized cytokines secreted during the first hour. After this initial burst, platelets synthesize and secrete additional proteins for the balance of their life (5–10 days).[21] The addition of thrombin and/or calcium chloride ($CaCl_2$) simulates natural clotting and, therefore, causes the release of several cytokines, in particular transforming growth factor beta (TGF-β), platelet-derived growth factor (PDGF), and vascular endothelial growth factor (VEGF), as well as microbicidal molecules beneficial to wound healing. Thus, the principal therapeutic advantage of platelet concentrate over isolated growth factors is that it represents a natural mixture of stimulatory and inhibitory mediators designed to have synergistic biologic effects within the environment of a wound. Indeed, recent *in vitro* studies have shown that PRP promotes proliferation of human dermal fibroblasts and causes differentiation of the fibroblast into contractile myofibroblasts, thereby promoting wound contraction.[22] Moreover, activated equine platelets, such as those found in PRF, are capable of releasing reactive oxygen species that can assist in killing bacteria,[23] including methicillin-resistant *Staphylococcus aureus*.[24]

The optimal content of platelets and leukocytes required to achieve a desired biologic effect in horses has not been determined and no doubt varies according to the intended therapeutic purpose. Change in fold of platelet numbers, compared to numbers in whole blood, and absolute platelet numbers are used to estimate adequacy of platelet concentration, with the latter being the best approximation of the concentration of cytokines expected within a tissue after platelet degranulation.[25] Platelet concentrations in human PRP commonly range from a 3- to 5-fold increase over whole blood[26] or a minimum concentration of 300 000 to 1 000 000 platelets/μL. Extrapolating appropriate concentrations from the human literature may be inappropriate because of differences in average platelet counts and platelet physiology between species, and, consequently, the most appropriate concentration of platelets in equine PRP has yet to be established. Thus, the current "clinically acceptable" value of 250 000 platelets/μL[25] is merely a suggestion. A study has shown that at least four different methods of counting platelets are suitable for quantifying platelets in equine PRP, including optical scatter, impedance, hand counting, and fluorescent antibody flow cytometry.[27]

When anticoagulated blood is centrifuged, three layers become evident: the bottom layer, comprised of red blood cells; the middle layer, comprised of platelets and white blood cells (the buffy coat); and the top, plasma layer.

Tip

- Use a solution of sodium citrate or acid-citrate-dextrose as an anticoagulant,[28] as well as low G forces during centrifugation, to preserve the integrity of the platelet membrane, thereby deferring degranulation and release of active mediators, until therapeutic use of the platelet concentrate is needed.

Numerous systems to produce autologous platelet concentrates, originally developed for human patients, are commercially available but often expensive.[29] Moreover, given the substantial interspecies differences in platelets, clinicians should not rely on the manufacturers' data relating to human patients to select the most appropriate method for horses.[30]

In an effort to improve accessibility to this therapy for all horse owners, inexpensive methods of tube centrifugation have been developed and tested; these appear sufficient to generate an autologous product, free from bacterial contamination, when conducted in a clean environment.[31] Dahlgren's team found that the use of a sterile, skirted, polypropylene, 50-mL conical centrifuge tube, spun for 15 minutes at 720 Xg, concentrates the platelets by more than 2.5-fold.[25] The yield of PRP using a method of tube centrifugation is approximately 10% of the volume of whole blood drawn. After the PRP is prepared it is stable, in the anticoagulated state, for 8 hours or longer.

Tip

- Because clotting induces immediate release of secretory proteins, the platelets should be activated just prior to delivering PRP to the wound's surface.

It was recently shown that, regardless of the stimulus, release of PDGF and TGF-β is maximal by 0.5–1 hour after clotting and very little release is observed after 24 hours.[32] The most effective and inexpensive method of activating PRP for use in horses seems to be the addition of 23 mM of $CaCl_2$.[33] Using autologous thrombin is not recommended in horses because it is less effective than $CaCl_2$ in eliciting release of cytokines from the platelets. That said, intrinsic factors, such as the breed, gender, and age of the horse, may affect the cellular content and release of cytokines from concentrates of equine platelets.[34]

Platelet concentrate can be delivered to the wound with a commercial spray applicator or with a dual-injection system (one syringe contains the PRP and the other contains the clotting agent), or it can be activated directly in the centrifuge tube after which the resulting gel (PRF) is applied to the wound.

What to avoid

- Avoid using the spray applicator or the dual-injection system when treating vertical wounds (i.e., limb wounds) because clotting does not occur instantaneously, resulting in the PRP runing off the wound before it has a chance to form an adherent, gel-like substance.[35]

Tip

- Activate then apply 0.25 mL of PRP/cm^2 of wound surface at the time of injury and again 1week later (the interval between treatments is based on the platelets' lifespan).[35]

A recent review of controlled studies (nine randomized, six prospective, and two retrospective) assessing the clinical outcome of acute wounds in humans treated with platelet-rich plasma found that PRP accelerates healing of acute wounds.[36] A handful of studies have measured the therapeutic effect of platelet concentrate on experimental wounds in horses. Platelet-rich plasma gel accelerated epithelial differentiation and enhanced collagen organization in wounds on the neck healing by primary intention,[37] and accelerated repair, induced fibrosis, and may have provided antibacterial activity in deep, second-degree burns on the rump.[38]

In our experience, PRP gel applied topically to acute, full-thickness skin wounds on the distal aspect of the limb favors fibroplasia, and therefore, we recommend applying PRP gel to acute wounds in which a large deficit must be filled with new granulation tissue.[35] Moreover, based on our experience, we conjecture that application of PRP to chronic wounds, after the wound has been thoroughly debrided, might also be beneficial.

What to do

- Discontinue the use of PRP as soon as a healthy bed of granulation tissue fills the defect, to avoid the development of EGT.

In conclusion, scientific data supporting the use of autologous platelet concentrate in horses to assist repair and regeneration of injured tissues is promising. That said, one must keep in mind that platelet concentrates are biologic products, rather than drugs, and therefore, their uniformity cannot be guarenteed, especially given the wide range of methods whereby they are prepared. In an effort to ensure maximum therapeutic efficacy, clinicians should verify the quality of the product by measuring its platelet concentration after it has been prepared and prior to using it on a wound. Because this technology necessitates minimal investment or expertise, it should be considered as part of an equine practitioner's armamentarium for wound management.

Honey

Another approach shown to positively modulate the inflammatory response to wounding involves the therapeutic use of honey. Wild honey combined with animal fats and lint was used to promote second-intention wound healing as far back in time as ancient Egypt.[39] Since then, in many parts of the world, different varietals of honey have been used to enhance wound healing. The appeal of honey as a therapeutic agent faded after the introduction of modern antimicrobial agents. More recently, the appearance of antibiotic resistance has revived interest in the antimicrobial properties of honey. Although most research has focused specifically on the antibacterial activity of different varietals of honey, honey appears to have a wider therapeutic scope in wound management.[40,41]

Honey has a broad range of bioactivities, including antimicrobial activity, osmotic and antioxidant activity, and an ability to modulate the inflammatory response to wounding. These combined bioactivities result in enhanced autolytic wound debridement, a deodorizing action, and an immunomodulation, that together reduce pain, edema, and exudate. Ultimately, the effect is to promote wound healing and minimize scarring.[40]

Despite the reported range of bioactivities of honey, a recent review of clinical trials in humans showed limited evidence of any consistent effects across different types of wounds.[42] Dismissing the value of honey as a wound healing agent is premature, however, because new bioactive components of honey are still being discovered.[43–45] The diverse spectrum and concentrations of these bioactive components within different varietals of honey means all honeys do not behave equally.[43–45] Whether or not different varietals of honey have variable effects when applied to dissimilar wounds during the various phases of healing has yet to be elucidated.

To date, research has focused predominantly on the antimicrobial properties of honey used for wound management in humans. Honey has a broad spectrum of activity against bacteria and fungi, but emerging evidence highlights a remarkable variability in antimicrobial potency between varietals of honey.[40,46] A high sugar content and low pH are common to all honeys. Many bacteria cannot thrive in an acidic environment, and the low pH of honey also reduces the activity of bacterial proteases within the wound,[47] thereby protecting cytokines and growth factors important to healing. The high sugar content of honey creates an osmotic gradient causing fluid shifts that: (1) shrink the bacterial cell wall and inhibit growth; and (2) provide a moist environment and nutrients required by healing tissues as fluids inflow from adjacent tissues and the circulation.[40] Glucose oxidase, produced by bees, is present in most honeys. Its antibacterial activity, via the production of hydrogen peroxide,[48,49] increases exponentially when it is diluted with wound exudate.[48,50] Damaged cells and some bacteria can produce substantial amounts of catalase that destroys hydrogen peroxide, thereby contributing to the variable antibacterial activity of honey in different types of wounds.[51] Encouragingly, there are currently no clinical reports of acquired antimicrobial resistance to honey; this is probably due to the multiple synergistic activities that give honey its antimicrobial properties.[45] Nevertheless, a recent *in vitro* study demonstrated that suboptimal concentrations of Manuka honey can allow resistant bacterial wound pathogens to emerge,[43] highlighting the need to maintain adequate concentrations of an efficacious honey at the wound–dressing interface.

Honey derived from the *Leptospermum* species of plants has been found to have superior antibacterial activity compared to other honeys, even in the presence of inhibitory concentrations of catalase.[51,52] The *Leptospermum* species include approximately 80 plants growing primarily in Australia and New Zealand. Honey from the Manuka bush (*L. scoparium*) found in New Zealand is the most extensively studied, and its antibacterial activity has been standardized for commercial production.

Hydrogen peroxide is not responsible for the antibacterial activity of Manuka-derived honey. Rather, this honey's antibacterial activity is attributed to methylglyoxal (MGO), derived from dihydroacetone in the nectar of the Manuka flower and referred to as the Unique Manuka Factor (UMF), displayed on commercial Manuka honey products.[53,54] The UMF is an antibacterial rating, determined by comparing the antibacterial activity of a honey to a standard concentration of phenol: the higher the UMF rating, the greater the spectrum and efficacy of the antibacterial properties of the honey. Generally speaking, honey with a UMF rating greater than 10 is associated with better therapeutic outcomes,[55–57] but as the UMF rating increases, so does the cost of treatment. Although biofilms appear to interfere with the antibacterial activity of many honeys, the MGO in Manuka honey is effective in preventing formation of biofilms and disrupting those that are established,[58–60] although higher concentrations are required to achieve the latter.[61]

Veterinary protocols of wound management that incorporate the use of honey describe using products that range from inexpensive honeys intended for human consumption to standardized, medical-grade, sterilized Manuka honey (Figure 22.5). Carnwath *et al.* recently measured the antimicrobial activity of various varietals of honey against 10 common equine wound bacterial isolates, including methicillin-resistant *Staphylococcus aureus* and *Pseudomonas aeruginosa*.[45] Of 29 tested products, over 60% were found to be contaminated with aerobic bacteria or fungi, emphasizing the importance of using only sterilized honey for wound treatment. Sterilization can be achieved with gamma-irradiation, which has no significant effect on the antibacterial properties of honey, as opposed to heat treatment, which does.[62] Eight products were effective against all 10 bacterial isolates at concentrations varying from <2% to 16% (v/v); these products included Manuka honey (UMF rating greater than 10), commercial wound products and dressings incorporating medical-grade Manuka honey, and some commercially available monoculture honey from local suppliers.[45]

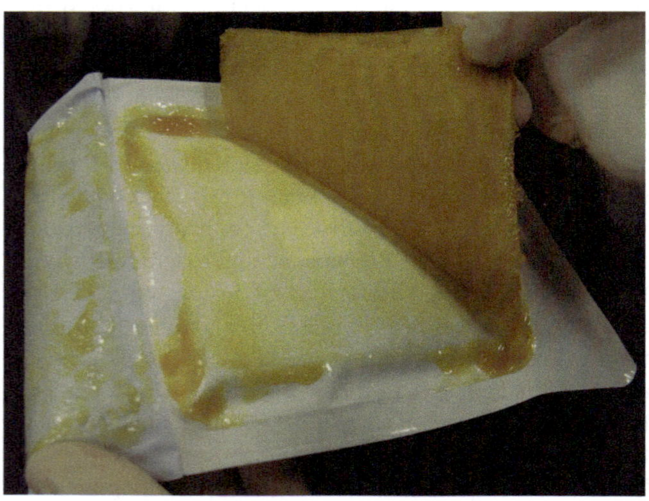

Figure 22.5 Manuka honey-impregnated tulle dressing from Advancis Medical. Courtesy of Dr. D. Knottenbelt.

Other areas of research have focused on the healing properties of honey, in particular its ability to modulate the inflammatory response to ultimately promote repair.[63] Some varietals of honey were shown to stimulate inflammation of acute wounds, thereby up-regulating the production of cytokines governing proliferation of fibroblasts and endothelial cells necessary for fibroplasia and angiogenesis.[64] For example, a component of Manuka honey was shown to stimulate the release of tumor necrosis factor (TNF)-α, interleukin (IL)-1β, and IL-6.[65,66] Conversely, other varietals of honey may inhibit the same cytokines, thereby diminishing the inflammatory response in microenvironments where inflammation is uncontrolled, as is the case in chronic wounds.[63,67] The immunomodulatory activity of different varietals of honey is complex and requires more study if honey is to be used strategically for the treatment of diverse types of wounds.[63] Moreover, the effects of gamma-irradiation on the healing properties of honey are unknown.

Three studies were recently conducted to investigate the effects of UMF 20 Manuka honey on second-intention healing of experimental, non-contaminated and contaminated wounds on the distal aspect of limbs of horses.[56,68,69] A 100% UMF 20 Manuka honey and a 66% UMF 20 Manuka honey/34% water-based gel were shown to equally decrease wound retraction when compared to no treatment; wounds remained significantly smaller than untreated wounds up to day 35 of healing (Figure 22.6).[56,68] Manuka honey gel decreased inflammation and increased angiogenesis, organization of collagen, and epithelialization in contaminated wounds, as determined histologically.[69] The investigators concluded that contaminated wounds on the distal aspect of the limb treated with 66% Manuka honey gel developed a more organized and mature bed of granulation tissue earlier than untreated wounds, although the mechanism underlying this acceleration was unclear.[69] When applied daily throughout healing, 66% Manuka honey gel decreased the overall time required for healing by approximately 10%.[68] Surprisingly, while experimental contamination of wounds produced the expected transient increase in aerobic and anaerobic bacterial counts, these counts were unaltered by the topical application of Manuka honey.[69] The degree of tissue damage and wound contamination achieved using an experimental model is likely not representative of many naturally occurring wounds on the distal aspect of the limb, causing the antibacterial and immunomodulatory effects of honey to be underestimated.[69]

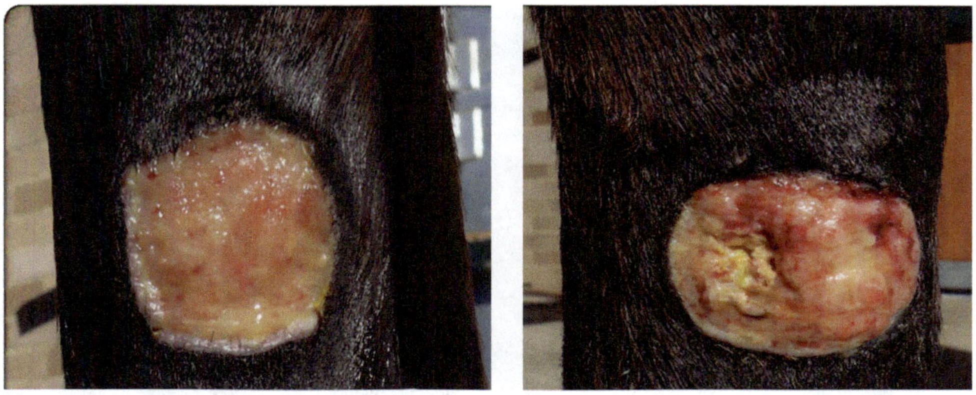

Figure 22.6 Surgically created wounds on the left and right metacarpi of a horse, 5 days after wound creation. Both wounds were bandaged and bandages were changed daily. **(a)** This wound was treated daily with Manuka honey. It is filled with healthy granulation tissue and is flush with the skin. **(b)** This wound received no treatment other than the bandage and shows irregular granulation tissue with areas of persistent fibrin deposits. The wound treated with honey appears to have a more mature and healthy granulation bed compared to the untreated wound. Courtesy of Dr. A. Dart.

Using honey

1. Begin treatment with commercially available, pure Manuka honey as soon as possible after wounding, ideally during the inflammatory phase of healing, particularly if the wound is contaminated. **Tip:** Additional beneficial effects can be achieved by continuing application until the wound has healed.[68]
2. Prior to applying honey, clean and debride the wound to remove as much necrotic tissue and debris as possible (Figure 22.7) (see Chapter 4 for more information on wound cleansing and debridement methods).
3. Where bacterial contamination is substantial or infection is a concern, use Manuka honey with UMF ≥15. Honey with a lower UMF can be used in mildly contaminated wounds, thereby reducing costs. **Tip:** Although Manuka honey is currently the only source of medical-grade honey available in dressings and wound treatment products, a recent study showed that several varietals of honey have antimicrobial properties and may, therefore, also be effective in the treatment of infected wounds of horses.[45] Consequently, locally sourced honey may provide an inexpensive and accessible alternative for treating contaminated wounds.
4. Honey is most easily and effectively applied when it has an ointment-like consistency; consider refrigerating prior to use if the consistency is too runny.
5. Consider using bandages when applying Manuka honey in the early phase of repair to improve honey–wound contact.
6. If not using a bandage, apply a thin film of honey at regular intervals (two to three times daily) to increase contact time and optimize efficacy. **Tip:** More honey is not necessarily better!
7. If using a bandage, apply 30 mL of Manuka honey to each 100 cm^2 area of dressing. Change bandages daily or every other day; frequency of changes can be reduced as the amount of exudate decreases.
8. Minimize the total period of bandaging (preferably ≤10 days), to reduce the risk of formation of EGT. Surgically excise EGT as it arises and continue applying Manuka honey.

Negative-pressure wound therapy

Since the middle of the 20th century, our greatest asset in the management of traumatic wounds and burns has been an improved understanding of the cellular and subcellular events of wound healing, including recognition of the highly interactive role of the extracellular matrix (ECM). Newly developed adjunctive therapies aimed at enhancing biologic processes (e.g., angiogenesis, fibroplasia) and reducing negative events (e.g., edema, infection) can now be used successfully in a variety of ways through pharmacologic, biologic, and mechanical interventions. One of the most commonly used adjuncts in human wound care today is negative-pressure wound therapy (NPWT); also termed "vacuum-assisted closure," "topical negative-pressure therapy," and "sub-atmospheric pressure dressings."[70,71]

In the few decades since the original publications on NPWT, the penetrance of this modality in human medicine has been astonishing. Although originally designed (and still used) for chronic wounds, this treatment modality has become the first line of treatment for acute traumatic wounds, including degloving injuries, shear trauma, high-energy soft-tissue wounds, and open fractures, as well as for dehisced surgical wounds, skin flaps, free grafts, and abdominal sepsis.[72–74]

The modality involves sealing the wound from the environment and delivering a controlled sub-atmospheric pressure to the entire wound. This is accomplished by trimming sterile, open-cell polyurethane ether foam to the dimensions of the wound, placing it directly on to the wound bed, and covering both wound and foam with an occlusive, adhesive drape. The drape establishes a closed-wound environment by adhering to the skin surrounding the wound, the hair of which has been closely clipped. A small hole is then cut through the adhesive drape over the foam and connected to a programmable vacuum pump via a fenestrated suction pad and evacuation tubing (Figure 22.8). Once activated, the pump provides continuous or intermittent suction, typically not exceeding −125 mmHg. Fluid produced by the wound is collected into a disposable reservoir

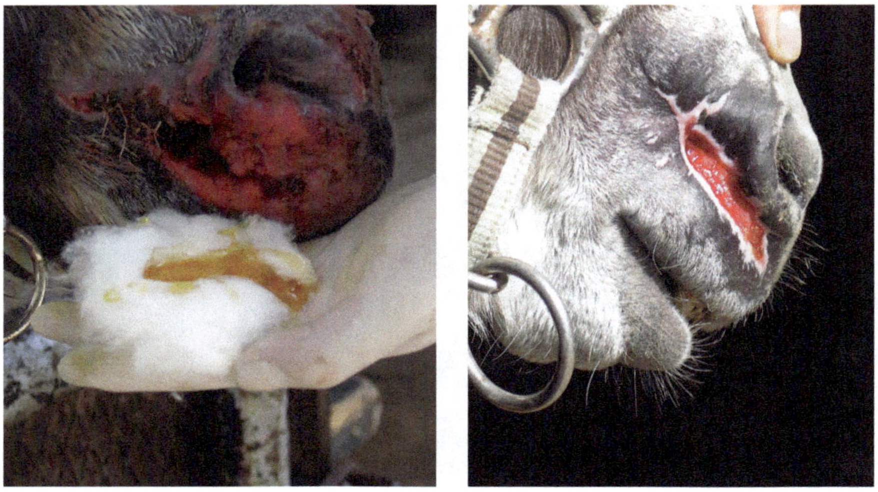

(a) (b)

Figure 22.7 This donkey was presented with a deep bite wound to the nostril/lip area. The wound was initially treated by sharp surgical debridement then irrigated. **(a)** In view of massive contamination and the presence of residual necrotic tissue, the wound was subsequently treated with locally sourced honey to encourage continued autolytic debridement. **(b)** Same wound, 22 days later. Courtesy of Dr. D. Frappier.

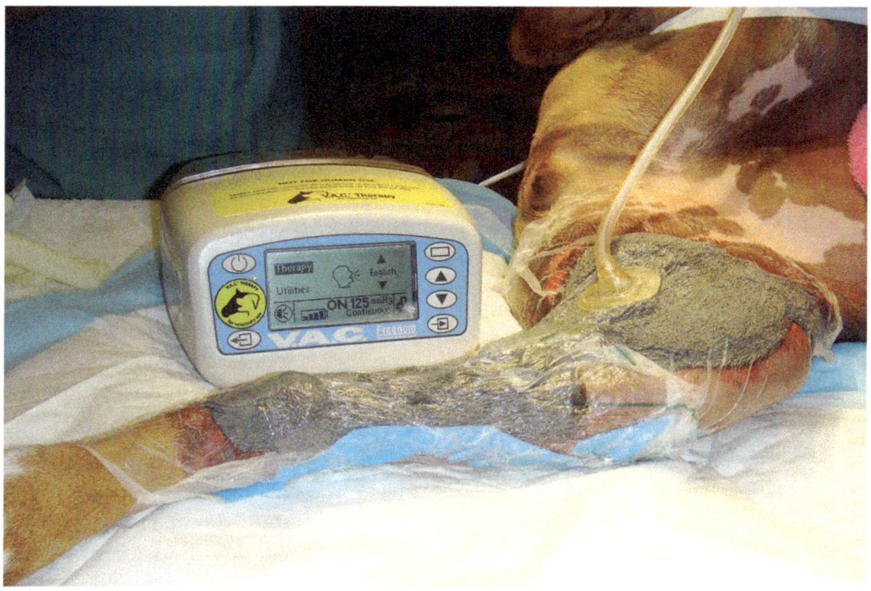

Figure 22.8 An extensive wound on the medial surface of the thigh and crus of a dog has been dressed with proprietary open cell foam and sealed from the environment by the placement of an adhesive drape. Vacuum is achieved through the fenestrated suction pad that is connected to the vacuum pump by tubing. There is a replaceable canister for collection of wound fluid at the back of the pump (not visible in photograph). Courtesy of Dr. B. Stanley.

canister attached to the pump. The open cell nature of the foam and the cell size (400–600 microns) ensure even distribution of negative pressure to the entire surface of the wound.

Early studies on animal models showed that NPWT stimulates the rapid formation of granulation tissue, reduces the size of the wound, and effectively removes fluid from the wound.[75,76] NPWT is currently used in all 6000 primary care hospitals in the USA, and is applied to over 90% of wounds of the extremity, encountered in the military arena.[77] The widespread use of NPWT is largely due to its huge clinical impact because not all mechanisms of action have been fully elucidated.[71] The early appearance of granulation tissue is remarkably consistent with the use of NPWT and concurs with observed increases in fibroblast activity and angiogenesis.[75,78] Other identified and validated mechanisms of NPWT include the removal of interstitial fluid (thus reducing wound edema), altered blood flow to the wound and up-regulated gene expression of cytokines associated with wound healing.[70,79–81] Using finite element analysis, the extracellular and cellular components of the wound treated with NPWT have been shown to be subjected to the same degree of micromechanical strain as that which promotes cellular (fibroblast) proliferation *in vitro*.[82] Nevertheless, certain claims of mechanisms of action, such as increased bacterial clearance, remain to be clarified.[70,83] More recent developments with this modality include the introduction of different types of foam, including a silver-impregnated polyurethane foam, and units that allow controlled delivery of topical solutions by alternating instillation and soak periods with the negative-pressure therapy (referred to as NPWTi).[84] These dressings and units are designed to be used to treat severely contaminated wounds, and thus may be of interest to the equine practitioner. A recent study conducted on an equine perfused *ex vivo* wound model determined that a polyvinyl alcohol foam dressing should be used as the primary dressing when performing NPWT for treating contaminated wounds healing by second intention in horses.[85]

Similar positive outcomes using NPWT have been documented in veterinary medicine, although the literature is far less extensive. A small number of case reports describe the use of NPWT in single animals of several species, including the horse; the authors of these reports concluded, based on subjective assessment, that NPWT facilitated second-intention healing and substantially shortened the time to healing. Several case series and reviews on the use of NPWT in various domestic animals and some experimental studies examining the use of NPWT in dogs, have provided a higher level of evidence of the effectiveness of NPWT used to treat wounded animals.[86–93] Most recently, a retrospective multicenter study of 50 dogs undergoing open wound management established that time to healing was halved in patients treated with NPWT compared to those treated with a highly absorbent foam dressing (Allevyn Cavity, Smith & Nephew), which in turn healed faster than patients treated with conventional non-adherent gauze dressing.[94] It is clear from these studies that not only is the use of NPWT feasible in veterinary medicine, but, as in wounds of human patients, it also leads to the early appearance of superior-quality granulation tissue and thus shortens the time to reconstruction (Figure 22.9). Indications for the use of NPWT in veterinary medicine include traumatic wounds (avulsions, degloving, shear injuries), full-thickness burns, dehiscence of surgical incisions, myofascial compartment syndrome, and chronic non-healing wounds.[86,90,92] NPWT is also excellent for enhancing acceptance of free grafts,[87] and it can be used effectively over sutured incisions to splint closures under tension, prevent formation of a seroma, particularly in closed incisional wounds with underlying dead space,[95] and minimize edema.[92] Negative-pressure wound therapy is used in all veterinary schools and many specialist facilities in North America.

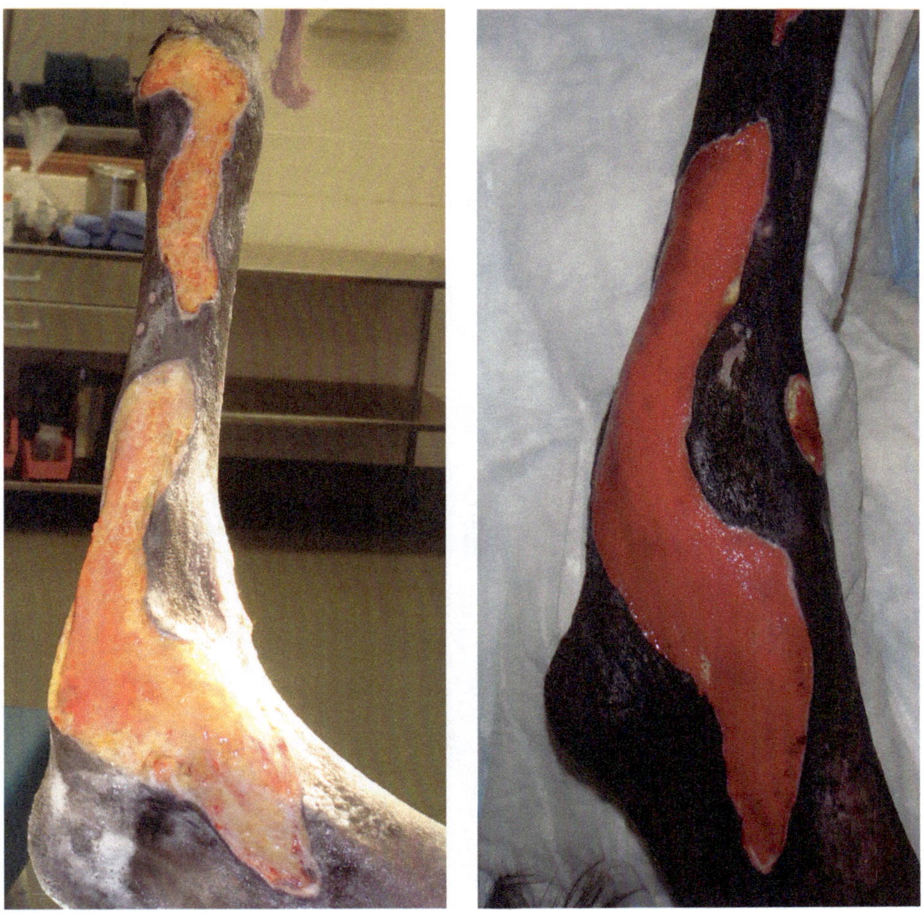

(a) (b)

Figure 22.9 Full-thickness frostbite injury on the lateral surface of the distal aspect of the hindlimb (beginning at the hock) in a foal. (**a**) Prior to application of NPWT. (**b**) Appearance of the wound having received NPWT, after 2 dressing changes, 7 days later. Courtesy of Dr. B. Stanley.

What to do

- Although NPWT can be used for prolonged periods (up to 36 days has been reported in a horse), it appears to have most benefit during the inflammatory phase of healing (less than 8–10 days in small animals).[86,90]

Several notable effects of NPWT may be particularly useful to the practitioner in the management of wounds of horses healing by second intention. NPWT prevents retraction of the wound, decreases the size of the wound, reduces wound edema, and stimulates early onset of fibroplasia. Granulation tissue forms earlier in wounded tissue treated by NPWT and is smoother, non-exuberant, and has well-organized collagen fibers, as demonstrated histologically (Figure 22.10).[89] This makes wounds treated with NPWT less likely to develop "proud flesh" and more amenable to early reconstructive procedures, such as skin grafting. Furthermore, NPWT increases the likelihood of acceptance of a free skin graft by immobilizing grafts at the wound.[87,96] Although NPWT should not replace basic tenets of wound management, such as cleansing, debridement, irrigation, and treatment for infection, its use as a dressing in an infected wound is likely to stimulate fibroplasia and increase resistance to infection early in the post-wounding period.[93]

Benefits of NPWT are as follows:

- One of the most appreciated advantages of NPWT is the elimination of frequent dressing changes and wound cleasing. Dressings of wounds treated with NPWT need be changed only every 48–72 hours.
- The dressing does not strike through (because exudate is collected in the disposable canister), thus protecting the wound from flies and other insects.
- Granulation tissue develops rapidly and is smooth.
- NPWT is excellent for securing all types of skin grafts and enhancing graft acceptance.

How to apply NPWT

1. Ensure the pump's battery is fully charged or that a power source can be permanently connected to the pump.
2. The reservoir canister and tubing are placed on the pump, ready to receive the tubing from the dressing.
3. Closely clip hair or otherwise thoroughly depilate skin for at least 10 cm around the wound.
4. Cleanse, debride, and thoroughly irrigate the wound. **Tip:** The skin surrounding the wound must also be cleansed and must be completely dry before applying the dressing, because moisture weakens adhesion of the drape.
5. Apply a skin adhesive, as a spray or liquid, to the skin surrounding the wound, and allow the adhesive to dry for several minutes. **Tip:** Applying an ostomy paste is useful to fill depressions or crevices and to facilitate adhesion of the drape.
6. Cut the foam dressing to the dimensions of the wound and place the dressing on to the wound. Pack all tunnels and crevices with foam. **Tip:** Securing the foam dressing with several skin staples is sometimes useful. Allow no foam to overlap on to the skin.
7. Apply the adhesive drape smoothly over the foam and the skin surrounding the wound. Cut a 2-cm diameter hole in the drape and apply the fenestrated suction pad directly to the foam.
8. Immediately connect the suction pad's evacuation tubing to the canister tubing and power the machine on, setting the pressure between −80 and −125 mmHg. Successful placement of the dressing is confirmed as the dressing shrinks, taking on a hard, wrinkled appearance. If the dressing is on a limb, a soft padded bandage is usually applied over the NPWT dressing. **Tip:** In horses, the vacuum pump can be attached to a surcingle (Figure 22.11) or suspended from an overhead beam, via coiled tubing and a swivel attachment.[89]

Also see Videos 22.1–22.4 on the supplementary website: www.wiley.com/go/theoret/wound.

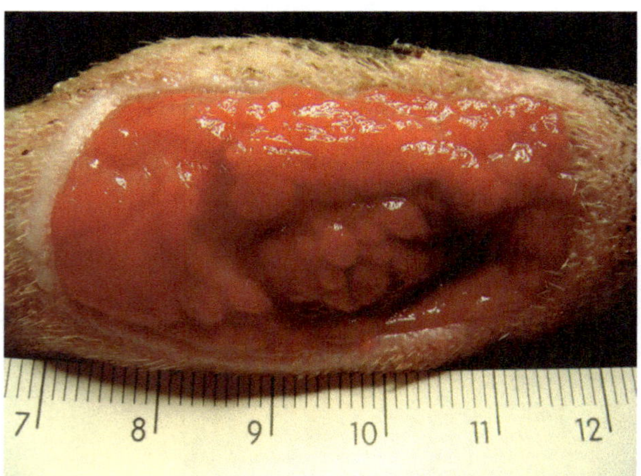

(a)

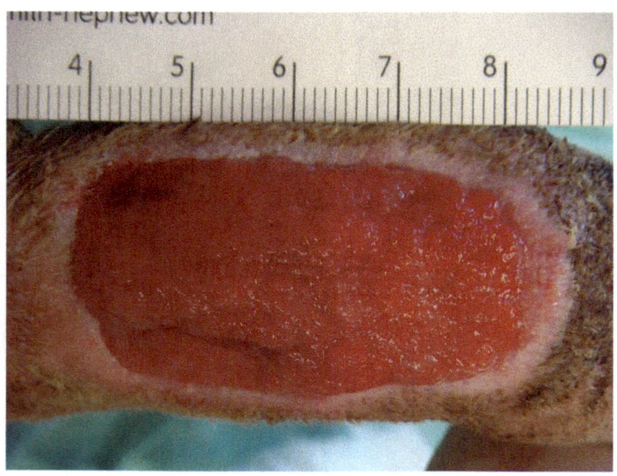

(b)

Figure 22.10 Appearance of granulation tissue in a 14-day-old open experimental wound in a dog, treated with a semi-occlusive, non-adherent dressing (a) or NPWT (b). Note the smooth and less exuberant appearance of the granulation tissue in the wound treated with NPWT. Courtesy of Dr. B. Stanley.

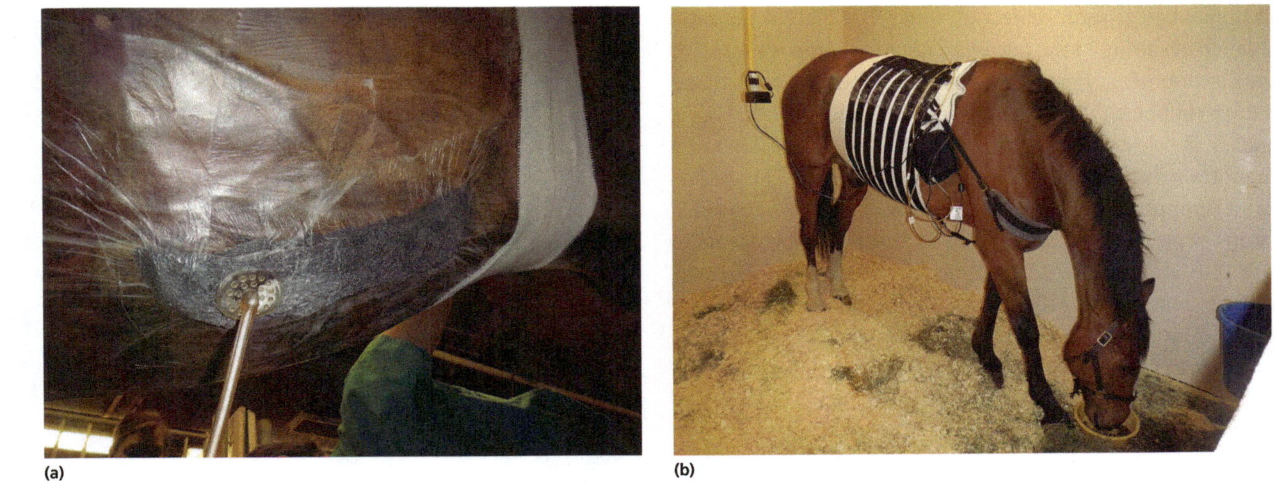

Figure 22.11 Incisional dehiscence of a midline celiotomy in a horse, not involving the abdominal cavity. **(a)** Following cleansing, NPWT has been applied. **(b)** The pump has been attached to the surcingle bandage. Note that the pump does not need to be connected to the power source if the battery is fully charged. Courtesy of Dr. B. Stanley.

Observe the following to avoid pitfalls when using NPWT:
- Meticulous attention to the clipping or depilation of the skin surrounding the wound is essential, as is careful application of the adhesive drape. A major issue when first learning to use NPWT is loss of vacuum due to inadequate adhesion of the drape to skin surrounding the wound.
- There is a learning curve to using this modality,[86] but complications associated with NPWT are minor after clinicians and technicians gain experience in using the device.
- To avoid loss of vacuum in large and irregular wounds, the adhesive drape can be applied in several broad strips; this facilitates manipulation and application.
- To facilitate dressing changes, only the foam need be removed. It is removed by cutting the adhesive drape at the wound's edge. The drape adhering to the skin surrounding the wound can remain in place. After the replacement foam dressing is in place, a new adhesive drape is placed on top of the original drape.

Contraindications include:[97]
- exposed vessels, nerves, tendons or ligaments within the wound;
- unexplored fistulas;
- unexplored wounds that could connect with the thoracic or abdominal cavity.

NPWT is an exciting and promising adjunct for the management of open wounds and grafted wounds of horses. After the practitioner is familiar with the device and the application procedure has been learned, treatment of the wound can be greatly facilitated, and healing times substantially shortened. Randomized, controlled clinical studies are indicated to determine if NPWT increases the rate of wound healing, decreases the likelihood of formation of EGT and improves graft acceptance in horses.

Extra-corporeal shockwave therapy

Another adjunctive therapy aimed at enhancing repair via mechanical and biologic manipulation of the wound's environment is extra-corporeal shockwave therapy (ESWT). The use of extra-corporeal shockwaves in medicine was first reported for the treatment of kidney stones (lithotripsy) and then for the treatment of various musculoskeletal conditions, but unanticipated positive responses of healing wounds to treatment with shockwaves led researchers and clinicians to expand the application of ESWT to acute and chronic wounds.[98]

Shockwaves are produced using an electrohydraulic, electromagnetic, or piezoelectric generator. Regardless of the mode of generation, the waves are "bundled" through a reflector in the applicator, or treatment head. For focused shockwaves, used mainly for lithotripsy and some orthopedic applications, the half-ellipsoid reflector within the applicator generates a high-energy focal point deep within the body. Conversely, unfocused shockwaves are bundled by a parabolic reflector that allows delivery of nearly parallel waves without a focal point; these waves have low energy density and a broad acoustic field that stimulates large superficial areas. In recent years, unfocused (also known as soft-focused) ESWT has been developed and successfully used to treat many soft tissue injuries, particularly wounds.[98] A meta-analysis of 13 clinical trials involving 919 patients recently concluded that ESWT is non-invasive, mostly painless, and safe for use as adjunct therapy for wound management and that it promotes faster wound closure.[99]

Shockwaves are short acoustic pulses characterized by a very rapid (nanoseconds) rise to a high peak pressure.[100] The total energy, consisting of a positive compression portion and a tensile portion, is measured in millijoules (mJ), and the energy flux density (EFD) is measured in mJ per square millimeter (mJ/mm^2). The energy flux density, the number of pulses, the pulse repetition frequency, and the number and interval of repeat treatments are important values for any therapy.[101]

Shockwaves emitted from a generator are sent through an applicator covered with electric coupling gel and held against the area to be treated. These pulsed high-energy pressure waves, when applied to tissues, deflect at zones of different acoustic impedance, resulting in the release of kinetic energy responsible for the development of pressure and shear forces as well as tissue cavitation (bubbles).[100] Cavitation bubbles collapse, releasing a secondary shockwave or jet stream that causes shear stress or mechanotransduction on cellular membranes.[102] This influences a complex spectrum of cellular and biomolecular functions promoting repair of injured tissues.[103] For example, VEGF, TGF, and nitric oxide synthase (NOS) are up-regulated in wounds treated with ESWT,[101] leading to faster neovascularization and lasting angiogenesis, as well as speedier epithelialization.[101,104] In wounded rats, ESWT triggered cellular release of adenosine triphosphate (ATP), leading to increased cellular proliferation and accelerated healing.[105]

Electrohydraulic shockwave generators with an unfocused/soft-focused applicator are used in human medicine mainly for the treatment of wounds with delayed healing, such as decubital ulcers, cast sores, and diabetic ulcers, as well as for the treatment of burns. The reported EFD ranges from 0.03–0.15 mJ/mm^2, when 100 pulses/cm^2 of wound area at an untreated frequency of 4–5 pulses/sec is used. This therapy has been shown to substantially accelerate epithelialization and decrease healing time.[101]

Two prospective clinical studies evaluated the effect of unfocused ESWT on healing of wounds in the distal aspect of the limb of horses.[106,107] In one study, five, 6.25-cm^2 wounds were created on each metacarpus of six horses (Figure 22.12). Wounds on one limb were randomly assigned to receive ESWT, while those on the other limb served as sham-treated controls. Electrohydraulically generated ESWT with an unfocused applicator was used, routine ultrasound transmission gel was applied, and the applicator was gently moved to make contact with the entire wound area. One hundred pulses/cm^2 (625 per wound) at an EFD of 0.11 mJ/mm^2 and a frequency of 5 pulses/sec were used at 7-day intervals for four treatments.[107] In the other study, one, 3–4-cm diameter circular wound was created on each metacarpal area of six horses and one wound per horse was randomly assigned to receive ESWT with a similar setting as in the former study while the wound on the other forelimb served as an untreated control. Wounds were treated weekly for 6–9 weeks until healing was complete.[106]

Both studies found that ESW-treated wounds were less inflamed, developed less EGT,[107] and healed significantly faster,[106] although neither study found differences in histologic or immunohistochemical variables.[106,107]

Another study examining the effect of ESWT on wounds on the distal aspect of the limb of horses by measuring gene expression of selected growth factors found that gene expression of TGF-β1 was significantly weaker in the ESW-treated wounds over time and until healing was complete.[108] The authors speculated that intervention with ESWT suppresses expression of TGF-β1, and by doing so may curb excessive fibroplasia, thereby improving healing of wounds of horses, predisposed to the developing EGT.

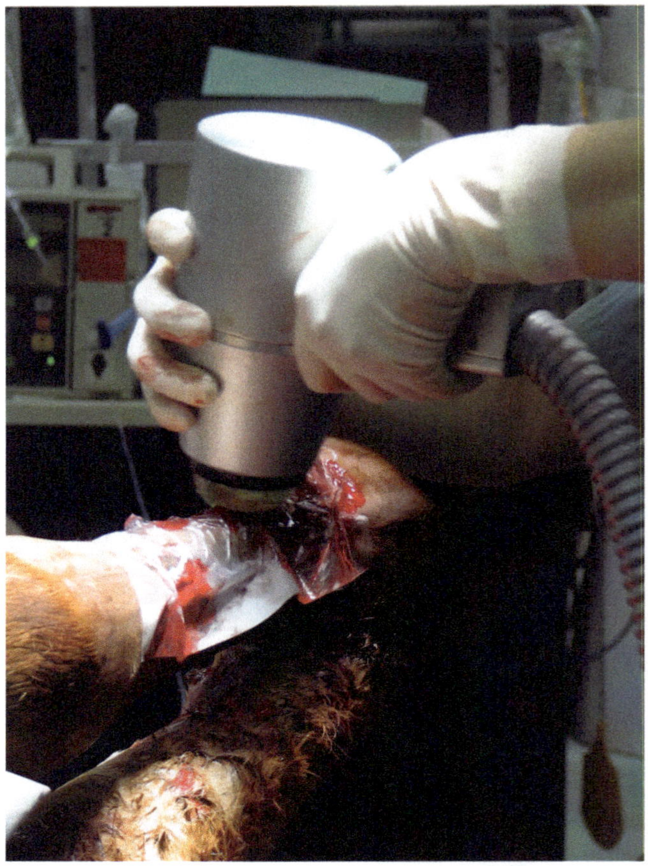

Figure 22.12 Use of unfocused shockwave therapy immediately after surgical creation of full-thickness wounds using an EFD of 0.11 mJ/mm^2 and 100 pulses/cm^2 of wound area. Ultrasound coupling gel is needed to cover the applicator, however the sterile barrier shown in this image is not required. Courtesy of Dr. J. Koenig.

What to do

- Use an unfocused applicator, applied with plenty of ultrasound coupling gel, at an EFD of 0.11 mJ/mm^2, 100 pulses/cm^2 of wound surface area, and a frequency of 5 pulses/sec, at weekly intervals, until the wound has healed (Figure 22.13).

Regenerative medicine

This section has been reprinted, in part, from a review published in *Veterinary Surgery* by CL Theoret.[109]

Skin has a considerable potential for efficient and functional repair, but even though cutaneous repair is a regenerative process in the fetus, inflammation and scarring predominate in mammals as of late gestation.[110] The ECM of scar tissue is poorly organized, and the neoepidermis is weak and fails to develop appendages, so that repair substitutes for regeneration during postnatal wound healing.[111]

The historical gold standard for the replacement of lost skin is the autologous skin graft. Free skin grafting is advocated to

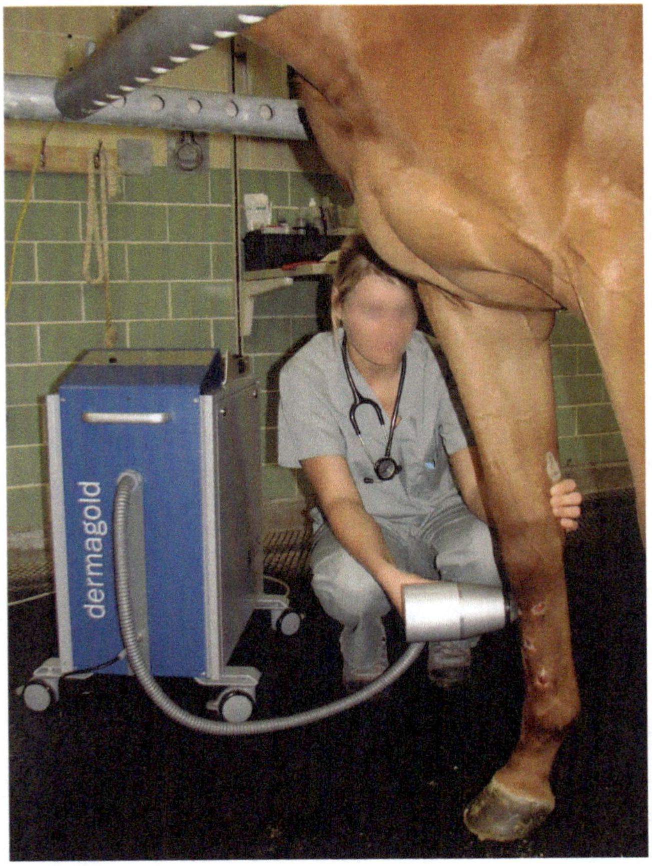

Figure 22.13 Use of unfocused shockwave therapy, 21 days after wounds were created experimentally, using an EFD of 0.11 mJ/mm^2 and 100 pulses/cm^2 of wound area. The horse was only lightly sedated for treatment. Courtesy of Dr. J. Koenig.

speed repair of full-thickness defects that cannot be closed using conventional suturing or reconstructive techniques or that cannot heal by secondary intention via contraction and epithelialization (for more information on skin grafting, readers are referred to Chapter 18). Unfortunately, conventional skin grafting in horses is limited by the scarcity of donor skin, as well as the risk of infection and loss of the graft.

A promising alternative to traditional skin grafting hails from the rapidly emerging field of regenerative medicine that incorporates knowledge of materials science, regeneration biology, and current advances in proteomics and genomics into a multidisciplinary translational research approach.[112] The aim is to design and construct, in the laboratory, a living component that can be used to maintain, repair, or replace malfunctioning or lost tissues.[113] In the case of skin, the ultimate goal is to rapidly generate a construct that effects the complete regeneration of functional skin, including all its layers and appendages, as well as an operational vascular and nervous network, that integrates, scar-free, into the surrounding host tissue. In addition to being available "off the shelf," such a construct should fulfill the usual functions of skin: barrier formation, defense against UV irradiation, thermoregulation, mechanical support, and protection. For this to be achieved, regenerative medicine relies on approaches such as: (1) administration of stem cells, referred to as "cell therapies"; (2) use of bioactive molecules, with or without cells, referred to as "immunomodulation therapies"; (3) strategies for *in situ* tissue regeneration, focusing on proliferation and migration of host stem or progenitor cells into target-specific scaffolds/biomaterials; and (4) transplantation of tissues or organs, grown in the laboratory, referred to as "tissue engineering."

Although the concept of regenerative medicine is relatively new to veterinary medicine, the body of work aiming to incorporate it into standard care is increasing monthly, in particular with regards to cellular therapies. The remainder of this section provides the reader with current information on the potential use of scaffolds/biomaterials, tissue-engineered skin substitutes, and stem cells for the management of skin wounds in horses.

Scaffolds/biomaterials for *in situ* tissue regeneration

Over the past three decades, extraordinary advances and improved understanding in cellular and molecular biology have led to achievements in the regeneration of skin for wound management.[114] Tissue engineering has enabled the production of "skin substitutes," both acellular and cellular, that incorporate bioactive elements to promote neovascularization and tissue regeneration. Acellular products are three-dimensional scaffolds intended to recreate the microenvironment to "instruct" or guide adhesion, growth, and differentiation of host cells into target tissue lineages during wound healing. Materials used for scaffolding are highly variable and include those derived from naturally occurring polymers, such as collagen, hyaluronan, glycosaminoglycan, fibronectin, silk, chitosan, and alginates, and those manufactured synthetically, such as polyglycolide, polylactide, polylactide coglycolide, polytetrafluoroethylene, and polyethylene terephthalate, among others. An ideal scaffold is compatible with the host's immune system, biodegrades in a controlled fashion to match the rate of neotissue growth, and has versatile options for processing to alter structure and morphology related to tissue-specific needs. A discussion of the various scaffold materials and fabrication techniques is beyond the scope of this chapter, and these have been extensively reviewed elsewhere.[115,116] It is, however, noteworthy that a recent study comparing the characteristics of an equine platelet-rich fibrin gel (PRFG) to those of a more traditionally used natural scaffold, the acellular fibrin gel, showed that inclusion of platelets in fibrin gel alters the architecture and increases the content of growth factors in the resulting scaffold.[117] The autologous, biodegradable PRFG may provide the cues required for cells involved in wound healing to migrate, proliferate, differentiate, and orient themselves correctly within the regenerating tissues.

Although a number of acellular scaffolds are commercially available for the management of wounds in human medicine, no new studies specifically investigating the use of these in the management of cutaneous wounds healing by second intention and/or in dermal reconstruction in horses have been conducted

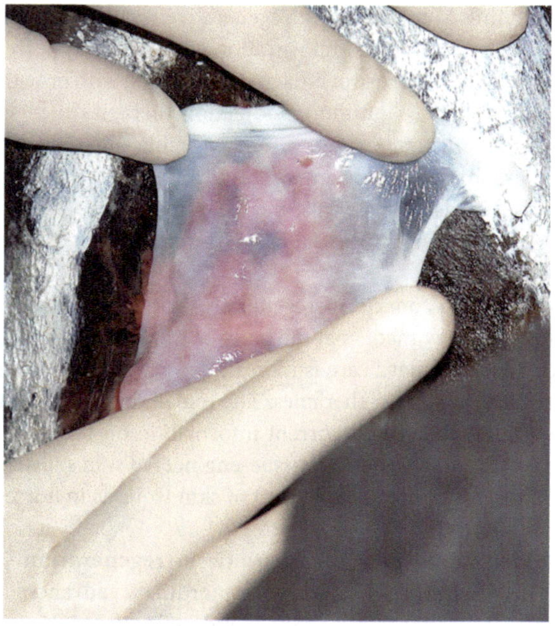

Figure 22.14 ACell Vet scaffold (lyophilized sheet) being applied to a wound in a horse. Courtesy of Dr. T. Stashak.

since the publication of the second edition of this textbook. At the time of writing, porcine urinary bladder matrix was marketed as an acellular biologic scaffold in the form of a powder, a lyophilized sheet, or a disc (Acell Vet; Acell) for use in the horse (Figure 22.14). A cross-linked acellular scaffold of hyaluronic acid (EquitrX® wound healing spray gel, Bayer Healthcare LLC Animal Health Division) was also commercially available to the equine practitioner.

Tissue-engineered skin substitutes

Skin substitutes grown *ex vivo*, with/without matrix, can be broadly divided into epidermal, dermal, and dermoepidermal (composite) tissue-engineered constructs. Although equine tissue-engineered skin products are not yet commercially available, the human market gives evidence that such constructs are possible, practical, and commercially successful; among the leading products are Apligraf, Alloderm, SureDerm, Integra, Dermagraft, MySkin, and CellSpray.[118]

Two recently published veterinary studies show that producing an equine skin substitute, using cell-culturing techniques developed in laboratory animals and humans, may be possible. The first study produced a construct with epidermal-like architecture by seeding explant-derived equine keratinocytes into a three-dimensional acellular scaffold (Matrigel, which contains solubilized basement membrane proteins). Ultrastructural, immunohistochemical, and biochemical analyses revealed that keratinocytes within the scaffolds were able to proliferate, differentiate, and form basal and suprabasal layers of epidermis.[119] The second study went one step further by producing a dermoepidermal construct out of cultures of pure equine keratinocytes and dermal fibroblasts obtained by enzymatic digestion of samples of horse skin. Fibroblasts were embedded into a type I-collagen matrix to obtain a dermal scaffold, the surface of which was seeded with keratinocytes. The three-dimensional cultures were then exposed to the air–liquid interface to induce epidermal stratification so that the product resembled horse skin grossly, histologically, ultrastructurally, and immunohistochemically.[120] Nevertheless, as is the case with human, canine, and murine skin substitutes, this tissue-engineered equine skin was incomplete due to an absence of appendages, blood vessels, and nerves.

For skin substitutes to become attractive, sophisticated alternatives to autografts, a focus on true regeneration, rather than replacement, is crucial. Unfortunately, in spite of recent advances, the skin substitutes presently available in human medicine are costly, may be unsuitable in terms of immunogenicity (because they contain non-autologous adult cells), and do not promote true regeneration. The latter limitation relates to the failure of keratinocyte performance (due to prolonged *in vitro* culture that reduces the number of highly proliferative units) and delayed vascularization, that collectively lead to the formation of weak scar tissue devoid of critical skin appendages.[121]

The unique features of stem cells, such as self-renewal and potential for differentiation, make them an attractive alternative for augmenting tissue repair and regeneration. Thus, current research is increasingly integrating the concept of engineering dermal scaffolds that promote regeneration by incorporating stem cells and biomolecules (usually growth factors) to recreate a favorable cellular microenvironment.[115] Likewise, the area that has garnered the most attention in equine regenerative medicine of late is, undisputably, that of stem-cell therapy.[122–125]

Stem cells

A stem cell is defined as an undifferentiated cell that can divide for an indefinite period of time and with the capacity to give rise to other undifferentiated stem cells (a process referred to as "self-renewal"), as well as to more committed descendants, including fully functional mature cells, through differentiation. "Stemness" is therefore a cellular property determined by two main hallmarks: (1) the ability for self-renewal and (2) the capability to differentiate into mature cell types. Cell potency, on the other hand, is a measure of the number and range of cell types into which a stem cell can develop.[126] "Potency" runs the gamut from unipotent (ability to give rise only to cells of its own type), to multipotent (ability to differentiate into a closely related family of cells), to pluripotent (ability to give rise to many or almost all cell types) all the way to totipotent (ability to give rise to all cell types and thus to an entire organism).[127] In mammals, only the zygote and subsequent blastomeres are totipotent. Pluripotent cells include embryonic stem cells (ESC) and induced pluripotent stem cells (iPSC). Examples of multipotent cells are mesenchymal stem cells (MSC), and examples of unipotent cells are some types of epithelial/keratinocyte stem cells (Figure 22.15). For more information on pluripotency, the reader is referred to the International Stem Cell

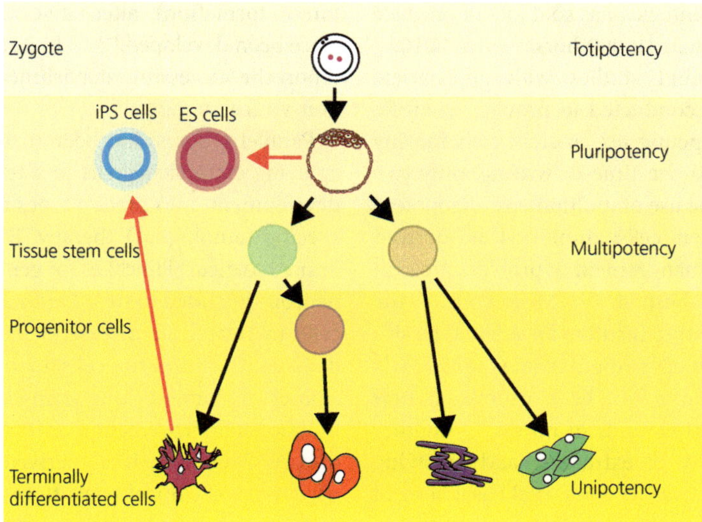

Figure 22.15 Cell potency is a cell's ability to differentiate into other cell types. *Totipotent* cells can give rise to all cell types; in mammals, only the zygote and subsequent blastomeres are totipotent. *Pluripotent* cells can give rise to many or almost all cell types; these include embryonic stem cells (ES cells) and induced pluripotent stem cells (iPS cells) that have the potential to differentiate into any of the three germ layers (endoderm, mesoderm, or ectoderm). *Multipotent* cells are progenitor cells able to differentiate into a closely related family of cells; for example, a multipotent blood stem cell (i.e. hematopoietic cell), shown as a pink circle, can differentiate into several types of blood cells. Finally, a *unipotent* cell can give rise only to cells of its own type; examples of unipotent cells (from left to right) are neurons, red blood cells, muscle cells, or epithelial cells. Figure drawn by Marco Langlois, Faculté de médecine vétérinaire, Université de Montréal.

Banking Initiative (ISCBI) that lists the irrefutable hallmarks of pluripotency.[128]

The therapeutic potential of stem cells appears to derive not only from their ability to contribute healthy, differentiated cells to injured tissue, but also from their chemotactic recruitment of native reparative cells and production of beneficial growth-promoting factors.[129,130] Consequently, even stem cells with limited potency, such as MSCs traditionally associated with differentiation into osteoblasts, chondrocytes, and adipocytes, have been shown to positively influence the outcome of cutaneous wound healing.[131]

Mesenchymal stem cells

Mesenchymal stem cells are found in a variety of adult tissues, including bone marrow, adipose tissue, and synovial fluid. They have also been derived from fetal tissues, such as amniotic fluid, amniotic membrane,[132] and umbilical cord. At present, there is no evidence that MSCs from a particular tissue origin are superior for use in wound management.[133] A systematic analysis of recent preclinical and clinical research concludes that "studies provide evidence that MSCs demonstrate chemotaxis toward a variety of wound healing cytokines, accelerate wound closure by modulating the inflammatory environment, promote the formation of a well-vascularized granulation tissue, encourage the migration of keratinocytes and attenuate the formation of fibrotic scar tissue."[134] Recent data implicate paracrine signaling as the primary mechanism for these regenerative effects; practically, this means that the conditioned medium obtained from MSC cultures may be used as a "stem cell-free therapy."[135]

In spite of the therapeutic promise of exogenously administered MSCs in the wound-management arena, at the time of writing, only two active clinical trials pertaining to the treatment of dermal wounds in humans with MSCs were registered at ClinicalTrials.gov. This may relate to the fact that MSCs are plagued by low survival and the lack of sustained engraftment,[136] possibly due to uncertainty as to the best mode of cell delivery. Systemic administration of MSCs is an attractive option, assuming the cells will home to the site of injury to impart their regenerative effects.[137] Cells applied topically require an appropriate carrier and/or scaffold to ensure that they remain viable and can efficiently migrate within the wound.[138,139] Alternatively, cell microencapsulation provides a supportive microenvironment for the cells, in which they can proliferate and release bioactive factors while being shielded from the external environment.[140] A team from the Baker Institute for Animal Health at Cornell University recently demonstrated that microencapsulation of equine MSCs does not interfere with the release of bioactive factors shown to positively contribute to wound healing.[141] The other major roadblock to the use of MSCs to enhance cutaneous wound healing concerns the restricted ability of MSCs to regenerate normal skin appendages (e.g., hair follicles, sweat and sebaceous glands), given their limited potency.

The therapeutic use of MSCs by veterinarians has exploded in the United States during the past decade in spite of the absence of FDA approval.[142] As an indication of their popularity, Vet-Stem, a company based in California, has provided stem-cell treatments to more than 5000 horses since 2004 and

Medi-Vet America, based in Kentucky, has sold kits to produce stem-cell injections for more than 10 000 horses since 2010.[142] Nevertheless, large, double-blind studies with appropriate control groups have yet to be conducted to provide scientific evidence to endorse the therapeutic use of stem cells for any clinical condition in horses. At the time of writing, only two anecdotal reports describing the use of multipotent/oligopotent stem cells (peripheral blood stem cells; amniotic fluid-derived MSC seeded in PRPG) for the management of problematic skin wounds in horses have been published.[143,144] Meanwhile, in the laboratory, the team from the Baker Institute for Animal Health demonstrated that the conditioned medium from equine MSCs isolated from peripheral blood might be a promising new therapy for impaired cutaneous wounds of horses.[141] Another study confirmed the feasability of extracting and purifying epidermal stem cells (EpSCs) from the epidermal basal layer of horse skin, then inducing their differentiation into keratinocytes and adipocytes (bipotent). EpSCs were subsequently placed into a PRP scaffold and used allogeneically, in full-thickness experimental skin wounds on a single horse to assess the ability of this combination to reduce scarring.[145] Although the authors felt this novel approach using adult somatic stem cells is auspicious, rigorous testing is pending. In an effort to overcome the limited ability of multipotent stem cells to regenerate all the components of normal skin, researchers have recently turned to pluripotent stem cells, on account of their potential to differentiate into most cell types of the body.

Embryonic stem cells and induced pluripotent stem cells

Both ESCs and iPSCs display a limitless capacity for self-renewal and the ability to differentiate into cells of all three germ layers (endoderm, mesoderm, and ectoderm). Embryonic stem cells from mice were established in 1981[146] and from humans in 1998 by veterinarian James Thomson.[147] Ethical and legislative issues associated with the harvest from embryonic sources, however, have hindered investigations for human applications. Moreover, in veterinary species, attempts to establish ESCs have proven elusive in spite of decades of trials. The problem faced by laboratories worldwide is loss of pluripotency over a short number of passages and *in vivo*.[148] In spite of the difficulty and costs associated with recovering embryos, two groups have reported the derivation of equine ES-like cell lines,[149,150] but these failed to give rise to teratomas when transplanted into immune-deficient mice (a test for pluripotency), and hence their genuine pluripotent nature is contested.

Induced pluripotent stem cells, on the other hand, are somatic cells that have been genetically reprogrammed to an ESC-like state by being forced to express specific genes that allow them to become pluripotent.[151] They, therefore, provide a novel renewable source of pluripotent cells engineered without destroying an embryo, thus circumventing ethical issues. Initially, reprogramming was achieved by transduction through viral vectors carrying the Oct4, Klf4, cMyc, and Sox2 transgenes.[152] To avoid the apparent drawbacks of the viral system (such as the risk of tumor formation), alternative reprogramming methods have since been developed.[153–155] In 2011, Nagy *et al.* were the first to report the successful establishment of iPSC from horses using a non-viral system.[156]

Parallel progress has been made in differentiating iPSCs, by applying extrinsic signals in a temporal sequence that mimics development, into precise types of cells to be used for patient-specific (autologous) therapy. Examples include, but are not limited to, neural lineages for generation of midbrain dopamine neurons intended to treat Parkinson's disease,[157] hepatocyte-like cells to treat liver disease,[158] insulin-producing cells to treat diabetes,[159] and germ cells to treat infertility.[160] All of these studies document long-term *in vivo* survival, as well as functional improvement in at least one relevant animal model of disease. Moreover, iPSC-derived retinal epithelium has been approved for clinical trials to restore sight to people suffering from macular degeneration, implying that iPSC-derived grafts are not far from the clinic.[161]

Regarding the possibility of one day using iPSC-based therapies to manage chronic wounds, a forward leap was recently achieved when murine and human iPSCs were differentiated into keratinocytes, then shown to successfully reconstitute a stratified epidermis and its appendages when grafted into the skin of mice[162] or used to populate a three-dimensional construct of human skin.[163] Although the complexity of *bona fide* skin has not yet been entirely reproduced, the essential components for a pigmented, three-dimensional skin equivalent have become available from the aforementioned studies and others differentiating iPSC into hair follicles[164] and melanocytes.[165]

An efficient protocol to drive equine iPSC to commit to a keratinocyte lineage in view of generating the cells required to engineer a stem cell-based skin equivalent for horses was recently designed and validated by Aguiar *et al.*[166] This protocol should be particularly interesting to equine practitioners given the prevalence of chronic wounds of horses that lack the epidermal cover vital for healing. The proof of concept study provided evidence that a differentiation protocol similar to that used for murine and human iPSCs drives equine iPSC towards ectodermal specification and that the keratinocytes thereby obtained exhibit morphologic and functional characteristics comparable to those of primary equine keratinocytes.

Although iPSCs, unlike ESCs, can be used in a patient-specific (autologous) manner, safety concerns related to incomplete reprogramming and genetic instability, in addition to tumorigenic potential persist.[167] In an effort to protect against these possible flaws, extensive screening is required, which is both costly and time consuming, particularly given the already tedious process of generating iPSCs. A simpler, quicker, and cheaper option entails the use of allogeneic cells that could be fully characterized, screened, and banked, allowing an "off-the-shelf" approach tailored to specific injuries.[168,169] Consequently, the immunogenicity of allogeneic iPSCs must be thoroughly studied and compared to that of autogenous iPSCs in an effort to validate this proposed approach.

Preliminary data from the horse suggest that, although intradermal transplantation of allogeneic, undifferentiated iPSCs into immunocompetent horses elicits a moderate cellular response, it does not cause acute rejection.[170] This study must now be repeated to test multiple lines of iPSCs differentiated into specific lineages, such as keratinocytes, in an effort to rigorously examine immunogenicity of equine iPSC before envisaging clinical uses for these cells.

Regulatory considerations

In spite of the enthusiasm generated by its therapeutic promise, veterinary regenerative medicine is a new product concept in terms of regulation. While it appears that, in the USA, the FDA is asserting primary and exclusive regulatory authority over veterinary regenerative therapies and products (cellular and tissue-based), intending to treat them as drugs for regulatory purposes, this was not yet officialized at the time of writing.[125] Consequently, as of 2015 there were no published regulations specific to veterinary stem cell-based products and treatments in the USA. Conversely, in the UK, the collection, storage, processing, production, and administration of equine stem cells for use as an autologous treatment for non-food-producing horses are regulated by the Veterinary Medicines Directorate (VMD) through Equine Stem Cell Centre Authorisations (PCDOCS #431064-v3-VMGN 15 Manufacturing Authorisations).[122] Irrespective of the legal connotations, products for clinical use must be safe and efficacious, and the welfare of animals used in the collection of stem cells (either autologous or allogeneic) must be respected.

Conclusion on the use of regenerative medicine as an adjunct to traditional wound management

It remains premature to recommend the use of scaffolds/biomaterials and/or cells for the management of skin wounds in horses due to the paucity of well-designed preclinical and clinical trials in equine patients to support an evidence-based approach. Moreover, because the products used in regenerative medicine are biologics, there can be tremendous inconsistencies in their production, as well as the response of the host, such that each product is likely to have a very specific range of activity that is animal, tissue, and injury dependent.

Conclusion

A dynamic, multimodal approach using local and systemic strategies to stimulate repair may be the key to successful wound management. Equine practitioners must thoroughly understand the mechanisms and complications of repair to critically assess the novel therapies that hit the market, and, consequently, to better advise their clients and serve their patients. Continued research in the field of equine wound repair and skin regeneration will lead to the development and implementation of rational therapeutic approaches targeted at the complications specific to the horse.

References

1. *Wound Care Market by Type - Global Forecast to* 2019.http://www.marketsandmarkets.com/Market-Reports/wound-care-market-371.html?gclid=CMf9jfvk88ECFZd6vQodNHgAaw (accessed November 12, 2014).
2. *The Global Market for Advanced Wound Care Products* 2014. http://www.reportsnreports.com/reports/280674-the-global-market-for-advanced-wound-care-products-2014.html (accessed November 12, 2014).
3. Wilmink JM, van Weeren PR. Treatment of exuberant granulation tissue. *Clin Tech Equine Pract* 2004; **3**: 141.
4. Jurga F, Morrison SE. Maggot debridement therapy. Alternative therapy for hoof infection and necrosis. *Hoofcare and Lameness* 2004; **78**: 28.
5. Dumville JC, Worthy G, Bland JM, *et al.* Larval therapy for leg ulcers (VenUS II): randomised controlled trial. *British Medical J* 2009; **338**: b773.
6. Lepage OM. La biochirurgie chez les equidés: utilisation de larves stériles dans le traitement des plaies. *Prat Vét Eq* 2012; **44**: 111.
7. Casu RE, Pearson RD, Jamey JM, *et al.* Excretory/secretory chymotrypsin from *Lucilia cuprina*: purification, enzymatic specificity and amino acid sequence deduced from mRNA. *Insect Mol Biol* 1994; **3**: 201.
8. Li P-N, Li H, Zhong L-X, *et al.* Molecular events underlying maggot extract promoted rat *in vivo* and human *in vitro* skin wound healing. *Wound Repair Reg* 2015; **23**: 65.
9. Daeschlein G, Mumcuoglu KY, Assadia O, *et al. In vitro* antibacterial activity of *Lucilia sericata* maggot secretions. *Skin Pharmacol Physiol* 2007; **20**: 112.
10. Cazander G, van de Veerdonk M, Vandenbroucke-Grauls C, *et al.* Maggot excretions inhibit biofilm formation on biomaterials. *Clin Orthop Relat Res* 2010; **468**: 2789.
11. Evans R, Dudley E, Nigam Y. Detection and partial characterization of antifungal bioactivity from the secretions of the medicinal maggot, Lucilia sericata. *Wound Repair Regen* 2015; **23**: 361
12. Bexfield A, Nigam Y, Thomas S, *et al.* Detection and partial characterization of two antibacterial factors from the excretions/secretions of the medicinal maggot *Lucilia sericata* and their activity against methicillin-resistant *Staphylococcus aureus* (MRSA). *Microbes Infect* 2004; **6**: 1297.
13. Grassberger M and Fleischmann W. The Biobag – a new device for the application of medicinal maggots. *Dermatol* 2002; **204**: 306.
14. Steenvoorde P, Jacobi CE, Oskam J. Maggot debridement therapy: free-range or contained? An *in-vivo* study. *Adv Skin Wound Care* 2005; **18**: 430.
15. Lepage OM, Doumbia A, Perron Lepage M-F, *et al.* The use of maggot debridement therapy in 41 equids. *Equine Vet J* 2012; **43**: 120.
16. Bras RJ, Morrison S. Retrospective case series of 20 horses (2002–2009) sustaining puncture wounds to the navicular bursa with maggot debridement therapy as an adjunctive therapy. *Proceedings 55th Congress of AAEP* 2009; **55**: 241.
17. Sun X, Jiang K, Chen J, *et al.* Systematic review of maggot debridement therapy for chronically infected wounds and ulcers. *Int J Inf Disease* 2014; **25**: 32.
18. Barrientos S, Brem H, Stojadinovic O, *et al.* Clinical application of growth factors and cytokines in wound healing. *Wound Repair Regen* 2014; **22**: 569.

19. Dohan Ehrenfest DM, Rasmusson L, Albrektsson T. Classification of platelet concentration: from pure platelet-rich plasma (P-PRP) to leucocyte- and platelet-rich fibrin (L-PRF). *Trends Biotechnol* 2009; **27**: 158.
20. Boudreaux M, Ebbe S. Comparison of platelet number, mean platelet volume and platelet mass in five mammalian species. *Comp Haematol Int* 1998; **8**: 16.
21. Pietrzak WS, Eppley BL. Platelet rich plasma: biology and new technology. *J Craniofac Surg* 2005; **16**: 1043.
22. Kushida S, Kakudo N, Suzuki K, *et al.* Effects of platelet-rich plasma on proliferation and myofibroblastic differentiation in human dermal fibroblasts. *Ann Plast Surg* 2013; **71**: 219.
23. Aktan I, Dunkel B, Cunningham FM. Equine platelets inhibit *E. coli* growth and can be activated by bacterial lipopolysaccharide and lipoteichoic acid although superoxide anion production does not occur and platelet activation is not associated with enhanced production by neutrophils. *Vet Immunol Immunopathol* 2013; **152**: 209.
24. Álvarez M, López C, Giraldo C, *et al. In vitro* bactericidal activity of equine platelet concentrates, platelet poor plasma, and plasma against methicillin-resistant *Staphylococcus aureus*. *Arch Med Vet* 2011; **43**: 155.
25. Fontenot RL, Sink CA, Werre SR, *et al.* Simple tube centrifugation for processing platelet-rich plasma in the horse. *Can Vet J* 2012; **53**: 1266.
26. Gonshor A. Technique for producing platelet-rich plasma and platelet concentrate: background and process. *Int J Periodontics Restorative Dent* 2002; **22**: 547.
27. O'Shea CM, Werre SR, Dahlgren LA. Comparison of platelet counting technologies in equine platelet concentrates. *Vet Surg* 2015; **44**: 304.
28. Giraldo CE, Álvarez ME, Carmona JU. Effects of sodium citrate and acid citrate dextrose solutions on cell counts and growth factor release from equine pure-platelet rich plasma and pure-platelet rich gel. *BMC Vet Res* 2015; **11**: 60.
29. Sutter WW, Kaneps AJ, Bertone AL. Comparison of hematologic values and transforming growth factor-β and insulin-like growth factor concentrations in platelet concentrates obtained by use of buffy coat and apheresis methods from equine blood. *Am J Vet Res* 2004; **65**: 924.
30. Hessel LN, Bosch G, van Weeren PR, *et al.* Equine autologous platelet concentrates: a comparative study between different available systems. *Equine Vet J* 2015; **47**: 319.
31. Álvarez ME, Giraldo CE, Carmona JU. Monitoring bacterial contamination in equine platelet concentrates obtained by the tube method in a clean laboratory environment under three different technical conditions. *Equine Vet J* 2010; **42**: 63.
32. Dunkel B, Bolt DM, Smith RK, *et al.* Stimulus-dependent release of tissue-regenerating factors by equine platelets. *Equine Vet J* 2012; **44**: 346.
33. Textor JA, Tablin F. Activation of equine platelet-rich plasma: comparison of methods and characterization of equine autologous thrombin. *Vet Surg* 2012; **41**: 784.
34. Giraldo CE, López C, Álvarez ME, *et al.* Effects of the breed, sex and age on cellular content and growth factor release from equine pure-platelet rich plasma and pure-platelet rich gel. *BMC Vet Res* 2013; **9**: 29.
35. Monteiro SO, Lepage OM, Theoret CL. Effects of platelet-rich plasma on the repair of wounds on the distal aspect of the forelimb in horses. *Am J Vet Res* 2009; **70**: 277.
36. Picard F, Hersant B, Bosc R, *et al.* Should we use platelet-rich plasma as an adjunct therapy to treat acute wounds, burns and laser therapies: A review and a proposal of a quality criteria checklist for further studies. *Wound Repair Regen* 2015; **23**: 163.
37. deRossi R, Coelho AC, Mello GS, *et al.* Effects of platelet-rich plasma gel on skin healing in surgical wound in horses. *Acta Cir Bras* 2009; **24**: 276.
38. Maciel FB, DeRossi R, Módolo TJ, *et al.* Scanning electron microscopy and microbiological evaluation of equine burn wound repair after platelet-rich plasma gel treatment. *Burns* 2012; **38**: 1058.
39. Majno G. Grease honey and lint. In: Majno G (ed). *The Healing Hand; Man and Wound in the Ancient World.* First Harvard University Press: Cambridge, 1975: 115.
40. Molan PC. The evidence and the rationale for the use of honey as a wound dressing. *Wound Pract Res* 2011; **19**: 204.
41. Lee DS, Sinno S, Khachemoune A. Honey and wound healing an overview. *Am J Clin Dermatol* 2011; **12**: 181.
42. Jull AB, Walker N, Deshpande S. Honey as a topical treatment for wounds. *Cochrane Database Syst Rev* 2013 Feb 28; (**2**): CD005083.
43. Cooper RA, Jenkins L. A comparison between medical grade honey and table honeys in relation to antimicrobial efficacy. *Wounds* 2009; **21**: 29.
44. Kwakman P, te Velde AA, de Boer L, *et al.* Two major medicinal honeys have different mechanisms of bactericidal activity. *PLoS One* 2011; **6**: e17709.
45. Carnwath R, Graham EM, Reynolds K, *et al.* The antimicrobial activity of honey against common equine bacterial isolates. *Vet J* 2014; **199**: 110.
46. Blair SE, Carter DA. The potential for honey in the management of wound and infection. *J Aust Inf Control* 2009; **28**: 1199.
47. Gethin GT. The impact of manuka honey dressings on the surface of chronic wounds. *Int Wound J* 2008; **5**: 185.
48. Bang LM, Buntting C, Molan P. The effect of dilution on the rate of hydrogen peroxide production in honey and its implications for wound healing. *J Altern Complement Med* 2003; **9**: 267.
49. Moore OA, Smith LA, Campbell F, *et al.* Systematic review of the use of honey as a wound dressing. *BMC Complement Altern Med* 2001; **1**: 1.
50. White JW, Schepartz AI, Subers MH. Identification of inhibine, the antibacterial factor in honey, as hydrogen peroxide and its origin in a honey glucose-oxidase system. *Biochim Biophysica Acta* 1963; **73**: 57.
51. Chelikani P, Fita I, Loewen PC. Diversity of structures and properties among catalases. *Cellular Molec Life Sci* 2004; **61**: 192.
52. Allen KL, Molan PC, Reid GM. A survey of the antibacterial activity of some New Zealand honeys. *J Pharm Pharmacol* 1991; **43**: 817.
53. Snow MJ, Manley-Harris M. On the nature of non-peroxide antibacterial activity in New Zealand manuka honey. *Food Chem* 2004; **84**: 145.
54. Mavric E, Wittmann S, Barth G, *et al.* constituent of Manuka (*Leptospermum scoparium*) honeys from New Zealand. *Molec Nutrit Food Res* 2008; **52**: 483.
55. Molan P. Why honey is effective as a medicine. 2. The scientific explanation of its effects. *Bee World* 2001; **82**: 22.
56. Bischofberger AS, Dart CM, Perkins NR, *et al.* A preliminary study on the effect of manuka honey on second-intention healing of contaminated wounds on the distal aspect of the forelimbs of horses. *Vet Surg* 2011; **40**: 898.

57. Henriques AF, Jenkins RG, Burton WF, *et al.* The effect of manuka honey on the structure of *Pseudomonas aeruginosa*. *Eur J Clin Microbiol Infect Dis* 2011; **30**: 167.
58. Jervis-Bardy J, Foreman A, Boase S, *et al.* What is the origin of *Staphylococcus aureus* in the early postoperative sinonasal cavity? *Int Forum Allergy Rhinol* 2001; **4**: 308.
59. Maddocks SE, Lopez MS, Rowlands RS, *et al.* Manuka honey inhibits the development of Streptococcus pyogenes biofilms and causes reduced expression of two fibronectin binding proteins. *Microbiol* 2012; **58**: 781.
60. Roberts A, Maddocks SE, Cooper RA. Manuka honey is bactericidal against *Pseudomonas aeruginosa* and results in differential expression of OprF and algD. *Microbiol* 2012; **158**: 3005.
61. Merckoll P, Jonasson TO, Vad ME, *et al.* Bacteria, biofilm and honey: a study of the effects of honey on 'planktonic' and biofilm-embedded chronic wound bacteria. *Scand J Inf Dis* 2009; **41**: 341.
62. Molan PC, Allen KL. The effect of gamma-irradiation on the antibacterial activity of honey. *J Pharm Pharmacol* 1996; **48**: 1206.
63. Matjan J. Honey: an immunomodulator in wound healing. *Wound Repair Regen* 2014; **22**: 187.
64. Tonks AJ, Cooper RA, Jones KP, *et al.* Honey stimulates inflammatory cytokine production from monocytes. *Cytokine* 2003; **21**: 242.
65. Tonks A, Cooper RA, Price AJ, *et al.* Stimulation of TNF-alpha release in monocytes by honey. *Cytokine* 2001; **14**: 240.
66. Tonks AJ, Dudley E, Porter NG, *et al.* 5.8-kDa component of manuka honey stimulates immune cells via TLR4. *J Leukoc Biol* 2007; **82**: 1147.
67. Matjan J, Bohova J, Garcia-Villalba R, *et al.* Fir honeydew honey flavanoids inhibit TNF-α-induced MMP-9 expression in human keratinocytes: a new action of honey in wound healing. *Arch Dermatol Res* 2013; **305**: 619.
68. Bischofberger AS, Dart CM, Perkins NR, *et al.* The effect of short- and long-term treatment with manuka honey on second intention healing of contaminated and non-contaminated wounds on the distal aspect of the forelimbs in horses. *Vet Surg* 2013; **42**: 154.
69. Bischofberger AS, Dart CM, Horadagoda N, *et al.* The effect of manuka honey gel on the transforming growth factor β1 and β3 concentration, bacterial counts and histomorphology of contaminated full thickness skin wounds in equine distal limbs. *Aust Vet J* 2016; **94**: 27.
70. Glass GE, Nanchahal J. The methodology of negative pressure wound therapy: separating fact from fiction. *J Plast Reconstr Aesthet Surg* 2012; **65**: 989.
71. Suissa D, Danino A, Nikolis A. Negative-pressure therapy versus standard wound care: a meta-analysis of randomized trials. *Plast Reconstr Surg* 2011; **128**: 498e.
72. Kanakaris NK, Thanasas C, Keramaris N, *et al.* The efficacy of negative pressure wound therapy in the management of lower extremity trauma: review of clinical evidence. *Injury* 2007; **38**: S9.
73. Moisidis E, Heath T, Boorer C, Ho K, *et al.* A prospective, blinded, randomized, controlled clinical trial of topical negative pressure use in skin grafting. *Plast Reconstr Surg* 2004; **114**: 917.
74. Schlatterer D, Hirshorn K. Negative pressure wound therapy with reticulated open cell foam-adjunctive treatment in the management of traumatic wounds of the leg: a review of the literature. *J Orthop Trauma* 2008; **22**: S152.
75. Morykwas MJ, Argenta LC, Shelton-Brown EI, *et al.* Vacuum-assisted closure: a new method for wound control and treatment: animal studies and basic foundation. *Ann Plast Surg* 1997; **38**: 553.
76. Argenta LC, Morykwas MJ. Vacuum-assisted closure: a new method for wound control and treatment: clinical experience. *Ann Plast Surg* 1997; **38**: 563; discussion 577.
77. Geiger S, McCormick F, Chou R, *et al.* War wounds: lessons learned from Operation Iraqi Freedom. *Plast Reconstr Surg* 2008; **122**: 146.
78. Morykwas MJ, Faler BJ, Pearce DJ, *et al.* Effects of varying levels of subatmospheric pressure on the rate of granulation tissue formation in experimental wounds in swine. *Ann Plast Surg* 2001; **47**: 547.
79. Morykwas MJ, Simpson J, Punger K, *et al.* Vacuum-assisted closure: state of basic research and physiologic foundation. *Plast Reconstr Surg* 2006; **117**: 121S.
80. Xie X, McGregor M, Dendukuri N. The clinical effectiveness of negative pressure wound therapy: a systematic review. *J Wound Care* 2010; **19**: 490.
81. Glass GE, Murphy GF, Esmaeili A, *et al.* Systematic review of molecular mechanism of action of negative-pressure wound therapy. *British J Surg* 2014; **101**: 1627.
82. Saxena V, Hwang CW, Huang S, *et al.* Vacuum-assisted closure: microdeformations of wounds and cell proliferation. *Plast Reconstr Surg* 2004; **114**: 1086; discussion 1097–1098.
83. Moues CM, Heule F, Hovius SE. A review of topical negative pressure therapy in wound healing: sufficient evidence? *Am J Surg* 2011; **201**: 544.
84. Kim PJ, Attinger CE, Steinberg JS, *et al.* The impact of negative-pressure wound therapy with instillation compared with standard negative-pressure wound therapy: a retrospective, historical, cohort, controlled study. *Plast Reconstr Surg* 2014; **133**: 709.
85. Van Hecke L, Haspeslagh M, Martens A. The antibacterial effect of vacuum-assisted closure (VAC) using 3 different foams in an equine perfused *ex vivo* wound model. *European College of Veterinary Surgeons Proceedings* 2015; **61**.
86. Pitt KA, Stanley BJ. Negative pressure wound therapy: experience in 45 dogs. *Vet Surg* 2014; **43**: 380.
87. Stanley BJ, Pitt KA, Weder CD, *et al.* Effects of negative pressure wound therapy on healing of free full-thickness skin grafts in dogs. *Vet Surg* 2013; **42**: 511.
88. Cioffi KM, Schmiedt CW, Cornell KK, *et al.* Retrospective evaluation of vacuum-assisted peritoneal drainage for the treatment of septic peritonitis in dogs and cats: 8 cases (2003–2010). *J Vet Emerg Crit Care (San Antonio)* 2012; **22**: 601.
89. Demaria M, Stanley BJ, Hauptman JG, *et al.* Effects of negative pressure wound therapy on healing of open wounds in dogs. *Vet Surg* 2011; **40**: 658.
90. Ben-Amotz R, Lanz OI, Miller JM, *et al.* The use of vacuum-assisted closure therapy for the treatment of distal extremity wounds in 15 dogs. *Vet Surg* 2007; **36**: 684.
91. Kirkby KA, Wheeler JL, Farese JP, *et al.* Vacuum-assisted wound closure: application and mechanism of action. *Compendium* 2009; E1–E7.
92. Kirkby KA, Wheeler JL, Farese JP, *et al.* Surgical views: vacuum-assisted wound closure: clinical applications. *Compendium* 2010; **32**: E1; quiz E7.

93. Orsini JA, Elce Y, Kraus B. Management of severely infected wounds in the equine patient. *Clin Tech Equine Pract* 2004; **3**: 225.
94. Nolff MC, Fehr M, Bolling A, *et al.* Negative pressure wound therapy, silver coated foam dressing and conventional bandages in open wound treatment in dogs; a retrospective comparison of 50 paired cases. *Vet Comp Orthop Traumatol* 2015; **28**: 30.
95. Suh H, Lee A-Y, Park EJ, *et al.* Negative pressure wound therapy on closed surgical wounds with dead space. *Ann Plast Surg* 2016; **76**: 717.
96. Rijkenhuizen ABM, van den Boom R, Cornelissen BPM. Can Vacuum assisted wound management enhance graft acceptance? *Pferdeheilkunde* 2005; **21**: 413.
97. Howe LM. Current concepts in negative pressure wound therapy. *Vet Clin Small Anim* 2015; **45**: 565.
98. Schaden W, Thiele R, Kölpl C, *et al.* Shock wave therapy for acute and chronic soft tissue wounds: a feasibility study. *J Surg Res* 2007; **143**: 1.
99. Dymarek R, Halski T, Ptaszkowski K, *et al.* Extracorporeal shock wave therapy as an adjunct wound treatment: a systematic review of the literature. *Ostomy Wound Manage* 2014; **60**: 26.
100. Ogden JA, Toth-Kischkat A, Schultheiss R. Principle of shock wave therapy. *Clin Orthop Relat Res* 2001; **387**: 8.
101. Mittermayr R, Antonic V, Hartinger J, *et al.* Extracorporeal shock wave therapy (ESWT) for wound healing: Technology, mechanisms, and clinical efficacy. *Wound Repair Reg* 2012; **20**: 456.
102. Mariotto S, Cercereri de Prati A, *et al.* Extracorporeal shockwave therapy in inflammatory diseases: molecular mechanism that triggers anti-inflammatory action. *Curr Med Chem* 2009; **16**: 2366.
103. Mittermayr R, Hartinger J, Antonic V, *et al.* Extracorporeal shock wave therapy (ESWT) minimizes ischemic tissue necrosis irrespective of application time and promotes tissue revascularization by stimulating angiogenesis. *Ann Surg* 2011; **253**: 1024.
104. Haupt G, Chvapil M. Effect of shock waves on the healing of partial-thickness wounds in piglets. *J Surg Res* 1990; **49**: 45.
105. Weihs AM, Fuchs C, Teuschl AH, *et al.* Shock wave treatment enhances cell proliferation and improves wound healing by ATP release-coupled extracellular signal-regulated kinase (ERK) activation. *J Biol Chem* 2014; **289**: 27090.
106. Morgan DD, McClure S, Yaeger MJ, *et al.* Effects of extracorporeal shock wave therapy on wounds of the distal portion of the limbs in horses. *J Am Vet Med Assoc* 2009; **234**: 1154.
107. Silveira A, Koenig JB, Arroyo LG, *et al.* Effects of unfocused extracorporeal shock wave therapy on healing of wounds of the distal portion of the forelimb in horses. *Am J Vet Res* 2010; **71**: 229.
108. Link KA, Koenig JB, Silveira A, *et al.* Effect of unfocused extracorporeal shock wave therapy on growth factor gene expression in wounds and intact skin of horses. *Am J Vet Res* 2013; **74**: 324.
109. Theoret CL. Tissue engineering in wound repair: the three "R"s – repair, replace, regenerate. *Vet Surg* 2009; **38**: 905.
110. Larson BJ, Longaker MT, Lorenz HP. Scarless fetal wound healing: a basic science review. *Plast Reconstr Surg* 2010; **126**: 1172.
111. Gurtner GC, Werner S, Barrandon Y *et al.* Wound repair and regeneration. *Nature* 2008; **453**: 314.
112. Metcalfe AD, Ferguson MWJ. Tissue engineering of replacement skin: the crossroads of biomaterials, wound healing, embryonic development, stem cells and regeneration. *J Royal Soc Interface* 2007; **4**: 413.
113. Sun X, Fu X, Sheng Z. Cutaneous stem cells something new and something borrowed. *Wound Repair Regen* 2007; **15**: 775.
114. Falanga V, Faria K, Robert L, *et al.* Bioengineered skin constructs. In: Lanza R, Langer R, Vacanti J (eds). *Principles of Tissue Engineering*, 3rd edn. Academic Press: Burlington, 2007: 1167.
115. Yildirimer L, Thanh NT, Seifalian AM. Skin regeneration scaffolds: a multimodal bottom-up approach. *Trends Biotechnol* 2012; **30**: 638.
116. Zhong SP, Zhang YZ, Lim CT. Tissue scaffolds for skin wound healing and dermal reconstruction. *Wiley Interdiscip Rev Nanomed Nanobiotechnol* 2010; **2**: 510.
117. Textor JA, Murphy KC, Leach JK, *et al.* Ultrastructure and growth factor content of equine platelet-rich fibrin gels. *Am J Vet Res* 2014; **75**: 392.
118. Harman RJ. Stem cell therapy in veterinary dermatology. *Vet Dermatol* 2013; **24**: 90.
119. Sharma R, Barakzai SZ, Taylor SE, *et al.* Epidermal-like architecture obtained from equine keratinocytes in three-dimensional cultures. *J Tissue Eng Regen Med* 2013 Jul 30. doi: 10.1002/term.1788. [Epub ahead of print]
120. Cerrato S, Ramió-Lluch L, Brazís P, *et al.* Development and characterization of an equine skin-equivalent model. *Vet Dermatol* 2014; **25**: 475.
121. Cerqueira MT, Marques AP, Reis RL. Using stem cells in skin regeneration: possibilities and reality. *Stem Cells Dev* 2012; **21**: 1201.
122. Lopez MJ, Jarazo J. State of the art: stem cells in equine regenerative medicine. *Equine Vet J* 2015; **47**: 145.
123. Borjesson DL, Peroni JF. The regenerative medicine laboratory: facilitating stem cell therapy for equine disease. *Clin Lab Med* 2011; **31**: 109.
124. Burk J, Badylak SF, Kelly J, *et al.* Equine cellular therapy – from stall to bench to bedside? *Cytometry Part A* 2013; **83A**: 103.
125. Schnabel LV, Fortier LA, McIlwraith CW, *et al.* Therapeutic use of stem cells in horses: which type, how, and when? *Vet J* 2013; **197**: 570.
126. Robey PG. Stem cells near the century mark. *J Clin Invest* 2000; **105**: 1489.
127. Koch TG, Berg LC, Betts DH. Current and future regenerative medicine-principles, concepts, and therapeutic use of stem cell therapy and tissue engineering in equine medicine. *Can Vet J* 2009; **50**: 155.
128. Crook JM, Hei D, Stacey G. The International Stem Cell Banking Initiative (ISCBI): raising standards to bank on. *In Vitro Cell Dev Biol Anim* 2010; **46**: 169.
129. De Schauwer C, Van de Walle GR, Van Soom A, *et al.* Mesenchymal stem cell therapy in horses: useful beyond orthopedic injuries? *Vet Q* 2013; **33**: 234.
130. Chen L, Tredget EE, Wu PY, *et al.* Paracrine factors of mesenchymal stem cells recruit macrophages and endothelial lineage cells and enhance wound healing. *PLoS One* 2008; **3**: e1886.
131. Teng M, Huang Y, Zhang H. Application of stem cells in wound healing – an update. *Wound Repair Regen* 2014; **22**: 151.
132. Seo MS, Park SB, Kim HS, *et al.* Isolation and characterization of equine amniotic membrane-derived mesenchymal stem cells. *J Vet Sci* 2013; **14**: 151.
133. Maxson S, Lopez EA, Yoo D, *et al.* Concise review: role of mesenchymal stem cells in wound repair. *Stem Cells Transl Med* 2012; **1**: 142.

134. Jackson WM, Nesti LJ, Tuan RS. Concise review: clinical translation of wound healing therapies based on mesenchymal stem cells. *Stem Cells Transl Med* 2012; **1**: 44.
135. Madrigal M, Rao KS, Riordan NH. A review of therapeutic effects of mesenchymal stem cell secretions and induction of secretory modification by different culture methods. *J Transl Med* 2014; **12**: 260.
136. Nakamura Y, Ishikawa H, Kawai K, *et al.* Enhanced wound healing by topical administration of mesenchymal stem cells transfected with stromal cell-derived factor-1. *Biomaterials* 2013; **34**: 9393.
137. Dabiri G, Heiner D, Falanga V. The emerging use of bone marrow-derived mesenchymal stem cells in the treatment of human chronic wounds. *Expert Opin Emerg Drugs* 2013; **18**: 405.
138. Sorrell JM, Caplan AI. Topical delivery of mesenchymal stem cells and their function in wounds. *Stem Cell Res Ther* 2010; **1**: 30.
139. Mansilla E, Spretz R, Larsen G, *et al.* Outstanding survival and regeneration process by the use of intelligent acellular dermal matrices and mesenchymal stem cells in a burn pig model. *Transplant Proc* 2010; **42**: 4275.
140. Orive G, Santos E, Pedraz JL, *et al.* Application of cell encapsulation for controlled delivery of biological therapeutics. *Adv Drug Deliv Rev* 2014; **67–68**: 3.
141. Bussche L, Harman RM, Syracuse BA, *et al.* Microencapsulated equine mesenchymal stromal cells promote cutaneous wound healing *in vitro*. *Stem Cell Res Ther* 2015; **6**: 66.
142. Cyranoski D. Stem cells boom in vet clinics. *Nature* 2013a; **496**: 148.
143. Spaas JH, Broeckx S, Van de Walle GR, *et al.* The effects of equine peripheral blood stem cells on cutaneous wound healing: a clinical evaluation in four horses. *Clin Dermatol* 2013; **38**: 280.
144. Iacono E, Merlo B, Pirrone A, *et al.* Effects of mesenchymal stem cells isolated from amniotic fluid and platelet-rich plasma gel on severe decubitus ulcers in a septic neonatal foal. *Res Vet Sci* 2012; **93**: 1439.
145. Broeckx SY, Maes S, Martinello T, *et al.* Equine epidermis: a source of epithelial-like stem/progenitor cells with in vitro and in vivo regenerative capacities. *Stem Cells Dev* 2014; **23**: 1134.
146. Evans MJ, Kaufman MH. Establishment in culture of pluripotential cells from mouse embryos. *Nature* 1981; **292**: 154.
147. Thomson JA, Itskovitz-Eldor J, Shapiro SS, *et al.* Embryonic stem cell lines derived from human blastocysts. *Science* 1998; **282**: 1145.
148. Volk SW, Theoret C. Translating stem cell therapies: the role of companion animals in regenerative medicine. *Wound Repair Regen* 2013; **21**: 382.
149. Guest DJ, Smith MR, Allen WR. Equine embryonic stem-like cells and mesenchymal stromal cells have different survival rates and migration patterns following their injection into damaged superficial digital flexor tendon. *Equine Vet J* 2010; **42**: 636.
150. Desmarais JA, Demers SP, Suzuki J Jr, *et al.* Trophoblast stem cell marker gene expression in inner cell mass-derived cells from parthenogenetic equine embryos. *Reproduction* 2011; **141**: 321.
151. Aguiar C. Immune potential and differentiation of equine induced pluripotent stem cells (eiPSC). PhD thesis. Université de Montréal. Copyright December 2014.
152. Takahashi K, Yamanaka S. Induction of pluripotent stem cells from mouse embryonic and adult fibroblast cultures by defined factors. *Cell* 2006; **126**: 663.
153. Okita K, Nakagawa M, Hyenjong H, *et al.* Generation of mouse induced pluripotent stem cells without viral vectors. *Science* 2008; **322**: 949.
154. Stadtfeld M, Nagaya M, Utikal J, *et al.* Induced pluripotent stem cells generated without viral integration. *Science* 2008; **322**: 945.
155. Bao X, Zhu X, Liao B, *et al.* MicroRNAs in somatic cell reprogramming. *Curr Opin Cell Biol* 2013; **25**: 208.
156. Nagy K, Sung HK, Zhang P, *et al.* Induced pluripotent stem cell lines derived from equine fibroblasts. *Stem Cell Rev* 2011; **7**: 693.
157. Kriks S, Shim JW, Piao J, *et al.* Dopamine neurons derived from human ES cells efficiently engraft in animal models of Parkinson's disease. *Nature* 2011; **480**: 547.
158. Aravalli RN, Cressman EN, Steer CJ. Hepatic differentiation of porcine induced pluripotent stem cells *in vitro*. *Vet J* 2012; **194**: 369.
159. Zhu FF, Zhang PB, Zhang DH, *et al.* Generation of pancreatic insulin-producing cells from rhesus monkey induced pluripotent stem cells. *Diabetologia* 2011; **54**: 2325.
160. Niu Z, Hu Y, Chu Z, *et al.* Germ-like cell differentiation from induced pluripotent stem cells (iPSCs). *Cell Biochem Funct* 2013; **31**: 12.
161. Cyranoski D. Stem cells cruise to clinic. *Nature* 2013b; **494**: 413.
162. Bilousova G, Chen J, Roop DR. Differentiation of mouse induced pluripotent stem cells into a multipotent keratinocyte lineage. *J Invest Dermatol* 2011; **131**: 857.
163. Itoh M, Kiuru M, Cairo MS, *et al.* Generation of keratinocytes from normal and recessive dystrophic epidermolysis bullosa-induced pluripotent stem cells. *Proc Natl Acad Sci U S A* 2011; **108**: 8797.
164. Veraitch O, Kobayashi T, Imaizumi Y, *et al.* Human induced pluripotent stem cell-derived ectodermal precursor cells contribute to hair follicle morphogenesis in vivo. *J Invest Dermatol* 2013; **133**: 1479.
165. Nissan X, Larribere L, Saidani M, *et al.* Functional melanocytes derived from human pluripotent stem cells engraft into pluristratified epidermis. *Proc Natl Acad Sci U S A* 2011; **108**: 14861.
166. Aguiar C, Therrien J, Lemire P, *et al.* Differentiation of equine induced pluripotent stem cells into a keratinocyte lineage. *Equine Vet J* 2016; **48**: 338.
167. Zhao T, Zhang ZN, Rong Z, *et al.* Immunogenicity of induced pluripotent stem cells. *Nature* 2011; **474**: 212.
168. Schnabel LV, Abratte CM, Schimenti JC, *et al.* Induced pluripotent stem cells have similar immunogenic and more potent immunomodulatory properties compared with bone marrow-derived stromal cells *in vitro*. *Regen Med* 2014; **9**: 621.
169. Smith RKW, Garvican ER, Fortier LA. The current state of play of regenerative medicine in horses: what the horse can tell the human. *Regen Med* 2014; **9**: 673.
170. Aguiar C, Theoret C, Smith O, *et al.* Immune potential of allogeneic equine induced pluripotent stem cells. *Equine Vet J* 2015; **47**: 708.

Index

Page numbers in *italics* denote figures, those in **bold** denote tables.

Equine Wound Management, Third Edition. Edited by Christine Theoret and Jim Schumacher.

Companion website: www.wiley.com/go/theoret/wound

Printed in the USA/Agawam, MA
September 16, 2026

910661.204